Taylor's Clinical Nursing Skills

A NURSING PROCESS APPROACH

Taylor's Clinical Nursing Skills

A NURSING PROCESS APPROACH

Second Edition

Pamela Lynn, RN, MSN
Faculty
School of Nursing
Gwynedd-Mercy College
Gwynedd Valley, Pennsylvania

Wolters Kluwer | Lippincott Williams & Wilkins
Health
Philadelphia • Baltimore • New York • London
Buenos Aires • Hong Kong • Sydney • Tokyo

Acquisitions Editor: Jean Rodenberger
Development Editor: Megan Duttera
Senior Production Editor: Sandra Cherrey Scheinin
Director of Nursing Production: Helen Ewan
Senior Managing Editor/Production: Erika Kors
Design Coordinator: Holly Reid McLaughlin
Interior Designer: Karen Quigley
Cover Designer: Carol Tippit Woolworth
Senior Manufacturing Manager: William Alberti
Manufacturing Coordinator: Karin Duffield
Indexer: Victoria Boyle
Compositor: Circle Graphics
Printer: RR Donnelley/Willard

Second Edition

9 8 7 6 5 4 3 2

Library of Congress Cataloging-in-Publication Data

Lynn, Pamela Barbara, 1961-
Taylor's clinical nursing skills : a nursing process approach / Pamela Lynn.—2nd ed.
p. ; cm.
Rev. ed of: Taylor's clinical nursing skills / [edited by] Pamela Evans-Smith. c2005.
To accompany: Fundamentals of nursing / Carol Taylor. . . . [et al.]. 6th ed. c2008.
Includes bibliographical references and index.
ISBN-13: 978-0-7817-7465-9 (alk. paper)
ISBN-10: 0-7817-7465-9 (alk. paper)
1. Nursing. I. Taylor, Carol, CSFN. II. Fundamentals of nursing. III. Title. IV. Title: Clinical nursing skills.
[DNLM: 1. Nursing Process. 2. Nursing Care—methods. WY 100 L989† 2008]
RT41.T398 2008
610.73—dc22

2006026473

LWW.com

To past, present, and future nursing students and my family:
Each one of you helps me to continue learning and caring every day.

Contributors and Reviewers

CONTRIBUTOR TO THIS EDITION

Mary Hermann, BSN, MSN, EdD
Assistant Professor
Gwynedd Mercy College
Gwynedd Valley, Pennsylvania
Chapter 2: Assessment
Chapter 6: Perioperative Nursing
Chapter 8: Skin Integrity and Wound Care
Chapter 11: Nutrition
Chapter 15: Fluid, Electrolyte, and Acid–Base Balance

CONTRIBUTORS TO THE FIRST EDITION

Sheryl Kathleen Buckner, RN, MS, CM
Academic and Staff Developer, Case Manager,
Clinical Instructor
University of Oklahoma, College of Nursing
Oklahoma City, Oklahoma
Unit III: Integrated Case Studies

Pamela Evans-Smith, MSN, FNP
Clinical Nursing Instructor
University of Missouri
Columbia, Missouri

Connie J. Hollen, RN, MS
Adjunct Instructor
University of Oklahoma, College of Nursing
Oklahoma City, Oklahoma
Unit III: Integrated Case Studies

Loren Nell Melton Stein, RNC, MSN
Adjunct Instructor
University of Oklahoma, College of Nursing
Oklahoma City, Oklahoma
Unit III: Integrated Case Studies

REVIEWERS

Faisal Aboul-Enein, RN, MSN
Clinical Instructor
Texas Woman's University
Denton, Texas

Lyda Arevalo, RN, MSN
Clinical Assistant Professor
The University of Texas
Health Science Center at San Antonio School of Nursing
San Antonio, Texas

Jane Benedict, RN, MSN
Faculty, Medical Surgical Nursing Program
Pennsylvania College of Technology
Williamsport, Pennsylvania

Linda Berry, RN, PhD
Associate Professor
Eastern Michigan University, School of Nursing
Ypsilanti, Michigan

Nell Britton, RN, MSN, NHA
Nursing Instructor and New Student Coordinator
Trident Technical College
Charleston, South Carolina

Michelle Byrne, RN, MS, PhD, CNOR
Associate Professor of Nursing
North Georgia College and State University
Dahlonega, Georgia

Stephen Campbell, RN, MSN
Nursing Instructor
Polk Community College
Winter Haven/Lakeland, Florida

Amy Carter-Gallagher, RN
Nursing Specialist
The Christ Hospital of Nursing
Cincinnati, Ohio

Susan Chessa, RN, MSN
Instructional Technologist—Family and Community Nurse
Practitioner Program
Husson College
Bangor, Maine

Veronica A. Clarke-Tasker, RN, MBA, MPH, PhD
Associate Professor
Howard University College of Pharmacy,
Division of Nursing
Washington, District of Columbia

Sara Clutter, RN, MSN
Assistant Professor, Nursing
Waynesburg University
Waynesburg, Pennsylvania

Barbara Craig, BSN, MSN
Associate Professor of Nursing
Pasco-Hernando Community College
New Port Richey, Florida

Lora Cruz, RN, BSN, RNC
Instructor of Nursing
Davis & Elkins College
Elkins, West Virginia

Susan Erue, MS, BSN
Instructor in Nursing
Iowa Wesleyan College
Mount Pleasant, Iowa

Kathleen Evans, RN, MSN
Nursing Instructor
Midway College
Midway, Kentucky

Mary Ann Fiese, RN, MSN, BC
Assistant Professor of Nursing
Austin Peay State University
Clarksville, Tennessee

Jamie Flower, RN, MS, SANE
Assistant Professor
University of Arkansas, Fort Smith
Fort Smith, Arkansas

Roberta Forsch, RN, MSN
Nursing Instructor
Prairie View A&M University
Prairie View, Texas

Jean Forsha-Byrd, RN, MSN, CNE
Assistant Professor
Community College of Philadelphia
Philadelphia, Pennsylvania

Christine Frazer, RN, CNS, MSN, DNSc(c)
Nursing Instructor
Penn State University
Hershey, Pennsylvania

Mary Catherine Gebhard, RN, MSN, PhD
Clinical Assistant Professor
Georgia State University
Atlanta, Georgia

Alison Green, RN, MSN
Instructor
Neumann College
Aston, Pennsylvania

Deborah Greenwald, RN, MSN
Instructor
Alvernia College
Reading, Pennsylvania

Karen Hecomovich, MS, BSN
Nursing Faculty
Arapahoe Community College
Littleton, Colorado

Roberta Hochmuth, RN, MSN
Instructor
Cincinnati State Technical and Community College
Cincinnati, Ohio

Barbara Hoerst, PhD, RN
Assistant Professor
LaSalle University, School of Nursing
Philadelphia, Pennsylvania

Marshall Hollinger, RN, BSN, MBA
Nursing Instructor
Central Ohio Technical College
Newark, Ohio

Verna Inandan, RN, MSN
Assistant Professor
Darton College
Albany, Georgia

Chris Jarrell, MS
Instructor
Wesley College
Dover, Delaware

Vicki Johnson, RN, MSN, CNAA
Clinical Assistant Professor
Cleveland State University
Cleveland, Ohio

Laura Kearney Schenk, RN, CNNP, PhD
Assistant Professor
University of Mississippi Medical Center School of Nursing
Jackson, Mississippi

Tammy Keith, RN, MS
Professor
Hocking College
Nelsonville, Ohio

Rose Knapp, BSN, CAN-P, MSN
Adjunct Clinical Assistant Professor
New York University
New York, New York

Brandi Koehler, RN, BSN
Staff Nurse Intervention Cardiac Unit
Doylestown Hospital
Doylestown, Pennsylvania

Susan Lamanna, RN, MA, MSN, ANP
Associate Professor
Onondaga Community College
Syracuse, New York

Rebecca Lohmeyer, RN, MSN, CMSRN
Assistant Professor, Nursing
Frederick Community College
Frederick, Maryland

Donna Lukich, MSN, PhD
Interim Provost/Vice President of Academic Affairs
West Liberty State College
West Liberty, West Virginia

LaToya Marsh, RN, MSN
Clinical Assistant Professor
North Carolina Agriculture and Technology State University, School of Nursing
Greensboro, North Carolina

Janet Massoglia, RN-BC, FNP, MSN
Instructor
Delta College
University Center, Michigan

Barbara Maxwell, RN, MSN, MS
Program Coordinator, Associate Professor of Nursing
SUNY, Ulster
Stone Ridge, New York

Jacquelyn Mayer, RN, MS
Associate Professor
Good Samaritan College of Nursing and Health Science
Cincinnati, Ohio

Tammie McCoy, BSN, MSN, BA PhD
Assistant Professor
Mississippi University for Women
Columbus, Mississippi

Susan Miovich, RNC, PhD
Associate Professor
Holy Family University
Philadelphia, Pennsylvania

Pamela Moore, RN, C, MSN, CNS
Director
Division of Nursing, Louisiana Technical University
Ruston, Louisiana

Karen Moore Schaefer, DNSc, RN
Undergraduate Nursing
Temple University, Department of Nursing
Philadelphia, Pennsylvania

Susan Moore, RN, MSN
Professor
New Hampshire Community Technical College
Manchester, New Hampshire

Carol Morris, RN, MSN
Assistant Professor
Bellen College of Nursing
Green Bay, Wisconsin

Kathleen Reilly Dolin, RN, MSN
Assistant Professor, Nursing
Northampton Community College
Bethlehem, Pennsylvania

Virginia Ousley, RN
Instructor
Radford University
Radford, Virginia

Colleen Quinn, RN, MSN
Pediatric Nursing
Broward Community College
Fort Lauderdale, Florida

Carla Randall, RN, MSN
Assistant Professor of Nursing
University of Southern Maine, College of Nursing
Portland, Maine

Jill Ray, RN, MSN
Assistant Professor, Adult Health Nursing
Georgia Baptist College of Nursing of Mercer University
Atlanta, Georgia

Darrell Richardson, RN, BSN
Fundamentals and Psychiatric Nursing
St. Catherine College
St. Catherine, Kentucky

Wendy Robb, RN, BSN
Assistant Professor of Nursing
Cedar Crest College
Allentown, Pennsylvania

Linda Roy, MSN, CRNP
Assistant Professor of Nursing
Montgomery County Community College
Blue Bell, Pennsylvania

Judith Sadler, RN, CNAA, BC, PhD
Associate Professor
WMU Bronson School of Nursing
Kalamazoo, Michigan

Buckie Sasser, RN, MSN
Assistant Professor of Nursing
South Georgia College
Douglas, Georgia

Donna Scott Tilley, RN, CNE, PhD
Associate Professor
Texas Technical University, School of Nursing
Lubbock, Texas

Tamara Shields, RN, MSN
Instructor of Nursing
St. Elizabeth School of Nursing
Lafayette, Indiana

Nancy Simpson, RN, MSN, CNE
Assistant Professor
University of New England
Portland, Maine

Jacque Snyder, RN, BSN
Instructor
North Seattle Community College
Seattle, Washington

D. Shane Strickland, RN, MScN
Lecturer
Lake Head University, School of Nursing
Thunder Bay, Ontario

Dianna Tison, RN, PhD
Nursing Faculty
University of Incarnate Word
San Antonio, Texas

Elayne Trepel, BSN, MSN
Clinical Instructor
University of Illinois–Chicago
Chicago, Illinois

Peggy Sorrell Truemann, RN, MSN, EdD
Instructor, Adult Health Nursing
Gaston College
Dallas, North Carolina

Susan Warner, BSN, MSN, PhD
Director of the Department of Nursing Science
St. Cloud State University
St. Cloud, Minnesota

Dawn Weiler, RN, MS, ANP
Assistant Professor
Boise State University, Department of Nursing
Boise, Idaho

Gail Zell Serdoz, RN, MSN
Associate Professor of Nursing
Mountain State University
Beckley, West Virginia

Preface

Taylor's Clinical Nursing Skills: A Nursing Process Approach aims to help nursing students or graduate nurses incorporate cognitive, technical, interpersonal, and ethical/legal skills into safe and effective patient care. This book is written to meet the needs of novice to advanced nurses. Many of the skills shown in this book may not be encountered in nursing school but may be encountered once the graduate nurse has entered the workforce.

Because it emphasizes the basic principles of patient care, we believe this book can easily be used with any Fundamentals text. However, this Skills book was specifically designed to accompany *Fundamentals of Nursing: The Art and Science of Nursing Care,* sixth edition, by Taylor, Lillis, LeMone, and Lynn, to provide a seamless learning experience. Some of the Skills and Guidelines for Nursing Care from the Taylor Fundamentals book may also be found in this book, but the content has been embellished here to:

- Highlight the nursing process.
- Emphasize unexpected situations that the nurse may encounter, along with related interventions for how to respond to these unexpected situations.
- Draw attention to critical actions within skills.
- Illustrate specific actions within a skill through the use of more than 1000 four-color photographs and illustrations.

Additionally, this book contains numerous higher level skills that are not addressed in the Taylor Fundamentals book.

LEARNING EXPERIENCE

This text and the entire Taylor Suite have been created with the student's experience in mind. Care has been taken to appeal to all learning styles. The student-friendly writing style ensures that students will comprehend and retain information. The extensive art program enhances understanding of important actions. Free video clips clearly demonstrate and reinforce important skill steps; as students watch and listen to the videos comprehension increases. In addition, each element of the Taylor Suite, which is described later in the preface, coordinates to provide a consistent and cohesive learning experience.

ORGANIZATION

Taylor's Clinical Nursing Skills is organized into three units. Ideally, the text will be followed sequentially, but every effort has been made to respect the differing needs of diverse curricula and students. Thus, each chapter stands on its own merit and may be read independently of others.

Unit I, Actions Basic to Nursing Care

This unit introduces the foundational skills used by nurses: measuring vital signs, assessing health, promoting safety, maintaining asepsis, administering medication, and caring for surgical patients.

Unit II, Promoting Healthy Physiologic Responses

This unit focuses on the physiologic needs of patients: hygiene; skin integrity and wound care; activity; comfort; nutrition; urinary elimination; bowel elimination; oxygenation; fluid, electrolyte, and acid–base balance; neurologic care; cardiovascular care; and specimen collection.

Unit III, Integrated Case Studies

Although nursing skills textbooks generally present content in a linear fashion for ease of understanding, in reality, many nursing skills are performed in combination for patients with complicated health needs. The integrated case studies in this unit are designed to challenge the reader to think critically, think outside the norm, consider the multiple needs of patients, and prioritize care appropriately—ultimately preparing the student and graduate nurse for complex situations that may arise in everyday practice.

FEATURES

- **Focusing on Patient Care.** Each chapter in Units I and II begins with a description of three real-world case scenarios that put the skills into context. These scenarios provide a framework for the chapter content to be covered.
- **New! Fundamentals Review.** Because of the breadth and depth of nursing knowledge that must be absorbed, nursing students and graduate nurses can easily become overwhelmed. Thus, this book is designed to eliminate excessive content and redundancy and to better focus the reader's attention. To this end, each chapter in Units I and II includes several boxes, tables, or figures that summarize important concepts that should be understood before performing a skill. For a more in-depth study of these concepts, readers are encouraged to refer to their Fundamentals textbook.
- **Step-by-Step Skills.** Each chapter presents a host of related step-by-step skills. The skills are presented in a concise, straightforward, and simplified two-column format to facilitate competent performance of nursing skills.

- The **nursing process** framework is used to integrate related nursing responsibilities for each of the five steps.
- **Scientific rationales** accompany each nursing action to promote a deeper understanding of the basic principles supporting nursing care.
- **Nursing Alerts** (in red type) draw attention to crucial information.

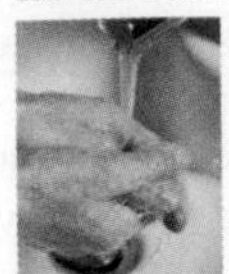

  - **New! Hand Hygiene** icons alert you to this crucial step that is the best way to prevent the spread of microorganisms.

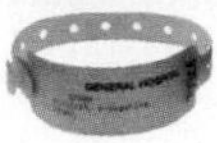

  - **New! Patient Identification** icons alert you to this crucial step ensuring the right patient receives the intervention and helping prevent errors.
- **New! Documentation Guidelines** direct students and graduate nurses in accurate documentation of the skill and their findings. **Sample Documentation** demonstrates proper documentation.
- **Infant, Child, and Older Adult Considerations** as well as **Home Health** and **Special Considerations** (eg, modifications and home care) appear throughout to explain the varying needs of patients across the lifespan and in various settings.
- **Unexpected Situations** are provided after the explanation of normal outcomes. Each situation is followed by an explanation of how best to react, with rationales. This feature serves as a starting point for group discussion.
- **New! Skill Variations** provide clear, start-to-finish instructions for variations in equipment or technique.

  - **New! Watch and Learn** icons direct students to free video clips that show students how to perform a skill.

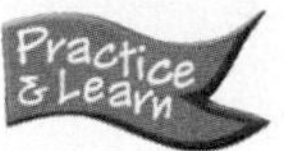

  - **New! Practice and Learn** icons direct students to free activities that allow students to apply skills to patient care.
- **Photo Atlas Approach.** When learning a new skill, it is often overwhelming to only *read* how to perform a skill. With more than 1000 photographs, this book offers a pictorial guide to performing each skill. The skill will not only be learned but also remembered through the use of text with pictures.
- **Developing Critical Thinking Skills.** Critical thinking questions at the end of the chapter reflect back to the opening scenarios for added cohesion throughout the chapters. Readers are challenged to apply the skills and use the new knowledge they have gained to "think through" learning exercises designed to show how critical thinking can impact patient care and possibly change outcomes.

TEACHING/LEARNING PACKAGE

To facilitate mastery of this text's content, a comprehensive teaching/learning package has been developed to assist faculty and students.

Instructor's Resource CD-ROM

This all-in-one resource features an Instructor's Manual and Image Bank.

- The Instructor's Manual contains a detailed step-by-step plan for setting up a skills course. The unique "Build-a-Skill" feature allows instructors to customize nursing skills. PowerPoint slides enhance lectures, providing key visuals and reinforcing content.
- The Image Bank provides free access to all of the textbook's illustrations and photos for use in PowerPoint, handouts, and so forth.

Student Resources

Student resources include a free front-of-book CD-ROM, Skill Checklists, and an Interactive CD-ROM (described later):

- FREE front-of-book CD-ROM features "Watch and Learn" video clips, "Practice and Learn" activities, an Alternate-Format NCLEX Tutorial, and a Spanish-English Audioglossary.
- *Skills Checklists to Accompany Taylor's Clinical Nursing Skills* is designed to accompany the Skills textbook and promote proper technique while increasing confidence.

thePoint

ThePoint (http://thepoint.lww.com/Lynn2E) is a web-based course and content-management system that provides every resource instructors and students need in one easy-to-use site. ThePoint . . . where teaching, learning, and technology click!

For Students

Students can visit thePoint to access supplemental multimedia resources to enhance their learning experience, check the course syllabus, download content, upload assignments, and join an online study group. ThePoint offers a variety of free student resources including Watch and Learn video clips, Practice and Learn activities, an Alternate-Format NCLEX tutorial, and a Spanish-English audioglossary. In addition, an online course is available, including many videos and interactive activities.

For Instructors

Advanced technology and superior content combine at thePoint to allow instructors to design and deliver online and offline courses, maintain grades and class rosters, and communicate with students. In addition to housing the material from the Instructor's Resource CD-ROM, thePoint also provides additional resources, including a syllabus, teaching plans, and strategies for effective teaching.

TAYLOR SUITE OF PRODUCTS

From traditional texts to video and interactive products, the Taylor Fundamentals/Skills suite is tailored to fit every learning style. This integrated suite of products offers students a seamless learning experience you won't find anywhere else. The following products accompany *Taylor's Clinical Nursing Skills:*

- ***Fundamentals of Nursing: The Art and Science of Nursing Care,*** sixth edition, by Carol Taylor, Carol Lillis, Priscilla LeMone, and Pamela Lynn. This traditional Fundamentals text promotes nursing as an evolving art and science, directed to human health and well-being. It challenges students to focus on the four blended skills of nursing care, which prepare students to combine the highest level of scientific knowledge and technologic skill with responsible, caring practice. The text includes engaging features to promote critical thinking and comprehension.
- ***Taylor's Video Guide to Clinical Nursing Skills.*** From reinforcing fundamental nursing skills to troubleshooting clinical problems on the fly, this dynamic 17-module video series follows a team of nursing students and their instructor as they perform a range of essential nursing procedures. Ideal as a stand-alone learning tool or as a companion to this book, these videos parallel the text, with each module corresponding to a book chapter for easy reference. The videos are available for purchase by your school. There are also student versions of the series, available on CD-ROM or DVD.
- ***Taylor's Interactive Nursing Skills (CD-ROM).*** This high-quality interactive electronic product provides a consistent learning structure for both Skills and Fundamentals. The two parts to *Taylor's Interactive Nursing Skills CD-ROM* are:
  - *Interactive Skills:* Students develop skills by answering critical thinking questions, as well as NCLEX-type questions.
  - *Interactive Tutorials:* Students engage in tutorials covering fundamentals concepts.
- ***Online Course to Accompany Taylor's Fundamentals of Nursing and Clinical Nursing Skills.*** Created specifically to match the texts, this dynamic course combines superior video with engaging interactive exercises. A perfect companion to any course, beginning students will find this an invaluable resource.

Contact your sales representative or check out LWW.com/Nursing for more details and ordering information.

Pamela Lynn, RN, MSN

Acknowledgments

This updated edition is the work of many talented people. I would like to acknowledge the hard work of all who have contributed to the completion of this project. Thanks to Carol Taylor, Carol Lillis, and Priscilla LeMone for inviting me to join them as an author for this teaching/learning suite and offering generous support and encouragement. You have been excellent mentors.

The work of this revision was skillfully coordinated by my dedicated Developmental Editor, Megan Duttera, in the Nursing Editorial division of Lippincott Williams & Wilkins. Megan, thank you for your patience, support, unending encouragement, and total commitment. My thanks to Danielle DiPalma, Senior Developmental Editor, for all her creativity, insight, and tireless work on the accompanying videos. My thanks to Jean Rodenberger, Executive Acquisitions Editor, and Joe Morita, Marketing Manager, for their hard work and guidance throughout the project. Thank you to the members of the production department, who patiently pulled everything together to form a completed book: Helen Ewan, Director of Nursing Production; Sandra Cherrey Scheinin, Senior Production Editor; Holly Reid McLaughlin, Design Coordinator; and Brett MacNaughton, Illustration Coordinator.

A special thanks to Mary Hermann, whose work on Chapters 2, 6, 8, 11, and 15 was invaluable and made meeting deadlines possible. Mary, you are an unbelievable role model. Also, thanks to Brenda Clapp, my wonderful colleague and friend, for her support and professional guidance.

Finally, I would like to gratefully acknowledge my family, for their love, understanding, and encouragement. Their support was essential during the long hours of research and writing.

Pamela Lynn

Contents

UNIT I

Actions Basic to Nursing Care

CHAPTER 1

Vital Signs

Focusing on Patient Care

This chapter will explain some of the skills needed to care for the following patients:

Tyrone Jeffries, age 5, is in the emergency department with a temperature of 101.3° F.

Toby White, age 26, has a history of asthma and is now breathing 32 times per minute.

Carl Glatz, age 58, has recently started taking medications to control his hypertension.

Learning Objectives

After studying this chapter, you will be able to:

1. Assess body temperature via the oral, rectal, tympanic, and axillary routes.
2. Assess peripheral pulses by palpation.
3. Assess an apical pulse by auscultation.
4. Assess peripheral pulses by ultrasound Doppler.
5. Assess respiration.
6. Assess blood pressure by auscultation or using an automatic blood pressure monitor.
7. Assess systolic blood pressure using an ultrasound Doppler.
8. Weigh a patient using a bed scale.
9. Monitor a newborn's temperature while using a radiant overhead warmer.

Key Terms

afebrile: a condition in which the body temperature is not elevated

apnea: absence of breathing

bell: (of stethoscope) hollowed, upright, curved portion used to auscultate low-pitched sounds such as murmurs

blood pressure: force of blood against arterial walls

bradycardia: slow heart rate

bradypnea: abnormally slow rate of breathing

diaphragm: (of stethoscope) large, flat disk on the stethoscope used to auscultate high-pitched sounds such as respiratory sounds

diastolic pressure: least amount of pressure exerted on arterial walls, which occurs when the heart is at rest between ventricular contractions

dyspnea: difficult or labored breathing

dysrhythmia: an abnormal cardiac rhythm; synonym is arrhythmia

eupnea: normal respirations

expiration: act of breathing out; synonym is exhalation

febrile: a condition in which the body temperature is elevated

hyperpyrexia: high fever, above 41°C

hypertension: blood pressure elevated above the upper limit of normal

hypotension: blood pressure below the lower limit of normal

hypothermia: body temperature below the lower limit of normal

inspiration: act of breathing in; synonym is inhalation

Korotkoff sounds: series of sounds that correspond to changes in blood flow through an artery as pressure is released

orthopnea: type of dyspnea in which breathing is easier when the patient sits or stands

orthostatic hypotension: temporary fall in blood pressure associated with assuming an upright position; synonym for postural hypotension

pulse deficit: difference between the apical and radial pulse rates

pulse pressure: difference between systolic and diastolic pressures

pyrexia: elevation above the upper limit of normal body temperature; synonym for fever

respiration: act of breathing and using oxygen in body cells

systolic pressure: highest point of pressure on arterial walls when the ventricles contract

tachycardia: rapid heart rate

tachypnea: abnormally rapid rate of breathing

vital signs: body temperature, pulse, and respiratory rates, and blood pressure; synonym for cardinal signs

Vital signs are a person's temperature, pulse, respiration, and blood pressure, abbreviated as T, P, R, and BP. Pain, often called the fifth vital sign, is discussed in Chapter 10, Comfort. Health status is reflected in these indicators of body function. A change in vital signs may indicate a change in health.

Vital signs are assessed and compared with accepted normal values and the patient's usual patterns in a wide variety of instances. Examples of appropriate times to measure vital signs include, but are not limited to, screenings at health fairs and clinics, in the home, upon admission to a healthcare setting, when certain medications are given, before and after diagnostic and surgical procedures, before and after certain nursing interventions, and in emergency situations. Nurses take vital signs as often as the condition of a patient requires such assessment.

Careful attention to the details of vital sign procedures and accuracy in the interpretation of the findings are extremely important. Although vital sign measurement may be delegated to other healthcare personnel, it is the nurse's responsibility to ensure accuracy of the data, interpret vital sign findings, and to report abnormal findings. Techniques for measuring each of the vital signs are presented in this chapter. Fundamental Review 1-1 outlines age-related variations in normal vital signs. Fundamental Review 1-2 provides guidelines for obtaining vital signs for infants and children.

Fundamentals Review 1-1

Age-Related Variations in Normal Vital Signs

Age	Temperature (°C)	Pulse (beats/min)	Respirations (breaths/min)	Blood Pressure (mm Hg)
Newborn	36.8 (Axillary)	80–180	30–60	73/55
1–3 yr	37.7 (Rectal)	80–140	20–40	90/55
6–8 yr	37 (Oral)	75–120	15–25	95/75
10 yr	37 (Oral)	75–110	15–25	102/62
Teens	37 (Oral)	60–100	15–20	102/80
Adults	37 (Oral)	60–100	12–20	120/80
>70 yr	36 (Oral)	60–100	15–20	120/80 (May normally be up to 160/95)

Fundamentals Review 1-2

Techniques for Obtaining Vital Signs of Infants and Children

- Due to the “fear factor” of blood pressure measurement, save the blood pressure for last. Children and infants often begin to cry during blood pressure assessment, and this may affect the respiration and pulse rate assessment.
- Perform as many tasks as possible while the child is sitting on the parent’s lap or in a chair next to the parent.
- Let the child see and touch the equipment before you begin to use it.
- Make measuring vital signs a game. For instance, if you are using a tympanic thermometer that makes a chirping sound, tell the child you are looking for “birdies” in the ear. While auscultating the pulse, tell the child you are listening for another type of animal.
- If the child has a doll or stuffed animal, pretend to take the doll’s vital signs first.

SKILL 1-1 Assessing Body Temperature

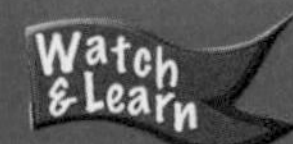

Body temperature is the heat of the body measured in degrees. Body temperature indicates the difference between production of heat and loss of heat. Heat is generated by metabolic processes in the core tissues of the body, transferred to the skin surface by the circulating blood, and then dissipated to the environment. Core body temperature is normally maintained within a range of 97.0°F (36.0°C) to 99.5°F (37.5°C). There are individual variations of these temperatures as well as normal changes during the day, with core body temperatures being lowest in the early morning and highest in the late afternoon (Porth, 2005). Table 1-1 outlines temperature equivalents in centigrade and Fahrenheit.

Temperatures differ in various parts of the body, with core body temperatures being higher than surface body temperatures. Core temperatures are measured at tympanic or rectal sites, but they may also be measured in the esophagus, pulmonary artery, or bladder by invasive monitoring devices. Surface body temperatures are measured at oral (sublingual) and axillary sites.

Several types of equipment and different procedures might be used to measure body temperature. To obtain an accurate measurement, the nurse must choose an appropriate site, the correct equipment, and the appropriate tool based on the patient's condition. If a temperature reading is obtained from a site other than the oral route, document the site used along with the measurement. If no site is listed, it is generally assumed to be the oral route.

It is important to note that glass thermometers with a mercury bulb have been used in the past for measuring body temperature. Most healthcare institutions have removed these thermometers from service and are phasing out mercury in any type of equipment, based on federal safety recommendations (U.S. Environmental Protection Agency [EPA], 2005a). However, many people still have mercury thermometers at home and may be continuing to use them. Information about the dangers of mercury, as well as how to handle a broken mercury thermometer, are important for nurses to know and share with their patients. Box 1-1 outlines important teaching points related to mercury thermometers. Many communities sponsor collection days for hazardous waste, including mercury thermometers. Encourage patients to use alternative devices to measure body temperature and to properly dispose of any mercury containing thermometers.

Equipment

- Digital or electronic thermometer
- Disposable probe covers
- Water-soluble lubricant for rectal temperature measurement
- Nonsterile gloves, if appropriate
- Toilet tissue, if needed
- Pencil or pen, paper or flow sheet

TABLE 1-1 Equivalent Centigrade and Fahrenheit Temperatures*

CENTIGRADE	FAHRENHEIT	CENTIGRADE	FAHRENHEIT
34.0	93.2	38.5	101.3
35.0	95.0	39.0	102.2
36.0	96.8	40.0	104.0
36.5	97.7	41.0	105.8
37.0	98.6	42.0	107.6
37.5	99.5	43.0	109.4
38.0	100.4	44.0	111.2

* To convert centigrade to Fahrenheit, multiply by 9/5 and add 32. To change Fahrenheit to centigrade, subtract 32 and multiply by 5/9.

SKILL 1-1 **Assessing Body Temperature** *(continued)*

BOX 1-1 Patient Teaching Related to Home Use of Mercury Thermometers

- Mercury is a heavy, odorless silver liquid.
- Mercury is toxic and a hazardous material that affects the central nervous system. The liquid and the vapors from the liquid are considered dangerous. Mercury is hazardous to people and the environment, especially if it gets into water. Mercury poisoning can lead to problems with mental development and learning disabilities.
- Glass thermometers containing mercury are easily broken.
- If a mercury glass thermometer breaks, **do not:**
  Sweep the area.
  Vacuum the area.
  Pour mercury down the drain.
  Wash mercury-contaminated clothes.
  Use household cleaning agents to clean the spill.
- If a mercury glass thermometer breaks, **do:**
  Open windows and close off the room from the rest of the house.
  Use fans for at least 24 hours.
- If the spill is on wood, linoleum, tile, or other like surfaces, it easily cleans up. **Do:**
  Use an eyedropper, a piece of heavy paper, or duct tape to scoop up the broken glass and beads of mercury.
  Put the mercury, broken glass, and any other materials used to scoop them up in a plastic zipper bag. Seal the bag tightly with tape. Place this bag into a second bag and seal with tape. Place the second bag into a third bag and seal with tape. Place the bags in a plastic wide-mouth sealable container.
- If the spill is on carpet, curtains, upholstery, or other like surfaces, throw material away. Cut out contaminated section. **Do:**
  Place the contaminated surfaces in a plastic zipper bag. Seal the bag tightly with tape. Place this bag into a second bag and seal with tape. Place the second bag into a third bag and seal with tape. Place the bags in a plastic wide-mouth sealable container.
- Throw everything away that was exposed to the mercury, including linens, clothing, and towels.
- Call local health department to find out about an approved disposal site.
- Wash hands with soap and water. Take a shower if you think any mercury touched other parts of your skin.

(U.S. Environmental Protection Agency [EPA]. [2005]. Safe mercury management: Cleanup instructions. Available at www.epa.gov/epaoswer/hazwaste/mercury/spills.hem#cleanmercuryspills.)

ASSESSMENT

Assess the patient to ensure that his or her cognitive functioning is intact. Taking an oral temperature of a patient unable to follow directions can result in injury if the patient would bite down on the thermometer. Assess whether the patient can close his or her lips around the thermometer; if the patient cannot, the oral method is not appropriate. Oral temperature measurement is contraindicated in patients with diseases of the oral cavity and those who have had surgery of the nose or mouth. Ask the patient if he or she has recently smoked, has been chewing gum, or was eating and drinking immediately before assessing temperature. If any of these have occurred, wait 15 to 30 minutes before taking an oral temperature because of the possible direct influence on the patient's temperature.

If you are taking a rectal temperature, review the patient's most recent platelet count. Do not insert a rectal thermometer into a patient who has a low platelet count. The rectum is very vascular, and a thermometer could cause rectal bleeding. Measuring rectal temperature is contraindicated in newborns, small children, and in patients who have had rectal surgery, or have diarrhea or disease of the rectum. Insertion of the thermometer into the rectum can slow the heart rate by stimulating the vagus nerve. Measurement of a rectal temperature for patients with certain heart diseases or after cardiac surgery is contraindicated in some institutions.

If a patient has an earache, do not use the affected ear to take a tympanic temperature. The movement of the tragus may cause severe discomfort. Assess the patient for significant ear drainage or a scarred tympanic membrane. These conditions can provide inaccurate results and could cause problems for the patient. However, an ear infection or the presence of earwax in the canal will not significantly affect a tympanic thermometer reading. If the

(continued)

SKILL 1-1 Assessing Body Temperature *(continued)*

patient has been sleeping with the head turned to one side, take a tympanic temperature in the other ear. Heat may be increased on the side that was against the pillow, especially if it is a plastic-covered pillow. Otherwise, either ear may be used.

NURSING DIAGNOSIS

Determine the related factors for the nursing diagnoses based on the patient's current status. Appropriate nursing diagnoses may include:

- Risk for Trauma
- Hyperthermia
- Hypothermia
- Risk for Imbalanced Body Temperature
- Ineffective Thermoregulation

OUTCOME IDENTIFICATION AND PLANNING

The expected outcomes to achieve when performing temperature assessment are that the patient's temperature is assessed accurately without injury and the patient experiences minimal discomfort. Other outcomes may be appropriate depending on the patient's nursing diagnosis.

IMPLEMENTATION

ACTION	RATIONALE
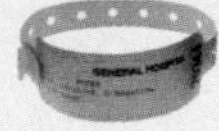 1. Check physician's order or nursing care plan for frequency and route. More frequent temperature measurement may be appropriate based on nursing judgment.	Provides for patient safety
2. Identify the patient. Discuss procedure with patient and assess patient's ability to assist with the procedure.	Identifying the patient ensures the right patient receives the intervention and helps prevent errors. This discussion promotes reassurance and provides knowledge about the procedure. Dialogue encourages patient participation and allows for individualized nursing care.
3. Ensure the electronic or digital thermometer is in working condition.	Improperly functioning thermometer may not give an accurate reading.
4. Close curtains around bed and close door to room if possible.	Provides for patient privacy
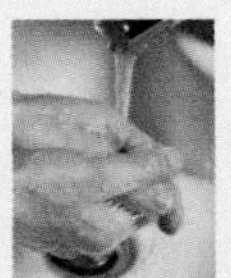 5. **Perform hand hygiene and put on gloves if appropriate or indicated.**	Hand hygiene deters the spread of microorganisms. Gloves prevent contact with blood and body fluids. Gloves are usually not required for an oral, axillary, or tympanic temperature measurement, unless contact with blood or body fluids is anticipated. Gloves should be worn for rectal temperature measurement.
6. Select the appropriate site based on previous assessment data.	Ensures safety and accuracy of measurement
7. Follow the steps as outlined below for the appropriate type of thermometer.	
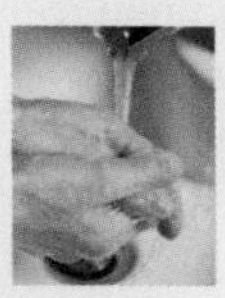 8. When measurement is completed, remove gloves, if worn. Perform hand hygiene.	Hand hygiene deters the spread of microorganisms.

SKILL 1-1

Assessing Body Temperature *(continued)*

ACTION | **RATIONALE**

Measuring a Tympanic Membrane Temperature

1. If necessary, push the "on" button and wait for the "ready" signal on the unit (Figure 1).

For proper function, thermometer must be turned on and warmed up.

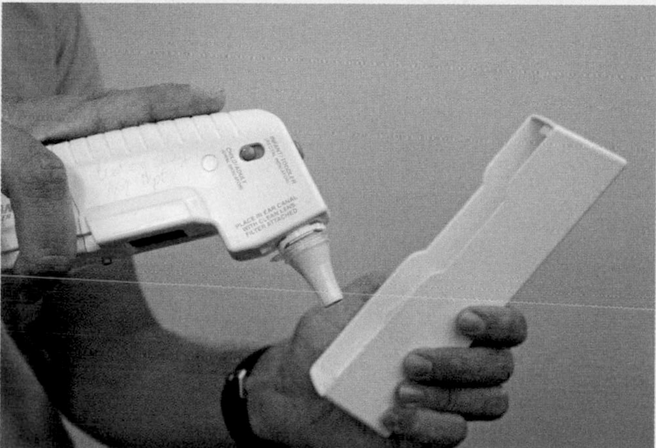

Figure 1. Turning unit on and awaiting the ready signal.

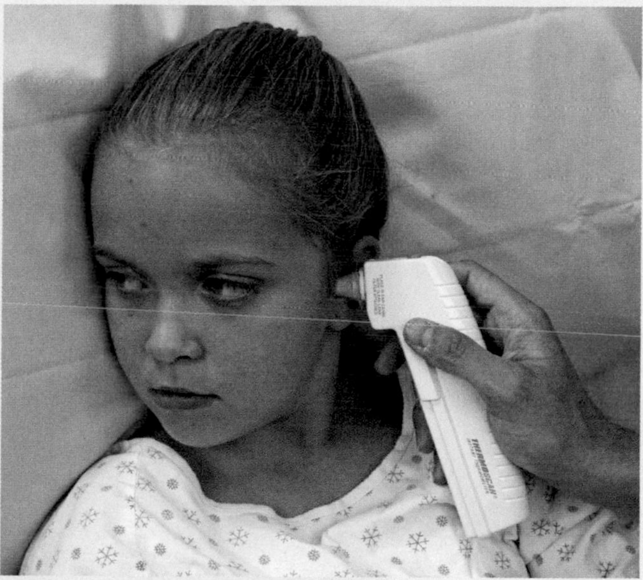

Figure 2. Inserting tympanic thermometer into the patient's ear.

2. Attach tympanic probe covering.

Use of the covering deters the spread of microorganisms.

3. **Insert the probe snugly into the external ear using gentle but firm pressure, angling the thermometer toward the patient's jaw line (Figure 2). Pull pinna up and back to straighten the ear canal in an adult.**

If the probe is not inserted correctly, the patient's temperature may be noted as lower than normal.

4. Activate the unit by pushing the trigger button. The reading is immediate (usually within 2 seconds). Note the reading.

The digital thermometer must be activated to record the temperature.

5. Discard the probe cover in an appropriate receptacle by pushing the probe-release button or use rim of cover to remove from probe (Figure 3). Replace the thermometer in its charger, if necessary.

Discarding the probe cover ensures that it will not be reused accidentally on another patient. Proper disposal prevents the spread of microorganisms. If necessary, the thermometer should stay on the charger so that it is ready to use at all times.

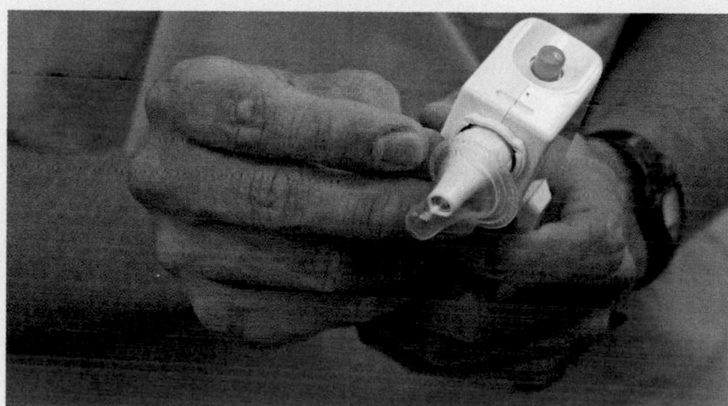

Figure 3. Disposing of probe cover.

(continued)

SKILL 1-1

Assessing Body Temperature *(continued)*

ACTION | RATIONALE

Assessing Oral Temperature

1. Remove the electronic unit from the charging unit, and remove the probe from within the recording unit.

   Electronic unit must be taken into the patient's room to assess the patient's temperature. On some models, by removing the probe the machine is already turned on.

2. Cover thermometer probe with disposable probe cover and slide it on until it snaps into place (Figure 4).

   Using a cover prevents contamination of the thermometer probe.

3. **Place the probe beneath the patient's tongue in the posterior sublingual pocket (Figure 5). Ask the patient to close his or her lips around the probe.**

   When the probe rests deep in the posterior sublingual pocket, it is in contact with blood vessels lying close to the surface.

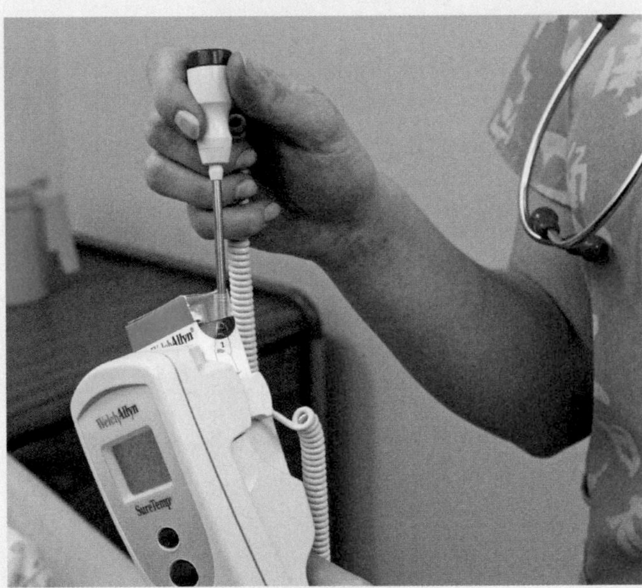

Figure 4. Putting probe cover on the thermometer.

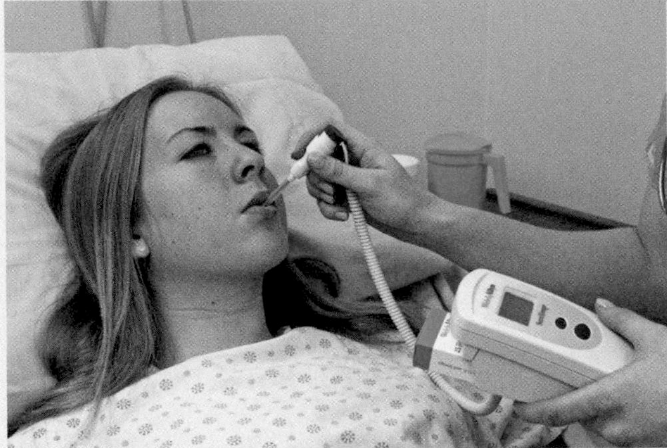

Figure 5. Inserting thermometer under the tongue in the posterior sublingual pocket.

4. **Continue to hold the probe until you hear a beep (Figure 6). Note the temperature reading.**

   If left unsupported, the weight of the probe tends to pull it away from the correct location. The signal indicates the measurement is completed. The electronic thermometer provides a digital display of the measured temperature.

5. Remove the probe from the patient's mouth. Dispose of the probe cover by holding the probe over an appropriate receptacle and pressing the probe release button (Figure 7).

   Disposing of the probe cover ensures that it will not be reused accidentally on another patient. Proper disposal prevents spread of microorganisms.

6. Return the thermometer probe to the storage place within the unit. Return the electronic unit to the charging unit, if appropriate.

   The thermometer needs to be recharged for future use. If necessary, the thermometer should stay on the charger so that it is ready to use at all times.

SKILL 1-1 Assessing Body Temperature *(continued)*

ACTION | RATIONALE

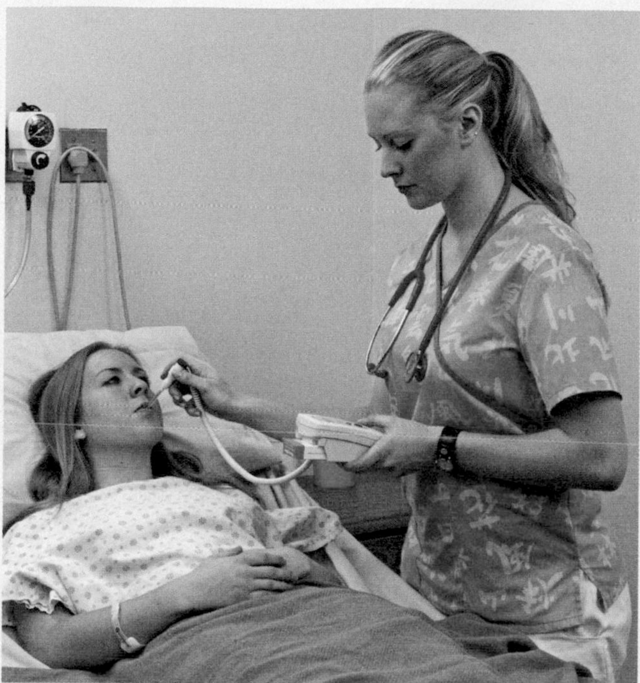

Figure 6. Holding probe in the patient's mouth.

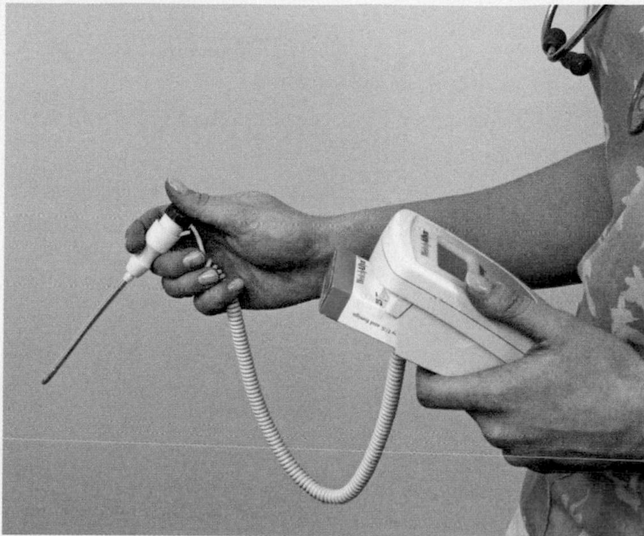

Figure 7. Pushing button to dispose of cover.

Assessing Rectal Temperature

1. Place the bed at an appropriate working height. Put on nonsterile gloves.

   Having the bed at the right height reduces strain on the nurse's back.

2. Assist the patient to a side-lying position. Pull back the covers enough to expose only the buttocks.

   The side-lying position allows the nurse to visualize the buttocks. Exposing only the buttocks keeps the patient warm and maintains his or her dignity.

3. Remove the rectal probe from within the recording unit of the electronic thermometer. Cover the probe with a disposable probe cover and slide it into place until it snaps in place (Figure 8).

   Using a cover prevents contamination of the thermometer.

4. **Lubricate about 1″ of the probe with a water-soluble lubricant (Figure 9).**

   Lubrication reduces friction and facilitates insertion, minimizing the risk of irritation or injury to the rectal mucous membranes.

5. Reassure the patient. Separate the buttocks until the anal sphincter is clearly visible.

   If not placed directly into the anal opening, the thermometer probe may injure adjacent tissue or cause discomfort.

6. **Insert the thermometer probe into the anus about 1.5″ in an adult or 1″ in a child (Figure 10).**

   Depth of insertion must be adjusted based on the patient's age. Rectal temperatures are not normally taken in an infant.

7. Hold the probe in place until you hear a beep, then carefully remove the probe. Note the temperature reading on the display.

   If left unsupported, movement of the probe in the rectum could cause injury and/or discomfort. The signal indicates the measurement is completed. The electronic thermometer provides a digital display of the measured temperature.

(continued)

SKILL 1-1

Assessing Body Temperature *(continued)*

ACTION | RATIONALE

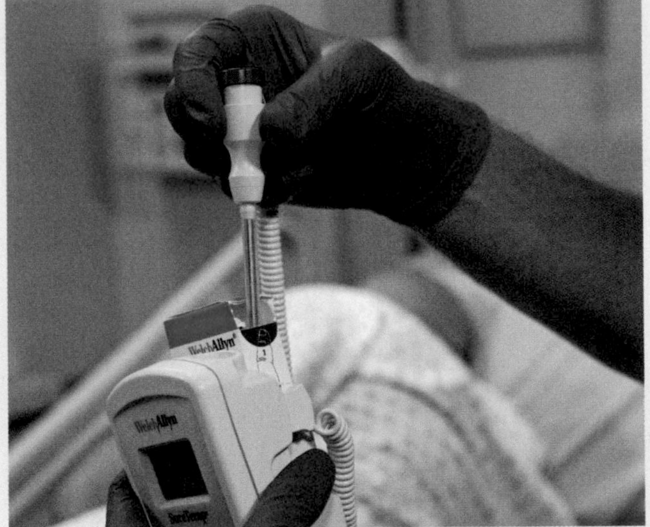

Figure 8. Removing appropriate probe and attaching disposable probe cover.

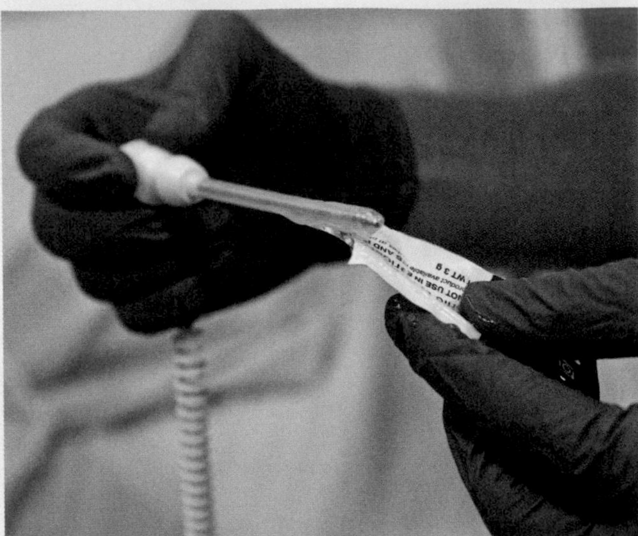

Figure 9. Lubricating thermometer tip.

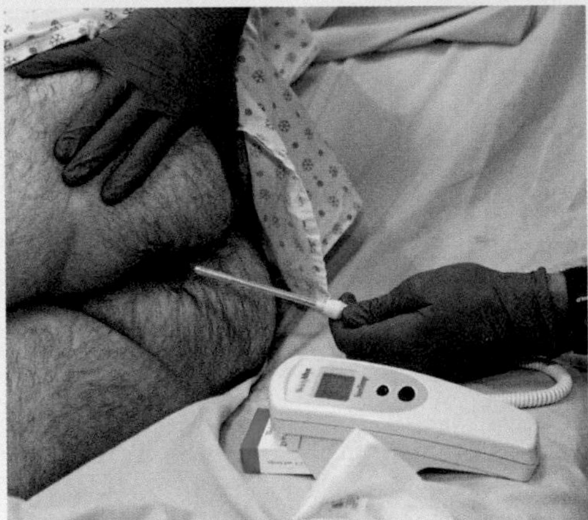

Figure 10. Inserting thermometer into the anus.

Action	Rationale
8. Dispose of the probe cover by holding the probe over an appropriate waste receptacle and pressing the release button.	Proper probe cover disposal reduces risk of microorganism transmission.
9. Using toilet tissue, wipe the anus of any feces or excess lubricant. Dispose of the toilet tissue.	Wiping promotes cleanliness. Disposing of the toilet tissue avoids transmission of microorganisms.
10. Cover the patient and help him or her to a position of comfort.	Ensures patient comfort.
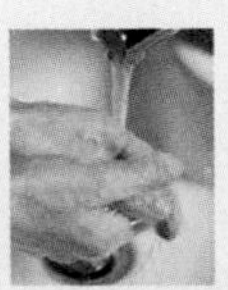 11. Remove gloves and discard them. Perform hand hygiene.	Hand hygiene avoids transmission of microorganisms.
12. Place the bed in the lowest position; elevate rails as needed.	These actions provide for the patient's safety.
13. Return the thermometer to the charging unit.	The thermometer needs to be recharged for future use.

SKILL 1-1 Assessing Body Temperature *(continued)*

ACTION	RATIONALE
Assessing Axillary Temperature	
1. Place the bed at an appropriate working height.	Having the bed at the right height reduces strain on the nurse's back.
2. Move the patient's clothing to expose only the axilla (Figure 11).	The axilla must be exposed for placement of the thermometer. Exposing only the axilla keeps the patient warm and maintains his or her dignity.
3. Remove the probe from the recording unit of the electronic thermometer. Place a disposable probe cover on by sliding it on and snapping it securely.	Using a cover prevents contamination of the thermometer probe.
4. **Place the end of the probe in the center of the axilla (Figure 12). Have the patient bring the arm down and close to the body.**	The deepest area of the axilla provides the most accurate measurement; surrounding the bulb with skin surface provides a more reliable measurement.

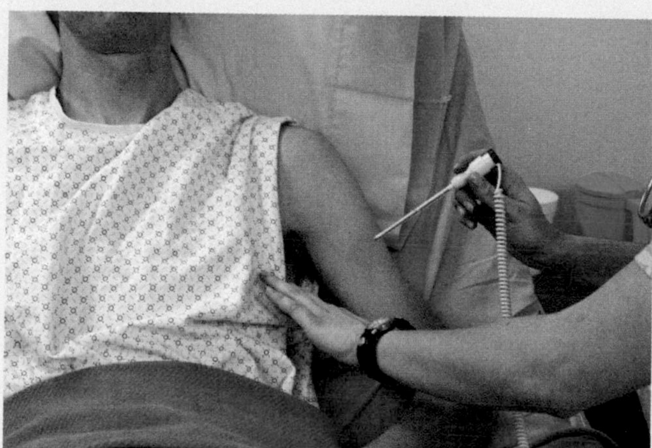

Figure 11. Exposing axilla to assess temperature.

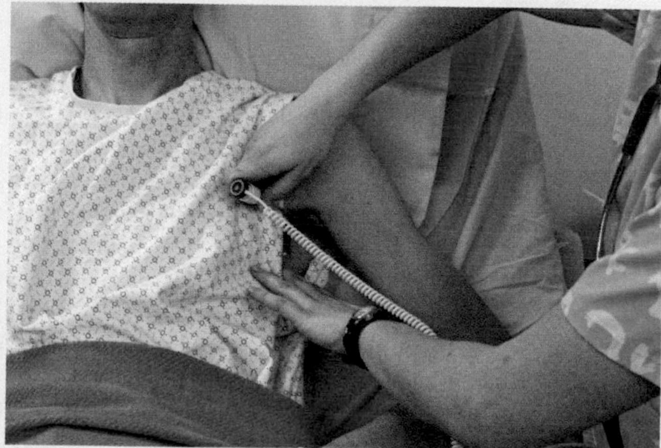

Figure 12. Placing thermometer in center of axilla.

ACTION	RATIONALE
5. Hold the probe in place until you hear a beep, and then carefully remove the probe. Note the temperature reading.	Axillary thermometers must be held in place to obtain an accurate temperature.
6. Cover the patient and help him or her to a position of comfort.	Ensures patient comfort
7. Dispose of the probe cover by holding the probe over an appropriate waste receptacle and pushing the release button.	Discarding the probe cover ensures that it will not be reused accidentally on another patient.
8. Place the bed in the lowest position and elevate rails as needed. Leave the patient clean and comfortable.	Low bed position and elevated side rails provide for patient safety.
9. Return the electronic thermometer to the charging unit.	Thermometer needs to be recharged for future use.

EVALUATION

The expected outcomes are met when the patient's temperature is assessed accurately without injury and the patient experiences minimal discomfort.

(continued)

SKILL 1-1

Assessing Body Temperature *(continued)*

DOCUMENTATION

Guidelines

Record temperature on paper, flow sheet, or computerized record. Report abnormal findings to the appropriate person. Identify the site of assessment if other than oral.

Sample Documentation

10/20/09 0800 Tympanic temperature assessed. Temperature 102.5° F. Physician notified. Received order to give 650 mg PO acetaminophen now. Incentive spirometer × 10 q 2 hours.—M. Evans, RN

Unexpected Situations and Associated Interventions

- *Temperature reading is higher or lower than expected based your assessment:* Reassess temperature with a different thermometer. The thermometer may not be calibrated correctly. If using a tympanic thermometer, you will get lower readings if the probe is not inserted far enough into the ear.
- *During rectal temperature assessment, the patient reports feeling lightheaded or passes out:* Remove the thermometer immediately. Quickly assess the patient's blood pressure and heart rate. Notify the physician. Do not attempt to take another rectal temperature on this patient.

Special Considerations

General Considerations

- When using a tympanic thermometer, make sure to insert the probe into the ear canal tightly enough to seal the opening to ensure an accurate reading.
- Non-mercury glass thermometers used for oral readings commonly have long, thin bulbs. Those for rectal readings have a blunt bulb to prevent injury. See the accompanying Skill Variation for information on assessing temperature with a non-mercury glass thermometer.
- Axillary temperatures are generally about one degree less than oral temperatures; rectal temperatures are generally about one degree higher.
- If the patient smoked, chewed gum, or consumed hot or cold food or fluids, wait 15 to 30 minutes before taking an oral temperature to allow the oral tissues to return to baseline temperature.
- Nasal oxygen is not thought to affect oral temperature readings. Oral temperatures should not be assessed for patients receiving oxygen by mask. Removal of the mask for the time period required for assessment could result in a serious drop in the patient's blood oxygen level.
- If the patient's axilla has been recently washed, wait 15 to 30 minutes before taking an axillary temperature to allow the skin to return to baseline temperature.

Infant and Child Considerations

- Small children have a limited attention span and have difficulty keeping their lips closed long enough to obtain an accurate oral temperature reading. For children younger than 6 years, use the axillary or tympanic site or use a temperature-sensitive tape (although research is ongoing to determine the accuracy of the measurements).
- Children with a high-grade fever (over 38.5 Celsius) should have their temperatures re-checked at a different site (Rush & Wetherall, 2003).
- Chemical dot thermometers (liquid crystal skin contact thermometers) are sometimes used as alternatives in pediatric settings. These single-use, disposable, flexible thermometers have specific chemical mixtures in circles on the thermometer that change color to measure temperature increments of two tenths of a degree. Keep this type of thermometer in the mouth for 1 minute, in the axilla 3 minutes, and the rectum 3 minutes. Read the color change 10 to 15 seconds after removing the thermometer. Read away from any heat source. Wearable, continuous-use chemical dot thermometers are available. These are placed under the axilla. Must be in place at least 2 to 3 minutes before taking first reading; continuously thereafter. Replace thermometer and assess underlying skin every 48 hours (Hockenberry, 2005).

SKILL 1-1 Assessing Body Temperature *(continued)*

Home Care Considerations

- Teach patients using electronic or digital thermometers to clean the probe after use to prevent transmission of microorganisms between family members. Clean according to manufacturer's directions.
- Teach patients using non-mercury glass thermometers to clean the thermometer after use in lukewarm soapy water and rinse in cool water. Store in an appropriate place to prevent breakage and injury from the glass.

SKILL VARIATION Assessing Temperature with a Non-Mercury Glass Thermometer

- If the thermometer is stored in a chemical solution, wipe the thermometer dry with a soft tissue, using a firm twisting motion. Wipe from the bulb toward the fingers.
- Grasp the thermometer firmly with the thumb and the forefinger and, using strong wrist movements, shake it until the chemical line reaches at least 96°F.
- Read the thermometer by holding it horizontally at eye level (Figure A). Rotate it between your fingers until you can see the chemical line. Verify the reading is less than or equal to 96°F.
- Place a disposable cover on the thermometer.
- **For oral use, place the bulb of the thermometer within the back of the right or left pocket under the patient's tongue and tell the patient to close the lips around the thermometer.**
- **For rectal use, place the thermometer bulb in the rectum as described when using an electronic thermometer.**
- **For axillary use, place the thermometer bulb in the center of the axilla. Move the patient's arm against the chest wall (Figure B).**
- **Leave the thermometer in place for 3 minutes (for oral use); 2 to 3 minutes (for rectal use); and 10 minutes (for axillary use); or according to agency protocol.**
- Remove the thermometer. Remove the disposable cover and place in a receptacle for contaminated items.
- Read the thermometer to the nearest tenth of a degree.
- Wash thermometer in lukewarm, soapy water. Rinse it in cool water. Dry and replace the thermometer in its container.

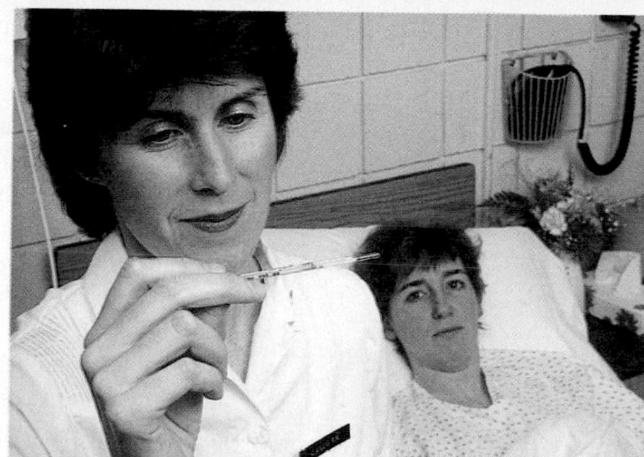

Figure A. Reading thermometer.

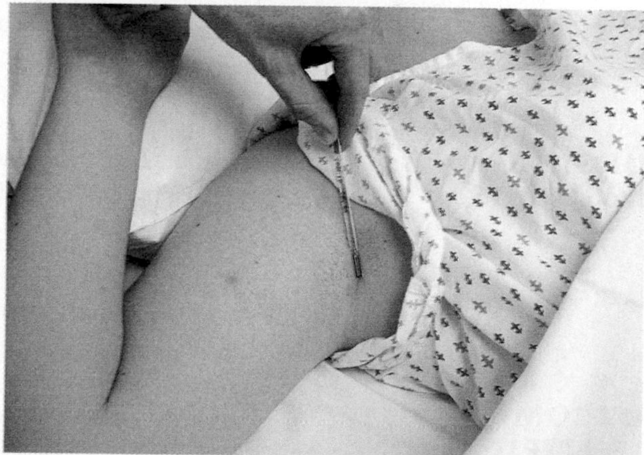

Figure B. Place thermometer in the center of the axilla.

SKILL 1-2 Assessing a Peripheral Pulse by Palpation

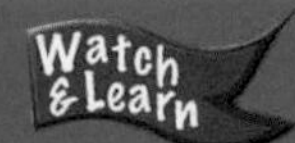

The pulse is a throbbing sensation that can be palpated over a peripheral artery or auscultated (listened to) over the apex of the heart. It results from a wave of blood being pumped into the arterial circulation by the contraction of the left ventricle. Each time the left ventricle contracts to eject blood into an already full aorta, the arterial walls in the cardiovascular system expand to compensate for the increase in pressure of the blood. Characteristics of the pulse, including rate, quality (amplitude), and rhythm provide information about the effectiveness of the heart as a pump and the adequacy of peripheral blood flow. Pulse rates are measured in beats per minute. Pulse amplitude describes the quality of the pulse in terms of its fullness. It is assessed by the feel of the blood flow through the vessel. Pulse rhythm is the pattern of the pulsations and the pauses between them. Pulse rhythm is normally regular; the pulsations and the pauses between occur at regular intervals. An irregular pulse rhythm occurs when the pulsations and pauses between beats occur at unequal intervals.

The pulse may be assessed by palpating peripheral arteries, by auscultating the apical pulse with a stethoscope, or by using a portable Doppler ultrasound (see the accompanying Skill Variation). To assess the pulse accurately, you need to know which site to choose and what method is most appropriate for the patient.

The most commonly used sites to palpate peripheral pulses and a scale used to describe pulse amplitude are illustrated in Box 1-2. Place your fingers over the artery so that the ends of your fingers are flat against the patient's skin when palpating peripheral pulses. Do not press with the tip of the fingers only (Refer to Figure 1, Step 8).

Equipment

- Watch with second hand or digital readout
- Pencil or pen, paper or flow sheet
- Nonsterile gloves, if appropriate

ASSESSMENT

Choose a site to assess the pulse. For an adult patient, the most common site is the radial or apical pulse. For a child older than 2 years, the radial pulse may be palpated. In infants and young children, the brachial pulse may be palpated. Assess for factors that could affect pulse characteristics, such as the patient's age, amount of exercise, fluid balance, and medications. Note baseline or previous pulse measurements.

NURSING DIAGNOSIS

Determine the related factors for the nursing diagnoses based on the patient's current status. Appropriate nursing diagnoses may include:

- Decreased Cardiac Output
- Ineffective Tissue Perfusion
- Deficient Fluid Volume
- Acute Pain

OUTCOME IDENTIFICATION AND PLANNING

The expected outcomes to achieve when measuring a pulse rate are that the patient's pulse is assessed accurately without injury and the patient's experiences minimal discomfort. Other outcomes may be appropriate depending on the patient's nursing diagnosis.

SKILL 1-2

Assessing a Peripheral Pulse by Palpation *(continued)*

BOX 1-2 Pulse Sites and Pulse Amplitude

Pulse Sites

Arteries commonly used for assessing the pulse include the temporal, carotid, brachial, radial, femoral, popliteal, posterior tibial, and dorsalis pedis.

Pulse Amplitude

Pulse amplitude typically is graded as 0 to 4:

0 (absent pulse): pulse cannot be felt, even with the application of extreme pressure
1+ (thready pulse): pulse is very difficult to feel, and applying slight pressure causes pulse to disappear
2+ (weak pulse): pulse is stronger than a thready pulse, but applying light pressure causes pulse to disappear
3+ (normal pulse): pulse is easily felt and requires moderate pressure to make it disappear
4+ (bounding pulse): pulse is strong and does not disappear with moderate pressure

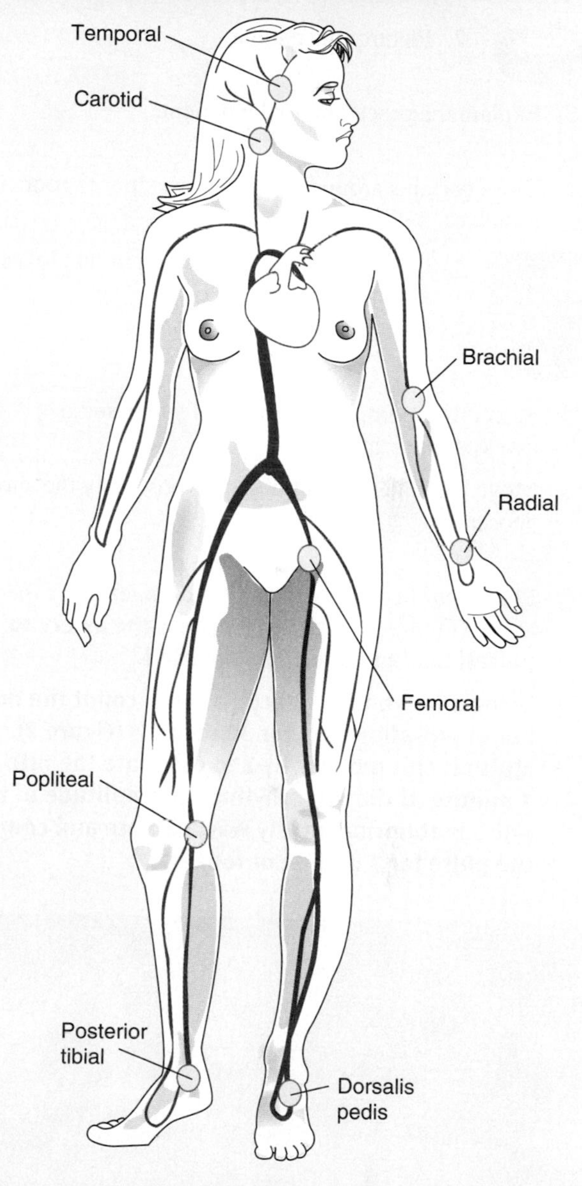

IMPLEMENTATION

ACTION	RATIONALE
1. Check physician's order or nursing care plan for frequency of pulse assessment. More frequent pulse measurement may be appropriate based on nursing judgment.	Provides for patient safety

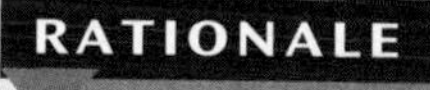

(continued)

SKILL 1-2 Assessing a Peripheral Pulse by Palpation *(continued)*

ACTION	RATIONALE
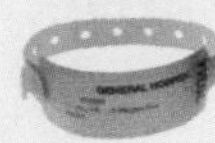 2. Identify the patient.	Identifying the patient ensure patient safety.
3. Explain the procedure to the patient.	Explanation reduces apprehension and encourages cooperation.
4. Close curtains around bed and close door to room if possible.	Provides for patient privacy
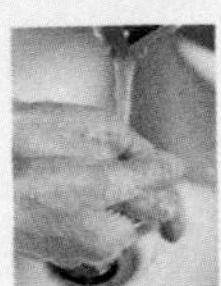 5. Perform hand hygiene and put on gloves as appropriate.	Hand hygiene deters the spread of microorganisms. Gloves are not usually worn to obtain a pulse measurement unless contact with blood or body fluids is anticipated. Gloves prevent contact with blood and body fluids.
6. Select the appropriate peripheral site based on assessment data.	Ensures safety and accuracy of measurement
7. Move the patient's clothing to expose only the site chosen.	The site must be exposed for pulse assessment. Exposing only the site keeps the patient warm and maintains his or her dignity.
8. Place your first, second, and third fingers over the artery (Figure 1). **Lightly compress the artery so pulsations can be felt and counted.**	The sensitive fingertips can feel the pulsation of the artery.
9. **Using a watch with a second hand, count the number of pulsations felt for 30 seconds (Figure 2). Multiply this number by 2 to calculate the rate for 1 minute. If the rate, rhythm, or amplitude of the pulse is abnormal in any way, palpate and count the pulse for 1 minute or longer.**	Ensures accuracy of measurement and assessment

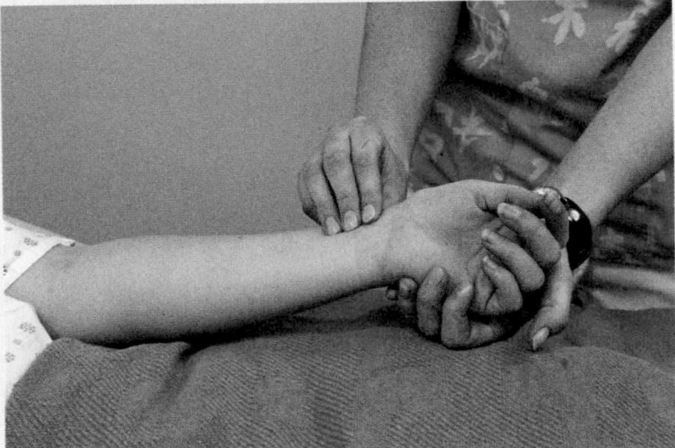

Figure 1. Palpating the radial pulse.

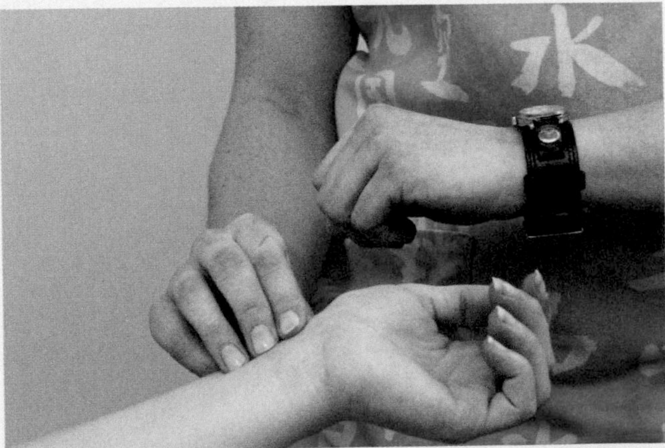

Figure 2. Counting the pulse.

ACTION	RATIONALE
10. **Note the rhythm and amplitude of the pulse.**	Provides additional assessment data regarding patient's cardiovascular status
11. Cover the patient and help him or her to a position of comfort.	Ensures patient comfort

SKILL 1-2

Assessing a Peripheral Pulse by Palpation *(continued)*

ACTION	RATIONALE
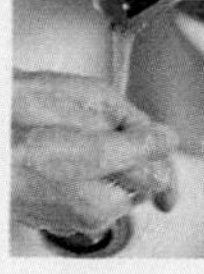 12. Remove gloves, if necessary. Perform hand hygiene.	Hand hygiene deters the spread of microorganisms.

EVALUATION

The expected outcomes are met when the patient's pulse is assessed accurately without injury and the patient experiences minimal discomfort

DOCUMENTATION

Guidelines

Record pulse rate, amplitude and rhythm on paper, flow sheet, or computerized record. Report abnormal findings to the appropriate person. Identify site of assessment.

Sample Documentation

2/6/08 1000 Pulses regular, 2+ and equal in radial, popliteal, and dorsalis pedis sites.—M. Evans, RN

Unexpected Situations and Associated Interventions

- *The pulse is irregular:* Monitor the pulse for a full minute. If this is a change for the patient, notify the physician.
- *The pulse is palpated easily but then disappears:* Apply only moderate pressure to the pulse. Applying too much pressure may obliterate the pulse.
- *You cannot palpate a pulse:* Use a portable ultrasound Doppler to assess the pulse. If this is a change in assessment, notify the physician. If you cannot find the pulse using an ultrasound Doppler, notify the physician. If you can find the pulse using an ultrasound Doppler, place a small X over the spot where the pulse is located. This can make palpating the pulse easier since the exact location of the pulse is known.

Special Considerations

General Considerations

- The normal heart rate varies by age. Refer to Fundamental Review 1-1.
- When palpating a carotid pulse, lightly press only one side of the neck at a time. Never attempt to palpate both carotid arteries at the same time.
- If a peripheral pulse is difficult to assess accurately because it is irregular, feeble, or extremely rapid, the apical rate should be assessed.

Infant and Child Considerations

- The apical pulse is the most reliable for infants and small children.

Home Care Considerations

- Teach the patient and family members how to take the patient's pulse, if appropriate.
- Inform the patient and family about digital pulse monitoring devices.
- Teach family members how to locate and monitor peripheral pulse sites, if appropriate.

(continued)

SKILL 1-2 Assessing a Peripheral Pulse by Palpation *(continued)*

SKILL VARIATION Assessing Peripheral Pulse Using a Portable Doppler Ultrasound Device

- Check physician's order or nursing care plan for frequency of pulse assessment. More frequent pulse measurement may be appropriate based on nursing judgment. Determine the need to use a Doppler ultrasound device for pulse assessment.
- Identify the patient.
- Explain the procedure to the patient.
- Close curtains around bed and close door to room if possible.
- Perform hand hygiene and put on gloves as appropriate.
- Select the appropriate peripheral site based on assessment data.
- Move the patient's clothing to expose only the site chosen.
- Remove Doppler from charger and turn it on. Make sure that volume is set at low.
- **Apply conducting gel to the site where you are auscultating the pulse.**
- Hold the Doppler base in your nondominant hand. With your dominant hand, place the Doppler probe tip in the gel. Adjust the volume as needed. Move the Doppler tip around until the pulse is heard.
- **Using a watch with a second hand, count the heartbeat for 1 minute.**
- Remove the Doppler tip and turn the Doppler off. Wipe excess gel off of the patient's skin with tissue.
- Place a small X over the spot where the pulse is located with an indelible pen. Marking the site allows for easier future assessment. It can also make palpating the pulse easier since the exact location of the pulse is known.
- Cover the patient and help him or her to a position of comfort.
- Wipe any gel remaining on the Doppler probe off with a tissue.
- Return the Doppler to the charge base.
- Record pulse rate, rhythm, and site.

SKILL 1-3 Assessing the Apical Pulse by Auscultation

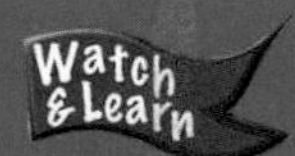

The pulse is a throbbing sensation that can be palpated over a peripheral artery or auscultated (listened to) over the apex of the heart. It results from a wave of blood being pumped into the arterial circulation by the contraction of the left ventricle. Each time the left ventricle contracts to eject blood into an already full aorta, the arterial walls in the cardiovascular system expand to compensate for the increase in pressure of the blood. Characteristics of the pulse, including rate, quality, rhythm, and amplitude, provide information about the effectiveness of the heart as a pump and the adequacy of peripheral blood flow. Pulse rates are measured in beats per minute. Pulse rhythm is the pattern of the pulsations and the pauses between them. Pulse rhythm is normally regular; the pulsations and the pauses between occur at regular intervals. An irregular pulse rhythm occurs when the pulsations and pauses between beats occur at unequal intervals.

The pulse may be assessed by palpating peripheral arteries, by auscultating the apical pulse with a stethoscope, or by using a portable Doppler ultrasound. To assess the pulse accurately, you need to know which site to choose and what method is most appropriate for the patient.

An apical pulse is assessed when giving medications that alter heart rate and rhythm. If a peripheral pulse is difficult to assess accurately because it is irregular, feeble, or extremely rapid, the apical rate should be assessed. In adults, the apical rate is counted for 1 full minute by listening with a stethoscope over the apex of the heart.

Equipment

- Watch with second hand or digital readout
- Stethoscope
- Alcohol swab
- Pencil or pen, paper or flow sheet

SKILL 1-3 Assessing the Apical Pulse by Auscultation *(continued)*

ASSESSMENT

Assess for factors that could affect apical pulse rate and rhythm, such as the patient's age, amount of exercise, fluid balance, and medications. Note baseline or previous apical pulse measurements. Assess the pulse rate and rhythm.

NURSING DIAGNOSIS

Determine the related factors for the nursing diagnoses based on the patient's current status. Appropriate nursing diagnoses may include:

- Decreased Cardiac Output
- Ineffective Tissue Perfusion
- Deficient Fluid Volume
- Acute Pain

OUTCOME IDENTIFICATION AND PLANNING

The expected outcomes to achieve when measuring an apical pulse rate are that the patient's pulse is assessed accurately without injury and the patient experiences minimal discomfort. Other outcomes may be appropriate depending on the patient's nursing diagnosis.

IMPLEMENTATION

ACTION	RATIONALE
1. Check physician's order or nursing care plan for frequency of pulse assessment. More frequent pulse measurement may be appropriate based on nursing judgment. Identify the need to obtain an apical pulse measurement.	Provides for patient safety and appropriate care
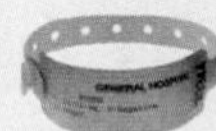 2. Identify the patient.	Identifying the patient ensures patient safety.
3. Explain the procedure to the patient.	Explanation reduces apprehension and encourages cooperation.
4. Close curtains around bed and close door to room if possible.	Provides for patient privacy
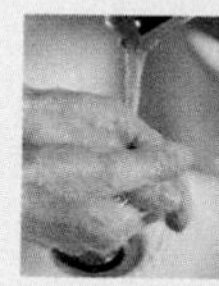 5. Perform hand hygiene and put on gloves as appropriate.	Hand hygiene deters the spread of microorganisms. Gloves are not usually worn to obtain an apical pulse measurement unless contact with blood or body fluids is anticipated. Gloves prevent contact with blood and body fluids.
6. Use alcohol swab to clean the diaphragm of the stethoscope. Use another swab to clean the earpieces if necessary.	Cleaning with alcohol deters transmission of microorganisms.
7. Assist patient to a sitting or reclining position and expose chest area.	This position facilitates identification of site for stethoscope placement.
8. Move the patient's clothing to expose only the apical site.	The site must be exposed for pulse assessment. Exposing only the apical site keeps the patient warm and maintains his or her dignity.
9. Hold the stethoscope diaphragm against the palm of your hand for a few seconds.	Warming the diaphragm promotes patient comfort.
10. **Palpate the space between the fifth and sixth ribs (fifth intercostal space), and move to the left mid-clavicular line.** Place the diaphragm over the apex of the heart (Figure 1 and Figure 2).	Positions stethoscope over the apex of the heart, where the heartbeat is best heard

(continued)

SKILL 1-3 Assessing the Apical Pulse by Auscultation *(continued)*

ACTION | RATIONALE

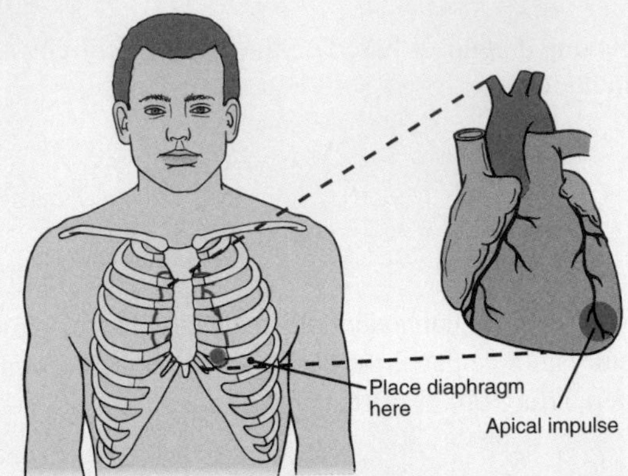

Figure 1. Locating the apical pulse: apex area.

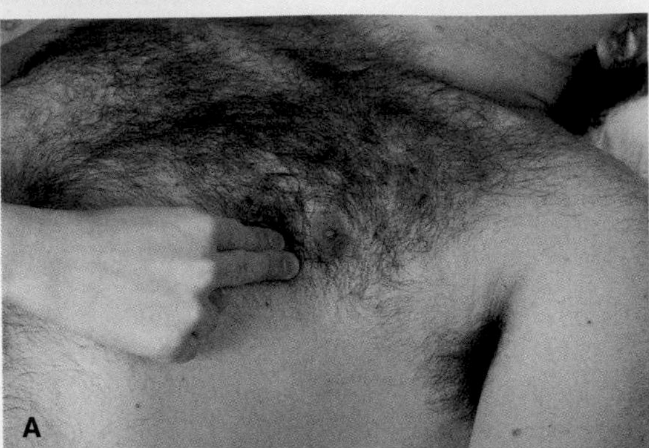

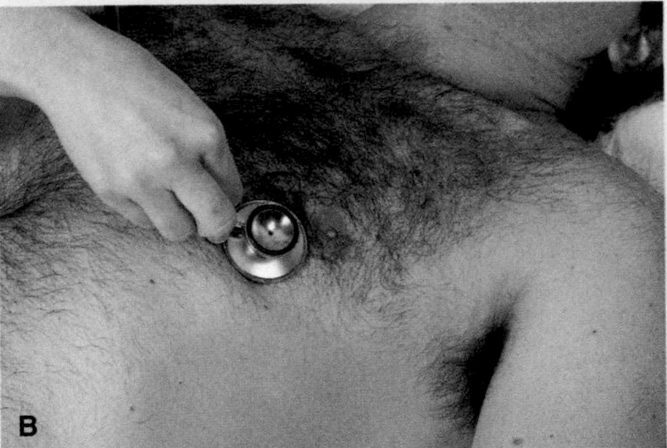

Figure 2. The apical pulse is usually found at (**A**) the fifth intercostal space just inside the midclavicular line and can be heard (**B**) over the apex of the heart.

11. Listen for heart sounds ("lub-dub"). Each "lub-dub" counts as one beat.

    These sounds occur as the heart valves close.

12. **Using a watch with a second hand, count the heartbeat for 1 minute.**

    Counting for a full minute increases the accuracy of assessment.

13. Cover the patient and help him or her to a position of comfort.

    This ensures patient comfort.

14. Clean diaphragm of the stethoscope with an alcohol swab.

    Cleaning with alcohol deters transmission of microorganisms.

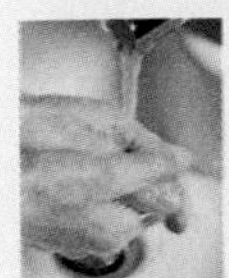

15. Remove gloves, if necessary. Perform hand hygiene.

    Hand hygiene deters the spread of microorganisms.

EVALUATION

The expected outcomes are met when the patient's apical pulse is assessed accurately without injury and the patient experiences minimal discomfort.

DOCUMENTATION

Guidelines

Record pulse rate and rhythm on paper, flow sheet, or computerized record. Report abnormal findings to the appropriate person. Identify site of assessment.

SKILL 1-3 Assessing the Apical Pulse by Auscultation *(continued)*

Sample Documentation

2/6/08 1000 Apical pulse 82 and regular. Digoxin 0.125 mg administered per order. Patient verbalized understanding of actions and untoward effects of medication. —B. Clapp, RN

Unexpected Situations and Associated Interventions

- If apical rate is irregular, assess patient for other symptoms, such as lightheadedness, dizziness, shortness of breath, or palpitations. Notify appropriate healthcare provider of findings.

Special Considerations

Infant and Child Considerations

- The apical pulse is the most reliable for infants and small children. Rate should be counted for 1 full minute in infants and children because of possible rhythm irregularities. (Hockenberry, 2005).
- Apical rate of infants is easily palpated with the fingertips.

SKILL 1-4 Assessing Respiration

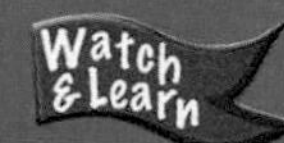

Under normal conditions, healthy adults breathe about 12 to 20 times per minute. Infants and children breathe more rapidly. Fundamental Review 1-1 outlines respiratory rate ranges for different age groups. The depth of respirations normal varies from shallow to deep. The rhythm of respirations is normally regular, with each inhalation/exhalation and the pauses between occurring at regular intervals. An irregular respiratory rhythm occurs when inhalation/exhalation and pauses between occur at unequal intervals. Table 1-2 outlines various respiratory patterns.

The nurse assesses respiratory rate, depth, and rhythm by inspection (observing and listening) or by listening with the stethoscope. The nurse determines the rate by counting the number of breaths per minute. If respirations are very shallow and difficult to visually detect, observe the sternal notch, where respiration is more apparent. With an infant or young child, assess respirations before taking the temperature so the child is not crying, which would alter the respiratory status.

Move right from the pulse assessment to counting the respiratory rate to avoid letting the patient know you are counting respirations. Patients should be unaware of the respiratory assessment because if they are conscious of the procedure, they might alter their breathing patterns or rate.

Equipment

- Watch with second hand or digital readout
- Pencil or pen, paper, or flow sheet

ASSESSMENT

Assess the patient for factors that could affect respirations, such as exercise, medications, smoking, chronic illness or conditions, neurologic injury, pain, and anxiety. Note baseline or previous respiratory measurements. Assess patient for any signs of respiratory distress, which include retractions, nasal flaring, grunting, orthopnea (breathing more easily in an upright position), or tachypnea (rapid respirations).

(continued)

SKILL 1-4

Assessing Respiration *(continued)*

TABLE 1-2 Patterns of Respiration

	DESCRIPTION	PATTERN	ASSOCIATED FEATURES
Normal	12–20 breaths/min Regular		Normal pattern
Tachypnea	>24 breaths/min Shallow		Fever, anxiety, exercise, respiratory disorders
Bradypnea	<10 breaths/min Regular		Depression of the respiratory center by medications, brain damage
Hyperventilation	Increased rate and depth		Extreme exercise, fear, diabetic ketoacidosis (Kussmaul's respirations), overdose of aspirin
Hypoventilation	Decreased rate and depth; irregular		Overdose of narcotics or anesthetics
Cheyne-Strokes respirations	Alternating periods of deep, rapid breathing followed by periods of apnea; regular		Drug overdose, heart failure, increased intracranial pressure, renal failure
Biot's respirations	Varying depth and rate of breathing, followed by periods of apnea; irregular		Meningitis, severe brain damage

NURSING DIAGNOSIS

Determine the related factors for the nursing diagnoses based on the patient's current status. Appropriate nursing diagnoses may include:

- Ineffective Breathing Pattern
- Impaired Gas Exchange
- Risk for Activity Intolerance
- Ineffective Airway Clearance
- Excess Fluid Volume
- Ineffective Tissue Perfusion

OUTCOME IDENTIFICATION AND PLANNING

The expected outcomes to achieve when assessing respirations are that the patient's respirations are assessed accurately without injury and the patient experiences minimal discomfort. Other outcomes may be appropriate depending on the patient's nursing diagnosis.

IMPLEMENTATION

ACTION	RATIONALE
1. **While your fingers are still in place for the pulse measurement, after counting the pulse rate, observe the patient's respirations (Figure 1).**	The patient may alter the rate of respirations if he or she is aware they are being counted.
2. Note the rise and fall of the patient's chest.	A complete cycle of an inspiration and an expiration composes one respiration.

SKILL 1-4 Assessing Respiration *(continued)*

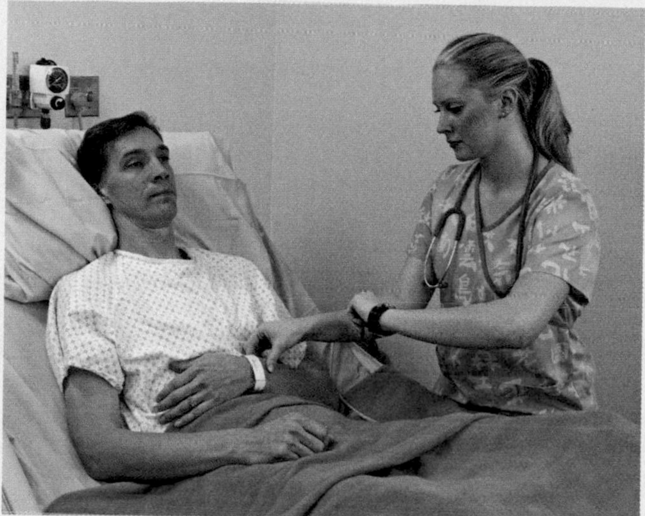

Figure 1. Assessing respirations.

3. Using a watch with a second hand, count the number of respirations for 30 seconds. Multiply this number by 2 to calculate the respiratory rate per minute.
   Sufficient time is necessary to observe the rate, depth, and other characteristics.
4. If respirations are abnormal in any way, count the respirations for at least 1 full minute.
   Increased time allows the detection of unequal timing between respirations.
5. Note the depth and rhythm of the respirations.
   Provides additional assessment data regarding patient's respiratory status

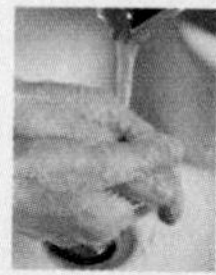

6. Perform hand hygiene.
   Hand hygiene deters the spread of microorganisms.

EVALUATION

The expected outcome is met when the patient's respirations are assessed without the patient altering the rate, rhythm, or depth.

DOCUMENTATION

Guidelines

Document respiratory rate, depth, and rhythm on paper, flow sheet, or computerized record. Report any abnormal findings to the appropriate person.

Sample Documentation

10/23/08 0830 Patient breathing at a rate of 16 respirations per minute. Respirations regular and unlabored—M. Evans, RN

Unexpected Situations and Associated Interventions

- *The patient is breathing with such shallow respirations that you cannot count the rate:* Sometimes it is easier to count respirations by auscultating the lung sounds. Auscultate lung sounds and count respirations for 30 seconds. Multiply by 2 to calculate the respiratory rate per minute. Notify the physician of respiratory rate and the shallowness of the respirations.

(continued)

SKILL 1-4 Assessing Respiration *(continued)*

Special Considerations

General Considerations

- If respiratory rate is irregular, count respirations for 1 minute.

Infant and Child Considerations

- In infants, count respirations for 1 full minute due to a normally irregular rhythm.

SKILL 1-5 Assessing a Brachial Artery Blood Pressure

Blood pressure refers to the force of the blood against arterial walls. Systolic pressure is the highest point of pressure on arterial walls when the ventricles contract. When the heart rests between beats during diastole, the pressure drops. The lowest pressure present on arterial walls during diastole is the diastolic pressure (Taylor et al., 2008). Blood pressure is measured in millimeters of mercury (mm Hg) and is recorded as a fraction. The numerator is the systolic pressure; the denominator is the diastolic pressure. The difference between the two is called the pulse pressure. For example, if the blood pressure is 120/80 mm Hg, 120 is the systolic pressure and 80 is the diastolic pressure. The pulse pressure, in this case, is 40. Table 1-3 outlines categories of blood pressure levels for adults.

TABLE 1-3 Categories for Blood Pressure Levels in Adults (Ages 18 and Older)

	BLOOD PRESSURE LEVEL (MM HG)	
Category	**Systolic**	**Diastolic**
Normal	<120	<80
Prehypertension	120–139	80–89
High Blood Pressure		
Stage 1	140–159	90–99
Stage 2	≥160	≥100

(These categories are from the National High Blood Pressure Education Program; National Heart, Lung, and Blood Institute; National Institutes of Health; and are available at www.nhlbi.nih.gov/hbp/detect/categ.htm.)

To get an accurate assessment of blood pressure, you should know what equipment to use, which site to choose, and how to identify the sounds you hear. Routine measurement should be taken after the patient has rested for a minimum of 5 minutes. In addition, the patient should not have any caffeine or nicotine 30 minutes before the blood pressure is measured.

The series of sounds for which the nurse listens when assessing blood pressure are called Korotkoff sounds. Table 1-4 describes and illustrates these sounds. Blood pressure may be assessed with different types of devices. Commonly, it is assessed by using a stethoscope and sphygmomanometer. Blood pressure may also be estimated with a Doppler ultrasound, estimated by palpation, and assessed with electronic or automated devices. It is very important to use correct technique and properly functioning equipment when assessing blood pressure to avoid errors in measurement. Use of a cuff of the correct size for the patient, correct limb placement, recommended deflation rate, and correct interpretation of the sounds heard are also necessary to ensure accurate blood pressure measurement (Armstrong, 2002; Porth, 2005; and Smeltzer et al., 2008). Table 1-5 outlines common errors in blood pressure measurement. It is important to

SKILL 1-5 **Assessing a Brachial Artery Blood Pressure** *(continued)*

TABLE 1-4 Korotkoff Sounds

PHASE	DESCRIPTION	ILLUSTRATION
Phase I	Characterized by the first appearance of faint but clear tapping sounds that gradually increase in intensity; the first tapping sound is the systolic pressure	
Phase II	Characterized by muffled or swishing sounds; these sounds may temporarily disappear, especially in hypertensive people; the disappearance of the sound during the latter part of phase I and during phase II is called the *auscultatory gap* and may cover a range of as much as 40 mm Hg; failing to recognize this gap may cause serious errors of underestimating systolic pressure or overestimating diastolic pressure.	
Phase III	Characterized by distinct, loud sounds as the blood flows relatively freely through an increasingly open artery	
Phase IV	Characterized by a distinct, abrupt, muffling sound with a soft, blowing quality; in adults, the onset of this phase is considered to be the first diastolic figure	
Phase V	The last sound heard before a period of continuous silence; the pressure at which the last sound is heard is the second diastolic measurement	

TABLE 1-5 Blood Pressure Assessment Errors and Contributing Causes

ERROR	CONTRIBUTING CAUSES
Falsely low assessments	• Hearing deficit • Noise in the environment • Viewing the meniscus from above eye level • Applying too wide a cuff • Inserting eartips of stethoscope incorrectly • Using cracked or kinked tubing • Releasing the valve rapidly • Misplacing the bell beyond the direct area of the artery • Failing to pump the cuff 20 to 30 mm Hg above the disappearance of the pulse
Falsely high assessments	• Using a manometer not calibrated at the zero mark • Assessing the blood pressure immediately after exercise • Viewing the meniscus from below eye level • Applying a cuff that is too narrow • Releasing the valve too slowly • Reinflating the bladder during auscultation

(continued)

SKILL 1-5 Assessing a Brachial Artery Blood Pressure *(continued)*

note that sphygmomanometers with mercury have been used in the past for measuring blood pressure. Most healthcare institutions have removed these devices from service and are phasing out mercury in any type of equipment, based on federal safety recommendations (EPA, 2005).

At times, it is necessary to assess a patient for orthostatic hypotension (postural hypotension). Orthostatic hypotension is a low blood pressure; it is defined as a drop of at least 20 mm Hg systolic or 10 mm Hg diastolic in blood pressure when the patient rises to an erect position, either supine to sitting, supine to standing, or sitting to standing (Rushing, 2005; Taylor et al, 2008). Box 1-3 outlines the procedure for blood pressure measurement to assess for orthostatic hypotension.

BOX 1-3 Blood Pressure Measurement to Assess for Orthostatic Hypotension

Throughout the procedure, assess for signs and symptoms of hypotension, such as dizziness, light-headedness, pallor, diaphoresis, or syncope. If the patient is attached to a cardiac monitor, assess for arrhythmias. Immediately return the patient to a supine position if symptoms appear during the procedure. Don't have the patient stand if symptoms of hypotension occur when the patient is sitting.

- Lower the head of the bed. Place the bed in a low position.
- Ask the patient to lie in a supine position for 3 to 10 minutes. At the end of this time, take an initial blood pressure and pulse measurement.
- Assist the patient to a sitting position on the side of the bed with the legs dangling. After 1 to 3 minutes, take another blood pressure and pulse measurement.
- Assist the patient to stand, unless standing is contraindicated. Wait 2 to 3 minutes, then take a blood pressure and pulse measurement.
- Record the measurements for each position, noting the position with the readings. An increase of 40 beats in the pulse rate or a decrease in blood pressure of 30 mm Hg are abnormal.

(Adapted from Taylor, C., Lillis, C., LeMone, P., et al. [2008]. *Fundamentals of Nursing* (6th ed.). Philadelphia:Lippincott Williams & Wilkins; and Rushing, J. [2005]. Assessing for orthostatic hypotension. *Nursing, 35*[1], 30.)

Various sites may be used to assess blood pressure. The brachial artery and the popliteal artery are most commonly used. This skill discusses using the brachial artery site to obtain a blood pressure measurement. The skill begins with the procedure for estimating systolic pressure. Estimation of systolic pressure prevents inaccurate readings in the presence of an auscultatory gap (a pause in the auscultated sounds). To identify the first Korotkoff sound accurately, the cuff must be inflated to a pressure above the point at which the pulse can no longer be felt.

Equipment

- Stethoscope
- Sphygmomanometer
- Blood pressure cuff of appropriate size
- Pencil or pen, paper or flow sheet
- Alcohol swab

ASSESSMENT

Assess the brachial pulse, or pulse appropriate for site being used. Assess for an intravenous infusion, and breast or axilla surgery on the side of the body corresponding to the arm used. Assess for the presence of a cast, arteriovenous shunt, or injured or diseased limb. If any of these conditions are present, do not use the affected arm to monitor blood pressure. Assess the size of the limb so that the appropriate-sized blood pressure cuff can be used. Assess for factors that could affect blood pressure reading, such as the patient's age, exercise, position, weight, fluid balance, smoking, and medications. Note baseline or previous blood pressure measurements. Assess the patient for pain. If the patient reports pain, give pain medication as ordered before assessing blood pressure. If the blood pres-

SKILL 1-5

Assessing a Brachial Artery Blood Pressure *(continued)*

sure is taken while the patient is in pain, make a notation concerning the pain if the blood pressure is elevated.

NURSING DIAGNOSIS

Determine the related factors for the nursing diagnoses based on the patient's current status. Appropriate nursing diagnoses may include:

- Decreased Cardiac Output
- Ineffective Health Maintenance
- Effective Therapeutic Regimen Management
- Risk for Falls

OUTCOME IDENTIFICATION AND PLANNING

The expected outcome to achieve when measuring blood pressure is that the patient's blood pressure is measured accurately without injury. Other outcomes may be appropriate depending on the patient's nursing diagnosis.

IMPLEMENTATION

ACTION	RATIONALE
1. Check physician's order or nursing care plan for frequency of blood pressure measurement. More frequent measurement may be appropriate based on nursing judgment.	Provides for patient safety
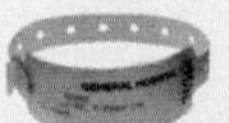 2. Identify the patient.	Identifying the patient ensures patient safety.
3. Explain the procedure to the patient.	Explanation reduces apprehension and encourages cooperation.
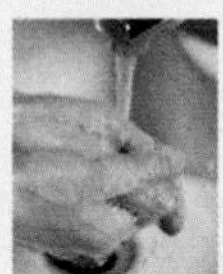 4. Perform hand hygiene and put on gloves if appropriate or indicated.	Hand hygiene deters the spread of microorganisms. Gloves prevent contact with blood and body fluids. Gloves are usually not required for an oral temperature measurement, unless contact with blood or body fluids is anticipated.
5. Close curtains around bed and close door to room if possible.	Provides for patient privacy
6. **Select the appropriate arm for application of cuff.**	Measurement of blood pressure may temporarily impede circulation to the extremity.
7. Have the patient assume a comfortable lying or sitting position with the forearm supported at the level of the heart and the palm of the hand upward (Figure 1).	This position places the brachial artery on the inner aspect of the elbow so that the bell or diaphragm of the stethoscope can rest on it easily.
8. Expose the brachial artery by removing garments, or move a sleeve, if it is not too tight, above the area where the cuff will be placed.	Clothing over the artery interferes with the ability to hear sounds and may cause inaccurate blood pressure readings. A tight sleeve would cause congestion of blood and possibly inaccurate readings.

(continued)

SKILL 1-5

Assessing a Brachial Artery Blood Pressure *(continued)*

ACTION

9. Palpate the location of the brachial artery. **Center the bladder of the cuff over the brachial artery, about midway on the arm, so that the lower edge of the cuff is about 2.5 to 5 cm (1″–2″) above the inner aspect of the elbow. Line the artery marking on the cuff up with the patient's brachial artery. The tubing should extend from the edge of the cuff nearer the patient's elbow (Figure 2).**

RATIONALE

Pressure in the cuff applied directly to the artery provides the most accurate readings. If the cuff gets in the way of the stethoscope, readings are likely to be inaccurate. A cuff placed upside down with the tubing toward the patient's head may give a false reading.

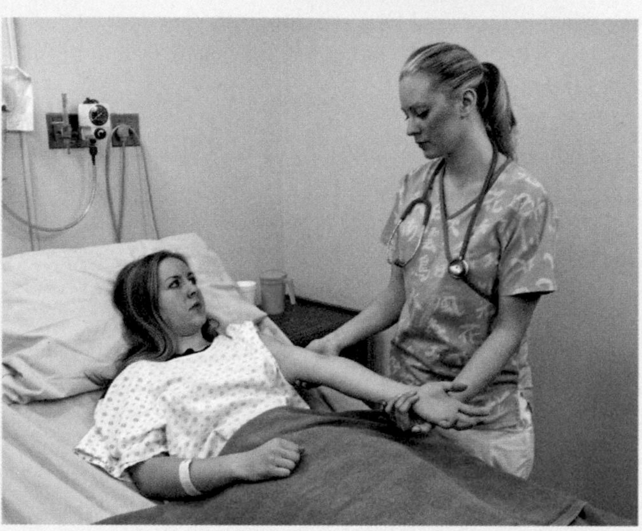

Figure 1. Proper positioning for blood pressure assessment using brachial artery.

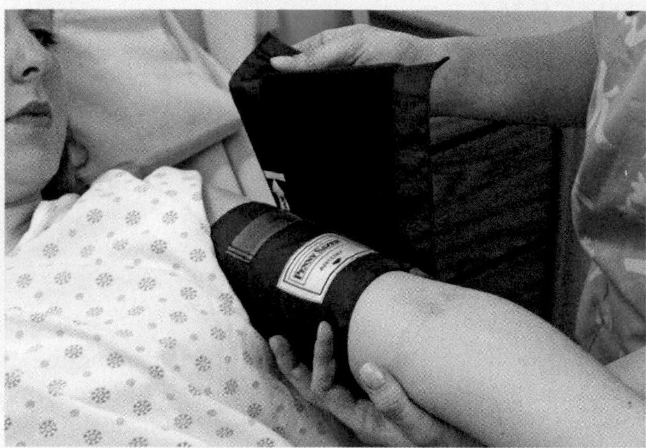

Figure 2. Placing the blood pressure cuff.

10. Wrap the cuff around the arm smoothly and snugly, and fasten it. Do not allow any clothing to interfere with the proper placement of the cuff.

A smooth cuff and snug wrapping produce equal pressure and help promote an accurate measurement. A cuff too loosely wrapped results in an inaccurate reading.

11. Check that the needle on the aneroid gauge is within the zero mark (Figure 3). If using a mercury manometer, check to see that the manometer is in the vertical position and that the mercury is within the zero level with the gauge at eye level.

If the needle is not in the zero area, the blood pressure may not be accurate. Tilting a mercury manometer, inaccurate calibration, or improper height for reading the gauge can lead to errors in determining the pressure measurements.

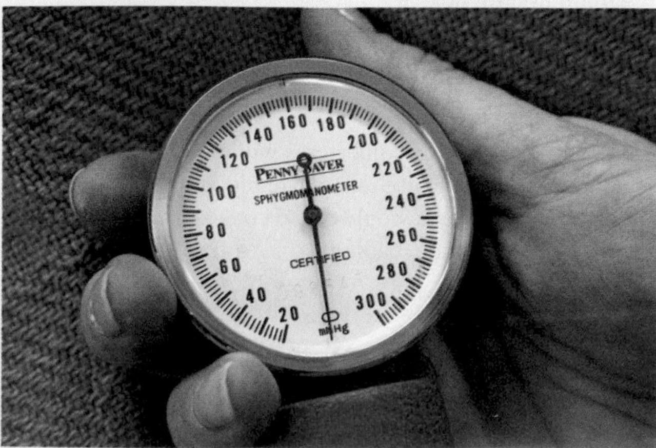

Figure 3. Ensuring gauge starts at zero.

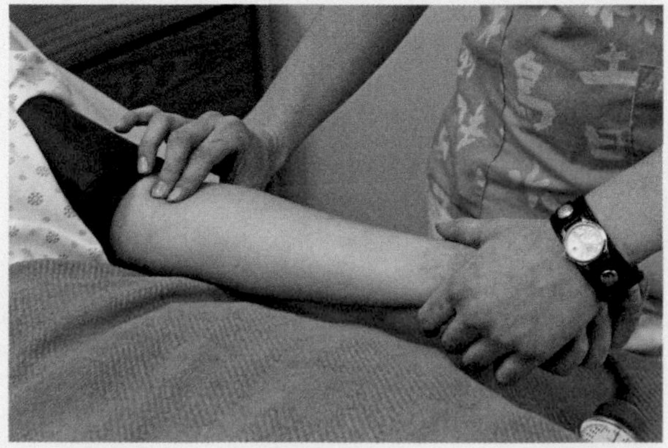

Figure 4. Palpating the brachial pulse.

SKILL 1-5

Assessing a Brachial Artery Blood Pressure *(continued)*

Estimating Systolic Pressure

12. **Palpate the pulse at the brachial or radial artery by pressing gently with the fingertips (Figure 4).**

Palpation allows for measurement of the approximate systolic reading.

13. Tighten the screw valve on the air pump.

The bladder within the cuff will not inflate with the valve open.

14. **Inflate the cuff while continuing to palpate the artery. Note the point on the gauge where the pulse disappears.**

The point where the pulse disappears provides an estimate of the systolic pressure. To identify the first Korotkoff sound accurately, the cuff must be inflated to a pressure above the point at which the pulse can no longer be felt.

15. Deflate the cuff and wait 15 seconds.

Allowing a brief pause before continuing permits the blood to refill and circulate through the arm.

Obtaining Blood Pressure Measurement

16. **Assume a position that is no more than 3 feet away from the gauge.**

A distance of more than about 3 feet can interfere with accurate readings of the numbers on the gauge.

17. Place the stethoscope earpieces in your ears. Direct the earpieces forward into the canal and not against the ear itself.

Proper placement blocks extraneous noise and allows sound to travel more clearly.

18. **Place the bell or diaphragm of the stethoscope firmly but with as little pressure as possible over the brachial artery (Figure 5). Do not allow the stethoscope to touch clothing or the cuff.**

Having the bell or diaphragm directly over the artery allows more accurate readings. Heavy pressure on the brachial artery distorts the shape of the artery and the sound. Placing the bell or diaphragm away from clothing and the cuff prevents noise, which would distract from the sounds made by blood flowing through the artery.

19. Pump the pressure 30 mm Hg above the point at which the systolic pressure was palpated and estimated. Open the valve on the manometer and allow air to escape slowly (allowing the gauge to drop 2–3 mm per heartbeat).

Increasing the pressure above the point where the pulse disappeared ensures a period before hearing the first sound that corresponds with the systolic pressure. It prevents misinterpreting phase II sounds as phase I.

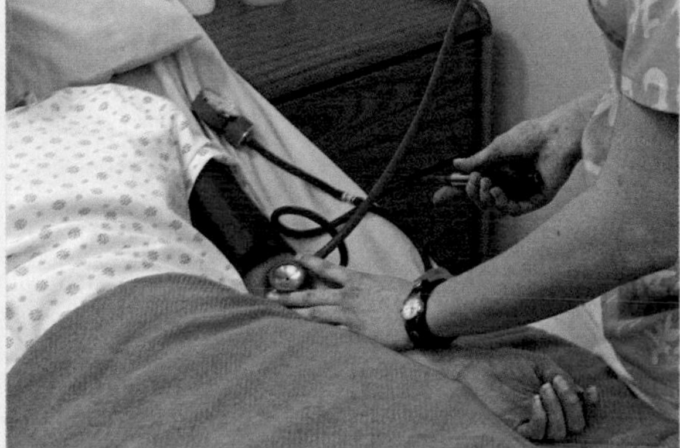

Figure 5. Proper placement of diaphragm of stethoscope.

(continued)

SKILL 1-5 Assessing a Brachial Artery Blood Pressure *(continued)*

ACTION	RATIONALE
20. **Note the point on the gauge at which the first faint, but clear, sound appears that slowly increases in intensity. Note this number as the systolic pressure (Figure 6).**	Systolic pressure is the point at which the blood in the artery is first able to force its way through the vessel at a similar pressure exerted by the air bladder in the cuff. The first sound is phase I of Korotkoff sounds.
21. Read the pressure to the closest even number.	It is common practice to read blood pressure to the closest even number.
22. Do not reinflate the cuff once the air is being released to recheck the systolic pressure reading.	Reinflating the cuff while obtaining the blood pressure is uncomfortable for the patient and may cause an inaccurate reading. Reinflating the cuff causes congestion of blood in the lower arm, which lessens the loudness of Korotkoff sounds.
23. **Note the pressure at which the sound first becomes muffled. Also observe the point at which the sound completely disappears (Figure 7). These may occur separately or at the same point.**	The point at which the sound changes corresponds to phase IV Korotkoff sounds and is considered the first diastolic pressure reading. According to the American Heart Association, this is used as the diastolic pressure recording in children. The last sound heard is the beginning of phase V and is the second diastolic measurement in adults.

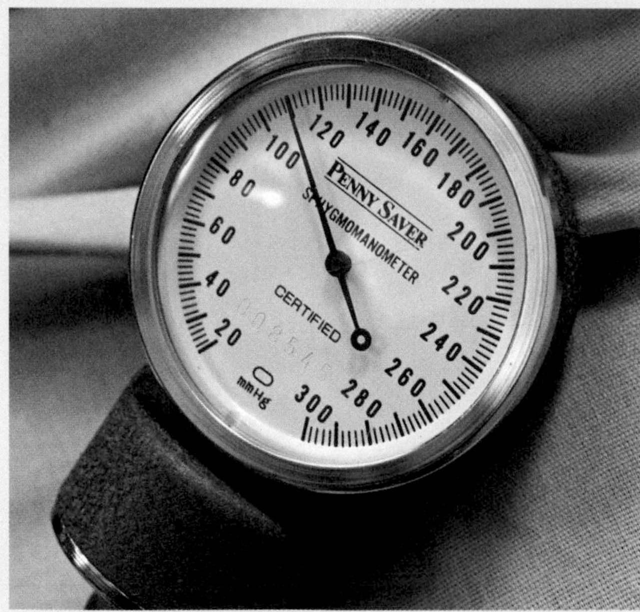

Figure 6. Measuring systolic blood pressure.

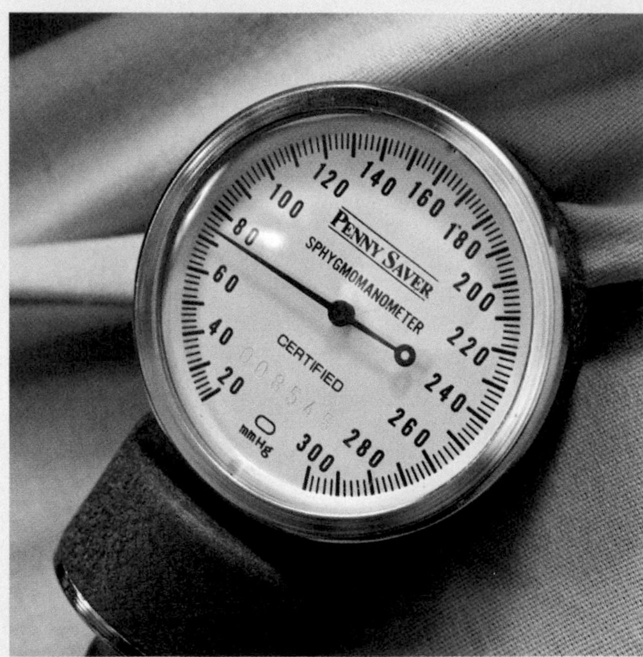

Figure 7. Measuring diastolic blood pressure.

ACTION	RATIONALE
24. Allow the remaining air to escape quickly. Repeat any suspicious reading, but wait 30 to 60 seconds between readings to allow normal circulation to return in the limb. Deflate the cuff completely between attempts to check the blood pressure.	False readings are likely to occur if there is congestion of blood in the limb while obtaining repeated readings.
25. Remove the cuff, and clean and store the equipment.	Equipment should be left ready for use.

SKILL 1-5

Assessing a Brachial Artery Blood Pressure *(continued)*

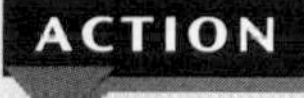

ACTION	RATIONALE
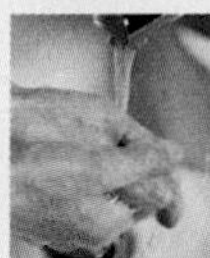 26. Remove gloves, if worn. Perform hand hygiene.	Deters the spread of microorganisms

EVALUATION

The expected outcome is met when the blood pressure is measured accurately without injury.

DOCUMENTATION

Guidelines

Record the findings on paper, flow sheet, or computerized record. Report abnormal findings to the appropriate person. Identify arm used and site of assessment if other than brachial.

Sample Documentation

10/18/09 0945 Blood pressure taken in right arm 180/100/88. Physician notified. Ordered Captopril 25 PO mg BID. Blood pressure to be repeated 30 minutes after administering medication.—M. Evans, RN

Special Considerations

General Considerations

- If this is the initial nursing assessment of a patient, take the blood pressure on both arms. It is normal to have a 5- to 10-mm Hg difference in the systolic reading between arms. Use the arm with the higher reading for subsequent pressures.
- If you have difficulty hearing the blood pressure sounds, raise the patient's arm, with cuff in place, over his or her head for 15 seconds before rechecking the blood pressure. Inflate the cuff while the arm is elevated, and then gently lower the arm while continuing to support it. Position the stethoscope and deflate the cuff at the usual rate while listening for Korotkoff sounds. Raising the arm over the head helps relieve congestion of blood in the limb, increases pressure differences, and makes the sounds louder and more distinct when blood enters the lower arm.
- Blood pressure may be assessed using an electronic device or Doppler ultrasound (see the accompanying Skill Variation).
- Many electronic devices are not recommended for patients with irregular heart rates, tremors, or the inability to hold the extremity still. The machine will continue to inflate, causing pain for the patient.

Infant and Child Considerations

- In infants and small children, the lower extremities are commonly used for blood pressure monitoring. The more common sites are the popliteal, dorsalis pedis, and posterior tibial. Blood pressures obtained in the lower extremities are generally higher than if taken in the upper extremities.
- In newborns, take blood pressure in all four extremities and document. Large differences among blood pressure readings can indicate heart defects.

Home Care Considerations

- Use a cuff size appropriate for limb circumference. Inform the patient that cuff sizes range from a pediatric cuff to a large thigh cuff and that a poorly fitting cuff may result in an inaccurate measurement.
- Inform patient about digital blood pressure monitoring equipment. Though costly, most provide an easy-to-read recording of systolic and diastolic measurements.

(continued)

SKILL 1-5 **Assessing a Brachial Artery Blood Pressure** *(continued)*

SKILL VARIATION Assessing Blood Pressure Using an Electronic Device

Automatic, electronic equipment is often used to monitor blood pressure in acute care settings, during anesthesia, postoperatively, or any time frequent assessments are necessary (Figure A). This unit determines blood pressure by analyzing the sounds of blood flow or measuring oscillations. The machine can be set to take and record blood pressure readings at preset intervals. Irregular heart rates, excessive patient movement, and environmental noise can interfere with the readings. Because electronic equipment is more sensitive to outside interference, these readings are susceptible to error. The cuff is applied in the same manner as the auscultatory method, with the microphone or pressure sensor positioned directly over the artery. When using an automatic blood pressure device for serial readings, check the cuffed limb frequently. Incomplete deflation of the cuff between measurements can lead to inadequate arterial perfusion and venous drainage, compromising the circulation in the limb.

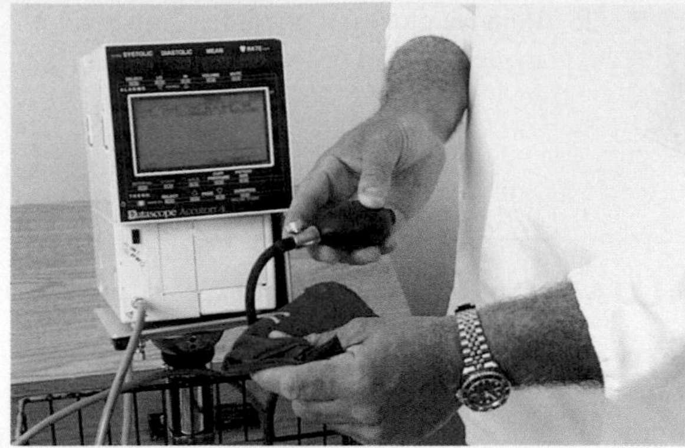

Figure A. Electronic blood pressure machine.

- Check physician's order or nursing care plan for frequency of blood pressure measurement. More frequent measurement may be appropriate based on nursing judgment.
- Identify the patient.
- Explain the procedure to the patient.
- Perform hand hygiene and put on gloves if appropriate or indicated.
- Close curtains around bed and close door to room if possible.
- **Select the appropriate limb for application of cuff.**
- Have the patient assume a comfortable lying or sitting position with the limb exposed.
- **Center the bladder of the cuff over the artery, lining the artery mark on the cuff up with the limb artery.**
- Wrap the cuff around the limb smoothly and snugly, and fasten it. Do not allow any clothing to interfere with the proper placement of the cuff.
- Turn the machine on. **If the machine has different settings for infants, children, and adults, select the appropriate setting. Push the start button. Instruct the patient to hold the limb still.**
- Wait until the machine beeps and the blood pressure reading appears. Remove the cuff from the patient's limb and clean and store the equipment.
- Remove gloves, if worn. Perform hand hygiene.
- Record the findings on paper, flow sheet, or computerized record. Report abnormal findings to the appropriate person. Identify arm used and site of assessment if other than brachial.

SKILL VARIATION Assessing Blood Pressure Using a Doppler Ultrasound

Blood pressure may be measured with an ultrasound or Doppler device, which amplifies sound. It is especially useful if the sounds are indistinct or inaudible with a regular stethoscope. This method only provides an estimate of systolic blood pressure.

- Check physician's order or nursing care plan for frequency of blood pressure measurement. More frequent measurement may be appropriate based on nursing judgment.
- Identify the patient.
- Explain the procedure to the patient.
- Perform hand hygiene and put on gloves if appropriate or indicated.
- Close curtains around bed and close door to room if possible.
- **Select the appropriate limb for application of cuff.**
- Have the patient assume a comfortable lying or sitting position with the appropriate limb exposed.
- **Center the bladder of the cuff over the artery, lining the artery marker on the cuff up with the artery.**
- Wrap the cuff around the limb smoothly and snugly, and fasten it. Do not allow any clothing to interfere with the proper placement of the cuff.
- Check that the needle on the aneroid gauge is within the zero mark. If using a mercury manometer, check to see that the manometer is in the vertical position and that the mercury is within the zero level with the gauge at eye level.
- Place a small amount of conducting gel over the artery.
- Hold the Doppler in your nondominant hand. Using your dominant hand, place the Doppler tip in the gel. Adjust the volume as needed. Move the Doppler tip around until you hear the pulse.
- Once the pulse is found using the Doppler, close the valve to the sphygmomanometer. Tighten the screw valve on the air pump.

SKILL 1-5 Assessing a Brachial Artery Blood Pressure *(continued)*

SKILL VARIATION Assessing Blood Pressure Using a Doppler Ultrasound *(continued)*

- **Inflate the cuff while continuing to use the Doppler on the artery. Note the point on the gauge where the pulse disappears.**
- Open the valve on the manometer and allow air to escape quickly. Repeat any suspicious reading, but wait 30 to 60 seconds between readings to allow normal circulation to return in the limb. Deflate the cuff completely between attempts to check the blood pressure.
- Remove the Doppler tip and turn the Doppler off. Wipe excess gel off of the patient's skin with tissue. Remove the cuff.
- Wipe any gel remaining on the Doppler probe off with a tissue.
- Return the Doppler to the charge base.
- Remove gloves, if worn. Perform hand hygiene.
- Record the findings on paper, flow sheet, or computerized record. Report abnormal findings to the appropriate person. Identify arm used and site of assessment if other than brachial.

SKILL 1-6 Using a Bed Scale

Obtaining a patient's weight is an important component of assessment. In addition to providing baseline information of the patient's overall status, weight is a valuable indicator of nutritional status and fluid balance. Changes in a patient's weight can provide clues to underlying problems, such as nutritional deficiencies or fluid excess or deficiency, or indicate the development of new problems, such as fluid overload. Weight also can be used to evaluate a patient's response to treatment. For example, if a patient was receiving nutritional supplementation, obtaining daily or biweekly weights would be used to determine achievement of the expected outcome (that is, weight gain).

Typically, weight is measured by having the patient stand on an upright scale. However, doing so requires that the patient is mobile and can maintain his or her balance. For patients who are confined to the bed, have limited mobility, or cannot maintain a balanced standing position for a short period of time, a bed scale can be used. With a bed scale, the patient is placed in a sling and raised above the bed. To ensure safety, a second nurse should be on hand to assist with weighing the patient. Many facilities are providing beds for patient use with built-in scales. The following procedure explains how to weigh the patient with a portable bed scale.

Equipment

- Bed scale with sling
- Cover for sling
- Sheet or bath blanket

ASSESSMENT

Assess the patient's ability to stand for a weight measurement. If patient cannot stand, assess the patient's ability to lie still for a weight measurement. Assess the patient for pain; medication may be given for pain or sedation before placing the patient on a bed scale. Assess for the presence of any material, such as tubes, drains, or IV tubing, that could become entangled in the scale or pulled during the weighing procedure.

NURSING DIAGNOSIS

Determine the related factors for the nursing diagnoses based on the patient's current status. Appropriate nursing diagnoses may include:

- Risk for Injury
- Impaired Physical Mobility

(continued)

SKILL 1-6 Using a Bed Scale *(continued)*

- Imbalanced Nutrition: Less Than Body Requirements
- Imbalanced Nutrition: More Than Body Requirements
- Risk for Injury

OUTCOME IDENTIFICATION AND PLANNING

The expected outcomes to achieve when weighing a patient using a bed scale are that the patient's weight is assessed accurately, without injury, and the patient experiences minimal discomfort. Other outcomes may be appropriate depending on the patient's nursing diagnosis.

IMPLEMENTATION

ACTION	RATIONALE
1. Check physician's order or nursing care plan for frequency of weight measurement. More frequent pulse measurement may be appropriate based on nursing judgment. Obtain the assistance of a second caregiver, based on patient's mobility and ability to cooperate with procedure.	This provides for patient safety and appropriate care.
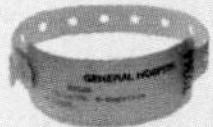 2. Identify the patient.	Identifying the patient provides patient safety.
3. Explain the procedure to the patient.	Explanation reduces apprehension and encourages cooperation.
4. Close curtains around bed and close door to room if possible.	Provides for patient privacy
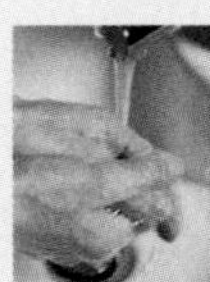 5. Perform hand hygiene.	Hand hygiene deters the spread of microorganisms.
6. Place a cover over the sling of the bed scale.	Using a cover deters the spread of microorganisms.
7. Attach the sling to the bed scale. Lay the sheet or bath blanket in the sling. Turn the scale on. **Adjust the dial so that weight reads 0.0.**	Scale will add the sling into the weight unless it is zeroed with the sling, blanket, and cover.
8. Raise bed to a comfortable working level. Position one caregiver on each side of the bed, if two caregivers are present. Raise side rail on the opposite side of the bed from where the scale is located, if not already in place. Cover the patient with the sheet or bath blanket. Remove other covers and any pillows.	Raising the bed to the appropriate height prevents strain to the nurse's back. Having one caregiver on each side of the bed provides for patient safety and appropriate care. Blanket maintains patient's dignity and provides warmth.
9. Turn patient onto side facing side rail, keeping his or her body covered with the sheet or blanket. Remove the sling from the scale. Roll sling long ways. Place rolled sling under patient, making sure the patient is centered in the sling.	Rolling the patient onto his or her side facilitates placing the patient onto the sling. Blanket maintains patient's dignity and provides warmth.
10. Roll patient back over sling and onto other side. Pull sling through, as if placing sheet under patient, unrolling sling as it is pulled through.	This facilitates placing patient onto sling.

SKILL 1-6 Using a Bed Scale *(continued)*

ACTION	RATIONALE
11. Roll scale over the bed so that arms of scale are directly over patient. **Spread the base of the scale.** Lower arms of the scale and place arm hooks into holes on the sling.	By spreading the base, you are giving the scale a wider base, thus preventing the scale from toppling over with the patient. Hooking sling to scale provides secure attachment to the scale and prevents injury.
12. Once scale arms are hooked onto the sling, begin to crank scale so that patient is lifted up off of the bed. **Assess all tubes and drains, making sure that none have tension placed on them as the scale is lifted. Once the sling is no longer touching the bed, ensure that nothing else is hanging onto the sling (eg, ventilator tubing, IV tubing). If any tubing is connected to the patient, raise it up so that it is not adding any weight to the patient.**	Scale must be hanging free to obtain an accurate weight. Any tubing that is hanging off the scale will add weight to the patient.
13. Note weight reading on the scale. Slowly and gently, lower patient back onto the bed. Disconnect scale arms from sling. Close base of scale and pull it away from the bed.	Lowering patient slowly does not alarm patient. Closing the base of the scale facilitates moving the scale.
14. Raise side rail. Turn patient to side rail. Roll the sling up against the patient's backside.	Raising the side rail is a safety measure.
15. Raise the other side rail. Roll patient back over the sling and up facing the other side rail. Remove sling from bed.	Patient needs to be removed from sling before it can be removed from the bed.
16. Cover the patient and help him or her to a position of comfort. **Place the bed in the lowest position.**	Ensures patient comfort and safety.
17. Remove disposable cover from sling and discard in appropriate receptacle. Replace scale and sling in appropriate spot. Plug scale into electrical outlet.	Using a cover deters spread of microorganisms. Scale should be ready for use at any time.
18. Document weight and scale used.	Reporting and recording ensure accurate documentation and communication.

EVALUATION

The expected outcome is met when the patient is weighed accurately without injury using the bed scale.

DOCUMENTATION

Guidelines

Document weight and scale used.

Sample Documentation

10/15/09 0230 Patient reports pain in legs 5/10. Premedicated with Percocet 2 tabs PO before obtaining weight per order. Patient weighed using bed scale. 75.2 kg.
—M. Evans, RN

(continued)

SKILL 1-6 Using a Bed Scale *(continued)*

Unexpected Situations and Associated Interventions

- *As the patient is being lifted, the scale begins to tip over:* Stop lifting the patient. Slowly lower the patient back to the bed. Ensure that the base of the scale is spread before attempting to weigh the patient.
- *Weight differs from the previous day's weight by more than 1 kg:* Weigh the patient using the same scale at the same time each day. Check calibration of the scale. Make sure that the patient is wearing the same clothing. Make sure that no tubes or containers are hanging on the scale. If the patient is incontinent, make sure undergarments are clean and dry.
- *Patient becomes agitated as the sling is raised into the air:* Stop lifting the patient and reassure him or her. If the patient continues to be agitated, lower him or her back to the bed. Reevaluate necessity of obtaining weight at that exact time. If appropriate, obtain an order for sedation before attempting to obtain another weight.

SKILL 1-7 Monitoring Temperature Using an Overhead Radiant Warmer

Neonates, infants who are exposed to stressors or chilling (eg, from undergoing numerous procedures), and infants who have an underlying condition that interferes with thermoregulation (eg, prematurity) are highly susceptible to heat loss.

An overhead radiant warmer warms the air to provide a neutral thermal environment, one that is neither too warm nor too cool for the patient. Typically, radiant warmers are used for infants who have trouble maintaining body temperature. In addition, use of a radiant warmer minimizes the oxygen and calories that the infant would expend to maintain body temperature, thereby minimizing the effects of body temperature changes on metabolic activity.

Equipment

- Overhead warmer
- Temperature probe
- Aluminum foil probe cover

ASSESSMENT

Assess the patient's temperature using the axillary route and assess the patient's fluid intake and output.

NURSING DIAGNOSIS

Determine the related factors for the nursing diagnoses based on the patient's current status. Appropriate nursing diagnoses may include:

- Hyperthermia
- Hypothermia
- Risk for Imbalanced Body Temperature
- Ineffective Thermoregulation

OUTCOME IDENTIFICATION AND PLANNING

The expected outcomes to achieve when using an overhead warmer are that the infant's temperature is maintained within normal limits without injury.

IMPLEMENTATION

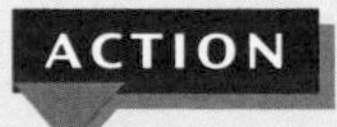

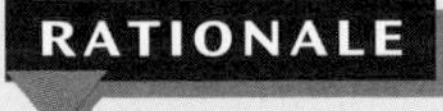

ACTION	RATIONALE
1. Check physician's order or nursing care plan for the use of a radiant warmer.	Provides for patient safety and appropriate care

SKILL 1-7 Monitoring Temperature Using an Overhead Radiant Warmer *(continued)*

ACTION	RATIONALE
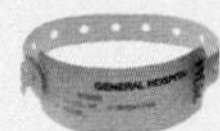 2. Identify the patient.	Identifying the patient provides for patient safety.
3. Explain the procedure to the family.	Explanation reduces the family's apprehension and encourages family cooperation.
4. Gather equipment.	Having all equipment on hand provides for an organized approach to the task.
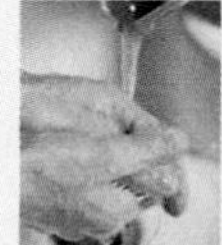 5. Perform hand hygiene.	Hand hygiene deters the spread of microorganisms.
6. Plug the warmer in. Turn the warmer to the manual setting. Allow the blankets to warm before placing the infant under the warmer.	By allowing the blankets to warm before placing the infant under the warmer, you are preventing heat loss through conduction. By placing the warmer on the manual setting, you are keeping the warmer at a set temperature no matter how warm the blankets become.
7. **Switch the warmer setting to automatic.** Place the infant under the warmer. Attach probe to the infant's skin but not on a bony area. Cover with a foil patch (Figure 1).	The automatic setting ensures that the warmer will regulate the amount of radiant heat depending on the temperature of the infant's skin. The foil patch prevents direct warming of the probe, allowing the probe to read only the infant's temperature.

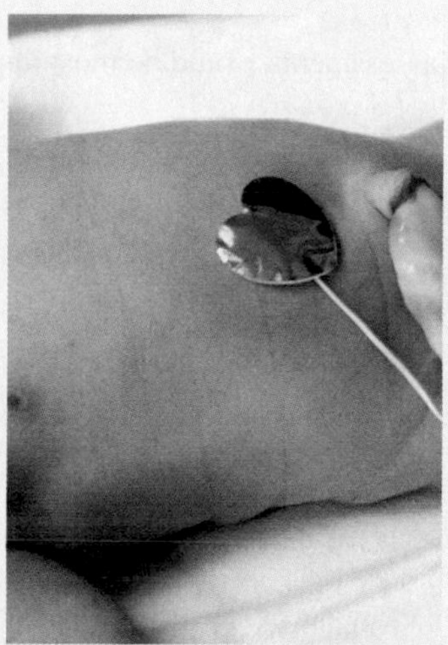
Figure 1. Probe in place with foil cover (Photo by Joe Mitchell).

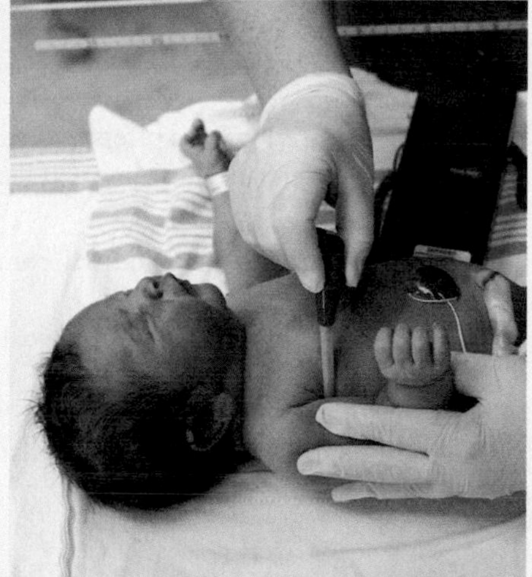
Figure 2. Taking infant's axillary temperature (Photo by Joe Mitchell).

ACTION	RATIONALE
8. **Adjust the temperature as ordered.**	The temperature should be adjusted so that the infant does not become too warm or too cold.
9. **Continue to monitor the axillary temperature as ordered (Figure 2).** The temperature may need to be monitored more frequently in the beginning.	By monitoring the infant's axillary temperature, you are watching for signs of fever or hypothermia.
10. Adjust the warmer's temperature as needed according to the axillary temperatures.	This prevents the infant from becoming too warm or too cool.

(continued)

SKILL 1-7 Monitoring Temperature Using an Overhead Radiant Warmer *(continued)*

EVALUATION

The expected outcomes are met when the infant is placed under a radiant warmer, the temperature is well controlled, and the infant experiences no injury.

DOCUMENTATION

Guidelines

Document initial assessment of the infant, including body temperature, the placement of the infant under the radiant warmer and the settings of the radiant warmer.

Sample Documentation

10/13/08 1110 Infant placed under radiant warmer. Warmer on automatic setting 36.7, baby's skin temperature 36.8.—M. Evans, RN

Unexpected Situations and Associated Interventions

- *The infant become febrile under the radiant warmer:* Do not turn the warmer off and leave the infant naked. This could cause cold stress and even death. Leave the warmer on automatic and dial the set temperature. Notify the physician.
- *The warmer's temperature is fluctuating constantly or is inaccurate:* Change the probe cover. If this does not improve the temperature variations, change the probe as well.

Special Considerations

- Radiant warmers increase insensible water loss in low-birthweight babies in the newborn period. This water loss needs to be taken into account when daily fluid requirements are calculated.
- Many times, plastic surgeons order overhead radiant warmers to be used for patients who have undergone extremity or digit reattachment surgery. In this case, judge the heat by the probe's reading of the skin temperature.

The Taylor Suite offers these additional resources to enhance learning and facilitate understanding of this chapter:

- thePoint online resource, http://thepoint.lww.com/Lynn2E
- Student CD-ROM included with the book
- Skills Checklist to Accompany Taylor's Clinical Nursing Skills
- Taylor's Interactive Nursing: *Vital Signs*
- Taylor's Video Guide to Clinical Nursing Skills: *Vital Signs*

Developing Critical Thinking Skills

1. Tyrone Jeffries, the 5-year-old with a fever of 38.9°C, is suspected of having a middle-ear infection. You need to obtain another set of vital signs for him. As you approach with the electronic thermometer, Tyrone begins to scream, saying, "Get away from me with that thing. You're not going to put that thing in me!" How would you respond?
2. Toby White, who is 26 years old with a history of asthma, has a respiratory rate of 32 breaths per minute. What other assessments would be most important to make?
3. Carl Glatz, the 58-year-old man receiving medications for hypertension, asks you about how he should monitor his blood pressure at home. What information would you suggest?

Bibliography

Armstrong, R. (2002). Nurses' knowledge of error in blood pressure measurement technique. *International Journal of Nursing Practice, 8*(3), 118–126.

Baue, W. (2003). Phase-out of mercury thermometers continues to rise. SocialFunds.com. Available at www.socialfunds.com/news/article.cgi?sfArticleId=752.

Bauer, J. (2002). Blood pressure cuffs. *RN, 65*(8), 61–62.

Bauer, J. (2002). Vital signs monitors. *RN, 65*(7), 61–62.

Bauer, J. (Ed.). (2003). Thermometers. *RN, 66*(3), 63–64.

Faria, S. (1999). Assessment of peripheral arterial pulses. *Home Care Provider, 4*(4), 140–141.

Flenady, V. J., & Woodgate, P. G. (2003). Radiant warmers versus incubators for regulating body temperature in newborn infants. *The Cochrane Database of Systematic Reviews,* Issue 4, Article : CD000435.DOI:10.1002/14651858.CD000435.

Gall, G. (2002). A useful screening tool. *RN, 65*(9), 41–43.

Hockenberry, M. (2005). *Wong's essentials of pediatric nursing* (7th ed.). St. Louis, MO: Elsevier Mosby.

Lanham, D., Walker, B., Klocke, E., & Jennings, M. (1999). Accuracy of tympanic temperature readings in children under 6 years of age. *Pediatric Nursing, 25*(1), 39–42.

Mehta, M. (2003). Assessing respiratory status. *Nursing, 33*(2), 54–56.

NANDA International. (2003). *Nursing diagnoses: Definitions & classification.* Philadelphia: Author.

National Heart, Lung, and Blood Institute. National Institutes of Health. (2006). Categories for Blood Pressure Levels in Adults. Available at www.nhlbi.gov/hbp/detect/categ.htm.

Porth, C. M. (2005). *Pathophysiology: Concepts of altered health states* (7th ed.). Philadelphia: Lippincott Williams & Wilkins.

Rush, M., & Wetherall, A. (2003). Temperature measurement: Practice guidelines. *Paediatric Nursing, 15*(9), 25–28.

Rushing, J. (2005). Assessing for orthostatic hypotension. *Nursing, 35*(1), 30.

Smeltzer, S., Bare, B., Hinkle, J. H., & Cheever, K. H. (2008). *Brunner & Suddarth's textbook of medical-surgical nursing* (11th ed.). Philadelphia: Lippincott Williams & Wilkins.

Taylor, C., Lillis, C., LeMone, P., et al. (2008). *Fundamentals of Nursing* (6th ed.). Philadelphia: Lippincott Williams & Wilkins

Trim, J. (2005). Monitoring pulse. *Nursing Times, 101*(21), 30–31.

Trim, J. (2005). Respirations. *Nursing Times, 101*(22), 30–31.

U.S. Department of Health and Human Services. (2003, May). *The seventh report of the Joint National Committee on Prevention, Detection, Evaluation, and Treatment of High Blood Pressure* (NIH Publication 03-5233). National Institutes of Health, National Heart, Lung, and Blood Institute.

U.S. Environmental Protection Agency (EPA). (2005a). Reducing mercury use in healthcare. Promoting a healthier environment. Available at www.epa.gov/ghpo/bnsdocs/merchealth/index.html.

U.S. Environmental Protection Agency (EPA). (2005b). Safe mercury management: Cleanup Instructions. Available at www.epa.gov/epaoswer/hazwaste/mercury/spills.hem#cleanmercuryspills.

Woodrow, P. (2003). Assessing pulse in older people. *Nursing Older People, 15*(6), 38–40.

Woodrow, P. (2003). Assessing temperature in older people. *Nursing Older People, 15*(1), 29–31.

CHAPTER 2

Health Assessment

Focusing on Patient Care

This chapter will help you develop some of the physical assessment skills related to health assessment necessary to care for the following patients:

William Lincoln comes to the clinic for a routine checkup.

Lois Felker, age 30, has a history of type 1 diabetes. She is a patient in the hospital.

Bobby Williams, a teenager brought to the emergency department by his parents, is suspected of having appendicitis.

Learning Objectives

After studying this chapter, you will be able to:

1. Use the appropriate equipment while performing a head-to-toe physical assessment.
2. Assist in positioning the patient in the correct position to perform the head-to-toe physical assessment.
3. Verbalize the appropriate rationale for performing the specific head-to-toe assessment techniques.
4. Assess the integumentary system.
5. Assess the head and neck.
6. Assess the thorax and lungs.
7. Assess the cardiovascular system.
8. Assess the abdomen.
9. Assess the neurologic, musculoskeletal, and peripheral vascular systems.

Key Terms

adventitious breath sounds: sounds that are not normally heard in the lungs on auscultation

auscultation: act of listening with a stethoscope to sounds produced within the body

bruits: abnormal "swooshing" sounds heard on auscultation indicating turbulent blood flow

cyanosis: bluish or grayish discoloration of the skin in response to inadequate oxygenation

ecchymosis: a collection of blood in the subcutaneous tissues, causing purplish discoloration

edema: excess fluid in the tissues, characterized by swelling

erythema: redness of the skin

inspection: process of performing deliberate, purposeful observations in a systematic manner

jaundice: yellow color of the skin resulting from liver and gallbladder diseases, some types of anemia, and hemolysis

pallor: paleness of the skin

palpation: an assessment technique that uses the sense of touch

percussion: the act of striking one object against another to produce sound

petechiae: small hemorrhagic spots caused by capillary bleeding

precordium: the area on the anterior chest corresponding to the aortic, pulmonic, tricuspid, and apical areas and Erb's point

turgor: fullness or elasticity of the skin

Assessment is the first step of the nursing process; health assessments reveal important information about the client's health status and healthcare needs. Data collected guide the overall plan of care. This plan of care is directed at promoting an optimal level of health through interventions to prevent illness, restore health, and facilitate the patient's coping with disabilities or death.

Health assessments are a part of nursing care for patients across the lifespan and are performed in a variety of settings. The scope and type of assessment that is conducted varies based on the setting, the patient's healthcare needs, and the acuity of the health problem. A health assessment may be a comprehensive, ongoing and focused, or emergency assessment. A comprehensive assessment with a detailed health history and complete physical examination is usually conducted when a patient enters a healthcare setting; information is used as a baseline for comparing later assessment. An ongoing and focused assessment is one that is conducted at regular intervals (such as at the beginning of each home health visit or each hospital shift) during patient care. This type of assessment focuses on updating baseline assessment data as well as identifying any changes in the health status of the patient. A focused assessment can be conducted to assess a specific problem, identify new problems, or evaluate the effectiveness of interventions. An emergency assessment is a type of rapid focused assessment conducted to determine potentially fatal situations. Health assessment consists of the health history and the physical examination. A health history is a collection of subjective data that provides a detailed profile of the patient's health status (Fundamentals Review 2-1 summarizes major components of a comprehensive health history). Nurses use therapeutic communication skills including interviewing techniques during the health history to gather data to identify actual and potential health problems as well as sources of patient strength. Additionally, during the health history, the establishment of an effective nurse–patient relationship is initiated. Generally, a physical assessment is performed after the health history. Physical assessment is the systematic collection of objective data that is directly observed or is elicited through examination techniques such as inspection, palpation, percussion and auscultation (Fundamentals Review 2-2). Performing a physical examination requires knowledge of anatomy and physiology, the equipment being used, and proper patient positioning and draping (Fundamentals Review 2-3). In addition, laboratory and diagnostic tests provide crucial information about a patient's health. These results become a part of the total health assessment.

This chapter will cover skills to assist the nurse in performing a physical assessment. However, in reality, examiners are often gathering the history of a problem or symptom (subjective data) while examining the patient. For a comprehensive assessment, the nurse integrates assessment of individual assessments following a systematic head-to-toe format. Fundamentals Review 2-4 summarizes components of a head-to-toe examination.

Fundamentals Review 2-1

Components of a Health History

Biographic Data

Biographic information is often collected during admission to a healthcare facility or agency and documented on a specific form; it helps to identify the patient. Biographic data include:

- Name
- Address
- Gender
- Marital status
- Race
- Ethnicity
- Occupation
- Religious preference
- Advance directives/living will
- Healthcare financing
- Primary healthcare provider

Reason for Seeking Care

The patient's reason for seeking care helps to focus the rest of the assessment. Present an open-ended question, such as "Tell me why you are here today." **Be sure to document in the patient's own words.** For example, if Nina Dunning comes into the clinic and states, "I'm having trouble sleeping. At night, I can't seem to stop my thoughts. All I do is worry."

Incorrect documentation: Patient complains of insomnia and anxiety.

Correct documentation: "I'm having trouble sleeping. At night, I can't seem to stop my thoughts. All I do is worry."

History of Present Health Concern

When taking the patient's history of present health concern, be sure to explore the symptoms thoroughly. The mnemonic "PQRST" is a helpful guide to analyze a patient's symptoms:

Provocative or palliative: What causes the symptom? What makes it better or worse?

- What were you doing when you first noticed it?
- What seems to trigger it? Stress? Position? Certain activities? An argument? (For a sign such as an eye discharge: What seems to cause it or make it worse? For a psychological symptom such as depression: Does the depression occur after specific events?)
- What relieves the symptom? Changing diet? Changing position? Taking medication? Being active?
- What makes the symptom worse?

Quality or quantity: How does the symptom feel, look, or sound? How much of it are you experiencing now?

- How would you describe the symptom—how it feels, looks, or sounds?
- How much are you experiencing now? Is it so much that it prevents you from performing any activities? Is it more or less than you experienced at any other time?

Region or radiation: Where is the symptom located? Does it spread?

- Where does the symptom occur?
- In the case of pain, does it travel down your back or arms, up your neck, or down your legs?

Severity: How does the symptom rate on a scale of 1 to 10, with 10 being the most severe?

- How bad is the symptom at its worst? Does it force you to lie down, sit down, or slow down?
- Does the symptom seem to be getting better, getting worse, or staying about the same?

Timing: When did the symptom begin? Did it occur suddenly or gradually? How often does it occur?

- On what date and time did the symptom first occur?
- How did the symptom start? Suddenly? Gradually?
- How often do you experience the symptom? Hourly? Daily? Weekly? Monthly?
- When do you usually experience the symptom? During the day? At night? In the early morning? Does it awaken you? Does it occur before, during, or after meals? Does it occur seasonally?
- How long does an episode of the symptom last?

Past Medical History

A patient's past medical history may provide insight into causes of current symptoms. It also alerts the nurse to certain risk factors. Past medical history includes past illnesses, chronic health problems and treatment, and previous surgeries or hospitalizations. Sample questions include:

- "Tell me about the childhood illnesses, such as measles or mumps, that you had."

(continued)

Fundamentals Review 2-1

Components of a Health History *(continued)*

- "Are your immunizations up to date?"
- "Do you have any chronic illnesses?"
- "What are you allergic to?"
- "Describe any accidents, injuries, and surgeries you have had."
- "What prescribed or over-the-counter medications do you use? Do you take any herbal or dietary supplements?"

Family History

Certain disorders have genetic links. For example, a family history of cancer is a risk factor for cancer. Sample family history questions include:

- "How old are the members of your family?"
- "If any members of your family are not living, what caused their death?"
- "Is there any history of this health problem you have in other family members?"
- "Do any family members have chronic illnesses?"

Lifestyle

A patient's lifestyle contributes to his or her overall health and well-being. For example, smoking is related to many health problems. Sample lifestyle questions include:

- "Do you smoke, drink, or use drugs? If so, for how long and how much?"
- "Describe the foods you eat during a typical day."
- "Tell me about how well you sleep."
- "How much exercise do you get each day?"
- "Who in your family or community is available to help you with health problems if you need it?"

Fundamentals Review 2-2

Assessment Techniques

Inspection is the process of performing deliberate, purposeful observations in a systematic manner. It uses the senses of smell, hearing, and sight.

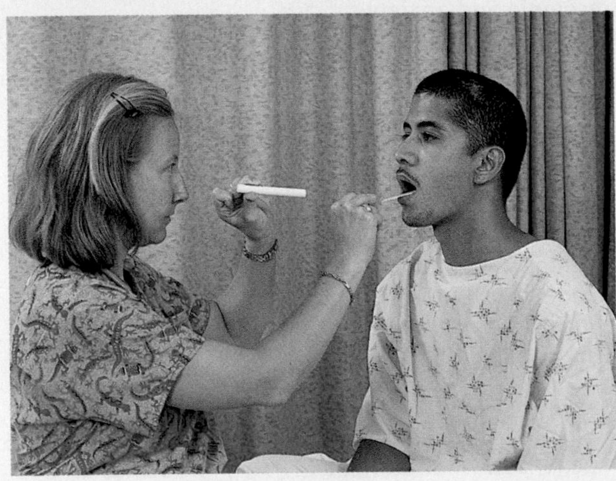

Inspection

Fundamentals Review 2-2

Assessment Techniques *(continued)*

Palpation is an assessment technique that uses the sense of touch. The hands and fingers are sensitive tools and can assess temperature, turgor, texture, moisture, pulsations, vibrations, shape and masses, and organs. For light palpation, apply light pressure with the dominant hand, using a circular motion to feel the surface structure; press down less than 1 cm (0.5″). For deep palpation, position your dominant hand on the skin surface and your nondominant hand on top of the dominant hand to apply pressure. This technique permits the examiner to feel more deeply to a depth of 2.5 to 5 cm (1″–2″).

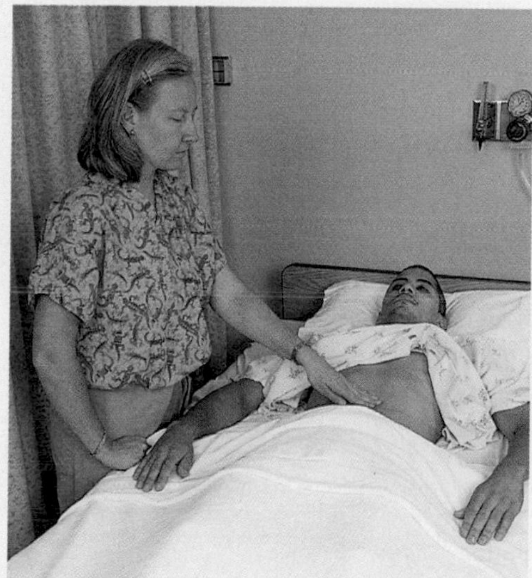

Light palpation

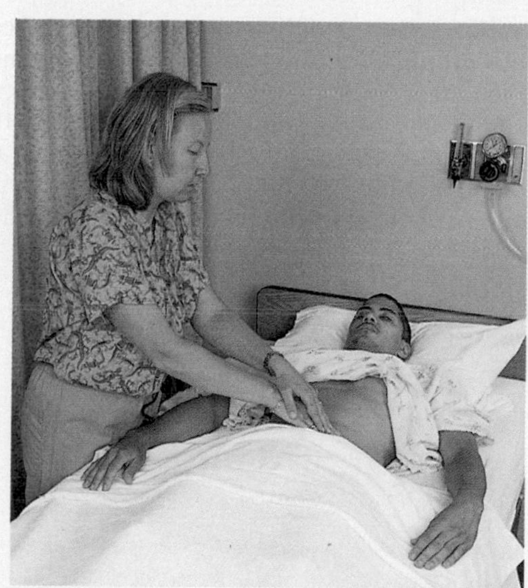

Deep palpation

Percussion is the act of striking one object against another to produce sound. The sound waves or vibrations produced by the striking action over body tissues are known as percussion tones. Percussion is used to assess the location, shape, size of organs, and density of other underlying structures or tissues.

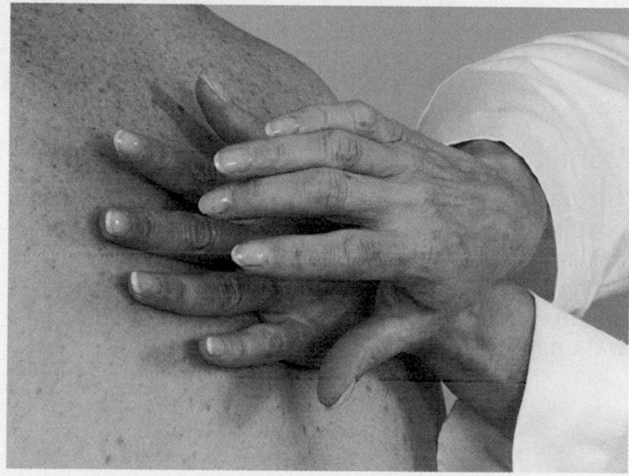

Percussion

(continued)

Fundamentals Review 2-2

Assessment Techniques *(continued)*

This technique is also used to elicit deep-tendon reflexes. Percussion tones include the following:

Tone	Relative Intensity	Sample Location
Flat	Soft	Thigh
Dull	Medium	Liver
Resonance	Loud	Normal lung
Hyperresonance	Very Loud	Emphysematous lung
Tympany	Loud	Gastric air bubble

Auscultation is the act of listening with a stethoscope to sounds produced within the body. This technique is used to listen for blood pressure, heart sounds, lung sounds, and bowel sounds. Four characteristics of sound are assessed by auscultation: (1) pitch (ranging from high to low); (2) loudness (ranging from soft to loud); (3) quality (eg, gurgling or swishing); and (4) duration (short, medium, or long).

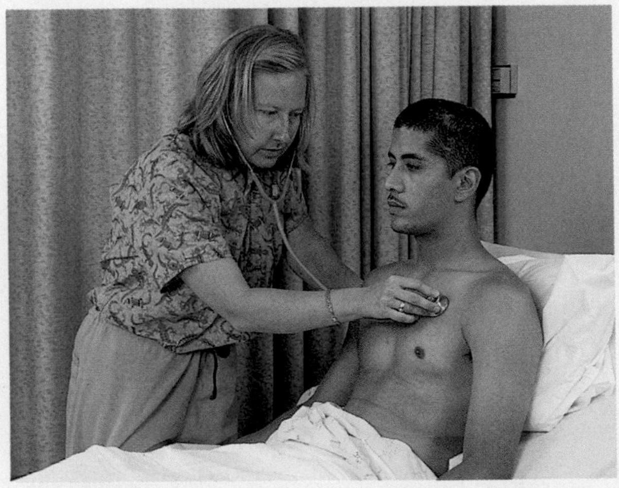

Auscultation. (Photos © B. Proud.)

Fundamentals Review 2-3

Positions Used in Physical Assessment

Standing

The patient stands erect. This position should not be used for patients who are weak, dizzy, or prone to fall. It is used to assess posture, balance, and gait (while walking upright).

Standing

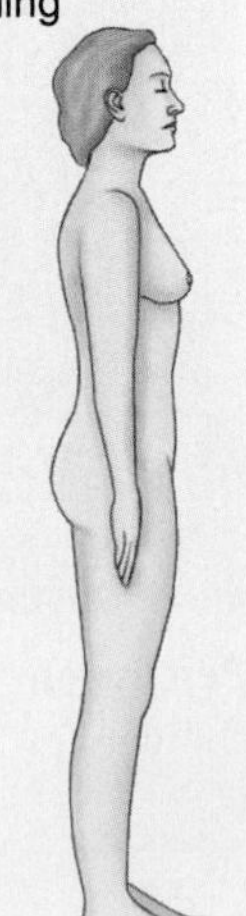

Sitting

The patient may sit in a chair or on the side of the bed or examining table, or remain in bed with the head elevated. It allows visualization of the upper body and facilitates full lung expansion, and is used to assess vital signs and the head, neck, anterior and posterior thorax and lungs, heart, breasts, and upper extremities.

Sitting

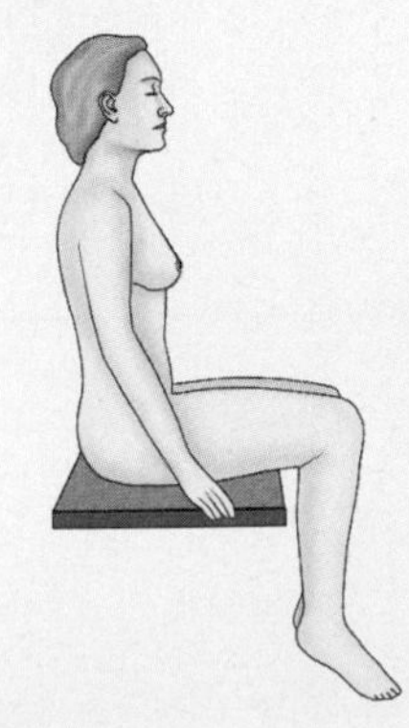

Fundamentals Review 2-3

Positions Used in Physical Assessment *(continued)*

Supine

The patient lies flat on the back with legs extended and knees slightly flexed. It facilitates abdominal muscle relaxation and is used to assess vital signs and the head, neck, anterior thorax and lungs, heart, breasts, abdomen, extremities, and peripheral pulses.

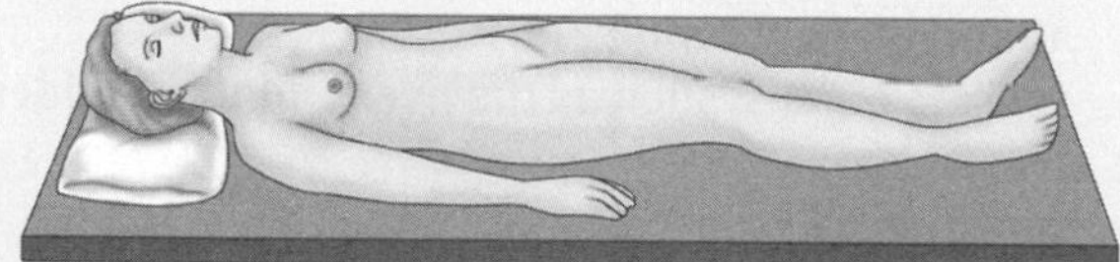
Supine

Dorsal Recumbent

The patient lies on the back with legs separated, knees flexed, and soles of the feet on the bed. It should not be used for abdominal assessment as it causes contraction of the abdominal muscles. It is used to assess the head, neck, anterior thorax and lungs, heart, breasts, extremities, and peripheral pulses.

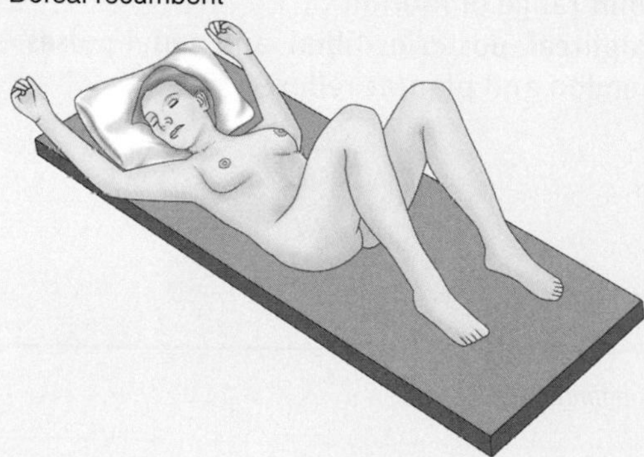
Dorsal recumbent

Sims' Position

The patient lies on either side with the lower arm below the body and the upper arm flexed at the shoulder and elbow. Both knees are flexed, with the upper leg more acutely flexed. It is used to assess the rectum or vagina.

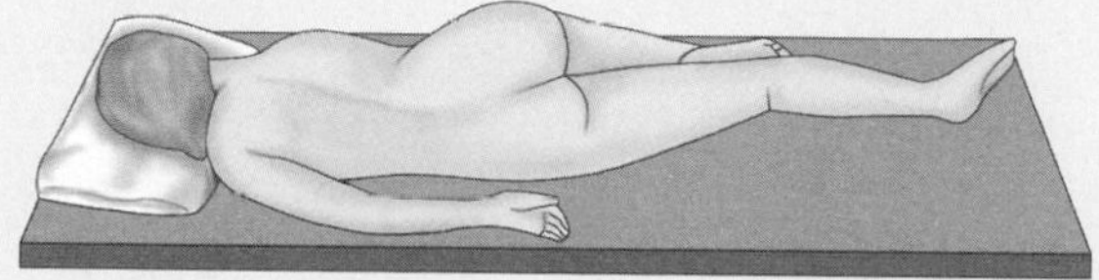
Sims

Prone

The patient lies flat on the abdomen with the head turned to one side. It is used to assess the hip joint and the posterior thorax.

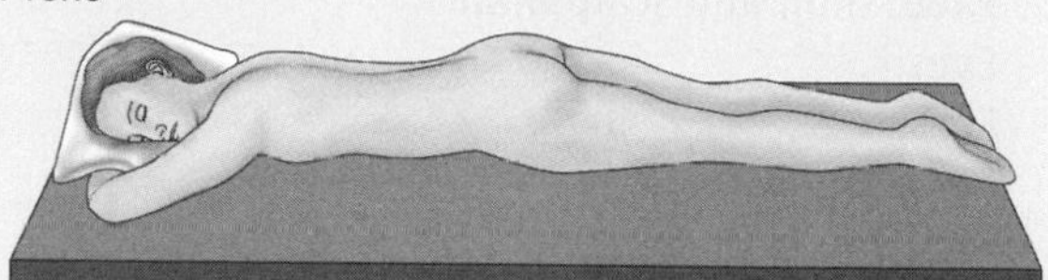
Prone

Lithotomy

The patient is in the dorsal recumbent position with the buttocks at the edge of the examining table and the heels in stirrups. It is used to assess female genitalia and rectum.

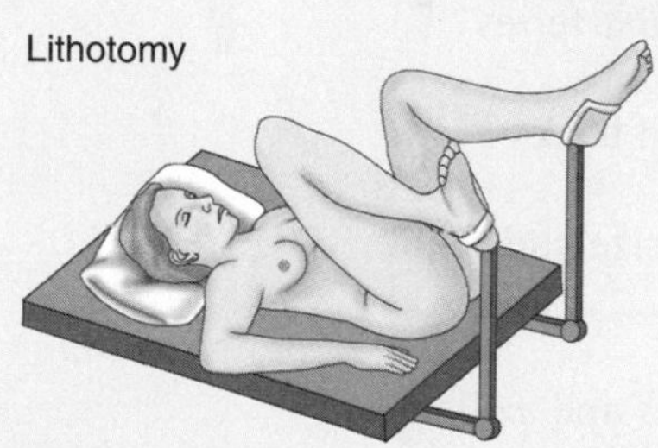
Lithotomy

Knee-Chest

The patient kneels, with the body at a 90-degree angle to the hips, back straight, and arms above the head. It is used to assess the anus and rectum.

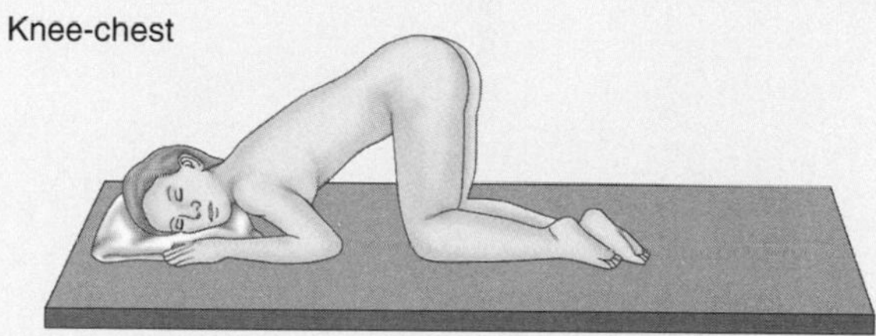
Knee-chest

Fundamentals Review 2-4

Outline of a Head-to-Toe Physical Assessment

- General survey
- Height and weight
- Vital signs
- Head
  - Skin
  - Face, skull and scalp, hair
  - Eyes
  - Ears
  - Nose and sinuses
  - Mouth and oropharynx
  - Cranial nerves
- Neck
  - Skin
  - Lymph nodes
  - Muscles
  - Thyroid
  - Trachea
  - Carotid arteries
  - Neck veins
- Chest and back
  - Skin
  - Chest size and shape
  - Heart
  - Lungs
  - Breasts and axilla
  - Spine
- Upper extremities
  - Skin, hair, and fingernails
  - Sensation
  - Muscle size, strength, and tone
  - Joint range of motion
  - Radial and brachial pulses
  - Tendon reflexes
- Abdomen
  - Skin
  - Bowel sounds
  - Vascular sounds
  - Abdominal contents
  - Specific organs, such as the liver and the bladder
- Genitalia
  - Skin and hair
  - Urethra
  - Males: penis and testes
  - Females: vagina*
  - Males: prostate*
- Anus and rectum*
- Lower extremities
  - Skin, hair, and toenails
  - Gait and balance
  - Muscle size, strength, and tone
  - Joint range of motion
  - Popliteal, posterior tibial, and pedal pulses
  - Tendon and plantar reflexes

**These internal structures are usually deferred during a routine health screening examination.*

SKILL 2-1 Performing Integumentary Assessment

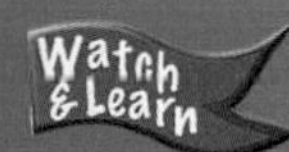

The integumentary system includes the skin, hair, nails, sweat glands, and sebaceous glands. Assessment of the skin, hair, and nails provides information about the nutritional and hydration status and overall health of the patient. Additionally, this assessment can provide information associated with certain systemic diseases, infection, immobility, excessive sun exposure, and allergic reactions. Assessment often begins with an overall inspection of the skin's condition. Assessment of specific regions is usually integrated into specific body system assessments.

Equipment

- Gloves
- Measuring tape or ruler
- Good light source

ASSESSMENT

Complete a health history, focusing on the integumentary system. Identify risk factors by asking about the following:

- History of rashes, lesions, change in color, or itching
- History of bruising or bleeding in the skin
- History of allergies to medications, plants, foods, or other substances
- Exposure to the sun and sunburn history
- Presence of lesions (wounds, bruises, abrasions, or burns)
- Change in the color, size, or shape of a mole
- Recent chemotherapy or radiation therapy
- Exposure to chemicals that may be harmful to the skin, hair, or nails
- Degree of mobility
- Types of food eaten and liquids consumed each day
- Recent falls or injury
- Lifestyle choices: tattoos, body piercing
- Cultural practices related to skin

NURSING DIAGNOSIS

Determine the related factors for the nursing diagnoses based on the client's current health status. An appropriate nursing diagnosis is Impaired Skin Integrity. Other nursing diagnoses related to the integument may include:

- Acute Pain related to pressure ulcers
- Disturbed Body Image related to illness (lesions associated with lupus)
- Hyperthermia related to inability or decreased ability to perspire
- Hypothermia related to malnutrition
- Impaired Skin Integrity related to surgical incision
- Impaired Tissue Integrity related to chemical irritants
- Risk for Latex Allergy Response
- Risk for Infection related to broken skin
- Self-mutilation related to irresistible urge to cut/hurt self

OUTCOME IDENTIFICATION AND PLANNING

The expected outcome to achieve in performing an integumentary assessment is that the assessment is completed without the patient experiencing anxiety or discomfort, the findings are documented, and the appropriate referral is made to the physician as needed for further evaluation. Other specific outcomes will be expected depending on the identified nursing diagnosis.

(continued)

SKILL 2-1 Performing Integumentary Assessment *(continued)*

IMPLEMENTATION

ACTION	RATIONALE
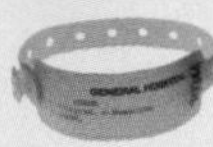 1. Identify the patient.	Identification of the patient ensures that the assessment will be performed on the right patient.
2. Explain the purpose of the integumentary examination and answer any questions.	Explanation helps to alleviate anxiety, promotes cooperation, and facilitates the examination.
3. Ask the patient to remove all clothing and put on an examination gown (if appropriate). The patient remains in the sitting position for most of the examination but will need to stand or lie on the side when the posterior part of the body is examined exposing only the body part being examined.	Only exposing the body part being examined provides privacy for the patient. During the initial part of the examination, assess the skin areas that are exposed (eg, the face, arms, and hands). As the different assessments are completed, incorporate skin examination within these systems.
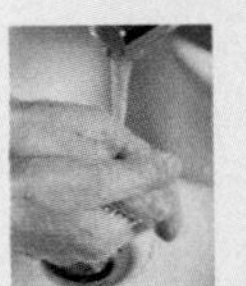 4. Perform hand hygiene.	Hand hygiene deters the risk of microorganism transmission.
5. Inspect the overall skin coloration (Figure 1).	Overall coloration is a good indication of health status. Skin color varies among races and individuals; individual skin color should be relatively consistent across the body. Abnormal findings include cyanosis, pallor, jaundice, and erythema.

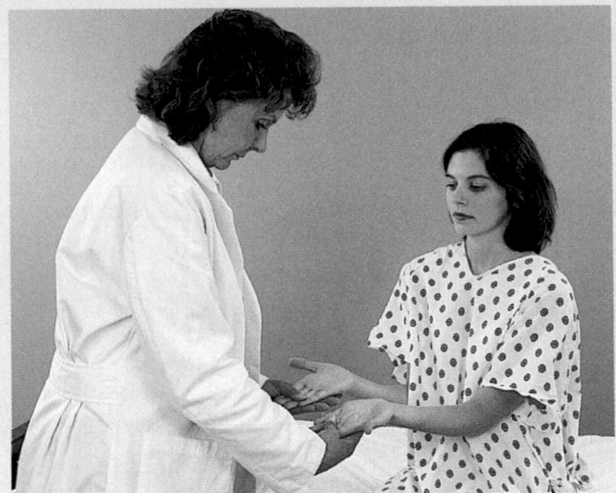

Figure 1. Inspecting overall skin coloration. (© B. Proud.)

ACTION	RATIONALE
6. Inspect skin for vascularity, bleeding, or bruising.	These signs may relate to injury or cardiovascular, hematologic, or liver dysfunction.
7. Inspect the skin for lesions. Note bruises, scratches, cuts, inspect bites, and wounds (see wound assessment in Chapter 8). If present, note size, shape, color, exudates, and distribution/pattern.	Lesions can be normal variations such as a macule or freckle or an abnormal lesion such as a melanoma.

SKILL 2-1 Performing Integumentary Assessment *(continued)*

ACTION	RATIONALE
8. Palpate skin using the backs of your hands to assess temperature. Wear gloves when palpating any potentially open area of the skin. (Figure 2).	The back of the hand is more sensitive to temperature. Increase in skin temperature may indicate elevated body temperature.
9. Palpate for texture and moisture.	In a dehydrated patient, skin is dry, loose, and wrinkled. Elevated body temperature may result in increased perspiration.
10. Assess for skin turgor by gently pinching the skin under thc clavicle (Figure 3).	This technique provides information about the patient's hydration status as well as mobility and elasticity of the skin. Decreased elasticity may be present in dehydrated patients.

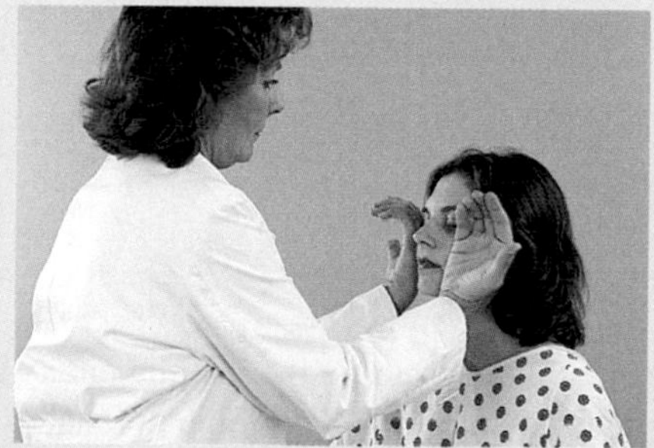

Figure 2. Assessing temperature. (© B. Proud.)

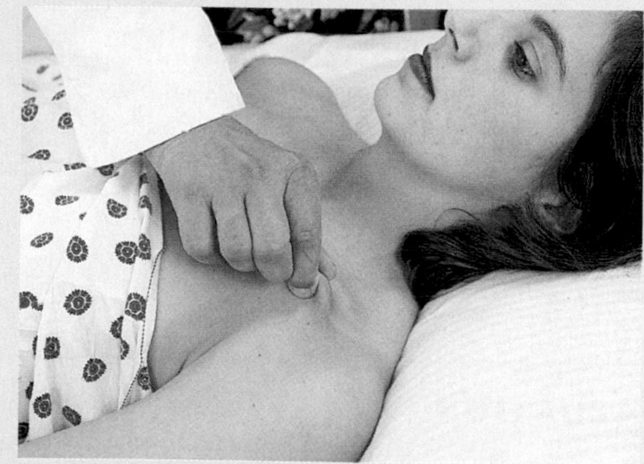

Figure 3. Palpating to assess turgor. (© B. Proud.)

ACTION	RATIONALE
11. Palpate for edema (which is characterized by swelling, with taut and shiny skin over the edematous area).	Edema may be the result of overhydration, heart failure, kidney dysfunction, or peripheral vascular disease.
12. If lesions are present, put on gloves and palpate the lesion.	Palpation of lesions may result in drainage, which provides clues to the type or cause of the lesion.
13. Inspect the nail angle noting if any clubbing is present, as well as the shape, and color of the nails.	Nail condition provides information about underlying illness and oxygenation status. Nails are normally convex and the cuticle is pink and intact. The angle of attachment of the nail is 160 degrees. Clubbing is present when the angle of the nail base exceeds 180 degrees.
14. Palpate nails for texture and capillary refill.	Normally, nails are firm and smooth and capillary refill should be brisk, 4 seconds.

(continued)

SKILL 2-1 Performing Integumentary Assessment *(continued)*

ACTION	RATIONALE
15. Inspect the hair and scalp (Figure 4). Wear gloves for palpation if lesions or infestation is suspected or if hygiene is poor.	Hair condition provides information about nutritional and oxygenation status. Hair should be evenly distributed over the scalp. There are variations in hair color. Scalp should feel mobile and nontender.

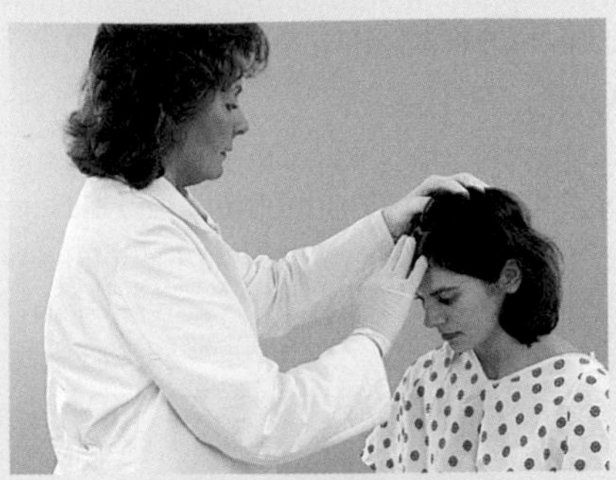

Figure 4. Inspecting the scalp and hair. (© B. Proud)

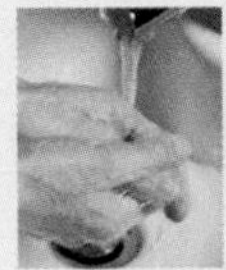

ACTION	RATIONALE
16. If wearing gloves, discard gloves. Perform hand hygiene.	This prevents the spread of microorganisms.

EVALUATION

The expected outcome is met when the patient participates in the integumentary assessment, displays decreased anxiety, and verbalizes understanding of integumentary assessment techniques as appropriate.

DOCUMENTATION

Guidelines

When documenting skin assessment, be sure to describe specific findings, including coloration, texture, moisture, temperature, turgor, and edema. Note hair distribution and texture. Describe condition of nails, including any abnormal findings. If lesions are present, document specifics, describing type, size, shape (use tape measure if necessary), elevation, coloring, location, drainage, distribution, and patterns.

Sample Documentation

5/2/08 Examined skin of Ms. Michaels. Patient reports history of atopic dermatitis. Uniform skin coloring (white) with pink undertones. Skin on all areas but the hands is soft and warm. Skin returns to position when pinched. Multiple lesions, consistent with dermatitis, observed on the hands. Lesions are red, scaly, and dry. Brown hair, shiny and evenly distributed. Nails are firm and the cuticle is pink and intact and without ridging or pitting.—B. Gentzler, RN

Unexpected Outcomes and Associated Interventions

- *While assessing the skin of a dark-skinned individual, you are unsure if the change in coloration in a particular area of the body is normal or abnormal:* It is especially important when assessing dark-skinned patients to conduct the assessment with natural light rather then artificial lighting. When an abnormal condition is present, first examining an area of the skin that is not affected by the dermatological disorder provides a comparison for identifying abnormal color conditions. Also, lesions that look red or brown on light skin may present as black or purple on dark skin.

SKILL 2-1 Performing Integumentary Assessment *(continued)*

Special Considerations

Older Adult Considerations

- In the elderly patient, expect to find overall thinning of the skin, reduced sweating and oil, and reduced skin turgor.

Cultural Considerations

- Pallor in dark-skinned individuals appears as absence of the "glow" of brown or black skin. Lighter skin appears more yellowish brown; darker skin looks ashen. Cyanosis can be assessed in darker individuals by examining the oral mucosa, the lips, nail beds, and the conjunctiva. Jaundice is assessed by observing the sclera of the eyes, the palms of the hands, and soles of the feet for a yellowish discoloration.
- In the infant, Mongolian spots (hyperpigmented bluish areas found on the lower back) are normal findings commonly found in some populations, such as African Americans, Filipinos, Turkish, and Asian groups. These could be mistaken for child abuse.
- Asian patients may exhibit normal variations in physical features such as a decrease in body hair and coarse head hair.

SKILL 2-2 Assessing the Head and Neck

The examination of the head and neck region includes the assessment of multiple structures and body systems. The eyes, ears, nose, mouth, and throat are located within the facial structures. Anterior neck structures include the trachea, esophagus, and the thyroid gland, as well as the arteries, veins, and lymph nodes. Posterior neck areas involve the upper portion of the spine.

Equipment

- Stethoscope
- Gloves
- Lighting, including a penlight
- Laryngeal mirror
- Tongue blades
- Otoscope
- Tuning fork
- Visual acuity chart
- Ophthalmoscope

ASSESSMENT

Complete a health history, focusing on the head and neck. Identify risk factors by asking about the following:

- Changes with aging in vision or hearing
- History of use of corrective lenses or hearing aids
- Loss of an eye (use of artificial eye)
- History of allergies
- History of disturbances in vision or hearing
- History of chronic illnesses, such as hypertension, diabetes mellitus, or thyroid disease
- Exposure to harmful substances or loud noises
- Exposure to ultraviolet light
- History of smoking, chewing tobacco, or cocaine use
- History of eye or ear infections

(continued)

SKILL 2-2 Assessing the Head and Neck *(continued)*

- History of head trauma
- History of persistent hoarseness
- Oral and dental care practices

NURSING DIAGNOSIS

Determine the related factors for the nursing diagnoses based on the client's current health status. An appropriate nursing diagnosis is Impaired Oral Mucous Membrane. Other nursing diagnoses related to the head and neck may include:

- Disturbed Sensory Perception (Visual, Auditory, Olfactory)
- Hygiene Self-care Deficit
- Impaired Dentition related to ineffective oral hygiene
- Impaired Swallowing
- Impaired Verbal Communication related to hearing loss
- Risk for Aspiration related to impaired swallowing
- Risk for Infection
- Risk for Disturbance in Body Image

OUTCOME IDENTIFICATION AND PLANNING

The expected outcome to achieve in performing an examination of the structures in the head and neck region is that the assessment is completed, the findings are documented, and the appropriate referral is made to the physician, as needed, for further evaluation. Other specific outcomes will be formulated depending on the identified nursing diagnosis.

IMPLEMENTATION

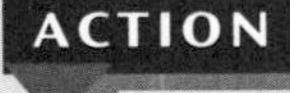

RATIONALE

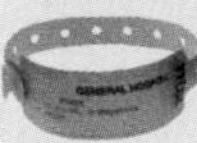

1. Identify the patient.

Identification of the patient ensures that the assessment will be performed on the right patient.

2. Explain the purpose of the head and neck examination and answer any questions.

Explanation helps to alleviate anxiety, promotes cooperation, and facilitates the examination.

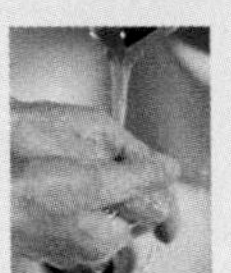

3. Perform hand hygiene.

Hand hygiene deters the risk of microorganism transmission.

4. Inspect the head and then the face for color, symmetry, lesions, and distribution of facial hair. Note facial expression. Palpate the skull.

Generally the shape of the head is normocephalic and symmetric Abnormal findings include a lack of symmetry or unusual size or contour of the head, which may be a result of trauma or disease. Facial expression is appropriate. Skull should be mobile and nontender.

5. Inspect the external eye structures (eyelids, eyelashes, eyeball, eyebrows), cornea, conjunctiva, and sclera. Note color, edema, symmetry, and alignment.

Inspection detects abnormalities such as ptosis, styes, conjunctivitis, or scleral color. Some abnormalities are associated with systemic disorders.

6. **Examine the pupils for equality of size, shape, reaction to light by darkening the room and using a penlight to shine the light on each pupil (Figure 1).**

Testing pupillary response to light and accommodation assesses cranial nerve III, the oculomotor nerve. The normal and consensual pupillary response is constriction.

SKILL 2-2 Assessing the Head and Neck *(continued)*

ACTION	RATIONALE
7. To test for pupillary accommodation and convergence, ask the patient to focus on an object as you bring it closer to the nose.	The normal pupillary response is constriction and convergence when focusing on a near object.
8. Using an ophthalmoscope, check the red reflex (Figure 2).	Presence of the red reflex indicates that the cornea, anterior chamber, and lens are free of opacity and clouding.

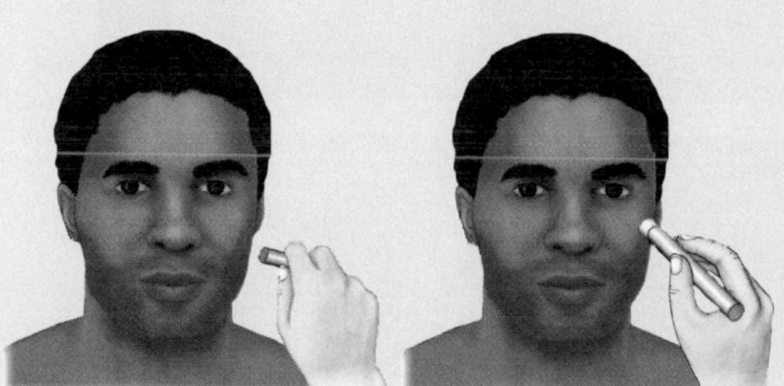

Figure 1. Assessing pupillary reaction.

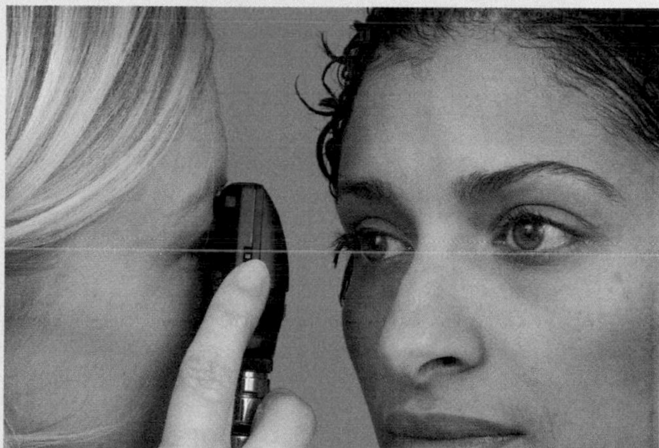

Figure 2. Checking red reflex using an ophthalmoscope. (Photo by B. Proud.)

ACTION	RATIONALE
9. Test the patient's visual acuity with a Snellen chart. Ask the patient to read the smallest possible line of letters, first with both eyes and then with one eye at a time.	This testing evaluates the patient's distance vision and function of cranial nerve II (optic nerve). Additional tools are used to test for color perception.
10. With the patient about 2 feet away, ask the patient to focus on your finger and move the patient's eyes through the six cardinal positions of gaze (Figure 3).	This evaluates the function of each of the six extraocular eye muscles (EOM) and tests cranial nerves III, IV, and VI (oculomotor, trochlear, and abducens nerves).
11. Inspect the external ear bilaterally for shape, size, and lesions. Palpate the ear and mastoid process.	Inspection may reveal abnormalities, such as uneven color, size, drainage or lesions; palpation may reveal inflammation (edema) or infection, nodules, lesions or tenderness.
12. Perform an otoscopic examination (Figure 4). For an adult, pull the auricle up and back; for a child, pull the auricle down and back. Note cerumen (wax), edema, discharge, or foreign bodies and condition of the tympanic membrane.	The ear canal should be smooth and pinkish and the tympanic membrane intact, shiny, and pearly gray with no bulging. Redness, discharge, and perforation of the tympanic membrane are all abnormal.
13. Use a whispered voice to test hearing. Stand about 1 to 2 feet away from the patient, out of her line of vision. Ask the patient to cover the ear not being tested. Perform test on each ear.	This testing provides a gross assessment of cranial nerve VII (acoustic nerve).
14. Use a tuning fork to perform Weber's test and Rinne's test if the patient reports diminished hearing in either ear (Figure 5).	These tests help to differentiate conductive from sensorineural hearing loss.

(continued)

SKILL 2-2 Assessing the Head and Neck *(continued)*

ACTION

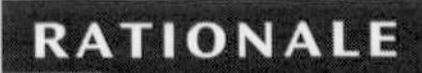

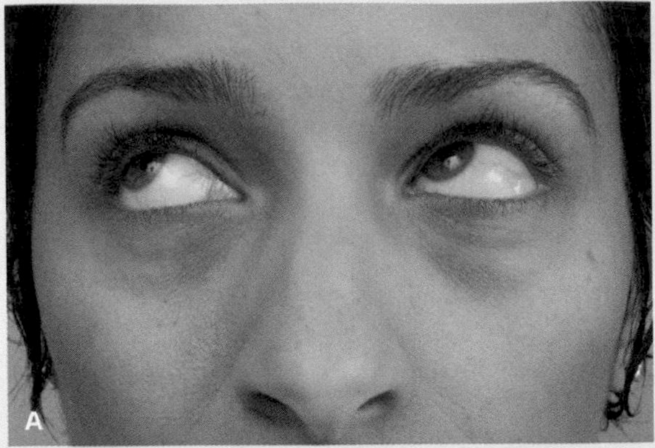

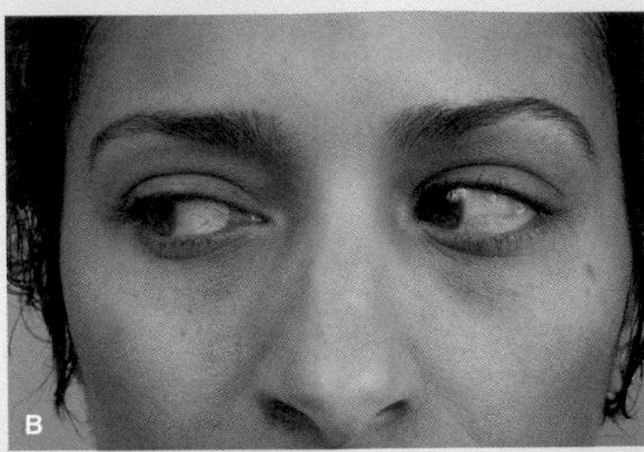

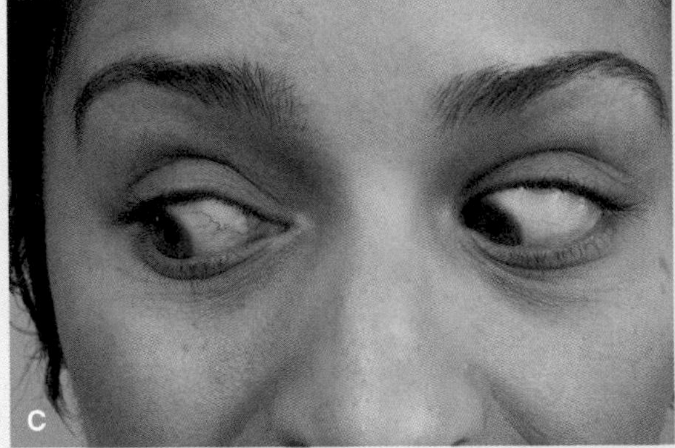

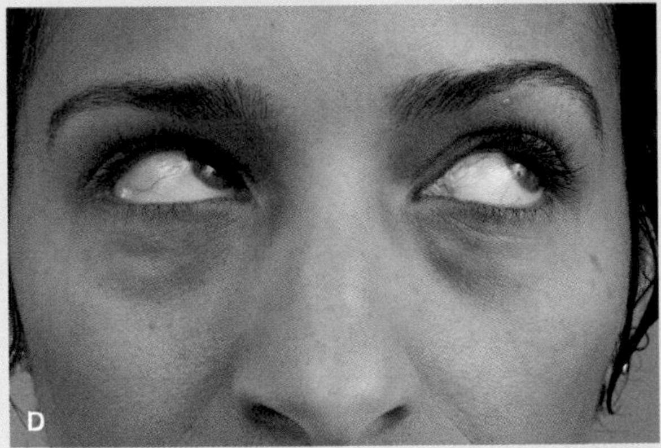

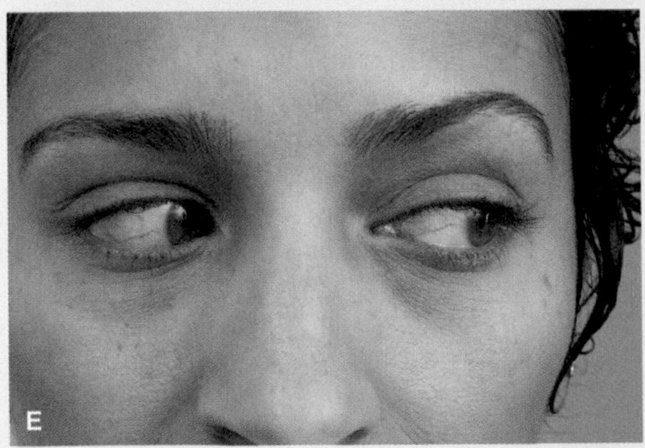

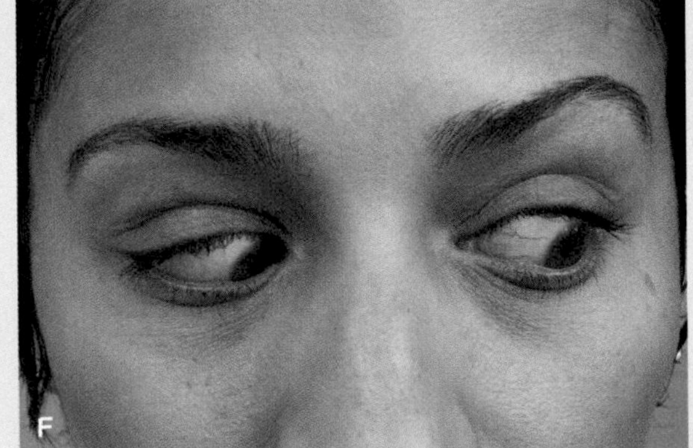

Figure 3. Six cardinal positions of gaze. (Photos by B. Proud.)

15. Inspect and palpate the external nose (Figure 6).

These actions assess for the color, shape, consistency and tenderness of the nose.

16. Palpate and lightly percuss over the frontal and maxillary sinuses (Figure 7). Transilluminate the sinuses if the patient reports tenderness.

Sinus palpation and percussion are used to elicit tenderness and/or crepitus, which may indicate sinus congestion or infection. Transillumination may show fluid in the sinuses.

17. Occlude one nostril externally with a finger while patient breathes through the other; repeat for the other side.

This technique checks the patency of the nasal passages.

SKILL 2-2

Assessing the Head and Neck *(continued)*

ACTION | **RATIONALE**

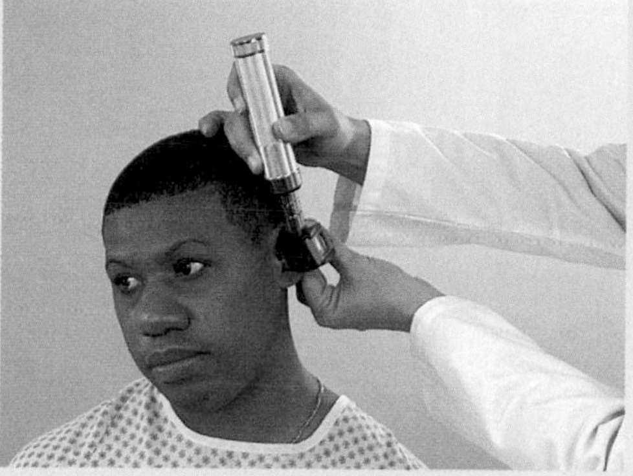

Figure 4. Inspecting the external canal and tympanic membrane. (© B. Proud)

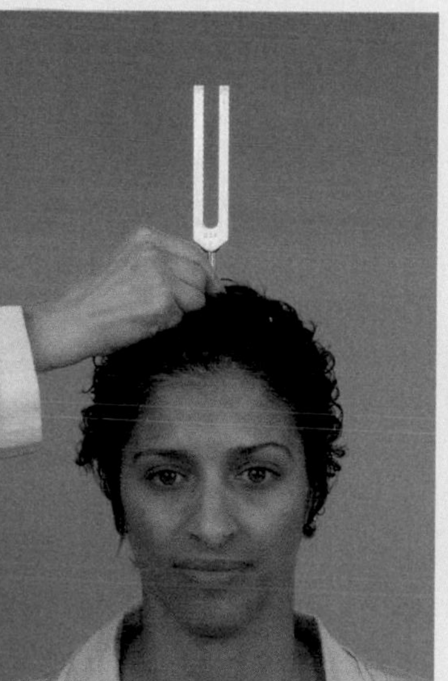

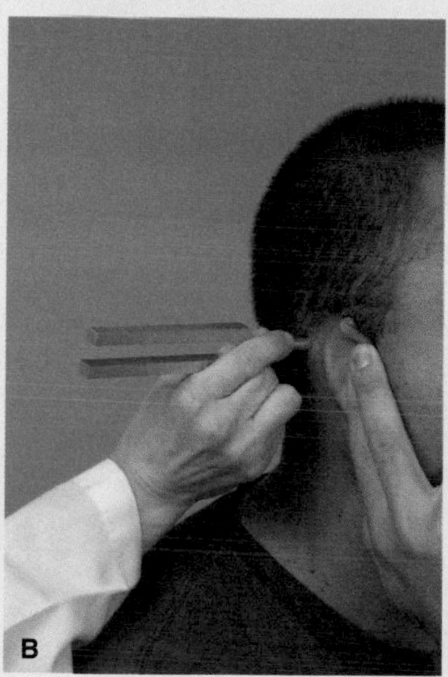

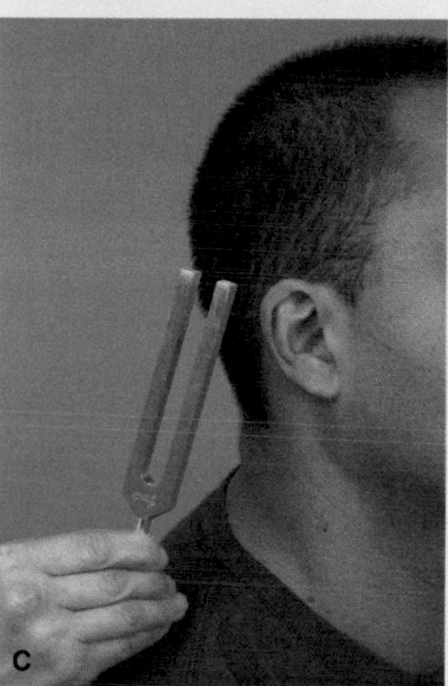

Figure 5. Testing hearing with the tuning fork. For both tests, hold the tuning fork at its base with one hand and then strike it against your opposite palm so it vibrates. (**A**) Performing a Weber's test. Place the base of the tuning fork on the center of the top of the patient's head. Ask the patient where sound is heard best. (**B** and **C**) Performing the Rinne test. First, place the tuning fork base on the mastoid process and ask the patient when the sound can no longer be heard (**B**), then immediately move the prongs to the front of the external auditory canal (**C**) and ask the patient if he can hear the sound; the normal ear will do so. (Photos by B. Proud.)

18. Inspect the internal nostrils using an otoscope with a nasal speculum attachment. (Figure 8).

This technique can detect edema, inflammation, and excessive drainage.

19. Palpate the temporomandibular joint by placing your index finger over the front of each ear as you ask the patient to open and close the mouth.

The action evaluates the temporomandibular joint and the motor portion of cranial nerve V (trigeminal nerve).

20. Perform hand hygiene and don gloves. Inspect the lips, oral mucosa, hard and soft palates, gingivae, teeth, and salivary gland openings by asking the patient to open the mouth wide using a tongue blade and penlight. (Figure 9).

This technique evaluates the condition of the oral structures and hydration level of the patient.

(continued)

SKILL 2-2 Assessing the Head and Neck *(continued)*

ACTION | **RATIONALE**

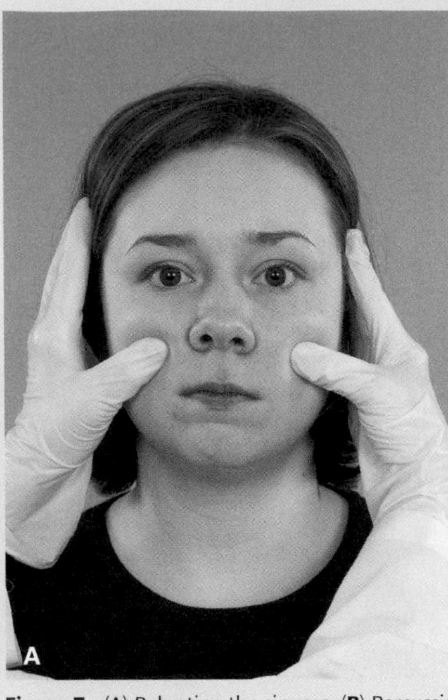

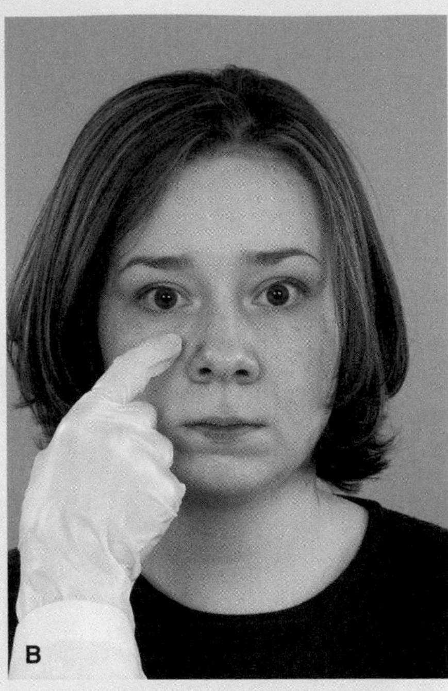

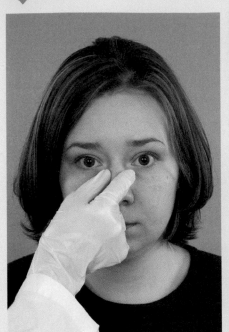

Figure 6. Palpating the nose. (Photo by B. Proud.)

Figure 7. (**A**) Palpating the sinuses. (**B**) Percussing the sinuses. (Photos by B. Proud.)

21. Inspect the tongue. Ask the patient to stick out the tongue. Place a tongue blade at the side of the tongue while patient pushes it to the left and right with the tongue. Inspect the uvula by asking the patient to say "ahh" while sticking out the tongue. Palpate the tongue for muscle tone and tenderness. Remove gloves.

Sticking out the tongue evaluates the function of cranial nerve XII (hypoglossal nerve). Saying "ahh" checks for movement of the uvula and soft palate.

Tongue should feel soft and positive muscle tone and be nontender.

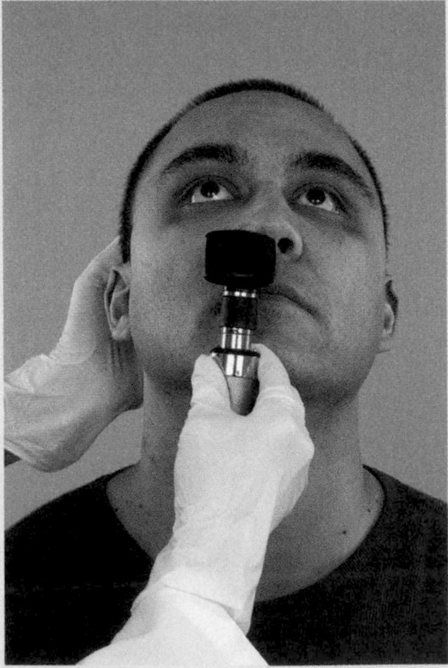

Figure 8. Inspecting the internal nostrils. (Photo by B. Proud.)

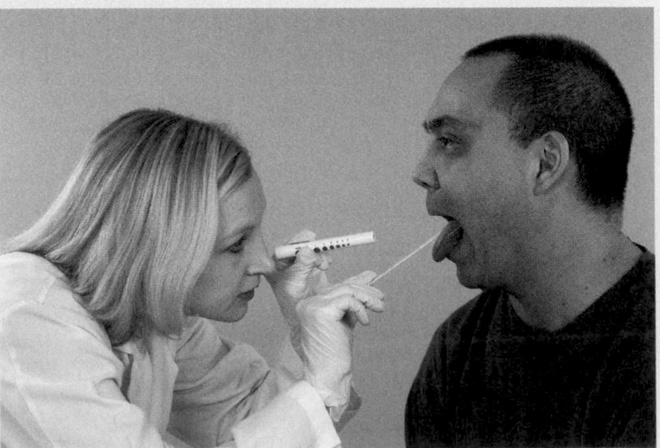

Figure 9. Inspecting the mouth using a tongue blade and penlight. (Photo by B. Proud.)

SKILL 2-2

Assessing the Head and Neck *(continued)*

ACTION	RATIONALE
22. Palpate from the forehead to the posterior triangle of the neck for the posterior cervical lymph nodes using the fingerpads in a slow, circular motion.	Inspection can detect asymmetry of the head and hair variations. Palpation can determine size, shape, mobility, consistency, and/or tenderness of enlarged lymph nodes.
23. Inspect and the palpate in front of and behind the ears, under the chin, and in the anterior triangle for the anterior cervical lymph nodes.	This technique can detect enlarged lymph nodes, lumps and masses.
24. Inspect and palpate (Figure 10) the left and then the right carotid arteries. **Only palpate one carotid artery at a time.** Use the bell of the stethoscope to auscultate the arteries.	Palpation of this area evaluates circulation through the arteries. **Palpating both arteries at once can obstruct blood flow to the brain.** Auscultation can detect a bruit.

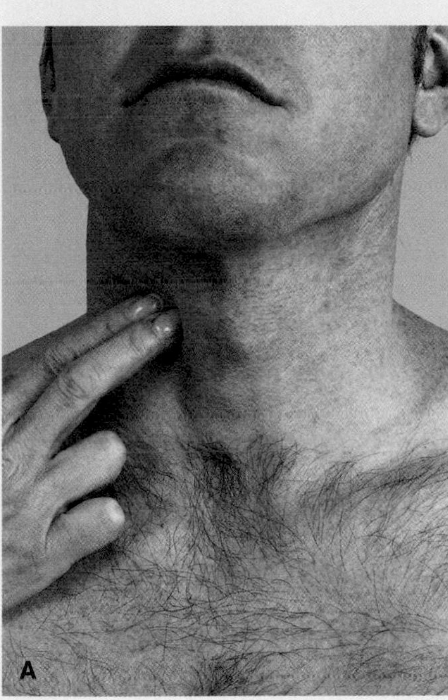

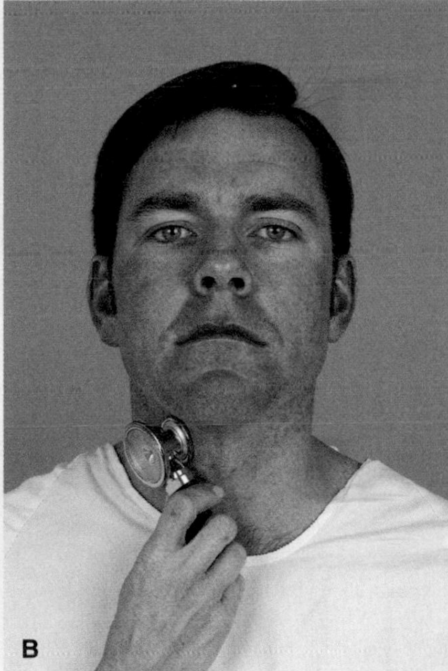

Figure 10. Palpating (**A**) and auscultating (**B**) carotid artery. (Photos by B. Proud.)

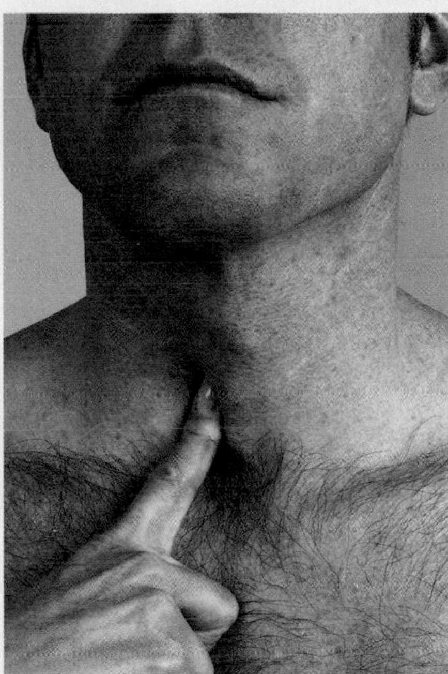

Figure 11. Palpating to determine position of trachea. (Photo by B. Proud.)

ACTION	RATIONALE
25. Inspect and palpate for the trachea (Figure 11).	Inspection of the neck and tracheal palpation evaluates its midline position.
26. Palpate the thyroid gland (Figure 12 illustrates the two techniques). Then, if enlarged, auscultate the thyroid gland using the bell of the stethoscope (Figure 13).	Palpation can reveal thyroid enlargement, tenderness, or nodules; auscultation identifies bruits.
27. Inspect and palpate the supraclavicular area (Figure 14).	This technique can detect enlarged lymph nodes.
28. Inspect the ability of the patient to move his neck. Ask the patient to touch his chin to chest and to each shoulder, each ear to the corresponding shoulder, and then tip head back as far as possible.	These actions assess neck range of motion, which is normally smooth and controlled.

(continued)

SKILL 2-2 Assessing the Head and Neck *(continued)*

ACTION | **RATIONALE**

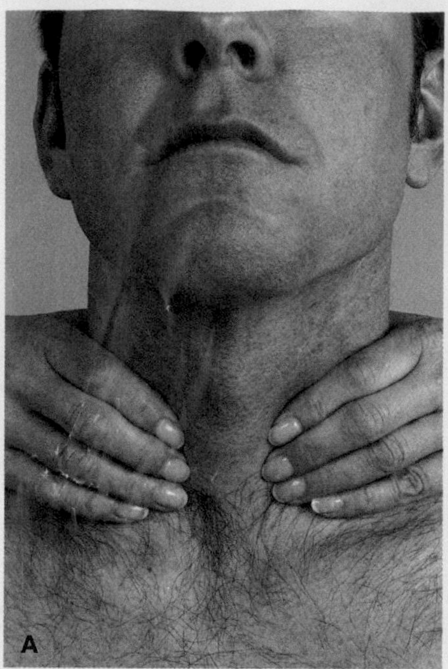

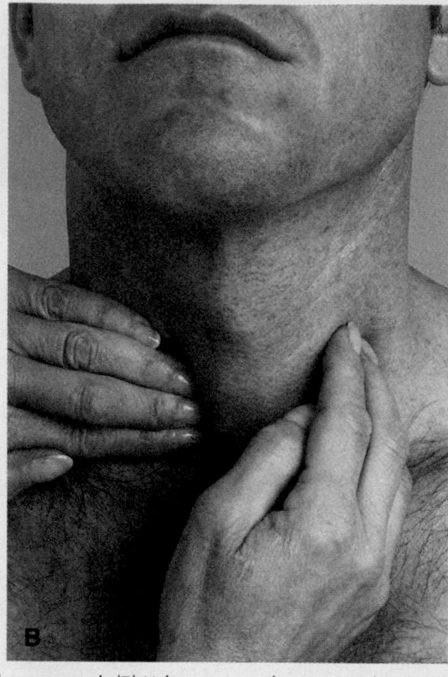

Figure 12. Palpating the thyroid. (**A**) Using a posterior approach (**B**) Using an anterior approach. (Photos by B. Proud.)

Figure 13. Auscultating the thyroid. (Photo by B. Proud.)

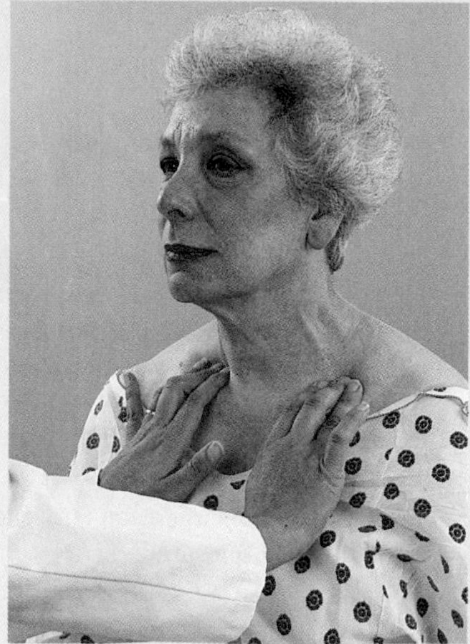

Figure 14. Palpating the supraclavicular nodes. (Photo © B. Proud.)

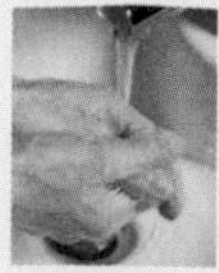

Action	Rationale
29. Perform hand hygiene.	This helps deter the spread of microorganisms.

SKILL 2-2

Assessing the Head and Neck *(continued)*

EVALUATION

The expected outcome is met when the patient participates in the head and neck assessment including the face, eyes, ears, nose and throat, displays decreased anxiety, and verbalizes understanding of these assessments as appropriate.

DOCUMENTATION

Guidelines

When documenting head and neck assessment, be sure to describe specific findings. For the head and face, document symmetry, coloration, and presence of lesions or edema. Note visual acuity, pupillary reaction, condition of the external eye, and red reflex. Document results of tests for accommodation, convergence, and extraocular muscles. Describe condition of external and internal ear, noting any lesions or discharge. Document results of any hearing tests. Note condition of internal and external nose and sinuses. Describe condition of lips, gums, tongue, and buccal mucosa. Document quality of carotid pulse. Note position of trachea and any enlargement of the thyroid. Describe quality of any lymph nodes palpable. Note range of motion of the neck. Document presence of pain or discomfort.

Sample Documentation

6/10/09 Examined head and neck of Mr. Edgars. Patient denies history of any sensory changes or sensory difficulties, but states "I have some sores in my mouth." Overall skin coloring consistent, with pink undertones. Head symmetric and normal in size. Eyes are symmetric. No lesions or redness noted. Red reflex intact. Pupils are equal and reactive to light. Accommodation and convergence normal. Visual acuity 20/20 in both eyes. Eyes move smoothly through 6 fields of gaze. External and internal ears free of discharge, lesions, or tenderness. Whisper test negative for hearing loss. Nose and sinuses are nontender. Minimal clear discharge is present in the nostrils, but nostrils are patent. Lips are free of lesions. Multiple white lesions approximately 1 cm in diameter noted on buccal mucosa and tongue. Uvula rise is normal. Carotid pulse strong bilaterally. No bruits auscultated. Trachea is midline. Thyroid not enlarged. No lymph nodes are palpable.—B. Gentzler, RN

Unexpected Situations and Associated Interventions

- *While you are testing a patient's visual acuity, the patient tells you he can't see anything without his glasses:* Stop the test. Instruct the patient to put on his glasses, and then resume testing.
- *While performing an examination of the regional lymph nodes in the neck area, you palpate a lymph node that feels hard and fixed:* Ask the patient if he have felt this node before and if so, for how long has it been present and is it painful. Refer the patient to a physician or nurse practitioner for follow-up care.

Special Considerations

General Considerations

- Ensure that a patient wears corrective lenses (if needed) when testing visual acuity.
- Cerumen may be dark orange, brown, yellow, gray or black and soft, moist, dry or hard.
- When assessing the ROM of the neck, the preferred approach is one movement at a time rather than a full rotation of the neck, to avoid dizziness on movement.

Infant and Child Considerations

- When examining the head of an infant, inspect and gently palpate the fontanels and sutures.
- Use a penlight to inspect an infant's or toddler's nostrils; a nasal speculum is too sharp.
- An infant's nose is usually slightly flattened.
- For a child under age 8 years, do not assess the frontal sinuses; they are usually too small to assess.

(continued)

SKILL 2-2 Assessing the Head and Neck *(continued)*

- Lymph nodes may be palpable in children under age 12 years, which is considered a normal variation.
- When performing an otoscopic exam on a young child, pull the pinna down and back (Figure 15).
- Note the number of teeth in a child; a child may have up to 20 temporary teeth.

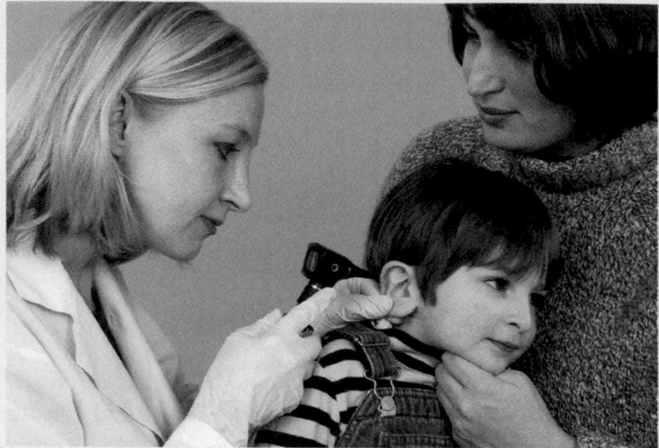

Figure 15. Performing an otoscopic examination on a young child. The pinna is pulled down and back. (Photo by B. Proud.)

Older Adult Considerations

- Look for a thin, grayish ring in the cornea (arcus senilis). This may be a normal finding in an older adult.
- In the elderly patient, when evaluating the neurologic system, expect to find normal age-related sensory changes such as a decrease in vision, hearing, olfaction, taste, proprioception, and touch.

Cultural Considerations

- Exophthalmos, protrusion of the eyeball, can be a normal finding in an African American patient.

SKILL 2-3 Assessing the Thorax and Lungs

A thorough examination of the respiratory system is essential as the primary purpose of this vital system is to supply oxygen and remove carbon dioxide from the body. The thorax comprises the lungs, rib cage, cartilage, and intercostal muscles. To perform a comprehensive respiratory assessment, all four physical examination techniques will be used. Recognizing and identifying normal and abnormal breath sounds, a crucial component of lung assessment, takes practice (Tables 2-1 and 2-2).

Equipment

- Draping
- Gloves
- Gown
- Light source
- Stethoscope
- Centimeter ruler

SKILL 2-3

Assessing the Thorax and Lungs *(continued)*

ASSESSMENT

Complete a health history, focusing on the thorax and lungs. Identify risk factors by asking about the following:

- History of trauma to the ribs or lung surgery
- Number of pillows used when sleeping
- History of chest pain with deep breathing
- History of persistent cough with or without producing sputum
- History of allergies
- Environmental exposure to chemicals, asbestos, or smoke
- History of smoking (including pack-years)
- History of lung disease in family members or self
- History of frequent or chronic respiratory infections

NURSING DIAGNOSIS

Determine the related factors for the nursing diagnoses based on the client's current health status. An appropriate nursing diagnosis is Ineffective Airway Clearance. Other nursing diagnoses related to the lungs may include:

- Disturbed Sleep Pattern related to shortness of breath
- Ineffective Breathing Pattern related to respiratory muscle fatigue
- Impaired Gas Exchange related to ventilation perfusion imbalance
- Ineffective Tissue Perfusion related to hypoventilation
- Anxiety related to difficulty in breathing
- Activity Intolerance related to decreased oxygenation

TABLE 2-1 **Normal Breath Sounds**

TYPE AND DESCRIPTION	LOCATION	RATIO OF INSPIRATION TO EXPIRATION
Bronchial or Tubular		
Blowing, hollow sounds	Auscultated over the trachea	Expiration is longer, lower, and higher pitched than inspiration.
Bronchovesicular		
Medium-pitched, medium intensity, blowing sounds	Auscultated over the first and second interspaces anteriorly and the scapula posteriorly	Inspiration and expiration have similar pitch and duration
Vesicular		
Soft, low-pitched sounds	Auscultated over the lung periphery	Inspiration is longer, louder, and higher pitched than expiration.

(continued)

SKILL 2-3 Assessing the Thorax and Lungs *(continued)*

TABLE 2-2 Abnormal Breath Sounds

TYPE AND CHARACTERISTICS	ILLUSTRATION
Wheeze (Sibilant) • Musical or squeaking • High-pitched, continuous sounds • Auscultated during inspiration and expiration • Occurs in small air passages	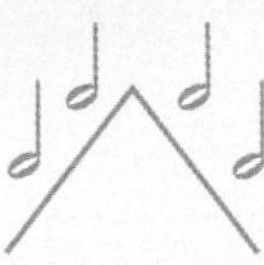
Wheeze (Sonorous) • Sonorous or course • Low-pitched, continuous sounds • Auscultated during inspiration and expiration • Occurs in large air passages • Coughing may clear the sound	
Crackles • Bubbling, crackling, popping • Low- to high-pitched, discontinuous sounds • Auscultated during inspiration • Occurs in small air passages, alveoli, bronchioles, bronchi, and trachea	
Friction Rub • Rubbing or grating • Loudest over lower lateral anterior surface • Auscultated during inspiration and expiration	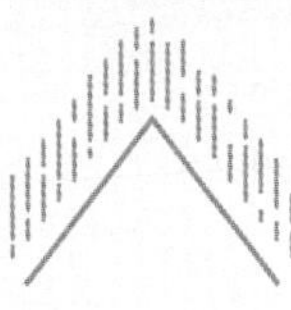

OUTCOME IDENTIFICATION AND PLANNING

The expected outcome to achieve in performing an examination of the structures of the respiratory system is that the assessment is completed without causing the patient to experience anxiety or discomfort, the findings are documented, and the appropriate referral is made to the physician, as needed, for further evaluation. Other specific outcomes will be formulated depending on the identified nursing diagnosis.

IMPLEMENTATION

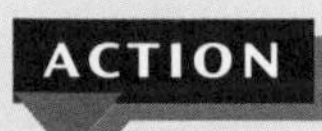

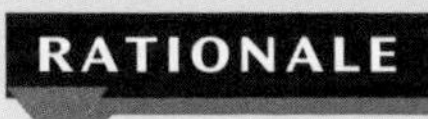

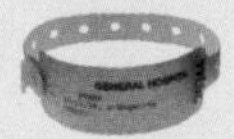

ACTION	RATIONALE
1. Identify the patient.	Positive identification of the patient is essential to ensure the assessment is performed on the right patient.

SKILL 2-3

Assessing the Thorax and Lungs *(continued)*

ACTION	RATIONALE
2. Explain the purpose of the respiratory system examination and answer any questions.	Explanation helps to alleviate anxiety, promotes cooperation, and facilitates the examination. Any anxiety may alter the patient's breathing pattern.
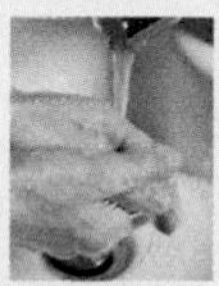 3. Perform hand hygiene.	Hand hygiene deters the risk of microorganism transmission.
4. Help the patient undress if needed and provide a patient gown. Assist the patient to a sitting position and expose the posterior thorax.	Having the patient wear a gown facilitates examination of the thorax.
5. Inspect the posterior thorax. Examine the skin (Figure 1), bones, and muscles of the spine, shoulder blades, and back as well as symmetry of expansion and accessory muscle use during respirations.	Examination provides information about lung expansion and accessory muscle use during respiration. Inspection of skin reveals color, presence of lesions, rashes, or masses.

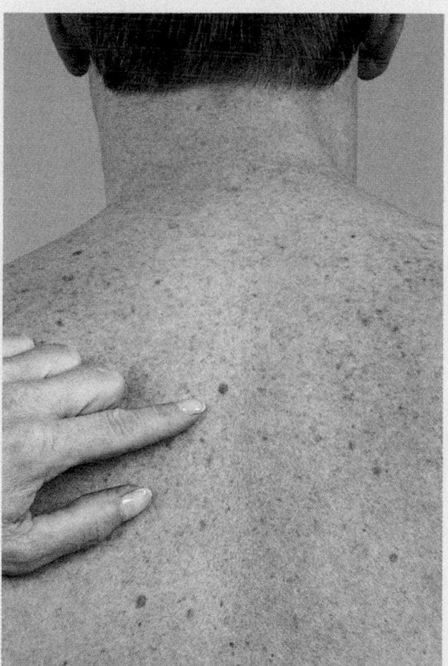

Figure 1. Inspecting the skin for abnormalities and variations. Any lesion or mole noted during inspection of the patient's back should be documented in the patient's medical record for follow-up evaluation. (Photos © B. Proud.)

ACTION	RATIONALE
6. Assess the anteroposterior and lateral diameters of the thorax.	This assessment helps to detect deformities, such as a barrel chest. Normally, the anteroposterior is less than the transverse diameter (1:2 ratio).

(continued)

SKILL 2-3 Assessing the Thorax and Lungs *(continued)*

ACTION	RATIONALE
7. Palpate over the spine and posterior thorax (Figure 2).	
a. Use the palmar surface of the hand to palpate for temperature, tenderness, muscle development, and masses.	Palpation may reveal abnormal findings, such as excessively dry or moist skin, muscle asymmetry, masses, or tenderness.
b. Instruct patient to take a deep breath. Assess for tactile fremitus by using the ball of the hands to palpate over the posterior thorax and while the patient says "ninety-nine" (Figure 3).	Assessing tactile fremitus provides information about the density of the lungs through vibratory sensation (vibrations increase over consolidated areas such as in pneumonia).

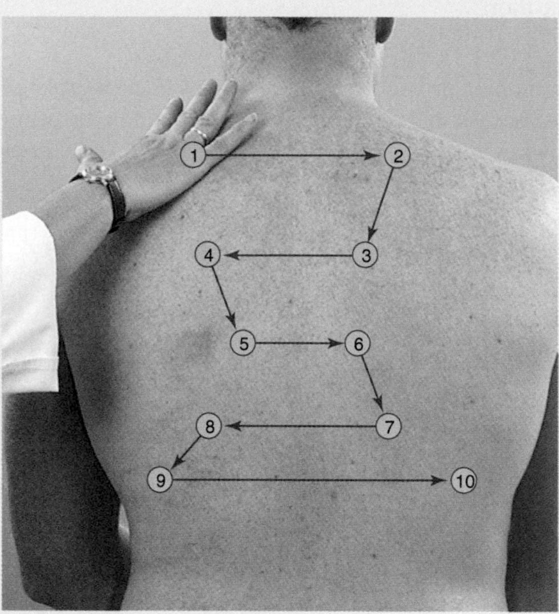

Figure 2. Sequence for palpating posterior thorax.

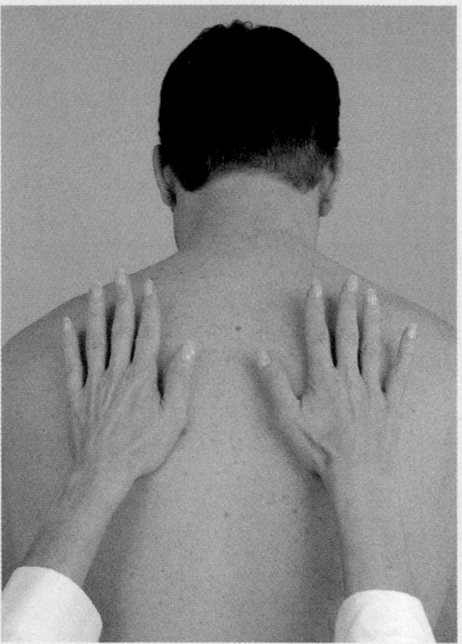

Figure 3. Palpating the posterior thorax for vocal or tactile fremitus. The examiner uses the palms of the hands to detect vibrations through the chest wall. (Photos © B. Proud.)

ACTION	RATIONALE
8. Assess thoracic expansion by standing behind the patient, placing both thumbs on either side of the patient's spine at the level of T9 or T10 (Figure 4). Ask the patient to take a deep breath and note movement of examiner's hands.	Movement should be symmetric bilaterally.
9. Percuss over the posterior and lateral lung fields for tone using a zigzag pattern, starting above the scapulae to the bases of the lungs (Figure 5). Note intensity, pitch, duration, and quality of sounds produced. Percuss for diaphragmatic excursion on each side of the posterior thorax.	Percussion over the lung fields helps identify the density and location of the lungs, diaphragm, and other anatomic structures. When the normal air-filled lung is percussed, the sound is hollow, loud, low in pitch, and long in durations. Diaphragmatic excursion provides information about diaphragm movement during respiration. Excursion usually measures 3 to 5 cm.

SKILL 2-3 **Assessing the Thorax and Lungs** *(continued)*

ACTION	RATIONALE
10. **Auscultate the lungs across and down the posterior thorax to the bases of lungs as the patient breathes slowly and deeply through the mouth (Figure 6).**	Lung auscultation assesses for normal breath sounds and for abnormal (adventitious) breath sounds. Abnormal breath sounds indicate respiratory compromise or diseases such as asthma or bronchitis.

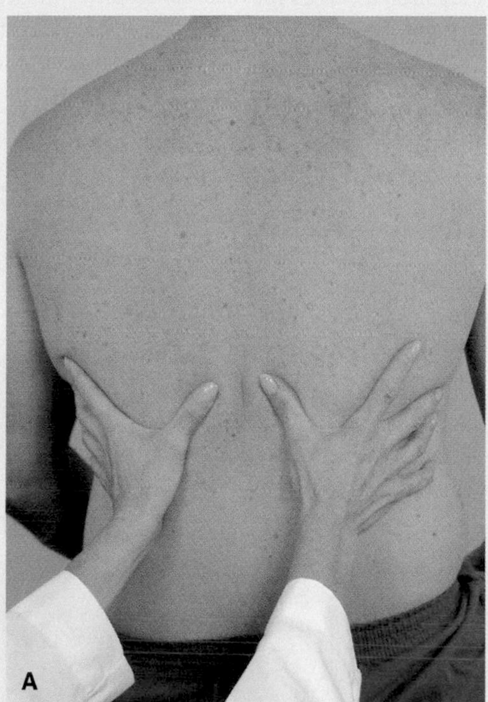

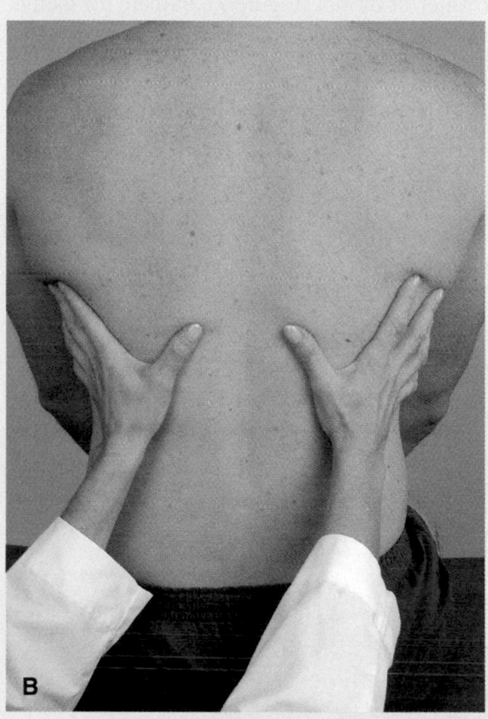

Figure 4. Palpating posterior thoracic excursion. (**A**) The examiner's hands are placed symmetrically on the patient's back. (**B**) As the patient inhales, the examiner's hands should move apart symmetrically. (Photos © B. Proud.)

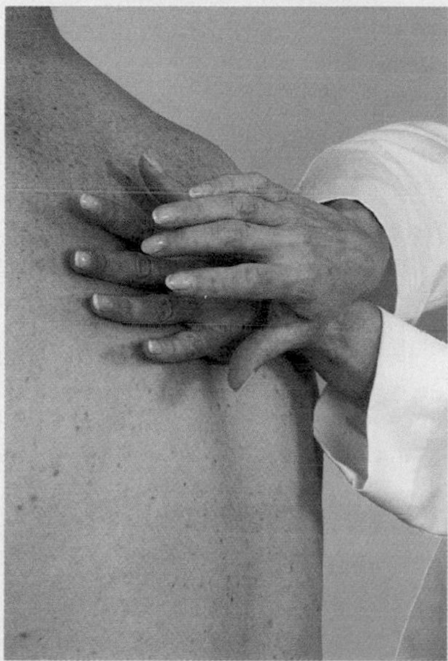

Figure 5. Percussing posterior thorax. (Photos © B. Proud.)

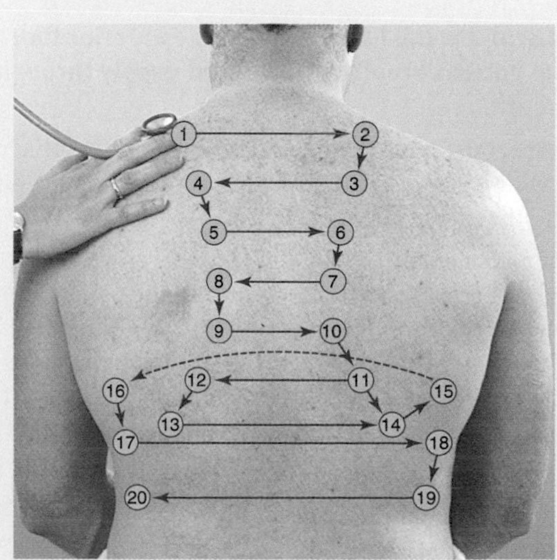

Figure 6. Sequence for auscultating posterior thorax.

(continued)

SKILL 2-3 Assessing the Thorax and Lungs *(continued)*

ACTION	RATIONALE
11. Examine the anterior thorax. With the patient sitting, rearrange the gown so the anterior chest is exposed. Inspect the skin, bones, and muscles, as well as symmetry of lung expansion and accessory muscle use.	Inspection provides information about lung expansion, use of accessory muscle, respiratory effort, and presence of deformities.
12. Palpate the anterior thorax (Figure 7). Palpate for tactile fremitus (as the patient repeats the word "ninety-nine").	Palpation assesses for masses, crepitus, muscle development, and tenderness. Assessing tactile fremitus provides information about lung density.
13. Percuss over the anterior thorax (Figure 8).	Percussion over the lung fields helps identify the density and location of the lungs, diaphragm, and other anatomic structures.

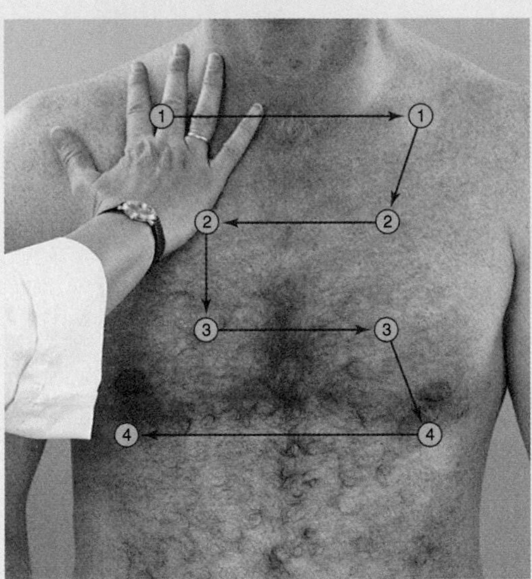

Figure 7. Sequence for palpating anterior thorax.

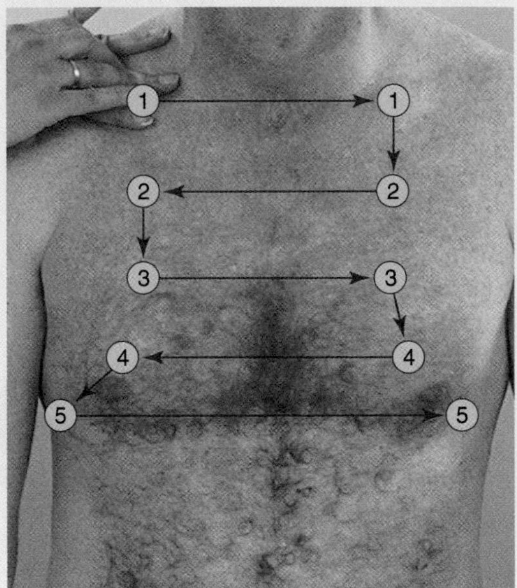

Figure 8. Sequence for percussing and auscultating anterior thorax.

ACTION	RATIONALE
14. **Auscultate the lungs through the anterior thorax as the patient breathes slowly and deeply through the mouth.**	Lung auscultation assesses for normal breath sounds and abnormal (adventitious) breath sounds.
15. Inspect the breasts and axillae with the patient's hands resting on both sides of the body, placed on the hips, and then raised above the head.	This technique evaluates the general condition of the breasts and helps to identify any abnormalities
16. Palpate the axillae with the patient's arms resting against the side of the body. Assist the patient into a supine position. Place a small pillow or towel under the patient's back. Palpate the breasts and nipples (Figure 9). Wear gloves if there is any discharge from the nipples or if a lesion is present.	Palpating the axillae helps to detect nodular enlargement, tenderness and other abnormalities; palpating the breasts evaluates the consistency and elasticity of breast tissue and nipples and for presence of lumps or masses.

SKILL 2-3 **Assessing the Thorax and Lungs** *(continued)*

ACTION

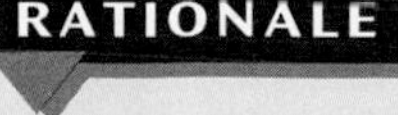

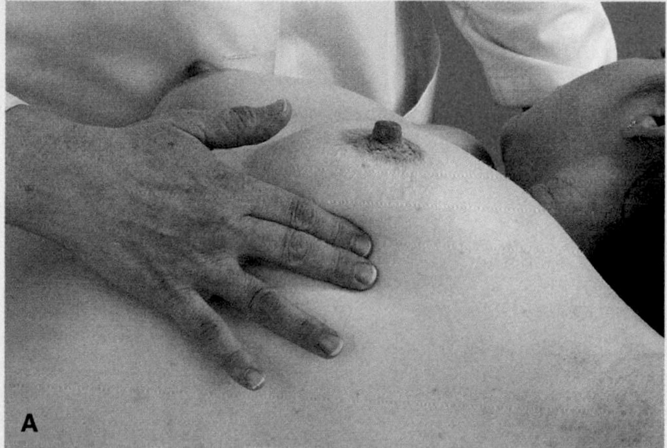

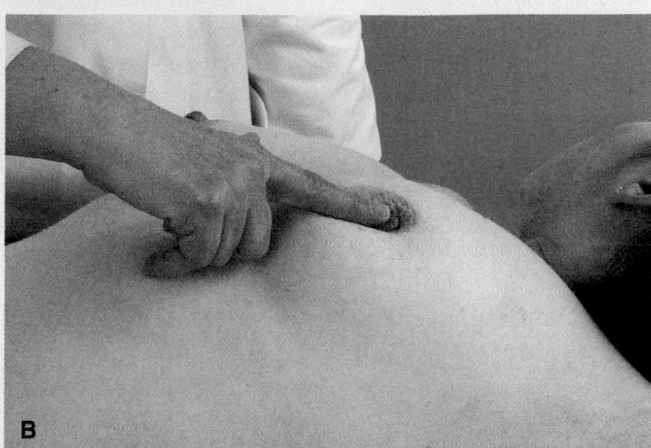

Figure 9. Palpating the breasts (**A**) and nipples (**B**). (Photos © B. Proud.)

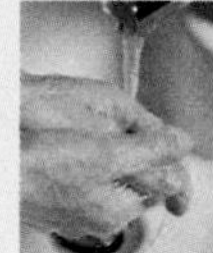

17. Assist the patient in replacing the gown. Perform hand hygiene.

Hand hygiene deters the risk of microorganism transmission.

EVALUATION

The expected outcome is met when the patient participated in the respiratory assessment, displays decreased anxiety, and verbalizes understanding of respiratory assessment techniques as appropriate.

DOCUMENTATION

Guidelines

When documenting respiratory assessment, be sure to describe both subjective and objective data. For example, ask the patient if he/she is experiencing any difficulty breathing, shortness of breath, or cough. Include specific findings on all four assessment techniques performed. For findings, document where they were elicited (eg, decreased breath sounds over left lower lobe of the lung). For breast assessment, clock position is often used to describe the location of findings (eg, palpation reveals a hard mass approximately 1 cm in diameter at the 2 o'clock position on the left breast).

Sample Documentation

6/10/08 P.L. states that she "has a dry cough for the past week and feels weak." Skin pale. RR is 30. Breathing effort moderately labored; right-sided intercostal retraction noted. Barrel-shaped chest. Tactile fremitus increased on right anterior and posterior chest. Resonant tone on percussion. Sonorous wheezes auscultated in RUL, RML, and RLL of lung fields.—B. Gentzler, RN

Unexpected Situations and Associated Interventions

- *When assessing a patient's lungs, you hear short, high-pitched popping sounds on inspiration:* Ask the patient to cough and auscultate again. If the sounds remain, suspect fine crackles and ask the patient if he/she is experiencing any difficulty in breathing or shortness of breath (SOB). Crackles may indicate disease such as pneumonia or heart failure. Continue to assess the patient and notify the physician if the condition worsens.

(continued)

SKILL 2-3 Assessing the Thorax and Lungs *(continued)*

Special Considerations

General Guidelines

- Always warm equipment such as a stethoscope before using it to prevent chilling the patient.
- Attempt to reduce the noise level in the room while auscultating for breath sounds to ensure accuracy in listening. Also, the presence of chest hair may mimic the sound of crackles and bumping the stethoscope against clothing may distort the sound.
- Always obtain the patient's subjective data as well as the physical examination findings. For example, the physical data may be normal; however, the patient may verbalize that he or she is having difficulty breathing. In this case, the patient needs to be monitored closely to assess for possible complications.

Infant and Child Considerations

- Avoid anterior thorax chest percussion in an infant because it is often unreliable due to the infant's small chest size.
- Auscultate a child's lungs before performing other assessment techniques that may cause crying.
- Expect to hear breath sounds that are harsher or more bronchial than those of an adult.

Older Adult Considerations

- In the elderly patient, expect to find a reduction in respiratory effort due to age-related changes. A common finding in the elderly is kyphoscoliosis, a skeletal deformity affecting the spinal column which causes the AP diameter to increase and the thorax to shorten. Also, the alveoli of the lung tissue decreases, which reduces the amount of alveolar surface area available for gas exchange.

SKILL 2-4 Assessing the Cardiovascular System

The cardiovascular system transports oxygen, nutrients, and other substances to the body tissues and removes metabolic waste products to the kidneys and lungs. Careful assessment of this vital system is essential. In the following section, assessment data associated with the heart will be presented. The peripheral vascular system assessment is included in Skill 2-6, because peripheral vascular, neurologic, and musculoskeletal systems are usually combined when performing a head-to-toe assessment.

While assessing the heart, careful auscultation is important. Identifying heart sounds takes practice; Box 2-1 provides a review of normal and abnormal heart sounds.

Equipment

- Draping
- Gown
- Stethoscope
- Centimeter ruler

ASSESSMENT

Complete a health history, focusing on the heart. Identify risk factors for altered health during the health history by asking about the following:

- History of chest pain, tightness, palpitations, dizziness, or fatigue
- Swelling in the ankles and feet
- Number of pillows used to sleep
- Type and amount of medications taken daily

SKILL 2-4 **Assessing the Cardiovascular System** *(continued)*

- History of heart defect, rheumatic fever, or chest or heart surgery
- Family history of hypertension (high blood pressure), myocardial infarction (heart attack), coronary artery disease, high blood cholesterol levels, or diabetes mellitus
- History of smoking (including pack-years)
- History of alcohol use
- Type and amount of exercise
- Usual foods eaten each day

NURSING DIAGNOSIS

Determine the related factors for the nursing diagnoses based on the client's current health status. An appropriate nursing diagnosis is Decreased Cardiac Output related to altered heart rhythm. Other nursing diagnoses related to the heart may include:

- Risk for Activity Intolerance
- Risk for Peripheral Neurovascular Dysfunction
- Risk for Impaired Gas Exchange
- Risk for Sexual Dysfunction
- Risk for Ineffective Denial
- Fatigue related to decreased cardiac output
- Acute Pain related to decreased oxygen supply
- Ineffective Tissue Perfusion related to inadequate circulation

OUTCOME IDENTIFICATION AND PLANNING

The expected outcome to achieve in performing an examination of the cardiovascular structures is that the assessment is completed without causing the patient to experience anxiety or discomfort, the findings are documented, and the appropriate referral for further evaluation is made to the physician as needed. Other specific outcomes will be formulated depending on the identified nursing diagnosis.

BOX 2-1 Heart Sounds

Normal Heart Sounds

During auscultation, the first heart sound, called S_1, is heard as the "lub" of "lub-dub." This sound occurs when the mitral and tricuspid valves close and corresponds to the onset of ventricular contraction. The sound, low-pitched and dull, is heard best at the apical area. The second heart sound, S_2, occurs at the termination of systole and corresponds to the onset of ventricular diastole. The "dub" of "lub-dub," it represents the closure of the aortic and pulmonic valves. The sound of S_2 is higher pitched and shorter than S_1. The two sounds occur within 1 second or less, depending on the heart rate.

Normal findings include S_1 that is louder at the tricuspid and apical areas, with S_2 louder at the aortic and pulmonic areas.

Abnormal Heart Sounds

Abnormal findings include extra heart sounds at any of the cardiac landmarks and abnormal rate or rhythm. Extra heart sounds are often heard when the patient has anemia or heart disease. A wide variety of conditions may alter the normal heart rate or rhythm, including serious infections, diseases of the heart muscle or conducting system, dehydration or overhydration, endocrine disorders, respiratory disorders, and head trauma. Extra heart sounds may be S_3, S_4, murmurs, or bruits.

S_3, known as the third heart sound, is often represented by a "lub-dub-dee" pattern ("dee" being S_3); this sound is best heard with the stethoscope bell at the mitral area, with the patient lying on the left side. S_3 is considered normal in children and young adults and abnormal in middle-aged and older adults.

S_4 is the fourth heart sound, represented by "dee-lub-dub." S_4 is considered normal in older adults but abnormal in children and adults.

Heart murmurs are extra heart sounds caused by some disruption of blood flow through the heart. The characteristics of a murmur depend on the adequacy of valve function, rate of blood flow, and size of the valve opening. Grading of heart murmurs:

Grade	*Description*
I	A murmur so faint that it can only be heard with great effort
II	A faint murmur but one that can be easily detected
III	A moderately loud murmur
IV	A very loud murmur that is usually associated with a thrill sound
V	An extremely loud murmur
VI	An exceptionally loud murmur that can be heard while the stethoscope is lifted off the skin

(continued)

SKILL 2-4 Assessing the Cardiovascular System *(continued)*

IMPLEMENTATION

ACTION	RATIONALE
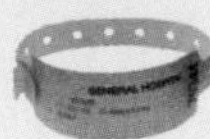 1. Identify the patient.	Identification of the patient ensures that the assessment will be performed on the right patient.
2. Explain the purpose of the cardiovascular examination and answer any questions.	Explanation helps to alleviate anxiety, promotes cooperation, and facilitates the examination.
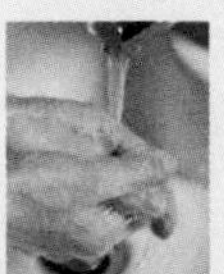 3. Perform hand hygiene.	Hand hygiene deters the risk of microorganism transmission.
4. Assist the patient to a supine position with the head elevated about 30 to 45 degrees and expose anterior chest.	Having the patient wear a gown facilitates examination of the chest. Provide privacy when exposing the chest of the female patient.
5. Inspect and palpate the left and then the right carotid arteries. **Only palpate one carotid artery at a time.** Use the bell of the stethoscope to auscultate the arteries.	Palpation of this area evaluates circulation through the arteries. **Palpating both arteries at once can obstruct blood flow to the brain.** Auscultation can detect a bruit.
6. **Inspect the neck for jugular vein distention, observing for pulsations.**	This technique helps to detect right-sided heart pressure.
7. Inspect the precordium for contour, pulsations, and heaves. Observe for the apical impulse at the 4th to 5th intercostal spaces (ICS).	Precordium inspection helps detect pulsations. There are normally no pulsations, except for a slight apical impulse.
8. Using the palmar surface with the four fingers held together, palpate the precordium gently for pulsations. Remember that hands should be warm. Palpation proceeds in a systematic manner, with assessment of specific cardiac landmarks—the aortic, pulmonic, tricuspid, and mitral areas and Erb's point (Figure 1). **Palpate the apical impulse in the mitral area (Figure 2).** Note size, duration, force, and location in relationship to the midclavicular line.	This helps identify any precordial thrills, which are fine, palpable, rushing vibrations over the right or left second intercostal space, and any lifts or heaves, which involve a rise along the border of the sternum with each heartbeat. Normal findings include no pulsation palpable over the aortic and pulmonic areas, with a palpable apical impulse.
9. **Use systematic auscultation, beginning at the aortic area, moving to the pulmonic area, then to Erb's point, then to the tricuspid area, and finally to the mitral area (Figure 3).** Ask the patient to breathe normally. The stethoscope diaphragm is first used to listen to high-pitched sounds, followed by use of the bell to listen to low-pitched sounds. Focus on the overall rate and rhythm of the heart and the normal heart sounds.	Auscultation evaluates heart rate and rhythm and assesses for normal sounds (the lub, S_1; the dub, S_2) and abnormal heart sounds (S_3 and S_4). The normal heart sounds (S_1 and S_2) are generated by the closing of the valves (the aortic, pulmonic, tricuspid, mitral). S_3 could be a normal finding in a pregnant woman in the third trimester due to increased cardiac output.
10. Replace the patient's gown and assist the patient to a comfortable position.	This ensures the patient's comfort.
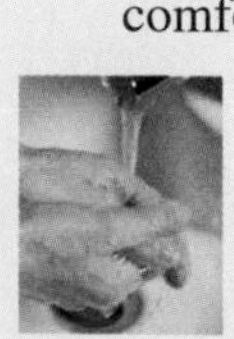 11. Perform hand hygiene.	This deters the spread of microorganisms.

SKILL 2-4

Assessing the Cardiovascular System *(continued)*

ACTION | RATIONALE

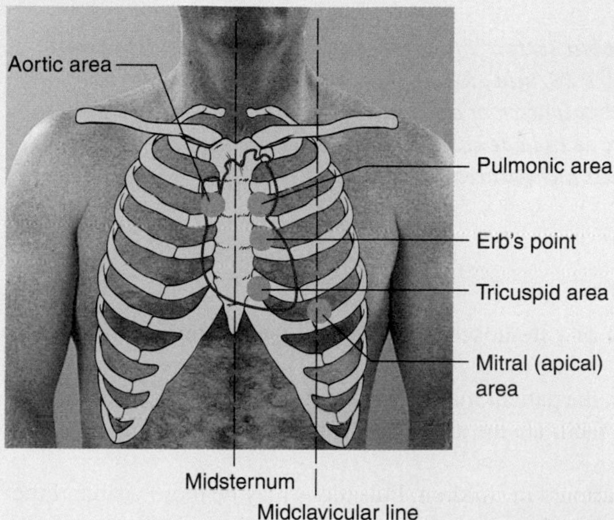

Figure 1. Traditional areas of auscultation.

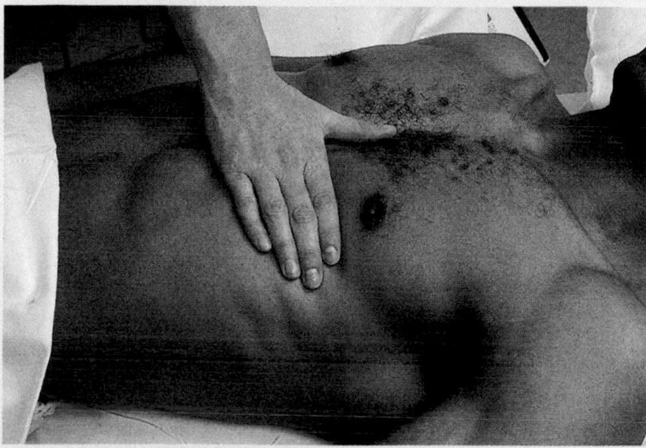

Figure 2. Palpating the apical impulse.

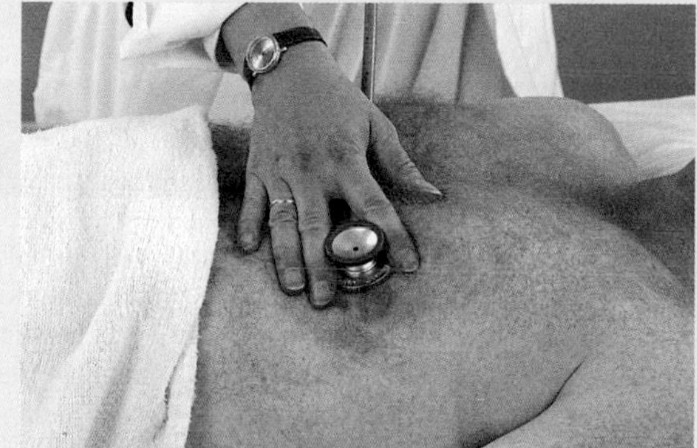

Figure 3. Auscultating the mitral area. (© B. Proud.)

EVALUATION

The expected outcome is met when the patient participated in the cardiovascular assessment, displays decreased anxiety, and verbalizes understanding of cardiovascular assessment, as appropriate.

DOCUMENTATION

Guidelines

When documenting cardiac assessment, be sure to describe data. Include assessment techniques performed, along with specific findings. It is important to ask the patient if he or she is experiencing any symptoms such as chest pain, dizziness, or palpitations. Vital signs, which provide insight into cardiovascular function, are usually included in this documentation note. Note assessment data related to color and temperature of the skin as well as capillary refill of nails. Record inspection findings related to the carotid arteries, jugular veins, and anterior chest wall area. Be sure to document findings related to palpation of the sternoclavicular area, as well as anterior chest wall for presence of pulsations, thrills, lifts, and heaves. Note auscultation findings, including rate, rhythm, pitch, and location of sounds. Record the normal heart sounds (S_1 and S_2) as well as the abnormal sounds (S_3 and S_4).

(continued)

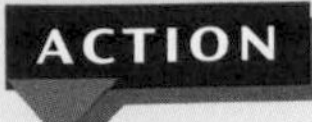

SKILL 2-4 Assessing the Cardiovascular System *(continued)*

ACTION | **RATIONALE**

Sample Documentation

5/10/09 B.K. denies chest pain but states, "I have palpitations occurring about once a week." T. 98.6 F., B.P. 140/92, P 88/min, RR20. Skin pale, cool to touch, brisk capillary refill. Inspection and palpation of chest: no lifts, pulsations, heaves were noted. Auscultation: S_1 loudest at the apex; S_2 loudest at the base; no S_3 or S_4 auscultated. No carotid bruits auscultated.—S. Moses, RN

Special Considerations

General Considerations

- Always warm equipment such as a stethoscope before using it to prevent chilling the patient.
- In auscultation of heart sounds, the patient may have to assume varied position such as lying on the left lateral side, to facilitate the auscultation of the cardiac sounds.

Infant and Child Considerations

- Be alert for functional heart murmurs in children. Pulsations may be more visible if the chest wall is thin. S_3 may be present in young children.

SKILL 2-5 Assessing the Abdomen

The abdominal cavity, the largest cavity in the body, contains the stomach, the small intestine, the large intestine, the liver, the gallbladder, the pancreas, the spleen, the kidneys, the urinary bladder, adrenal gland and major blood vessels (Figure 1). In women, the uterus, fallopian tubes, and ovaries are also located in the abdomen. Not all of these organs can be assessed. For identification/documentation purposes, the abdomen can be divided into four quadrants (Figure 2).

For the abdominal assessment, the order of the techniques differs from the other systems. The nurse should start with inspection, then auscultation, percussion, and palpation. This is the preferred approach because palpation and percussion before auscultation may alter the sounds heard on auscultation. Also, before beginning the abdominal assessment, the patient should be asked to empty his/her bladder since a full bladder may cause discomfort during the exam or affect the findings.

Equipment

- Draping
- Gown
- Stethoscope
- Penlight
- Centimeter ruler

ASSESSMENT

Complete a health history, focusing on the abdomen. Identify risk factors for altered health during the health history by asking about the following:

- History of abdominal pain
- History of indigestion, nausea or vomiting, constipation or diarrhea
- History of food allergies or lactose intolerance
- Appetite and usual food and fluid intake

SKILL 2-5 **Assessing the Abdomen** *(continued)*

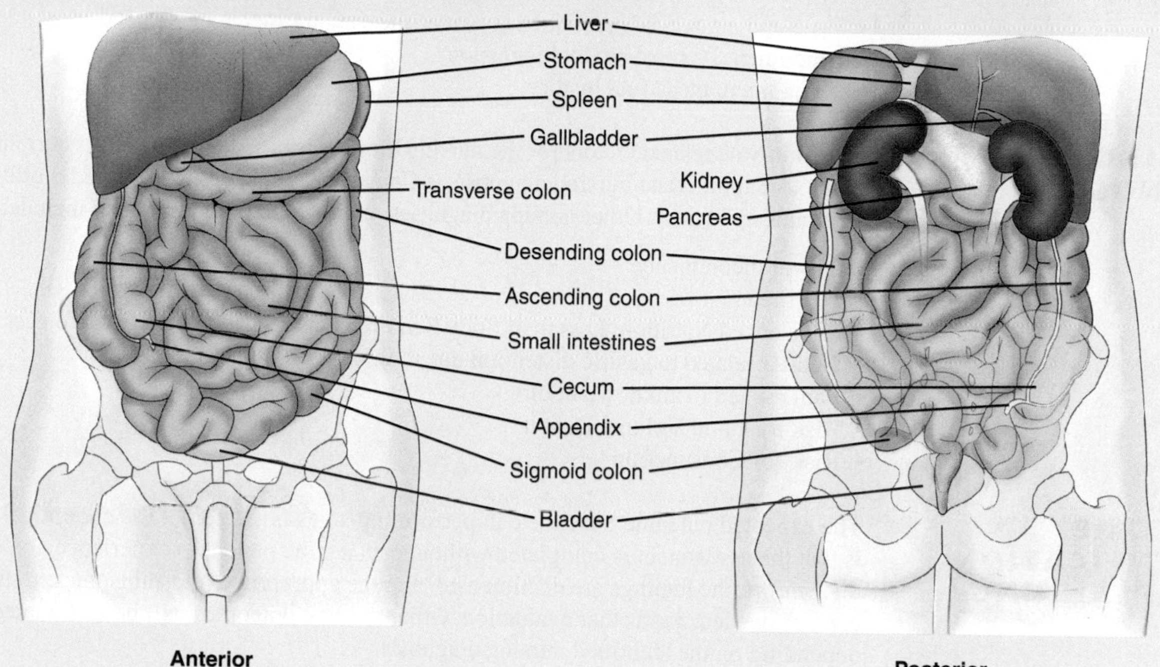

Figure 1. Organs of the abdominal cavity.

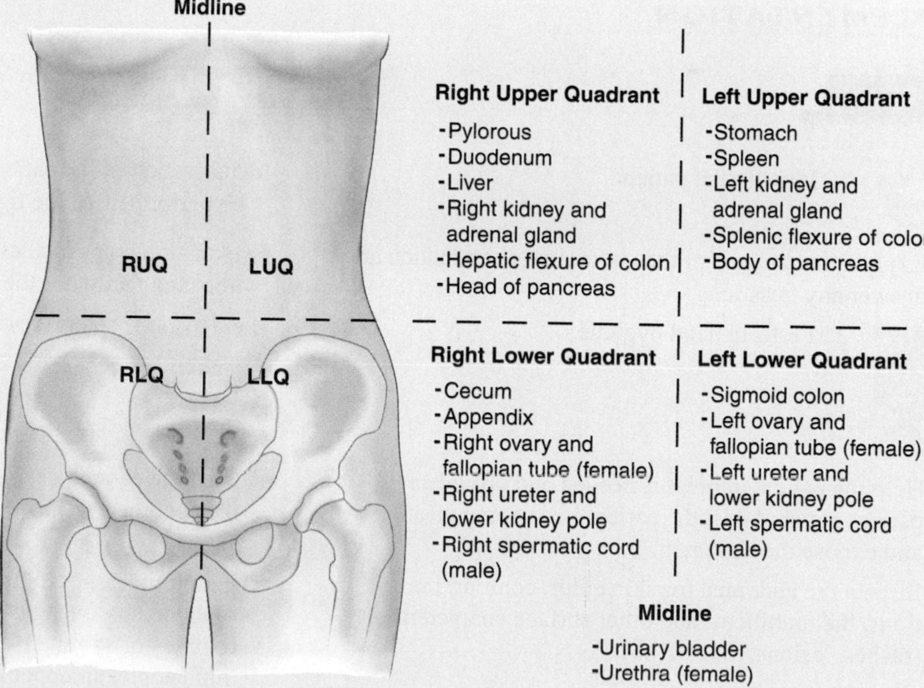

Figure 2. Diagram of abdominal quadrants and outline of underlying organs.

- Usual bowel and bladder elimination patterns
- History of gastrointestinal disorders, such as peptic ulcer disease, bowel disease, gallbladder disease, liver disease, or appendicitis
- History of urinary tract disorders, such as infections, kidney stones, or kidney disease
- History of abdominal surgery or trauma

(continued)

SKILL 2-5 Assessing the Abdomen *(continued)*

- Type and amount of prescribed and over-the-counter medications used
- Amount and type of alcohol ingestion
- For women, menstrual history

NURSING DIAGNOSIS

Determine the related factors for the nursing diagnoses based on the client's current health status. An appropriate nursing diagnosis is Constipation related to decreased motility of the gastrointestinal tract. Other nursing diagnoses related to the abdomen may include:

- Bowel Incontinence
- Diarrhea
- Imbalanced Nutrition: Less than Body Requirements related to inability to digest nutrients
- Nausea related to gastric distention due to upper bowel stasis
- Pain related to unknown etiology
- Risk for Fluid Volume Deficit
- Risk for Constipation

OUTCOME IDENTIFICATION AND PLANNING

The expected outcome to achieve in performing an examination of the abdominal cavity is that the assessment is completed without causing the patient to experience anxiety or discomfort, the findings are documented, and the appropriate referral is made to the physician, as needed, for further evaluation. Other specific outcomes will be formulated depending on the identified nursing diagnosis.

IMPLEMENTATION

ACTION	RATIONALE
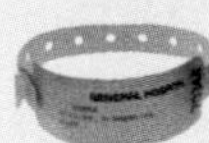 1. Identify the patient.	Identification of the patient ensures that the assessment will be performed on the right patient.
2. Explain the purpose of the abdominal examination and answer any questions.	Explanation helps to alleviate anxiety, promotes cooperation, and facilitates the examination.
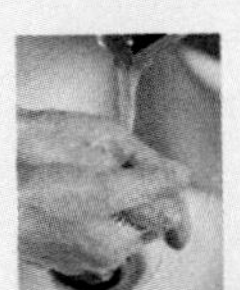 3. Perform hand hygiene.	Hand hygiene deters the risk of microorganism transmission.
4. Help the patient undress if needed and provide a patient gown. Assist the patient to a supine position and expose the abdomen.	Having the patient wear a gown facilitates examination of the abdomen.
5. Inspect the abdomen for skin color, contour, pulsations, the umbilicus, and other surface characteristics (rashes, lesions, masses, scars).	The umbilicus should be centrally located and may be flat, rounded, or concave. The abdomen should be evenly rounded or symmetric, without visible peristalsis. In thin people, an upper midline pulsation may normally be visible.
6. **Auscultate all four quadrants of the abdomen for bowel sounds by using the diaphragm of the stethoscope.** Use a systematic method.	Performing auscultation before percussion or palpation prevents percussion and palpation techniques from interfering with findings. Auscultation detects the presence of bowel sounds, which indicate peristalsis.
7. **Auscultate the abdomen for vascular sounds by using the bell of the stethoscope (Figure 3).**	A bruit on auscultation suggests an aneurysm or arterial stenosis.

SKILL 2-5 Assessing the Abdomen *(continued)*

ACTION	RATIONALE
8. Percuss the abdomen for tones (Figure 4).	Percussion assesses for the density of the abdominal contents, organs, or possible masses. Tympany over more air-filled regions (eg, stomach and intestines) and dullness over a solid organ (eg, liver) are the predominant tones elicited. Percussion on the right side helps evaluate the size of the liver; on the left side, it helps to evaluate the spleen; percussion over the symphysis pubis helps to evaluate the bladder for fullness.

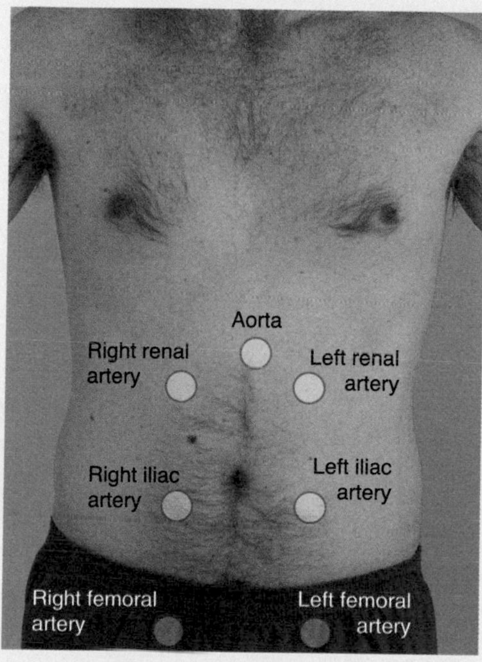

Figure 3. Locations to auscultate for bruits. (Photo by B. Proud.)

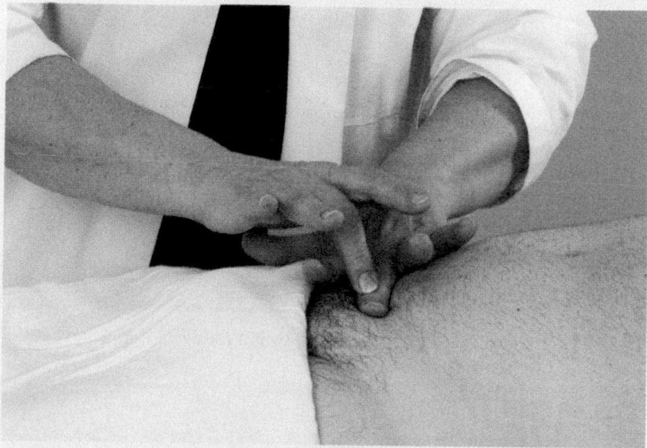

Figure 4. Percussing the area over the symphysis pubis. (Photo by B. Proud.)

ACTION	RATIONALE
9. Palpate the abdomen lightly in all four quadrants and then palpate using deep palpation technique (Figure 5). If the patient complains of pain or discomfort in a particular area of the abdomen, palpate that area last.	Palpation provides information about the location, size, tenderness, and condition of the underlying structures.

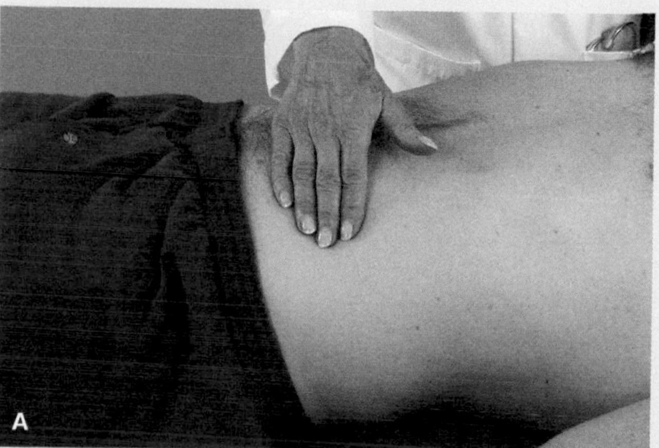

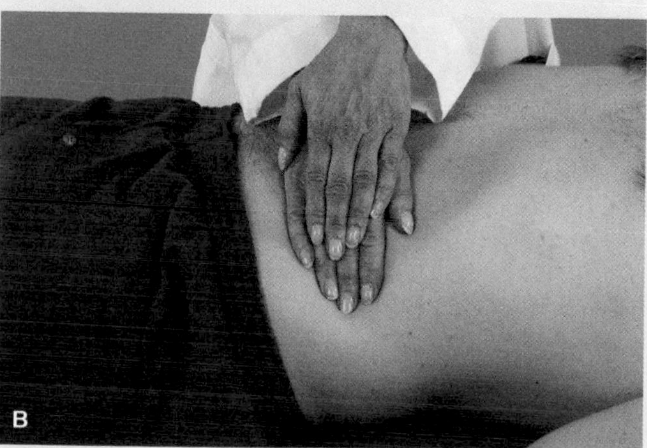

Figure 5. Palpating the abdomen: (**A**) Light palpation; (**B**) Deep palpation. (Photos by B. Proud.)

(continued)

SKILL 2-5

Assessing the Abdomen *(continued)*

ACTION / **RATIONALE**

10. Palpate for the kidneys on each side of the abdomen (Figure 6). Palpate the liver at the right costal border (Figure 7). Palpate for the spleen at the left costal border (Figure 8).

A normal liver, spleen, and kidneys are often not palpable. Palpation helps detect enlarged organs.

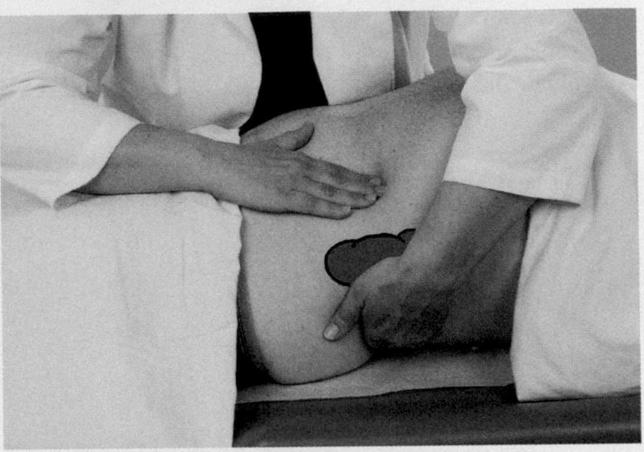

Figure 6. Palpating the kidney. (Photo by B. Proud.)

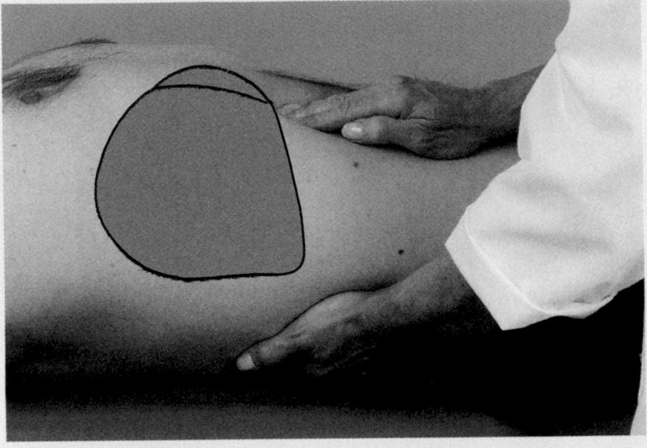

Figure 7. Palpating the liver. (Photo by B. Proud.)

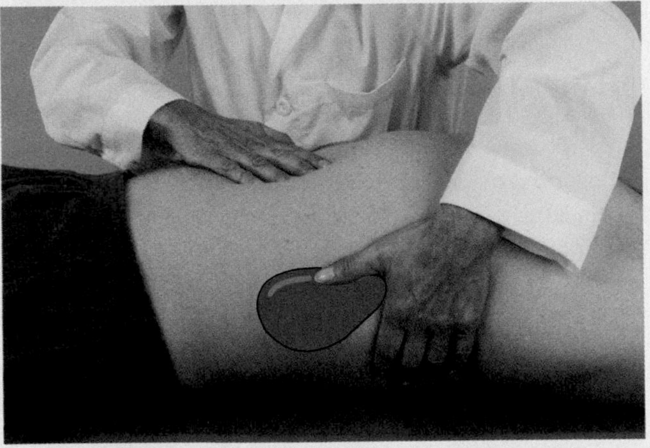

Figure 8. Palpating the spleen. (Photo by B. Proud.)

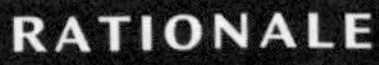

11. **Assess for rebound tenderness last if the patient reports pain by pressing deeply and gently into the abdomen with the hand and fingers downward and then withdrawing the hand rapidly (Figure 9).**

Rebound tenderness is present when the patient indicates that there is increased pain upon withdrawal of the examiner's hand.

Rebound tenderness indicates peritoneal irritation, such as from appendicitis. This assessment is performed last because it can cause pain and muscle spasm that could interfere with the rest of the examination. Continued palpation for rebound tenderness could lead to rupture of the appendix.

12. **Palpate and then auscultate the femoral pulses in the groin (Figure 10).**

This technique assesses vascular patency.

SKILL 2-5 Assessing the Abdomen *(continued)*

ACTION | **RATIONALE**

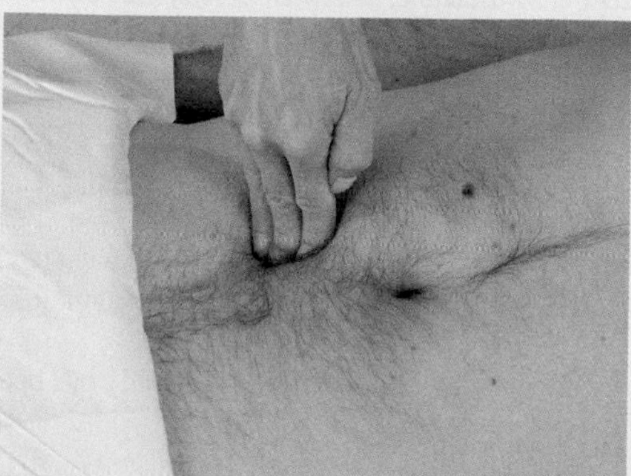
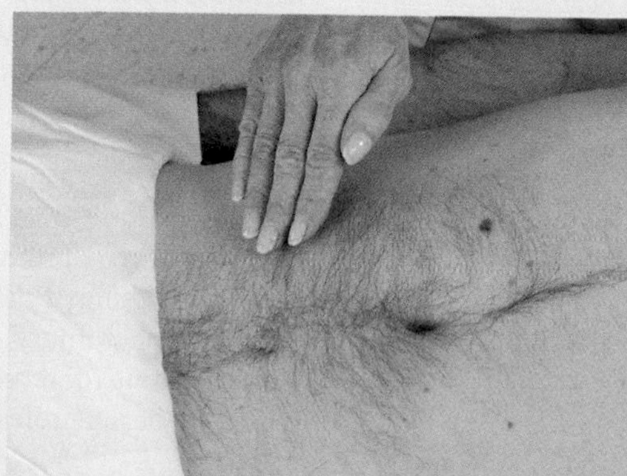

Figure 9. Palpating for rebound tenderness. (Photos by B. Proud.)

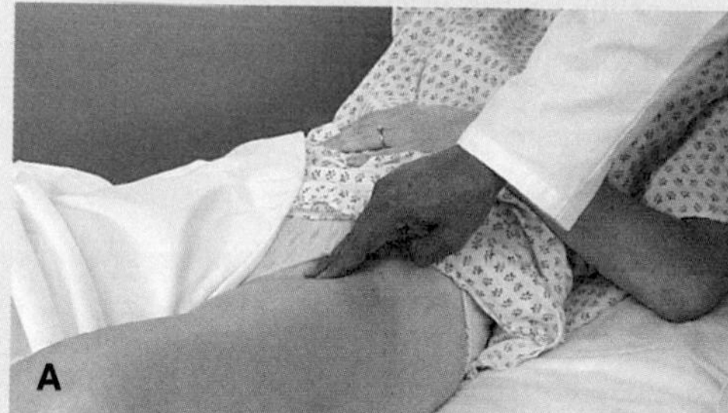

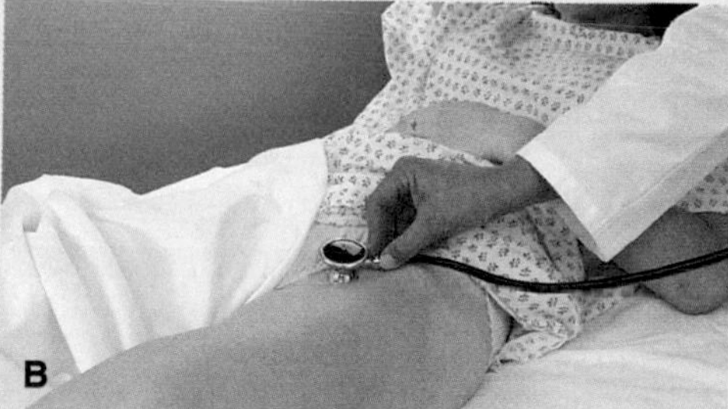

Figure 10. Palpating (**A**) and auscultating (**B**) the femoral pulses. (Photos © B. Proud.)

13. Replace the patient's gown and assist the patient to a comfortable position. — This ensures the patient's comfort.

14. Perform hand hygiene. — This deters the spread of microorganisms.

EVALUATION

The expected outcome is met when the patient participates in the abdominal assessment, displays decreased anxiety, and verbalizes understanding of abdominal assessment techniques as appropriate.

DOCUMENTATION

Guidelines

When documenting abdominal assessment, be sure to describe both subjective and objective data. For example, document if the patient has experienced nausea or any kind of abdominal pain. If pain is present, refer to the PQRST in analyzing the pain. Include the physical examination techniques that are used. For inspection, include a description of the color, presence of lesions, rashes, scars, distention, or masses. For auscultation, note the character of the bowel sounds and if any bruits are present. For percussion, note the percussion tones of the quadrants such as dullness noted in right upper quadrant; tympany percussed in the stomach and intestinal areas. For palpation, note the overall softness or hardness of the abdomen, presence of palpable masses, and if the patient is experiencing any pain. Also, include whether any abdominal organs could be palpated, eg, the liver in the RUQ or the spleen in the LUQ.

(continued)

SKILL 2-5 Assessing the Abdomen *(continued)*

Sample Documentation

3/30/09 Patient states, "I have been nauseated over the past 24 hours." Denies any abdominal pain. On physical examination, abdomen is soft, slightly distended, umbilicus midline, no scars, bowel sounds present in all four quadrants but decreased. Liver, spleen, and kidneys are nonpalpable.—B. Gentzler, RN

Special Considerations

General Considerations

- Always warm equipment such as a stethoscope before using it to prevent chilling the patient.
- Avoid percussing or palpating the spleen of a patient if there is suspicion of splenic engorgement or injury.
- Avoid retesting for rebound tenderness of the abdomen if it already has been documented by another health professional.

Infant and Child Considerations

- In infants, expect a large abdomen in relation to the pelvis.
- Note the number of teeth in a child; a child may have up to 20 temporary teeth.
- Avoid percussion or palpation of the spleen in a child.
- Some children may be unable to tolerate abdominal palpation due to a ticklish sensation.

SKILL 2-6 Assessing the Neurologic, Musculoskeletal, and Peripheral Vascular Systems

The focus of the following assessment is integration of the findings from the neurologic, musculoskeletal, and peripheral vascular systems. In assessing the neurologic system, the patient will be asked to respond to a series of questions that will enable the nurse to obtain data related to overall cognitive function. In addition, sensation will be evaluated in different areas of the body as well as selected cranial nerves and deep tendon reflexes (DTR). Musculoskeletal examination will provide information concerning the condition and functioning of certain muscles and joints throughout the body.

The peripheral vascular system assessment will identify the condition of the arteries and veins in the extremities as gained through inspection and palpation of the skin. The four physical examinations techniques will be used in this section.

Equipment

- Patient gown
- Gloves
- Sheet, bath blanket, or towel, as needed for draping
- Tongue blades
- Percussion (reflex) hammer
- Test tubes of hot and cold water
- Containers of odorous materials (eg, coffee or chocolate) and substances for taste assessment (sugar, salt, vinegar)
- Miscellaneous items such as coin, pin, cotton, or paper clip
- Cotton-tipped applicators

ASSESSMENT

Complete a health history, focusing on the neurologic, musculoskeletal, and peripheral vascular systems. Identify risk factors for altered health during the health history by asking about the following:

SKILL 2-6

Assessing the Neurologic, Musculoskeletal, and Peripheral Vascular Systems *(continued)*

- History of numbness, tingling, or tremors
- History of seizures
- History of headaches
- History of dizziness
- History of trauma to the head or spine
- History of infections of the brain
- History of stroke
- Changes in the ability to hear, see, taste, or smell
- Loss of ability to control bladder and bowel
- History of smoking
- History of chronic alcohol use
- History of diabetes mellitus
- Use of prescription and over-the-counter medications
- Family history of Alzheimer's disease, epilepsy, cancer, or Huntington's chorea, hypertension (high blood pressure), myocardial infarction (heart attack), coronary artery disease, high blood cholesterol levels, or diabetes mellitus
- Frequency of blood cholesterol tests and results
- Exposure to environmental hazards (eg, lead, insecticides)
- History of trauma, arthritis, or neurologic disorder
- History of pain or swelling in the joints
- History of pain in the muscles
- Frequency and type of usual exercise
- Dietary intake of calcium
- Changes in color or temperature of the extremities
- History of pain in the legs when sleeping or pain that is worsened by walking
- History of blood clots or sores on the legs that do not heal

NURSING DIAGNOSIS

Determine the related factors for the nursing diagnoses based on the client's current health status. An appropriate nursing diagnosis is Risk for Falls. Other nursing diagnoses related to the abdomen may include:

- Chronic Confusion related to Alzheimer's disease
- Impaired Verbal Communication related to brain tumor
- Delayed Growth and Development
- Risk for Delayed Development
- Impaired Environmental Interpretation Syndrome related to dementia
- Impaired Physical Mobility related to musculoskeletal/neuromuscular impairment
- Risk for Peripheral Neurovascular Dysfunction
- Bathing/Hygiene Self-care Deficit related to musculoskeletal/neuromuscular impairment
- Social Isolation related to alterations in mental status
- Wandering related to cognitive impairment
- Risk for Ineffective Tissue Perfusion
- Risk for Activity Intolerance

OUTCOME IDENTIFICATION AND PLANNING

The expected outcome to achieve in performing an examination of the neurologic, musculoskeletal, and peripheral systems is that the assessment is completed, the findings are documented, and the appropriate referral for further evaluation is made to the physician, as needed. Other specific outcomes will be formulated depending on the identified nursing diagnoses.

(continued)

SKILL 2-6

Assessing the Neurologic, Musculoskeletal, and Peripheral Vascular Systems *(continued)*

IMPLEMENTATION

ACTION	RATIONALE
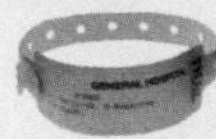 1. Identify the patient.	Identification of the patient ensures that the assessment will be performed on the right patient.
2. Explain the purpose of the neurologic, musculoskeletal, and peripheral vascular examination and answer any questions.	Explanation helps to alleviate anxiety, promotes cooperation, and facilitates the examination.
3. Instruct the patient to void if possible. Collect a urine specimen if ordered.	Emptying the bladder increases patient comfort during the examination.
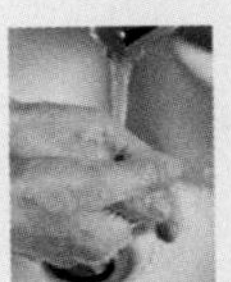 4. Perform hand hygiene.	Hand hygiene deters the risk of microorganism transmission.
5. Help the patient undress if needed and provide a patient gown. Assist the patient to a sitting position.	Having the patient wear a gown facilitates examination of the various body areas.
6. Begin with a survey of the patient's overall hygiene and physical appearance.	This provides initial impressions of the patient. Hygiene and appearance can provide clues about the patient's mental state and comfort level.
7. Assess the patient's mental status.	
a. Evaluate the patient's orientation to person, place, and time.	This helps identify the patient's level of awareness.
b. Evaluate level of consciousness.	The patient should be awake and alert. Patients with altered level of consciousness may be lethargic, stuporous, or comatose.
c. Assess memory (immediate recall and past memory).	Memory problems may indicate neurologic impairment.
d. Assess abstract reasoning by asking the patient to explain a proverb, such as "The early bird catches the worm."	If intellectual ability is impaired, the patient usually gives a literal interpretation or repeats the phrase.
e. Evaluate the patient's ability to understand spoken and written word.	This helps assess for aphasia.
8. Test cranial nerve (CN) function.	
a. Ask the patient to close the eyes, occlude one nostril, and then identify the smell of different substances, such as coffee, chocolate, or alcohol. Repeat with other nostril.	This action tests the function of CN I (olfactory nerve).
b. Test visual acuity and pupillary constriction.	This tests function of CN II and III (optic and oculomotor nerves).
c. Move the patient's eyes through the six cardinal positions of gaze.	This testing evaluates the function of tests CN III, IV, and VI (oculomotor, trochlear, and abducens nerves).
d. Ask the patient to smile, frown, wrinkle forehead, and puff out cheeks (Figure 1).	This maneuver evaluates the motor function of cranial nerve VII (facial nerve).
e. Test hearing.	This evaluates function of CN VIII (acoustic nerve).

SKILL 2-6 Assessing the Neurologic, Musculoskeletal, and Peripheral Vascular Systems *(continued)*

ACTION	RATIONALE
f. **Test the gag reflex by touching the posterior pharynx with the tongue depressor. Explain to patient that this may be uncomfortable.**	An intact gag reflex indicates normal functioning of cranial nerves IX and X (glossopharyngeal and vagus).
g. Place your hands on the patient's shoulders (Figure 2) while he or she shrugs against resistance. Then place your hand on the patient's left cheek, then the right cheek, and have the patient push against it.	These actions check cranial nerve XI (spinal accessory nerve) function and trapezius and sternocleidomastoid muscle strength.

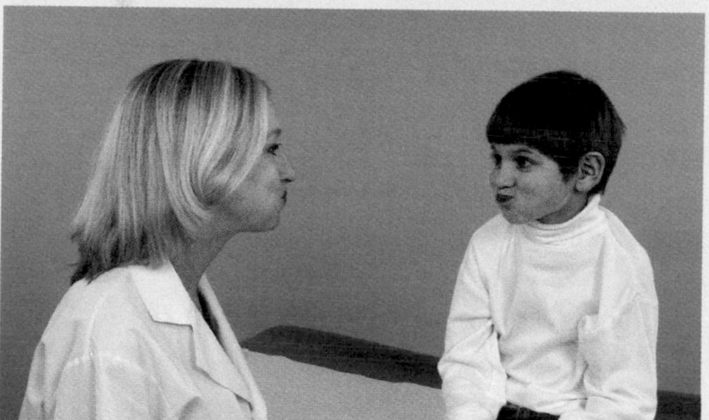

Figure 1. Evaluating motor function of facial nerve. The patient puffs out cheeks as instructed. (Photo by B. Proud.)

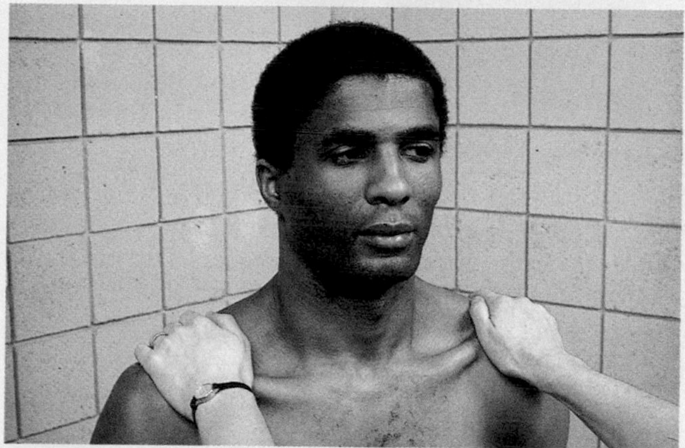

Figure 2. Testing accessory nerve. The patient shrugs his shoulders against the resistance of the nurse's hands. (Photo © Ken Kasper.)

ACTION	RATIONALE
9. Inspect the ability of the patient to move his neck. Ask the patient to touch his or her chin to chest and to each shoulder, each ear to the corresponding shoulder, and then tip head back as far as possible.	These actions assess neck range of motion, which is normally smooth and controlled.
10. Inspect the upper extremities Observe for skin color, presence of lesions, rashes, and muscle mass. Palpate for skin temperature, texture, and presence of masses.	Examination of the upper extremities provides information about the circulatory, integumentary, and musculoskeletal systems.
11. Ask patient to extend arms forward and then rapidly turn palms up and down.	This maneuver tests proprioception and cerebellar function.
12. Ask patient to flex upper arm and to resist examiner's opposing force.	This technique assesses the muscle strength of the upper extremities.
13. Inspect and palpate the hands, fingers, wrists (Figure 3), and elbow joints; palpate the hands.	Inspection and palpation provide information about abnormalities, tenderness, and range of motion.
14. Palpate the radial and brachial pulses.	Pulse palpation evaluates the peripheral vascular status of the upper extremities.
15. Have the patient squeeze two of your fingers (Figure 4).	This maneuver tests the muscle strength of the hands.

(continued)

SKILL 2-6 Assessing the Neurologic, Musculoskeletal, and Peripheral Vascular Systems *(continued)*

ACTION | **RATIONALE**

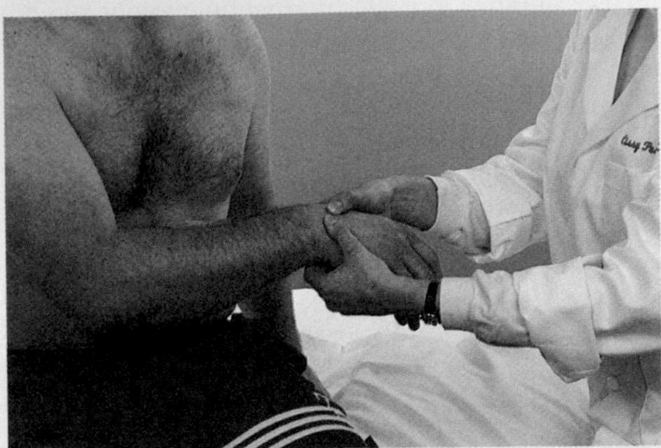

Figure 3. Palpating the wrist. (Photo by B. Proud.)

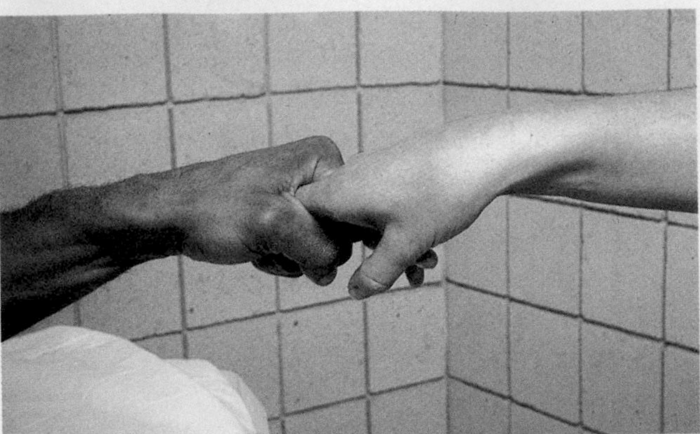

Figure 4. Testing grip. Patient squeezes nurse's index and middle fingers.

16. Ask the patient to close his/her eyes. Using your finger or applicator, trace a one-digit number on the patient's palm and ask him or her to identify the number. Repeat on the other hand with a different number (Figure 5).

This test evaluates tactile discrimination, specifically graphesthesia.

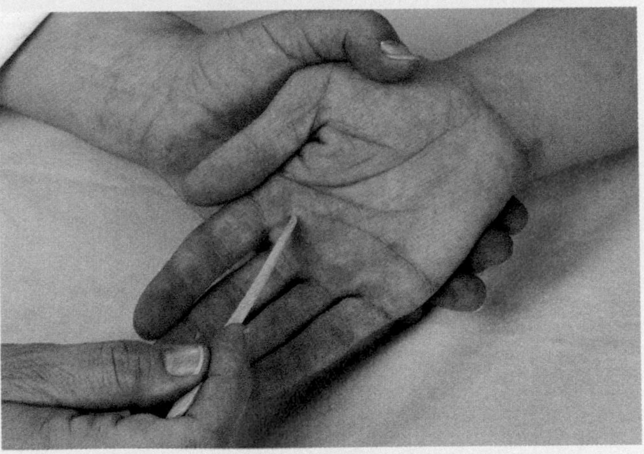

Figure 5. Testing tactile discrimination (graphesthesia). (Photo by B. Proud.)

17. Ask the patient to close his/her eyes. Place a familiar object such as a key in the patient's hand and ask him or her to identify the object. Repeat using another object for the other hand.

This test evaluates tactile discrimination specifically stereognosis.

18. Assist the patient to a supine position. Examine the lower extremities. Inspect the legs and feet for color, lesions, varicosities, hair growth, nail growth, edema, and muscle mass.

Inspection provides information about peripheral vascular function.

19. Test for pitting edema in the pretibial area by pressing fingers into the skin of the pretibial area. If an indentation remains in the skin after the fingers have been lifted, pitting edema is present.

This technique reveals information about excess interstitial fluid. Nurses refer to a "pitting edema scale" in assessing the amount of edema; 1+ about 2mm deep to 4+ about 8mm deep.

SKILL 2-6

Assessing the Neurologic, Musculoskeletal, and Peripheral Vascular Systems *(continued)*

ACTION	RATIONALE
20. Palpate for pulses and skin temperature at the posterior tibial, dorsalis pedis, and popliteal areas.	Pulses and skin temperature provide information about the patient's peripheral vascular status.
21. Have the patient perform the straight leg test with one leg at a time (Figure 6).	This test checks for vertebral disk problems.
22. Ask the patient to move one leg laterally with the knee straight to test abduction and medially to test adduction of the hips.	This maneuver assesses range of motion and provides information about joint problems.
23. Ask the patient to raise the thigh against the resistance of your hand (Figure 7); next have the patient push outward against the resistance of your hand; then have the patient pull backward against the resistance of your hand. Repeat on the opposite side.	These measures assess motor strength of the upper and lower legs.

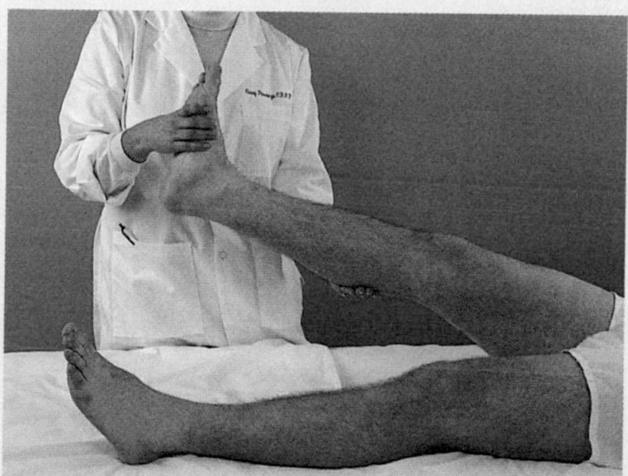

Figure 6. Performing straight leg test. (Photo © B. Proud)

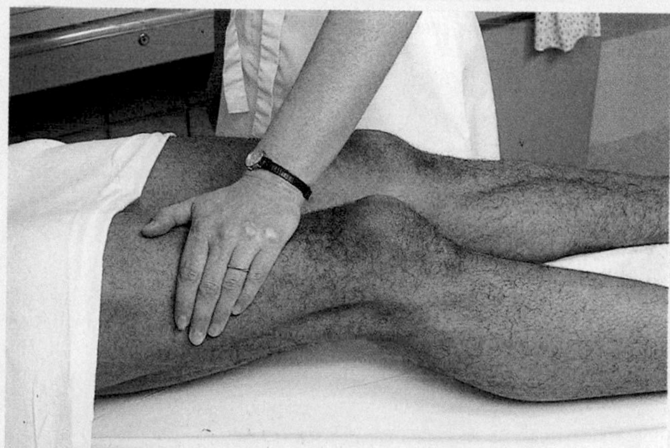

Figure 7. Testing motor strength of upper leg. Patient attempts to raise thigh against nurse's resistance.

ACTION	RATIONALE
24. Assess the patient's deep tendon reflexes (DTRs).	
a. Place your fingers above the patient's wrist and tap with a reflex hammer; repeat on the other arm (Figure 8). b. Place your fingers over the antecubital area and tap with a reflex hammer; repeat on the other side (Figure 9). c. Place your fingers over the triceps tendon area and tap with a reflex hammer; repeat on the other side (Figure 10). d. Tap just below the patella with a reflex hammer; repeat on the other side (Figure 11). e. Tap over the Achilles tendon area with reflex hammer; repeat on the other side (Figure 12).	These tests evaluate the brachioradialis, biceps, triceps, patellar, and Achilles DTRs, respectively.
25. Stroke the sole of the patient's foot with the end of a reflex hammer handle (Figure 13) or other hard object such as a key; repeat on the other side.	Plantar flexion of all the toes is considered a normal finding in an individual 18 months and older; a negative Babinski reflex

(continued)

SKILL 2-6

Assessing the Neurologic, Musculoskeletal, and Peripheral Vascular Systems *(continued)*

ACTION | RATIONALE

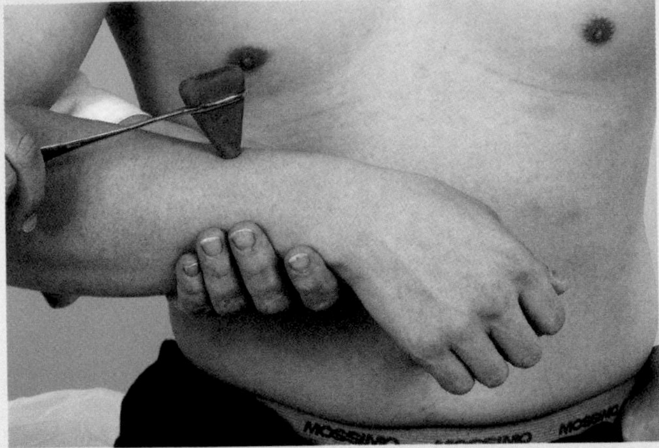

Figure 8. Assessing the brachioradialis reflex. (Photo by B. Proud.)

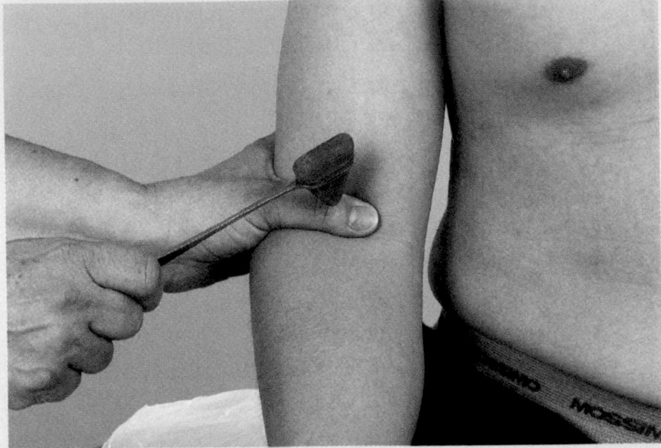

Figure 9. Assessing the biceps reflex. (Photo by B. Proud.)

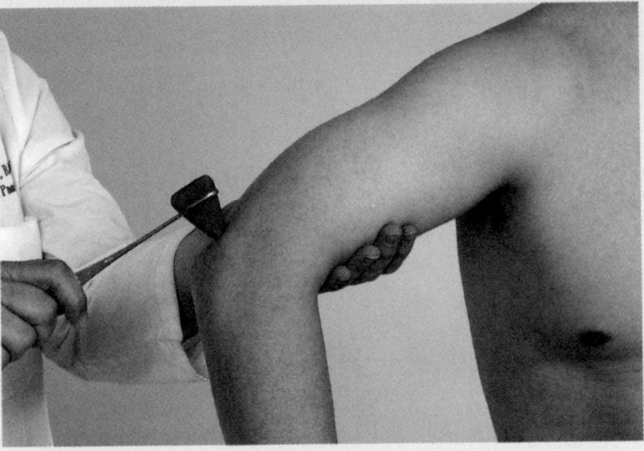

Figure 10. Assessing the triceps reflex. (Photo by B. Proud.)

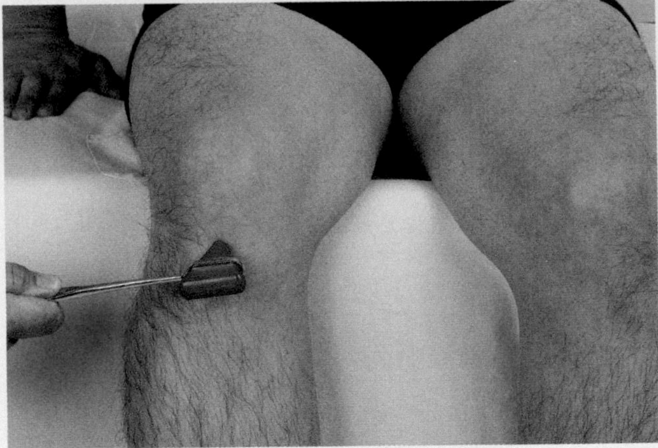

Figure 11. Assessing the patellar reflex. (Photo by B. Proud.)

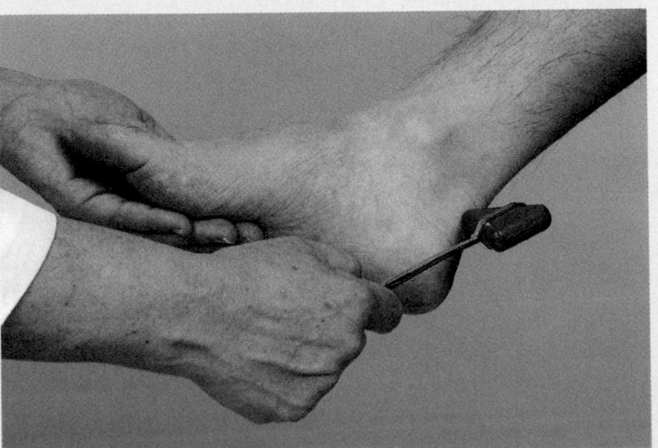

Figure 12. Assessing the Achilles' reflex. (Photo by B. Proud.)

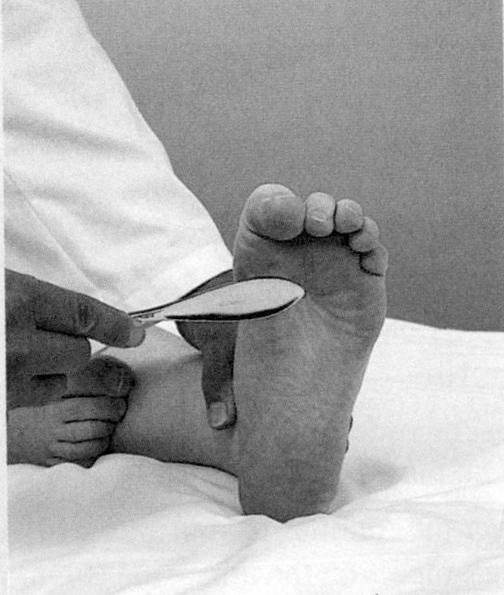

Figure 13. Eliciting plantar reflex.

26. Ask patient to dorsiflex and then plantarflex both feet against opposing resistance (Figure 14).

These measures test foot strength and range of motion.

SKILL 2-6

Assessing the Neurologic, Musculoskeletal, and Peripheral Vascular Systems *(continued)*

ACTION	RATIONALE

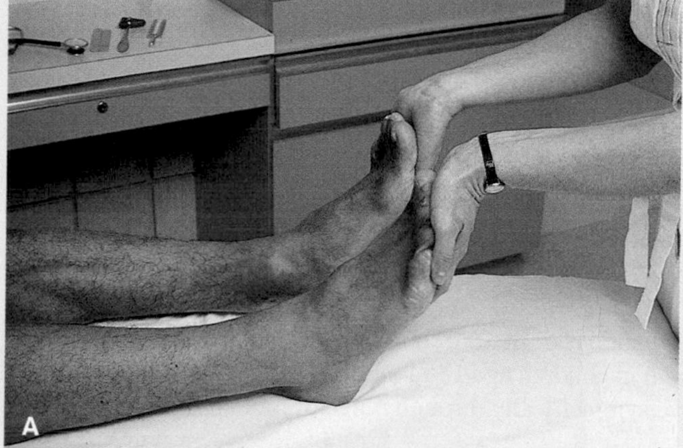

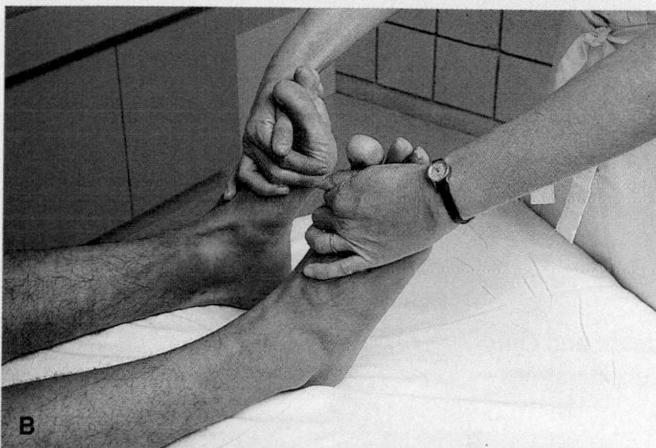

Figure 14. Testing ankle flexion and dorsiflexion. The patient first pushes the balls of the feet against resistance of the nurse's hands (**A**), the attempts to pull against nurse's resistance (**B**).

ACTION	RATIONALE
27. As needed, assist the patient to a standing position. Observe the patient as he or she walks with a regular gait, on the toes, on the heels, and then heel to toe.	This procedure evaluates cerebellar and motor function.
28. Perform the Romberg's test; ask the patient to stand straight with feet together, both eyes closed with arms at side. Wait 20 seconds and observe for patient swaying and ability to maintain balance. Nurse must be alert to prevent patient fall or injury related to losing balance during this assessment.	This test checks cerebellar functioning and evaluates balance, equilibrium, and coordination. Slight swaying is normal but patient should be able to maintain balance.
29. Assist the patient to a comfortable position.	This ensures the patient's comfort.
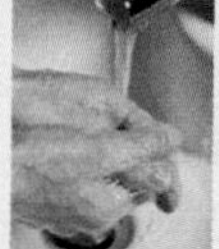 30. Perform hand hygiene.	This deters the spread of microorganisms.

EVALUATION

The expected outcome is met when the patient participated in the neurologic, musculoskeletal, and peripheral vascular assessment, displays decreased anxiety, and verbalizes understanding of the assessment techniques as appropriate.

DOCUMENTATION

Guidelines

When documenting neurologic, musculoskeletal, and peripheral vascular assessment, be sure to describe specific data. Include assessment techniques performed, along with specific findings. Note the cognitive responses of the patient, the tested cranial nerves, sensation and motor responses, and reflex testing data. Document any patient statements of pain, muscle weakness or joint abnormality. Record inspection findings, including color, turgor, temperature, pulses, capillary refill, hair distribution, and presence of lesions.

(continued)

SKILL 2-6 Assessing the Neurologic, Musculoskeletal, and Peripheral Vascular Systems *(continued)*

Sample Documentation

4/4/09 B.H. alert, oriented, cognitively appropriate. CNs intact. Sensation intact. DTR +2 throughout. Full ROM of all joints. Muscles soft, firm, nontender, no atrophy. B.H. states pain in Right calf. R calf skin paler tone, slightly cooler, pulses slightly weaker compared to L calf.—S. Moses, RN

Special Considerations

General Considerations

- Before asking questions related to the mini-mental examination, inform the patient that some of the questions may seem unusual, but the nurse is attempting to evaluate overall cognitive function.

Infant and Child Considerations

- In an infant, jerky and brief twitchings of the extremities may be noted.
- Expect to elicit Babinski's sign in children age 18 months and younger.
- The infant's extremities move symmetrically through range of motion but lack full extension.
- Use Barlow-Orolani's maneuver to assess hip abduction and adduction in an infant.
- Before age 5 years, sensory function is normally not tested.
- Coordination of movement varies according to developmental level of the young child.

Older Adult Considerations

- Short-term memory, such as recall of recent events, may diminish with age, as well as slowed reaction time.
- In the elderly patient, expect to find decreased musculoskeletal function such as loss of muscle strength.
- Keep in mind that older adults may take longer to perform certain actions such as completing activities for testing coordination.

The Taylor Suite offers these additional resources to enhance learning and facilitate understanding:

- thePoint online resource, http://thepoint.lww.com/Lynn2E
- Student CD-ROM included with the book
- Skills Checklist to Accompany Taylor's Clinical Nursing Skills

Developing Critical Thinking Skills

1. When obtaining the history from Mr. Lincoln, he reports having a stuffed-up nose, postnasal drip, and a cough that sometimes produces mucus. He has smoked about one and a half packs of cigarettes a day for the past 20 years. Which areas of his physical examination would be most important?
2. Bobby Williams is suspected of having appendicitis. Which aspects of the physical examination would the nurse use to help confirm this diagnosis?
3. Lois Felker, who has a history of type 1 diabetes mellitus, has arrived for her appointment with the physician. Due to this patient's diagnosis, what systems will be most important to include in the routine checkup?

Bibliography

Barkauskas, V., Baumann, L., & Darling-Fisher, C. (2002). *Health & physical assessment* (3rd ed.). Philadelphia: Mosby.

Best practices: A guide to excellence in nursing care. (2002). Philadelphia: Lippincott Williams & Wilkins.

Bickley, L. (2007). *Bates' guide to physical examination and history taking* (9th ed.). Philadelphia: Lippincott Williams & Wilkins.

Black, J. & Hawks, J. (2005). *Medical-surgical nursing* (7th ed.). St. Louis, MO: Elsevier Saunders.

Hockenberry, M. (2005). *Wong's essentials of pediatric nursing* (7th ed.). St. Louis, MO: Elsevier Mosby.

Ladewig, P., London, M., & Davidson, M. (2006). *Contemporary maternal-newborn nursing care.* (6th ed.). Upper Saddle River, NJ: Pearson Prentice Hall.

Lyneham, J. (2001). Physical examination (abdomen, thorax and lungs): A review. *Australian Journal of Advanced Nursing, 18*(3), 31.

Manning, J. (2004). The assessment of dark skin and dermatological disorders. *Nursing Times, 100*(22), 48–51.
Nursing procedures (4th ed.). (2004). Philadelphia: Lippincott Williams & Wilkins.
Purnell, L. & Paulanka, B. (2005). *Guide to culturally competent health care.* Philadelphia: F. A. Davis.
Stanley, M., Blair, K., & Beare, P. (2005). *Gerontological nursing: Promoting successful aging with older adults* (3rd ed.). Philadelphia: F. A. Davis.
Taylor, C., Lillis, C., LeMone, P., & Lynn, P. (2008). *Fundamentals of nursing: The art and science of nursing care* (6th ed.). Philadelphia: Lippincott Williams & Wilkins.
Watson, R. (2001). Assessing the musculoskeletal system in older people. *Nursing Older People, 13*(5), 29–30.
Weber, K. & Kelley, J. (2007). *Health assessment in nursing* (3rd ed.). Philadelphia: Lippincott Williams & Wilkins.
Wilson, S. & Giddens, J. (2005). *Health assessment for nursing practice* (3rd ed.). St. Louis, MO: Elsevier Mosby.

CHAPTER 3

Safety

Focusing on Patient Care

This chapter will help you develop some of the skills related to safety issues for monitoring and interventions that may be necessary to care for the following patients:

Megan Lewis, an 18-month-old who has an IV access in her left forearm.

Kevin Mallory, a 35-year-old professional body builder admitted with a severe closed head injury. He is intubated and is constantly reaching for his endotracheal tube.

John Frawley, a 72-year-old diagnosed with Alzheimer's disease who continues to try to get out of bed after falling and breaking a hip.

Learning Objectives

After studying this chapter, you will be able to:

1. Identify nursing interventions related to fall prevention.
2. Identify nursing interventions to be used as alternatives to restraints.
3. Identify guidelines for the use of physical restraints.
4. Apply an extremity restraint correctly and safely.
5. Apply a jacket or vest restraint correctly and safely.
6. Apply an elbow restraint correctly and safely.
7. Apply a mummy restraint correctly and safely.
8. Use leather restraints correctly and safely.

Key Terms

event report: documentation that describes any injury or potential for injury sustained by a patient in a healthcare agency

restraint: any method, physical or mechanical, of restricting a person's freedom of movement, physical activity, or normal access to his or her body (JCAHO, 2001)

Safety and security are basic human needs. Safety is a paramount concern that underlies all nursing care, and patient safety is a responsibility of all healthcare providers. It is a focus in all healthcare facilities as well as the home, workplace, and community. Nursing strategies that identify potential hazards and promote wellness evolve from an awareness of factors that affect safety in the environment.

This chapter will cover the skills to assist the nurse in monitoring and intervening for patients with issues involving safety. The first skill discusses fall prevention. Subsequent skills discuss safe and correct use of several types of physical restraints. Physical restraints are any physical method of restricting a person's freedom of movement, physical activity or normal access to his or her body (JCAHO, 2001). An item used to restrict movement is considered a restraint; however, that same item is not considered a restraint if/when it enables a person in some way (McBeth, 2004). For example, bed rails are considered a restraint if used to keep a patient from getting out of bed. If used to assist mobility in and out of bed, bed rails are not considered a restraint.

Physical restraints should be considered as a last resort after other care alternatives have been unsuccessful. Fundamentals Review 3-1 outlines possible alternatives to restraints. Alternatives must be tried, and their use documented.

When it is necessary to apply a restraint, the least restrictive method should be used and it should be removed at the earliest possible time (Letizia, Babler & Cockrell, 2004). Consider the laws regulating the use of restraints and facility regulations and policies. Ensure compliance with ordering, assessment, and maintenance procedures. Fundamentals Review 3-2 provides general guidelines for restraint use and Fundamentals Review 3-3 defines the R-E-S-T-R-A-I-N-T acronym aimed at promoting effective use. Always treat patients with respect and protect their dignity. Several skills in this chapter review the appropriate techniques for applying different types of physical restraints. Many skills require quick-release knots for securing restraints to bed frame or chair; Figure 3-1 shows appropriate knots.

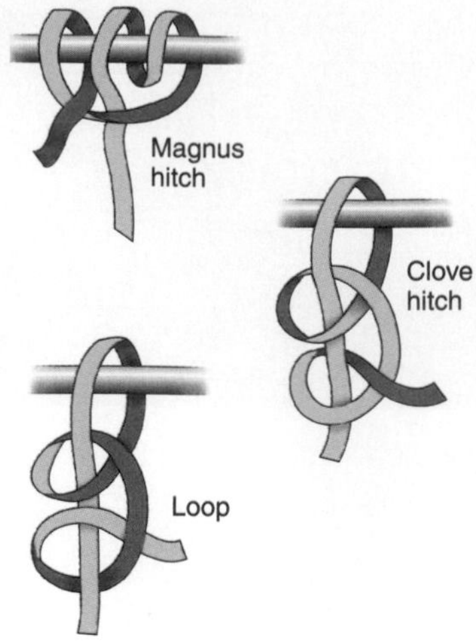

Figure 3-1. Appropriate quick-release knots for securing restraint to bed frame.

Choosing Alternatives to Restraints

- Determine whether behavior pattern exists.
- Assess for pain and treat appropriately.
- Rule out physical causes for agitation. Assess respiratory status, vital signs, blood glucose level, fluid and electrolyte issues, and medications.
- Involve the family/significant others in the plan of care.
- Ask family members or significant other to stay with the patient.
- Reduce stimulation, noise, and light.
- Distract and redirect, using a calming voice.
- Use simple, clear explanations and directions.
- Check environment for hazards.
  - Provide for basic needs relative to nutrition, fluids, and toileting.
  - Institute bowel and bladder programs.
  - Provide frequent orientation and explanations of care.
- Use night light.
- Use an alarm system (eg, bed or position-sensitive alarms) to warn of unassisted activity.
- Allow restless patient to walk after ensuring that environment is safe.
- Use a large plant or piece of furniture as a barrier to limit wandering from designated area.
- Use low-height beds.
- Place floor mats on each side of the bed.
- Ensure the use of glasses and hearing aids, if necessary.
- Use full-length body pillows.
- Arrange for a bedside commode.
- Make the environment as homelike as possible; provide familiar objects.
- Provide a warm beverage.
- Provide comfortable rocking chairs.
- Use therapeutic touch.
- Play music or video selections of the patient's choice.

Fundamentals Review 3-1

Choosing Alternatives to Restraints *(continued)*

- Offer diversional activities, such as games, television, and books.
- Encourage daily exercise/provide exercise and activities or relaxation techniques.
- Consider relocation of the patient room closer to the nursing station.
- Conceal tubes and tubing necessary for care. Anchor tubing securely. Conceal tubing with gauze wrap; unwrap regularly to assess site for complications.
- Investigate possibility of discontinuing bothersome treatment devices (eg, IV line, catheter, feeding tube).

(Adapted from Letizia, M., Babler, C. & Cockrell, A. [2004]. Repeating the call for restraint reduction. MEDSURG Nursing, *13(1), 9–12, and Napierkowski, D. [2002]. Using restraints with restraint.* Nursing, *32[11], 58–62.)*

Fundamentals Review 3-2

General Guidelines for Restraint Use

- The patient has the right to be free from restraints that aren't medically necessary. Restraints are not used for the convenience of staff or to punish a patient.
- The patient's family must be involved in the plan of care. They must be consulted when the decision is made to use restraints. The family must be instructed regarding the facility's restraint policy and alternatives to restraints that are available.
- Alternatives to restraints and less restrictive interventions must have been implemented and failed. All alternatives used must be documented.
- The benefit gained from using a restraint must outweigh the known risks for that patient.
- The restraints must be ordered by a physician or other licensed independent practitioner. The order can never be for use on an 'as needed' basis.
- Once in place, the patient must be monitored and reassessed. Adult patients must be reassessed within 4 hours; children (9–17 years) within 2 hours; and children younger than 9 within 1 hour.
- A physician or licensed independent practitioner must reevaluate and assess the patient every 24 hours (in the medical–surgical setting).
- Assess the patient's vital signs and visually observe the patient every 2 hours for medical patients.
- Personal needs must be met. Provide fluids, nutrition, and toileting assistance every 2 hours.
- Assess skin integrity every 2 hours and provide range-of-motion exercises.
- Documentation regarding why, how, where, and for how long the restraints were placed, and patient monitoring are vital.

(Modified from Kleen, K. [2004]. Restraint regulation: The tie that binds. Nursing Management, *35(11), 36–38; and Napierkowski, D. [2002]. Using restraints with restraint.* Nursing, *32[11], 58–62.)*

Fundamentals Review 3-3

R-E-S-T-R-A-I-N-T Acronym

The following R-E-S-T-R-A-I-N-T acronym prompts effective use of restraints (DiBartolo, 1998).

- **R**espond to the present, not the past. The patient's current condition, not his or her past history, must determine the need for restraints. This includes assessment of physical condition and mental and behavior status.
- **E**valuate the potential for injury. Determine whether the patient is at increased risk for harming self or others.
- **S**peak with family members or caregivers. Ask them for insights into the patient's behavior, and enlist their help in making a decision.
- **T**ry alternative measures first. Also, investigate the patient's medication regimen and attempt to discuss options with the patient.
- **R**eassess the patient to determine whether alternatives are successful. Agency policy dictates the frequency of assessments and documentation.
- **A**lert the physician and the patient's family if restraints are indicated. Agency policy, JCAHO, and state and federal guidelines require an order from a physician or other healthcare professional licensed to prescribe in the state. The order should include the type of restraint, justification, criteria for removal, and intended duration of use.
- **I**ndividualize restraint use. Choose the least restrictive device.
- **N**ote important information on the chart. Document the date and time the restraint is applied, the type of restraint, alternatives that were attempted and their results, and notification of the patient's family and physician. Include frequency of assessment, your findings, regular intervals when the restraint is removed, and nursing interventions.
- **T**ime-limit the use of restraints. Release the patient from the restraint as soon as he or she is no longer a risk to self or others. Restraints should be used no longer than 24 hours on nonpsychiatric patients. After 24 hours, a new order is required.

(Modified from DiBartolo, V. [1998]. 9 steps to effective restraint use. RN, 61*[12], 23–24.)*

SKILL 3-1 Fall Prevention

Falls are associated with physical and psychological trauma, especially in older people. Fall-related injuries are often serious and can be fatal. Falls are caused by and associated with multiple factors. Box 3-1 outlines the primary causes of falls. Many of these causes are within the realm of nursing responsibility. Identifying at-risk patients is crucial to planning appropriate interventions to prevent a fall. The combination of an assessment tool with a care plan sets the stage for best practice (Kelly & Dowling, 2004). Accurate assessment and use of appropriate fall interventions leads to maximum prevention. Refer to Table 3-1 for examples of fall-prevention strategies based on fall risk assessment. Providing patient education and a safer patient environment can reduce the incidence and severity of falls. The ultimate goal is to reduce the physical and psychological trauma experienced by patients and their significant others.

BOX 3-1 Primary Causes of Falls

- Change in balance or gait disturbance
- Muscle weakness
- Dizziness, syncope, and vertigo
- Cardiovascular changes such as postural hypotension
- Change in vision or vision impairment
- Physical environment/Environmental hazards
- Acute illness
- Neurologic disease, such as dementia or depression
- Language disorders that impair communication
- Polypharmacy

(Adapted from Rao, S. [2005]. Prevention of falls in older patients. *American Family Physician, 72*[1], 81–88 and from Kelly, A. & Dowling, M. [2004]. Reducing the likelihood of falls in older people. *Nursing Standard, 18*[49], 33–40.)

Equipment

- Fall-risk assessment tool, if available

ASSESSMENT

Assess the patient and the medical record for factors that increase the patient's risk for falling. The use of an objective, systematic fall assessment is made easier by the use of a fall assessment tool (Kelly & Dowling, 2004). Figure 3-1 provides an example of a fall assessment tool. Assess for a history of falls. If the patient has experienced a previous fall, assess the circumstances surrounding the fall and any associated symptoms. Review the patient's medication history and medication record for medications that may increase the risk for falls. Assess for the following additional risk factors for falls (Kelly & Dowling, 2004; Rao, 2005):

- Lower extremity muscle weakness
- Gait or balance deficits
- Use of an assistive device
- Visual deficit
- Arthritis
- Presence of intravenous therapy
- History of cerebrovascular accident
- Impaired activities of daily living
- Depression
- Cognitive impairment
- Age older than 80 years
- Secondary diagnosis/chronic disease
- Use of four or more medications
- Urinary alterations

(continued)

SKILL 3-1 Fall Prevention *(continued)*

TABLE 3-1 Recommended Fall-Prevention Strategies by Fall Risk Level

LOW FALL RISK	MODERATE FALL RISK	HIGH FALL RISK
Fall Risk Score: 0–5 Points	Fall Risk Score: 6–10 Points Color Code: Yellow	Fall Risk Score: >10 Points Color Code: Red
Maintain safe unit environment including: • Remove excess equipment/supplies/furniture from rooms and hallways. • Coil and secure excess electrical and telephone wires. • Clean all spills in patient room or in hallway immediately. Place signage to indicate wet floor danger. • Restrict window openings. The following are examples of basic safety interventions: • Orient patient to surroundings, including bathroom location, use of bed, and location of call light. • Keep bed in lowest position during use unless impractical (as in ICU nursing or specialty beds). • Keep top 2 side rails up (excludes box beds). In ICUs, keep all side rails up. • Secure locks on beds, stretchers, and wheelchairs. • Keep floors clutter/obstacle free (with attention to path between bed and bathroom/commode). • Place call light and frequently needed objects within patient reach. Answer call light promptly. • Encourage patients/families to call for assistance when needed. • Display special instructions for vision and hearing. • Assure adequate lighting, especially at night. • Use properly fitting nonskid footwear. • Encourage patients/families to call for assistance when needed.	• Institute flagging system yellow card outside room and yellow sticker on medical record. Hill ROM flag (if available), assignment board/electronic board. In addition to measures listed under low fall risk: • Monitor and assist patient in following daily schedules. • Supervise and/or assist bedside sitting, personal hygiene, and toileting as appropriate. • Reorient confused patients as necessary. • Establish elimination schedule, including use of bedside commode, if appropriate. • PT consult if patient has a history of fall and/or mobility impairment Evaluate need for: • OT consult • Slip-resistant chair mat (do *not* use in shower chair) • Use of seat belt, when in wheelchair	• Institute flagging system: red card outside room and red sticker on medical record, assignment board/electronic board: nurse call system flag if available. In addition to measures listed under moderate and low fall risk: • Remain with patient while toileting. • Observe q 60 min unless patient is on activated bed/chair alarm. • If patient requires an air overlay, remove mattress (unless contraindicated by overlay type) or use side rail protectors. • When necessary, transport throughout hospital with assistance of staff or trained caregivers. Consider alternatives, for example, bedside procedure. Notify receiving area of high fall risk. Evaluate need for the following, starting with less restrictive to more restrictive measures in the listed order: • Moving patient to room with best visual access to nursing station • Bed/chair alarm • Specialty fall-prevention bed • 24-h supervision/sitter • Physical restraint/enclosed bed (only if less restrictive alternatives have been considered and found to be ineffective)

(Recommended fall-prevention strategies by fall risk level. Reprinted with permission. Copyright 2003, The Johns Hopkins Hospital.)

SKILL 3-1 Fall Prevention *(continued)*

Fall risk factor category * (NA If comatose, complete paralysis, or completely immobilized)	Points
Age • 70–79 y (2 points) • ≥80 y (3 points)	
Fall history • Fall within 3 months before admission (5 points) • Fall during this hospitalization (11 points)	
Mobility • Ambulates or transfers with unsteady gait and **NO** assistance or assistive devices (2 points) • Ambulates or transfers with assistance or assistive device (2 points) • Visual or auditory impairment affecting mobility (4 points)	
Elimination • Urgency/nocturia (2 points) • Incontinence (5 points)	
Mental status changes • Affecting awareness of environment (2 points) • Affecting awareness of one's physical limitations (4 points)	
Medications: One present (3 points); 2 or more present; or sedated procedure within the past 24 h (5 points) Psychotropics (antidepressants, hypnotics, antipsychotics, sedatives, benzodiazepines, some antiemetics) Anticonvulsants Diuretics/cathartics PCS/narcotics/opiates Antihypertensives	
Patient care equipment: One present (1 point); ≥ 2 present (2 points) (IV, chest tube, indwelling catheter, SCDs, etc)	
Total points	

***Moderate risk = 6–10 Total points, High risk > 10 Total points**

Figure 1. The Johns Hopkins Fall Risk Assessment Tool. Reprinted with permission. *©2003, The Johns Hopkins Hospital.*

NURSING DIAGNOSIS

Determine the related factors for nursing diagnoses based on the patient's current status. Appropriate nursing diagnoses may include:

- Risk for Falls
- Risk for Injury
- Activity Intolerance
- Impaired Home Maintenance
- Impaired Urinary Elimination
- Deficient Knowledge Related to Safety Precautions
- Impaired Physical Mobility

(continued)

SKILL 3-1 Fall Prevention *(continued)*

OUTCOME IDENTIFICATION AND PLANNING

The expected outcome to achieve is that the patient does not experience a fall and remains free of injury. Other outcomes that may be appropriate include the following: the patient's environment is free from hazards; the patient and/or caregiver demonstrates an understanding of appropriate interventions to prevent falls; the patient uses assistive devices correctly; the patient uses safe transfer procedures; and appropriate precautions are implemented related to the use of medications that increase the risk for falls.

IMPLEMENTATION

ACTION	RATIONALE
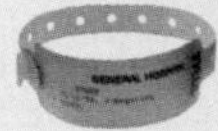 1. Identify the patient. Explain the rationale for fall prevention interventions to the patient and family/significant others.	Identifying the patient ensures the right patient receives the intervention and helps prevent errors. Explanation helps reduce anxiety and promotes compliance and understanding.
2. Provide adequate lighting.	Good lighting reduces accidental tripping over and bumping into objects that may not be seen. Reduces falling over objects that may not be seen.
3. Remove excess equipment, supplies, furniture, and other objects from rooms and walkways. Pay particular attention to high traffic areas and the route to the bathroom.	All are possible hazards.
4. Orient patient and significant others to new surroundings, including use of the telephone, call signal, patient bed, and room illumination. Indicate the location of the patient bathroom.	Knowledge of proper use of equipment relieves anxiety and promotes compliance.
5. Provide nonskid footwear (Figure 2).	Prevents slipping when ambulating or transferring

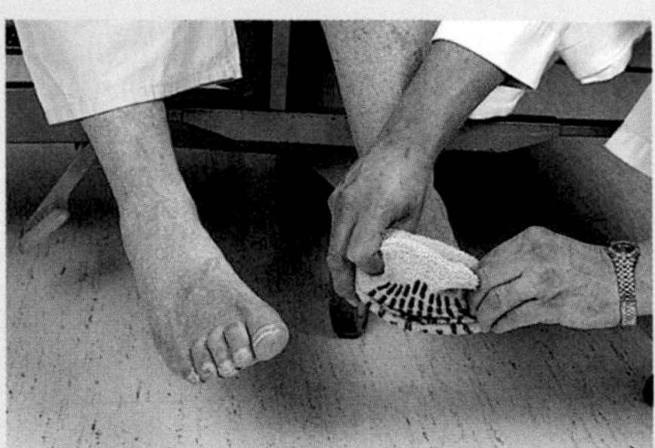

Figure 2. Providing nonskid footwear.

ACTION	RATIONALE
6. Provide a bedside commode, if appropriate. Ensure that it is near the bed at all times.	This prevents falls related to incontinence.
7. Ensure that the call signal, bedside table, telephone, and other personal items are within the patient's reach at all times.	This prevents the patient from having to overreach for device or items, and/or possibly attempt ambulation or transfer unassisted.
8. Confer with physician or primary care provider regarding appropriate exercise and physical therapy.	Exercise programs such as muscle strengthening, balance training, and walking plans decrease falls and fall-related injuries.

SKILL 3-1 Fall Prevention *(continued)*

ACTION	RATIONALE
9. Encourage the patient to rise or change position slowly and sit for several minutes before standing.	Reduces risk of falls related to orthostatic hypotension
10. Evaluate the appropriateness of elastic stockings for lower extremities.	Minimizes venous pooling
11. Review medications for potential hazards.	Certain medications and combinations of medications have been associated with increased risk for falls.
12. Keep the bed in the lowest position during use. If elevated to provide care (to reduce caregiver strain), ensure that it is lowered when care is completed.	Keeping bed in lowest position reduces risk of fall-related injury.
13. Make sure locks on the bed or wheelchair are secured at all times (Figure 3).	Prevents the bed from moving out from under the patient

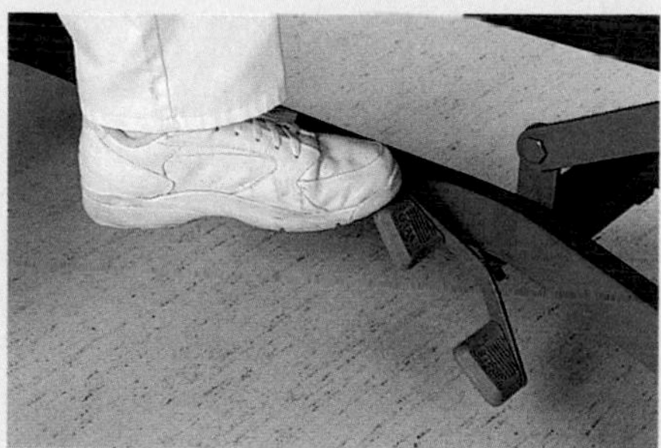

Figure 3. Engaging bed locks.

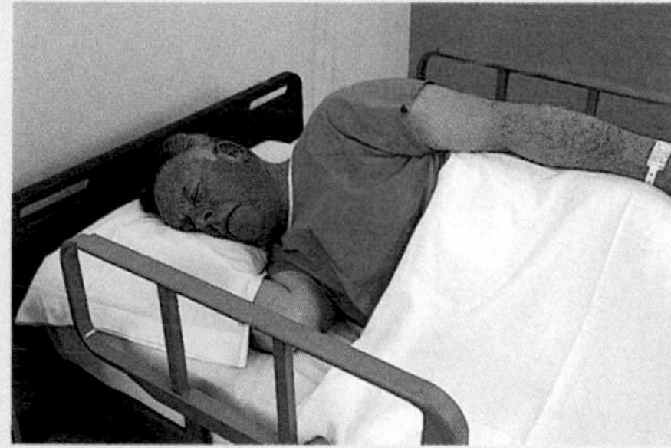

Figure 4. Raising side rails on bed at the patient's request; patient must be able to raise and lower rails himself.

ACTION	RATIONALE
14. Use bed rails according to facility policy, when appropriate (Figure 4).	Inappropriate bed-rail use has been associated with patient injury and increased fall risk. Side rails may be considered a restraint when used to prevent an ambulatory patient from getting out of bed.
15. Anticipate patient needs and provide assistance with activities instead of waiting for the patient to ask.	Patients whose needs are met sustain fewer falls.
16. Consider the use of an electronic bed or chair alarm (Figure 5).	Alert staff to unassisted changes in position by the patient.

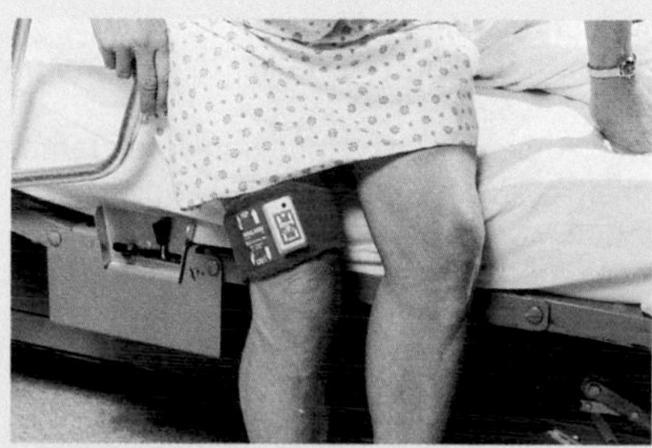

Figure 5. Wearing an Ambularm device.

ACTION	RATIONALE
17. Include the patient's family and/or significant others in the plan of care.	This promotes continuity of care and cooperation.

(continued)

SKILL 3-1 Fall Prevention *(continued)*

EVALUATION

The expected outcomes are met when the patient remains free of falls, and injury interventions to minimize risk factors that might precipitate a fall are implemented; patient's environment is free from hazards; patient and/or caregiver demonstrates an understanding of appropriate interventions to prevent falls; the patient uses assistive devices correctly; the patient uses safe transfer procedures; and appropriate precautions are implemented related to use of medications that increase the risk for falls.

DOCUMENTATION

Guidelines

Document patient fall-risk assessment. Include appropriate interventions to reduce fall risk in nursing care plan. Document patient and family teaching relative to fall-risk reduction. Document interventions included in care.

Sample Documentation

11/1/08 1730 Patient admitted to room 650W. Fall assessment low risk (5 pts). Basic safety interventions in place per facility Fall Prevention Guidelines. Will continue to monitor and reevaluate.—B. Clapp, RN

Unexpected Situations and Associated Interventions

- *Patient experiences a fall:* Immediately assess the patient's condition. Provide care and interventions appropriate for status/injuries. Notify the patient's physician or primary caregiver of incident and your assessment of the patient. Ensure prompt follow-through for any orders for diagnostic tests, such as x-rays or CT scans, as ordered. Evaluate circumstances of the fall and the patient's environment and institute appropriate measures to prevent further incidents. Document incident, assessments, and interventions in the patient's medical record. Complete an event report per facility policy.

Special Considerations

Home Care Considerations

Patients are at risk for falls in their home settings. Assess for risk factors and home environment. See Box 3-2 for possible interventions for the home setting.

BOX 3-2 Patient Education for Preventing Falls in the Home

- Talk with your doctor about a plan for an exercise program. Regular exercise helps maintain strength and flexibility, and can help slow bone loss.
- Have regular hearing and vision testing. Always wear glasses and hearing aids, if prescribed. Even small changes in sight and hearing can affect stability.
- Wear low-heeled rubber-soled shoes. Avoid wearing only socks or shoes with smooth soles.
- Have hand rails on both sides of stairs and make use of them when using the stairs. Try not to carry things when using the steps. When necessary, hold item in one hand and use the hand rail with the other hand.
- Avoid using chairs and tables as ladders to reach items that are too high to reach.
- Keep electrical and telephone cords against the wall and out of walkways.
- Rails next to the toilet and in the shower or tub and raised toilet seats should be considered.
- Know the possible side effects of medications used. Some can affect coordination and balance.
- Use a cane, walking stick, or walker to help improve stability
- Keep home temperature at a moderate level. Temperatures too hot or too cold can contribute to dizziness.
- Stand up slowly after eating, lying down, or resting. Standing too quickly can cause fainting or dizziness.
- Make sure there is good lighting, particularly at the stairs.
- Remove clutter from walkways inside and outside the house.
- Carpets should be fixed firmly to the floor to prevent slipping. Use no-slip strips on uncarpeted surfaces.
- Use nonskid mats, strips, or carpet on surfaces that get wet.

(Adapted from National Institute on Aging. [2004]. Age Page: Preventing Falls and Fractures. Available at http://www.niapublications.org/engagepages/falls.asp.)

SKILL 3-2

Applying an Extremity Restraint

Cloth extremity restraints immobilize one or more extremity. They may be indicated after other measures have failed to prevent a patient from removing therapeutic devices such as intravenous access devices, endotracheal tubes, oxygen, or other treatment interventions. Restraints can be applied to the hands, wrists, or ankles. Restraints should be used only after less restrictive methods have failed. Ensure compliance with ordering, assessment, and maintenance procedures. **Look over general guidelines for using restraints in the chapter introduction and Fundamentals Review 3-1 and 3-2.**

Equipment

- Appropriate cloth restraint for the extremity that is to be immobilized
- Padding, if necessary, for bony prominences

ASSESSMENT

Assess the patient's physical condition and assess for the potential for injury to self or others. A confused patient who might remove devices needed to sustain life is considered at risk for injury to self and may require the use of restraints. Assess the patient's behavior, including the presence of confusion, agitation, combativeness, and ability to understand and follow directions. Evaluate the appropriateness of the least restrictive restraint device. For example, if the patient has had a stroke and cannot move the left arm, a restraint may be needed only on the right arm. Inspect the extremity where the restraint will be applied. Baseline skin condition should be established for comparison at future assessments while the restraint is in place. Consider using another form of restraint if the restraint may cause further injury at the site. Before application, assess for adequate circulation in the extremity to which the restraint is to be applied, including capillary refill and proximal pulses.

NURSING DIAGNOSIS

Determine the related factors for nursing diagnoses based on the patient's current status. Appropriate nursing diagnoses may include:

- Risk for Injury
- Risk for Impaired Skin Integrity
- Anxiety
- Impaired Physical Mobility
- Acute Confusion
- Bathing/Hygiene Self-Care Deficit
- Feeding Self-Care Deficit
- Toileting Self-Care Deficit

OUTCOME IDENTIFICATION AND PLANNING

The expected outcome to achieve is that the patient is constrained by the restraint, remains free from injury, and the restraint does not interfere with therapeutic devices. Other outcomes that may be appropriate include the following: the patient does not experience impaired skin integrity; the patient does not injure himself or herself due to the restraints; and the patient's family will demonstrate an understanding about the use of the restraint and their role in the patient's care.

IMPLEMENTATION

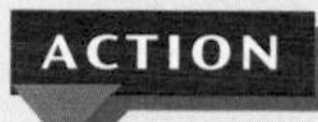

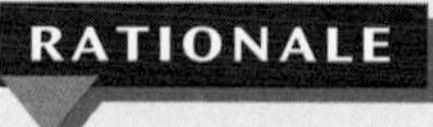

ACTION	RATIONALE
1. Determine need for restraints. Assess patient's physical condition, behavior, and mental status. Refer to the review boxes at the beginning of the chapter.	Restraints should be used only as a last resort when alternative measures have failed and the patient is at increased risk for harming himself or others.

(continued)

SKILL 3-2 Applying an Extremity Restraint *(continued)*

ACTION	RATIONALE
2. Confirm agency policy for application of restraints. **Secure a physician's order, or validate that the order has been obtained within the past 24 hours.**	Policy protects the patient and the nurse and specifies guidelines for application as well as type of restraint and duration. **Joint Commission on Accreditation of Healthcare Organizations (JCAHO) standards require that a new order for restraints must be written every 24 hours.**
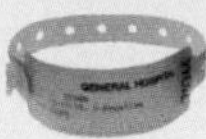 3. Identify the patient.	Identifying the patient ensures the right patient receives the intervention and helps prevent errors.
4. Explain reason for use to patient and family. Clarify how care will be given and how needs will be met. Explain that restraint is a temporary measure.	Explanation to patient and family may lessen confusion and anger and provide reassurance. A clearly stated agency policy on application of restraints should be available for patient and family to read. In a long-term care facility, the family must give consent before a restraint is applied.
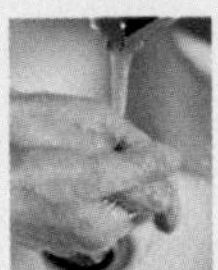 5. Perform hand hygiene.	Hand hygiene deters the spread of microorganisms.
6. Apply restraint according to manufacturer's directions:	Proper application prevents injury.
a. Choose the least restrictive type of device that allows the greatest possible degree of mobility.	This provides minimal restriction.
b. Pad bony prominences.	Padding helps prevent skin injury.
c. Wrap the restraint around the extremity with the soft part in contact with the skin. If hand mitt is being used, pull over hand with cushion to the palmar aspect of hand (Figure 1). Secure in place with the Velcro® straps or reverse clove hitch (Figure 2).	This prevents excess pressure on extremity. A quick-release knot ensures that restraint will not tighten when pulled and can be removed quickly in an emergency.

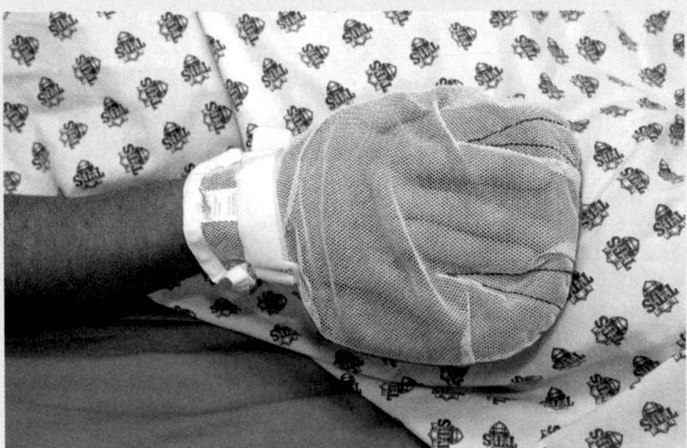

Figure 1. Using a hand mitt.

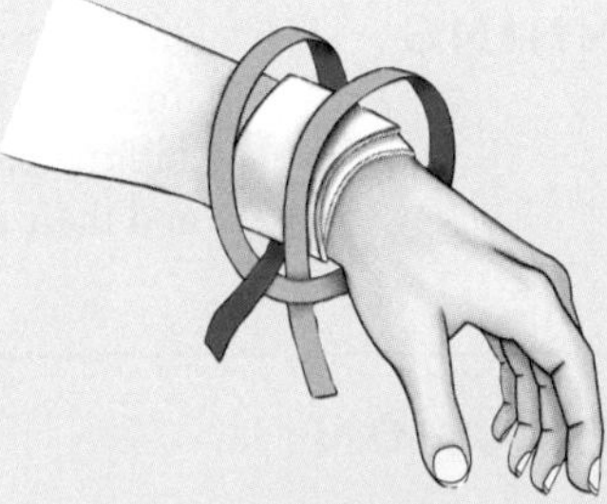

Figure 2. Securing a cloth wrist restraint using a quick-release reverse clove hitch.

SKILL 3-2

Applying an Extremity Restraint *(continued)*

ACTION	RATIONALE
7. **Ensure that two fingers can be inserted between the restraint and patient's wrist or ankle (Figure 3).**	Proper application ensures that there is no interference with patient's circulation.

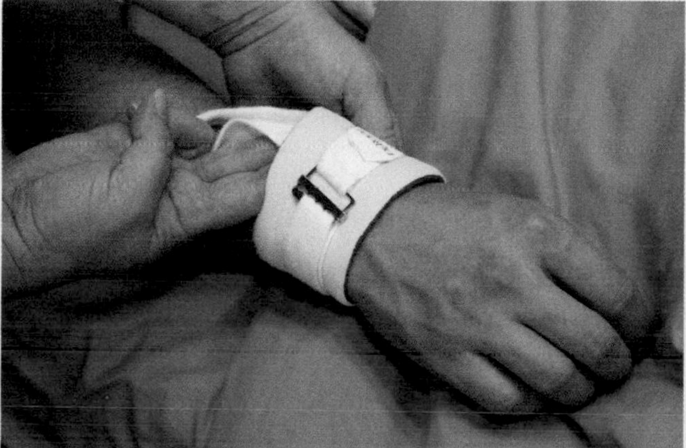

Figure 3. Ensuring that two fingers can be inserted between the restraint and the patient's wrist.

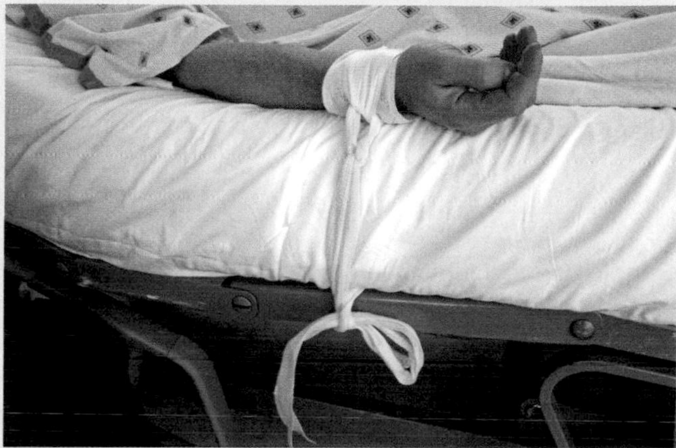

Figure 4. Securing restraint to bed frame.

ACTION	RATIONALE
8. Maintain restrained extremity in normal anatomic position. **Use a quick-release knot to tie the restraint to the bed frame, not side rail (Figure 4). Refer to chapter introduction for examples of knots. The restraint may also be attached to chair frame. The site should not be readily accessible to patient.**	Maintaining a normal position lessens possibility of injury. A quick-release knot ensures that restraint will not tighten when pulled and can be removed quickly in an emergency. Securing the restraint to a side rail may injure the patient when the side rail is lowered. Tying restraint out of patient's reach promotes security.
9. Assess the patient at least every hour or according to facility policy. Assessment should include: the placement of the restraint, neurovascular assessment of the affected extremity, and skin integrity. In addition, assess for signs of sensory deprivation, such as increased sleeping, daydreaming, anxiety, panic, and hallucinations.	Improperly applied restraints may cause skin tears, abrasions, or bruises. Decreased circulation may result in paleness, coolness, decreased sensation, tingling, numbness, or pain in extremity. Use of restraints may decrease environmental stimulation and result in sensory deprivation.
10. **Remove restraint at least every 2 hours, or according to agency policy and patient need.** Perform range-of-motion exercises.	Removal allows nurse to assess patient and reevaluate need for restraint. It also allows interventions for toileting, provision of nutrition and liquids, exercise, and change of position. Exercise increases circulation in restrained extremity.
11. Evaluate patient for continued need of restraint. Reapply restraint only if continued need is evident and order is still valid.	Continued need must be documented for reapplication.
12. Reassure patient at regular intervals. Provide continued explanation of rationale for interventions, reorientation if necessary, and plan of care. **Keep call bell within easy reach.**	Reassurance demonstrates caring and provides opportunity for sensory situation as well as ongoing assessment and evaluation. Patient can use call bell to summon assistance quickly.
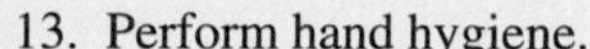 13. Perform hand hygiene.	Hand hygiene deters the spread of microorganisms.

(continued)

SKILL 3-2 Applying an Extremity Restraint *(continued)*

EVALUATION

The expected outcomes are met when the patient remains free of injury to self or others, circulation to extremity remains adequate, skin integrity is not impaired under the restraint, and family is aware of rationale for restraints.

DOCUMENTATION

Guidelines

Document alternative measures attempted before applying restraint. Document patient assessment before application. Record patient and family education and understanding regarding restraint use. Document family consent if necessary, according to facility policy. Document reason for restraining patient, date and time of application, type of restraint, times when removed, and result and frequency of nursing assessment. Obtain a new order after 24 hours if restraints are still necessary.

Sample Documentation

7/10/07 0830 Patient disoriented and combative. Attempting to remove tracheostomy and indwelling urinary catheter. Sitting at bedside, patient continued to tug at catheter and pull on tracheostomy. Family unwilling to sit with patient. Wrist restraints applied bilaterally as ordered.—K. Urhahn, RN

7/10/07 1030 Patient continues to be disoriented and combative. Wrist restraints removed for 30 minutes during patient's bath; skin intact, passive and active range of motion completed. Wrist restraints reapplied.—K. Urhahn, RN

Unexpected Situations and Associated Interventions

- *Patient has an IV catheter in the right wrist and is trying to remove drain from wound:* The left wrist may have a cloth restraint applied. Due to the IV in the right wrist, alternative forms of restraints should be tried, such as a cloth mitt or an elbow restraint.
- *Patient cannot move left arm:* Do not apply restraint to an extremity that is immobile. If patient cannot move the extremity, there is no need to apply a restraint. Restraint may be applied to right arm after obtaining a physician's order.

Special Considerations

General Considerations

- Do not position patient flat in a supine position with wrist restraints. If patient vomits, aspiration may occur.
- Extremity restraints are available in different sizes. Check restraint for correct size before applying. If restraint is too large, patient may free the extremity. If restraint is too small, circulation may be affected.
- Consider keeping a pair of scissors with emergency supplies in case the restraints cannot be untied quickly.

SKILL 3-3

Applying a Jacket or Vest Restraint

Jacket and vest restraints are a form of restraint that is applied to the patient's torso. They are applied over the patient's clothes, gown, or pajamas. When using a jacket or vest restraint, patients can move their extremities but cannot get out of the chair or bed. Ensure compliance with ordering, assessment, and maintenance procedures. Review general guidelines for using restraints in the chapter introduction and Fundamentals Review 3-1 and 3-2.

Equipment

- Vest restraint
- Additional padding as needed

ASSESSMENT

Assess the patient's physical condition and for the potential for injury to self or others. A confused patient who might remove devices needed to sustain life is considered at risk for injury to self and may require the use of restraints. Assess the patient's behavior, including the presence of confusion, agitation, combativeness and ability to understand and follow directions. Evaluate the appropriateness of the least restrictive restraint device. For example, if the patient has had a stroke and cannot move the left arm, a restraint may be needed only on the right arm. Inspect patient's torso for any wounds or therapeutic devices that may be affected by the vest. Consider using another form of restraint if the restraint may cause further injury at the site. Assess the patient's respiratory effort. If applied incorrectly, the vest can restrict the patient's ability to breathe.

NURSING DIAGNOSIS

Determine the related factors for nursing diagnoses based on the patient's current status. Appropriate nursing diagnoses may include:

- Risk for Injury
- Risk for Impaired Skin Integrity
- Anxiety
- Impaired Physical Mobility
- Acute Confusion
- Bathing/Hygiene Self-Care Deficit
- Feeding Self-Care Deficit
- Toileting Self-Care Deficit
- Wandering

OUTCOME IDENTIFICATION AND PLANNING

The expected outcome to achieve is that the patient is constrained by the restraint, remains free from injury, and the restraint does not interfere with therapeutic devices. Other outcomes that may be appropriate include the following: the patient does not experience impaired skin integrity; the patient does not injure himself or herself due to the restraints; and the patient's family will demonstrate an understanding about the use of the restraint and their role in the patient's care.

IMPLEMENTATION

ACTION	RATIONALE
1. Determine need for restraints. Assess patient's physical condition, behavior, and mental status. Refer to Fundamentals Review material in the beginning of the chapter.	Restraints should be used only as a last resort when alternative measures have failed and the patient is at increased risk for harming himself or others.

(continued)

SKILL 3-3

Applying a Jacket or Vest Restraint *(continued)*

ACTION	RATIONALE
2. Confirm agency policy for application of restraints. **Secure a physician's order, or validate that the order has been obtained within the past 24 hours.**	Policy protects the patient and the nurse and specifies guidelines for application as well as type of restraint and duration. **Joint Commission on Accreditation of Healthcare Organizations (JCAHO) standards require that a new order for restraints must be written every 24 hours.**
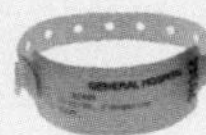 3. Identify the patient.	Identifying the patient ensures the right patient receives the intervention and helps prevent errors.
4. Explain reason for use to patient and family. Clarify how care will be given and how needs will be met. Explain that restraint is a temporary measure.	Explanation to patient and family may lessen confusion and anger and provide reassurance. A clearly stated agency policy on application of restraints should be available for patient and family to read. In a long-term care facility, the family must give consent before a restraint is applied.
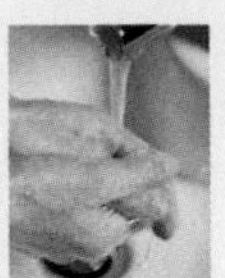 5. Perform hand hygiene.	Hand hygiene deters the spread of microorganisms.
6. Apply restraint according to manufacturer's directions:	Proper application prevents injury. Proper application ensures that there is no interference with patient's respiration.
a. Choose the correct size of the least restrictive type of device that allows the greatest possible degree of mobility.	This provides minimal restriction.
b. Pad bony prominences that may be affected by the vest.	Padding helps prevent injury.
c. Assist patient to a sitting position, if not contraindicated.	This will assist the nurse in helping the patient into the vest.
d. **Place vest on patient over gown, with flaps crisscrossing over the abdomen if appropriate. The V opening should be on the patient's front (Figure 1).**	Placing the V in the back may cause the patient to choke.
e. Pull the tabs secure (Figure 2). **Ensure that there are no wrinkles in the vest behind the patient.**	Wrinkles in the vest behind the patient may lead to skin impairment.

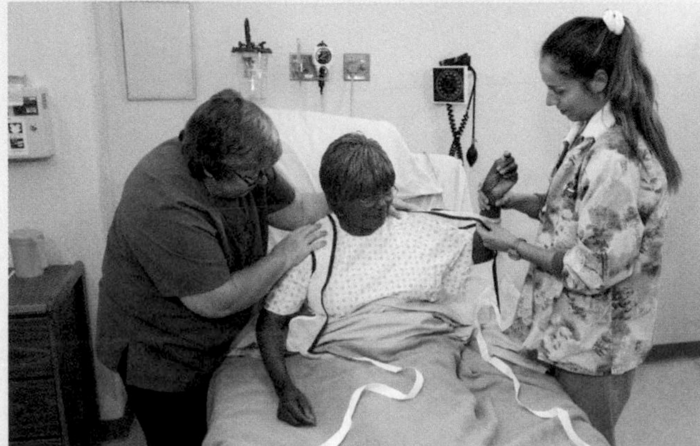

Figure 1. Applying vest restraint with V opening in front.

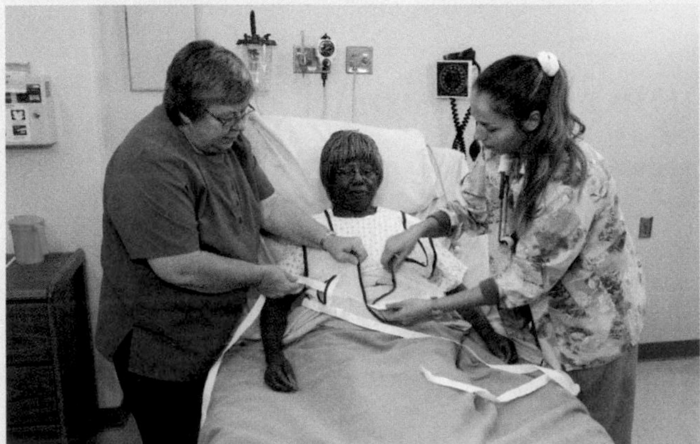

Figure 2. Pulling tabs secure.

SKILL 3-3 Applying a Jacket or Vest Restraint *(continued)*

ACTION	RATIONALE
f. **Insert fist between restraint and patient to ensure that breathing is not constricted. Assess respirations after restraint is applied.**	This prevents impaired respirations.
7. **Use a quick-release knot to tie the restraint to the bed frame, not side rail (Figure 3).** Refer to chapter introduction for examples of knots. If patient is in a wheelchair, lock the wheels and place the restraints under the arm rests and tie behind the chair (Figure 4). Site should not be readily accessible to the patient.	A quick-release knot ensures that restraint will not tighten when pulled and can be removed quickly in an emergency. Securing the restraint to a side rail may injure the patient when the side rail is lowered. Tying restraint out of patient's reach promotes security.

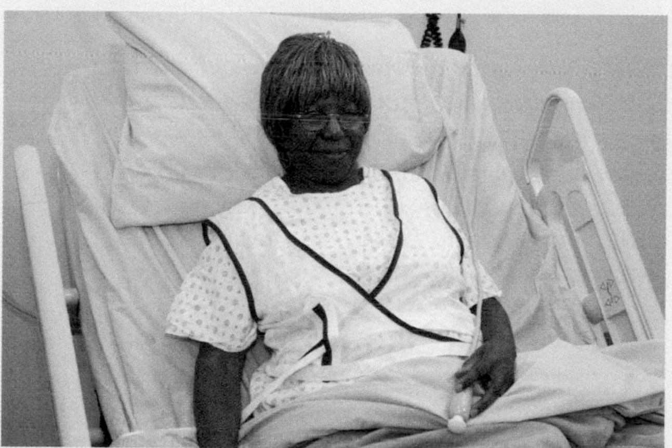

Figure 3. Vest restraint in place, tied to bed frame with quick-release knots.

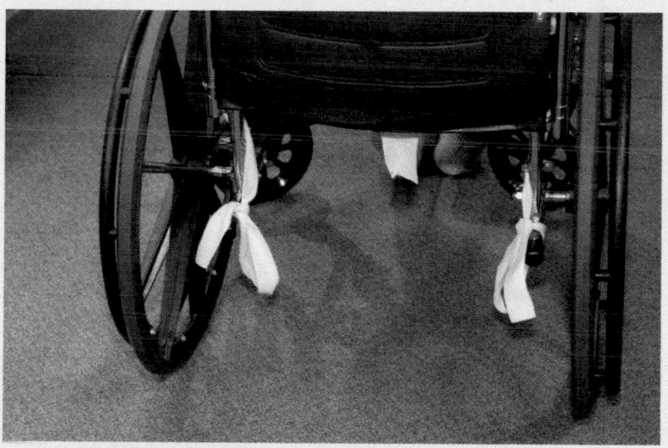

Figure 4. Restraint secured behind chair, out of the patient's reach.

ACTION	RATIONALE
8. Assess the patient at least every hour or according to facility policy is required. An assessment should include: the placement of the restraint, respiratory assessment, and skin integrity. Assess for signs of sensory deprivation, such as increased sleeping, daydreaming, anxiety, panic, and hallucinations.	Improperly applied restraints may cause difficulty breathing, skin tears, abrasions, or bruises. Decreased circulation may result in impaired skin integrity. Use of restraints may decrease environmental stimulation and result in sensory deprivation.
9. **Remove restraint at least every 2 hours or according to agency policy and patient need.** Perform range-of-motion exercises.	Removal allows nurse to assess patient and reevaluate need for restraint. Allows interventions for toileting, provision of nutrition and liquids, exercise, and change of position. Exercise increases circulation in restrained extremity.
10. Evaluate patient for continued need of restraint. Reapply restraint only if continued need is evident and order is still valid.	Continued need must be documented for reapplication.
11. Reassure patient at regular intervals. Provide continued explanation of rationale for interventions, reorientation if necessary, and plan of care. **Keep call bell within easy reach.**	Reassurance demonstrates caring and provides opportunity for sensory situation as well as ongoing assessment and evaluation. Patient can use call bell to summon assistance quickly.
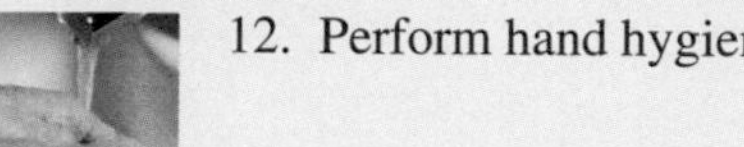 12. Perform hand hygiene.	Hand hygiene deters the spread of microorganisms.

(continued)

SKILL 3-3 Applying a Jacket or Vest Restraint *(continued)*

EVALUATION

The expected outcomes are met when the patient remains free of injury; the restraints prevent injury to the patient or others; respirations are easy and effortless; skin integrity is maintained under the restraint; and the family demonstrates understanding of the rationale for using the restraints.

DOCUMENTATION

Guidelines

Document alternative measures attempted before applying restraint. Document patient assessment before application. Record patient and family education and understanding regarding restraint use. Document family consent if necessary, according to facility policy. Document reason for restraining patient, date and time of application, type of restraint, times when removed, and result and frequency of nursing assessment. Obtain a new order after 24 hours if restraints are still necessary.

Sample Documentation

9/30/09 2130 Patient continues to attempt to get out of bed without assistance. Vest restraint applied at night as ordered when family leaves. Bed height low; side rails up × 2.—B. Clapp, RN

9/30/09 2300 Vest removed; skin intact; patient ambulated to restroom with assistance. Patient requested to ambulate to kitchen for snack; patient assisted to kitchen; graham crackers and milk obtained. Patient returned to bed and vest reapplied after snack.—B. Clapp, RN

Unexpected Situations and Associated Interventions

- *Patient slides down and neck is caught in restraint:* Immediately release restraint. Determine alternate methods for restraining.
- *Patient slides down and out of restraint:* Apply smaller vest restraint. Vest restraints come in various sizes, and the patient should not be able to slide out of vest.
- *Patient is exhibiting signs of respiratory distress:* Release vest. Vest may be applied too tightly and cause difficulty with chest expansion.

Special Considerations

General Considerations

- Consider keeping a pair of scissors with emergency supplies in case the restraints cannot be untied quickly.

SKILL 3-4 Applying an Elbow Restraint

Elbow restraints are generally used on infants and children. They prevent the child from bending the elbows and reaching incisions or therapeutic devices. The child can move all joints and extremities except the elbow. Restraints should be used only after less restrictive methods have failed. Ensure compliance with ordering, assessment, and maintenance procedures. Review general guidelines for using restraints in the chapter introduction and Fundamentals Review 3-1 and 3-2.

Equipment

- Elbow restraint
- Padding as necessary

SKILL 3-4 Applying an Elbow Restraint *(continued)*

ASSESSMENT

Assess the patient's physical condition and for the potential for injury to self or others. A confused patient who might remove devices needed to sustain life is considered at risk for injury to self and may require the use of restraints. Assess the patient's behavior, including the presence of confusion, agitation, combativeness, and ability to understand and follow directions. Evaluate the appropriateness of the least restrictive restraint device. Inspect the arm where the restraint will be applied. Baseline skin condition should be established for comparison at future assessments while the restraint is in place. Consider using another form of restraint if the restraint may cause further injury at the site. Assess capillary refill and proximal pulses in the arm to which the restraint is to be applied. This helps to determine the circulation in the extremity before applying the restraint. The restraint should not interfere with circulation. Measure the distance from the patient's shoulder to wrist to determine which size of elbow restraint to apply.

NURSING DIAGNOSIS

Determine the related factors for nursing diagnoses based on the patient's current status. Appropriate nursing diagnoses may include:

- Risk for Injury
- Risk for Impaired Skin Integrity
- Anxiety
- Impaired Physical Mobility
- Bathing/Hygiene Self-Care Deficit
- Feeding Self-Care Deficit
- Toileting Self-Care Deficit

OUTCOME IDENTIFICATION AND PLANNING

The expected outcome to achieve when applying an extremity restraint is that the patient is constrained by the restraint, remains free from injury, and the restraint does not interfere with therapeutic devices. Other outcomes that may be appropriate include the following: the patient does not experience impaired skin integrity; the patient does not injure himself or herself due to the restraints; and the patient's family will demonstrate an understanding about the use of the restraint and their role in the patient's care.

IMPLEMENTATION

ACTION	RATIONALE
1. Determine need for restraints. Assess patient's physical condition, behavior, and mental status. Refer to review material in the chapter introduction.	Restraints should be used only as a last resort when alternative measures have failed and the patient is at increased risk for harming himself or others.
2. Confirm agency policy for application of restraints. **Secure a physician's order, or validate that the order has been obtained within the past 24 hours.**	Policy protects the patient and the nurse and specifies guidelines for application as well as type of restraint and duration. **Joint Commission on Accreditation of Healthcare Organizations (JCAHO) standards require that a new order for restraints must be written every 24 hours.**
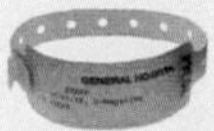 3. Identify the patient.	Identifying the patient ensures the right patient receives the intervention and helps prevent errors.
4. Explain reason for use to patient and family. Clarify how care will be given and how needs will be met. Explain that restraint is a temporary measure.	Explanation to patient and family may lessen confusion and anger and provide reassurance. A clearly stated agency policy on application of restraints should be available for patient and family to read.

(continued)

SKILL 3-4 Applying an Elbow Restraint *(continued)*

ACTION / **RATIONALE**

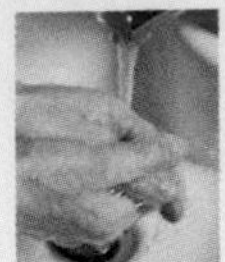

5. Perform hand hygiene. — Hand hygiene deters the spread of microorganisms.

6. Apply restraint according to manufacturer's directions: — Proper application prevents injury. Proper application ensures that there is no interference with patient's circulation.

   a. Choose the correct size of the least restrictive type of device that allows the greatest possible degree of mobility. — This provides minimal restriction.

   b. Pad bony prominences that may be affected by the restraint. — Padding helps prevent injury.

   c. Spread elbow restraint out flat. Place middle of elbow restraint behind patient's elbow. **The restraint should not extend below the wrist or place pressure on the axilla.** — Elbow restraint should be placed in middle of arm to ensure that child cannot bend the elbow. Child should be able to move wrist. Pressure on the axilla may lead to skin impairment.

   d. **Wrap restraint snugly around patient's arm, but make sure that two fingers can easily fit under restraint.** — Wrapping snugly ensures that child will not be able to remove the device. Being able to insert two fingers helps to prevent impaired circulation from restraint.

   e. Wrap Velcro straps around restraint (Figure 1). — Velcro straps will hold the restraint in place and prevent child from removing restraint.

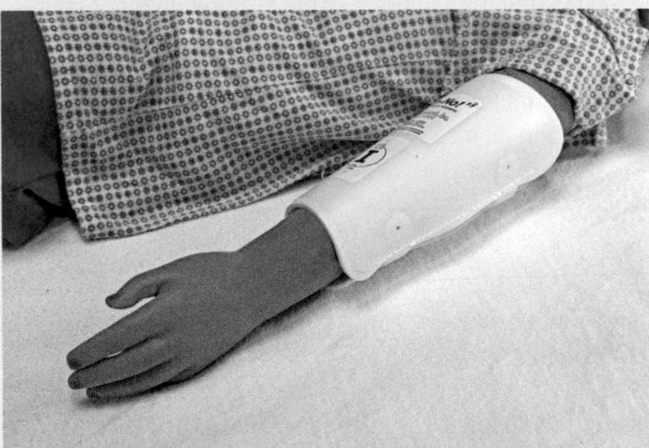

Figure 1. Child with elbow restraint in place.

   f. Apply restraint to opposite arm if patient can move arm. — Bilateral elbow restraints are needed if patient can move both arms.

   g. Thread Velcro strap from one elbow restraint across the back and into the loop on the opposite elbow restraint. — Strap across the back prevents child from wiggling out of elbow restraints.

7. **Assess circulation to fingers and hand.** — Circulation should not be impaired from elbow restraint.

8. Assess the patient at least every hour or according to facility policy is required. An assessment should include: the placement of the restraint, neurovascular assessment, and skin integrity. Assess for signs of sensory deprivation, such as increased sleeping, daydreaming, anxiety, inconsolable crying, and panic. — Improperly applied restraints may cause alterations in circulation, skin tears, abrasions, or bruises. Decreased circulation may result in impaired skin integrity. Use of restraints may decrease environmental stimulation and result in sensory deprivation.

SKILL 3-4 Applying an Elbow Restraint *(continued)*

ACTION	RATIONALE
9. **Remove restraint at least every 2 hours for children ages 9–17 years and at least every 1 hour for children under age 9, or according to agency policy and patient need.** Perform range-of-motion exercises.	Removal allows nurse to assess patient and reevaluate need for restraint. Allows interventions for toileting, provision of nutrition and liquids, exercise and change of position. Exercise increases circulation in restrained extremity
10. Evaluate patient for continued need of restraint. Reapply restraint only if continued need is evident.	Continued need must be documented for reapplication.
11. Reassure patient at regular intervals. **Keep call bell within easy reach.**	Reassurance demonstrates caring and provides opportunity for sensory situation as well as ongoing assessment and evaluation. Parent or child old enough to use call bell can use it to summon assistance quickly.
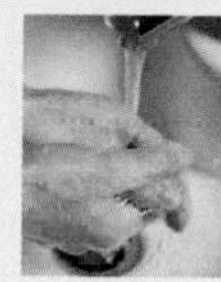 12. Perform hand hygiene.	Hand hygiene deters the spread of microorganisms.

EVALUATION

The expected outcome is met when the restraint prevents injury to self or others. In addition, the child cannot bend the elbow; skin integrity is maintained under the restraint; and the family demonstrates an understanding of the rationale for the elbow restraint.

DOCUMENTATION

Guidelines

Document alternative measures attempted before applying restraint. Document patient assessment before application. Record patient and family education regarding restraint use and their understanding. Document family consent if necessary, according to facility policy. Document reason for restraining patient, date and time of application, type of restraint, times when removed, and result and frequency of nursing assessment. Obtain a new order after 24 hours if restraints are still necessary.

Sample Documentation

9/1/07 0800 Elbow restraints removed while AM care performed (45 minutes). Patient moving arms appropriately. Continues to pick at colostomy bag. Distraction techniques used to no avail. Child removes abdominal binder when applied.—B. Clapp, RN

9/1/07 0855 Skin intact and warm. Elbow restraints reapplied. Will remove when family arrives at bedside or every 2 hours as per policy.—B. Clapp, RN

Unexpected Outcomes and Associated Interventions

- *Skin breakdown is noted on elbows:* Ensure that restraints are being removed routinely for at least 30 minutes and a skin inspection is done. If restraints are still needed, a padded dressing may be applied under the elbow restraint.
- *Patient cries when elbow is moved:* Restraints need to be removed more frequently, with active and/or passive range of motion. If elbow is not moved, it will become stiff and painful.

SKILL 3-5 Applying a Mummy Restraint

A mummy restraint is appropriate for short-term restraint of an infant or small child to control the child's movements during examination or to provide care for the head and neck. Restraints should be used only after less restrictive methods have failed. Ensure compliance with ordering, assessment, and maintenance procedures. Review general guidelines for using restraints in the chapter introduction and Fundamentals Review 3-1 and 3-2.

Equipment

- Small blanket or sheet

ASSESSMENT

Assess patient's behavior and need for restraint. Assess for wounds or therapeutic devices that may be affected by the restraint. Another form of restraint may be more appropriate to prevent injury.

NURSING DIAGNOSIS

Determine the related factors for nursing diagnoses based on the patient's current status. Appropriate nursing diagnoses may include:

- Risk for Injury
- Anxiety
- Impaired Physical Mobility

OUTCOME IDENTIFICATION AND PLANNING

The expected outcome to achieve is that the patient is contained by the restraint, remains free from injury, and that the restraint does not interfere with therapeutic devices. Other outcomes that may be appropriate include the following: examination and/or treatment is provided without incident and the patient's family will demonstrate an understanding about the use of the restraint and their role in the patient's care.

IMPLEMENTATION

ACTION	RATIONALE
1. Determine need for restraints. Assess patient's physical condition, behavior, and mental status. Refer to review material in the chapter introduction.	Restraints should be used only as a last resort when alternative measures have failed, and the patient is at increased risk for harming himself or others.
2. Confirm agency policy for application of restraints.	Policy protects the patient and the nurse and specifies guidelines for application as well as type of restraint and duration.
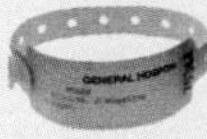 3. Identify the patient.	Identifying the patient ensures the right patient receives the intervention and helps prevent errors.
4. Explain reason for use to patient and family. Clarify how care will be given and how needs will be met. Explain that restraint is a temporary measure.	Explanation to patient and family may lessen confusion and anger and provide reassurance. A clearly stated agency policy on application of restraints should be available for patient and family to read.
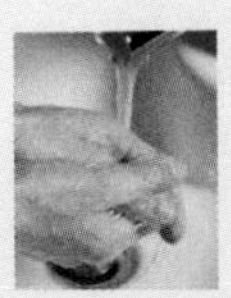 5. Perform hand hygiene.	Hand hygiene deters the spread of microorganisms.
6. Open the blanket or sheet. Fold one corner to the center. Place the child on the blanket, shoulders at the fold, and feet toward the opposite corner.	This positions child correctly on the blanket.

SKILL 3-5 Applying a Mummy Restraint *(continued)*

ACTION	RATIONALE
7. Position the child's right arm alongside his body. Left arm should not be constrained at this time. Pull the right side of the blanket tightly over the child's right shoulder and chest. Secure under the left side of his body (Figure 1).	Wrapping snugly ensures that child will not be able to wiggle out.

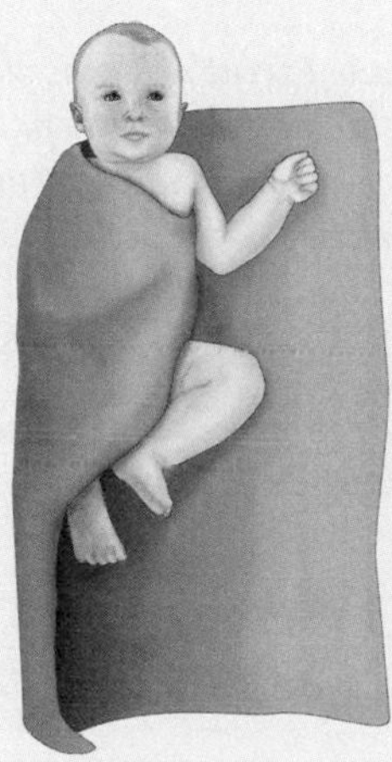

Figure 1. Pulling blanket over right shoulder and chest and securing under patient's left side.

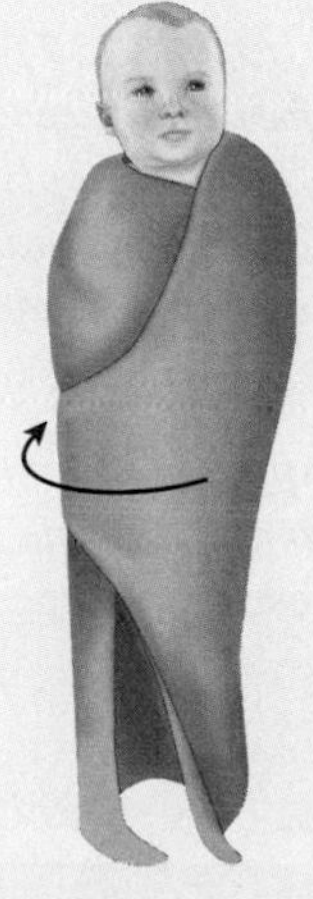

Figure 2. Securing blanket under right side of body.

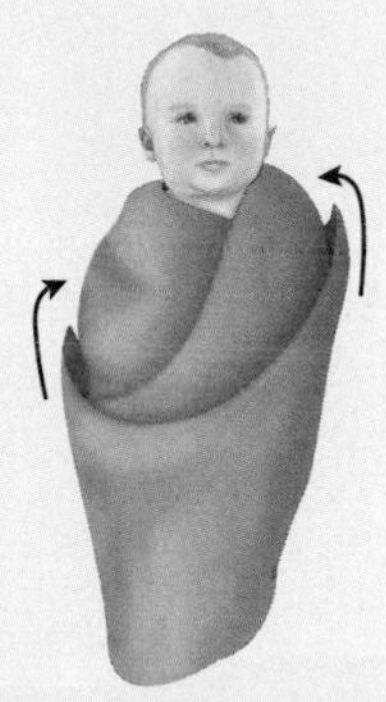

Figure 3. Securing lower corner of blanket under each side of patient's body.

ACTION	RATIONALE
8. Position the left arm along side the child's body. Pull the left side of the blanket tightly over the child's left shoulder and chest. Secure under the right side of his body (Figure 2).	Wrapping snugly ensures that child will not be able to wiggle out.
9. Fold the lower corner up and pull over the child's body. Secure under the child's body on each side or with safety pins (Figure 3).	This ensures that child will not be able to wiggle out.
10. Stay with child while mummy wrap is in place. Reassure child and parents at regular intervals. Once examination or treatment is completed, unwrap child.	Prevents injury. Reassurance demonstrates caring and provides opportunity for ongoing assessment and evaluation.
11. Perform hand hygiene.	Hand hygiene deters the spread of microorganisms.

EVALUATION

The expected outcome is met when the restraint prevents injury to self or others. In addition, the examination or treatment is provided without incident; and the family demonstrates an understanding of the rationale for the elbow restraint.

(continued)

SKILL 3-5 Applying a Mummy Restraint *(continued)*

DOCUMENTATION

Guidelines

Document alternative measures attempted before applying restraint. Document patient assessment before application. Record patient and family education and understanding regarding restraint use. Document family consent if necessary, according to facility policy. Document reason for restraining patient, date and time of application, type of restraint, times when removed, and result and frequency of nursing assessment. Obtain a new order after 24 hours if restraints are still necessary.

Sample Documentation

6/9/08 0230 Patient requires suturing of forehead. Parent attempted to hold child for procedure without success. Need to restrain child explained to parents. Mummy restraint applied with parents' consent. Restraint removed after 20 minutes; sutures intact. Wound care instructions (verbal and written) provided to parents; parents verbalize understanding.—D. Dunn, RN.

Unexpected Situation

- *Application of mummy wrap does not control the infant's or child's body movement to allow for needed examination or treatment:* Reassess situation and consider more restrictive type of restraint.

SKILL 3-6 Applying Leather Restraints

Leather restraints are used whenever cloth restraints are not strong enough to restrain the patient. Leather restraints come in a locking and a nonlocking version. If using the locking version, ensure that the key is available at all times. In an emergency situation, leather restraints cannot be cut easily. Restraints should be used only after less restrictive methods have failed. Ensure compliance with ordering, assessment, and maintenance procedures. Review general guidelines for using restraints in the chapter introduction and Fundamentals Review 3-1 and 3-2.

Equipment

- Leather restraint
- Padding, if necessary, for bony prominences

ASSESSMENT

Assess the patient's physical condition and for the potential for injury to self or others. A confused patient who might remove devices needed to sustain life is considered at risk for injury to self and may require the use of restraints. Assess the patient's behavior, including the presence of confusion, agitation, combativeness, and ability to understand and follow directions. Evaluate the appropriateness of the least restrictive restraint device. Inspect the extremity where the restraint will be applied. Baseline skin condition should be established for comparison at future assessments while the restraint is in place. Consider using another form of restraint if the restraint may cause further injury at the site. Assess capillary refill and proximal pulses in the extremity to which the restraint is to be applied. This helps to determine the circulation in the extremity before applying the restraint.

NURSING DIAGNOSIS

Determine the related factors for nursing diagnoses based on the patient's current status. Appropriate nursing diagnoses may include:

- Risk for Injury
- Risk for Impaired Skin Integrity

SKILL 3-6 **Applying Leather Restraints** *(continued)*

- Anxiety
- Impaired Physical Mobility
- Acute Confusion
- Bathing/Hygiene Self-Care Deficit
- Feeding Self-Care Deficit
- Toileting Self-Care Deficit

OUTCOME IDENTIFICATION AND PLANNING

The expected outcome to achieve is that the patient is constrained by the restraint, remains free from injury, and the restraint does not interfere with therapeutic devices. Other outcomes that may be appropriate include the following: the patient does not experience impaired skin integrity; the patient does not injure himself or herself due to the restraints; and the patient's family will demonstrate an understanding about the use of the restraint and their role in the patient's care.

IMPLEMENTATION

ACTION	RATIONALE
1. Determine need for restraints. Assess patient's physical condition, behavior, and mental status. Refer to review material in the chapter introduction.	Restraints should be used only as a last resort when alternative measures have failed. and the patient is at increased risk for harming himself or others.
2. Confirm agency policy for application of restraints. **Secure a physician's order, or validate that the order has been obtained within the past 24 hours.**	Policy protects the patient and the nurse and specifies guidelines for application as well as type of restraint and duration. **Joint Commission on Accreditation of Healthcare Organizations (JCAHO) standards require that a new order for restraints must be written every 24 hours.**
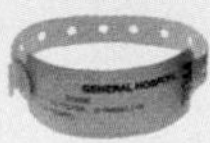 3. Identify the patient.	Identifying the patient ensures the right patient receives the medications and helps prevent errors.
4. Explain reason for use to patient and family. Clarify how care will be given and how needs will be met. Explain that restraint is a temporary measure.	Explanation to patient and family may lessen confusion and anger and provide reassurance. A clearly stated agency policy on application of restraints should be available for patient and family to read. In a long-term care facility, the family must give consent before a restraint is applied.
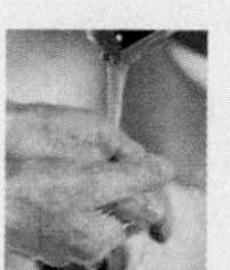 5. Perform hand hygiene.	Hand hygiene deters the spread of microorganisms.
6. Apply restraints according to manufacturer's directions:	Proper application ensures that there is no interference with patient's circulation.
a. Pad bony prominences.	This protects the skin and prevents breakdown.
b. Wrap the restraint around the extremity with the soft part in contact with the skin. Secure in place with the buckles.	This prevents excess pressure on extremity.
c. **Ensure that two fingers can be inserted between the restraint and patient's wrist or ankle.** Maintain restrained extremity in normal anatomic position.	Proper application ensures that there is no interference with patient's circulation. Maintaining a normal position lessens possibility of injury.

(continued)

SKILL 3-6 Applying Leather Restraints *(continued)*

ACTION	RATIONALE
d. **If using locking leather restraints, ensure that key is available at all times.**	Leather restraints cannot be cut easily in an emergency situation. Key must be available to release patient quickly if needed.
7. **Fasten restraint to bed frame, not side rail.** Leather restraints have leather straps with buckles to secure to the bed frame (Figure 1). Site should not be readily accessible to the patient.	Securing restraint to a side rail may cause injury to patient if side rail is lowered. Securing restraint out of patient's reach promotes security.

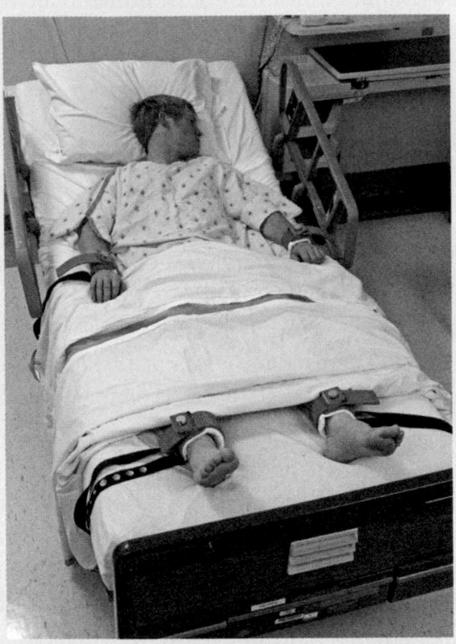

Figure 1. Patient secured in leather restraints on all four extremities.

ACTION	RATIONALE
8. Assessment of the patient at least every hour or according to facility policy is required. An assessment should include: the placement of the restraint, neurovascular assessment of the affected extremity, and skin integrity. Assess for signs of sensory deprivation, such as increased sleeping, daydreaming, anxiety, panic, and hallucinations.	Improperly applied restraints may cause skin tears, abrasions, or bruises. Decreased circulation may result in paleness, coolness, decreased sensation, tingling, numbness, or pain in extremity. Use of restraints may decrease environmental stimulation and result in sensory deprivation.
9. **Remove restraint at least every 2 hours, or according to agency policy and patient need.** Perform range-of-motion exercises.	Removal allows nurse to assess patient and reevaluate need for restraint. Allows interventions for toileting, provision of nutrition and liquids, exercise, and change of position. Exercise increases circulation in restrained extremity.
10. Evaluate patient for continued need of restraint. Reapply restraint only if continued need is evident and order is valid.	Continued need must be documented for reapplication.
11. Reassure patient at regular intervals. **Keep call bell within easy reach.**	Reassurance demonstrates caring and provides opportunity for sensory situation as well as ongoing assessment and evaluation. Patient can use call bell to summon assistance quickly.
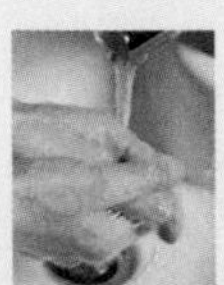 12. Perform hand hygiene.	Hand hygiene deters the spread of microorganisms.

SKILL 3-6 **Applying Leather Restraints** *(continued)*

EVALUATION

The expected outcome is met when the patient remains free of injury due to the application of restraints. In addition, injury to others is prevented; circulation to extremity remains adequate; skin integrity remains intact under the restraint; and the family verbalizes an awareness of the rationale for restraint use.

DOCUMENTATION

Guidelines

Document alternative measures attempted before applying restraint. Document patient assessment before application. Record patient and family education and understanding regarding restraint use. Document family consent if necessary, according to facility policy. Document reason for restraining patient, date and time of application, type of restraint, times when removed, and result and frequency of nursing assessment. Obtain a new order after 24 hours if restraints are still necessary.

Sample Documentation

9/13/08 0100 Patient threatening to injure self and others. De-escalating attempts to no effect; security called; patient subdued and placed in four-point leather restraints as ordered. Key kept in room at all times; patient placed on right side.—B. Clapp, RN
9/13/08 0200 With security at bedside, extremities released one at a time and range of motion performed; skin intact and warm; patient continuing to threaten harm to others.—B. Clapp, RN

Unexpected Outcomes and Associated Interventions

- *Patient is continually pulling on leather restraints and causing injury to extremities:* Notify physician. Patient may need sedation. Talk with patient to see if there is anything that can be done to help him or her relax.
- *Nurse is afraid for own safety when releasing restraints for inspection and range of motion:* Call for assistance. For their own safety, nurses should have assistance when releasing a combative or agitated patient from leather restraints. Security personnel should be available to assist, if necessary.

Special Considerations

General Considerations

- Do not position patient flat in a supine position with wrist restraints. If patient vomits, aspiration may occur.
- Have the key for locking leather restraints readily available at all times.

The Taylor Suite offers these additional resources to enhance learning and facilitate understanding:

- thePoint online resource, http://thepoint.lww.com/Lynn2E
- Student CD-ROM included with the book
- Skills Checklist to Accompany Taylor's Clinical Nursing Skills

Developing Critical Thinking Skills

1. Megan Lewis, an 18-month-old with an IV access in her left forearm, is continually picking at the IV and dressing. What interventions would be appropriate as alternatives to restraints? If unsuccessful, what restraints would be appropriate for Megan?
2. Kevin Mallory, a 35-year-old body builder with a closed head injury, is extremely strong. The nurse is afraid that he will rip the cloth restraints and extubate himself. What other type of restraints could the nurse try?
3. John Frawley, a 72-year-old patient with Alzheimer's disease, continually tries to get out of bed without assistance. He has an unsteady gait and has broken one hip due to a fall. What are the appropriate interventions to try with Mr. Frawley? If the use of a restraint becomes necessary, what is the least restrictive restraint for John?

Bibliography

Alexander, N. & Edelberg, H. (2002). Assessing mobility and preventing falls in older patients. *Patient Care, 36*(2), 19–29.

Bernardo, L. (2002). Emergency nurses' role in injury prevention. *Emergency Nursing, 37*(1), 135–142.

Brenner, Z. & Duffy-Durnin, K. (1998). Toward restraint-free care. *American Journal of Nursing, 98*(12), 16F–16I.

Centers for Disease Control and Prevention (2003). *Injury mortality reports, 1999–2000.* Available at http://webapp.cdc.gov/sasweb/ncipc/mortrate10.html.

Crawley-Coha, T. (2002). Childhood injury: A status report, part 2. *Journal of Pediatric Nursing, 17*(2), 133–136.

DiBartolo, V. (1998). 9 steps to effective restraint use. *RN, 61*(12), 23–24.

Dochterman, J., & Bulechek, G. (Eds.). (2004). *Nursing interventions classification (NIC)* (4th ed.). St. Louis, MO: Mosby.

Dunn, K. (2001). The effect of physical restraints on fall rates in older adults who are institutionalized. *Journal of Gerontological Nursing, 27*(10), 40–48.

Eliopoulos, C. (2003). *Gerontological nursing* (5th ed.). Philadelphia: Lippincott Williams & Wilkins.

Hockenberry, M. (2005). *Wong's essentials of pediatric nursing* (7th ed.). St. Louis, MO: Elsevier Mosby.

Joint Commission on Accreditation of Healthcare Organizations (JCAHO). (2001). Care of the patient: Restraint and seclusion standards. Comprehensive accreditation manual for hospitals, TX.7.1-TX.7.5.5.

Joint Commission on Accreditation of Healthcare Organizations. (2005). *Restraint and seclusion.* Available at www.jcaho.org/accredited+organizations/hospitals/standards/hospital+faqs/provision+of+care/restraint+and+seclusion/restraint_seclusion.htm. Accessed October 5, 2005.

Kelly, A. & Dowling, M. (2004). Reducing the likelihood of falls in older people. *Nursing Standard, 18*(49), 33–40.

Kleen, K. (2004). Restraint regulation: The tie that binds. *Nursing Management, 35*(11), 36–38.

Letizia, M., Babler, C. & Cockrell, A. (2004). Repeating the call for restraint reduction. *MEDSURG Nursing, 13*(1), 9–12.

London, M., Ladewig, P., Ball, J., et al. (2003). *Maternal-newborn & child nursing.* Upper Saddle River, NJ: Prentice Hall.

Mace, S., Gerardi, M., Dietrick, A., et al. (2001). Injury prevention and control in children. *Annals of Emergency Medicine, 38*(4), 405–413.

McBeth, S. (2004). Get a firmer grasp on restraints. *Nursing Management, 35*(10), 20, 22.

Melillo, K., & Futrell, M. (1998). Wandering and technology devices. *Journal of Gerontological Nursing, 24*(8), 32–38.

Mulryan, K., Cathers, P., & Fagin, A. (2000). Protecting the child. *Nursing, 30*(7), 39–45.

Napierkowski, D. (2002). Using restraints with restraint. *Nursing, 32*(11), 58–62.

National Institute on Aging. (2004). *Age page: Preventing falls and fractures.* Available at http://www.niapublications.org/engagepages/falls.asp. Accessed October 1, 2005.

North American Nursing Diagnosis Association. (2005). *NANDA nursing diagnoses: Definitions & classifications 2005–2006.* Philadelphia: Author.

Poe, S., Gartrell, D., Radzik, B., et al. (2005). An evidence-based approach to fall risk assessment, prevention, and management: Lessons learned. *Journal of Nursing Care Quality, 20*(2), 107–116.

Rao, S. (2005). Prevention of falls in older patients. *American Family Physician, 72*(1), 81–88.

Talerico, K., & Capezuti, E. (2001). Myths and facts about side rails. *American Journal of Nursing, 101*(7), 43–48.

Todd, J. (2002). When bed isn't a safe haven. *Nursing, 32*(12), 82.

U.S. Census Bureau (2002). *Statistical abstract of the United States, 2002* (122nd ed.). Washington, DC: Author.

CHAPTER 4

Asepsis and Infection Control

Focusing on Patient Care

This chapter will help you develop some of the skills related to asepsis and infection control necessary to care for the following patients:

Joe Wilson is scheduled to undergo a cardiac catheterization later this morning.

Sheri Lawrence has been ordered to have an indwelling urinary catheter inserted and is at risk for a nosocomial infection.

Edgar Barowski is suspected of having tuberculosis and requires infection-control precautions.

Learning Objectives

After studying this chapter, you will be able to:

1. Perform hand hygiene using soap and water (handwashing).
2. Perform hand hygiene using an alcohol-based hand rub.
3. Prepare a sterile field.
4. Add sterile items to a sterile field.
5. Put on and remove sterile gloves.
6. Put on and remove personal protective equipment safely.

Key Terms

healthcare-associated infection: infection not present on admission to healthcare agency, acquired during the course of treatment for other conditions

medical asepsis: clean technique; involves procedures and practices that reduce the number and transfer of pathogens

nosocomial infection: hospital-acquired infection

personal protective equipment (PPE): specialized clothing or equipment worn by a healthcare worker for protection against infectious materials

Standard Precautions: precautions used in the care of all hospitalized individuals regardless of their diagnosis or possible infection status; these precautions apply to blood, all body fluids, secretions and excretions (except sweat), nonintact skin, and mucous membranes

surgical asepsis: sterile technique; involves practices used to render and keep objects and areas free from microorganisms

Transmission-Based Precautions: precautions used in addition to Standard Precautions for patients in hospitals who are suspected of being infected with pathogens that can be transmitted by airborne, droplet, or contact routes; these precautions encompass all the diseases or conditions previously listed in the disease-specific or category-specific classifications

A major concern for all health practitioners is the danger of spreading microorganisms from person to person and from place to place. Prevention of infection is a major focus for nurses. As primary caregivers, nurses are involved in identifying, preventing, controlling, and teaching the patient about infection.

Healthcare-associated infections most commonly result from person-to-person transmission via the hands of healthcare workers (Sickbert-Bennett et al, 2005). Nurses and other healthcare workers have a key role in reducing the spread of disease, minimizing complications, and reducing adverse outcomes for their patients. Limiting the spread of microorganisms is accomplished by breaking the chain of infection. The practice of asepsis includes all activities to prevent infection or break the chain of infection. Medical asepsis, or clean technique, involves procedures and practices that reduce the number and transfer of pathogens (Fundamentals Review 4-1). Surgical asepsis, or sterile technique, includes practices used to render and keep objects and areas free from microorganisms (Fundamentals Review 4-2)

This chapter reviews procedures to assist nurses in preventing the spread of infection, including the use of sterile technique, personal protective equipment, and hand hygiene. Hand hygiene is the most effective way to help prevent the spread of organisms. Hand hygiene refers to handwashing with soap and water, the use of alcohol-based hand rubs, and surgical hand antisepsis (Centers for Disease Control and Prevention [CDC], 2002a). Refer to Fundamentals Review 4-3 for general guidelines regarding hand hygiene for healthcare workers. The CDC has reinforced previous guidelines that handwashing is the most effective way to help prevent disease transmission. However, it has looked at the use of other agents, and the guidelines now include the routine use of alcohol-based hand rubs. Improved compliance with hand hygiene has been shown to reduce overall infection rates in healthcare facilities (CDC, 2002b).

The use of Standard and Transmission-Based Precautions is another important part of protecting patients and healthcare providers and preventing the spread of infection. Fundamentals Review 4-4 and Fundamentals Review 4-5 outline a summary of CDC recommended practices for Standard and Transmission-Based Precautions.

Fundamentals Review 4-1

Basic Principles of Medical Asepsis in Patient Care

- Practice good hand hygiene techniques.
- Carry soiled items, including linens, equipment, and other used articles, away from the body to prevent them from touching the clothing.
- Do not place soiled bed linen or any other items on the floor, which is grossly contaminated. It increases contamination of both surfaces.
- Avoid having patients cough, sneeze, or breathe directly on others. Provide patients with disposable tissues, and instruct them, as indicated, to cover their mouth and nose to prevent spread by airborne droplets.
- Move equipment away from you when brushing, dusting, or scrubbing articles. This helps prevent contaminated particles from settling on your hair, face, and uniform.
- Avoid raising dust. Use a specially treated or a dampened cloth. Do not shake linens. Dust and lint particles constitute a vehicle by which organisms may be transported from one area to another.
- Clean the least soiled areas first and then move to the more soiled ones. This helps prevent having the cleaner areas soiled by the dirtier areas.
- Dispose of soiled or used items directly into appropriate containers. Wrap items that are moist from body discharge or drainage in waterproof containers, such as plastic bags, before discarding into the refuse holder so that handlers will not come in contact with them.
- Pour liquids that are to be discarded, such as bath water, mouth rinse, and the like, directly into the drain to avoid splattering in the sink and onto you.
- Sterilize items that are suspected of containing pathogens. After sterilization, they can be managed as clean items if appropriate.
- Use personal grooming habits that help prevent spreading microorganisms. Shampoo your hair regularly; keep your fingernails short and free of broken cuticles and ragged edges; do not wear false nails; and do not wear rings with grooves and stones that may harbor microorganisms.
- Follow guidelines conscientiously for infection-control or barrier techniques as prescribed by the agency.

Fundamentals Review 4-2

Basic Principles of Surgical Asepsis

- Only a sterile object can touch another sterile object. Unsterile touching sterile means contamination has occurred.
- Open sterile packages so that the first edge of the wrapper is directed away from the worker to avoid the possibility of a sterile surface touching unsterile clothing. The outside of the sterile package is considered contaminated.
- Avoid spilling any solution on a cloth or paper used as a field for a sterile setup. The moisture penetrates the sterile cloth or paper and carries organisms by capillary action to contaminate the field. A wet field is considered contaminated if the surface immediately below it is not sterile.
- Hold sterile objects above waist level. This will ensure keeping the object within sight and preventing accidental contamination.
- Avoid talking, coughing, sneezing, or reaching over a sterile field or object. This helps to prevent contamination by droplets from the nose and the mouth or by particles dropping from the worker's arm.
- Never walk away from or turn your back on a sterile field. This prevents possible contamination while the field is out of the worker's view.
- All items brought into contact with broken skin, used to penetrate the skin to inject substances into the body, or used to enter normally sterile body cavities should be sterile. These items include dressings used to cover wounds and incisions, needles for injection, and tubes (catheters) used to drain urine from the bladder.
- Use dry, sterile forceps when necessary. Forceps soaked in disinfectant are not considered sterile.
- Consider the outer 1″ edge of a sterile field to be contaminated.
- Consider an object contaminated if you have any doubt about its sterility.

Fundamentals Review 4-3

Hand Hygiene for Healthcare Workers

Hand Hygiene is Required:

- Before and after contact with each patient
- Before putting on sterile gloves
- Before performing any invasive procedure, such as placement of a peripheral vascular catheter
- After accidental contact with body fluids or excretions, mucous membranes, nonintact skin, and wound dressings, even if hands are not visibly soiled
- When moving from a contaminated body site to a clean body site during patient care
- After contact with inanimate objects near the patient
- After removal of gloves

Additional Guidelines:

- The use of gloves does not eliminate the need for hand hygiene.
- The use of hand hygiene does not eliminate the need for gloves.
- Natural fingernails should be kept less than 1/4″ long.
- Artificial fingernails or extenders should not be worn when having direct contact with patients at high risk.
- Gloves should be worn when contact with blood, infectious material, mucous membranes, and nonintact skin could occur.
- Hand lotions or creams are recommended to moisturize and protect skin related to the occurrence of irritant dermatitis associated with hand hygiene.

(Modified from Centers for Disease Control and Prevention [2002]. Guidelines for hand hygiene in health-care settings. Morbidity and Mortality Weekly Report, *51(RR16), 1–45.)*

Fundamentals Review 4-4

Standard Precautions

Standard Precautions are to be used for all patients receiving care in hospitals without regard to their diagnosis or presumed infection status. Standard Precautions apply to blood; all body fluids, secretions, and excretions except sweat, regardless of the presence of visible blood; nonintact skin; and mucous membranes. Standard Precautions reduce the risk of transmission of microorganisms that cause infections in hospitals.

Standard Precautions (Tier 1)

- Follow hand hygiene techniques.
- Wear clean nonsterile gloves when touching blood, body fluids, excretions of secretions, contaminated items, mucous membranes, and nonintact skin. Change gloves between tasks on the same patient as necessary and remove gloves promptly after use.
- Wear personal protective equipment such as mask, eye protection, face shield, or fluid-repellent gown during procedures and care activities that are likely to generate splashes or sprays of blood or body fluids. Use gown to protect skin and prevent soiling of clothing.
- Avoid recapping used needles. If you must recap, never use two hands. Use a needle-recapping device or the one-handed scoop technique. Place needles, sharps, and scalpels in appropriate puncture-resistant containers after use.
- Handle used patient-care equipment that is soiled with blood or identified body fluids, secretions, and excretions carefully to prevent transfer of microorganisms. Clean and reprocess items appropriately if used for another patient.
- Use adequate environmental controls to ensure that routine care, cleaning, and disinfection procedures are followed.
- Review room assignments carefully. Place patients who may contaminate the environment in private rooms (such as an incontinent patient).

(Adapted from Centers for Disease Control and Prevention. [1996]. Available at http://www.cdc.gov/ncidod/hip/ISOLAT/isopart2.htm)

Transmission-Based Precautions

Transmission-Based Precautions are used in addition to Standard Precautions for patients in hospitals with suspected infection with pathogens that can be transmitted by airborne, droplet, or contact routes. Any of the three types can be used in combination with the others.

Airborne Precautions

- Use these for patients who have infections that spread through the air, such as tuberculosis, varicella (chicken pox), and rubeola (measles).
- Place patient in private room that has monitored negative air pressure in relation to surrounding areas, 6 to 12 air changes per hour, and appropriate discharge of air outside or monitored filtration if air is recirculated. Keep door closed and patient in room.
- Use respiratory protection when entering room of patient with known or suspected tuberculosis. If patient has known or suspected rubeola or varicella, respiratory protection should be worn unless person entering room is immune to these diseases.
- Transport patient out of room only when necessary and place a surgical mask on the patient if possible.
- Consult CDC Guidelines for additional prevention strategies for tuberculosis.

Droplet Precautions

- Use these for patients with an infection that is spread by large-particle droplets, such as rubella, mumps, diphtheria, and the adenovirus infection in infants and young children.
- Use a private room, if available. Door may remain open.
- Wear a mask when working within 3 feet of the patient.
- Transport patient out of room only when necessary and place a surgical mask on the patient if possible.
- Keep visitors 3 feet from the infected person.

Contact Precautions

- Use these for patients who are infected or colonized by a microorganism that spreads by direct or indirect contact, such as MRSA, VRE, or VISA.
- Place patient in a private room if available.
- Wear gloves whenever you enter the room. Change gloves after having contact with infective material. Remove gloves before leaving the patient environment, and wash hands with an antimicrobial or waterless antiseptic agent.
- Wear a gown if contact with infectious agent is likely or patient has diarrhea, an ileostomy, colostomy, or wound drainage not contained by a dressing.
- Limit movement of the patient out of the room.
- Avoid sharing patient-care equipment.

(Adapted from Centers for Disease Control and Prevention. [1996]. Available at http://www.cdc.gov/ncidod/hip/ISOLAT/isopart2.htm)

SKILL 4-1 Performing Hand Hygiene Using Soap and Water (Handwashing)

Handwashing remains the best method to decontaminate hands. Handwashing, as opposed to hand hygiene with an alcohol-based rub, is required (CDC, 2002a).

- When hands are visibly dirty
- When hands are visibly soiled with or in contact with blood or other body fluids
- Before eating and after using the restroom
- If exposure to certain organisms, such as those causing anthrax or *Clostridium difficile,* is known or suspected. (Other agents have poor activity against these organisms.)

Equipment

- Antimicrobial or non-antimicrobial soap (if in bar form, soap must be placed on a soap rack)
- Paper towels
- Oil-free lotion (optional)

(continued)

SKILL 4-1

Performing Hand Hygiene Using Soap and Water (Handwashing) *(continued)*

ASSESSMENT

Assess for any of the above requirements for handwashing. If no requirements are fulfilled, the caregiver has the option of decontaminating hands with soap and water or using an alcohol-based hand rub.

NURSING DIAGNOSIS

Determine the related factors for the nursing diagnoses based on the patient's current status. An appropriate nursing diagnosis is Risk for Infection. Many other nursing diagnoses also may require the use of this skill.

OUTCOME IDENTIFICATION AND PLANNING

The expected outcome to achieve when performing handwashing is that the hands will be free of visible soiling and transient microorganisms will be eliminated. Other outcomes may be appropriate depending on the specific nursing diagnosis identified for the patient.

IMPLEMENTATION

ACTION	RATIONALE
1. Gather the necessary supplies. Stand in front of the sink. Do not allow your clothing to touch the sink during the washing procedure (Figure 1).	The sink is considered contaminated. Clothing may carry organisms from place to place.
2. Remove jewelry, if possible, and secure in a safe place. A plain wedding band may remain in place.	Removal of jewelry facilitates proper cleansing. Microorganisms may accumulate in settings of jewelry. If jewelry was worn during care, it should be left on during handwashing.

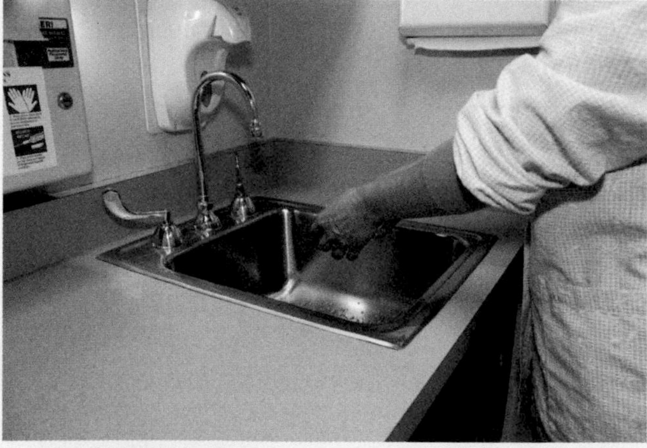

Figure 1. Standing in front of sink.

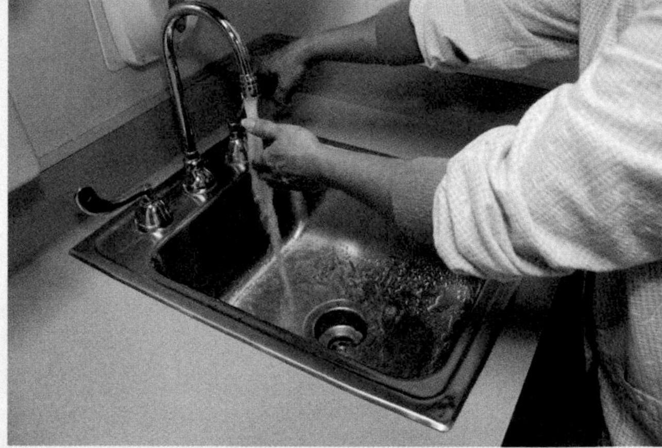

Figure 2. Turning on the water at the sink.

ACTION	RATIONALE
3. Turn on water and adjust force (Figure 2). Regulate the temperature until the water is warm.	Water splashed from the contaminated sink will contaminate clothing. Warm water is more comfortable and is less likely to open pores and remove oils from the skin. Organisms can lodge in roughened and broken areas of chapped skin.
4. Wet the hands and wrist area. Keep hands lower than elbows to allow water to flow toward fingertips (Figure 3).	Water should flow from the cleaner area toward the more contaminated area. Hands are more contaminated than forearms.

SKILL 4-1

Performing Hand Hygiene Using Soap and Water (Handwashing) *(continued)*

ACTION	RATIONALE
5. Use about 1 teaspoon liquid soap from dispenser or rinse bar of soap and lather thoroughly (Figure 4). Cover all areas of hands with the soap product. Rinse soap bar again and return to soap dish.	Rinsing the soap before and after use removes the lather, which may contain microorganisms.

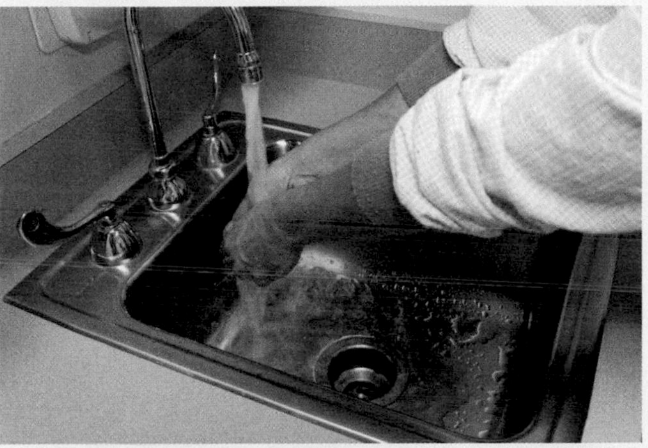

Figure 3. Wetting hands to the wrist.

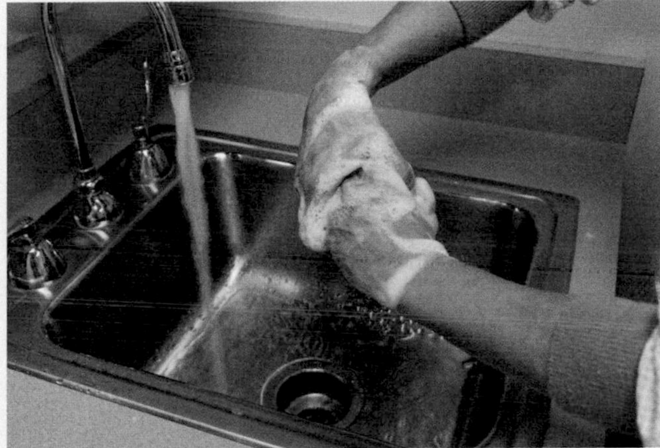

Figure 4. Lathering hands with soap and rubbing with firm circular motion.

ACTION	RATIONALE
6. With firm rubbing and circular motions, wash the palms and backs of the hands, each finger, the areas between the fingers (Figure 5), and the knuckles, wrists, and forearms. **Wash at least 1″ above area of contamination.** If hands are not visibly soiled, wash to 1″ above the wrists (Figure 6).	Friction caused by firm rubbing and circular motions helps to loosen dirt and organisms that can lodge between the fingers, in skin crevices of knuckles, on the palms and backs of the hands, and on the wrists and forearms. Cleaning less contaminated areas (forearms and wrists) after hands are clean prevents spreading microorganisms from the hands to the forearms and wrists.

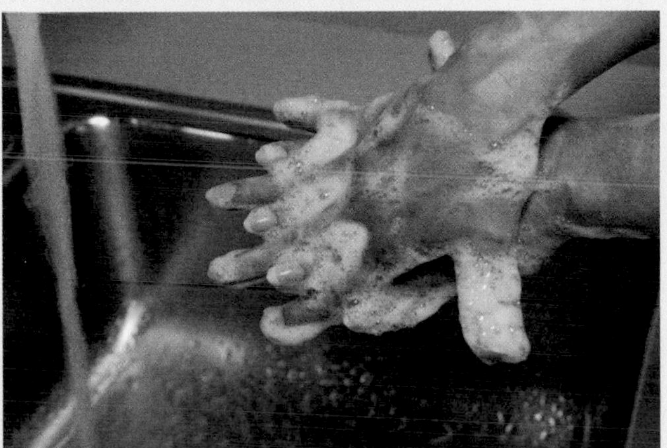

Figure 5. Washing areas between fingers.

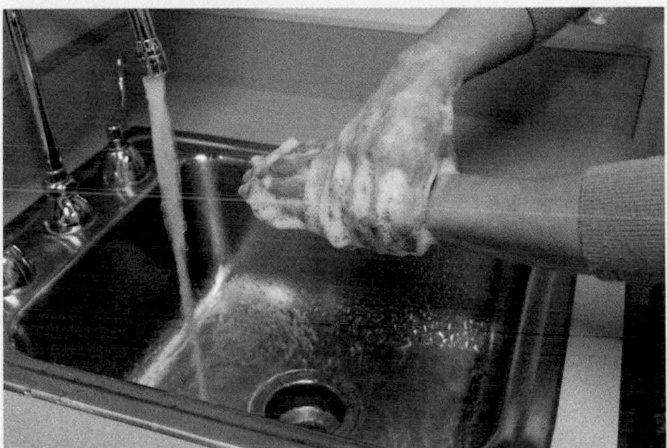

Figure 6. Washing to 1 inch above the wrist.

(continued)

SKILL 4-1 Performing Hand Hygiene Using Soap and Water (Handwashing) *(continued)*

ACTION	RATIONALE
7. Continue this friction motion for at least 15 seconds.	Length of handwashing is determined by degree of contamination.
8. Use fingernails of the opposite hand or a clean orange-wood stick to clean under fingernails (Figure 7).	Area under nails has a high microorganism count, and organisms may remain under the nails, where the organisms can grow and be spread to other persons.
9. Rinse thoroughly with water flowing toward fingertips (Figure 8).	Running water rinses microorganisms and dirt into the sink.

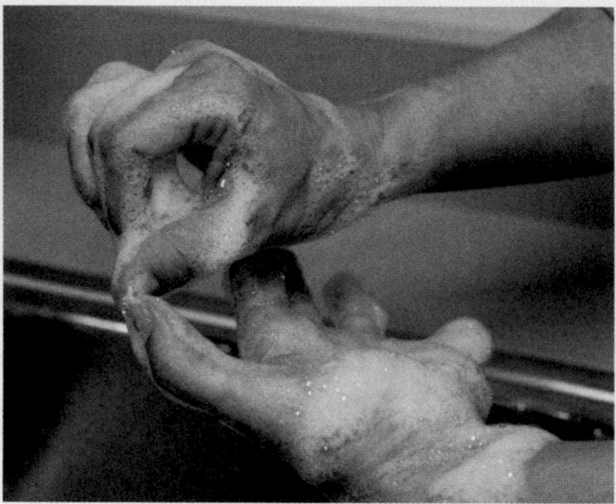

Figure 7. Using fingernails to clean under nails of opposite hand.

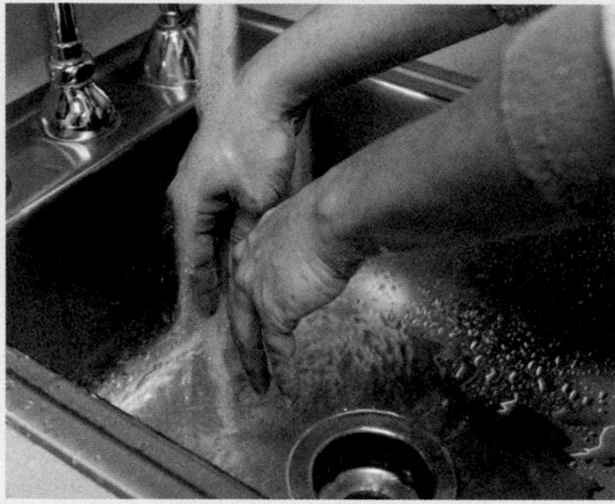

Figure 8. Rinsing hands under running water with water flowing toward fingertips.

ACTION	RATIONALE
10. Pat hands dry with a paper towel, beginning with the fingers and moving upward toward forearms, and discard it immediately. Use another clean towel to turn off the faucet. Discard towel immediately without touching other clean hand.	Patting the skin dry prevents chapping. Dry hands first because they are considered the cleanest and least contaminated area. Turning the faucet off with a clean paper towel protects the clean hands from contact with a soiled surface.
11. Use oil-free lotion on hands if desired.	Oil-free lotion helps to keep the skin soft and prevents chapping. It is best applied after patient care is complete and from small, personal containers. Oil-based lotions should be avoided because they can cause deterioration of gloves.

EVALUATION

The expected outcome is met when the hands are free of visible soiling and transient microorganisms are eliminated.

Special Considerations

- An antimicrobial soap product is recommended for use with handwashing before participating in an invasive procedure and after exposure to blood or body fluids. The length of the scrub will vary based on need.
- Liquid or bar soap, granules, or leaflets are all acceptable forms of non-antimicrobial soap.

SKILL 4-2 Performing Hand Hygiene Using an Alcohol-Based Hand Rub

Alcohol-based hand rubs can be used in the healthcare setting and take less time to use than traditional handwashing. When using these products, check the product labeling for correct amount of product needed. Alcohol-based hand rubs (CDC, 2002a; 2002b):

- May be used if hands are not visibly soiled, or have not come in contact with blood or body fluids
- Should be used before and after each patient contact, or contact with surfaces in the patient's environment
- Significantly reduce the number of microorganisms on skin, are fast acting, and cause less skin irritation.

Equipment

- Alcohol-based hand rub
- Oil-free lotion (optional)

ASSESSMENT

Assess hands for any visible soiling or contact with blood or body fluids. Alcohol-based hand rubs may be used if hands are not visibly soiled, or have not come in contact with blood or body fluids.

If food is to be eaten, or the nurse has used the restroom, hands must be washed with soap and water. If hands are visibly soiled, proceed with washing the hands with soap and water. If hands have been in contact with blood or body fluids, even if there is no visible soiling, proceed with washing the hands with soap and water.

NURSING DIAGNOSIS

Determine the related factors for the nursing diagnoses based on the patient's current status. An appropriate nursing diagnosis is Risk for Infection. Many other nursing diagnoses also may require the use of this skill.

OUTCOME IDENTIFICATION AND PLANNING

The expected outcome to achieve when performing hand decontamination with alcohol-based rubs is that transient microorganisms will be eliminated from the hands. Other outcomes may be appropriate depending on the specific nursing diagnosis identified for the patient.

IMPLEMENTATION

ACTION	RATIONALE
1. Remove jewelry, if possible, and secure in a safe place. A plain wedding band may remain in place.	Removal of jewelry facilitates proper cleansing. Microorganisms may accumulate in settings of jewelry. If jewelry was worn during care, it should be left on during handwashing.
2. Check the product labeling for correct amount of product needed (Figure 1).	Amount of product required to be effective varies from manufacturer to manufacturer.
3. Apply the correct amount of product to the palm of one hand. Rub hands together, covering all surfaces of hands and fingers.	Adequate amount of product is required to thoroughly cover hand surfaces. All surfaces must be treated to prevent disease transmission.
4. Rub hands together until they are dry.	Drying ensures antiseptic effect.

(continued)

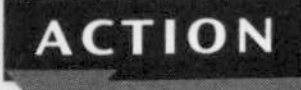

SKILL 4-2 Performing Hand Hygiene Using an Alcohol-Based Hand Rub *(continued)*

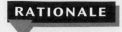

ACTION | **RATIONALE**

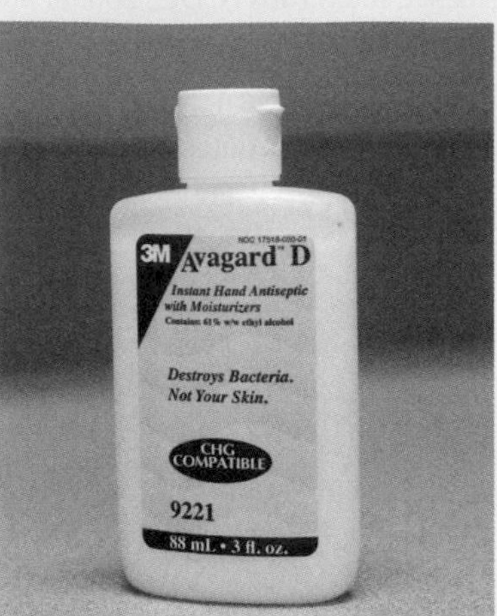

Figure 1. Checking product label for correct amount of product needed.

5. Use oil-free lotion on hands if desired.

Oil-free lotion helps to keep the skin soft and prevents chapping. It is best applied after patient care is complete and from small, personal containers. Oil-based lotions should be avoided because they can cause deterioration of gloves.

EVALUATION The expected outcome is met when transient microorganisms are eliminated from the hands.

SKILL 4-3 Preparing a Sterile Field Using a Packaged Sterile Drape

A sterile field is created to provide a surgically aseptic workspace. It should be considered a restricted area. A sterile drape may be used to establish a sterile field or to extend the sterile working area. The sterile drape should be waterproof on one side, with that side placed down on the work surface. After establishing the sterile field, other sterile items needed, including solutions, are added. Sterile items and sterile gloved hands are the only objects allowed in the sterile field. Refer to Fundamentals Review 4-2 to review basic principles of surgical asepsis.

Equipment

- Sterile wrapped drape
- Additional sterile supplies, such as dressings, containers, or solution, as needed

ASSESSMENT Assess the situation to determine the necessity for creating a sterile field. Then assess the area in which the sterile field is to be prepared. Move any unnecessary equipment out of the immediate vicinity.

SKILL 4-3 Preparing a Sterile Field Using a Packaged Sterile Drape *(continued)*

NURSING DIAGNOSIS

Determine the related factors for the nursing diagnoses based on the patient's current status. Appropriate nursing diagnoses may include:

- Risk for Infection
- Ineffective Protection

In addition, other nursing diagnoses also may require the use of this skill.

OUTCOME IDENTIFICATION AND PLANNING

The expected outcome to achieve when preparing a sterile field is that the sterile field is created without evidence of contamination and the patient remains free of exposure to potential infection-causing microorganisms.

IMPLEMENTATION

ACTION	RATIONALE
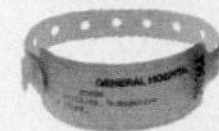 1. Identify the patient. Explain the procedure to the patient.	Identifying the patient ensures the right patient receives the intervention and helps prevent errors. An explanation encourages patient cooperation and reduces apprehension.
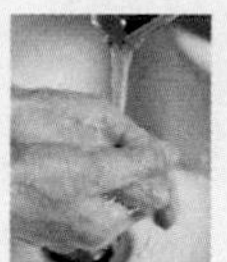 2. Perform hand hygiene.	Hand hygiene deters the spread of microorganisms.
3. Check that packaged sterile drape is dry and unopened. Also note expiration date, making sure that the date is still valid.	Moisture contaminates a sterile package. Expiration date indicates period that package remains sterile.
4. Select a work area that is waist level or higher.	Work area is within sight. Bacteria tend to settle, so there is less contamination above the waist.
5. Open the outer covering of the drape. Remove sterile drape, lifting it carefully by its corners. Hold away from body and above the waist and work surface.	Outer 1″ (2.5 cm) of drape is considered contaminated. Any item touching this area is also considered contaminated.
6. Continue to hold only by the corners. Allow the drape to unfold, away from your body and any other surface (Figure 1).	Touching outer side of wrapper maintains sterile field. Contact with any surface would contaminate the field.
7. Position the drape on the work surface with the moisture-proof side down (Figure 2). This would be the shiny or blue side. Avoid touching any other surface or object with the drape.	Moisture-proof side prevents contamination of the field if it becomes wet. The moisture penetrates the sterile cloth or paper and carries organisms by capillary action to contaminate the field. A wet field is considered contaminated if the surface immediately below it is not sterile.
8. Place additional sterile items on field as needed. Refer to Skill 4-5. Continue with the procedure as indicated.	Sterility of the field is maintained.

(continued)

SKILL 4-3

Preparing a Sterile Field Using a Packaged Sterile Drape *(continued)*

ACTION | **RATIONALE**

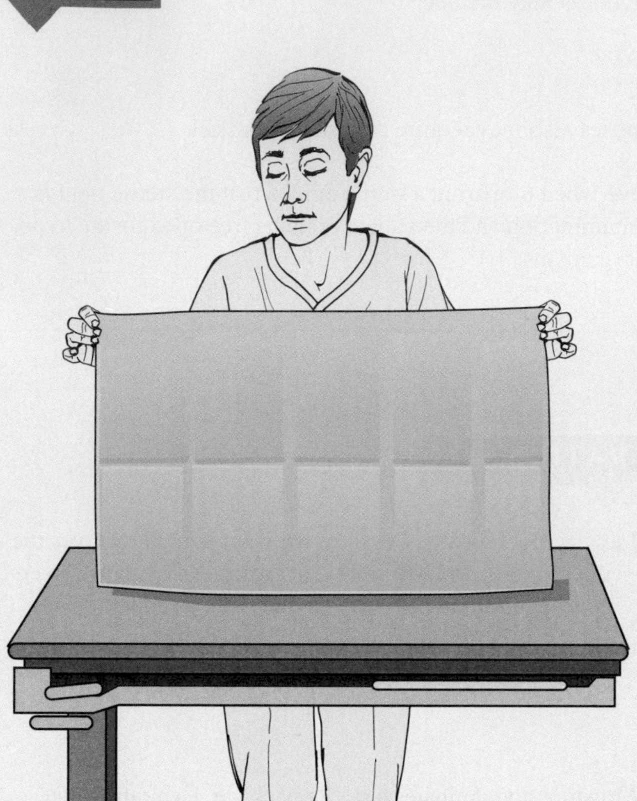

Figure 1. Holding drape by corners and allow it to unfold away from body and surfaces.

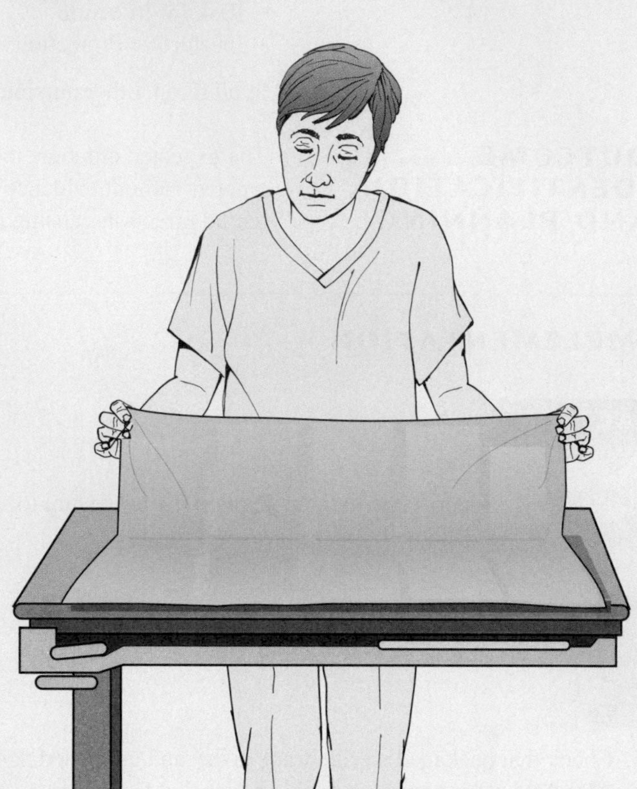

Figure 2. Positioning the drape on the work surface with the moisture-proof side down.

EVALUATION

The expected outcome is met when the sterile field is prepared without contamination and the patient has remained free of exposure to potentially infectious microorganisms.

DOCUMENTATION

It is not usually necessary to document the preparation of a sterile field. However, documentation should be recorded regarding the use of sterile technique for any procedure performed using sterile technique.

Unexpected Situations and Associated Interventions

- *A part of the sterile field becomes contaminated:* When any portion of the sterile field becomes contaminated, discard all portions of the sterile field and start over.
- *You realize you are missing a supply:* Call for help. Do not leave the sterile field unattended. If you are not able to visualize the sterile field at all times, it is considered contaminated.
- *The patient touches your hands or the sterile field:* If the patient touches your hands and nothing else, you may remove your contaminated gloves and don new, sterile gloves. It is always a good idea to bring two pairs of sterile gloves into the room. If the patient touches the sterile field, discard the supplies and prepare a new sterile field. If the patient is confused, it is a good idea to have someone assist you by holding the patient's hands or reinforcing what is happening.

SKILL 4-4 Preparing a Sterile Field Using a Commercially Prepared Sterile Kit or Tray

A sterile field is created to provide a surgically aseptic workspace. It should be considered a restricted area. Commercially prepared sterile kits and trays are wrapped in a sterile wrapper that, once opened, becomes the sterile field. Sterile items and sterile gloved hands are the only objects allowed in the sterile field. If the area is breached, the entire sterile field is considered contaminated. Refer to Fundamentals Review 4-2 for guidelines related to working with a sterile field.

Equipment

- Commercially prepared sterile package
- Additional sterile supplies, such as dressings, containers, or solution, as needed

ASSESSMENT

Assess the situation to determine the necessity for creating a sterile field. Then assess the area in which the sterile field is to be prepared. Move any unnecessary equipment out of the immediate vicinity.

NURSING DIAGNOSIS

Determine the related factors for the nursing diagnoses based on the patient's current status. Appropriate nursing diagnoses may include:

- Risk for Infection
- Ineffective Protection

In addition, other nursing diagnoses also may require the use of this skill.

OUTCOME IDENTIFICATION AND PLANNING

The expected outcome to achieve when opening a commercially packaged sterile kit or tray is that a sterile field is created without evidence of contamination, the contents of the package remain sterile, and the patient remains free of exposure to potential infection-causing microorganisms.

IMPLEMENTATION

ACTION	RATIONALE
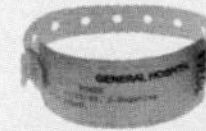 1. Identify the patient. Explain the procedure to the patient.	Identifying the patient ensures the right patient receives the intervention and helps prevent errors. An explanation encourages patient cooperation and reduces apprehension.
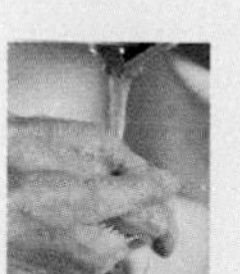 2. Perform hand hygiene.	Hand hygiene deters the spread of microorganisms.
3. Check that packaged kit or tray is dry and unopened. Also note expiration date, making sure that the date is still valid.	Moisture contaminates a sterile package. Expiration date indicates period that package remains sterile.
4. Select a work area that is waist level or higher.	Work area is within sight. Bacteria tend to settle, so there is less contamination above the waist.
5. Open the outside cover of the package and remove the kit or tray. Place in the center of the work surface.	This allows sufficient room for sterile field.
6. Reach around the package and grasp the outer surface of the end of the topmost flap, holding no more than one inch from the border of the flap. Pull open away from the body, keeping the arm outstretched and away from the inside of the wrapper (Figure 1). Allow the wrapper to lie flat on the work surface.	This maintains sterility of inside of wrapper, which is to become the sterile field. Outer surface of the wrapper is considered unsterile. Outer one inch border of the wrapper is considered contaminated.

(continued)

SKILL 4-4 Preparing a Sterile Field Using a Commercially Prepared Sterile Kit or Tray *(continued)*

ACTION	RATIONALE
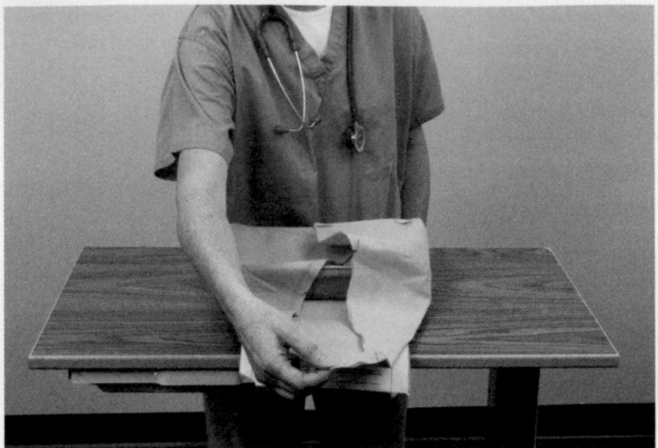 Figure 1. Pulling top flap open, away from body.	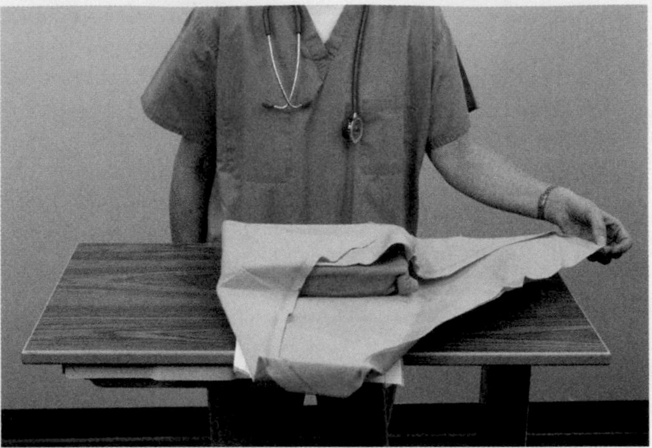 Figure 2. Pulling open the first side flap.
7. Reach around the package and grasp the outer surface of the first side flap, holding no more than one inch from the border of the flap. Pull open to the side of the package, keeping the arm outstretched and away from the inside of the wrapper (Figure 2). Allow the wrapper to lie flat on the work surface.	This maintains sterility of inside of wrapper, which is to become the sterile field. Outer surface of the wrapper is considered unsterile. Outer one inch border of the wrapper is considered contaminated.
8. Reach around the package and grasp the outer surface of the remaining side flap, holding no more than one inch from the border of the flap. Pull open to the side of the package, keeping the arm outstretched and away from the inside of the wrapper (Figure 3). Allow the wrapper to lie flat on the work surface.	This maintains sterility of inside of wrapper, which is to become the sterile field. Outer surface of the wrapper is considered unsterile. Outer one inch of border of the wrapper is considered contaminated.
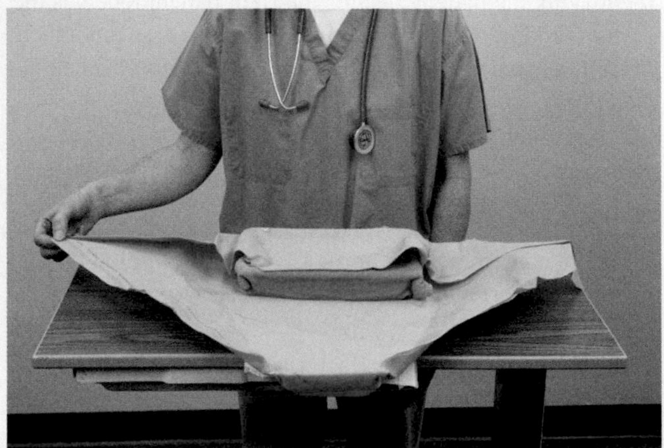 Figure 3. Pulling open the remaining side flap.	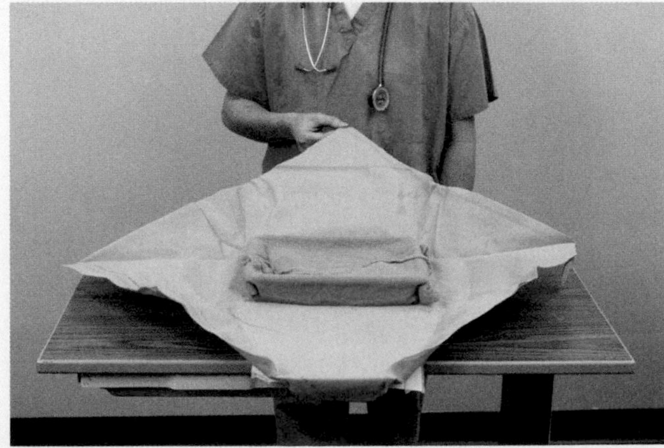 Figure 4. Pulling open flap closest to body.

SKILL 4-4 Preparing a Sterile Field Using a Commercially Prepared Sterile Kit or Tray *(continued)*

ACTION	RATIONALE
9. Stand away from the package and work surface. Grasp the outer surface of the remaining flap closest to the body, holding not more than one inch from the border of the flap. Pull the flap back toward the body, keeping arm outstretched and away from the inside of the wrapper (Figure 4). Allow the wrapper to lie flat on the work surface.	This maintains sterility of inside of wrapper, which is to become the sterile field. Outer surface of the wrapper is considered unsterile. Outer one-inch border of the wrapper is considered contaminated.
10. The outer wrapper of the package has become a sterile field with the packages supplies in the center. Do not touch or reach over the sterile field. Place additional sterile items on field as needed. Refer to Skill 4-5. Continue with the procedure as indicated.	Sterility of the field and contents are maintained.

EVALUATION

The expected outcome is met when the sterile field is prepared without contamination, the contents of the package remain sterile, and the patient remains free of exposure to potential infection-causing microorganisms.

DOCUMENTATION

It is not usually necessary to document the preparation of a sterile field. However, documentation should be recorded regarding the use of sterile technique for any procedure performed using sterile technique.

Unexpected Situations and Associated Interventions

- *A part of the sterile field becomes contaminated:* When any portion of the sterile field becomes contaminated, discard all portions of the sterile field and start over.
- *You realize you are missing a supply:* Call for help. Do not leave the sterile field unattended. If you are not able to visualize the sterile field at all times, it is considered contaminated.
- *The patient touches the sterile field:* If the patient touches the sterile field, discard the supplies and prepare a new sterile field. If the patient is confused, it is a good idea to have someone assist you by holding the patient's hands or reinforcing what is happening.

SKILL 4-5 Adding Sterile Items to a Sterile Field

A sterile field is created to provide a surgically aseptic workspace. It should be considered a restricted area. After establishing the sterile field, other sterile items needed, including solutions, are added. Items can be wrapped and sterilized within the agency or can be commercially prepared. Care must be taken to ensure that nothing unsterile touches the field or other items in the field, including hands or clothes. Refer to Fundamentals Review 4-2 for guidelines related to working with a sterile field.

Equipment

- Sterile field
- Sterile gauze, forceps, dressings, containers, solutions, or other sterile supplies as needed

(continued)

SKILL 4-5 Adding Sterile Items to a Sterile Field *(continued)*

ASSESSMENT

Assess the situation to determine the necessity for creating a sterile field. Assess the area in which the sterile field is to be prepared. Move any unnecessary equipment out of the immediate vicinity. Identify additional supplies needed for procedure.

NURSING DIAGNOSIS

Determine the related factors for the nursing diagnoses based on the patient's current status. Appropriate nursing diagnoses may include:

- Risk for Infection
- Ineffective Protection

In addition, other nursing diagnoses also may require the use of this skill.

OUTCOME IDENTIFICATION AND PLANNING

The expected outcome to achieve when adding items to a sterile field is that the sterile field is created without evidence of contamination, the sterile supplies are not contaminated, and the patient remains free of exposure to potential infection-causing microorganisms.

IMPLEMENTATION

ACTION	RATIONALE
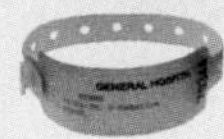 1. Identify the patient. Explain the procedure to the patient.	Identifying the patient ensures the right patient receives the intervention and helps prevent errors. An explanation encourages patient cooperation and reduces apprehension.
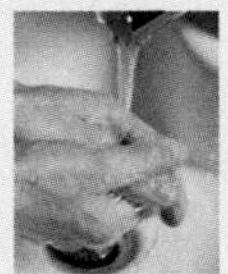 2. Perform hand hygiene.	Hand hygiene deters the spread of microorganisms.
3. Check that the sterile, packaged drape and supplies are dry and unopened. Also note expiration date, making sure that the date is still valid.	Moisture contaminates a sterile package. Expiration date indicates period that package remains sterile.
4. Select a work area that is waist level or higher.	Work area is within sight. Bacteria tend to settle, so there is less contamination above the waist.
5. Prepare sterile field as described in Skill 4-3 or Skill 4-4.	Proper technique maintains sterility.
6. Add sterile item:	
To Add an Agency-Wrapped and Sterilized Item:	
a. Hold agency-wrapped item in the dominant hand, with top flap opening away from the body. With other hand, reach around the package and unfold top flap and both sides.	Only sterile surface and item are exposed before dropping onto sterile field.
b. Keep a secure hold on item through the wrapper with the dominant hand. Grasp the remaining flap of the wrapper closest to the body, taking care not to touch the inner surface of the wrapper or the item. Pull the flap back toward the wrist, so the wrapper covers the hand and wrist.	Only sterile surface and item are exposed before dropping onto sterile field.

SKILL 4-5 Adding Sterile Items to a Sterile Field *(continued)*

ACTION	RATIONALE
c. Grasp all the corners of the wrapper together with the nondominant hand and pull back toward wrist, covering hand and wrist. Hold in place.	Only sterile surface and item are exposed before dropping onto sterile field.
d. Hold the item 6 inches above the surface of the sterile field and drop onto the field. Be careful to avoid touching the surface or other items or dropping onto the 1″ border.	Prevents contamination of the field and inadvertent dropping of the sterile item too close to the edge or off the field. Any items landing on 1″ border are considered contaminated.
To Add a Commercially Wrapped and Sterilized Item:	
a. Hold package in one hand. Pull back top cover with other hand. Alternately, carefully peel the edges apart using both hands (Figure 1).	Contents remain uncontaminated by hands.
b. After top cover or edges are partially separated, hold the item 6 inches above the surface of the sterile field. Continue opening the package and drop the item onto the field (Figure 2). Be careful to avoid touching the surface or other items or dropping onto the 1″ border.	This prevents contamination of the field and inadvertent dropping of the sterile item too close to the edge or off the field. Any items landing on 1″ border are considered contaminated.
c. Discard wrapper.	A neat work area promotes proper technique.

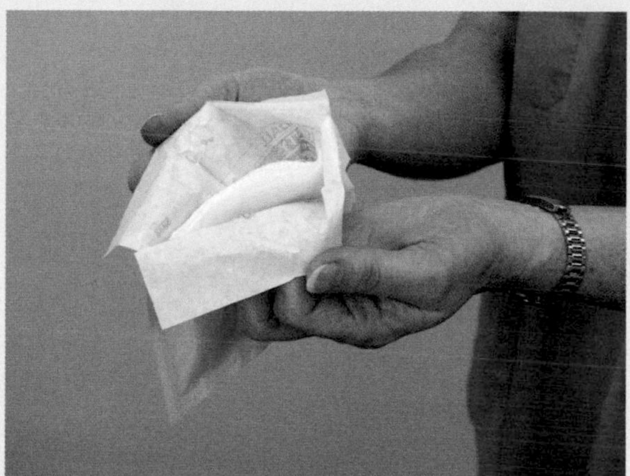

Figure 1. Carefully peeling edges apart.

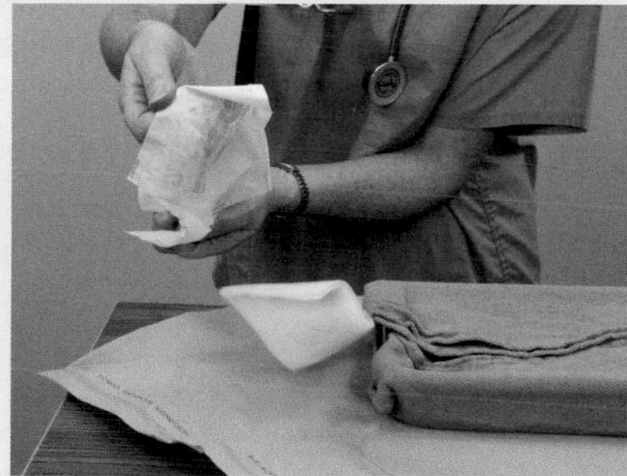

Figure 2. Dropping sterile item onto sterile field.

ACTION	RATIONALE
To Add a Sterile Solution:	
a. Obtain appropriate solution and check expiration date.	Once opened, a bottle should be labeled with date and time. Solution remains sterile for 24 hours once opened.
b. Open solution container according to directions and **place cap on table with edges up (Figure 3).**	Sterility of inside cap is maintained.
c. If bottle has previously been opened, "lip" it by pouring a small amount of solution into waste container (Figure 4).	This cleanses the lip of the bottle.
d. Hold bottle outside the edge of the sterile field with the label side facing the palm of your hand and prepare to pour from a height of 4″ to 6″ (10 to 15 cm). The tip of the bottle should never touch a sterile container or dressing (Figure 5).	Label remains dry, and solution may be poured without reaching across sterile field. Minimal splashing occurs from that height. Accidentally touching the tip of the bottle to a container or dressing contaminates them both.

(continued)

SKILL 4-5 Adding Sterile Items to a Sterile Field *(continued)*

ACTION	RATIONALE
e. Pour required amount of solution steadily into sterile container positioned at side of sterile field or onto dressings. **Avoid splashing any liquid.**	Moisture contaminates sterile field.
f. Touch only the outside of the lid when recapping. Label solution with date and time of opening.	Solution remains uncontaminated.
7. Continue with procedure as indicated.	

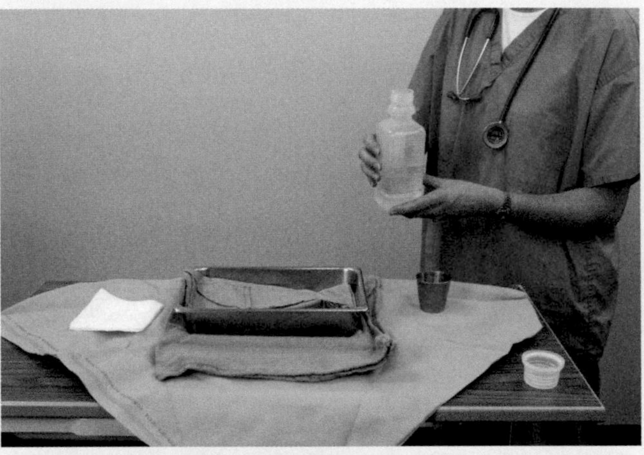

Figure 3. Opening bottle of sterile solution without contaminating the cap.

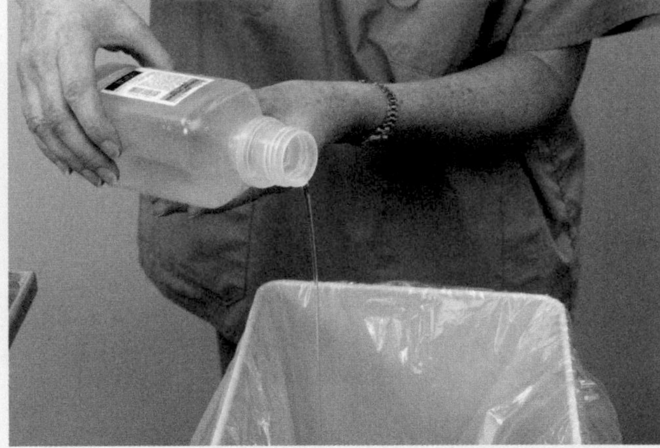

Figure 4. Pouring off a small amount of solution into a trash receptacle.

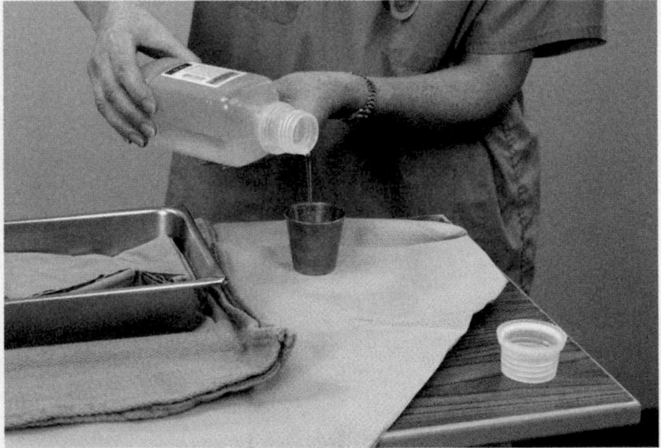

Figure 5. Pouring solution into sterile container.

EVALUATION

The expected outcome to achieve when adding items to a sterile field is that the sterile field is created without evidence of contamination, the sterile supplies are not contaminated, and the patient remains free of exposure to potential infection-causing microorganisms.

DOCUMENTATION

It is not usually necessary to document the addition of sterile items to a sterile field. However, documentation should be recorded regarding the use of sterile technique for any procedure performed using sterile technique.

SKILL 4-6 Putting on Sterile Gloves and Removing Soiled Gloves

While working within a sterile field, sterile gloves must be used. Applying, using, and disposing of sterile gloves requires specific skills to avoid contamination. When applying and wearing sterile gloves, keep your hands above waist level and away from nonsterile surfaces. Any item or hand that goes below your waist is considered contaminated. If this happens, replace your gloves or the item immediately. Also be prepared to replace your gloves if they develop an opening or tear, the integrity of the material becomes compromised, or the gloves come in contact with any unsterile surface or unsterile item. Refer to Fundamentals Review 4-2 for additional guidelines related to working with sterile gloves. It is a good idea to bring an extra pair of gloves when you gather your supplies, according to facility policy. That way, if the first pair is contaminated in some way and needs to be replaced, you won't have to leave the procedure to get a new pair.

Equipment

- Sterile gloves of the appropriate size

ASSESSMENT

Assess the situation to determine the necessity for sterile gloves. In addition, check the patient's chart for information about a possible latex allergy. Also, question the patient about any history of allergy, including latex allergy or sensitivity and signs and symptoms that have occurred. If the patient has a latex allergy, anticipate the need for latex-free gloves.

NURSING DIAGNOSIS

Determine the related factors for the nursing diagnoses based on the patient's current status. An appropriate nursing diagnosis is Risk for Infection. Other nursing diagnoses that may be appropriate include:

- Ineffective Protection
- Risk for Latex Allergy Response

Many other nursing diagnoses also may require the use of this skill.

OUTCOME IDENTIFICATION AND PLANNING

The expected outcome to achieve when putting on and removing sterile gloves is that the gloves are applied and removed without contamination. Other outcomes that may be appropriate include the following: the patient remains free of exposure to infectious microorganisms, and the patient does not exhibit signs and symptoms of a latex allergy response.

IMPLEMENTATION

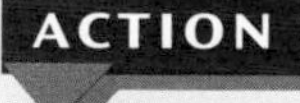

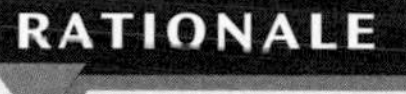

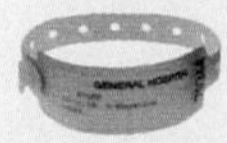

1. Identify the patient. Explain the procedure to the patient.

Identifying the patient ensures the right patient receives the intervention and helps prevent errors. An explanation encourages patient cooperation and reduces apprehension.

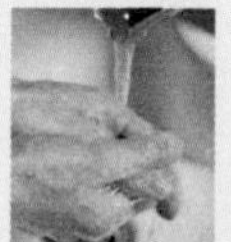

2. Perform hand hygiene.

Hand hygiene deters the spread of microorganisms.

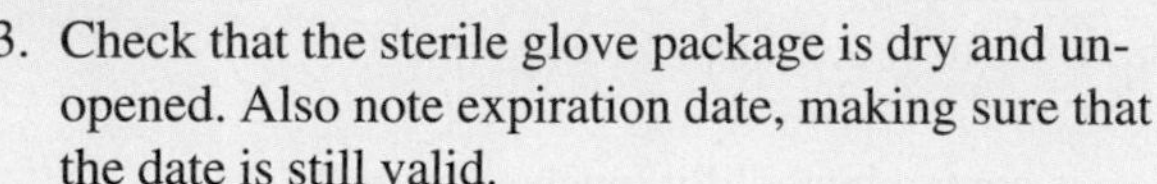

3. Check that the sterile glove package is dry and unopened. Also note expiration date, making sure that the date is still valid.

Moisture contaminates a sterile package. Expiration date indicates period that package remains sterile.

(continued)

SKILL 4-6 Putting on Sterile Gloves and Removing Soiled Gloves *(continued)*

ACTION	RATIONALE
4. Place sterile glove package on clean, dry surface at or above your waist.	Moisture could contaminate the sterile gloves. Any sterile object held below the waist is considered contaminated.
5. Open the outside wrapper by carefully peeling the top layer back (Figure 1). Remove inner package, handling only the outside of it.	This maintains sterility of gloves in inner packet.

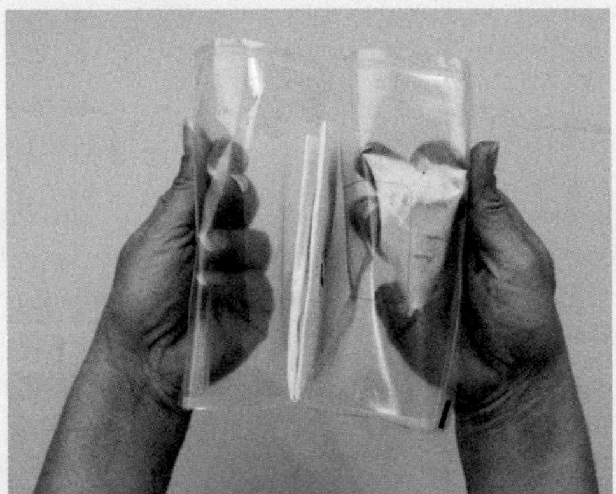

Figure 1. Pulling top layer of outside wrapper back.

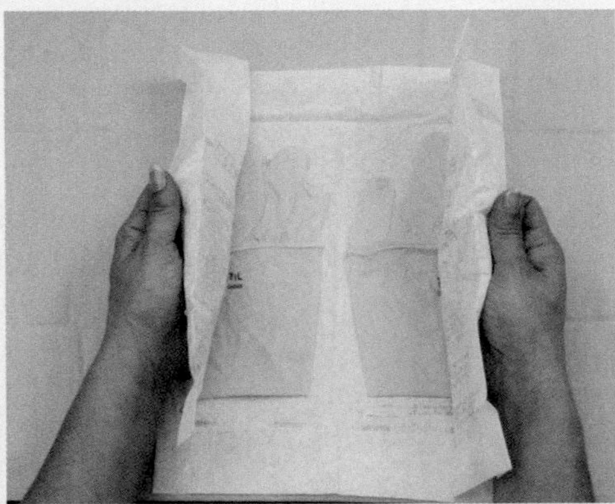

Figure 2. Folding back side flaps.

ACTION	RATIONALE
6. Place the inner package on the work surface with the side labeled 'cuff end' closest to the body.	Allows for ease of glove application.
7. Carefully open the inner package. Fold open the top flap, then the bottom and sides (Figure 2). Take care not to touch the inner surface of the package or the gloves.	The inner surface of the package is considered sterile. The outer 1″ border of the inner package is considered contaminated. The sterile gloves are exposed with the cuff end closest to the nurse.
8. With the thumb and forefinger of the nondominant hand, grasp the folded cuff of the glove for dominant hand, touching only the exposed inside of the glove (Figure 3).	Unsterile hand touches only inside of glove. Outside remains sterile.

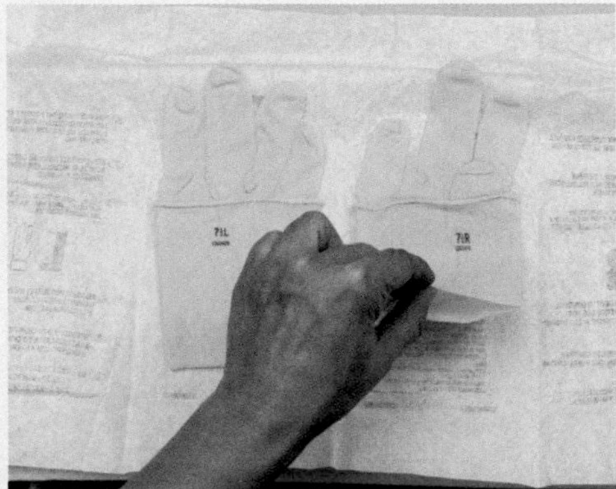

Figure 3. Grasping cuff of glove for dominant hand.

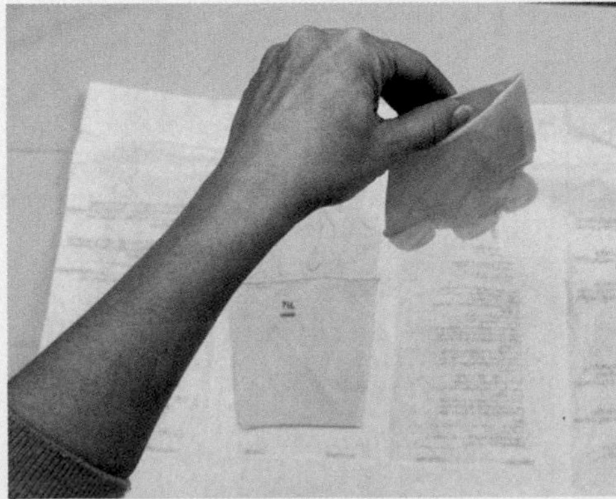

Figure 4. Lifting glove from package.

ACTION	RATIONALE
9. Keeping the hands above the waistline, lift and hold the glove up and off the inner package with fingers down (Figure 4). **Be careful it does not touch any unsterile object.**	Glove is contaminated if it touches unsterile object.

SKILL 4-6

Putting on Sterile Gloves and Removing Soiled Gloves *(continued)*

ACTION	RATIONALE
10. Carefully insert dominant hand palm up into glove (Figure 5) and pull glove on. Leave the cuff folded until the opposite hand is gloved.	Attempting to turn upward with unsterile hand may result in contamination of sterile glove.

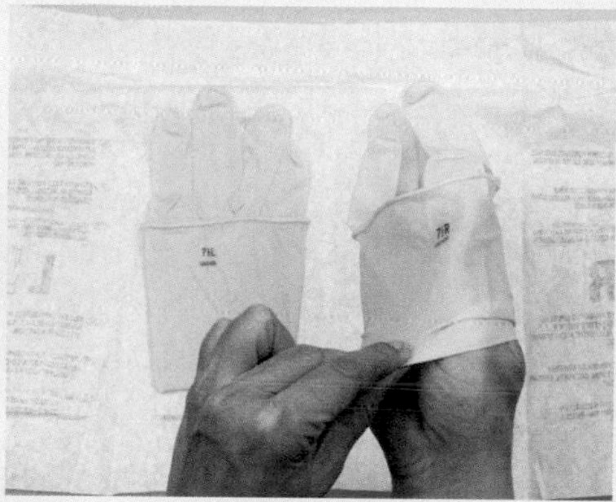

Figure 5. Inserting dominant hand into glove.

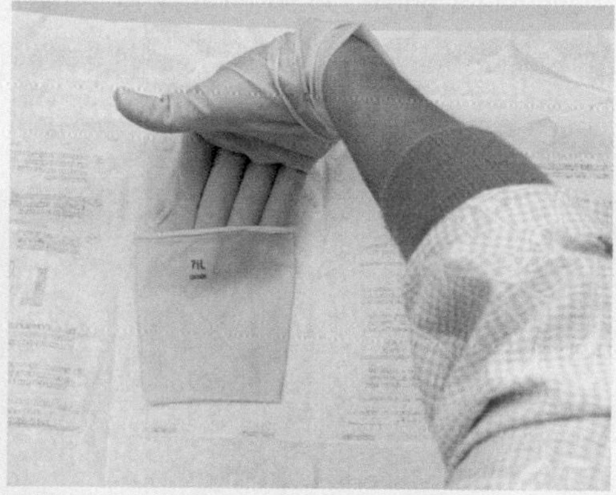

Figure 6. Sliding fingers under cuff of glove for nondominant hand.

ACTION	RATIONALE
11. Hold the thumb of the gloved hand outward. Place the fingers of the gloved hand inside the cuff of the remaining glove (Figure 6). Lift it from the wrapper, taking care not to touch anything with the gloves or hands.	Thumb is less likely to become contaminated if held outward. Sterile surface touching sterile surface prevents contamination.
12. Carefully insert nondominant hand into glove. Pull the glove on, taking care that the skin does not touch any of the outer surfaces of the gloves.	Sterile surface touching sterile surface prevents contamination.
13. **Slide the fingers of one hand under the cuff of the other and fully extend the cuff down the arm, touching only the sterile outside of the glove (Figure 7). Repeat for the remaining hand.**	Sterile surface touching sterile surface prevents contamination.

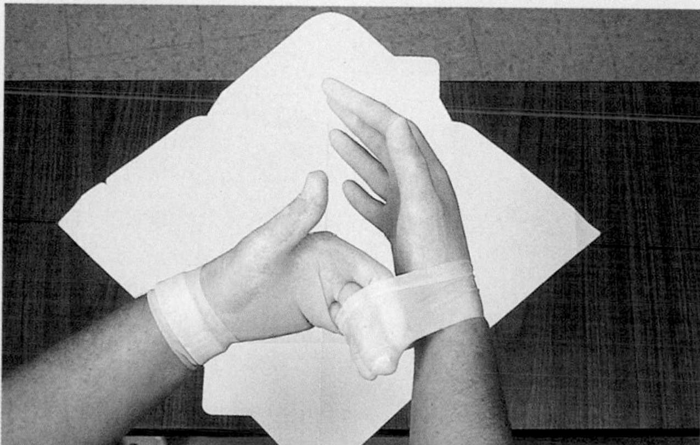

Figure 7. Sliding fingers of one hand under cuff of other hand and extending cuff down the arm.

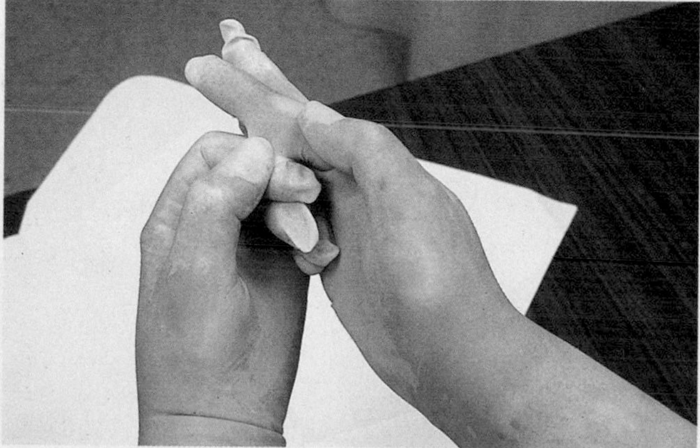

Figure 8. Adjusting gloves as necessary.

ACTION	RATIONALE
14. **Adjust gloves on both hands if necessary, touching only sterile areas with other sterile areas (Figure 8).**	Sterile surface touching sterile surface prevents contamination.

(continued)

SKILL 4-6 Putting on Sterile Gloves and Removing Soiled Gloves *(continued)*

ACTION	RATIONALE
15. Continue with procedure as indicated.	
Removing Soiled Gloves	
16. Use dominant hand to grasp the opposite glove near cuff end on the outside exposed area. Remove it by pulling it off, inverting it as it is pulled, keeping the contaminated area on the inside (Figure 9). Hold the removed glove in the remaining gloved hand.	Contaminated area does not come in contact with hands or wrists.

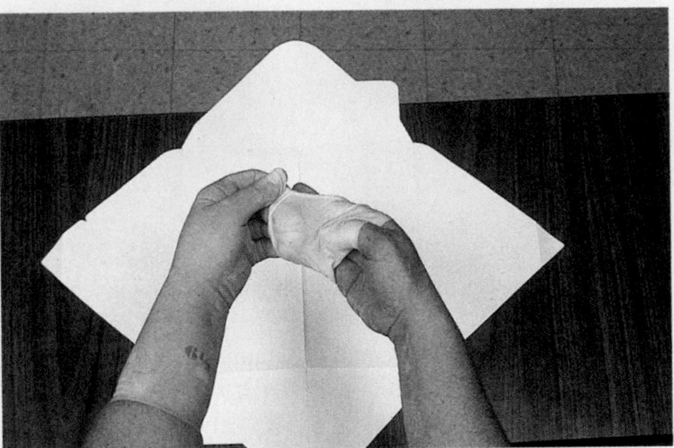

Figure 9. Inverting glove as it is removed.

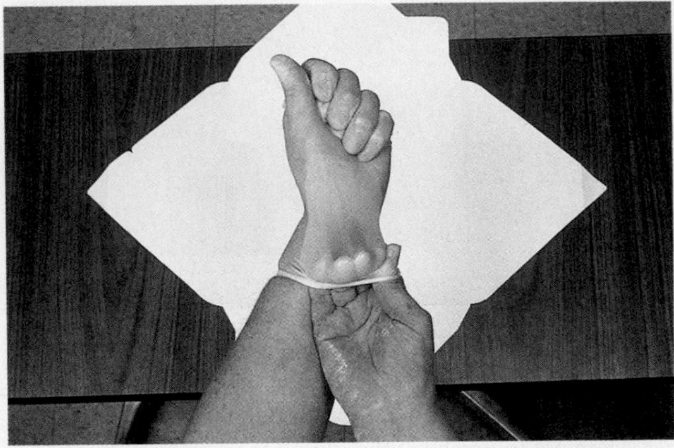

Figure 10. Sliding fingers of ungloved hand inside remaining glove.

ACTION	RATIONALE
17. Slide fingers of ungloved hand between the remaining glove and the wrist (Figure 10). Take care to avoid touching the outside surface of the glove. Remove it by pulling it off, inverting it as it is pulled, keeping the contaminated area on the inside, and securing the first glove inside the second (Figure 11).	Contaminated area does not come in contact with hands or wrists.

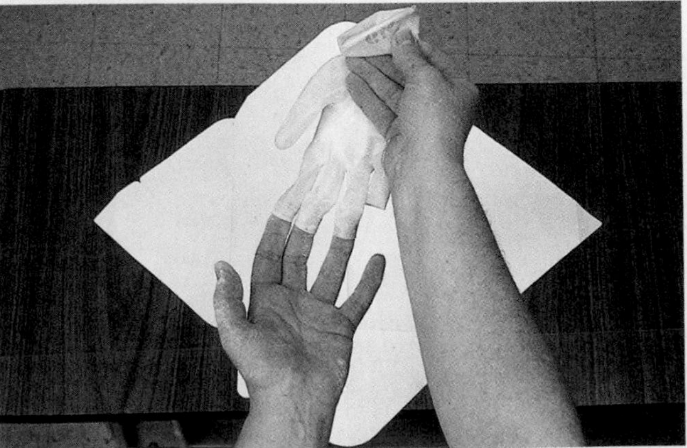

Figure 11. Inverting glove as it is removed, securing first glove inside it.

SKILL 4-6 Putting on Sterile Gloves and Removing Soiled Gloves *(continued)*

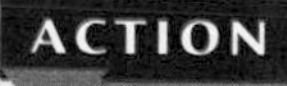

ACTION	RATIONALE
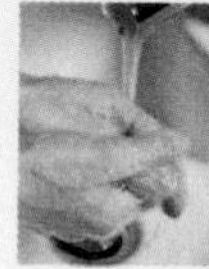 18. Discard gloves in appropriate container and perform hand hygiene.	Prevents transmission of microorganisms. Hand hygiene deters the spread of microorganisms.

EVALUATION

The expected outcome is met when gloves are applied and removed without any contamination. Other expected outcomes are met when the patient remains free of exposure to potential infection-causing microorganisms and does not exhibit any signs and symptoms of a latex allergy response.

DOCUMENTATION

It is not usually necessary to document the addition of sterile items to a sterile field. However, documentation should be recorded regarding the use of sterile technique for any procedure performed using sterile technique.

Unexpected Situations and Associated Interventions

- *Contamination occurs during application of the sterile gloves:* Discard gloves and open new package of sterile gloves.
- *A hole or tear is noticed in one of the gloves:* Discard gloves and open new package of sterile gloves.
- *A hole or tear is noticed in one of the gloves during the procedure:* Stop procedure. Remove damaged gloves. Wash hands or perform hand hygiene (depending on whether soiled or not) and put on new sterile gloves.
- *The patient touches your hands or the sterile field:* If the patient touches your hands and nothing else, you may remove your contaminated gloves and put on new, sterile gloves. It is always a good idea to bring two pairs of sterile gloves into the room, depending on facility policy. If the patient touches the sterile field, discard the supplies and prepare a new sterile field. If the patient is confused, it is a good idea to have someone assist you by holding the patient's hands or reinforcing what is happening.
- *Patient has a latex allergy:* Obtain latex-free sterile gloves.

SKILL 4-7 Using Personal Protective Equipment

Personal protective equipment (PPE) refers to specialized clothing or equipment worn by an employee for protection against infectious materials. PPE is used in healthcare settings to improve personnel safety in the healthcare environment through the appropriate use of PPE (CDC, 2004a). This equipment includes clean (unsterile) and sterile gloves, impervious gowns/aprons, surgical and high-efficiency particulate air (HEPA) masks, N95 disposable masks, face shields, and protective eyewear/goggles.

Understanding the potential contamination hazards related to the patient's diagnosis and condition and the institutional policies governing PPE is very important. The type of PPE used will vary based on the type of exposure anticipated and category of isolation precautions; Standard and Contact, Droplet, or Airborne Precautions. It is always your responsibility to enforce the proper wearing of PPE during patient care for members of the healthcare team. Refer to Fundamentals Review 4-4 and Fundamentals Review 4-5 for a summary of CDC-recommended practices for Standard and Transmission-based Precautions. Box 4-1 provides Guidelines for Effective Use of PPE.

(continued)

SKILL 4-7 **Using Personal Protective Equipment** *(continued)*

BOX 4-1 Guidelines for Effective Use of PPE

- Put on PPE before contact with the patient, preferably before entering the patient's room.
- Choose appropriate PPE based on the type of exposure anticipated and category of isolation precautions.
- When wearing gloves, work from 'clean' areas to 'dirty' ones.
- Touch as few surfaces and items with your PPE as possible.
- Avoid touching or adjusting other PPE.
- Keep gloved hands away from your face.
- If gloves become torn or heavily soiled, remove and replace. Perform hand hygiene before putting on the new gloves.
- Personal glasses are not a substitute for goggles.

(Adapted from Centers for Disease Control and Prevention. [2004a]. *PPE in healthcare settings.* [Slide presentation]. Available on-line: www.cdc.gov/ncidod/hip/ppe/default.htm. Accessed October 23, 2005)

Equipment

- Gloves
- Mask (surgical or particulate respirator)
- Impervious gown
- Protective eyewear (does not include eyeglasses)

Depending on the institution's policy, equipment for PPE may vary.

ASSESSMENT

Assess the situation to determine the necessity for PPE. In addition, check the patient's chart for information about a suspected or diagnosed infection or communicable disease. Determine the possibility of exposure to blood and body fluids and identify the necessary equipment to prevent exposure. Refer to the infection-control manual provided by your facility.

NURSING DIAGNOSIS

Determine the related factors for the nursing diagnoses based on the patient's current status. An appropriate nursing diagnosis is Risk for Infection. Many other nursing diagnoses also may require the use of this skill, including the following:

- Ineffective Protection
- Deficient Knowledge
- Bowel Incontinence
- Diarrhea
- Total Urinary Incontinence
- Impaired Skin Integrity

OUTCOME IDENTIFICATION AND PLANNING

The expected outcome to achieve when using PPE is that the transmission of microorganisms is prevented. Other outcomes that may be appropriate include the following: patient and staff remain free of exposure to potentially infectious microorganisms; patient verbalizes information about the rationale for use of PPE; episodes of bowel or urinary incontinence or diarrhea are controlled; and drainage from skin breakdown is contained.

IMPLEMENTATION

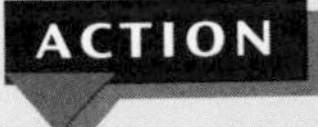

RATIONALE

ACTION	RATIONALE
1. Check physician's order for type of precautions and review precautions in infection-control manual.	Mode of transmission or organism determines type of precautions required.
2. Plan nursing activities before entering patient's room.	Organization facilitates performance of task and adherence to precautions.

SKILL 4-7 Using Personal Protective Equipment *(continued)*

ACTION	RATIONALE
3. Provide instruction about precautions to patient, family members, and visitors.	Explanation encourages cooperation of patient and family and reduces apprehension about precaution procedures.
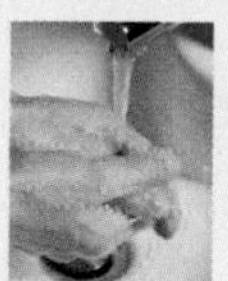 4. Perform hand hygiene.	Hand hygiene deters the spread of microorganisms.
5. Put on gown, gloves, mask, and protective eyewear, based on the type of exposure anticipated and category of isolation precautions.	Use of PPE interrupts chain of infection and protects patient and nurse. Gown should protect entire uniform. Gloves protect hands and wrists from microorganisms. Masks protect nurse or patient from droplet nuclei and large-particle aerosols. Eyewear protects mucous membranes in the eye from splashes.
a. Put on the gown, with the opening in the back. Tie gown securely at neck and waist (Figure 1).	Gown should fully cover the torso from the neck to knees, arms to the end of wrists, and wrap around the back.
b. Put on the mask or respirator over your nose, mouth and chin (Figure 2). Secure ties or elastic bands at the middle of the head and neck. If respirator is used, perform a fit check. Inhale; the respirator should collapse. Exhale; air should not leak out.	Masks protect nurse or patient from droplet nuclei and large-particle aerosols. Must fit securely to provide protection.
c. Put on goggles (Figure 3). Place over eyes and adjust to fit. Alternately, a face shield could be used to take the place of the mask and goggles (Figure 4).	Eyewear protects mucous membranes in the eye from splashes. Must fit securely to provide protection.
d. Put on clean disposable gloves. Extend gloves to cover wrists of gown (Figure 5).	Gloves protect hands and wrists from microorganisms.

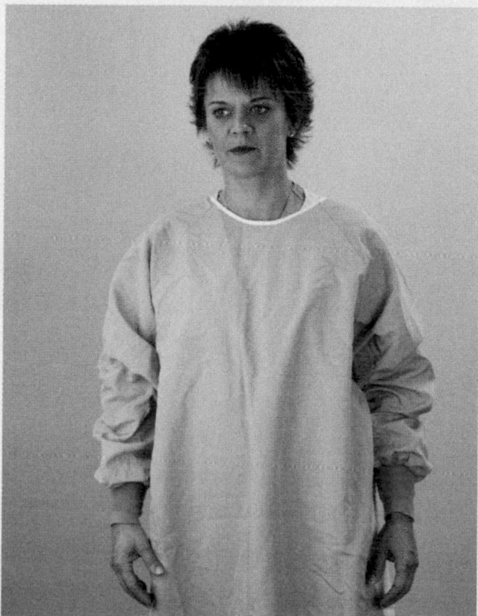

Figure 1. Gown tied at waist and neck.

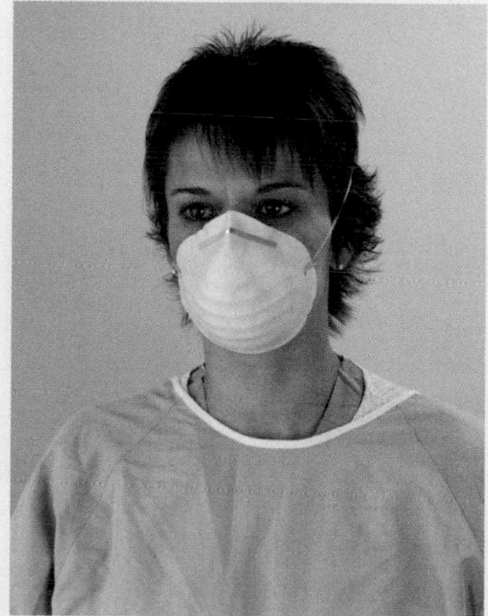

Figure 2. Mask applied over nose, mouth, and chin.

(continued)

SKILL 4-7 Using Personal Protective Equipment *(continued)*

ACTION | RATIONALE

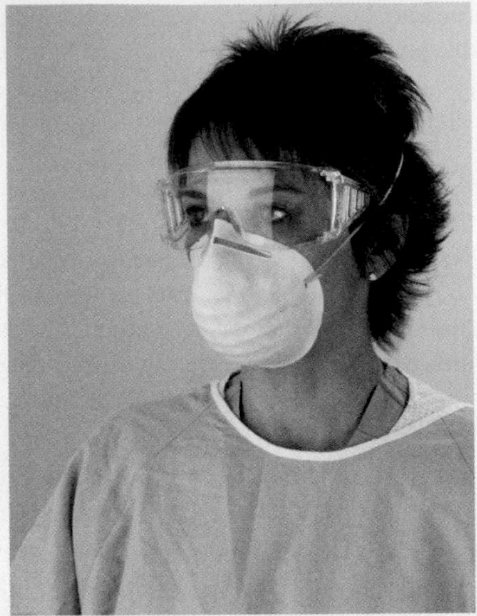

Figure 3. Goggles.

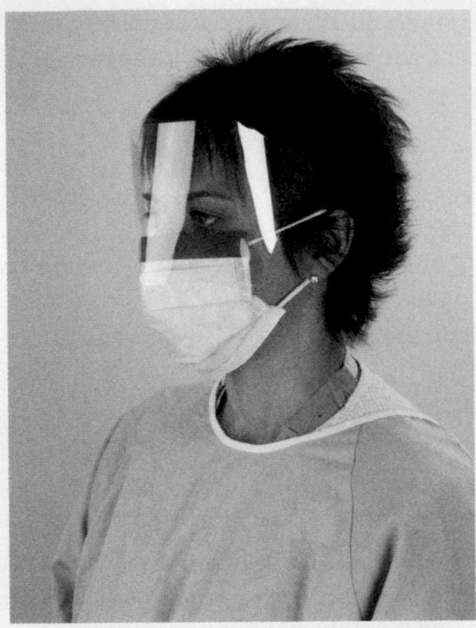

Figure 4. Face shield.

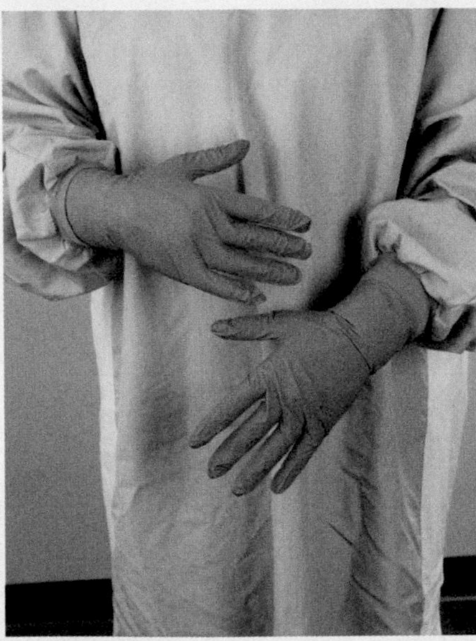

Figure 5. Glove cuffs covering wrists of gown.

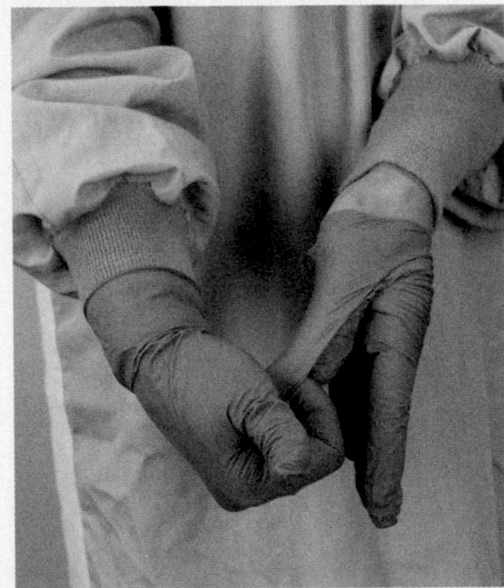

Figure 6. Grasping the outside of one glove and peeling off.

6. Remove PPE: Except for respirator, remove PPE at the doorway or in anteroom. Remove respirator after leaving the patient room and closing door.

Prevents contact with and the spread of microorganisms. Outside front of equipment is considered contaminated. The inside, outside back, ties on head and back, are considered clean; areas of PPE that are not likely to have been in contact with infectious organisms.

   a. If impervious gown has been tied in front of the body at the waistline, untie waist strings before removing gloves.

Front of gown, including waist strings, are contaminated. If tied in front of body, must be untied prior to removing gloves.

SKILL 4-7 Using Personal Protective Equipment *(continued)*

ACTION	RATIONALE
b. Grasp the outside of one glove with the opposite gloved hand and peel off, turning the glove inside out as you pull it off (Figure 6). Hold the removed glove in the remaining gloved hand.	Outside of gloves are contaminated.
c. Slide fingers of ungloved hand under the remaining glove at the wrist, taking care not to touch the outer surface of the glove (Figure 7).	Ungloved hand is clean and should not touch contaminated areas.
d. Peel off the glove over the first glove, containing the one glove inside the other (Figure 8). Discard in appropriate container.	Prevents transmission of microorganisms.
e. To remove the goggles: Handle by the head band or ear pieces. Lift away from the face. Place in designated receptacle for reprocessing or in an appropriate waste container.	Outside of goggles or face shield is contaminated. Prevents transmission of microorganisms.
f. To remove gown: Unfasten ties, if at the neck and back. Allow the gown to fall away from shoulders. Touching only the inside of the gown, pull away from the torso. Keeping hands on the inner surface of the gown, pull from arms. Turn gown inside out. Fold or roll into a bundle and discard.	Gown front and sleeves are contaminated. Prevents transmission of microorganisms.
g. To remove mask or respirator: Grasp the neck ties or elastic, then top ties or elastic and remove. Take care to avoid touching front of mask or respirator. Discard in waste container. If using a respirator, save for future use in the designated area.	Front of mask or respirator is contaminated; **Do Not Touch.** Prevents transmission of microorganisms

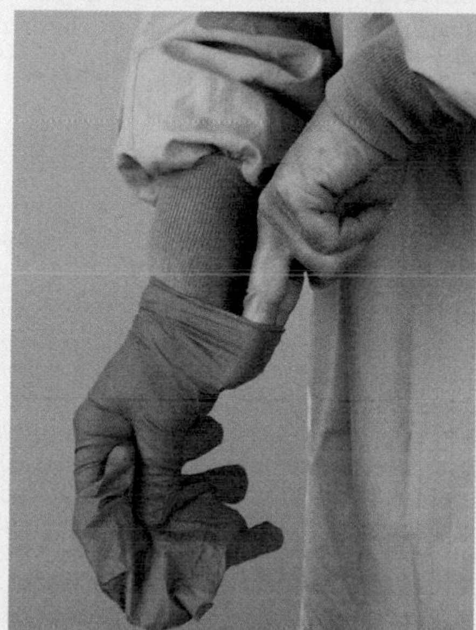

Figure 7. Sliding fingers of ungloved hand under the remaining glove at the wrist.

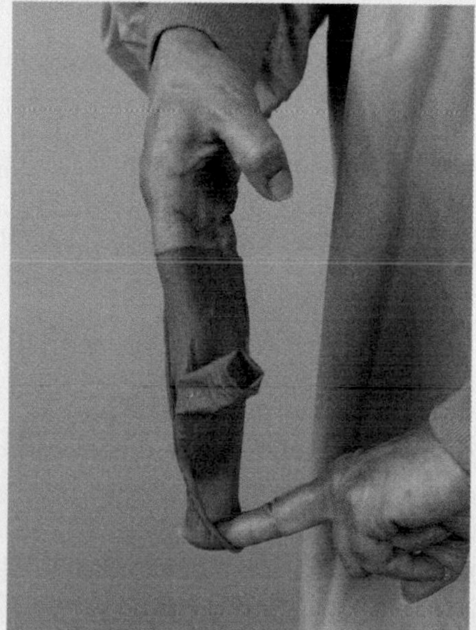

Figure 8. Pulling glove off the hand and over the other glove.

(continued)

SKILL 4-7 Using Personal Protective Equipment *(continued)*

ACTION	RATIONALE
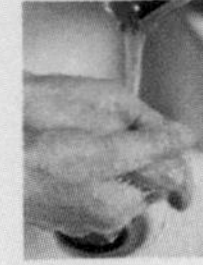 7. Perform hand hygiene immediately after removing all PPE.	Hand hygiene prevents spread of microorganisms.

EVALUATION

The expected outcome is met when the transmission of microorganisms is prevented; the patient and staff remain free from exposure to potentially infectious microorganisms; patient verbalizes an understanding about the rationale for use of PPE; episodes of bowel or urinary incontinence or diarrhea are controlled; and drainage from skin breakdown is contained.

DOCUMENTATION

It is not usually necessary to document the use of Standard Precautions or specific articles of PPE. However, documentation should be recorded regarding the implementation of specific Transmission-based Precautions.

Unexpected Situations and Associated Interventions

- *You did not realize the need for protective equipment at beginning of task:* Stop task and obtain appropriate protective wear.
- *You are accidentally exposed to blood and body fluids:* Stop task and immediately follow agency protocol for exposure, including reporting the exposure.

The Taylor Suite offers these additional resources to enhance learning and facilitate understanding of this chapter:

- thePoint online resource, http://thepoint.lww.com/Lynn2E
- Student CD-ROM included with the book
- Skills Checklist to Accompany Taylor's Clinical Nursing Skills
- Taylor's Interactive Nursing
- Taylor's Video Guide to Clinical Nursing Skills: Asepsis

Developing Critical Thinking Skills

1. While preparing the sterile table in the cardiac catheterization lab for Joe Wilson, you realize that you did not obtain a sterile bowl. How can you obtain a sterile bowl?
2. While you are putting on sterile gloves in preparation for an indwelling urinary catheter insertion, your patient, Sheri Lawrence, moves her leg. You do not *think* that Sheri's leg touched the glove, but you are not positive. What should you do?
3. Edgar Barowski's son is visiting and asks you why the masks that are outside Edgar's room are different from the ones that people wear in the operating room. What should you tell Edgar's son?

Bibliography

Advice, P. R. N. (2004). Hand hygiene: Rings on or off? *Nursing, 34*(12), 18.

Centers for Disease Control and Prevention. (1996a). *Airborne precautions. Excerpted from guideline for isolation precautions in hospitals.* Available at www.cdc.gov/ncidod/hip/isolat/isolat.html/. Accessed October 8, 2005.

Centers for Disease Control and Prevention. (1996b). *Contact precautions. Excerpted from guideline for isolation precautions in hospitals.* Available at www.cdc.gov/ncidod/hip/isolat/isolat.html/. Accessed October 8, 2005.

Centers for Disease Control and Prevention. (1996c). *Droplet precautions. Excerpted from guideline for isolation precautions in hospitals.* Available at www.cdc.gov/ncidod/hip/isolat/isolat.html/. Accessed October 8, 2005.

Centers for Disease Control and Prevention. (1996d). *Standard precautions. Excerpted from guideline for isolation precautions in hospitals.* Available at www.cdc.gov/ncidod/hip/isolat/isolat.html/. Accessed October 8, 2005.

Centers for Disease Control and Prevention. (2000). Monitoring hospital-acquired infections to promote patient safety—US, 1990–1999. *Morbidity and Mortality Weekly Report, 49*(08), 149–153.

Centers for Disease Control and Prevention. (2002a). Guidelines for hand hygiene in health-care settings. *Morbidity and Mortality Weekly Report, 51*(RR16), 1–45.

Centers for Disease Control and Prevention (CDC). (2002b). *Hand hygiene guidelines fact sheet.* Available at www.cdc.gov/od/oc/media/preswsrel/fs021025.htm. Accessed October 8, 2005.

Centers for Disease Control and Prevention. (2004a). *Guidance for the selection and use of personal protective equipment (PPE) in healthcare settings.* (Slide presentation). Available at www.cdc.gov/ncidod/hip/ppe/default.htm. Accessed October 23, 2005.

Centers for Disease Control and Prevention. (2004b). *Sequence for donning and removing personal protective equipment (PPE).* Poster. Available at www.cdc.gov/ncidod/hip/ppe/default.htm. Accessed October 8, 2005.

Duffy, J. (2002). Nosocomial infections: Important acute care nursing-sensitive outcomes indicators. *AACN Clinical Issues, 13*(3), 358–366.

Girard, N. (2003). OR masks: Safe practice or habit? *AORN Journal, 77*(1), 12–15.

Graves, P. & Twomey, C. (2002). The changing face of hand protection. *AORN Journal, 76*(2), 248–264.

Perry, J. & Jagger, J. (2004). Getting the most from your personal protective gear. *Nursing, 34*(12), 72.

Saiman, L., Lerner, A., Saal, L., et al. (2002). Banning artificial nails from health care settings. *American Journal of Infection Control, 30*(4), 252–254.

Sickbert-Bennett, E., Weber, D., Gergen-Teague, M., et al. (2005). Comparative efficacy of hand hygiene agents in the reduction of bacteria and viruses. *American Journal of Infection Control. 33*(2), 67–77.

Smeltzer, S., Bare, B., Hinkle, J. H., & Cheever, K. H. (2008). *Brunner & Suddarth's textbook of medical-surgical nursing* (11th ed.). Philadelphia: Lippincott Williams & Wilkins.

Storr, J. & Clayton-Kent, S. (2002). Hand hygiene. *Nursing Standard, 18*(4), 45–52.

White, C., Kolble, R., Carlson, R., et al. (2005). The impact of a health campaign on hand hygiene and upper respiratory illness among college students living in residence halls. *Journal of American College Health, 53*(4), 175–181.

Winslow, E., & Jacobson, A. (2000). Can a fashion statement harm the patient? *American Journal of Infection Control, 100*(9), 63, 65.

Worthington, K. (2002). Are your medical gloves really protecting you? Take an active role in purchasing the right glove for the job. *American Journal of Infection Control, 102*(10), 108.

CHAPTER 5

Medications

Focusing on Patient Care

This chapter will help you develop the skills needed to safely administer medications to the following patients:

Cooper Jackson, age 2 years, does not want to take his ordered oral antibiotic.

Erika Jenkins, age 20, is extremely afraid of needles and is at the clinic for her birth-control injection.

Jonah Dinerman, age 63, was recently diagnosed with diabetes and needs to be taught how to give himself insulin injections.

Learning Objectives

After studying this chapter, you will be able to:

1. Prepare medications for administration in a safe manner.
2. Administer oral medications.
3. Remove medication from an ampule.
4. Remove medication from a vial.
5. Mix medications from two vials in one syringe.
6. Identify appropriate needle size and angle of insertion for intradermal, subcutaneous, and intramuscular injections.
7. Locate appropriate sites for intradermal injection.
8. Administer an intradermal injection.
9. Locate appropriate sites for a subcutaneous injection.
10. Administer a subcutaneous injection.
11. Locate appropriate sites for an intramuscular injection.
12. Administer an intramuscular injection.
13. Apply an insulin pump.
14. Add medications to an intravenous (IV) solution container.
15. Administer medications by intravenous bolus or push through an intravenous infusion.
16. Administer a piggyback intermittent intravenous infusion of medication.
17. Administer an intermittent intravenous infusion of medication via a volume-control administration set.
18. Introduce drugs through a medication or drug-infusion lock using the saline flush.
19. Apply a transdermal patch.
20. Instill eye drops.
21. Administer an eye irrigation.
22. Instill eardrops.
23. Administer an ear irrigation.
24. Instill nose drops.

25. Administer a vaginal cream.
26. Administer medication via a metered-dose inhaler.
27. Administer medication via a small-volume nebulizer.
28. Administer medication via a dry-powder inhaler.
29. Administer medications via a gastric tube.
30. Administer a rectal suppository.

Key Terms

ampule: a glass flask that contains a single dose of medication for parenteral administration

inhalation: route to administer medications directly into the lungs or airway passages

intradermal injection: injection placed just below the epidermis; sites commonly used are the inner surface of the forearm, the dorsal aspect of the upper arm, and the upper back

intramuscular injection: injection placed into muscular tissue; sites commonly used are the ventrogluteal, vastus lateralis, deltoid, and dorsogluteal muscles

intravenous (IV) route: route to administer medications directly into the vein or venous system; the most dangerous route of medication administration

metered-dose inhaler (MDI): device to deliver a controlled dose of medication for inhalation

nebulizer: instrument that produces a fine spray or mist; in this case, passing air through a liquid medication to produce fine particles for inhalation

needle gauge: measurement of the diameter of a needle

subcutaneous injection: injection placed between the epidermis and muscle, into the subcutaneous tissue; sites commonly used are the outer aspect of the upper arm, the abdomen, the anterior aspects of the thigh, the upper back, and the upper ventral or dorsogluteal area

sublingually: under the tongue

suppository: oval or cone-shaped substance that is inserted into a body cavity and melts at body temperature

vial: a glass bottle with a self-sealing stopper through which medication is removed

Medication administration is a basic nursing function that involves skillful technique and consideration of the patient's development, health status, and safety. The nurse administering medications needs a knowledge base about drugs, including drug names, preparations, classifications, adverse effects, and physiologic factors that affect drug action (Fundamentals Review 5-1).

The nurse observes the Three Checks and the Rights of Medication Administration when administering medications to ensure medications are being administered safely (see Fundamentals Review 5-2 and 5-3 for these important tools). Another way to prevent medication errors is always to clarify a medication order that is:

- Illegible
- Incomplete
- Incorrect route or dosage
- Not expected for patient's current diagnosis

Nursing responsibilities for drug administration are summarized in Fundamentals Review 5-4. This chapter will cover skills that the nurse needs to safely administer medications via multiple routes. Proper use of equipment and technique is imperative. Fundamentals Review 5-5 and Figure 5-1 review important guidelines related to administering parenteral medications.

When administering medication, always remember age considerations. Older people are sensitive to medications because their bodies have experienced physiologic changes associated with the aging process, including decreased gastric motility, muscle mass, acid production, and blood flow, which affect drug absorption. They may also be more susceptible to certain side effects. The physiologic changes in older people that increase drug susceptibility are summarized in Fundamentals 5-6. Older adults are more likely to take multiple drugs, so drug interactions in the older adult are a very real and dangerous problem.

Fundamentals Review 5-1

Know Your Medications

Before administering any unfamiliar medications, know the following:

- Mode of action and purpose of medication (making sure that this medication is appropriate for the patient's diagnosis)
- Side effects of and contraindications for medication
- Antagonist of medication
- Safe dosage range for medication
- Interactions with other medications
- Precautions to take before administration
- Proper administration technique

Fundamentals Review 5-2

The Three Checks

"Three Checks" denotes that label on the medication package or container should be checked three times during medication preparation and administration. The label should be read:

(1) When the nurse reaches for the container or unit dose package,

(2) After retrieval from the drawer and compared with the MAR, or compared with the MAR immediately before pouring from a multidose container, and

(3) When replacing the container to the drawer or shelf or before giving the unit dose medication to the patient.

Fundamentals Review 5-3

Rights of Medication Administration

The "Rights of Medication Administration" help to ensure accuracy when administering medications. To prevent medication errors, always ensure that the:

(1) Right medication is given to the
(2) Right patient in the
(3) Right dosage through the
(4) Right route at the
(5) Right time.

Additional rights have been suggested to include ensuring (6) the right reason and (7) the right documentation (Balas et al, 2004; Pape, 2003). Validating the right reason requires the nurse to understand the rationale for administration and answer the question, 'Does it make sense?' The right documentation refers to accurate and timely documentation of administration.

Fundamentals Review 5-4

Nursing Responsibilities for Administering Drugs

- Assessment of the patient and clear understanding of why the patient is receiving a particular medication
- Ensuring the rights of medication administration: The (1) right medication is given to the (2) right patient in the (3) right dosage through the (4) right route at the (5) right time, ensuring (6) the right reason and (7) the right documentation.
- Preparing the medication to be administered (checking labels, preparing injections, observing proper asepsis techniques with needles and syringes)
- Accurate dosage calculations
- Administration of the medication (proper injection techniques, aids to help swallowing, topical methods)
- Documentation of medications given
- Monitoring the patient's reaction and evaluating the patient's response
- Educating the patient regarding his or her medications and medication regimen

Fundamentals Review 5-5

Needle/Syringe Selection Technique

- When looking at a needle package, the first number is the gauge or diameter of the needle (eg, 18, 20) and the second number is the length in inches (eg, 1, 1½).
- As the gauge number becomes larger, the size of the needle becomes smaller: for instance, a 24-gauge needle is smaller than an 18-gauge needle.
- When giving an injection, the viscosity of the medication directs the choice of gauge (diameter). A thicker medication such as a hormone is given through a bigger needle, such as a 20 gauge. A thinner-consistency medication, such as morphine, is given through a smaller needle, such as a 24 gauge.
- The size of the syringe is directed by the amount of medication to be given. If the amount is less than 1 mL, use a 1-mL syringe to administer the medication. In a 1-mL syringe, the amount of medication may be rounded to the 100th decimal place. In syringes larger than 1 mL, the amount is rounded to the 10th decimal place. If the amount of medication to be administered is less than 3 mL, use a 3-mL syringe. If the amount of medication is equal to the size of the syringe (eg, 1 mL and using a 1-mL syringe), you may go up to the next size syringe to prevent awkward movements when deploying the plunger.

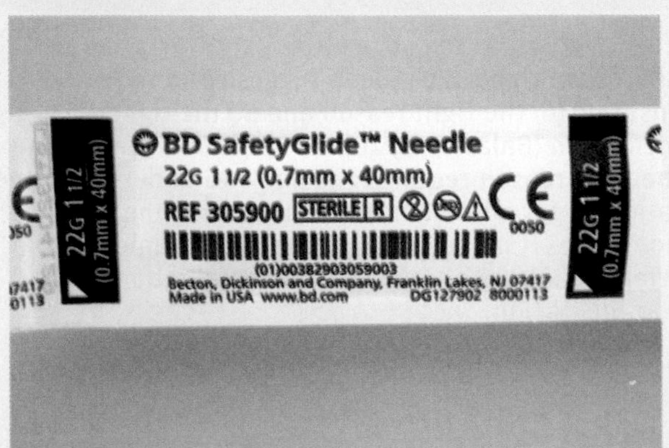

Needle package showing first number (gauge or diameter of the needle) and second number (length of the needle in inches).

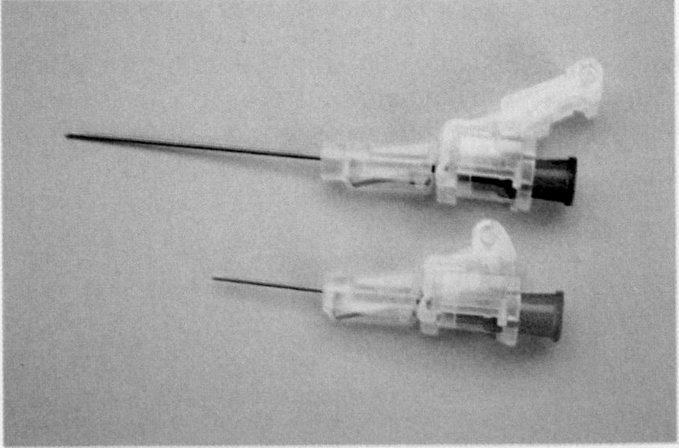

Different needle sizes. An 18-gauge needle (*top*) and a 24-gauge needle (*bottom*).

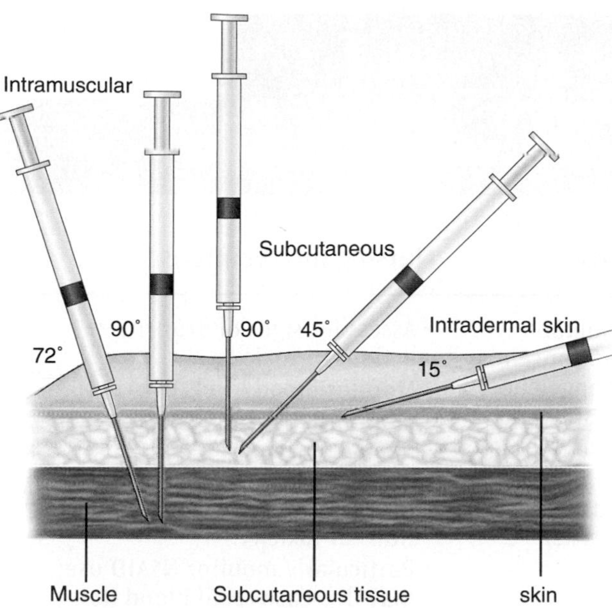

Figure 5-1. Comparison of the angles of insertion for intramuscular, subcutaneous, and intradermal injections.

Fundamentals Review 5-6

Altered Drug Response in Older People

Age-Related Changes	Implication or Response	Nursing Interventions
Decreased gastric motility; increased gastric pH	Stomach irritation; nausea; vomiting; gastric ulceration	• Assess for symptoms of gastrointestinal discomfort. • Assess stools for blood.
Decreased lean body mass; decreased total body water	Decreased distribution of water-soluble drugs and higher plasma concentrations, leading to increased possibility of drug toxicity	• Assess for signs of drug interactions or toxicity. • Monitor blood levels of drugs. • Monitor fluid balance; intake and output.
Increased adipose tissue	Accumulation of fat-soluble drugs; delay in elimination from and accumulation of drug in the body, leading to prolonged action and increased possibility of toxicity	• Assess for signs of drug interactions or toxicity. • Monitor blood levels of drugs.
Decreased number of protein-binding sites	Higher drug plasma concentrations, leading to increased possibility of drug toxicity	• Assess for signs of drug interactions or toxicity. • Monitor blood levels of drugs. • Monitor laboratory values—albumin and prealbumin.

(continued)

Fundamentals Review 5-6

Altered Drug Response in Older People *(continued)*

Age-Related Changes	Implication or Response	Nursing Interventions
Decreased liver function; decreased enzyme production for drug metabolism; decreased hepatic perfusion	Decreased rate of drug metabolism; higher drug plasma concentrations, leading to prolonged action and increased possibility of drug toxicity	• Assess for signs of drug interactions or toxicity. • Monitor blood levels of drugs. • Monitor laboratory values—hepatic enzymes.
Decreased kidney function, renal mass, and blood flow	Decreased excretion of drugs, leading to possible increased serum levels/toxicity	• Assess for signs of drug interactions or toxicity. • Particularly monitor NSAID use; may decrease renal blood flow and function. • Monitor blood levels of drugs. • Monitor laboratory values—creatinine clearance, blood urea nitrogen, serum creatinine.
Alterations in normal homeostatic responses; altered peripheral venous tone	Exacerbated response to cardiovascular drugs; more pronounced hypotensive effects from medications	• Assess for signs of drug interactions or toxicity. • Monitor blood levels of drugs. • Monitor vital signs. • Orthostatic hypotension precautions
Alterations in blood–brain barrier	Enhanced central nervous system penetration of fat-soluble drugs; increased possibility for alterations in mental status, dizziness, gait disturbances	• Assess for signs of drug interactions or toxicity. • Assess for dizziness and lightheadedness. • Fall safety precautions
Decreased central nervous system efficiency	Prolonged effect of drugs on the central nervous system; exacerbated response to analgesics and sedatives	• Assess for signs of drug interactions or toxicity. • Assess for alterations in neurologic status. • Monitor vital signs and pulse oximetry.
Decreased production of oral secretions; dry mouth	Difficulty swallowing oral medications	• Monitor ability to swallow medications, especially tablets and capsules. • Discuss changing medications to forms that can be crushed and/or liquid forms with prescribing practitioner.
Decreased lipid content in skin	Possible decrease in absorption of transdermal medications	• Monitor effectiveness of transdermal preparations.

(Adapted from Aschenbrenner, D. & Venable, S. [2006]. Drug therapy in nursing [2nd ed.]. *Philadelphia: Lippincott Williams & Wilkins; Tabloski, P. [2006].* Gerontological nursing. *Upper Saddle River, NJ: Pearson Prentice Hall; Porth, C. [2005].* Pathophysiology: Concepts of altered health states. [7th ed.]. *Philadelphia: Lippincott Williams & Wilkins; and Smeltzer, S., & Bare, B. [2008].* Brunner & Suddarth's textbook of medical-surgical nursing. [11th ed.]. *Philadelphia: Lippincott Williams & Wilkins.*

SKILL 5-1 Administering Oral Medications

Drugs given orally are intended for absorption in the stomach and small intestine. The oral route is the most commonly used route of administration. It is usually the most convenient and comfortable for the patient. After oral administration, drug action has a slower onset and a more prolonged but less potent effect than other routes.

Equipment

- Medication in disposable cup or oral syringe
- Liquid (water, juice, etc.) with straw if not contraindicated
- Medication cart or tray
- Medication Administration Record (MAR) or Computer-generated MAR (CMAR)

ASSESSMENT

Assess the appropriateness of the drug for the patient. Review medical history, allergy, assessment, and laboratory data that may influence drug administration. Assess the patient's ability to swallow medications. If the patient cannot swallow, is NPO, or is experiencing nausea or vomiting, the medication should be withheld, the physician notified, and proper documentation completed. Assess the patient's knowledge of the medication. If the patient has a knowledge deficit about the medication, this may be the appropriate time to begin education about the medication. If the medication may affect the patient's vital signs, assess them before administration. If the medication is for pain relief, assess the patient's pain level before and after administration. Verify the patient name, dose, route, and time of administration.

NURSING DIAGNOSIS

Determine related factors for the nursing diagnoses based on the patient's current status. Appropriate nursing diagnoses may include:

- Impaired Swallowing
- Risk for Aspiration
- Anxiety
- Deficient Knowledge
- Noncompliance

OUTCOME IDENTIFICATION AND PLANNING

The expected outcome to achieve when administering an oral medication is that the patient will swallow the medication. Other outcomes that may be appropriate include the following: the patient will experience the desired effect from the medication; the patient will not aspirate; the patient experiences decreased anxiety; the patient does not experience adverse effects; and the patient understands and complies with the medication regimen.

IMPLEMENTATION

ACTION	RATIONALE
1. Gather equipment. Check each medication order against the original physician's order according to agency policy. Clarify any inconsistencies. Check the patient's chart for allergies.	This comparison helps to identify errors that may have occurred when orders were transcribed. The physician's order is the legal record of medication orders for each agency.
2. Know the actions, special nursing considerations, safe dose ranges, purpose of administration, and adverse effects of the medications to be administered. Consider the appropriateness of the medication for this patient.	This knowledge aids the nurse in evaluating the therapeutic effect of the medication in relation to the patient's disorder and can also be used to educate the patient about the medication.

(continued)

SKILL 5-1 Administering Oral Medications *(continued)*

ACTION	RATIONALE
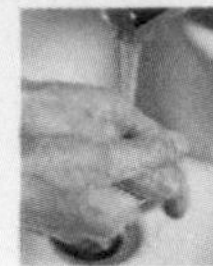 3. Perform hand hygiene.	Hand hygiene prevents the spread of microorganisms.
4. Move the medication cart to the outside of the patient's room or prepare for administration in the medication area.	Organization facilitates error-free administration and saves time.
5. Unlock the medication cart or drawer. Enter pass code and scan employee identification, if required.	Locking of the cart or drawer safeguards each patient's medication supply. Hospital accrediting organizations require medication carts to be locked when not in use. Entering pass code and scanning ID allows only authorized users into the system and identifies user for documentation by the computer.
6. **Prepare medications for one patient at a time.**	This prevents errors in medication administration.
7. Read the MAR and select the proper medication from the patient's medication drawer or unit stock.	This is the first check of the label.
8. Compare the label with the MAR (Figure 1). Check expiration dates and perform calculations, if necessary. Scan the bar code on the package, if required.	This is the second check of the label. Verify calculations with another nurse to ensure safety, if necessary.

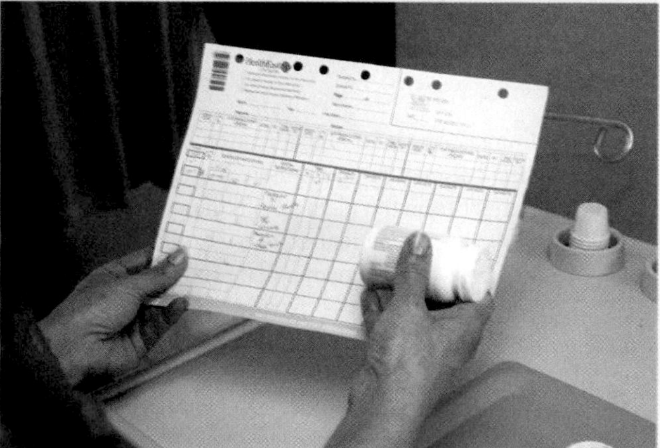

Figure 1. Comparing medication label with the MAR.

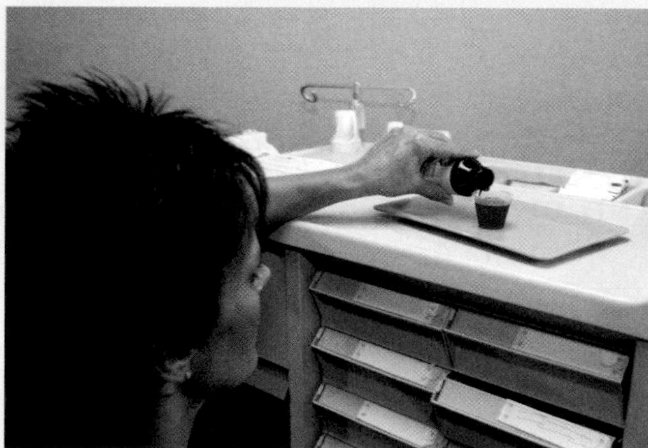

Figure 2. Measuring at eye level.

ACTION	RATIONALE
9. **Prepare the required medications:**	
a. *Unit dose packages:* Place unit dose-packaged medications in a disposable cup. **Do not open wrapper until at the bedside.** Keep narcotics and medications that require special nursing assessments in a separate container.	Wrapper is kept intact because the label is needed for an additional safety check. Special assessments may be required before giving certain medications. These may include assessing vital signs and checking laboratory test results.
b. *Multidose containers:* When removing tablets or capsules from a multidose bottle, pour the necessary number into the bottle cap and then place the tablets in a medication cup. Break only scored tablets, if necessary, to obtain the proper dosage. Do not touch tablets with hands.	Pouring medication into the cap allows for easy return of excess medication to bottle. Pouring tablets or capsules into the nurse's hand is unsanitary.

SKILL 5-1 Administering Oral Medications *(continued)*

ACTION	RATIONALE
c. *Liquid medication in multidose bottle:* When pouring liquid medications in a multidose bottle, hold the bottle so the label is against the palm. Use the appropriate measuring device when pouring liquids, and read the amount of medication at the bottom of the meniscus at eye level (Figure 2). Wipe the lip of the bottle with a paper towel.	Liquid that may drip onto the label makes the label difficult to read. Accuracy is possible when the appropriate measuring device is used and then read accurately.
10. **When all medications for one patient have been prepared, recheck the label with the MAR before taking them to the patient. Replace any multidose containers in the patient's drawer or unit stock. Lock the medication cart before leaving it.**	This is a *third* check to ensure accuracy and to prevent errors. Locking the cart or drawer safeguards the patient's medication supply. Hospital accrediting organizations require medication carts to be locked when not in use.
11. Transport medications to the patient's bedside carefully, and keep the medications in sight at all times.	Careful handling and close observation prevent accidental or deliberate disarrangement of medications.
12. **Ensure that the patient receives the medications at the correct time.**	Check agency policy, which may allow for administration within a period of 30 minutes before or 30 minutes after designated time.
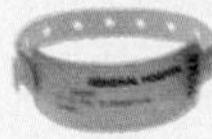 13. **Identify the patient.** Usually, the patient should be identified using two methods. Compare information with the MAR or CMAR.	Identifying the patient ensures the right patient receives the medications and helps prevent errors.
a. Check the name and identification number on the patient's identification band (Figure 3).	This is the most reliable method. Replace the identification band if it is missing or inaccurate in any way.
b. Ask the patient to state his or her name.	This requires a response from the patient, but illness and strange surroundings often cause patients to be confused.
c. If the patient cannot identify him or herself, verify the patient's identification with a staff member who knows the patient for the second source.	This is another way to double check identity. Do not use the name on the door or over the bed, because these may be inaccurate.

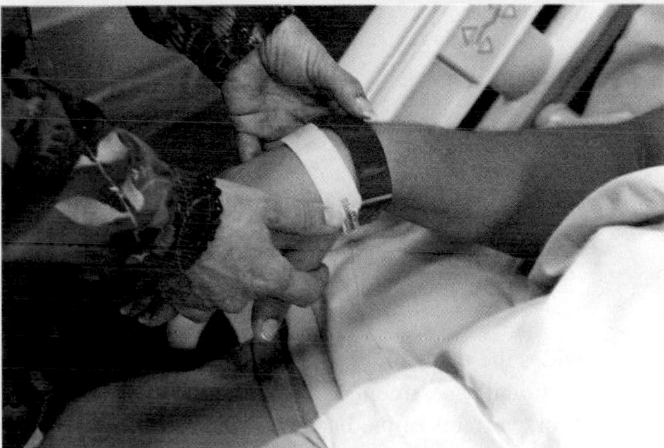

Figure 3. Checking patient's name and ID number.

(continued)

SKILL 5-1 Administering Oral Medications *(continued)*

ACTION	RATIONALE
14. **Complete necessary assessments before administering medications. Check allergy bracelet or ask patient about allergies. Explain the purpose and action of each medication to the patient.**	Assessment is a prerequisite to administration of medications.
15. Scan the patient's bar code on the identification band, if required.	The bar code provides an additional check to ensure that the medication is given to the right patient.
16. Assist the patient to an upright or lateral position.	Swallowing is facilitated by proper positioning. An upright or side-lying position protects the patient from aspiration.
17. Administer medications:	
a. Offer water or other permitted fluids with pills, capsules, tablets, and some liquid medications.	Liquids facilitate swallowing of solid drugs. Some liquid drugs are intended to adhere to the pharyngeal area, in which case liquid is not offered with the medication.
b. Ask whether the patient prefers to take the medications by hand or in a cup.	This encourages the patient's participation in taking the medications.
18. **Remain with the patient until each medication is swallowed. Never leave medication at the patient's bedside (Figure 4).**	Unless the nurse has seen the patient swallow the drug, the drug cannot be recorded as administered. The patient's chart is a legal record. Only with a physician's order can medications be left at the bedside.

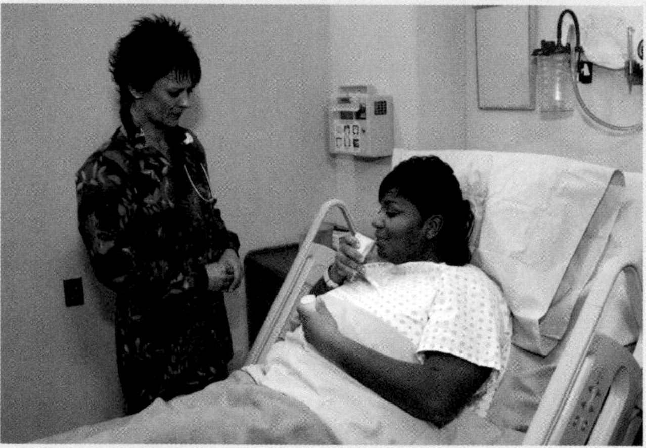

Figure 4. Remaining with the patient until each medication is swallowed.

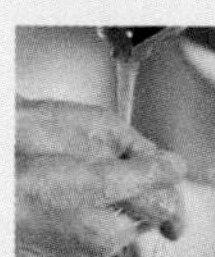

ACTION	RATIONALE
19. Perform hand hygiene. Leave the patient in a comfortable position.	Hand hygiene prevents the spread of microorganisms.
20. Check on the patient within 30 minutes, or time appropriate for drug(s), to verify response to medication.	This provides the opportunity for further documentation and additional assessment of effectiveness of pain relief and adverse effects of medications.

SKILL 5-1

Administering Oral Medications *(continued)*

EVALUATION

The expected outcomes are met when the patient swallows the medication, does not aspirate, verbalizes an understanding of the medication, experiences the desired effect from the medication, and does not experience adverse effects.

DOCUMENTATION

Guidelines

Record each medication given on the MAR or record using the required format immediately after it is administered, including date and time of administration (Figure 5). If using a bar-code system, medication administration is automatically recorded when scanned. PRN medications require documentation of the reason for administration. Prompt recording avoids the possibility of accidentally repeating the administration of the drug. If the drug was refused or omitted, record this in the appropriate area on the medication record and notify the physician. This verifies the reason medication was omitted and ensures that the physician is aware of the patient's condition. Recording of administration of a narcotic may require additional documentation on a narcotic record, stating drug count and other specific information. Record fluid intake if intake and output measurement is required.

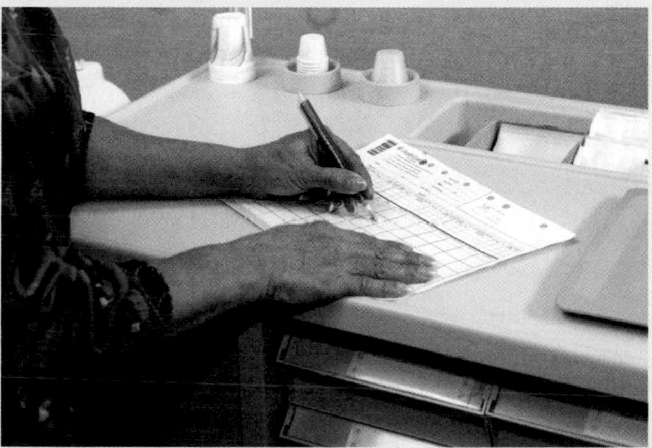

Figure 5. Recording each medication given on the MAR.

Sample Documentation

8/6/08 0835 Mr. Jones complaining of leg pains. Rates pain as an 8/10. Percocet 2 tabs administered.—K. Sanders, RN

8/6/08 0905 Mr. Jones resting comfortably. Rates leg pain as a 1/10.—K. Sanders, RN

8/6/08 1300 Mr. Jones refusing to take pain medication. States, "It made me feel woozy last time." Feelings discussed with patient. Patient agrees to take Percocet 1 tab at this time.—K. Sanders, RN

8/6/08 1320 Percocet, 1 tablet given P.O.—K. Sanders, RN

Unexpected Situations and Associated Interventions

- *Patient feels that medication is lodged in throat:* Offer patient more fluids to drink. If allowed, offer the patient bread or crackers to help move the medication to stomach.
- *It is unclear whether patient swallowed medication:* Check in the patient's mouth, under tongue, and between cheek and gum. Patients may "cheek" medications to avoid taking the medication or to save it for later use. This has been established with many medications, especially antidepressants and pain medication. Patients requiring suicide precautions should be watched closely to ensure that they are not "cheeking" the medication or hiding it in the mouth. These patients may be trying to accumulate a large amount of medication to take all at once in a suicide attempt. Substance abusers may cheek medication to accumulate a large amount to take all at once so that they may feel a high from medication.

(continued)

SKILL 5-1 Administering Oral Medications *(continued)*

- *Patient vomits immediately or shortly after receiving oral medication:* Assess vomit, looking for pills or fragments. Do not readminister medication without notifying physician. If a whole pill is seen and can be identified, physician may ask that medication be administered again. If a pill is not seen or medications cannot be identified, medication should not be readministered so that patient does not receive too large a dose.
- *Child refuses to take oral medications:* Some medications may be mixed in a small amount of food, such as pudding or ice cream. Do not add to liquid, because medication may alter the taste of liquids; if child then refuses to drink the rest of the liquid, you will not know how much of the medication was ingested. Creativity may be needed when devising ways to administer medications to a child. See below under "Infant and Child Considerations" for suggestions.
- *The capsule or tablet falls to the floor during administration.* Discard and obtain a new dose for administration. This prevents contamination and transmission of microorganisms.
- *Patient refuses medication.* Explore the reason for the patient's refusal. Review the rationale for using the drug and any other information that may be appropriate. If you are unable to administer the medication despite education and discussion, document the omission according to facility policy and notify the physician.

Special Considerations

General Considerations

- Some liquid medication preparations, such as suspensions, require agitation to ensure even distribution of medication in the solution. Be familiar with the specific requirements for medications you are administering.
- Medications intended for sublingual absorption should be placed under the patient's tongue. Instruct the patient to allow the medication to dissolve completely. Reinforce the importance of not swallowing the medication tablet.
- Some oral medications are provided in powdered forms. Verify the correct liquid to dissolve the medication in for administration. This information is usually included on the package; verify any unclear instructions with a pharmacist or medication reference. If there is more than one possible liquid to dissolve the medication in, include the patient in the decision process; patients may find one choice more palatable than another.
- Ongoing assessment is an important part of nursing care to evaluate patient response to administered medications and early detection of adverse effects. If an adverse effect is suspected, withhold further medication doses and notify the patient's primary healthcare provider. Additional intervention is based on type of reaction and patient assessment.
- If the patient questions a medication order or states the medication is different from the usual dose, always recheck and clarify with the original order or physician before giving medication.
- If the patient's level of consciousness is altered or his or her swallowing is impaired, check with the physician to clarify the route of administration or alternative forms of medication. This may also be a solution for a pediatric or a confused patient who is refusing to take a medication.
- Patients with poor vision can request large-type labels on medication containers. A magnifying lens also may be helpful.
- Provide written medication information to reinforce discussion and education, if the patient is literate. If the patient is unable to read, provide written information to family or significant other, if appropriate. Written information should be at a 5th-grade level to ensure ease of understanding.

SKILL 5-1 Administering Oral Medications *(continued)*

- If the patient has difficulty swallowing tablets, it may be appropriate to crush the medication to facilitate administration. Not all medications can be crushed or altered. Consult a medication reference and/or pharmacist. Long-acting and slow-release drugs are examples of medications that cannot be crushed. If the medication can be crushed, use a pill-crusher or mortar and pestle to grind the tablet into a powder. Crush each pill one at a time. Dissolve the powder with water or other recommended liquid in a liquid medication cup, keeping each medication separate from the others. Keep the package label with the medication cup for future comparison of information. The medication can then be combined with small amount of soft food, such as applesauce or pudding, to facilitate administration.

Infant and Child Considerations

- Special devices, such as oral syringes and calibrated nipples, are available in a pharmacy to ensure accurate dose calculations for young children and infants.
- Some creative ways to administer medications to children include: have a "tea party" with medicine cups; place syringe (without needle) or dropper in the space between the cheek and gum and slowly administer the medication; save a special treat for after the medication administration (eg, movie, playroom time, or a special food if allowed).
- The FDA has received reports of infants choking on the plastic caps that fit on the end of syringes when used to administer oral medications. They recommend the following: remove and dispose of caps before giving syringes to patients or families, caution family caregivers to dispose of caps on syringes they buy over the counter, and report any problems with syringe caps to the FDA. Companies have begun to manufacture syringes labeled "oral use" without the caps on them.

Older Adult Considerations

- Elderly patients with arthritis may have difficulty opening childproof caps. On request, the pharmacist can substitute a cap that is easier to open. A rubber band twisted around the cap may provide a more secure grip for older patients.
- Consider large-print written information when appropriate.

Home Care Considerations

- Encourage the patient to discard outdated prescription medications.
- Discuss safe storage of medications when there are children and pets in the environment.
- Discuss with parents the difference in over-the-counter medications made for infants and medications made for children. Many times parents do not realize that there are different strengths to the actual medications, leading to under- or overdosing.
- Encourage patients to carry a card listing all medications, dosage, and frequency in case of an emergency.
- Discuss the importance of using an appropriate measuring device for liquid medications. Patients should be cautioned not to use eating utensils for measuring medications. A liquid medication cup, oral syringe, or measuring spoon should be used to provide accurate dosing.

SKILL 5-2 Removing Medication From an Ampule

An ampule is a glass flask that contains a single dose of medication for parenteral administration. Because there is no way to prevent airborne contamination of any unused portion of medication after the ampule is opened, if not all the medication is used, the remainder must be discarded. Medication is removed from an ampule after its thin neck is broken.

Equipment

- Sterile syringe and filter needle
- Ampule of medication
- Small gauze pad
- Medication Administration Record (MAR) or Computer-generated MAR (CMAR)

ASSESSMENT

Assess the medication in the ampule for any particles or discoloration. Assess the ampule for any cracks or chips. Check expiration date before administering the medication. Verify patient name, dose, route, and time of administration. Assess the appropriateness of the drug for the patient. Review assessment and laboratory data that may influence drug administration.

NURSING DIAGNOSIS

Determine related factors for the nursing diagnoses based on the patient's current status. Appropriate nursing diagnoses may include:

- Risk for Infection
- Risk for Injury
- Anxiety
- Deficient Knowledge

OUTCOME IDENTIFICATION AND PLANNING

The expected outcome to achieve when removing medication from an ampule is that the medication will be removed in a sterile manner, be free from glass shards, and the proper dose is prepared.

IMPLEMENTATION

ACTION	RATIONALE
1. Gather equipment. Check the medication order against the original physician's order according to agency policy. Clarify any inconsistencies. Check the patient's chart for allergies.	This comparison helps to identify errors that may have occurred when orders were transcribed. The physician's order is the legal record of medication orders for each agency.
2. Know the actions, special nursing considerations, safe dose ranges, purpose of administration, and adverse effects of the medications to be administered. Consider the appropriateness of the medication for this patient.	This knowledge aids the nurse in evaluating the therapeutic effect of the medication in relation to the patient's disorder and can also be used to educate the patient about the medication.
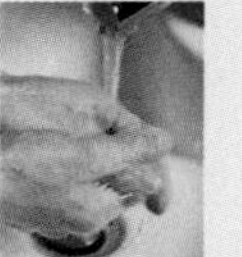 3. Perform hand hygiene.	Hand hygiene deters the spread of microorganisms.
4. Move the medication cart to the outside of the patient's room or prepare for administration in the medication area.	Organization facilitates error-free administration and saves time.

SKILL 5-2

Removing Medication From an Ampule *(continued)*

ACTION	RATIONALE
5. Unlock the medication cart or drawer. Enter pass code and scan employee identification, if required.	Locking of the cart or drawer safeguards each patient's medication supply. Hospital accrediting organizations require medication carts to be locked when not in use. Entering pass code and scanning ID allows only authorized users into the system and identifies user for documentation by the computer.
6. **Prepare medications for one patient at a time.**	This prevents errors in medication administration.
7. Read the MAR and select the proper medication from the patient's medication drawer or unit stock.	This is the first check of the label.
8. Compare the label with the MAR. Check expiration dates and perform calculations, if necessary. Scan the bar code on the package, if required.	This is the second check of the label. Verify calculations with another nurse to ensure safety, if necessary.
9. Tap the stem of the ampule (Figure 1) or twist your wrist quickly (Figure 2) while holding the ampule vertically.	This facilitates movement of medication in the stem to the body of the ampule.
10. **Wrap a small gauze pad around the neck of the ampule.**	This protects the nurse's fingers from the glass as the ampule is broken.
11. Use a snapping motion to break off the top of the ampule along the scored line at its neck (Figure 3). Always break away from your body.	This protects the nurse's face and fingers from any shattered glass fragments.

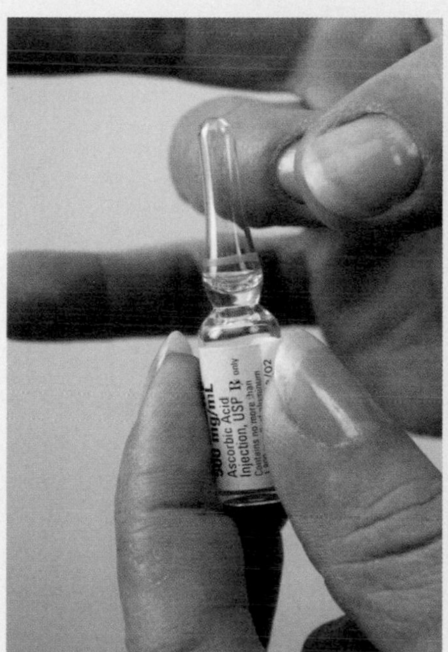

Figure 1. Tapping stem of the ampule.

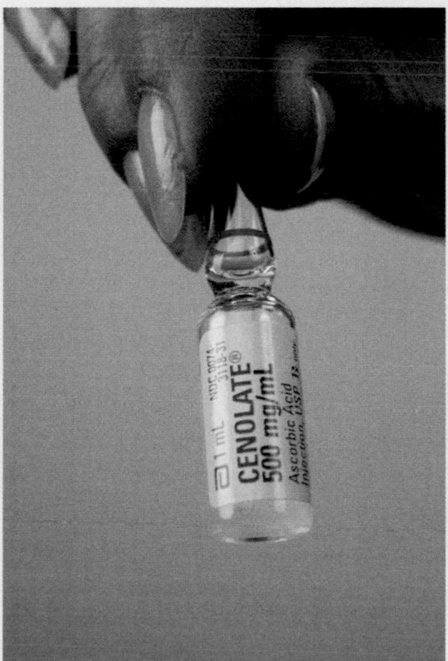

Figure 2. Twisting wrist quickly while holding the ampule vertically.

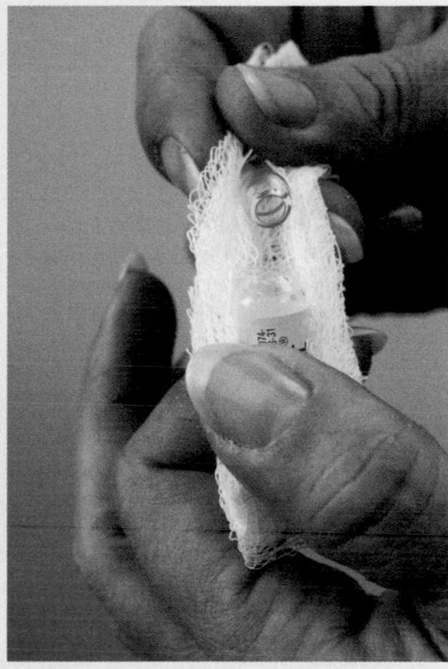
Figure 3. Using a snapping motion to break top of the ampule.

(continued)

SKILL 5-2 Removing Medication From an Ampule *(continued)*

ACTION	RATIONALE
12. Attach filter needle to syringe. **Remove the cap from the filter needle by pulling it straight off. Insert the filter needle into the ampule, being careful not to touch the rim.**	The rim of the ampule is considered contaminated. Use of a filter needle prevents the accidental withdrawing of small glass particles with the medication.
13. Withdraw medication in the amount ordered plus a small amount more (approximately 30%). **Do not inject air into the solution.** Use either of the following methods:	By withdrawing a small amount more of medication, any air bubbles in the syringe can be displaced once the syringe is removed and there will still be ample medication in the syringe.
a. Insert the tip of the needle into the ampule, which is upright on a flat surface, and withdraw fluid into the syringe (Figure 4). **Touch plunger at knob only.**	The contents of the ampule are not under pressure; therefore, air is unnecessary and will cause the contents to overflow. Handling plunger at knob only will keep shaft of plunger sterile.
b. Insert the tip of the needle into the ampule and invert the ampule (Figure 5). Keep the needle centered and not touching the sides of the ampule. Withdraw fluid into syringe. **Touch plunger at knob only.**	Surface tension holds the fluids in the ampule when inverted. If the needle touches the sides or is removed and then reinserted into the ampule, surface tension is broken, and fluid runs out. Handling plunger at knob only will keep shaft of plunger sterile.

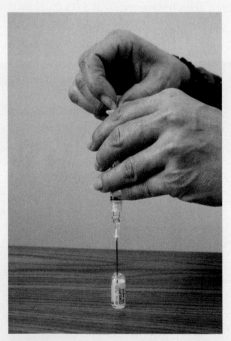

Figure 4. Withdrawing medication from upright ampule.

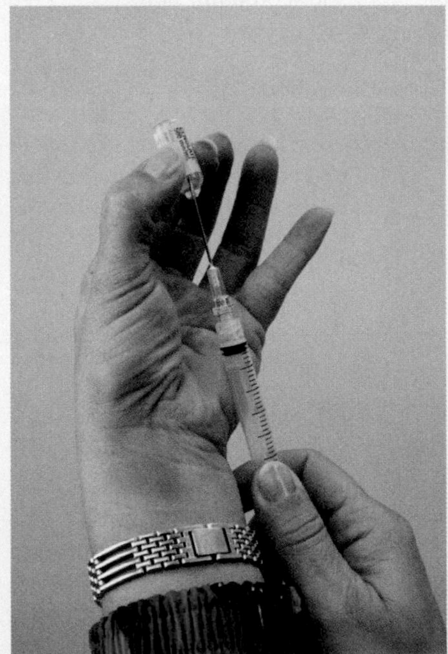

Figure 5. Withdrawing medication from inverted ampule.

ACTION	RATIONALE
14. **Wait until the needle has been withdrawn to tap the syringe and expel the air carefully by pushing on the plunger. Check the amount of medication in the syringe with the medication dose and discard any surplus according to facility policy.**	Ejecting air into the solution increases pressure in the ampule and can force the medication to spill out over the ampule. Ampules may have overfill. Careful measurement ensures that correct dose is withdrawn.
15. **Recheck the label with the MAR.**	This is the *third* check to ensure accuracy and to prevent errors.

SKILL 5-2 Removing Medication From an Ampule *(continued)*

ACTION	RATIONALE
16. Engage safety guard on filter needle and remove. Discard the filter needle in a suitable container. Attach appropriate administration device to syringe.	**Filter needle used to draw up medication should not be used to administer the medication, to prevent any glass shards from entering the patient.**
17. Discard the ampule in a suitable container.	Any medication that has not been removed from the ampule must be discarded because there is no way to maintain sterility of contents in an opened ampule.
18. Lock the medication cart before leaving it.	Locking the cart or drawer safeguards the patient's medication supply. Hospital accrediting organizations require medication carts to be locked when not in use.
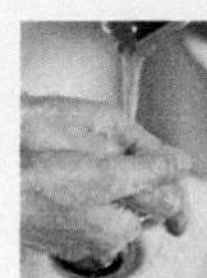 19. Perform hand hygiene.	Hand hygiene deters the spread of microorganisms.
20. Proceed with administration, based on prescribed route.	See appropriate skill for prescribed route.

EVALUATION

The expected outcome is met when the medication is removed from the ampule in a sterile manner, free from glass shards, and the proper dose is prepared.

Unexpected Situations and Associated Interventions

- *Nurse cuts self while trying to open ampule:* Discard ampule in case contamination has occurred. Bandage wound and obtain a new ampule. Report according to agency policy.
- *All of medication was not removed from the stem and there is not enough medication left in body of ampule for dose:* Discard ampule and drawn medication. Obtain a new ampule and start over. Medication in original ampule stem is considered contaminated once neck of ampule has been placed on a nonsterile surface.
- *Nurse injects air into inverted ampule, spraying medication:* Wash hands to remove any medication. If any medication has gotten into eyes, perform eye irrigation. Obtain a new ampule for medication dose. Report injury, if necessary, according to agency policy.
- *Medication is drawn up without using a filter needle:* Replace needle with a filter needle. Inject the medication through the filter needle into a new syringe and then administer to patient.
- *Plunger becomes contaminated before inserted into ampule:* Discard needle and syringe and start over. If plunger is contaminated after medication is drawn into the syringe, it is not necessary to discard and start over. The contaminated plunger will enter the barrel of the syringe when pushing the medication out and will not contaminate the medication.

SKILL 5-3 Removing Medication From a Vial

A vial is a glass bottle with a self-sealing stopper through which medication is removed. For safety in transporting and storing, the vial top is usually covered with a soft metal cap that can be removed easily. The self sealing stopper that is then exposed is the means of entrance into the vial. Single-dose vials are used once, then discarded, regardless of the amount of the drug that is used from the vial. Multidose vials contain several doses of medication and can be used multiple times. The medication contained in a vial can be in liquid or powder form. Powdered forms must be dissolved in an appropriate diluent before administration. The following skill reviews removing liquid medication from a vial. Refer to the accompanying Skill Variation for steps to reconstitute a powdered medication.

Equipment

- Sterile syringe and needle or blunt cannula (size depends on medication being administered and patient)
- Vial of medication
- Antimicrobial swab
- Second needle (optional)
- Filter needle (optional)
- Medication Administration Record (MAR) or Computer-generated MAR (CMAR)

ASSESSMENT

Assess the medication in vial for any discoloration or particles. Check expiration date before administering medication. Assess the appropriateness of the drug for the patient. Review assessment and laboratory data that may influence drug administration. Verify the patient name, dose, route, and time of administration.

NURSING DIAGNOSIS

Determine related factors for the nursing diagnoses based on the patient's current status. Appropriate nursing diagnoses include:

- Risk for Infection.
- Risk for Injury
- Anxiety
- Deficient Knowledge

OUTCOME IDENTIFICATION AND PLANNING

The expected outcome to achieve when removing medication from a vial is withdrawal of the medication into a syringe in a sterile manner and that the proper dose is prepared.

IMPLEMENTATION

ACTION	RATIONALE
1. Gather equipment. Check the medication order against the original physician's order according to agency policy.	This comparison helps to identify errors that may have occurred when orders were transcribed. The physician's order is the legal record of medication orders for each agency.
2. Know the actions, special nursing considerations, safe dose ranges, purpose of administration, and adverse effects of the medications to be administered. Consider the appropriateness of the medication for this patient.	This knowledge aids the nurse in evaluating the therapeutic effect of the medication in relation to the patient's disorder and can also be used to educate the patient about the medication.

SKILL 5-3 Removing Medication From a Vial *(continued)*

ACTION	RATIONALE
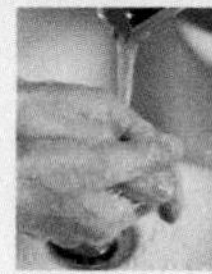 3. Perform hand hygiene.	Hand hygiene deters the spread of microorganisms.
4. Move the medication cart to the outside of the patient's room or prepare for administration in the medication area.	Organization facilitates error-free administration and saves time.
5. Unlock the medication cart or drawer. Enter pass code and scan employee identification, if required.	Locking of the cart or drawer safeguards each patient's medication supply. Hospital accrediting organizations require medication carts to be locked when not in use. Entering pass code and scanning ID allows only authorized users into the system and identifies user for documentation by the computer.
6. **Prepare medications for one patient at a time.**	This prevents errors in medication administration.
7. Read the MAR and select the proper medication from the patient's medication drawer or unit stock.	This is the first check of the label.
8. Compare the label with the MAR. Check expiration dates and perform calculations, if necessary. Scan the bar code on the package, if required.	This is the second check of the label. Verify calculations with another nurse to ensure safety, if necessary.
9. Remove the metal or plastic cap on the vial that protects the rubber stopper.	Needs to be removed to access medication in vial.
10. **Swab the rubber top with the antimicrobial swab and allow to dry.**	Antimicrobial swab removes surface bacteria contamination. Allowing the alcohol to dry prevents it from entering the vial on the needle.
11. Remove the cap from the needle or blunt cannula by pulling it straight off. Touch the plunger at the knob only. Draw back an amount of air into the syringe that is equal to the specific dose of medication to be withdrawn. Some agencies recommend use of a filter needle when withdrawing premixed medication from multidose vials.	Before fluid is removed, injection of an equal amount of air is required to prevent the formation of a partial vacuum, because a vial is a sealed container. If not enough air is injected, the negative pressure makes it difficult to withdraw the medication. Handling plunger at knob only will keep shaft of plunger sterile. Using filter needle prevents any solid material from being withdrawn through the needle.
12. Hold the vial on a flat surface. Pierce the rubber stopper in the center with the needle tip and inject the measured air into the space above the solution (Figure 1). Do not inject air into the solution.	Air bubbled through the solution could result in withdrawal of an inaccurate amount of medication.
13. **Invert the vial. Keep the tip of the needle or blunt cannula below the fluid level (Figure 2).**	This prevents air from being aspirated into the syringe.
14. Hold the vial in one hand and use the other to withdraw the medication. Touch the plunger at the knob only. **Draw up the prescribed amount of medication while holding the syringe vertically and at eye level (Figure 3).**	Holding the syringe at eye level facilitates accurate reading, and the vertical position makes removal of air bubbles from the syringe easy. Handling plunger at knob only will keep shaft of plunger sterile.

(continued)

SKILL 5-3

Removing Medication From a Vial *(continued)*

ACTION	RATIONALE

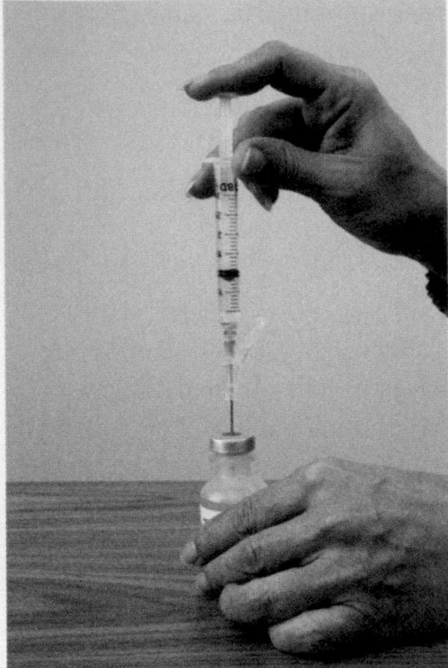

Figure 1. Injecting air with vial upright.

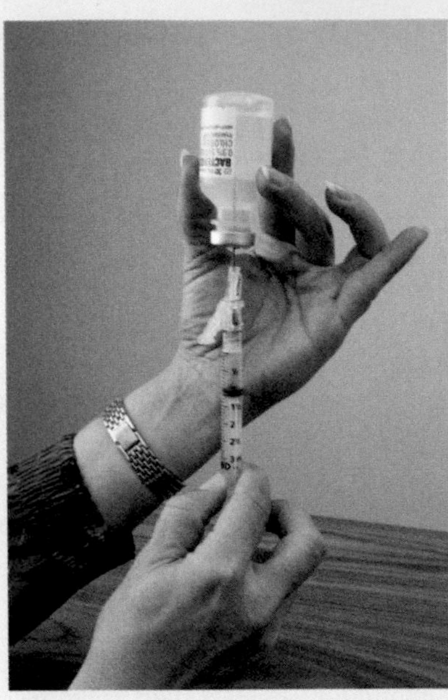

Figure 2. Positioning needle tip in solution.

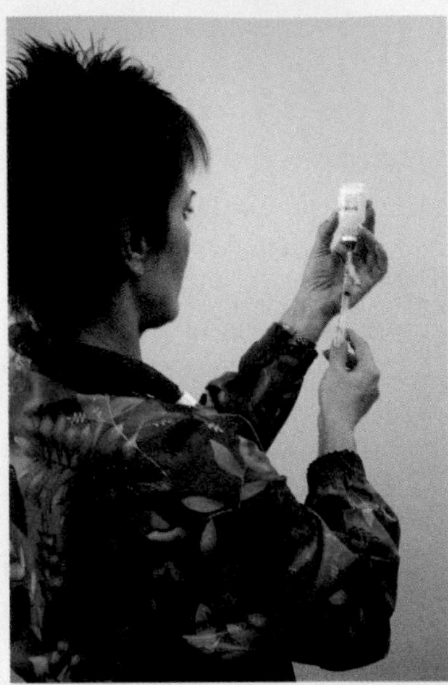

Figure 3. Withdrawing medication at eye level.

ACTION	RATIONALE
15. If any air bubbles accumulate in the syringe, tap the barrel of the syringe sharply and move the needle past the fluid into the air space to reinject the air bubble into the vial. Return the needle tip to the solution and continue withdrawal of the medication.	Removal of air bubbles is necessary to ensure accurate dose of medication.
16. After the correct dose is withdrawn, remove the needle from the vial and carefully replace the cap over the needle. If a filter needle has been used to draw up the medication, remove it and attach the appropriate administration device. Some agencies recommend changing the needle, if one was used to withdraw the medication, before administering the medication.	This prevents contamination of the needle and protects the nurse against accidental needlesticks. A one-handed recap method may be used as long as care is taken not to contaminate the needle during the process. Filter needle used to draw up medication should not be used to administer the medication to prevent any solid material from entering the patient.
17. **Check the amount of medication in the syringe with the medication dose and discard any surplus.**	Careful measurement ensures that correct dose is withdrawn.
18. **Recheck the label with the MAR.**	This is the *third* check to ensure accuracy and to prevent errors.
19. **If a multidose vial is being used, label the vial with the date and time opened, and store the vial containing the remaining medication according to agency policy.**	Because the vial is sealed, the medication inside remains sterile and can be used for future injections. Labeling the opened vials with a date and time limits its use after a specific time period.
20. Lock the medication cart before leaving it.	Locking the cart or drawer safeguards the patient's medication supply. Hospital accrediting organizations require medication carts to be locked when not in use.
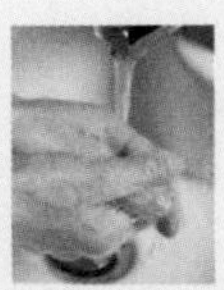 21. Perform hand hygiene.	Hand hygiene deters the spread of microorganisms.
22. Proceed with administration, based on prescribed route.	See appropriate skill for prescribed route.

SKILL 5-3

Removing Medication From a Vial *(continued)*

EVALUATION

The expected outcome is met when the medication is withdrawn into the syringe in a sterile manner and the proper dose is prepared.

Unexpected Situations and Associated Interventions

- *A piece of rubber stopper is noticed floating in medication in syringe:* Discard the syringe and needle and the vial. Obtain new vial and prepare dose as ordered.
- *As needle attached to syringe filled with air is inserted into vial, the plunger is immediately pulled down:* If possible to withdraw medication, continue steps as explained above. If such a vacuum has formed that this is impossible, remove syringe and inject more air into the vial. This is caused by previous withdrawal of medication without the addition of air into the vial.
- *Plunger is contaminated before injecting air into vial:* Discard needle and syringe and start over. If plunger is contaminated after medication is drawn into syringe, it is not necessary to discard and start over. The contaminated plunger will enter the barrel of the syringe when pushing the medication out and will not contaminate the medication.

SKILL VARIATION Reconstituting Powdered Medication in a Vial

Drugs that are unstable in solution form are often provided in a dry powder form. The powder must be mixed with the correct amount of appropriate solution to prepare medication for administration. Verify the correct amount and correct solution type for the specific medication prescribed. This information is found on the vial label, package insert, in a drug reference, or from the pharmacist. To reconstitute powdered medication:

- Gather equipment. Check the medication order against the original physician's order according to agency policy.
- Know the actions, special nursing considerations, safe dose ranges, purpose of administration, and adverse effects of the medications to be administered. Consider the appropriateness of the medication for this patient.
- Perform hand hygiene.
- Move the medication cart to the outside of the patient's room or prepare for administration in the medication area
- Unlock the medication cart or drawer. Enter pass code and scan employee identification, if required.
- Prepare medications for one patient at a time.
- Read the MAR and select the proper medication and diluent from the patient's medication drawer or unit stock.
- Compare the labels with the MAR. Check expiration dates and perform calculations, if necessary. Scan the bar code on the package, if required.
- Remove the metal or plastic cap on the medication vial and diluent vial that protects the self-sealing stoppers.
- Swab the self-sealing tops with the antimicrobial swab and allow to dry.
- **Draw up the appropriate amount of diluent into the syringe.**
- Insert the needle or blunt cannula through the center of the self-sealing stopper on the powdered medication vial.
- Inject the diluent into the powdered medication vial.
- Remove the needle or blunt cannula from the vial and replace cap.
- **Gently agitate the vial to mix the powdered medication and the diluent completely. Do not shake the vial.**
- **Draw up the prescribed amount of medication while holding the syringe vertically and at eye level.**
- After the correct dose is withdrawn, remove the needle from the vial and carefully replace the cap over the needle. If a filter needle has been used to draw up the medication, remove it and attach the appropriate administration device. Some agencies recommend changing the needle, if one was used to withdraw the medication, before administering the medication.
- **Check the amount of medication in the syringe with the medication dose and discard any surplus.**
- **Recheck the label with the MAR.**
- Lock the medication cart before leaving it.
- Perform hand hygiene.
- Proceed with administration, based on prescribed route.

SKILL 5-4 Mixing Medications From Two Vials in One Syringe

Preparation of medications in one syringe depends on how the medication is supplied. When using a single-dose vial and a multidose vial, air is injected into both vials and the medication in the multidose vial is drawn into the syringe first. This prevents the contents of the multidose vial from being contaminated with the medication in the single-dose vial.

When considering mixing two medications in one syringe, you must ensure that the two drugs are compatible. Nurses must be aware of drug incompatibilities when preparing medications in one syringe. Certain medications, such as diazepam (Valium), are incompatible with other drugs in the same syringe. Other drugs have limited compatibility and should be administered within 15 minutes of preparation. Incompatible drugs may become cloudy or form a precipitate in the syringe. Such medications are discarded and prepared again in separate syringes. Mixing more than two drugs in one syringe is not recommended. If it must be done, the pharmacist should be contacted to determine the compatibility of the three drugs, as well as the compatibility of their pH values and the preservatives that may be present in each drug. A drug-compatibility table should be available to nurses who are preparing medications.

Many types of insulin are available for use by patients with diabetes mellitus and are an example of medications that are often combined together in one syringe for injection, and are used as the example in the following procedure. Insulins vary in their onset and duration of action and are classified as short acting, intermediate acting, and long acting. Before administering any insulin, the nurse should be aware of the onset time, peak and duration of effects, and ensure that proper food is available. Refer to a drug reference for a listing of the different types of insulin and action specific to each type.

Insulin dosages are calculated in units. The scale commonly used is U100, which is based on 100 units of insulin contained in 1 mL of solution. Many cases of diabetes mellitus are regulated with a combination of two insulins (eg, regular and NPH insulin).

Equipment

- Two vials of medication (insulin in this example)
- Sterile syringe (insulin syringe in this example)
- Antimicrobial swabs
- Medication Administration Record (MAR) or Computer-generated MAR (CMAR)

ASSESSMENT

Determine the compatibility of the two medications. Not all insulins can be mixed together. Assess the contents of each vial of insulin. Preparations that are not modified typically appear as clear substances, so they should be without particles or foreign matter. Modified preparations are typically suspensions, so they do not appear as clear substances. It is no longer safe, however, to use the terms "clear" and "cloudy" to designate types of insulin preparation. Insulin Glargine (Lantus) is a clear but long-acting insulin (24-hour duration). It is very important to be familiar with the particular drug's properties to be able to assess the quality of the medication in the vial before withdrawal. Check expiration date before administering medication. Assess the appropriateness of the drug for the patient. Review assessment and laboratory data that may influence drug administration. Check the patient's blood glucose level if appropriate before administering the insulin. Verify patient name, dose, route, and time of administration.

NURSING DIAGNOSIS

Determine related factors for the nursing diagnoses based on the patient's current status. Appropriate nursing diagnoses include:

- Risk for Infection
- Risk for Injury
- Anxiety
- Deficient Knowledge

SKILL 5-4 Mixing Medications From Two Vials in One Syringe *(continued)*

OUTCOME IDENTIFICATION AND PLANNING

The expected outcome to achieve when mixing two different types of insulin in one syringe is the accurate withdrawal of the medication into a syringe in a sterile manner and that the proper dose is prepared.

IMPLEMENTATION

ACTION	RATIONALE
1. Gather equipment. Check medication order against the original physician's order according to agency policy.	This comparison helps to identify errors that may have occurred when orders were transcribed. The physician's order is the legal record of medication orders for each agency.
2. Know the actions, special nursing considerations, safe dose ranges, purpose of administration, and adverse effects of the medications to be administered. Consider the appropriateness of the medication for this patient.	This knowledge aids the nurse in evaluating the therapeutic effect of the medication in relation to the patient's disorder and can also be used to educate the patient about the medication.
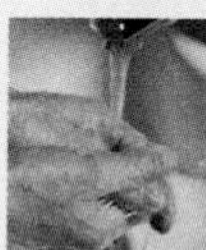 3. Perform hand hygiene.	Hand hygiene deters the spread of microorganisms.
4. Move the medication cart to the outside of the patient's room or prepare for administration in the medication area.	Organization facilitates error-free administration and saves time.
5. Unlock the medication cart or drawer. Enter pass code and scan employee identification, if required.	Locking of the cart or drawer safeguards each patient's medication supply. Hospital accrediting organizations require medication carts to be locked when not in use. Entering pass code and scanning ID allows only authorized users into the system and identifies user for documentation by the computer.
6. **Prepare medications for one patient at a time.**	This prevents errors in medication administration.
7. Read the MAR and select the proper medications from the patient's medication drawer or unit stock.	This is the first check of the labels.
8. Compare the labels with the MAR. Check expiration dates and perform calculations, if necessary. Scan the bar code on the package, if required.	This is the second check of the labels. Verify calculations with another nurse to ensure safety, if necessary.
9. If necessary, remove the cap that protects the rubber stopper on each vial.	The cap protects the rubber top.
10. **If insulin is a suspension (eg, NPH, Lente), roll and agitate the vial to mix it well.**	There is controversy regarding how to mix insulins in suspension. Some sources advise rolling the vial; others advise shaking the vial. Consult facility policy. Regardless of the method used, it is essential that the suspension be mixed well to avoid administering an inconsistent dose. Regular insulin, which is clear, does not need to be mixed before withdrawal.
11. Cleanse the rubber tops with antimicrobial swabs.	Antimicrobial swab removes surface contamination. Some sources question whether cleaning with alcohol actually disinfects or instead transfers resident bacteria from the hands to another surface.

(continued)

SKILL 5-4 Mixing Medications From Two Vials in One Syringe *(continued)*

ACTION	RATIONALE
12. Remove cap from needle by pulling it straight off. Touch the plunger at the knob only. Draw back an amount of air into the syringe that is equal to the dose of modified insulin to be withdrawn.	Before fluid is removed, injection of an equal amount of air is required to prevent the formation of a partial vacuum, because a vial is a sealed container. If not enough air is injected, the negative pressure makes it difficult to withdraw the medication. Handling plunger by knob only ensures sterility of shaft of plunger.
13. Hold the modified vial on a flat surface. Pierce the rubber stopper in the center with the needle tip and inject the measured air into the space above the solution (Figure 1). Do not inject air into the solution. Withdraw the needle.	Unmodified insulin should never be contaminated with modified insulin. Placing air in the modified insulin first without allowing the needle to contact the insulin ensures that the second vial entered (unmodified) insulin is not contaminated by the medication in the other vial. Air bubbled through the solution could result in withdrawal of an inaccurate amount of medication.
14. Draw back an amount of air into the syringe that is equal to the dose of unmodified insulin to be withdrawn.	Before fluid is removed, injection of an equal amount of air is required to prevent the formation of a partial vacuum, because a vial is a sealed container. If not enough air is injected, the negative pressure makes it difficult to withdraw the medication.
15. Hold the unmodified vial on a flat surface. Pierce the rubber stopper in the center with the needle tip and inject the measured air into the space above the solution (Figure 2). Do not inject air into the solution. Keep the needle in the vial.	Air bubbled through the solution could result in withdrawal of an inaccurate amount of medication.

Figure 1. Injecting air into modified insulin preparation.

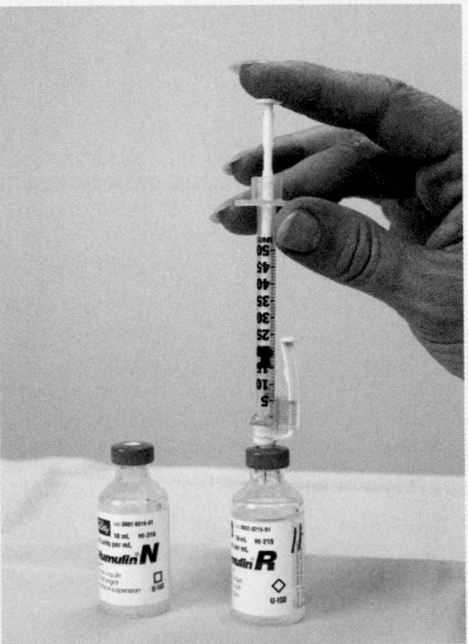

Figure 2. Injecting air into the unmodified insulin vial.

SKILL 5-4 Mixing Medications From Two Vials in One Syringe *(continued)*

ACTION	RATIONALE
16. Invert vial of unmodified insulin. Hold the vial in one hand and use the other to withdraw the medication. Touch the plunger at the knob only. **Draw up the prescribed amount of medication while holding the syringe at eye level and vertically (Figure 3).** Turn the vial over and then remove needle from vial.	Holding the syringe at eye level facilitates accurate reading, and the vertical position makes removal of air bubbles from the syringe easy. First dose is prepared and is not contaminated by insulin that contains modifiers.
17. Check that there are no air bubbles in the syringe.	The presence of air in the syringe would result in an inaccurate dose of medication.
18. **Check the amount of medication in the syringe with the medication dose and discard any surplus.**	Careful measurement ensures that correct dose is withdrawn.
19. **Recheck the vial label with the MAR.**	This is the *third* check to ensure accuracy and to prevent errors.
20. Calculate the endpoint on the syringe for the combined insulin amount by adding the number of units for each dose together.	Allows for accurate withdrawal of second dose.
21. Insert the needle into the modified vial and invert it, taking care not to push the plunger and inject medication from the syringe into the vial. Invert vial of modified insulin. Hold the vial in one hand and use the other to withdraw the medication. Touch the plunger at the knob only. **Draw up the prescribed amount of medication while holding the syringe at eye level and vertically (Figure 4). Take care to only withdraw the prescribed amount.** Turn the vial over and then remove needle from vial. Carefully recap the needle. Carefully replace the cap over the needle.	Previous addition of air eliminates need to create positive pressure. Holding the syringe at eye level facilitates accurate reading. Capping the needle prevents contamination and protects the nurse against accidental needlesticks. A one-handed recap method may be used as long as care is taken to ensure that the needle remains sterile.

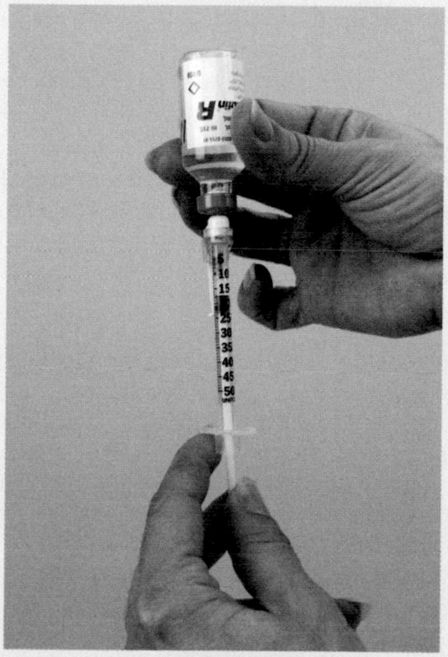

Figure 3. Withdrawing the prescribed amount of unmodified insulin.

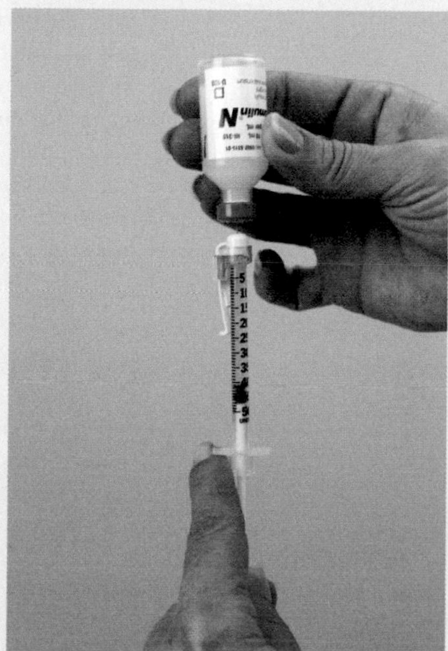

Figure 4. Withdrawing modified insulin.

(continued)

SKILL 5-4 Mixing Medications From Two Vials in One Syringe *(continued)*

ACTION	RATIONALE
22. **Check the amount of medication in the syringe with the medication dose.**	Careful measurement ensures that correct dose is withdrawn.
23. **Recheck the vial label with the MAR.**	This is the *third* check to ensure accuracy and to prevent errors.
24. **Label the vials with the date and time opened, and store the vials containing the remaining medication according to agency policy.**	Because the vial is sealed, the medication inside remains sterile and can be used for future injections. Labeling the opened vials with a date and time limits its use after a specific time period.
25. Lock medication cart before leaving it.	Locking the cart or drawer safeguards the patient's medication supply. Hospital accrediting organizations require medication carts to be locked when not in use.
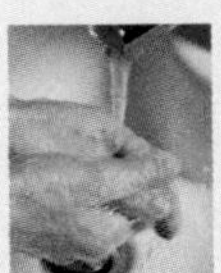 26. Perform hand hygiene.	Hand hygiene deters the spread of microorganisms.
27. Proceed with administration, based on prescribed route.	See appropriate skill for prescribed route.

EVALUATION

The expected outcome is met when the insulin is withdrawn into a syringe in a sterile manner, and the proper dose is prepared.

Unexpected Situations and Associated Interventions

- *Nurse contaminates plunger before injecting air into insulin vial:* Discard needle and syringe and start over. If plunger is contaminated after medication is drawn into the syringe, it is not necessary to discard and start over. The contaminated plunger will enter the barrel of the syringe when pushing the medication out and will not contaminate the medication.
- *Nurse allows modified insulin to come in contact with the needle before entering the unmodified insulin vial:* Discard needle and syringe and start over.
- *Nurse notices that the combined amount is not the ordered amount (eg, nurse has less or more units in combined syringe than ordered):* Discard syringe and start over. There is no way to know for sure which dosage is wrong or which medication would be expelled.
- *Nurse injects unmodified insulin into modified vial:* Discard vial and syringe and start over.

Special Considerations

General Considerations

- A diabetic patient who is visually impaired may find it helpful to use a magnifying apparatus that fits around the syringe.
- Before attempting to explain or demonstrate devices that help low-vision diabetic patients to prepare their medication, attempt to use the device yourself under similar circumstances. To detect any difficulties the patient may experience, practice using the aid with your eyes closed or in a poorly lit room.

Infant and Child Considerations

- School-age children are generally able to prepare and administer their own injections, such as insulin, with supervision (Hockenberry, 2005). Parents/significant others and the child should be involved in teaching.

SKILL 5-5 Administering an Intradermal Injection

Intradermal injections are administered into the dermis, just below the epidermis. The intradermal route has the longest absorption time of all parenteral routes. For this reason, intradermal injections are used for sensitivity tests, such as tuberculin and allergy tests, and local anesthesia. The advantage of the intradermal route for these tests is that the body's reaction to substances is easily visible, and degrees of reaction are discernible by comparative study.

Sites commonly used are the inner surface of the forearm and the upper back, under the scapula. Equipment used for an intradermal injection includes a tuberculin syringe calibrated in tenths and hundredths of a milliliter and a ¼″ to ½″, 26- or 27-gauge needle. The dosage given intradermally is small, usually less than 0.5 mL. The angle of administration for an intradermal injection is 10–15 degrees (see Figure 5-1 in the chapter opener.)

Equipment

- Prescribed medication
- Sterile syringe, usually a tuberculin syringe calibrated in tenths and hundredths, and needle, ¼″ to ½″, 26- or 27-gauge
- Antimicrobial swab
- Disposable gloves
- Small gauze square
- Medication Administration Record (MAR) or Computer-generated MAR (CMAR)

ASSESSMENT

Assess the patient for any allergies. Check expiration date before administering medication. Assess the appropriateness of the drug for the patient. Review assessment and laboratory data that may influence drug administration. Assess the site on the patient where the injection is to be given. Avoid areas of broken or open skin. Avoid areas that are highly pigmented, have lesions, bruises, or scars and are hairy. Assess the patient's knowledge of the medication. This may provide an opportune time for patient education. Verify the patient's name, dose, route, and time of administration.

NURSING DIAGNOSIS

Determine related factors for the nursing diagnoses based on the patient's current status. Appropriate nursing diagnoses may include:

- Deficient Knowledge
- Risk for Allergy Response
- Risk for Infection
- Risk for Injury
- Anxiety

OUTCOME IDENTIFICATION AND PLANNING

The expected outcome to achieve when administering an intradermal injection is appearance of a wheal at the site of injection. Other outcomes that may be appropriate include the following: the patient refrains from rubbing the site; the patient's anxiety is decreased; the patient does not experience adverse effects; and the patient understands and complies with the medication regimen.

IMPLEMENTATION

ACTION	RATIONALE
1. Gather equipment. Check each medication order against the original physician's order according to agency policy. Clarify any inconsistencies. Check the patient's chart for allergies.	This comparison helps to identify errors that may have occurred when orders were transcribed. The physician's order is the legal record of medication orders for each agency.

(continued)

SKILL 5-5 Administering an Intradermal Injection *(continued)*

ACTION	RATIONALE
2. Know the actions, special nursing considerations, safe dose ranges, purpose of administration, and adverse effects of the medications to be administered. Consider the appropriateness of the medication for this patient.	This knowledge aids the nurse in evaluating the therapeutic effect of the medication in relation to the patient's disorder and can also be used to educate the patient about the medication.
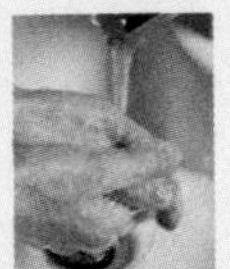 3. Perform hand hygiene.	Hand hygiene prevents the spread of microorganisms.
4. Move the medication cart to the outside of the patient's room or prepare for administration in the medication area.	Organization facilitates error-free administration and saves time.
5. Unlock the medication cart or drawer. Enter pass code and scan employee identification, if required.	Locking of the cart or drawer safeguards each patient's medication supply. Hospital accrediting organizations require medication carts to be locked when not in use. Entering pass code and scanning ID allows only authorized users into the system and identifies user for documentation by the computer.
6. **Prepare medications for one patient at a time.**	This prevents errors in medication administration.
7. Read the MAR and select the proper medication from the patient's medication drawer or unit stock.	This is the first check of the label.
8. Compare the label with the MAR. Check expiration dates and perform calculations, if necessary. Scan the bar code on the package, if required.	This is the second check of the label. Verify calculations with another nurse to ensure safety, if necessary.
9. If necessary, withdraw medication from an ampule or vial as described in Skills 5-2 and 5-3.	
10. **When all medications for one patient have been prepared, recheck the label with the MAR before taking them to the patient.**	This is a *third* check to ensure accuracy and to prevent errors.
11. Lock the medication cart before leaving it.	Locking the cart or drawer safeguards the patient's medication supply. Hospital accrediting organizations require medication carts to be locked when not in use.
12. Transport medications to the patient's bedside carefully, and keep the medications in sight at all times.	Careful handling and close observation prevent accidental or deliberate disarrangement of medications.
13. **Ensure that the patient receives the medications at the correct time.**	Check agency policy, which may allow for administration within a period of 30 minutes before or 30 minutes after designated time.
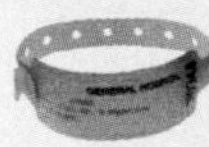 14. **Identify the patient.** Usually, the patient should be identified using two methods. Compare information with the MAR or CMAR.	Identifying the patient ensures the right patient receives the medications and helps prevent errors.
a. Check the name and identification number on the patient's identification band.	This is the most reliable method. Replace the identification band if it is missing or inaccurate in any way.
b. Ask the patient to state his or her name.	This requires a response from the patient, but illness and strange surroundings often cause patients to be confused.
c. If the patient cannot identify him or herself, verify the patient's identification with a staff member who knows the patient for the second source.	This is another way to double-check identity. Do not use the name on the door or over the bed, because these may be inaccurate.

SKILL 5-5

Administering an Intradermal Injection *(continued)*

ACTION	RATIONALE
15. Close the door to the room or pull the bedside curtain.	This provides patient privacy.
16. Complete necessary assessments before administering medications. Check allergy bracelet or ask patient about allergies. Explain the purpose and action of the medication to the patient.	Assessment is a prerequisite to administration of medications. Explanation provides rationale, increases knowledge, and reduces anxiety.
17. Scan the patient's bar code on the identification band, if required.	Provides additional check to ensure that the medication is given to the right patient.
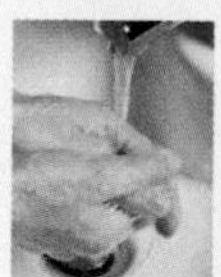 18. Perform hand hygiene and put on clean gloves.	Hand hygiene prevents the spread of microorganisms. Gloves help prevent exposure to contaminants.
19. Select an appropriate administration site. Assist the patient to the appropriate position for the site chosen. Drape as needed to expose only area of site to be used.	Appropriate site prevents injury and allows for accurate reading of the test site at the appropriate time.
20. Cleanse the site with an antimicrobial swab while wiping with a firm, circular motion and moving outward from the injection site. Allow the skin to dry.	Pathogens on the skin can be forced into the tissues by the needle. Moving from the center outward prevents contamination of the site. Allowing skin to dry prevents introducing alcohol into the tissue, which can be irritating and uncomfortable.
21. Remove the needle cap with the nondominant hand by pulling it straight off.	This technique lessens the risk of an accidental needlestick.
22. Use the nondominant hand to spread the skin taut over the injection site (Figure 1).	Taut skin provides an easy entrance into intradermal tissue.
23. Hold the syringe in the dominant hand, between the thumb and forefinger with the bevel of the needle up.	Using dominant hand allows for easy, appropriate handling of syringe. Having the bevel up allows for smooth piercing of the skin and introduction of medication into the dermis.
24. Hold the syringe at a 10 to 15 degree angle from the site. **Place the needle almost flat against the patient's skin (Figure 2), bevel side up, and insert the needle into the skin so that the point of the needle can be seen through the skin. Insert the needle only about ⅛″ with entire bevel under the skin.**	The dermis is entered when the needle is held as nearly parallel to the skin as possible and is inserted about ⅛″.

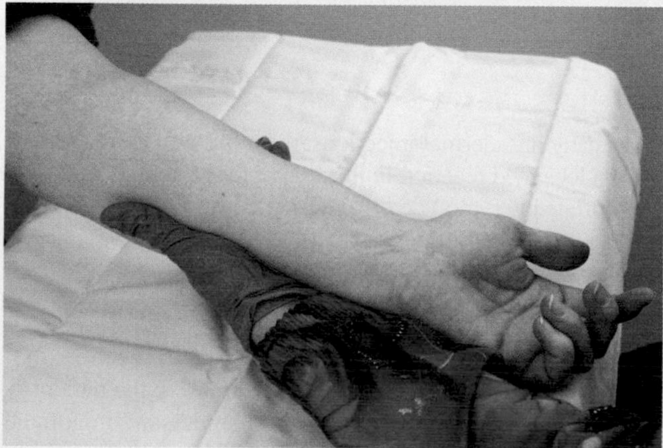

Figure 1. Spreading the skin taut over the injection site.

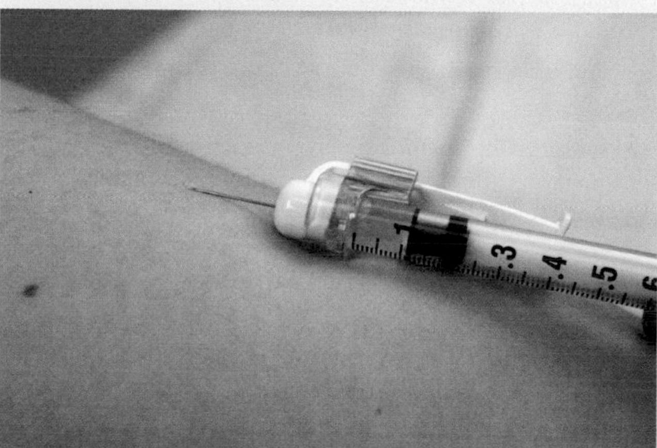

Figure 2. Inserting the needle almost level with the skin.

(continued)

SKILL 5-5

Administering an Intradermal Injection *(continued)*

ACTION	RATIONALE
25. Once the needle is in place, steady the lower end of the syringe. Slide your dominant hand to the end of the plunger.	Prevents injury and inadvertent advancement or withdrawal of needle.
26. Slowly inject the agent while watching for a small wheal or blister to appear (Figure 3).	The appearance of a wheal indicates the medication is in the dermis.

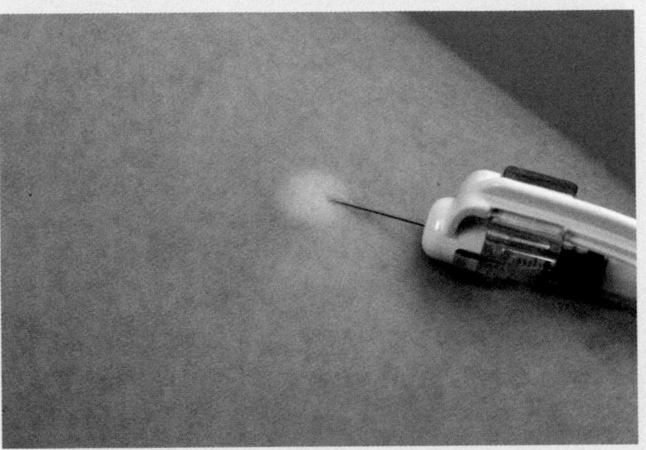

Figure 3. Observing for wheal while injecting medication.

ACTION	RATIONALE
27. Withdraw the needle quickly at the same angle that it was inserted.	Withdrawing the needle quickly and at the angle at which it entered the skin minimizes tissue damage and discomfort for the patient.
28. **Do not massage area after removing needle. Tell patient not to rub or scratch site. If necessary, gently blot the site with a dry gauze square. Do not apply pressure or rub the site.**	Massaging the area where an intradermal injection is given may spread the medication to underlying subcutaneous tissue.
29. Do not recap the used needle. Engage the safety shield or needle guard, if present. Discard the needle and syringe in the appropriate receptacle.	Proper disposal of the needle prevents injury.
30. Assist the patient to a position of comfort.	This provides for the well-being of the patient.
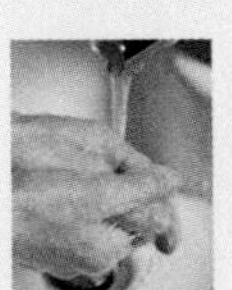 31. Remove gloves and dispose of them properly. Perform hand hygiene.	Hand hygiene deters the spread of microorganisms.
32. Observe the area for signs of a reaction at determined intervals after administration. Inform the patient of the need for inspection.	With many intradermal injections, the nurse will need to look for a localized reaction in the area of the injection at the appropriate interval(s) determined by the type of medication and purpose. Preparing the patient increases compliance.

EVALUATION

The expected outcomes are met when the nurse notes a wheal at site of injection; the patient refrains from rubbing the site; the patient's anxiety is decreased; the patient did not experience adverse effects; and the patient verbalizes an understanding of and complies with the medication regimen.

SKILL 5-5 **Administering an Intradermal Injection** *(continued)*

DOCUMENTATION

Guidelines

Record each medication given on the MAR or record using the required format, including date, time, and the site of administration, immediately after administration. Some agencies recommend circling the injection site with ink (Figure 4). Circling the injection site easily identifies the site of the intradermal injection and allows for careful observation of the exact area. If using a bar-code system, medication administration is automatically recorded when scanned. PRN medications require documentation of the reason for administration. Prompt recording avoids the possibility of accidentally repeating the administration of the drug. If the drug was refused or omitted, record this in the appropriate area on the medication record and notify the physician. This verifies the reason medication was omitted and ensures that the physician is aware of the patient's condition.

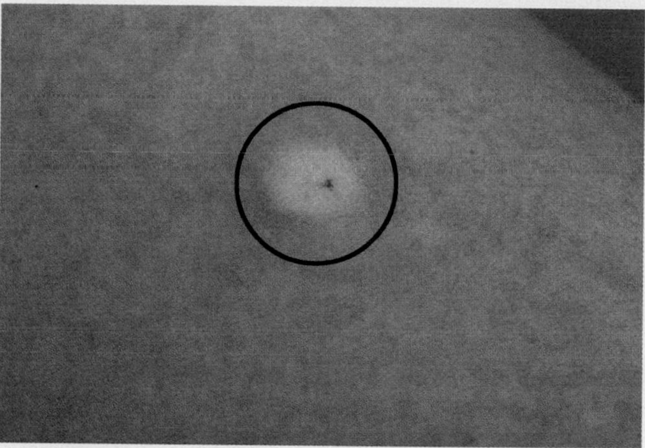

Figure 4. Drawing a circle around the wheal on skin.

Unexpected Situations and Associated Interventions

- *Nurse does not note wheal or blister at site of injection:* Medication has been injected subcutaneously. Document according to facility policy and inform the physician. Nurse may need to obtain order to repeat procedure.
- *Medication leaks out of injection site before needle is withdrawn:* Needle was inserted less than ⅛″. Document according to facility policy and inform the physician. Nurse may need to obtain order to repeat procedure.
- *Nurse sticks self with needle before injection:* Discard needle and syringe appropriately. Follow agency policy regarding needlestick injury. Prepare new syringe with medication and administer to patient. Complete appropriate paperwork and follow agency's policy regarding accidental needlesticks.
- *Nurse sticks self with needle after injection:* Discard needle and syringe appropriately. Follow agency policy regarding needlestick injury. Complete appropriate paperwork and follow agency's policy regarding accidental needlesticks.

Special Considerations

General Considerations

- Ongoing assessment is an important part of nursing care to evaluate patient response to administered medications and early detection of adverse effects. If an adverse effect is suspected, withhold further medication doses and notify the patient's primary healthcare provider. Additional intervention is based on type of reaction and patient assessment.
- Aspiration, pulling back on the plunger after insertion and before administration, is not recommended for an intradermal injection. The dermis does not contain large blood vessels.
- Some agencies recommend administering intradermal injections with the bevel down instead of the bevel up. Check facility policy.

SKILL 5-6 Administering a Subcutaneous Injection

Subcutaneous injections are administered into the adipose tissue layer just below the epidermis and dermis. This tissue has few blood vessels, so drugs administered here have a slow, sustained rate of absorption into the capillaries.

To correctly and effectively administer a subcutaneous injection, the nurse must choose the right equipment, select the appropriate location, use the correct technique, and deliver the correct dose.

It is important to choose the right equipment to ensure depositing the medication into the intended tissue layer and not the underlying muscle. Equipment used for a subcutaneous injection includes a syringe of appropriate volume for the amount of drug being administered. (An insulin pen may be used for subcutaneous injection of insulin; see the accompanying Skill Variation for technique). A 25-to 30-gauge, 3/8″ to 1″ needle can be used. The 3/8″ and 5/8″ needles are most commonly used. Some medications are packaged in prefilled cartridges with a needle attached. Confirm that the provided needle is appropriate for the patient before use. If not, the medication will have to be transferred to another syringe and the appropriate needle attached. Review the specifics of the particular medication before administrating. Various sites may be used for subcutaneous injections, including the outer aspect of the upper arm, the abdomen (from below the costal margin to the iliac crests), the anterior aspects of the thigh, the upper back, and the upper ventral or dorsogluteal area. Figure 1 shows the sites on the body where subcutaneous injections can be given. Absorption rates are different from the different sites. Injections in the abdomen are most rapidly absorbed, somewhat slower from the arms, even slower from the thighs, and slowest from the upper ventral or dorsogluteal areas (Caffrey, 2003).

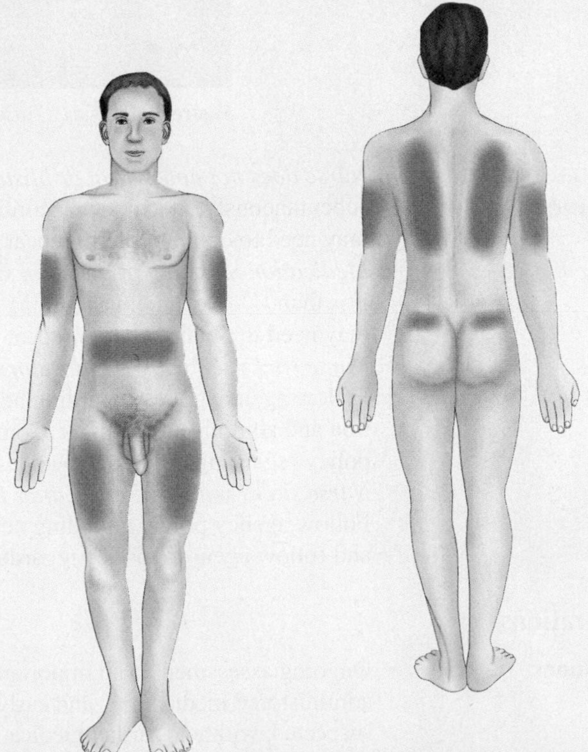

Figure 1. Sites on the body where subcutaneous injections can be given.

SKILL 5-6 Administering a Subcutaneous Injection *(continued)*

Subcutaneous injections are administered at a 45–90 degree angle. Choose the angle of needle insertion based on the amount of subcutaneous tissue present and the length of the needle. Generally, the shorter, 3/8″ needle should be inserted at a 90-degree angle and the longer, 5/8″ needle is inserted at a 45-degree angle. Figure 5-1 in the chapter opener shows the angles of insertion for subcutaneous injections.

Recommendations differ regarding pinching or bunching of a skin fold for administration. Pinching is advised for thinner patients and when a longer needle is used, to lift the adipose tissue away from underlying muscle and tissue. If pinching is used, once the needle is inserted, release the skin to avoid injecting into compressed tissue (King, 2003; Rushing, 2004; Stephens, 2003a).

Aspiration, or pulling back on the plunger to check that a blood vessel has been entered, is not necessary and has not proved to be a reliable indicator of needle placement. The likelihood of injecting into a blood vessel is small (Rushing, 2004; Stephens, 2003b). Aspiration is definitely contraindicated with administration of heparin because this action can result in hematoma formation.

Usually, no more than 1 mL of solution is given subcutaneously. Giving larger amounts adds to the patient's discomfort and may predispose to poor absorption

Equipment

- Prescribed medication
- Sterile syringe and needle. Needle size depends on the medication administered and patient body type (see previous discussion).
- Antimicrobial swab
- Disposable gloves
- Small gauze square
- Medication Administration Record (MAR) or Computer-generated MAR (CMAR)

ASSESSMENT

Assess the patient for any allergies. Check expiration date before administering medication. Assess the appropriateness of the drug for the patient. Verify patient name, dose, route, and time of administration. Review assessment and laboratory data that may influence drug administration. Assess the site on the patient where the injection is to be given. Avoid sites that are bruised, tender, hard, swollen, inflamed, or scarred. These conditions could affect absorption or cause discomfort and injury (Rushing, 2004). Assess the patient's knowledge of the medication. If the patient has deficient knowledge about the medication, this may be the appropriate time to begin education about the medication. If the medication may affect the patient's vital signs, assess them before administration. If the medication is for pain relief, assess the patient's pain level before and after administration.

NURSING DIAGNOSIS

Determine related factors for the nursing diagnoses based on the patient's current status. Appropriate nursing diagnoses may include:

- Deficient Knowledge
- Acute Pain
- Risk for Infection
- Risk for Injury
- Anxiety
- Risk for Allergy Response

OUTCOME IDENTIFICATION AND PLANNING

The expected outcome is that the patient receives medication via the subcutaneous route. Other outcomes that may be appropriate include the following: the patient's anxiety is decreased; the patient does not experience adverse effects; and the patient understands and complies with the medication regimen.

(continued)

SKILL 5-6 Administering a Subcutaneous Injection *(continued)*

IMPLEMENTATION

ACTION	RATIONALE
1. Gather equipment. Check each medication order against the original physician's order according to agency policy. Clarify any inconsistencies. Check the patient's chart for allergies.	This comparison helps to identify errors that may have occurred when orders were transcribed. The physician's order is the legal record of medication orders for each agency.
2. Know the actions, special nursing considerations, safe dose ranges, purpose of administration, and adverse effects of the medications to be administered. Consider the appropriateness of the medication for this patient.	This knowledge aids the nurse in evaluating the therapeutic effect of the medication in relation to the patient's disorder and can also be used to educate the patient about the medication.
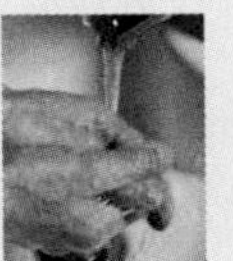 3. Perform hand hygiene.	Hand hygiene prevents the spread of microorganisms.
4. Move the medication cart to the outside of the patient's room or prepare for administration in the medication area.	Organization facilitates error-free administration and saves time.
5. Unlock the medication cart or drawer. Enter pass code and scan employee identification, if required.	Locking of the cart or drawer safeguards each patient's medication supply. Hospital accrediting organizations require medication carts to be locked when not in use. Entering pass code and scanning ID allows only authorized users into the system and identifies user for documentation by the computer.
6. **Prepare medications for one patient at a time.**	This prevents errors in medication administration.
7. Read the MAR and select the proper medication from the patient's medication drawer or unit stock.	This is the first check of the label.
8. Compare the label with the MAR. Check expiration dates and perform calculations, if necessary. Scan the bar code on the package, if required.	This is the second check of the label. Verify calculations with another nurse to ensure safety, if necessary.
9. If necessary, withdraw medication from an ampule or vial as described in Skills 5-2 and 5-3.	
10. **When all medications for one patient have been prepared, recheck the label with the MAR before taking them to the patient.**	This is a *third* check to ensure accuracy and to prevent errors.
11. Lock the medication cart before leaving it.	Locking the cart or drawer safeguards the patient's medication supply. Hospital accrediting organizations require medication carts to be locked when not in use.
12. Transport medications to the patient's bedside carefully, and keep the medications in sight at all times.	Careful handling and close observation prevent accidental or deliberate disarrangement of medications.
13. **Ensure that the patient receives the medications at the correct time.**	Check agency policy, which may allow for administration within a period of 30 minutes before or 30 minutes after designated time.

SKILL 5-6 Administering a Subcutaneous Injection *(continued)*

ACTION	RATIONALE
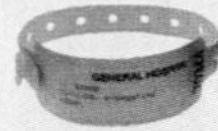 14. **Identify the patient.** Usually, the patient should be identified using two methods. Compare information with the MAR or CMAR.	Identifying the patient ensures the right patient receives the medications and helps prevent errors.
a. Check the name and identification number on the patient's identification band.	This is the most reliable method. Replace the identification band if it is missing or inaccurate in any way.
b. Ask the patient to state his or her name.	This requires a response from the patient, but illness and strange surroundings often cause patients to be confused.
c. If the patient cannot identify him or herself, verify the patient's identification with a staff member who knows the patient for the second source.	This is another way to double-check identity. Do not use the name on the door or over the bed, because these may be inaccurate.
15. Close the door to the room or pull the bedside curtain.	This provides patient privacy.
16. Complete necessary assessments before administering medications. Check allergy bracelet or ask patient about allergies. Explain the purpose and action of the medication to the patient.	Assessment is a prerequisite to administration of medications. Explanation provides rationale, increases knowledge, and reduces anxiety.
17. Scan the patient's bar code on the identification band, if required.	Scanning provides additional check to ensure that the medication is given to the right patient.
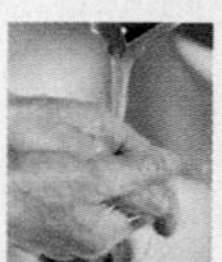 18. Perform hand hygiene and put on clean gloves.	Hand hygiene prevents the spread of microorganisms. Gloves help prevent exposure to contaminants.
19. Select an appropriate administration site.	Appropriate site prevents injury and allows for accurate reading of the test site at the appropriate time.
20. Assist the patient to the appropriate position for the site chosen. Drape as needed to expose only area of site to be used.	Draping helps maintain the patient's privacy.
21. Identify the appropriate landmarks for the site chosen.	Good visualization is necessary to establish the correct location of the site and to avoid damage to tissues.
22. Clean the area around the injection site with an antimicrobial swab. Use a firm, circular motion while moving outward from the injection site (Figure 2). Allow area to dry.	Pathogens on the skin can be forced into the tissues by the needle. Moving from the center outward prevents contamination of the site. Allowing skin to dry prevents introducing alcohol into the tissue, which can be irritating and uncomfortable.
23. Remove the needle cap with the nondominant hand, pulling it straight off.	The cap protects the needle from contact with microorganisms. This technique lessens the risk of an accidental needlestick.
24. Grasp and bunch the area surrounding the injection site or spread the skin taut at the site (Figure 3).	Decision to create a skin fold is based on the nurse's assessment of the patient and needle length used. Pinching is advised for thinner patients and when a longer needle is used, to lift the adipose tissue away from underlying muscle and tissue. If pinching is used, once the needle is inserted, release the skin to avoid injecting into compressed tissue. If skin is pulled taut, it provides easy, less painful entry into the subcutaneous tissue.

(continued)

SKILL 5-6

Administering a Subcutaneous Injection *(continued)*

ACTION	RATIONALE
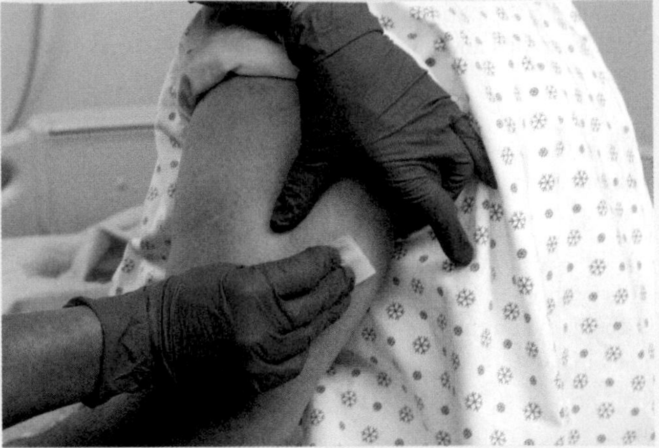 **Figure 2.** Cleaning injection site.	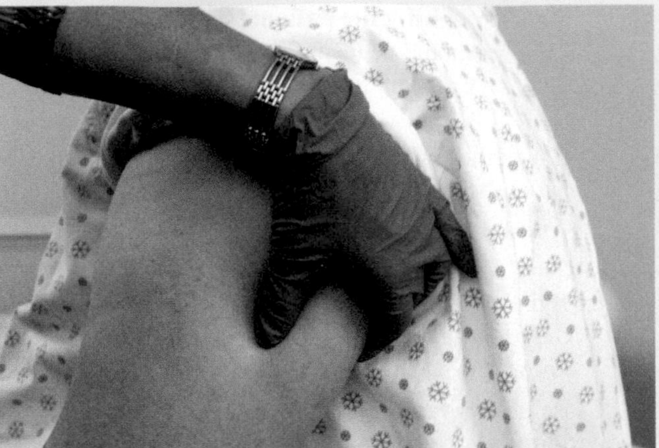 **Figure 3.** Bunching tissue around injection site.
25. **Hold the syringe in the dominant hand between the thumb and forefinger. Inject the needle quickly at a 45–90 degree angle (Figure 4).**	Inserting the needle quickly causes less pain to the patient. Subcutaneous tissue is abundant in well-nourished, well-hydrated people and spare in emaciated, dehydrated, or very thin persons. For a person with little subcutaneous tissue, it is best to insert the needle at a 45-degree angle.
26. After the needle is in place, release the tissue. If you have a large skin fold pinched up, ensure that the needle stays in place as the skin is released. Immediately move your nondominant hand to steady the lower end of the syringe. Slide your dominant hand to the end of the plunger. Avoid moving the syringe.	Injecting the solution into compressed tissues results in pressure against nerve fibers and creates discomfort. If there is a large skin fold, the skin may retract away from the needle. The nondominant hand secures the syringe. Moving the syringe could cause damage to the tissues and inadvertent administration into incorrect area.
27. Inject the medication slowly (at a rate of 10 seconds per milliliter).	Rapid injection of the solution creates pressure in the tissues, resulting in discomfort.
28. Withdraw the needle quickly at the same angle at which it was inserted, while supporting the surrounding tissue with your nondominant hand (Figure 5).	Slow withdrawal of the needle pulls the tissues and causes discomfort. Applying counter traction around the injection site helps to prevent pulling on the tissue as the needle is withdrawn. Removing the needle at the same angle at which it was inserted minimizes tissue damage and discomfort for the patient.
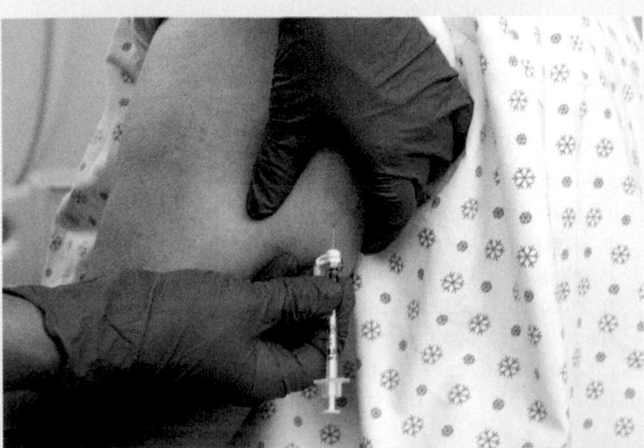 **Figure 4.** Inserting needle.	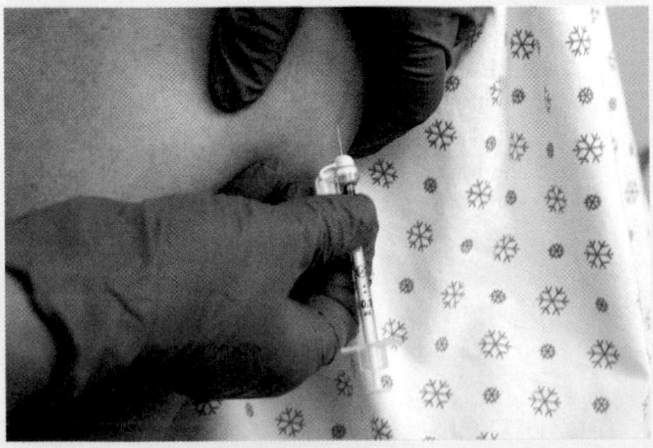 **Figure 5.** Withdrawing needle.

SKILL 5-6

Administering a Subcutaneous Injection *(continued)*

ACTION	RATIONALE
29. **Using a gauze square, apply gentle pressure to the site after the needle is withdrawn (Figure 6). Do not massage the site.**	Massaging the site is not necessary and can damage underlying tissue and increase the absorption of the medication. Massaging after heparin administration can contribute to hematoma formation. Massaging after an insulin injection may contribute to unpredictable absorption of the medication.

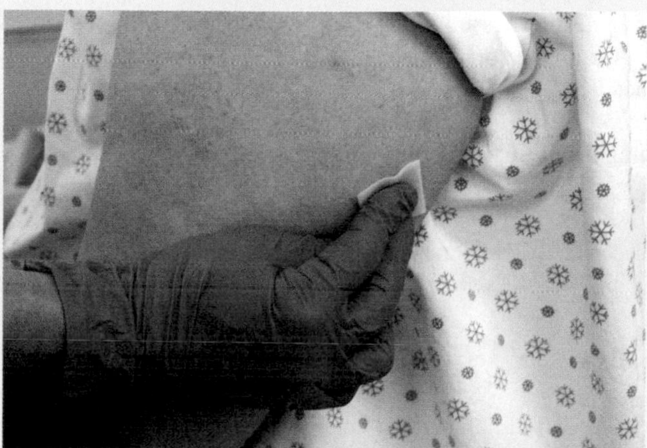

Figure 6. Applying pressure to the injection site.

ACTION	RATIONALE
30. Do not recap the used needle. Engage the safety shield or needle guard, if present. Discard the needle and syringe in the appropriate receptacle.	Proper disposal of the needle prevents injury.
31. Assist the patient to a position of comfort.	This provides for the well-being of the patient.
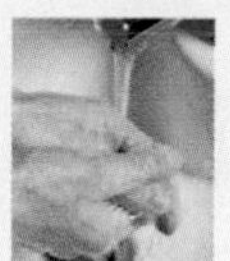 32. Remove gloves and dispose of them properly. Perform hand hygiene.	Hand hygiene deters the spread of microorganisms.
33. Evaluate the response of the patient to the medication within an appropriate time frame for the particular medication.	Evaluate effectiveness of drug and provides early detection of adverse effect.

EVALUATION

The expected outcomes are met when the patient receives the medication via the subcutaneous route; the patient's anxiety is decreased; the patient does not experience adverse effects; and the patient understands and complies with the medication regimen.

DOCUMENTATION

Guidelines

Record each medication given on the MAR or record using the required format, including date, dose, time, and the site of administration, immediately after administration. If using a bar-code system, medication administration is automatically recorded when scanned. PRN medications require documentation of the reason for administration. Prompt recording avoids the possibility of accidentally repeating the administration of the drug. If the drug was refused or omitted, record this in the appropriate area on the medication record and notify the physician. This verifies the reason medication was omitted and ensures that the physician is aware of the patient's condition.

(continued)

SKILL 5-6 Administering a Subcutaneous Injection *(continued)*

Unexpected Situations and Associated Interventions

- *When skin fold is released, needle pulls out of skin:* Remove and appropriately discard needle. Attach new needle to syringe and administer injection.
- *Patient refuses to let nurse administer medication in a different location:* Explain the rationale behind rotating injection sites. Discuss other available injection sites with patient. If patient will still not allow injection in another area, administer medication to patient, document patient's refusal and discussion, and notify physician.
- *Nurse sticks self with needle before injection:* Discard needle and syringe appropriately. Follow agency policy regarding needlestick injury. Prepare new syringe with medication and administer to patient. Complete appropriate paperwork and follow agency's policy regarding accidental needlesticks.
- *Nurse sticks self with needle after injection:* Discard needle and syringe appropriately. Follow agency policy regarding needlestick injury. Complete appropriate paperwork and follow agency's policy regarding accidental needlesticks.
- *During injection, patient pulls away from needle before medication is delivered fully:* Remove and appropriately discard needle. Attach a new needle to syringe and administer remaining medication at a different site. Document events and interventions according to facility policy.

Special Considerations

General Considerations

Ongoing assessment is an important part of nursing care to evaluate patient response to administered medications and early detection of adverse effects. If an adverse effect is suspected, withhold further medication doses and notify the patient's primary healthcare provider. Additional intervention is based on type of reaction and patient assessment.

Infant and Child Considerations

- Do not tell a child that an injection will not hurt. Describe the feel of the injection as a pinch or a sting. A child who believes you have been dishonest with him or her is less likely to cooperate with future procedures.

Older Adult Considerations

- Many elderly patients have less adipose tissue. Adjust the angle of the needle and angle of insertion accordingly. You do not want to inadvertently give a subcutaneous medication intramuscularly.

Home Care Considerations

- Reuse of syringes in the home setting is not recommended. Changes and improvements to insulin syringes to make injections painless have resulted in thinner, shorter, sharper, and better lubricated needles. As a result, after one injection the tip of the fine needles can bend and form a hook that can tear tissue if reused. These fine needles can break and leave fragments in the skin and tissue if reused. Reuse results in more painful injections related to a reduction in needle lubricant and tip damage (Caffrey, 2003; King, 2003).
- Encourage patients to consult the policies of their local government regarding contaminated and sharps waste disposal. Needles and syringes should be disposed of in a hard, plastic container. Liquid detergent or liquid fabric softener containers are good choices. Glass containers should not be used.

SKILL 5-6 Administering a Subcutaneous Injection *(continued)*

SKILL VARIATION Using an Insulin Pen to Administer Insulin via the Subcutaneous Route

- Perform hand hygiene.
- Remove the pen cap.
- Insert an insulin cartridge into the pen, following the manufacturer's directions.
- Clean the tip of the reservoir with alcohol.
- Invert the pen 20 times to mix if using an insulin suspension.
- Remove the protective tab from the needle.
- Screw the needle onto the reservoir.
- Remove the outer and inner needle caps.
- Hold the pen upright and tap to force any air bubbles to the top.
- Dial the dose selector to 2 units to perform an "air shot" to get rid of bubbles.
- Hold the pen upright and press the plunger firmly. Watch for a drop of insulin at the needle tip.
- Check the drug reservoir to make sure enough insulin is available for the dose.
- Check that the dose selector is at "0," and then dial the units of insulin for the dose.
- Clean the injection site and administer the subcutaneous injection, holding the pen like a dart. Push the button on the pen all the way in.
- Keep the button depressed and count to 6 before removing from the skin.
- Remove the needle from the pen and dispose in a sharps container. Perform hand hygiene.

(Adapted from Moshang, J. [2005]. Making a point about insulin pens. *Nursing, 35*[2], 46–47.)

SKILL 5-7 Administering an Intramuscular Injection

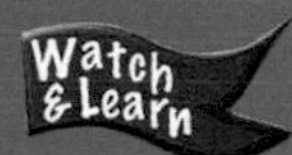

Intramuscular injections deliver medication through the skin and subcutaneous tissues into certain muscles. Muscles have larger and a greater number of blood vessels than subcutaneous tissue, allowing faster onset of action than with subcutaneous injections. Some medications administered intramuscularly are formulated to have a longer duration of effect. The deposit of medication creates a depot at the site of injection, designed to deliver slow, sustained release over hours, days, or weeks.

To correctly and effectively administer an intramuscular injection, the nurse must choose the right equipment, select the appropriate location, use the correct technique, and deliver the correct dose.

It is important to choose the right needle length for a particular intramuscular injection. Needle length should be based on the site for injection and the patient's age. See Table 5-1

TABLE 5-1 Intramuscular Injection Needle Length

SITE/AGE	NEEDLE LENGTH
Vastus lateralis	⅝″ to 1″
Deltoid (children)	⅝″ to 1¼″
Deltoid (adults)	1″ to 1½″
Ventrogluteal (adults)	1½″

(Adapted from Nicoll, L. & Hesby, A. [2002]. Intramuscular injection: An integrative research review and guideline for evidence-based practice. *Applied Nursing Research, 16*[2], 149–162.)

(continued)

SKILL 5-7

Administering an Intramuscular Injection *(continued)*

for intramuscular needle length recommendations. Patients who are obese may require a longer needle, and emaciated patients may require a shorter needle. Appropriate gauge is determined by the medication being administered. Generally, biologic agents and medications in aqueous solutions should be administered with a 20-to 25-gauge needle. Medications in oil-based solutions should be administered with an 18-to 25-gauge needle. Many medications come in prefilled syringe units. If a needle is provided on the prefilled unit, the nurse should ensure that the needle on the unit is the appropriate length for the patient and situation.

To avoid complications, the nurse must be able to identify anatomic landmarks and site boundaries. See Figure 1 for a depiction of anatomic landmarks and site boundaries

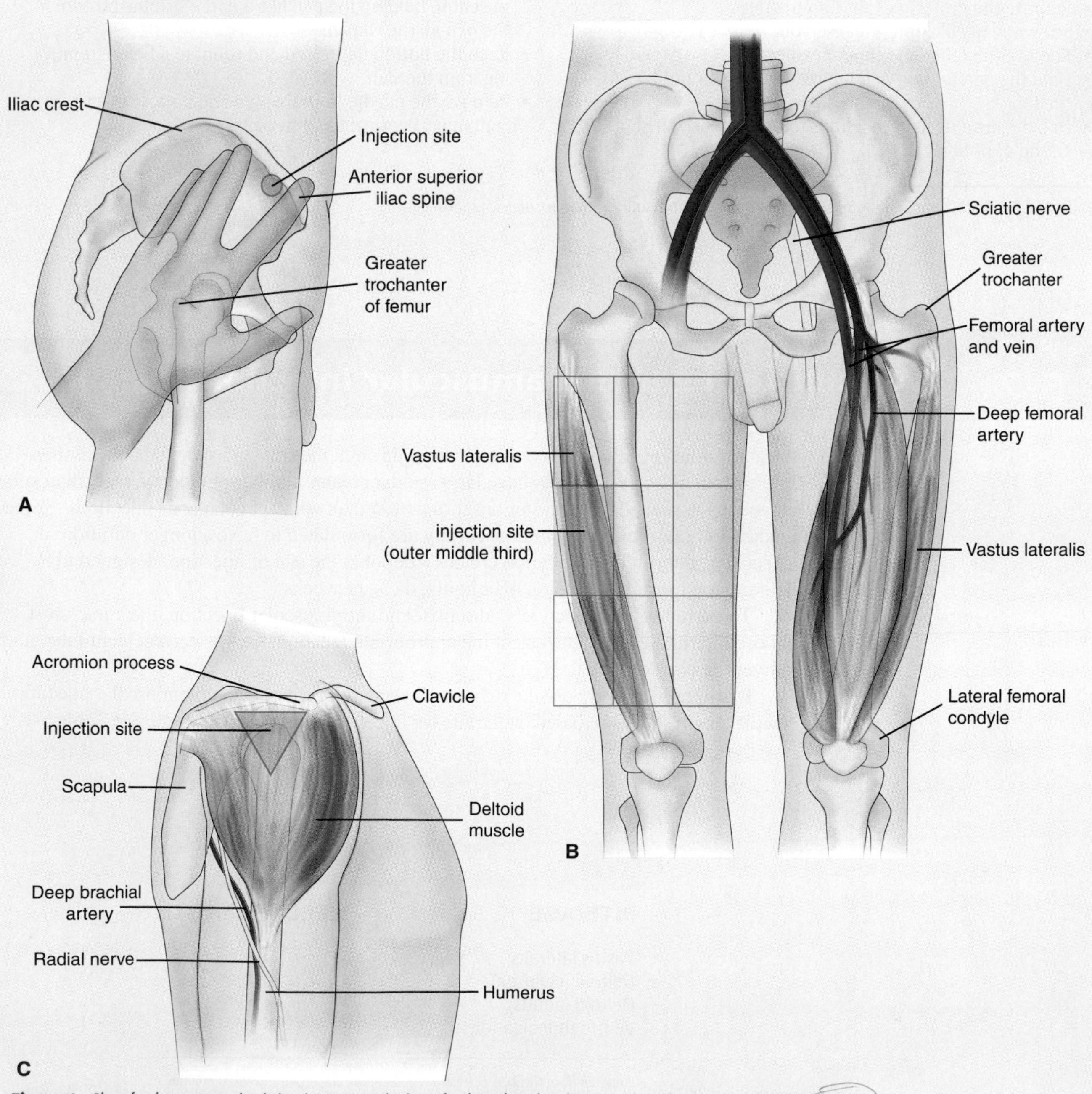

Figure 1. Sites for intramuscular injections. Descriptions for locating the sites are given in the text. (**A**) The ventrogluteal site is located by placing the palm on the greater trochanter and the index finger toward the anterosuperior iliac spine. (**B**) The vastus lateralis site is identified by dividing the thigh into thirds, horizontally and vertically. (**C**) The deltoid muscle site is located by palpating the lower edge of the acromion process.

SKILL 5-7

Administering an Intramuscular Injection *(continued)*

for potential intramuscular injection sites. The age of the patient, medication type, and medication volume should be considered when selecting a site for intramuscular injection. See Table 5-2 for information related to intramuscular site selection. The sites used to administer intramuscular medications should be rotated when therapy requires repeated injections. Whatever pattern of rotating sites is used, a description of it should appear in the patient's plan of nursing care. Depending on the site selected, the nurse may need to reposition the patient (see Table 5-3).

The nurse should use accurate, careful technique when administering intramuscular injections. If care is not taken, possible complications include abscesses, cellulites, injury to blood vessels, bones and nerves, lingering pain, tissue necrosis, and periostitis (inflammation of the membrane covering a bone). Administer the intramuscular injection so that the needle is perpendicular to the patient's body. This ensures it is given using an angle of injection between 72 to 90 degrees (Nicoll & Hesby, 2002). Figure 5-1 in the chapter opener shows the angles of insertion for intramuscular injections.

TABLE 5-2 Intramuscular Site Selection

	RECOMMENDED SITE
Age of Patient	
Infants	Vastus lateralis
Toddlers and children	Vastus lateralis or deltoid
Adults	Ventrogluteal or deltoid
Medication Type	
Biologicals (infants and young children)	Vastus lateralis
Biologicals (older children and adults)	Deltoid
Hepatitis B/Rabies	Deltoid
Depot formulations	Ventrogluteal
Medications that are known to be irritating, viscous, or oily solutions	Ventrogluteal

(Adapted from Nicoll, L. & Hesby, A. [2002]. Intramuscular injection: An integrative research review and guideline for evidence-based practice. *Applied Nursing Research, 16*[2], 149–162.)

TABLE 5-3 Patient Positioning

SITE OF INJECTION	PATIENT POSITION
Deltoid	Patient may sit or stand. A child may be held in an adult's lap.
Ventrogluteal	Patient may stand, sit, lay laterally, lay supine.
Vastus lateralis	Patient may sit or lay supine. Infants and young children may lay supine or be held in an adult's lap.

(Adapted from Nicoll, L. & Hesby, A. [2002]. Intramuscular injection: An integrative research review and guideline for evidence-based practice. *Applied Nursing Research, 16*[2], 149–162.)

The volume of medication that can be administered intramuscularly varies based on the intended site. Generally, 1 to 4 mL is the accepted volume range, with no more than 1 to 2 mL given at the deltoid site. The less-developed muscles of children and elderly people limit the intramuscular injection to 1 to 2 mL.

(continued)

SKILL 5-7 Administering an Intramuscular Injection *(continued)*

Equipment

- Disposable gloves
- Medication
- Sterile syringe and needle of appropriate size and gauge
- Antimicrobial swab
- Small gauze square
- Medication Administration Record (MAR) or Computer-generated MAR (CMAR)

ASSESSMENT

Assess the patient's knowledge of the medication. If the patient has a knowledge deficit about the medication, this may be an appropriate time to begin education about the medication. Assess the area where the injection is to be given. If the medication is for pain, assess the patient's level of pain. If the medication may affect the patient's vital signs or laboratory test results, check them before administering the medication. Assess the patient for any allergies. Check expiration date before administering medication. Assess the appropriateness of the drug for the patient. Verify patient name, medication dose, route, and time of administration. Review assessment and laboratory data that may influence drug administration. Assess the site on the patient where the injection is to be given. Avoid any site that is bruised, tender, hard, swollen, inflamed, or scarred. Assess the patient's knowledge of the medication. If the patient has a knowledge deficit about the medication, this may be the appropriate time to begin education about the medication. If the medication may affect the patient's vital signs, assess them before administration. If the medication is for pain relief, assess the patient's pain level before and after administration

NURSING DIAGNOSIS

Determine related factors for the nursing diagnoses based on the patient's current status. Appropriate diagnoses may include:

- Deficient Knowledge
- Acute Pain
- Risk for Allergy Response
- Anxiety
- Risk for Injury
- Risk for Impaired Skin Integrity

OUTCOME IDENTIFICATION AND PLANNING

The expected outcome to achieve when administering an intramuscular injection is that the patient receives the medication via the intramuscular route. Other outcomes that may be appropriate include the following: the patient's anxiety is decreased; the patient does not experience adverse effects; and the patient understands and complies with the medication regimen.

IMPLEMENTATION

ACTION	RATIONALE
1. Gather equipment. Check each medication order against the original physician's order according to agency policy. Clarify any inconsistencies. Check the patient's chart for allergies.	This comparison helps to identify errors that may have occurred when orders were transcribed. The physician's order is the legal record of medication orders for each agency.
2. Know the actions, special nursing considerations, safe dose ranges, purpose of administration, and adverse effects of the medications to be administered. Consider the appropriateness of the medication for this patient.	This knowledge aids the nurse in evaluating the therapeutic effect of the medication in relation to the patient's disorder and can also be used to educate the patient about the medication.

SKILL 5-7 Administering an Intramuscular Injection *(continued)*

ACTION	RATIONALE
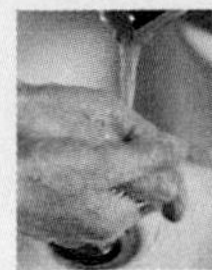 3. Perform hand hygiene.	Hand hygiene prevents the spread of microorganisms.
4. Move the medication cart to the outside of the patient's room or prepare for administration in the medication area.	Organization facilitates error-free administration and saves time.
5. Unlock the medication cart or drawer. Enter pass code and scan employee identification, if required.	Locking of the cart or drawer safeguards each patient's medication supply. Hospital accrediting organizations require medication carts to be locked when not in use. Entering pass code and scanning ID allows only authorized users into the system and identifies user for documentation by the computer.
6. **Prepare medications for one patient at a time.**	This prevents errors in medication administration.
7. Read the MAR and select the proper medication from the patient's medication drawer or unit stock.	This is the first check of the label.
8. Compare the label with the MAR. Check expiration dates and perform calculations, if necessary. Scan the bar code on the package, if required.	This is the second check of the label. Verify calculations with another nurse to ensure safety, if necessary.
9. If necessary, withdraw medication from an ampule or vial as described in Skills 5-2 and 5-3.	
10. **When all medications for one patient have been prepared, recheck the label with the MAR before taking them to the patient.**	This is a *third* check to ensure accuracy and to prevent errors.
11. Lock the medication cart before leaving it.	Locking the cart or drawer safeguards the patient's medication supply. Hospital accrediting organizations require medication carts to be locked when not in use.
12. Transport medications to the patient's bedside carefully, and keep the medications in sight at all times.	Careful handling and close observation prevent accidental or deliberate disarrangement of medications.
13. **Ensure that the patient receives the medications at the correct time.**	Check agency policy, which may allow for administration within a period of 30 minutes before or 30 minutes after designated time.
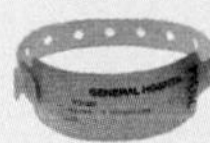 14. **Identify the patient.** Usually, the patient should be identified using two methods. Compare information with the MAR or CMAR.	Identifying the patient ensures the right patient receives the medications and helps prevent errors.
a. Check the name and identification number on the patient's identification band.	This is the most reliable method. Replace the identification band if it is missing or inaccurate in any way.
b. Ask the patient to state his or her name.	This requires a response from the patient, but illness and strange surroundings often cause patients to be confused.
c. If the patient cannot identify him or herself, verify the patient's identification with a staff member who knows the patient for the second source.	This is another way to double-check identity. Do not use the name on the door or over the bed, because these may be inaccurate.
15. Close the door to the room or pull the bedside curtain.	This provides patient privacy.
16. Complete necessary assessments before administering medications. Check allergy bracelet or ask patient about allergies. Explain the purpose and action of the medication to the patient.	Assessment is a prerequisite to administration of medications. Explanation provides rationale, increases knowledge, and reduces anxiety.

(continued)

SKILL 5-7 Administering an Intramuscular Injection *(continued)*

ACTION	RATIONALE
17. Scan the patient's bar code on the identification band, if required.	Provides additional check to ensure that the medication is given to the right patient.
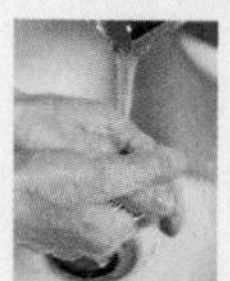 18. Perform hand hygiene and put on clean gloves.	Hand hygiene prevents the spread of microorganisms. Gloves help prevent exposure to contaminants.
19. Select an appropriate administration site.	Selecting the appropriate site prevents injury.
20. Assist the patient to the appropriate position for the site chosen. See Table 5-3. Drape as needed to expose only area of site to be used.	
21. **Identify the appropriate landmarks for the site chosen.**	Good visualization is necessary to establish the correct location of the site and avoid damage to tissues.
22. Clean the area around the injection site with an antimicrobial swab. Use a firm, circular motion while moving outward from the injection site. Allow area to dry.	Pathogens on the skin can be forced into the tissues by the needle. Moving from the center outward prevents contamination of the site. Allowing skin to dry prevents introducing alcohol into the tissue, which can be irritating and uncomfortable.
23. Remove the needle cap by pulling it straight off. Hold the syringe in your dominant hand between the thumb and forefinger.	This technique lessens the risk of an accidental needlestick and also prevents inadvertently unscrewing the needle from the barrel of the syringe.
24. Displace the skin in a Z-track manner by pulling the skin down or to one side about 1″ (2.5 cm) with your nondominant hand and hold the skin and tissue in this position (Figure 2). (See the accompanying Skill Variation for information on administering an intramuscular injection without using the Z-track technique.)	This ensures medication does not leak back along the needle track and into the subcutaneous tissue.

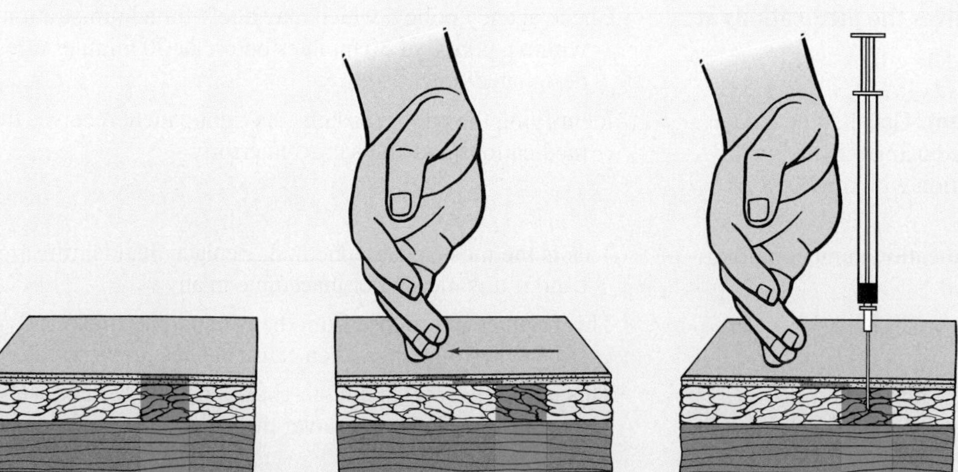
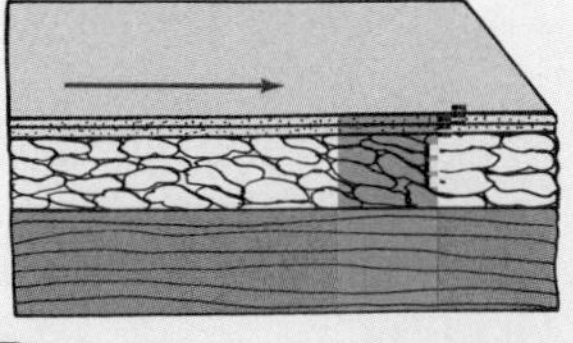

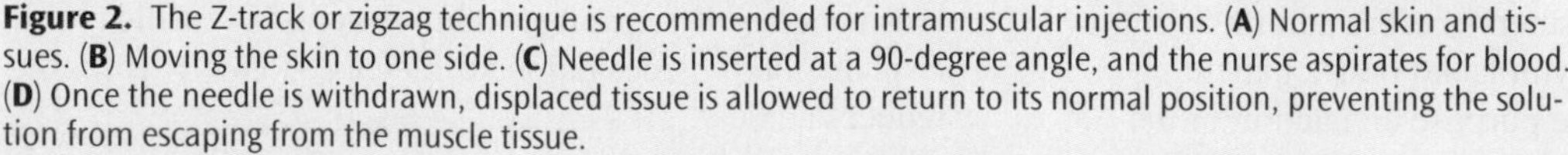
Figure 2. The Z-track or zigzag technique is recommended for intramuscular injections. (**A**) Normal skin and tissues. (**B**) Moving the skin to one side. (**C**) Needle is inserted at a 90-degree angle, and the nurse aspirates for blood. (**D**) Once the needle is withdrawn, displaced tissue is allowed to return to its normal position, preventing the solution from escaping from the muscle tissue.

SKILL 5-7

Administering an Intramuscular Injection *(continued)*

ACTION

RATIONALE

25. Quickly dart the needle into the tissue so that the needle is perpendicular to the patient's body (Figure 3). This should ensure that it is given using an angle of injection between 72 to 90 degrees.

A quick injection is less painful. Inserting the needle at a 72-to-90-degree angle facilitates entry into muscle tissue.

26. As soon as the needle is in place, use your thumb and forefinger of your nondominant hand to hold the lower end of the syringe. Slide your dominant hand to the end of the plunger.

Moving the syringe could cause damage to the tissues and inadvertent administration into incorrect area.

27. **Aspirate by slowly (for at least 5 seconds) pulling back on the plunger to determine whether the needle is in a blood vessel (Figure 4). Watch for a flash of pink or red in the syringe.**

Discomfort and possibly a serious reaction may occur if a drug intended for intramuscular use is injected into a vein. Allowing slow aspiration facilitates backflow of blood even if needle is in a small, low-flow blood vessel.

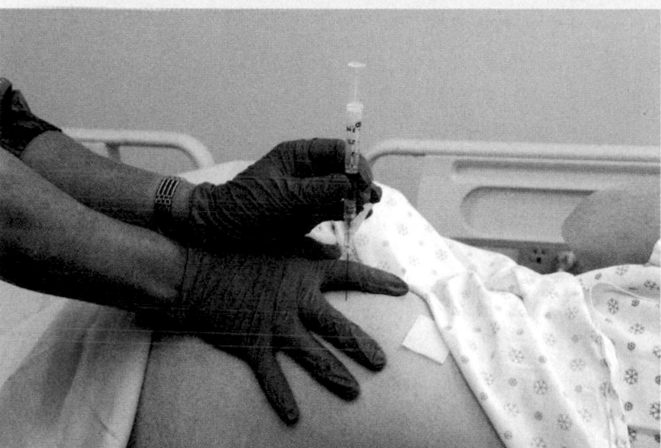

Figure 3. Darting the needle into the tissue.

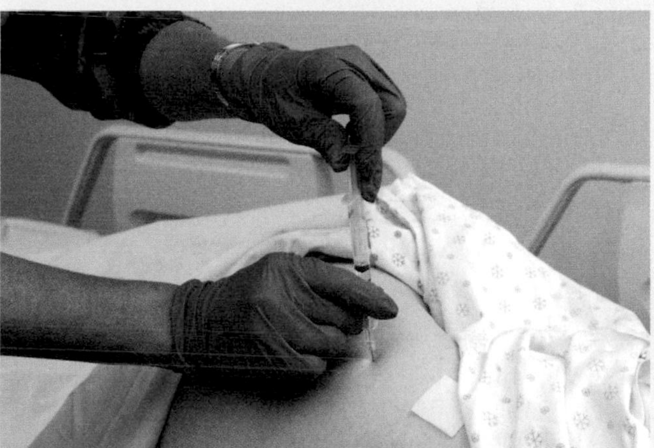

Figure 4. Aspirating.

28. If no blood is aspirated, inject the solution slowly (10 seconds per milliliter of medication).

Rapid injection of the solution creates pressure in the tissues, resulting in discomfort.

29. Once the medication has been instilled, wait 10 seconds before withdrawing the needle.

Allows medication to begin to diffuse into the surrounding muscle tissue (Nicoll & Hesby, 2002)

30. Withdraw the needle smoothly and steadily at the same angle at which it was inserted, supporting tissue around the injection site with your nondominant hand.

Slow withdrawal of the needle pulls the tissues and causes discomfort. Applying counter traction around the injection site helps to prevent pulling on the tissue as the needle is withdrawn. Removing the needle at the same angle at which it was inserted minimizes tissue damage and discomfort for the patient.

31. **Apply gentle pressure at the site with a dry gauze (Figure 5).**

Light pressure causes less trauma and irritation to the tissues. Massaging can force medication into subcutaneous tissues.

(continued)

SKILL 5-7 Administering an Intramuscular Injection *(continued)*

ACTION	RATIONALE
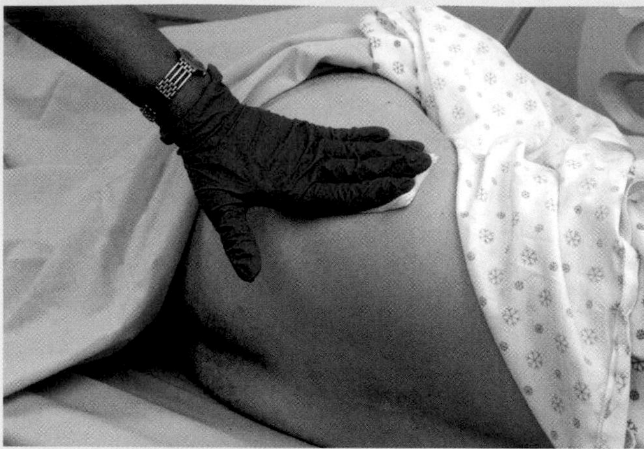 **Figure 5.** Applying pressure at the injection site.	
32. Do not recap the used needle. Engage the safety shield or needle guard, if present. Discard the needle and syringe in the appropriate receptacle.	Proper disposal of the needle prevents injury.
33. Assist the patient to a position of comfort.	This provides for the well-being of the patient.
34. Remove gloves and dispose of them properly. Perform hand hygiene.	Hand hygiene deters the spread of microorganisms.
35. Evaluate patient's response to medication within an appropriate time frame. Assess site, if possible, within 2 to 4 hours after administration.	Evaluates effectiveness of drug and provides early detection of adverse effect. Adverse reaction to medication given by the parenteral route is a possibility. Visualization of the site also allows for assessment of any untoward effects.

EVALUATION

The expected outcomes are met when the patient receives the medication via the intramuscular route; the patient's anxiety is decreased; the patient does not experience adverse effects or injury; and the patient understands and complies with the medication regimen.

Documentation

Guidelines

Record each medication given on the MAR or record using the required format, including date, time and the site of administration, immediately after administration. If using a bar-code system, medication administration is automatically recorded when scanned. PRN medications require documentation of the reason for administration. Prompt recording avoids the possibility of accidentally repeating the administration of the drug. If the drug was refused or omitted, record this in the appropriate area on the medication record and notify the physician. This verifies the reason medication was omitted and ensures that the physician is aware of the patient's condition.

Unexpected Situations and Associated Interventions

- *Nurse sticks self with needle before injection:* Discard needle and syringe appropriately. Follow agency policy regarding needlestick injury. Prepare new syringe with medication and administer to patient. Complete appropriate paperwork and follow agency's policy regarding accidental needlesticks.

SKILL 5-7 Administering an Intramuscular Injection *(continued)*

- *Nurse sticks self with needle after injection:* Discard needle and syringe appropriately. Follow agency policy regarding needlestick injury. Complete appropriate paperwork and follow agency's policy regarding accidental needlesticks.
- *During injection, patient pulls away from needle before medication is delivered fully:* Remove and appropriately discard needle. Attach a new needle to syringe and administer remaining medication at a different site. Document events and interventions according to facility policy.
- *While injecting needle into patient, nurse hits patient's bone:* Withdraw and discard the needle. Apply new needle to syringe and administer in alternate site. Document incident in patient's notes. Notify physician. Complete appropriate paperwork related to adverse events according to facility policy.

Special Considerations

General Considerations

Ongoing assessment is an important part of nursing care to evaluate patient response to administered medications and early detection of adverse effects. If an adverse effect is suspected, withhold further medication doses and notify the patient's primary healthcare provider. Additional intervention is based on type of reaction and patient assessment.

Infant and Child Considerations

- The vastus lateralis is the preferred site for infants.

Older Adult Considerations

- Muscle mass atrophies as a person ages. Take care to evaluate the patient's muscle mass and body composition. Use appropriate needle length and gauge for patient's body composition. Choose appropriate site based on the patient's body composition.

Home Care Considerations

- Encourage patients to consult the policies of their local government regarding contaminated and sharps waste disposal. Needles and syringes should be disposed of in a hard, plastic container. Liquid detergent or liquid fabric softener containers are good choices. Glass containers should not be used.

SKILL VARIATION Administering an Intramuscular Injection Without Using the Z-Track Technique

If the Z-Track technique is not used, the skin is stretched flat between two fingers and held taut for needle insertion. To administer the injection:

- Perform hand hygiene and put on clean gloves.
- Select an appropriate administration site.
- Assist the patient to the appropriate position for the site chosen. Drape as needed to expose only area of site to be used.
- Identify the appropriate landmarks for the site chosen with your nondominant hand.
- Clean the area around the injection site with an antimicrobial swab. Use a firm, circular motion while moving outward from the injection site. Allow area to dry.
- Remove the needle cap by pulling it straight off. Hold the syringe in your dominant hand between the thumb and forefinger.
- Stretch the skin flat between two fingers and hold taut for needle insertion.
- Quickly dart the needle into the tissue so that the needle is perpendicular to the patient's body. This should ensure that it is given using an angle of injection between 72 to 90 degrees.
- As soon as the needle is in place, use your thumb and forefinger of your nondominant hand to hold the lower end of the syringe. Slide your dominant hand to the end of the plunger.
- Aspirate by slowly (for at least 5 seconds) pulling back on the plunger to determine whether the needle is in a blood vessel. Watch for a flash of pink or red in the syringe.
- If no blood is aspirated, inject the solution slowly (10 seconds per mL of medication)
- Withdraw the needle smoothly and steadily at the same angle at which it was inserted, supporting tissue around the injection site with your nondominant hand.
- Apply gentle pressure at the site with a dry gauze.
- Do not recap the used needle. Engage the safety shield or needle guard, if present. Discard the needle and syringe in the appropriate receptacle.
- Assist the patient to a position of comfort.
- Remove gloves and dispose of them properly. Perform hand hygiene.
- Evaluate patient's response to medication within an appropriate time frame. Assess site, if possible, within 2 to 4 hours after administration.

SKILL 5-8 Administering Continuous Subcutaneous Infusion: Applying an Insulin Pump

Some medications, such as insulin, may be administered continuously via the subcutaneous route. Continuous subcutaneous insulin infusion (CSII or insulin pump) allows for multiple preset rates of insulin delivery. This system uses a small computerized reservoir that delivers insulin via tubing through a needle inserted into the subcutaneous tissue. The pump is programmed to deliver multiple preset rates of insulin delivery. The settings can be adjusted for exercise and illness, and bolus dose delivery can be timed in relation to meals. Change sites every two to three days to prevent tissue damage or absorption problems (Olohan & Zappitelli, 2003). Advantages of continuous subcutaneous medication infusion include the longer rate of absorption via the subcutaneous route and convenience for the patient.

Equipment

- Insulin pump
- Pump syringe
- Vial of insulin as ordered
- Sterile infusion set
- Insertion (triggering) device
- Needle (24 or 22 gauge, or blunt-ended needle)
- Antimicrobial swabs
- Sterile nonocclusive dressing
- Medication Administration Record (MAR) or Computer-generated MAR (CMAR)
- Clean gloves

ASSESSMENT

Assess the patient for any allergies. Check expiration date before administering medication. Assess the appropriateness of the drug for the patient. Review assessment and laboratory data that may influence drug administration. Verify patient name, dose, route, and time of administration. Assess skin in the area where the pump is to be applied. The pump should not be placed on skin that is irritated or broken down. Assess the patient's knowledge of the medication. If the patient has a knowledge deficit about the medication, this may be the appropriate time to begin education about the medication. If the medication may affect the patient's vital signs, assess them before administration. If the medication is for pain relief, assess the patient's pain level before and after administration. Assess the patient's blood glucose level as appropriate or as ordered.

NURSING DIAGNOSIS

Determine related factors for the nursing diagnoses based on the patient's current status. Appropriate nursing diagnoses may include:

- Deficient Knowledge
- Risk for Allergy Response
- Risk for Impaired Skin Integrity
- Acute Pain
- Risk for Infection

OUTCOME IDENTIFICATION AND PLANNING

The expected outcome is that the device is applied successfully and medication is administered. Other outcomes that may be appropriate include the following: patient understands the rationale for the pump use and mechanism of action; patient experiences no allergy response; patient's skin remains intact; pump is applied using aseptic technique; and patient does not experience adverse effect.

SKILL 5-8 Administering Continuous Subcutaneous Infusion: Applying an Insulin Pump *(continued)*

IMPLEMENTATION

ACTION	RATIONALE
1. Gather equipment. Check each medication order against the original physician's order according to agency policy. Clarify any inconsistencies. Check the patient's chart for allergies.	This comparison helps to identify errors that may have occurred when orders were transcribed. The physician's order is the legal record of medication orders for each agency.
2. Know the actions, special nursing considerations, safe dose ranges, purpose of administration, and adverse effects of the medications to be administered. Consider the appropriateness of the medication for this patient.	This knowledge aids the nurse in evaluating the therapeutic effect of the medication in relation to the patient's disorder and can also be used to educate the patient about the medication.
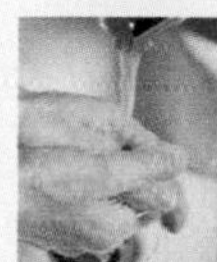 3. Perform hand hygiene.	Hand hygiene prevents the spread of microorganisms.
4. Move the medication cart to the outside of the patient's room or prepare for administration in the medication area.	Organization facilitates error-free administration and saves time.
5. Unlock the medication cart or drawer. Enter pass code and scan employee identification, if required.	Locking of the cart or drawer safeguards each patient's medication supply. Hospital accrediting organizations require medication carts to be locked when not in use. Entering pass code and scanning ID allows only authorized users into the system and identifies user for documentation by the computer.
6. **Prepare medications for one patient at a time.**	This prevents errors in medication administration.
7. Read the MAR and select the proper medication from the patient's medication drawer or unit stock.	This is the first check of the label.
8. Compare the label with the MAR. Check expiration dates and perform calculations, if necessary. Scan the bar code on the package, if required.	This is the second check of the label. Verify calculations with another nurse to ensure safety, if necessary.
9. Attach blunt-ended needle or small-gauge needle to syringe. Follow Skill 5-3 to remove insulin from vial. Remove enough insulin to last patient 2 to 3 days, plus 30 units for priming tubing.	Patient will wear pump for up to 3 days without changing syringe or tubing.
10. **When all medications for one patient have been prepared, recheck the label with the MAR before taking them to the patient.**	This is a *third* check to ensure accuracy and to prevent errors.
11. Lock the medication cart before leaving it.	Locking the cart or drawer safeguards the patient's medication supply. Hospital accrediting organizations require medication carts to be locked when not in use.
12. Transport medications to the patient's bedside carefully, and keep the medications in sight at all times.	Careful handling and close observation prevent accidental or deliberate disarrangement of medications.
13. **Ensure that the patient receives the medications at the correct time.**	Check agency policy, which may allow for administration within a period of 30 minutes before or 30 minutes after designated time.

(continued)

SKILL 5-8 Administering Continuous Subcutaneous Infusion: Applying an Insulin Pump *(continued)*

ACTION	RATIONALE
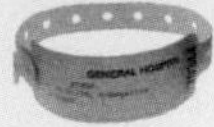 14. **Identify the patient.** Usually, the patient should be identified using two methods. Compare information with the MAR or CMAR.	Identifying the patient ensures the right patient receives the medications and helps prevent errors.
a. Check the name and identification number on the patient's identification band.	This is the most reliable method. Replace the identification band if it is missing or inaccurate in any way.
b. Ask the patient to state his or her name.	This requires a response from the patient, but illness and strange surroundings often cause patients to be confused.
c. If the patient cannot identify him or herself, verify the patient's identification with a staff member who knows the patient.	This is another way to double-check identity. Do not use the name on the door or over the bed, because these may be inaccurate.
15. Close the door to the room or pull the bedside curtain.	This provides patient privacy.
16. Complete necessary assessments before administering medications. Check allergy bracelet or ask patient about allergies. Explain the purpose and action of the medication to the patient.	Assessment is a prerequisite to administration of medications. Explanation provides rationale, increases knowledge, and reduces anxiety.
17. Scan the patient's bar code on the identification band, if required.	Provides additional check to ensure that the medication is given to the right patient.
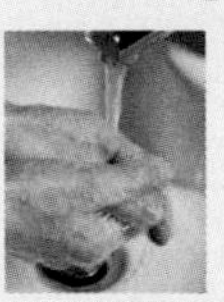 18. Perform hand hygiene.	Hand hygiene prevents the spread of microorganisms.
19. Attach sterile tubing to syringe. Prime the tubing by pushing the plunger of syringe until insulin is coming from introducer needle (Figure 1). **Check for any bubbles in tubing.**	Removing all air from tubing ensures that patient receives the correct dose of insulin.
20. Program pump according to manufacturer's recommendations following physician's orders. Open pump and place syringe in compartment according to manufacturer's directions (Figure 2). Close pump.	Syringe must be placed in pump correctly for delivery of insulin.

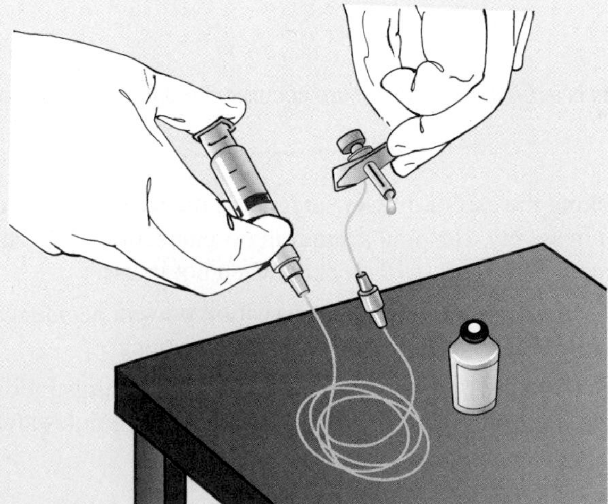

Figure 1. Priming insulin pump tubing.

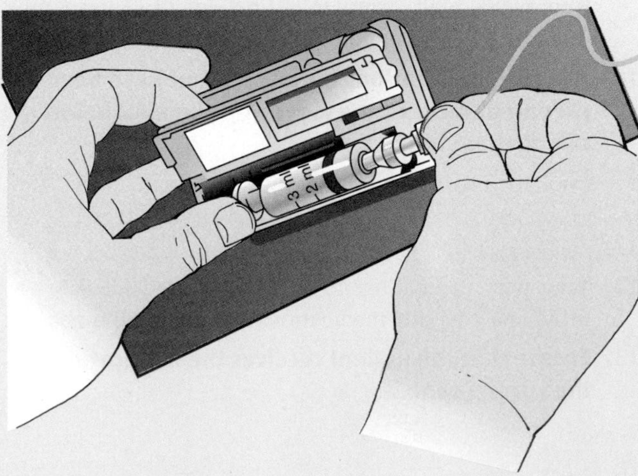

Figure 2. Placing syringe in compartment according to manufacturer's directions.

SKILL 5-8

Administering Continuous Subcutaneous Infusion: Applying an Insulin Pump *(continued)*

ACTION	RATIONALE
21. Activate delivery device. Place needle between prongs of insertion device with sharp edge facing out. Push insertion set down until click is heard.	To ensure correct placement of insulin pump needle, insertion device must be used.
22. Put on clean gloves.	Gloves help prevent exposure to contaminants.
23. Select an appropriate administration site.	Appropriate site prevents injury.
24. Assist the patient to the appropriate position for the site chosen. Drape as needed to expose only area of site to be used.	Maintains privacy and warmth.
25. Identify the appropriate landmarks for the site chosen.	Good visualization is necessary to establish the correct location of the site and avoid damage to tissues.
26. Clean area around injection site with antimicrobial swab. Use a firm, circular motion while moving outward from insertion site (Figure 3). Allow antiseptic to dry.	Pathogens on the skin can be forced into the tissues by the needle. Moving from the center outward prevents contamination of the site. Allowing skin to dry prevents introducing alcohol into the tissue, which can be irritating and uncomfortable.
27. Remove paper from adhesive backing. Remove needle guard. Pinch skin at insertion site, press insertion device on site, and press release button to insert needle (Figure 4). Remove triggering device.	To ensure delivery of insulin into subcutaneous tissue, a skin fold is made with a pinch *before* insertion of the medication.

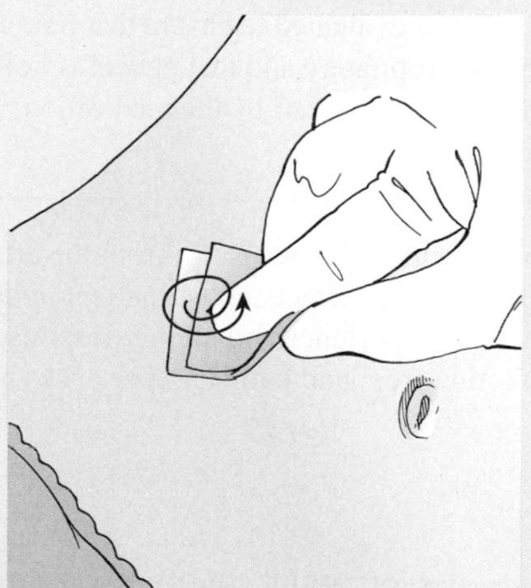

Figure 3. Cleaning area before insertion.

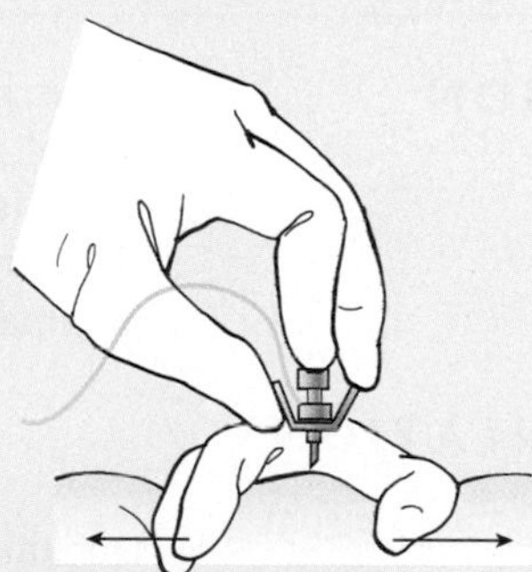

Figure 4. Inserting needle and delivery device.

ACTION	RATIONALE
28. **While holding needle hub, turn it a quarter-turn and remove needle (Figure 5).** Do not recap the used needle. Engage the safety shield or needle guard, if present.	The actual metal needle is removed and a plastic stylet is left in place to deliver the medication. If needle hub is not rotated, the stylet may be removed as well. Needle guards prevent injury.
29. Apply sterile occlusive dressing over insertion site (Figure 6). Attach the pump to patient's clothing.	Dressing prevents contamination of site. Pump can be dislodged easily if not attached securely to patient.

(continued)

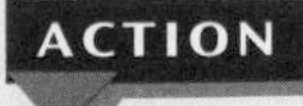

Administering Continuous Subcutaneous Infusion: Applying an Insulin Pump *(continued)*

ACTION | **RATIONALE**

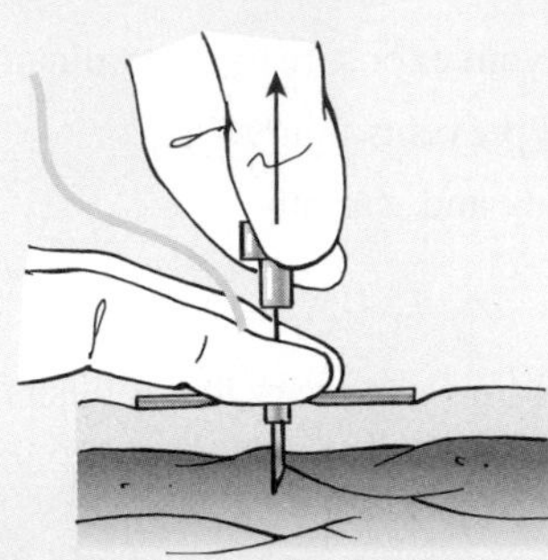

Figure 5. Removing needle from delivery device.

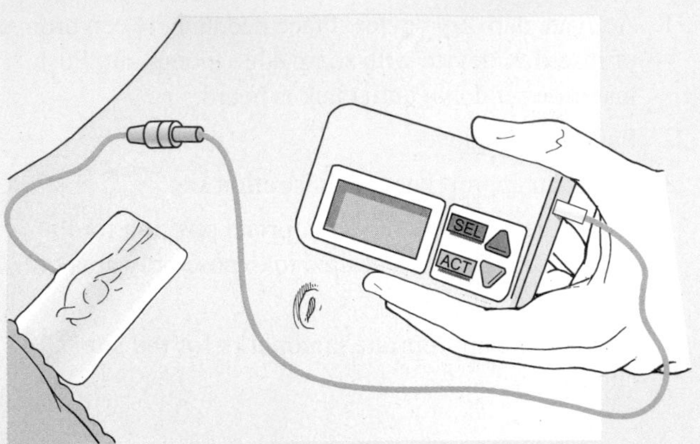

Figure 6. MiniMed insulin pump attached.

30. Discard the needle and syringe in the appropriate receptacle.

Proper disposal of the needle prevents injury.

31. Assist the patient to a position of comfort.

This provides for the well-being of the patient.

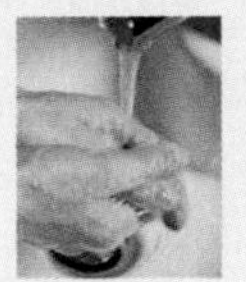

32. Remove gloves and dispose of them properly. Perform hand hygiene.

Hand hygiene deters the spread of microorganisms.

33. Evaluate patient's response to medication within appropriate time frame. Monitor the patient's blood glucose levels as appropriate or as ordered.

Patient needs to be evaluated to ensure that pump is delivering drug appropriately and that patient is not suffering any adverse affects caused by the medication.

EVALUATION

The expected outcomes are met when the patient receives insulin from the attached pump successfully without hypo- or hyperglycemic effects noted; patient understands the rationale for the pump attachment; patient experiences no allergy response; patient's skin remained intact; patient remains infection free; and patient experiences no or minimal pain.

DOCUMENTATION

Guidelines

Document the application of the pump, the type of insulin used, pump settings, insertion site, and any teaching done with patient on the MAR or record using the required format, including date, time and the site of administration, immediately after administration. If using a bar-code system, medication administration is automatically recorded when scanned. PRN medications require documentation of the reason for administration. Prompt recording avoids the possibility of accidentally repeating the administration of the drug. If the drug was refused or omitted, record this in the appropriate area on the medication record and notify the physician. This verifies the reason medication was omitted and ensures that the physician is aware of the patient's condition.

SKILL 5-8

Administering Continuous Subcutaneous Infusion: Applying an Insulin Pump *(continued)*

Sample Documentation

9/22/08 1000 Insulin pump inserted by patient on LUQ of abdomen with minimal assistance. Pump filled with 300 units (3 mL) of lispro insulin. Rate set at 1 unit per hour. Patient verbalizes desire to apply pump without assistance when site next changed.—B. Clapp, RN

Unexpected Situations and Associated Interventions

- *After pump is attached to patient, a large amount of air is noted in tubing:* Remove pump from patient. Obtain new sterile tubing with insertion needle. Prime tubing and reinsert.
- *Patient must rotate site more frequently than every 2 to 3 days due to insulin usage:* Check manufacturer's recommendations. Most pumps are initially set in a smaller mode but can be changed for a large amount of insulin delivery.
- *Patient is refusing to rotate site at least every 3 days:* Inform patient that absorption of medication decreases after 3 days, which may increase his or her need for insulin. Rotating sites prevents this decrease in absorption from developing.
- *Nurse notes that insertion site is now erythematous:* Remove the stylet, obtain a new pump setup, and insert at a different site at least 1″ from old site.
- *Occlusive dressing will not stick due to perspiration:* Apply deodorant around insertion site but not over insertion site. Alternately, apply skin barrier around insertion site but not over insertion site.

Special Considerations

General Considerations

- Assess infusion site areas routinely for inflammation, allergic reactions, infection, and lipodystrophy.
- Good hygiene and frequent catheter site changes reduce risk of site complications. Change catheter site every 2 to 3 days.
- Contact dermatitis is sometimes a problem at the catheter site area. The physician or healthcare provider may order topical antibiotics, aloe, vitamin E, or corticosteroids to treat a contact dermatitis.
- Insulin self-administered by the patient through the insulin pump should be communicated to the nurse at the time of administration. This allows for accurate documentation of insulin requirements.
- Ongoing assessment is an important part of nursing care to evaluate patient response to administered medications and early detection of adverse effects. If an adverse effect is suspected, withhold further medication doses and notify the patient's primary healthcare provider. Additional intervention is based on type of reaction and patient assessment.

Home Care Considerations

- Encourage patients to consult the policies of their local government regarding contaminated and sharps waste disposal. Needles and other sharps should be disposed of in a hard, plastic container. Liquid detergent or liquid fabric softener containers are good choices. Glass containers should not be used.

SKILL 5-9 Adding Medications to an Intravenous (IV) Solution Container

Medications may be added to the patient's infusion solution. The pharmacist commonly adds the prescribed drug to a large volume of IV solution, but sometimes the drug is added in the nursing unit, in which case sterile technique must be maintained.

When medication is administered by continuous infusion, the patient receives it slowly, over a long period. If the patient needs the medication quickly, this route/method should not be used. Consider also that if for some reason all of the solution cannot be infused, the patient will not receive the prescribed amount of the medication. Check a patient receiving medication by a continuous IV infusion for possible adverse effects at least every hour.

Equipment

- Prescribed medication
- Syringe with a 19- to 21-gauge needle, blunt needle, or needleless device (follow agency policy)
- IV fluid container (bag or bottle)
- Antimicrobial swab
- Label to be attached to the IV fluid container
- Medication Administration Record (MAR) or Computer-generated MAR (CMAR)

ASSESSMENT

Assess the patient for any allergies. Check expiration date before administering medication. Assess the appropriateness of the drug for the patient. Assess the compatibility of the ordered medication and the IV fluid. Review assessment and laboratory data that may influence drug administration. Verify patient name, dose, route, and time of administration. Assess the patient's knowledge of the medication. If the patient has a knowledge deficit about the medication, this may be the appropriate time to begin education about the medication. If the medication may affect the patient's vital signs, assess them before administration. Assess the IV insertion site, noting any swelling, coolness, leakage of fluid at site, redness, or pain.

NURSING DIAGNOSIS

Determine related factors for the nursing diagnoses based on the patient's current status. Appropriate nursing diagnoses may include:

- Risk for Injury
- Risk for Allergy Response
- Risk for Infection
- Deficient Knowledge
- Anxiety

OUTCOME IDENTIFICATION AND PLANNING

The expected outcome is that the medication is added to an adequate amount of compatible solution and mixed appropriately. Other outcomes that may be appropriate include the following: medication is delivered to the patient in a safe manner and at the appropriate infusion rate; patient experiences no allergy response; patient remains infection free; and the patient understands and complies with the medication regimen.

IMPLEMENTATION

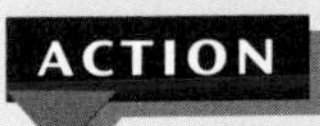

ACTION	RATIONALE
1. Gather equipment. Check medication order against the original physician's order according to agency policy. Clarify any inconsistencies. Check the patient's chart for allergies. Verify the compatibility of the medication and IV fluid. Calculate the infusion rate.	This comparison helps to identify errors that may have occurred when orders were transcribed. The physician's order is the legal record of medication orders for each agency. Compatibility of medication and solution prevents complications. Delivers the correct dose of medication as prescribed.

SKILL 5-9 Adding Medications to an Intravenous (IV) Solution Container *(continued)*

ACTION	RATIONALE
2. Know the actions, special nursing considerations, safe dose ranges, purpose of administration, and adverse effects of the medications to be administered. Consider the appropriateness of the medication for this patient.	This knowledge aids the nurse in evaluating the therapeutic effect of the medication in relation to the patient's disorder and can also be used to educate the patient about the medication.
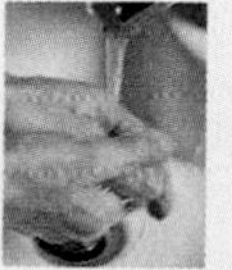 3. Perform hand hygiene.	Hand hygiene prevents the spread of microorganisms.
4. Move the medication cart to the outside of the patient's room or prepare for administration in the medication area.	Organization facilitates error-free administration and saves time.
5. Unlock the medication cart or drawer. Enter pass code and scan employee identification, if required.	Locking of the cart or drawer safeguards each patient's medication supply. Hospital accrediting organizations require medication carts to be locked when not in use. Entering pass code and scanning ID allows only authorized users into the system and identifies user for documentation by the computer.
6. **Prepare medication for one patient at a time.**	This prevents errors in medication administration.
7. Read the MAR and select the proper medication from the patient's medication drawer or unit stock.	This is the first check of the label.
8. Compare the label with the MAR. Check expiration dates and perform calculations, if necessary. Scan the bar code on the package, if required.	This is the second check of the label. Verify calculations with another nurse to ensure safety, if necessary.
9. If necessary, withdraw medication from an ampule or vial as described in Skills 5-2 and 5-3.	
10. **Recheck the label with the MAR before taking it to the patient.**	This is a *third* check to ensure accuracy and to prevent errors.
11. Lock the medication cart before leaving it.	Locking the cart or drawer safeguards the patient's medication supply. Hospital accrediting organizations require medication carts to be locked when not in use.
12. Transport medications and equipment to the patient's bedside carefully, and keep the medications in sight at all times.	Careful handling and close observation prevent accidental or deliberate disarrangement of medications. Having equipment available saves time and facilitates performance of the task.
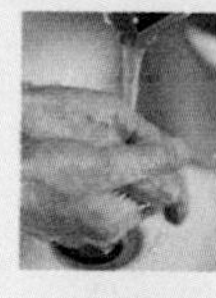 13. Perform hand hygiene.	Hand hygiene deters the spread of microorganisms.
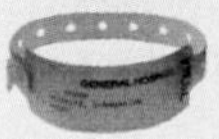 14. **Identify the patient.** Usually, the patient should be identified using two methods. Compare information with the MAR or CMAR.	Identifying the patient ensures the right patient receives the medications and helps prevent errors.
a. Check the name and identification number on the patient's identification band.	This is the most reliable method. Replace the identification band if it is missing or inaccurate in any way.

(continued)

SKILL 5-9 Adding Medications to an Intravenous (IV) Solution Container *(continued)*

ACTION	RATIONALE
b. Ask the patient to state his or her name.	This requires a response from the patient, but illness and strange surroundings often cause patients to be confused.
c. If the patient cannot identify him or herself, verify the patient's identification with a staff member who knows the patient for the second source.	This is another way to double-check identity. Do not use the name on the door or over the bed, because these may be inaccurate.
15. Close the door to the room or pull the bedside curtain.	This provides patient privacy.
16. Complete necessary assessments before administering medications. Check allergy bracelet or ask patient about allergies. Explain the purpose and action of the medication to the patient.	Assessment is a prerequisite to administration of medications. Explanation provides rationale, increases knowledge, and reduces anxiety.
17. Scan the patient's bar code on the identification band, if required.	Provides additional check to ensure that the medication is given to the right patient.
18. **Check that the volume in the current IV infusion is adequate.** (See the accompanying Skill Variation for information on adding medication to a new IV container.)	The volume should be sufficient to dilute the drug.
19. Close the clamp between the solution container and roller clamp on the infusion tubing (Figure 1) and pause the IV pump, if appropriate.	This prevents back-flow directly to the patient of improperly diluted medication.
20. Clean the medication port with an antimicrobial swab (Figure 2).	This deters entry of microorganisms when the port is punctured.

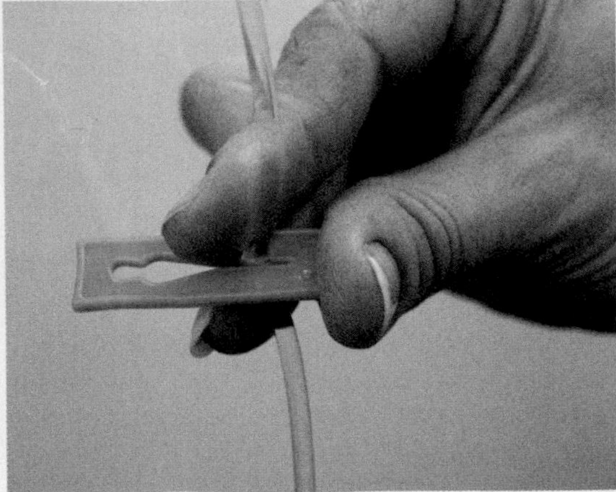

Figure 1. Closing the clamp on the infusion tubing.

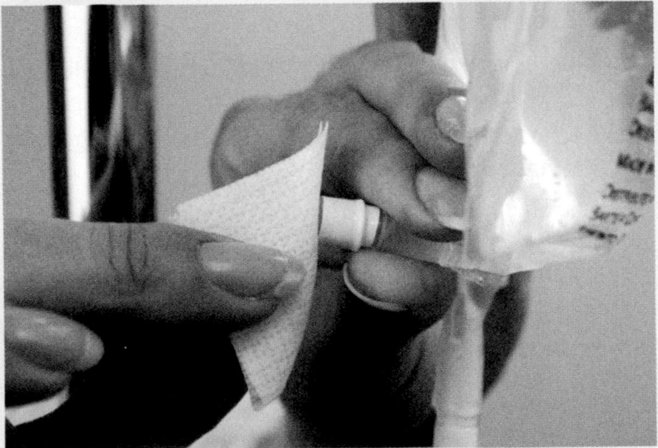

Figure 2. Cleaning the medication port.

ACTION	RATIONALE
21. Steady the container and uncap the needle or needleless device. Insert it into the port (Figure 3). Inject the medication. Withdraw the needle or needleless device. Do not recap the used needle. Engage the safety shield or needle guard, if present.	This ensures that the needle or needleless device enters the container and medication can be dispersed into the solution. Use of safety shield or needle guard prevents accidental injury.
22. Remove the container from the IV pole and gently rotate the container to mix the medication and solution (Figure 4).	This mixes the medication with the solution.

SKILL 5-9

Adding Medications to an Intravenous (IV) Solution Container *(continued)*

ACTION | RATIONALE

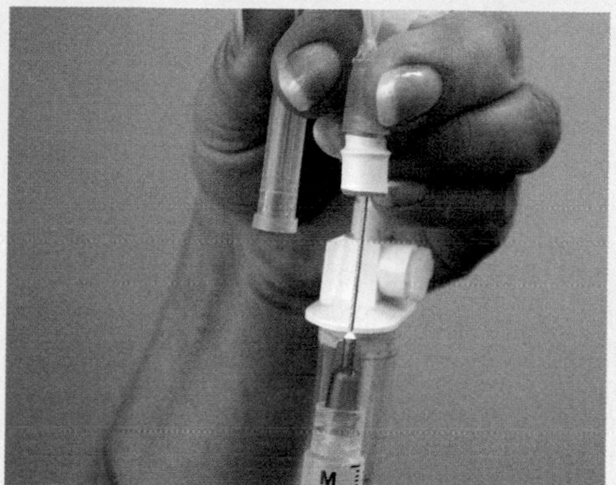

Figure 3. Inserting the needle into the port.

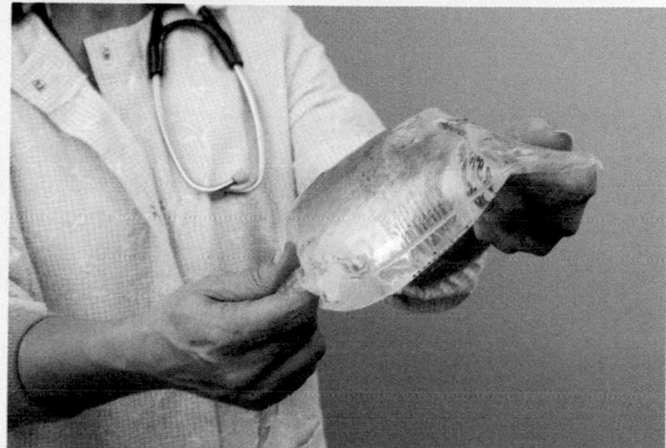

Figure 4. Rotating the container to mix the medication and solution.

23. Rehang the container on the pole. **Attach the label to the container so that the dose of medication that has been added is apparent (Figure 5).**

This confirms that the prescribed dose of medication has been added to the IV solution.

24. Open the clamp, and readjust the flow rate (Figure 6) or check the pump settings for correct infusion rate and restart pump.

Ensures the infusion of the IV with the medication at the prescribed rate.

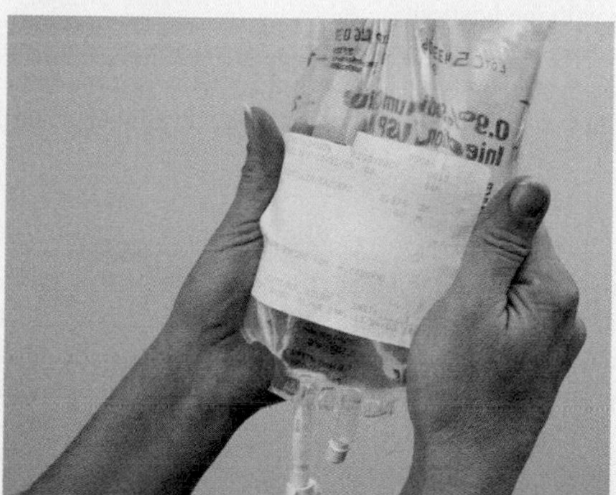

Figure 5. Labeling container to show medication addition.

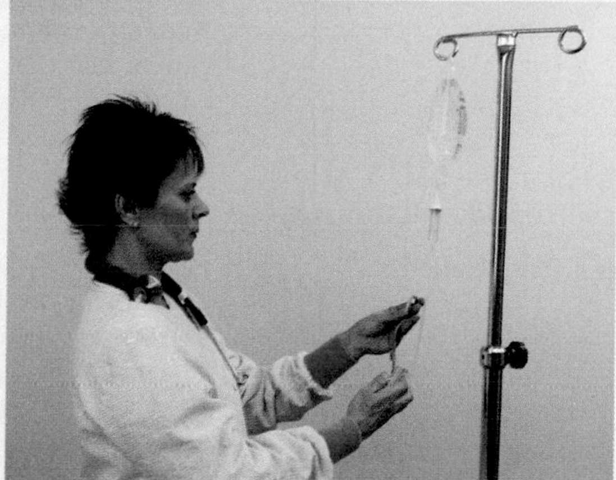

Figure 6. Readjusting flow rate.

25. Discard the needle and syringe in the appropriate receptacle.

Proper disposal of the needle prevents injury.

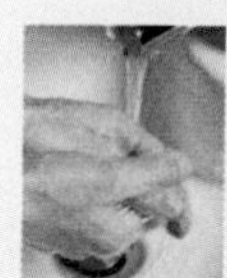

26. Perform hand hygiene.

This prevents spread of microorganisms.

27. Evaluate the patient's response to medication within the appropriate time frame.

Patients require careful observation because medications given by the IV route may have a rapid effect.

(continued)

SKILL 5-9

Adding Medications to an Intravenous (IV) Solution Container *(continued)*

EVALUATION

The expected outcomes are met when the medication is added to an adequate amount of IV solution and mixed appropriately; patient receives the medication in a safe and effective way; patient experiences no allergy response; patient experiences no infection; patient understands reasons for procedure; and patient experiences decreased anxiety regarding medication infusion.

DOCUMENTATION

Guidelines

Document the addition of the medication to the IV solution immediately after administration, including date, time, dose, route of administration, site of administration, and rate of administration on the MAR or record using the required format. If using a bar-code system, medication administration is automatically recorded when scanned. PRN medications require documentation of the reason for administration. Prompt recording avoids the possibility of accidentally repeating the administration of the drug. If the drug was refused or omitted, record this in the appropriate area on the medication record and notify the physician. This verifies the reason medication was omitted and ensures that the physician is aware of the patient's condition.

Unexpected Situations and Associated Interventions

- *There is not enough IV solution in container:* Obtain new IV fluid container from medication station and add medication. Remove current IV bag and replace with newly admixed IV fluid. (Some institutions would prefer that the pharmacy mix any new bags so that the process may be done in a sterile environment.)
- *Nurse realizes that wrong medication or wrong amount of medication was added to the IV bag:* Immediately stop infusion. Assess patient for any distress and notify physician. Follow agency policy for medication error. Remove bag of IV fluids and replace with IV containing ordered medication.
- *Nurse sticks self with needle while trying to inject medication into port:* Discard syringe and needle. Prepare new syringe with medication.
- *Needle goes through side of medication injection port:* Discard syringe, needle, and current bag of IV solution. Replace with newly mixed IV fluid. (Some institutions would prefer pharmacy mix any new bags so that the process may be done in a sterile environment.)

Special Considerations

General Considerations

- Ongoing assessment is an important part of nursing care to evaluate patient response to administered medications and early detection of adverse effects. If an adverse effect is suspected, withhold further medication doses and notify the patient's primary healthcare provider. Additional intervention is based on type of reaction and patient assessment.

SKILL 5-9 Adding Medications to an Intravenous (IV) Solution Container *(continued)*

SKILL VARIATION Adding Medication to a New Intravenous Container

- Check medication order against the original physician's order according to agency policy. Clarify any inconsistencies. Check the patient's chart for allergies. Verify the compatibility of the medication and IV fluid. Calculate the infusion rate.
- Know the actions, special nursing considerations, safe dose ranges, purpose of administration, and adverse effects of the medications to be administered. Consider the appropriateness of the medication for this patient.
- Perform hand hygiene.
- Move the medication cart to the outside of the patient's room or prepare for administration in the medication area.
- Unlock the medication cart or drawer. Enter pass code and scan employee identification, if required.
- Read the MAR and select the proper medication from the patient's medication drawer or unit stock.
- Compare the label with the MAR. Check expiration dates and perform calculations, if necessary. Scan the bar code on the package, if required.
- If necessary, withdraw medication from an ampule or vial as described in Skills 5-2 and 5-3.
- Recheck the label with the MAR before taking it to the patient.
- Lock the medication cart before leaving it.
- Transport medications and equipment to the patient's bedside carefully, and keep the medications in sight at all times.
- Perform hand hygiene.
- Identify the patient. Usually, the patient should be identified using two methods.
- Close the door to the room or pull the bedside curtain.
- Complete necessary assessments before administering medications. Check allergy bracelet or ask patient about allergies. Explain the purpose and action of the medication to the patient.
- Scan the patient's bar code on the identification band, if required.
- Carefully remove any protective cover and locate the injection port. Clean with an antimicrobial swab.
- Uncap the needle or needleless device and insert into the port. Inject the medication.
- Gently rotate the IV solution in the bag or bottle.
- Attach the label to the container so that the dose of medication that has been added is apparent.
- Do not recap the used needle. Engage the safety shield or needle guard, if present. Discard the needle and syringe in the appropriate receptacle.
- Perform hand hygiene.
- Prepare the IV infusion for administration according to facility policy.
- Evaluate the patient's response to medication within the appropriate time frame.

SKILL 5-10 Administering Medications by Intravenous Bolus or Push Through an Intravenous Infusion

A medication can be administered as an IV bolus or push. This involves a single injection of a concentrated solution directly into an IV line. Drugs given by IV push are used for intermittent dosing or to treat emergencies. The drug is administered very slowly over at least one minute. Exact administration times should be confirmed by consulting a pharmacist or drug reference.

Equipment

- Antimicrobial swab
- Watch with second hand, or stopwatch
- Clean gloves
- Prescribed medication
- Syringe with a needleless device or 23- to 25-gauge, 1″ needle (follow agency policy)
- Medication Administration Record (MAR) or Computer-generated MAR (CMAR)

ASSESSMENT

Assess the patient for any allergies. Check expiration date before administering medication. Assess the appropriateness of the drug for the patient. Assess the compatibility of the ordered medication and the IV fluid. Review assessment and laboratory data that may influence drug administration. Verify the patient's name, dose, route, and time of adminis-

(continued)

SKILL 5-10 Administering Medications by Intravenous Bolus or Push Through an Intravenous Infusion *(continued)*

tration. Assess patient's IV site, noting any swelling, coolness, leakage of fluid from IV site, or pain. Assess the patient's knowledge of the medication. If the patient has a knowledge deficit about the medication, this may be the appropriate time to begin education about the medication. If the medication may affect the patient's vital signs, assess them before administration.

NURSING DIAGNOSIS

Determine related factors for the nursing diagnoses based on the patient's current status. Appropriate nursing diagnoses may include:

- Acute Pain
- Risk for Allergy Response
- Deficient Knowledge
- Risk for Infection
- Anxiety
- Risk for Injury

OUTCOME IDENTIFICATION AND PLANNING

The expected outcome to achieve is that the medication is given safely. Other outcomes that may be appropriate include the following: patient experiences no adverse effect; patient experiences no allergy response; patient is knowledgeable about medication being added by bolus IV; patient remains infection free; and patient has no, or decreased, anxiety.

IMPLEMENTATION

ACTION	RATIONALE
1. Gather equipment. Check medication order against the original physician's order according to agency policy. Clarify any inconsistencies. Check the patient's chart for allergies. Verify the compatibility of the medication and IV fluid. Check a drug resource to clarify whether medication needs to be diluted before administration. Check the infusion rate.	This comparison helps to identify errors that may have occurred when orders were transcribed. The physician's order is the legal record of medication orders for each agency. Compatibility of medication and solution prevents complications. Delivers the correct dose of medication as prescribed.
2. Know the actions, special nursing considerations, safe dose ranges, purpose of administration, and adverse effects of the medications to be administered. Consider the appropriateness of the medication for this patient.	This knowledge aids the nurse in evaluating the therapeutic effect of the medication in relation to the patient's disorder and can also be used to educate the patient about the medication.
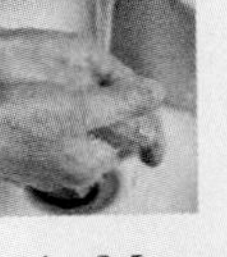 3. Perform hand hygiene.	Hand hygiene prevents the spread of microorganisms.
4. Move the medication cart to the outside of the patient's room or prepare for administration in the medication area.	Organization facilitates error-free administration and saves time.
5. Unlock the medication cart or drawer. Enter pass code and scan employee identification, if required.	Locking of the cart or drawer safeguards each patient's medication supply. Hospital accrediting organizations require medication carts to be locked when not in use. Entering pass code and scanning ID allows only authorized users into the system and identifies user for documentation by the computer.

SKILL 5-10 Administering Medications by Intravenous Bolus or Push Through an Intravenous Infusion *(continued)*

ACTION	RATIONALE
6. **Prepare medication for one patient at a time.**	This prevents errors in medication administration.
7. Read the MAR and select the proper medication from the patient's medication drawer or unit stock.	This is the first check of the label.
8. Compare the label with the MAR. Check expiration dates and perform calculations, if necessary. Scan the bar code on the package, if required.	This is the second check of the label. Verify calculations with another nurse to ensure safety, if necessary.
9. If necessary, withdraw medication from an ampule or vial as described in Skills 5-2 and 5-3.	
10. **Recheck the label with the MAR before taking it to the patient.**	This is a *third* check to ensure accuracy and to prevent errors.
11. Lock the medication cart before leaving it.	Locking the cart or drawer safeguards the patient's medication supply. Hospital accrediting organizations require medication carts to be locked when not in use.
12. Transport medications and equipment to the patient's bedside carefully, and keep the medications in sight at all times.	Careful handling and close observation prevent accidental or deliberate disarrangement of medications. Having equipment available saves time and facilitates performance of the task.
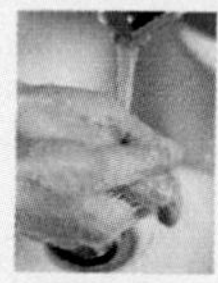 13. Perform hand hygiene.	Hand hygiene deters the spread of microorganisms.
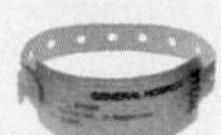 14. **Identify the patient.** Usually, the patient should be identified using two methods. Compare information with the MAR or CMAR.	Identifying the patient ensures the right patient receives the medications and helps prevent errors.
a. Check the name and identification number on the patient's identification band.	This is the most reliable method. Replace the identification band if it is missing or inaccurate in any way.
b. Ask the patient to state his or her name.	This requires a response from the patient, but illness and strange surroundings often cause patients to be confused.
c. If the patient cannot identify him or herself, verify the patient's identification with a staff member who knows the patient for the second source.	This is another way to double-check identity. Do not use the name on the door or over the bed, because these may be inaccurate.
15. Close the door to the room or pull the bedside curtain.	This provides patient privacy.
16. Complete necessary assessments before administering medications. Check allergy bracelet or ask patient about allergies. Explain the purpose and action of the medication to the patient.	Assessment is a prerequisite to administration of medications. Explanation provides rationale, increases knowledge, and reduces anxiety.
17. Scan the patient's bar code on the identification band, if required.	Provides additional check to ensure that the medication is given to the right patient.
18. **Assess IV site for presence of inflammation or infiltration.**	IV medication must be given directly into a vein for safe administration.
19. If IV infusion is being administered via an infusion pump, pause the pump.	Pausing prevents infusion of fluid during bolus administration and activation of pump occlusion alarms.
20. Put on clean gloves.	Gloves prevent contact with blood and body fluids.

(continued)

SKILL 5-10 Administering Medications by Intravenous Bolus or Push Through an Intravenous Infusion *(continued)*

ACTION	RATIONALE
21. Select injection port on tubing that is closest to venipuncture site. Clean port with antimicrobial swab (Figure 1).	Using port closest to needle insertion site minimizes dilution of medication. Cleaning deters entry of microorganisms when port is punctured.
22. Uncap syringe. Steady port with your nondominant hand while inserting syringe, needleless device, or needle into center of port (Figure 2).	This supports injection port and lessens risk for accidentally dislodging IV or entering port incorrectly.

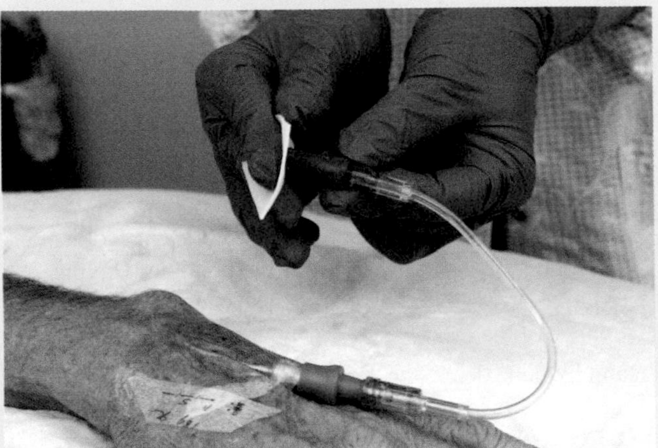

Figure 1. Cleaning injection port.

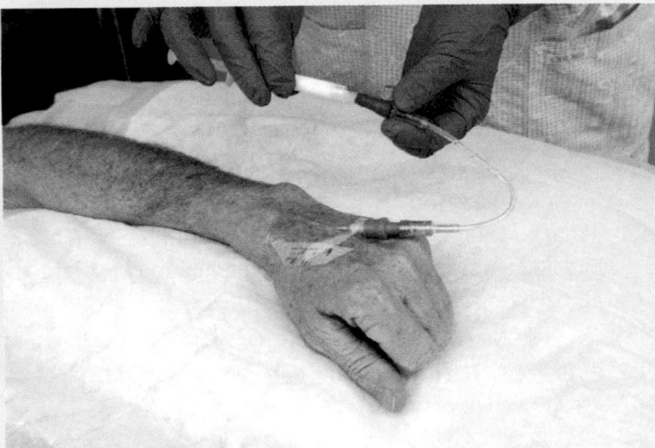

Figure 2. Inserting syringe into port.

ACTION	RATIONALE
23. Move your nondominant hand to section of IV tubing just above the injection port. Fold tubing between your fingers (Figure 3).	This temporarily stops flow of gravity IV infusion and prevents medication from backing up tubing.
24. Pull back slightly on plunger just until blood appears in tubing.	This ensures injection of medication into the bloodstream.
25. **Inject medication at recommended rate** (see Special Considerations below) (Figure 4).	This delivers correct amount of medication at proper interval according to manufacturer's directions.

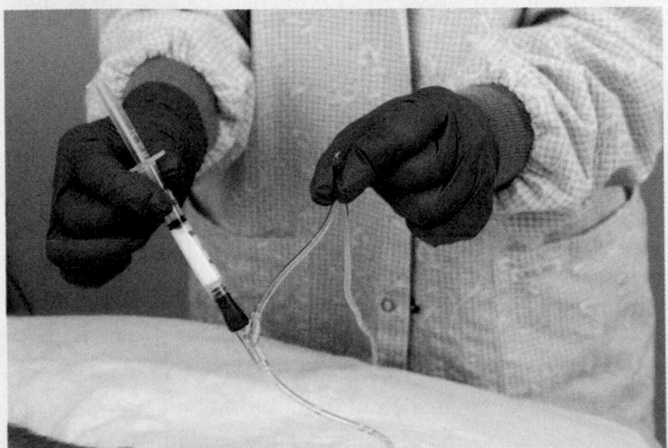

Figure 3. Folding tubing above port between fingers.

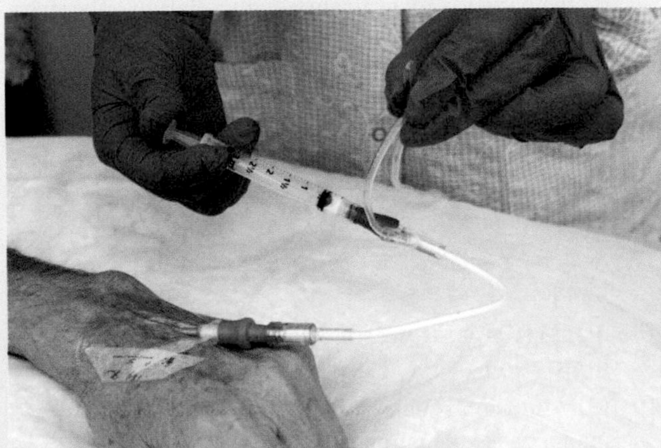

Figure 4. Injecting medication while interrupting IV flow.

SKILL 5-10

Administering Medications by Intravenous Bolus or Push Through an Intravenous Infusion *(continued)*

ACTION	RATIONALE
26. Release the tubing. Remove the syringe. Do not recap the used needle. Engage the safety shield or needle guard, if present. Release the tubing and allow the IV fluid to flow. Discard the needle and syringe in the appropriate receptacle.	Proper disposal of the needle prevents injury.
27. Check IV fluid infusion rate. Restart infusion pump, if appropriate.	Injection of bolus may alter rate of fluid infusion, if infusing by gravity.
28. Remove gloves and perform hand hygiene.	Hand hygiene deters spread of microorganisms.
29. Evaluate patient's response to medication within appropriate time frame.	Patient requires careful observation because medications given by IV bolus injection may have a rapid effect.

EVALUATION

The expected outcomes are met when the medication is safely administered via IV bolus; the patient's anxiety is decreased; the patient does not experience adverse effects; and the patient understands and complies with the medication regimen.

DOCUMENTATION

Guidelines

Document the administration of the medication immediately after administration, including date, time, dose, route of administration, site of administration, and rate of administration on the MAR or record using the required format. If using a bar-code system, medication administration is automatically recorded when scanned. PRN medications require documentation of the reason for administration. Prompt recording avoids the possibility of accidentally repeating the administration of the drug. If the drug was refused or omitted, record this in the appropriate area on the medication record and notify the physician. This verifies the reason medication was omitted and ensures that the physician is aware of the patient's condition.

Unexpected Situations and Associated Interventions

- *Upon assessing IV site before administering medication, no blood return is aspirated:* If IV appears patent, without signs of infiltration, and IV fluid infuses without difficulty, proceed with administration. Observe closely for signs and symptoms of infiltration during and after administration.
- *Upon assessing patient's IV site before administering medication, nurse notes that IV has infiltrated:* Stop IV fluid and remove IV from extremity. Restart IV in a different location. Continue to monitor new IV site as medication is administered.
- *While administering medication, nurse notes a cloudy, white substance forming in IV tubing:* Stop IV from flowing and stop administering medication. Clamp IV at site nearest to patient. Change administration tubing and restart infusion. Check literature or consult pharmacist regarding compatibility of medication and IV fluid.
- *While nurse is administering medication, patient begins to complain of pain at IV site:* Stop medication. Assess IV site for any signs of infiltration or phlebitis. You may want to flush the IV with normal saline to check for patency. If the IV site appears within normal limits, resume medication administration at a slower rate.

(continued)

SKILL 5-10 Administering Medications by Intravenous Bolus or Push Through an Intravenous Infusion *(continued)*

Special Considerations

General Considerations

- Agency policy may recommend the following variations when injecting a bolus IV medication:
  - Release folded tubing after each increment of the drug has been administered at prescribed rate to facilitate delivery of medication.
  - Use a syringe with 1 mL normal saline to flush tubing after an IV bolus is delivered to ensure that residual medication in tubing is not delivered too rapidly.
- Consider how fast IV fluid is flowing to determine whether a flush of normal saline is in order after administering medication. If IV fluid is flowing less than 50 mL per hour, it may take medication up to 30 minutes to reach patient. This depends on what type of tubing is being used in the agency.
- If the IV is a small gauge (22- to 24-gauge) placed in a small vein, a blood return may not occur even if IV is intact. Also, patient may complain of stinging and pain at site while medication is being administered due to irritation of vein. Placing a warm pack over vein or slowing the rate may relieve discomfort.
- If the medication and IV solution are incompatible, bolus may be given by flushing the tubing with normal saline before and after the medication bolus. Consult facility policy.
- Ongoing assessment is an important part of nursing care to evaluate patient response to administered medications and early detection of adverse effects. If an adverse effect is suspected, withhold further medication doses and notify the patient's primary healthcare provider. Additional intervention is based on type of reaction and patient assessment.

SKILL 5-11 Administering a Piggyback Intermittent Intravenous Infusion of Medication

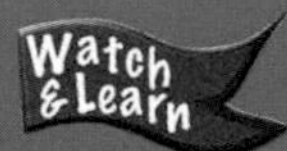

With intermittent IV infusion, the drug is mixed with a small amount of the IV solution, such as 50 to 100 mL, and administered over a short period at the prescribed interval (eg, every 4 hours). Medication may be administered by gravity infusion, which requires the nurse to calculate the infusion rate in drops per minute, or it may be administered using an IV infusion pump, which requires the nurse to program the infusion rate into the pump. 'Smart (computerized) pumps' are beginning to be used by many facilities for IV infusions, including intermittent infusions. 'Smart pumps' also requiring programming of infusion rates by the nurse, but, in addition, are able to identify dosing limits and practice guidelines to aid in safe administration. Needleless devices (recommended by the Centers for Disease Control and Prevention and the Occupational Safety and Health Administration) prevent needlesticks and provide access to the primary venous line. Either blunt-ended cannulas or recessed connection ports may be used to connect intermittent IV infusions.

The IV piggyback delivery system requires the intermittent or additive solution to be placed higher than the primary solution container. An extension hook provided by the manufacturer provides for easy lowering of the main IV container. The port on the primary IV line has a back-check valve that automatically stops the flow of the primary solution, allowing the secondary or piggyback solution to flow when connected. Because manufacturers' designs vary, the nurse should check the directions carefully for the systems used in the agency. The nurse is responsible for calculating and manually adjusting the flow rate of the IV intermittent infusion or regulating the infusion with an infusion pump or controller.

Equipment

- Medication prepared in labeled small-volume bag or bottle
- Short secondary infusion tubing (microdrip or macrodrip)

SKILL 5-11 Administering a Piggyback Intermittent Intravenous Infusion of Medication *(continued)*

- IV pump, if appropriate
- Needleless connector, stopcock, or sterile needle (21- to 23-gauge)
- Antimicrobial swab
- Tape (optional)
- Metal or plastic hook
- IV pole
- Date label for tubing
- Medication Administration Record (MAR) or Computer-generated MAR (CMAR)

ASSESSMENT

Assess the patient for any allergies. Check expiration date before administering medication. Assess the appropriateness of the drug for the patient. Assess the compatibility of the ordered medication, diluent, and the infusing IV fluid. Review assessment and laboratory data that may influence drug administration. Verify patient name, dose, route, and time of administration. Assess the patient's knowledge of the medication. If the patient has a knowledge deficit about the medication, this may be the appropriate time to begin education about the medication. If the medication may affect the patient's vital signs, assess them before administration. Assess the IV insertion site, noting any swelling, coolness, leakage of fluid at site, redness, or pain.

NURSING DIAGNOSIS

Determine related factors for the nursing diagnoses based on the patient's current status. Appropriate nursing diagnoses include:

- Acute Pain
- Risk for Allergy Response
- Risk for Injury
- Risk for Infection
- Deficient Knowledge

OUTCOME IDENTIFICATION AND PLANNING

The expected outcome to achieve is that the medication is delivered via the parenteral route using sterile technique. Other outcomes that may be appropriate include the following: medication is delivered to the patient in a safe manner and at the appropriate infusion rate; patient experiences no allergy response; patient remains infection free; and the patient understands and complies with the medication regimen.

IMPLEMENTATION

ACTION	RATIONALE
1. Gather equipment. Check each medication order against the original physician's order according to agency policy. Clarify any inconsistencies. Check the patient's chart for allergies.	This comparison helps to identify errors that may have occurred when orders were transcribed. The physician's order is the legal record of medication orders for each agency.
2. Know the actions, special nursing considerations, safe dose ranges, purpose of administration, and adverse effects of the medications to be administered. Consider the appropriateness of the medication for this patient.	This knowledge aids the nurse in evaluating the therapeutic effect of the medication in relation to the patient's disorder and can also be used to educate the patient about the medication.
3. Perform hand hygiene.	Hand hygiene prevents the spread of microorganisms.

(continued)

SKILL 5-11 Administering a Piggyback Intermittent Intravenous Infusion of Medication *(continued)*

ACTION	RATIONALE
4. Move the medication cart to the outside of the patient's room or prepare for administration in the medication area.	Organization facilitates error-free administration and saves time.
5. Unlock the medication cart or drawer. Enter pass code and scan employee identification, if required.	Locking of the cart or drawer safeguards each patient's medication supply. Hospital accrediting organizations require medication carts to be locked when not in use. Entering pass code and scanning ID allows only authorized users into the system and identifies user for documentation by the computer.
6. **Prepare medications for one patient at a time.**	This prevents errors in medication administration.
7. Read the MAR and select the proper medication from the patient's medication drawer or unit stock.	This is the first check of the label.
8. Compare the label with the MAR. Check expiration dates. Confirm the prescribed or appropriate infusion rate. Calculate the drip rate if using gravity system. Scan the bar code on the package, if required.	This is the second check of the label. Verify calculations with another nurse to ensure safety, if necessary. Infusing medication at appropriate rate prevents injury.
9. **When all medications for one patient have been prepared, recheck the label with the MAR before taking them to the patient.**	This is a *third* check to ensure accuracy and to prevent errors.
10. Lock the medication cart before leaving it.	Locking the cart or drawer safeguards the patient's medication supply. Hospital accrediting organizations require medication carts to be locked when not in use.
11. Transport medications to the patient's bedside carefully, and keep the medications in sight at all times.	Careful handling and close observation prevent accidental or deliberate disarrangement of medications.
12. **Ensure that the patient receives the medications at the correct time.**	Check agency policy, which may allow for administration within a period of 30 minutes before or 30 minutes after designated time.
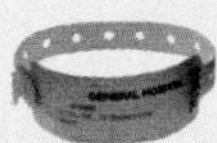 13. **Identify the patient.** Usually, the patient should be identified using two methods. Compare information with the MAR or CMAR.	Identifying the patient ensures the right patient receives the medications and helps prevent errors.
a. Check the name and identification number on the patient's identification band.	This is the most reliable method. Replace the identification band if it is missing or inaccurate in any way.
b. Ask the patient to state his or her name.	This requires a response from the patient, but illness and strange surroundings often cause patients to be confused.
c. If the patient cannot identify him or herself, verify the patient's identification with a staff member who knows the patient for the second source.	This is another way to double-check identity. Do not use the name on the door or over the bed, because these may be inaccurate.
14. Close the door to the room or pull the bedside curtain.	This provides patient privacy.
15. Perform hand hygiene.	This prevents transmission of microorganisms.

SKILL 5-11 Administering a Piggyback Intermittent Intravenous Infusion of Medication *(continued)*

ACTION	RATIONALE
16. Complete necessary assessments before administering medications. Check allergy bracelet or ask patient about allergies. Explain the purpose and action of the medication to the patient.	Assessment is a prerequisite to administration of medications. Explanation provides rationale, increases knowledge, and reduces anxiety.
17. Scan the patient's bar code on the identification band, if required.	Scanning provides an additional check to ensure that the medication is given to the right patient.
18. Assess the IV site for the presence of inflammation or infiltration.	IV medication must be given directly into a vein for safe administration.
19. Close the clamp on the short secondary infusion tubing. Using aseptic technique, remove the cap on the tubing spike and the cap on the port of the medication container, taking care to not contaminate either end.	Closing the clamp prevents fluid from entering system until the nurse is ready. Maintaining sterility of tubing and medication port prevents contamination.
20. Attach infusion tubing to the medication container by inserting the tubing spike into the port with a firm push and twisting motion, taking care to not contaminate either end.	Maintaining sterility of tubing and medication port prevents contamination.
21. **Hang piggyback container on IV pole, positioning it higher than primary IV according to manufacturer's recommendations (Figure 1).** Use metal or plastic hook to lower primary IV fluid container. (See the accompanying Skill Variation for information on administering an intermittent IV medication using a tandem piggyback set-up)	Position of containers influences the flow of IV fluid into primary setup.
22. Place label on tubing with appropriate date.	Tubing for piggyback setup may be used for 48 to 72 hours, depending on agency policy. Label allows for tracking of the next date to change.
23. Squeeze drip chamber and release. Fill to the line or about half full. Open clamp and prime tubing. Close clamp. Place needleless connector or needle on the end of the tubing, using sterile technique, if required.	This removes air from tubing and preserves sterility of setup.
24. Use an antimicrobial swab to clean the access port or stopcock above the roller clamp on the primary IV infusion tubing (Figure 2).	This deters entry of microorganisms when piggyback setup is connected to port.
25. Connect piggyback setup to the access port or stopcock (Figure 3). If using, turn the stopcock to the open position.	Needleless systems and stopcock setup eliminate the need for a needle and are recommended by the Centers for Disease Control and Prevention.
26. Use strip of tape to secure secondary tubing to primary infusion tubing, if a needle is used to connect.	Tape stabilizes needle in infusion port and prevents it from slipping out. Backflow valve in primary line secondary port stops flow of primary infusion while piggyback solution is infusing. Once completed, backflow valves opens and flow of primary solution resumes.
27. Open clamp on the secondary tubing. Use the roller clamp on the primary infusion tubing to regulate flow at prescribed delivery rate (Figure 4) or set rate for secondary infusion on infusion pump (Figure 5). Monitor medication infusion at periodic intervals.	Backflow valve in primary line secondary port stops flow of primary infusion while piggyback solution is infusing. Once completed, backflow valves opens and flow of primary solution resumes. It is important to verify the safe administration rate for each drug to prevent effects.

(continued)

SKILL 5-11 Administering a Piggyback Intermittent Intravenous Infusion of Medication *(continued)*

ACTION | **RATIONALE**

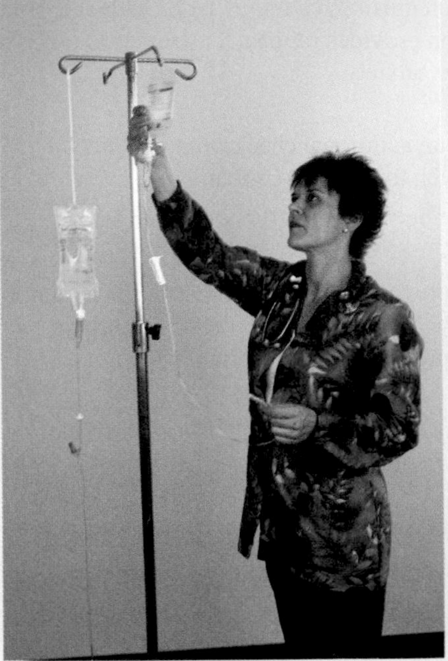

Figure 1. Positioning piggyback container on IV pole.

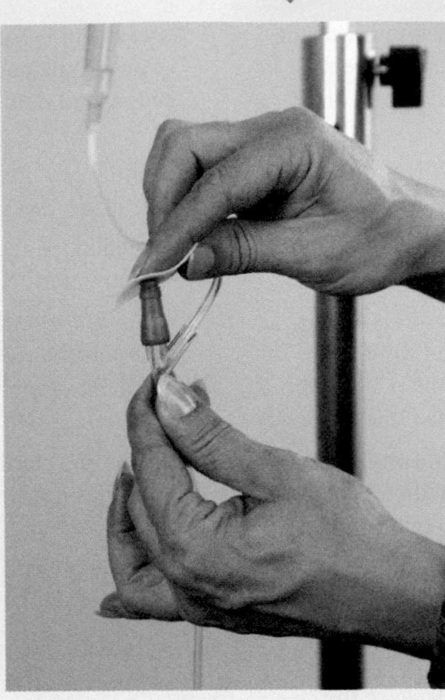

Figure 2. Cleaning access port.

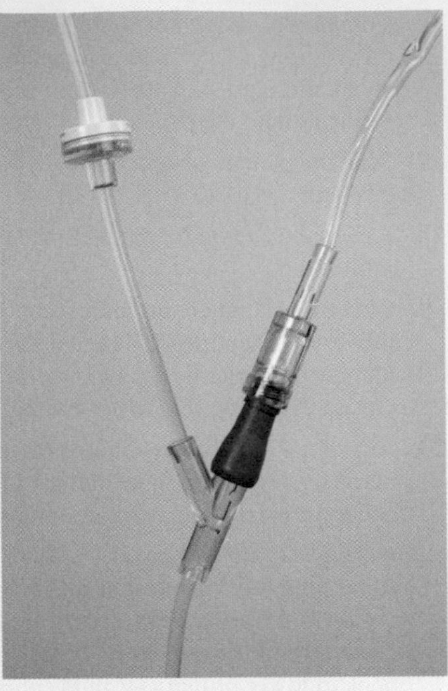

Figure 3. Connecting piggyback setup to access port.

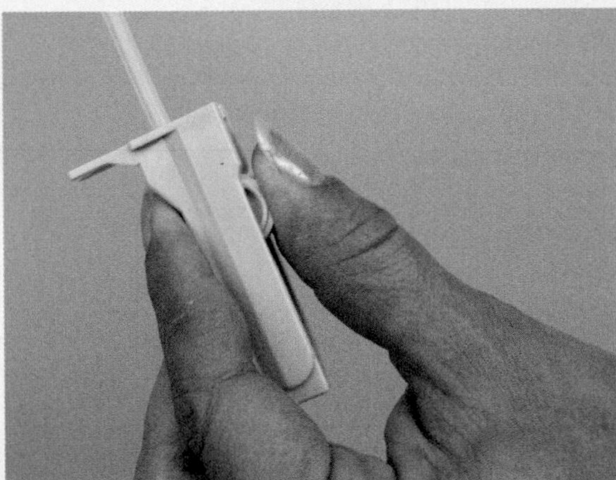

Figure 4. Using roller clamp on primary infusion tubing to regulate flow.

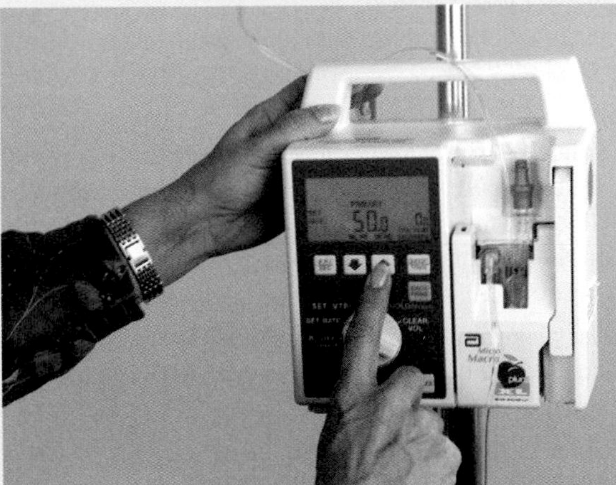

Figure 5. Adjusting pump rate.

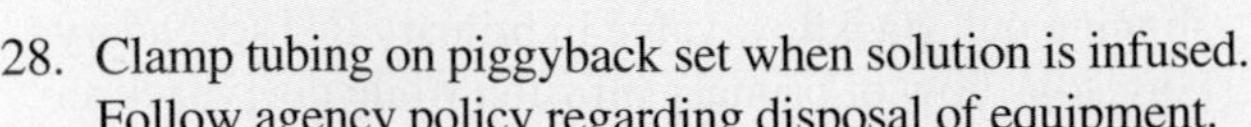

28. Clamp tubing on piggyback set when solution is infused. Follow agency policy regarding disposal of equipment.

Most facilities allow the reuse of tubing for 48 to 72 hours. This reduces risk for contaminating primary IV setup.

29. Replace primary IV fluid container to original height. **Readjust flow rate of primary IV or check primary infusion rate on infusion pump.**

Piggyback medication administration may interrupt normal flow rate of primary IV. Rate readjustment may be necessary. Many infusion pumps automatically restart primary infusion at previous rate after secondary infusion is completed.

SKILL 5-11 Administering a Piggyback Intermittent Intravenous Infusion of Medication *(continued)*

ACTION	RATIONALE
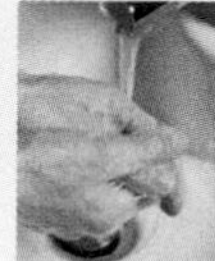 30. Perform hand hygiene.	Hand hygiene deters spread of microorganisms.
31. Evaluate patient's response to medication within appropriate time frame. Monitor IV site at periodic intervals.	Evaluate effectiveness of drug and provides early detection of adverse effect. Adverse reaction to medication given by the parenteral route is a possibility. Visualization of the site also allows for assessment of any untoward effects.

EVALUATION

The expected outcomes are met when the medication is delivered via the parenteral route using sterile technique; the medication is delivered to the patient in a safe manner and at the appropriate infusion rate; patient experiences no allergy response; patient remains infection free; and the patient understands and complies with the medication regimen.

DOCUMENTATION

Guidelines

Document the administration of the medication immediately after administration, including date, time, dose, route of administration, site of administration, and rate of administration on the MAR or record using the required format. If using a bar-code system, medication administration is automatically recorded when scanned. PRN medications require documentation of the reason for administration. Prompt recording avoids the possibility of accidentally repeating the administration of the drug. If the drug was refused or omitted, record this in the appropriate area on the medication record and notify the physician. This verifies the reason medication was omitted and ensures that the physician is aware of the patient's condition. Document the volume of fluid administered on the intake and output record, if necessary.

Unexpected Situations and Associated Interventions

- *Upon assessing the IV site before administering medication, the nurse notes that the IV has infiltrated:* Stop IV fluid and remove the IV from the extremity. Restart the IV in a different location. Continue to monitor the new IV site as medication is administered.
- *While administering medication, the nurse notes a cloudy, white substance forming in the IV tubing:* Stop the IV from flowing and stop administering the medication to prevent precipitate from entering the patient's circulation. Clamp the IV at the site nearest to the patient. Replace tubing on primary and secondary infusions. Check the literature regarding incompatibilities of medications before administering. Medication infusion may require second IV site or flushing of tubing before and after administration, using tandem system.
- *While nurse is administering medication, the patient begins to complain of pain at the IV site:* Stop the medication. Assess the IV site for any signs of infiltration or phlebitis. You may want to flush the IV with normal saline to check for patency. If the IV site appears within normal limits, resume medication administration at a slower rate.

Special Considerations

General Considerations

- An alternate way to prime the secondary tubing, particularly if administration set is in place from previous infusion, is to "backfill" the secondary tubing. Attach the medication bag to the secondary infusion tubing. Lower the medication bag below the main IV solution container and open the clamp on the secondary infusion tubing. This allows the primary IV solution to flow up the secondary tubing to the drip chamber, "backfilling" the tubing. Allow the solution to enter the drip chamber until the drip chamber is half full.

(continued)

SKILL 5-11 Administering a Piggyback Intermittent Intravenous Infusion of Medication *(continued)*

Close the clamp on the secondary tubing and hang the medication container on the IV pole. Proceed with administration by lowering the primary IV container, as described above. This "backfill" method keeps the infusion system intact, preventing introduction of microorganisms and prevents loss of medication when the tubing is primed.

- Ongoing assessment is an important part of nursing care to evaluate patient response to administered medications and early detection of adverse effects. If an adverse effect is suspected, withhold further medication doses and notify the patient's primary healthcare provider. Additional intervention is based on type of reaction and patient assessment.

Infant and Child Considerations

- Small infants and children with fluid restrictions may not tolerate the added IV fluid needed for administration with piggyback or volume-control systems. For these children, consider using the mini-infusion pump.

SKILL VARIATION Tandem Piggyback Setup

A tandem delivery setup allows for simultaneous infusion of the primary and secondary IV solutions. Both solution containers are hung at the same height. The tubing for the secondary infusion is attached to an access port below the roller clamp on the primary tubing. There is no back-check valve at the secondary port on the primary line. This type of setup is used infrequently because the solution from the primary IV line will back up into the tandem line if this intermittent infusion is not clamped immediately after it is infused.

- Check medication order against the original physician's order according to agency policy. Clarify any inconsistencies. Check the patient's chart for allergies. Verify the compatibility of the medication and IV fluid.
- Know the actions, special nursing considerations, safe dose ranges, purpose of administration, and adverse effects of the medications to be administered. Consider the appropriateness of the medication for this patient.
- Perform hand hygiene.
- Move the medication cart to the outside of the patient's room or prepare for administration in the medication area.
- Unlock the medication cart or drawer. Enter pass code and scan employee identification, if required.
- Read the MAR and select the proper medication from the patient's medication drawer or unit stock.
- Compare the label with the MAR. Check expiration dates. Confirm the prescribed or appropriate infusion rate. Calculate the drip rate if using gravity system. Scan the bar code on the package, if required.
- Recheck the label with the MAR before taking it to the patient.
- Lock the medication cart before leaving it.
- Transport medications and equipment to the patient's bedside carefully, and keep the medications in sight at all times.
- Perform hand hygiene.
- Identify the patient. Usually, the patient should be identified using two methods.
- Close the door to the room or pull the bedside curtain.
- Complete necessary assessments before administering medications. Check allergy bracelet or ask patient about allergies. Explain the purpose and action of the medication to the patient.
- Scan the patient's bar code on the identification band, if required.
- Assess the IV site for the presence of inflammation or infiltration.
- Close the clamp on the secondary infusion tubing. Using aseptic technique, remove the cap on the tubing spike and the cap on the port of the medication container, taking care to not contaminate either end.
- Attach infusion tubing to the medication container by inserting the tubing spike into the port with a firm push and twisting motion, taking care to not contaminate either end.
- Hang secondary container on IV pole, positioning it at the same height as the primary IV.
- Place label on tubing with appropriate date and attach needle or needleless device to end of tubing according to manufacturer's directions.
- Squeeze drip chamber and release. Fill to the line or about half full. Open clamp and prime tubing. Close clamp. Place needleless connector or needle on the end of the tubing, using sterile technique, if required.
- Use antimicrobial swab to clean the access port or stopcock below the roller clamp on the primary IV infusion tubing, usually the port closest to the IV insertion site.
- Connect secondary setup to the access port or stopcock. If using, turn the stopcock to the open position.
- Use strip of tape to secure secondary tubing to primary infusion tubing if a needle is used to connect.
- Use the roller clamp on the secondary infusion tubing to regulate flow at prescribed delivery rate. Monitor medication infusion at periodic intervals.
- Clamp tubing on secondary set when solution is infused. Remove secondary tubing from access port and replace connector or needle with a new capped one, if reusing. Follow agency policy regarding disposal of equipment.
- Check primary infusion rate.
- Perform hand hygiene.
- Evaluate patient's response to medication within appropriate time frame. Monitor IV site at periodic intervals.

SKILL 5-12 Administering an Intermittent Intravenous Infusion of Medication via a Mini-Infusion Pump

With intermittent IV infusion, the drug is mixed with a small amount of the IV solution, such as 50 to 100 mL, and administered over a short period at the prescribed interval (eg, every 4 hours). Medication administration using an IV infusion pump requires the nurse to program the infusion rate into the pump. "Smart (computerized) pumps" are beginning to be used by many facilities for IV infusions, including intermittent infusions. "Smart pumps" also requiring programming of infusion rates by the nurse, but, in addition, are able to identify dosing limits and practice guidelines to aid in safe administration. Needleless devices (recommended by the Centers for Disease Control and Prevention and the Occupational Safety and Health Administration) prevent needlesticks and provide access to the primary venous line. Either blunt-ended cannulas or recessed connection ports may be used to connect intermittent IV infusions.

The mini-infusion pump (syringe pump) for intermittent infusion is battery or electrical operated and allows medication mixed in a syringe to be connected to the primary line and delivered by mechanical pressure applied to the syringe plunger (Figure 1).

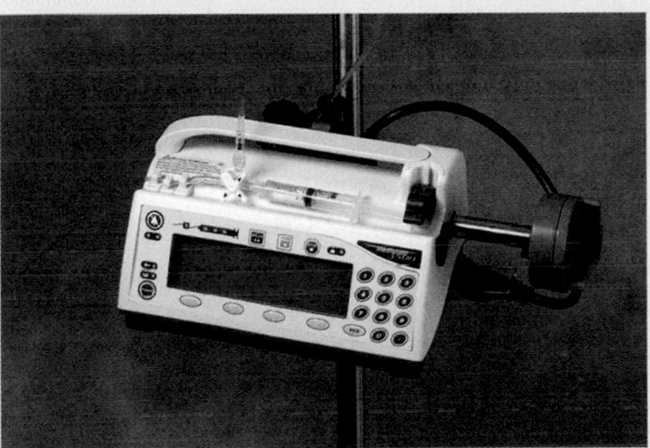

Figure 1. Syringe infusion pump.

Equipment

- Medication prepared in labeled syringe
- Mini-infusion pump and tubing
- Needleless connector, stopcock, or sterile needle (21- to 23-gauge)
- Antimicrobial swab
- Tape (optional)
- Date label for tubing
- Medication Administration Record (MAR) or Computer-generated MAR (CMAR)

ASSESSMENT

Assess the patient for any allergies. Check expiration date before administering medication. Assess the appropriateness of the drug for the patient. Assess the compatibility of the ordered medication, diluent, and the infusing IV fluid. Review assessment and laboratory data that may influence drug administration. Verify patient name, dose, route, and time of administration. Assess the patient's knowledge of the medication. If the patient has a knowledge deficit about the medication, this may be the appropriate time to begin education about the medication. If the medication may affect the patient's vital signs, assess them before administration. Assess the IV insertion site, noting any swelling, coolness, leakage of fluid at site, redness, or pain.

(continued)

SKILL 5-12 Administering an Intermittent Intravenous Infusion of Medication via a Mini-Infusion Pump *(continued)*

NURSING DIAGNOSIS

Determine related factors for the nursing diagnoses based on the patient's current status. Appropriate nursing diagnoses include:

- Acute Pain
- Risk for Allergy Response
- Risk for Injury
- Risk for Infection
- Deficient Knowledge

OUTCOME IDENTIFICATION AND PLANNING

The expected outcome is that the medication is delivered via the parenteral route using sterile technique. Other outcomes that may be appropriate include the following: medication is delivered to the patient in a safe manner and at the appropriate infusion rate; patient experiences no allergy response; patient remains infection free; and the patient understands and complies with the medication regimen.

IMPLEMENTATION

ACTION	RATIONALE
1. Gather equipment. Check each medication order against the original physician's order according to agency policy. Clarify any inconsistencies. Check the patient's chart for allergies.	This comparison helps to identify errors that may have occurred when orders were transcribed. The physician's order is the legal record of medication orders for each agency.
2. Know the actions, special nursing considerations, safe dose ranges, purpose of administration, and adverse effects of the medications to be administered. Consider the appropriateness of the medication for this patient.	This knowledge aids the nurse in evaluating the therapeutic effect of the medication in relation to the patient's disorder and can also be used to educate the patient about the medication.
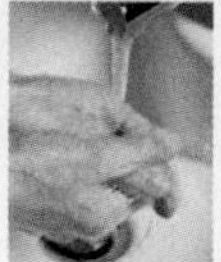 3. Perform hand hygiene.	Hand hygiene prevents the spread of microorganisms.
4. Move the medication cart to the outside of the patient's room or prepare for administration in the medication area.	Organization facilitates error-free administration and saves time.
5. Unlock the medication cart or drawer. Enter pass code and scan employee identification, if required.	Locking of the cart or drawer safeguards each patient's medication supply. Hospital accrediting organizations require medication carts to be locked when not in use. Entering pass code and scanning ID allows only authorized users into the system and identifies user for documentation by the computer.
6. **Prepare medications for one patient at a time.**	This prevents errors in medication administration.
7. Read the MAR and select the proper medication from the patient's medication drawer or unit stock.	This is the first check of the label.
8. Compare the label with the MAR. Check expiration dates. Confirm the prescribed or appropriate infusion rate. Calculate the drip rate if using gravity system. Scan the bar code on the package, if required.	This is the second check of the label. Verify calculations with another nurse to ensure safety, if necessary. Infusing medication at appropriate rate prevents injury.

SKILL 5-12 Administering an Intermittent Intravenous Infusion of Medication via a Mini-Infusion Pump *(continued)*

ACTION	RATIONALE
9. **When all medications for one patient have been prepared, recheck the label with the MAR before taking them to the patient.**	This is the *third* check to ensure accuracy and to prevent errors.
10. Lock the medication cart before leaving it.	Locking the cart or drawer safeguards the patient's medication supply. Hospital accrediting organizations require medication carts to be locked when not in use.
11. Transport medications to the patient's bedside carefully, and keep the medications in sight at all times.	Careful handling and close observation prevent accidental or deliberate disarrangement of medications.
12. **Ensure that the patient receives the medications at the correct time.**	Check agency policy, which may allow for administration within a period of 30 minutes before or 30 minutes after designated time.
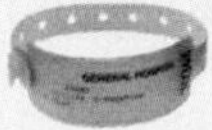 13. **Identify the patient.** Usually, the patient should be identified using two methods. Compare information with the MAR or CMAR.	Identifying the patient ensures the right patient receives the medications and helps prevent errors.
a. Check the name and identification number on the patient's identification band.	This is the most reliable method. Replace the identification band if it is missing or inaccurate in any way.
b. Ask the patient to state his or her name.	This requires a response from the patient, but illness and strange surroundings often cause patients to be confused.
c. If the patient cannot identify him or herself, verify the patient's identification with a staff member who knows the patient for the second source.	This is another way to double-check identity. Do not use the name on the door or over the bed, because these may be inaccurate.
14. Close the door to the room or pull the bedside curtain.	Provides patient privacy.
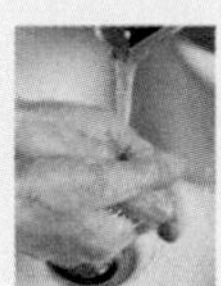 15. Perform hand hygiene.	Prevents transmission of microorganisms.
16. Complete necessary assessments before administering medications. Check allergy bracelet or ask patient about allergies. Explain the purpose and action of the medication to the patient.	Assessment is a prerequisite to administration of medications. Explanation provides rationale, increases knowledge, and reduces anxiety.
17. Scan the patient's bar code on the identification band, if required.	Provides additional check to ensure that the medication is given to the right patient.
18. Assess the IV site for the presence of inflammation or infiltration.	IV medication must be given directly into a vein for safe administration.
19. Using aseptic technique, remove the cap on the tubing and the cap on the syringe, taking care to not contaminate either end.	Maintaining sterility of tubing and syringe prevents contamination.
20. Attach infusion tubing to the syringe, taking care to not contaminate either end.	Maintaining sterility of tubing and medication port prevents contamination.
21. Place label on tubing with appropriate date and attach needle or needleless device to end of tubing according to manufacturer's directions.	Tubing for piggyback setup may be used for 48 to 72 hours, depending on agency policy. Label allows for tracking of the next date to change.

(continued)

SKILL 5-12 Administering an Intermittent Intravenous Infusion of Medication via a Mini-Infusion Pump *(continued)*

ACTION	RATIONALE
22. Fill tubing with medication by applying gentle pressure to syringe plunger. Place needleless connector or needle on the end of the tubing, using sterile technique, if required.	This removes air from tubing and maintains sterility.
23. Insert syringe into mini-infusion pump according to manufacturer's directions.	Syringe must fit securely in pump apparatus for proper operation.
24. Use antimicrobial swab to clean the access port or stopcock below the roller clamp on the primary IV infusion tubing, usually the port closest to the IV insertion site.	This deters entry of microorganisms when piggyback setup is connected to port. Proper connection allows IV medication to flow into primary line.
25. Connect the secondary infusion to the primary infusion at the cleansed port.	Allows for delivery of medication.
26. Program pump to the appropriate rate and begin infusion. Set alarm if recommended by manufacturer.	Pump delivers medication at controlled rate. Alarm is recommended for use with IV lock apparatus.
27. Clamp tubing on secondary set when solution is infused. Remove secondary tubing from access port and replace connector or needle with a new, capped one, if reusing. Follow agency policy regarding disposal of equipment.	Many facilities allow reuse of tubing for 48 to 72 hours. Replacing connector or needle with a new, capped one maintains sterility of system.
28. Check rate of primary infusion.	Administration of secondary infusion may interfere with primary infusion rate.
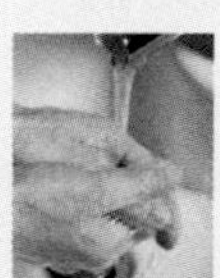 29. Perform hand hygiene.	Hand hygiene deters spread of microorganisms.
30. Evaluate patient's response to medication within appropriate time frame. Monitor IV site at periodic intervals.	Evaluate effectiveness of drug and provides early detection of adverse effect. Adverse reaction to medication given by the parenteral route is a possibility. Visualization of the site also allows for assessment of any untoward effects.

EVALUATION

The expected outcomes are met when the medication is delivered via the parenteral route using sterile technique; the medication is delivered to the patient in a safe manner and at the appropriate infusion rate; patient experiences no allergy response; patient remains infection free; and the patient understands and complies with the medication regimen.

DOCUMENTATION

Guidelines

Document the administration of the medication immediately after administration, including date, time, dose, route of administration, site of administration, and rate of administration on the MAR or record using the required format. If using a bar-code system, medication administration is automatically recorded when scanned. PRN medications require documentation of the reason for administration. Prompt recording avoids the possibility of accidentally repeating the administration of the drug. If the drug was refused or omitted, record this in the appropriate area on the medication record and notify the physician. This verifies the reason medication was omitted and ensures that the physician is aware of the patient's condition. Document the volume of fluid administered on the intake and output record, if necessary.

SKILL 5-12 Administering an Intermittent Intravenous Infusion of Medication via a Mini-Infusion Pump *(continued)*

Special Considerations

General Considerations

- Ongoing assessment is an important part of nursing care to evaluate patient response to administered medications and early detection of adverse effects. If an adverse effect is suspected, withhold further medication doses and notify the patient's primary healthcare provider. Additional intervention is based on type of reaction and patient assessment.

SKILL 5-13 Administering an Intermittent Intravenous Infusion of Medication via a Volume-Control Administration Set

With intermittent IV infusion, the drug is mixed with a small amount of the IV solution, such as 50 to 100 mL, and administered over a short period at the prescribed interval (eg, every 4 hours). Administration is achieved by gravity infusion, which requires the nurse to calculate the infusion rate in drops per minute. This skill discusses using a volume-control administration set for intermittent IV infusion. The medication is diluted with a small amount of solution and administered through the patient's IV line. This type of equipment is commonly used for infusing solutions into children, critically ill, and older patients when the volume of fluid infused is a concern. Needleless devices (recommended by the Centers for Disease Control and Prevention and the Occupational Safety and Health Administration) prevent needlesticks and provide access to the primary venous line. Either a blunt-ended cannula or a recessed connection port may be used to connect intermittent IV infusions.

Equipment

- Prescribed medication
- Syringe with a 19- to 21-gauge needle, blunt needle or needleless device (follow agency policy)
- Volume-control set (Volutrol®, Buretrol®, Burette®)
- Needleless connector, stopcock, or sterile needle (21- to 23-gauge)
- Antimicrobial swab
- Tape (optional)
- Date label for tubing
- Medication label
- Medication Administration Record (MAR) or Computer-generated MAR (CMAR)

ASSESSMENT

Assess the patient for any allergies. Check expiration date before administering medication. Assess the appropriateness of the drug for the patient. Assess the compatibility of the ordered medication, diluent, and the infusing IV fluid. Review assessment and laboratory data that may influence drug administration. Assess the patient's knowledge of the medication. If the patient has a knowledge deficit about the medication, this may be the appropriate time to begin education about the medication. If the medication may affect the patient's vital signs, assess them before administration. Assess the IV insertion site, noting any swelling, coolness, leakage of fluid at site, redness, or pain.

NURSING DIAGNOSIS

Determine related factors for the nursing diagnoses based on the patient's current status. Appropriate nursing diagnoses include:

- Acute Pain
- Risk for Allergy Response
- Risk for Injury
- Risk for Infection
- Deficient Knowledge

(continued)

SKILL 5-13

Administering an Intermittent Intravenous Infusion of Medication via a Volume-Control Administration Set *(continued)*

OUTCOME IDENTIFICATION AND PLANNING

The expected outcome to achieve when administering an intermittent IV infusion of medication via a volume control set is that the medication is delivered via the parenteral route using sterile technique. Other outcomes that may be appropriate include the following: medication is delivered to the patient in a safe manner and at the appropriate infusion rate; patient experiences no allergy response; patient remains infection free; and the patient understands and complies with the medication regimen.

IMPLEMENTATION

ACTION	RATIONALE
1. Gather equipment. Check medication order against the original physician's order according to agency policy. Clarify any inconsistencies. Check the patient's chart for allergies. Verify the compatibility of the medication and IV fluid.	This comparison helps to identify errors that may have occurred when orders were transcribed. The physician's order is the legal record of medication orders for each agency. Compatibility of medication and solution prevents complications.
2. Know the actions, special nursing considerations, safe dose ranges, purpose of administration, and adverse effects of the medications to be administered. Consider the appropriateness of the medication for this patient.	This knowledge aids the nurse in evaluating the therapeutic effect of the medication in relation to the patient's disorder and can also be used to educate the patient about the medication.
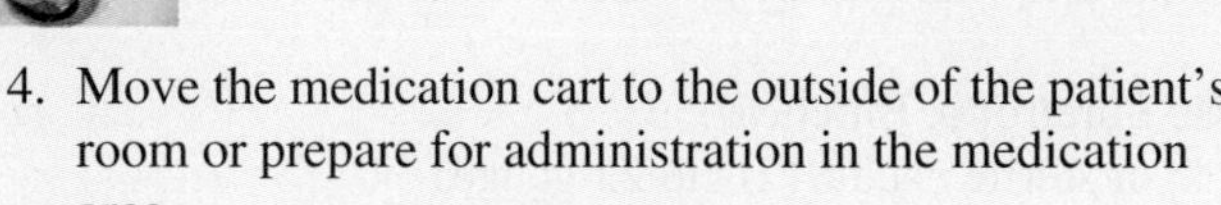 3. Perform hand hygiene.	Hand hygiene prevents the spread of microorganisms.
4. Move the medication cart to the outside of the patient's room or prepare for administration in the medication area.	Organization facilitates error-free administration and saves time.
5. Unlock the medication cart or drawer. Enter pass code and scan employee identification, if required.	Locking of the cart or drawer safeguards each patient's medication supply. Hospital accrediting organizations require medication carts to be locked when not in use. Entering pass code and scanning ID allows only authorized users into the system and identifies user for documentation by the computer.
6. **Prepare medication for one patient at a time.**	This prevents errors in medication administration.
7. Read the MAR and select the proper medication from the patient's medication drawer or unit stock.	This is the first check of the label.
8. Compare the label with the MAR. Check expiration dates and perform calculations, if necessary. Scan the bar code on the package, if required. Check the infusion rate.	This is the second check of the label. Verify calculations with another nurse to ensure safety, if necessary. Delivers the correct dose of medication as prescribed.
9. If necessary, withdraw medication from an ampule or vial as described in Skills 5-2 and 5-3. Attach needleless connector or needle to end of syringe, if necessary.	Allows for entry into the volume-control administration set chamber.
10. **Recheck the label with the MAR before taking it to the patient.**	This is a *third* check to ensure accuracy and to prevent errors.

SKILL 5-13 Administering an Intermittent Intravenous Infusion of Medication via a Volume-Control Administration Set *(continued)*

ACTION	RATIONALE
11. Prepare medication label including name of medication, dose, total volume, including diluent, and time of administration.	Allows for accurate identification of medication.
12. Lock the medication cart before leaving it.	Locking the cart or drawer safeguards the patient's medication supply. Hospital accrediting organizations require medication carts to be locked when not in use.
13. Transport medications and equipment to the patient's bedside carefully, and keep the medications in sight at all times.	Careful handling and close observation prevent accidental or deliberate disarrangement of medications. Having equipment available saves time and facilitates performance of the task.
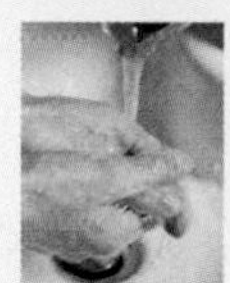 14. Perform hand hygiene.	Hand hygiene deters the spread of microorganisms.
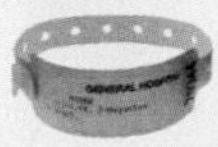 15. **Identify the patient.** Usually, the patient should be identified using two methods. Compare information with the MAR or CMAR.	Identifying the patient ensures the right patient receives the medications and helps prevent errors.
a. Check the name and identification number on the patient's identification band.	This is the most reliable method. Replace the identification band if it is missing or inaccurate in any way.
b. Ask the patient to state his or her name.	This requires a response from the patient, but illness and strange surroundings often cause patients to be confused.
c. If the patient cannot identify him or herself, verify the patient's identification with a staff member who knows the patient for the second source.	This is another way to double-check identity. Do not use the name on the door or over the bed, because these may be inaccurate.
16. Close the door to the room or pull the bedside curtain.	This provides patient privacy.
17. Complete necessary assessments before administering medications. Check allergy bracelet or ask patient about allergies. Explain the purpose and action of the medication to the patient.	Assessment is a prerequisite to administration of medications. Explanation provides rationale, increases knowledge, and reduces anxiety.
18. Scan the patient's bar code on the identification band, if required.	Provides additional check to ensure that the medication is given to the right patient.
19. **Assess IV site for presence of inflammation or infiltration.**	IV medication must be given directly into a vein for safe administration.
20. Fill the volume-control administration set (Figure 1) with the prescribed amount of IV fluid by opening the clamp between IV solution and the volume-control administration set. Follow manufacturer's instructions and fill with prescribed amount of IV solution (Figure 2). Close clamp.	This dilutes the medication in the minimal amount of solution. Reclamping prevents the continued addition of fluid to the volume to be mixed with medication.
21. Check to make sure the air vent on the volume-control administration set chamber is open.	Air vent allows fluid in the chamber to flow at a regular rate.
22. Use antimicrobial swab to clean access port on volume-control administration set chamber (Figure 3).	This deters entry of microorganisms when the syringe enters chamber.

(continued)

SKILL 5-13 Administering an Intermittent Intravenous Infusion of Medication via a Volume-Control Administration Set *(continued)*

ACTION | **RATIONALE**

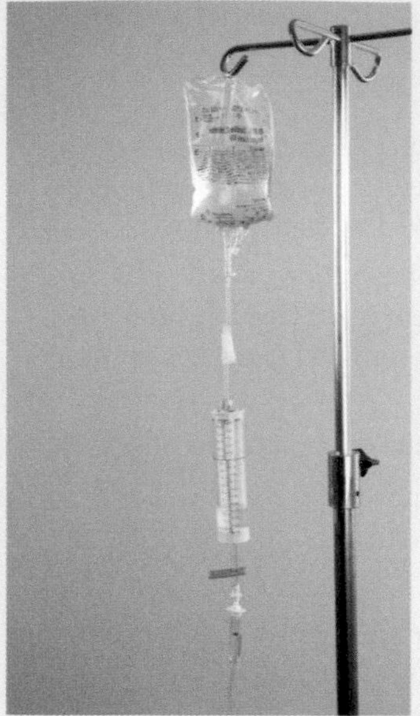

Figure 1. Volume-control administration set and IV solution for dilution of medication.

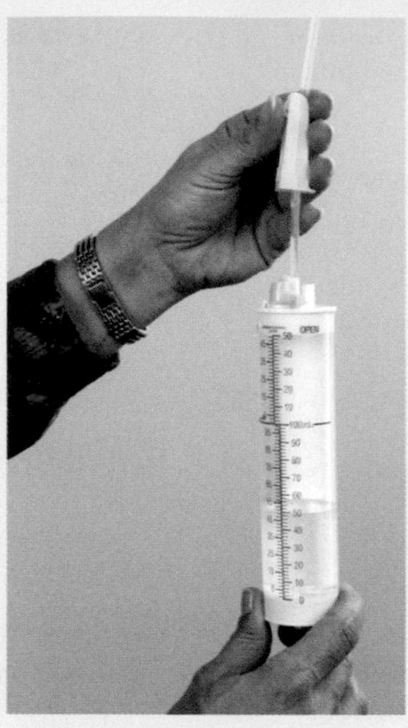

Figure 2. Opening clamp between IV solution and volume-control administration set to fill chamber with prescribed amount of solution.

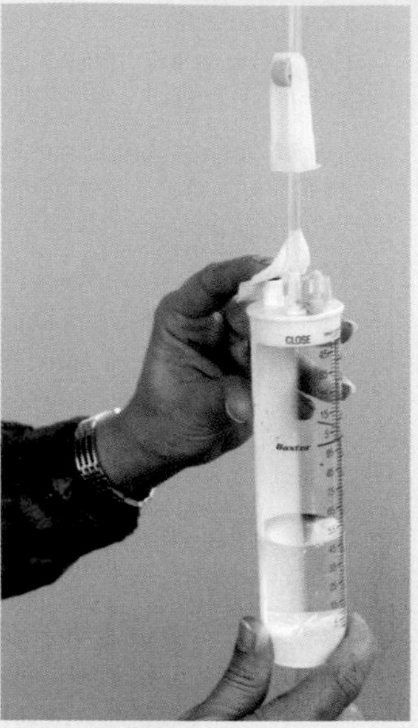

Figure 3. Cleaning access port.

23. Insert the needle or blunt needleless device into port while holding syringe steady (Figure 4). Inject medication into the chamber (Figure 5). Gently rotate the chamber.

This ensures that medication is evenly mixed with solution.

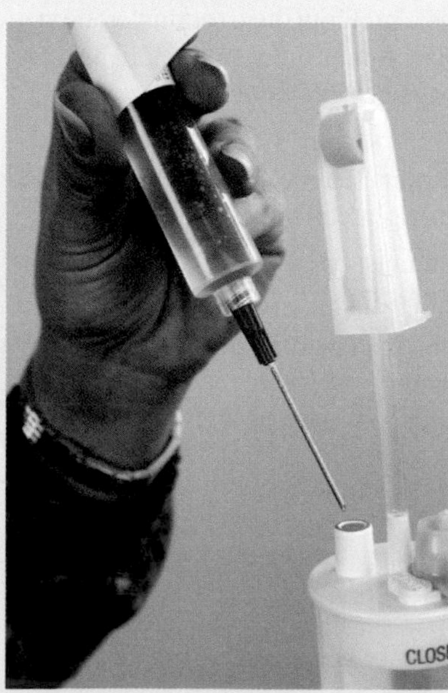

Figure 4. Inserting needleless device into port.

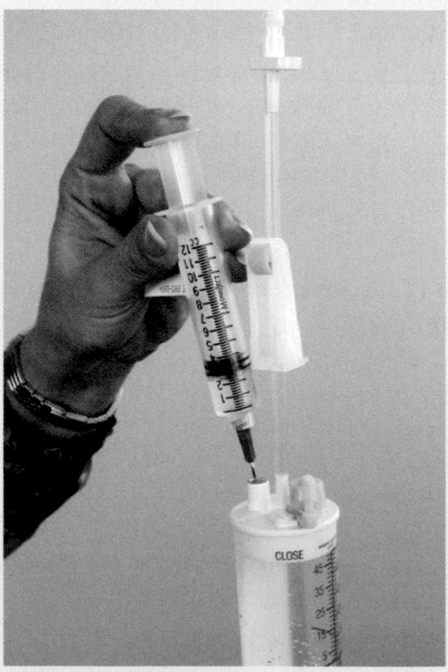

Figure 5. Injecting the medication into the volume-control device.

SKILL 5-13

Administering an Intermittent Intravenous Infusion of Medication via a Volume-Control Administration Set *(continued)*

ACTION	RATIONALE
24. Attach the medication label to the volume-control device (Figure 6).	This identifies contents of the set and prevents medication error.
25. Use antimicrobial swab to clean the access port or stopcock below the roller clamp on the primary IV infusion tubing, usually the port closest to the IV insertion site.	This deters entry of microorganisms when piggyback setup is connected to port. Proper connection allows IV medication to flow into primary line.
26. Connect the secondary infusion to the primary infusion at the cleansed port.	This allows for delivery of medication.
27. Use the roller clamp on the volume-control administration set tubing to adjust the infusion to the prescribed rate (Figure 7).	Delivery over a 30- to 60-minute interval is a safe method of administering IV medication.

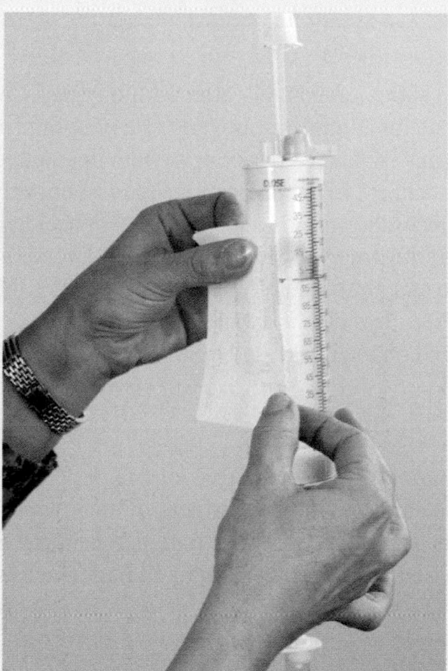

Figure 6. Applying medication label to volume-control device.

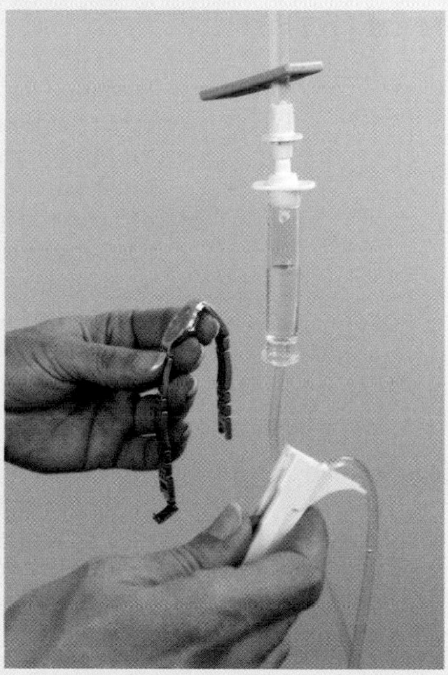

Figure 7. Using roller clamp on volume-control administration set to adjust medication infusion rate.

ACTION	RATIONALE
28. Do not recap the used needle. Engage the safety shield or needle guard, if present. Discard the needle and syringe in the appropriate receptacle.	Proper disposal of the needle prevents injury.
29. Clamp tubing on secondary set when solution is infused. Remove secondary tubing from access port and replace connector or needle with a new, capped one, if reusing. Follow agency policy regarding disposal of equipment.	Many facilities allow reuse of tubing for 48 to 72 hours. Replacing connector or needle with a new, capped one maintains sterility of system.
30. Check rate of primary infusion.	Administration of secondary infusion may interfere with primary infusion rate.
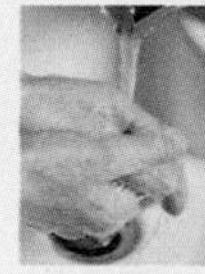 31. Perform hand hygiene.	Hand hygiene deters spread of microorganisms.

(continued)

SKILL 5-13 Administering an Intermittent Intravenous Infusion of Medication via a Volume-Control Administration Set *(continued)*

ACTION	RATIONALE
32. Evaluate patient's response to medication within appropriate time frame. Monitor IV site at periodic intervals.	Evaluates effectiveness of drug and provides early detection of adverse effect. Adverse reaction to medication given by the parenteral route is a possibility. Visualization of the site also allows for assessment of any untoward effects.

EVALUATION

The expected outcomes are met when the medication is delivered via the parenteral route using sterile technique; the medication is delivered to the patient in a safe manner and at the appropriate infusion rate; patient experiences no allergy response; patient remains infection free; and the patient understands and complies with the medication regimen.

DOCUMENTATION

Guidelines

Document the administration of the medication immediately after administration, including date, time, dose, route of administration, site of administration, and rate of administration on the MAR or record using the required format. If using a bar-code system, medication administration is automatically recorded when scanned. PRN medications require documentation of the reason for administration. Prompt recording avoids the possibility of accidentally repeating the administration of the drug. If the drug was refused or omitted, record this in the appropriate area on the medication record and notify the physician. This verifies the reason medication was omitted and ensures that the physician is aware of the patient's condition. Document the volume of fluid administered on the intake and output record, if necessary.

Special Considerations

General Considerations

- Ongoing assessment is an important part of nursing care to evaluate patient response to administered medications and early detection of adverse effects. If an adverse effect is suspected, withhold further medication doses and notify the patient's primary healthcare provider. Additional intervention is based on type of reaction and patient assessment.

SKILL 5-14 Introducing Drugs Through a Medication or Drug-Infusion Lock Using the Saline Flush (Intermittent Peripheral Venous Access Device)

A medication or drug-infusion lock, also known as an intermittent peripheral venous access device, is used for patients who require intermittent IV medication but not a continuous IV infusion. This device consists of a needle or catheter connected to a short length of tubing capped with a sealed injection port. After the catheter is in place in the patient's vein, the catheter and tubing are anchored to the patient's arm so that the catheter remains in place until the patient no longer requires the repeated medication intravenously.

A peripheral venous access device allows the patient more freedom than a continuous IV infusion. The patient is connected to the IV line when it is time to receive the medication and disconnected when the medication is completed. The device is kept patent (working) by flushing with small amounts of saline or heparin pushed through the device on a routine basis. Using saline eliminates any possible systemic effects on coagulation,

SKILL 5-14 Introducing Drugs Through a Medication or Drug-Infusion Lock Using the Saline Flush (Intermittent Peripheral Venous Access Device) *(continued)*

development of a heparin allergy, and drug incompatibility, which may occur when a heparin solution is used. The intermittent infusion is not started until the nurse confirms IV placement. The saline lock is flushed before the infusion is begun and after the infusion is completed to clear the vein of any medication and to prevent clot formation in the needle. If infiltration or phlebitis occurs, the lock is removed and replaced in a new site.

Equipment

- Medication
- Saline flushes (2), volume according to facility policy, usually 2 to 3 mL
- Sterile syringe with needleless device or 25-gauge needle
- Antimicrobial swabs
- Watch with second hand or stopwatch feature
- Gloves
- Medication Administration Record (MAR) or Computer-generated MAR (CMAR)

ASSESSMENT

Assess the patient for any allergies. Check expiration date before administering medication. Assess the appropriateness of the drug for the patient. Assess the compatibility of the ordered medication and the IV fluid. Review assessment and laboratory data that may influence drug administration. Assess patient's IV site, noting any swelling, coolness, leakage of fluid from IV site, or pain. Assess the patient's knowledge of the medication. If the patient has a knowledge deficit about the medication, this may be the appropriate time to begin education about the medication. If the medication may affect the patient's vital signs, assess them before administration.

NURSING DIAGNOSIS

Determine related factors for the nursing diagnoses based on the patient's current status. Appropriate nursing diagnoses may include:

- Acute Pain
- Risk for Allergy Response
- Risk for Infection
- Deficient Knowledge
- Risk for Injury

OUTCOME IDENTIFICATION AND PLANNING

The expected outcome to achieve when administering an intermittent IV infusion of medication via a volume-control set is that the medication is delivered via the parenteral route using sterile technique. Other outcomes that may be appropriate include the following: medication is delivered to the patient in a safe manner and at the appropriate infusion rate; patient experiences no adverse effect; and the patient understands and complies with the medication regimen.

IMPLEMENTATION

ACTION	RATIONALE
1. Gather equipment. Check medication order against the original physician's order according to agency policy. Clarify any inconsistencies. Check the patient's chart for allergies. Verify the compatibility of the medication and IV fluid. Check a drug resource to clarify whether medication needs to be diluted before administration. Check the infusion rate.	This comparison helps to identify errors that may have occurred when orders were transcribed. The physician's order is the legal record of medication orders for each agency. Compatibility of medication and solution prevents complications. Delivers the correct dose of medication as prescribed.

(continued)

SKILL 5-14

Introducing Drugs Through a Medication or Drug-Infusion Lock Using the Saline Flush (Intermittent Peripheral Venous Access Device) *(continued)*

ACTION	RATIONALE
2. Know the actions, special nursing considerations, safe dose ranges, purpose of administration, and adverse effects of the medications to be administered. Consider the appropriateness of the medication for this patient.	This knowledge aids the nurse in evaluating the therapeutic effect of the medication in relation to the patient's disorder and can also be used to educate the patient about the medication.
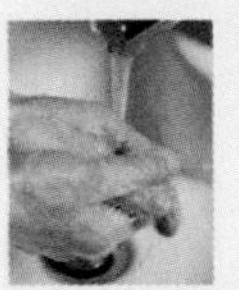 3. Perform hand hygiene.	Hand hygiene prevents the spread of microorganisms.
4. Move the medication cart to the outside of the patient's room or prepare for administration in the medication area.	Organization facilitates error-free administration and saves time.
5. Unlock the medication cart or drawer. Enter pass code and scan employee identification, if required.	Locking of the cart or drawer safeguards each patient's medication supply. Hospital accrediting organizations require medication carts to be locked when not in use. Entering pass code and scanning ID allows only authorized users into the system and identifies user for documentation by the computer.
6. **Prepare medication for one patient at a time.**	This prevents errors in medication administration.
7. Read the MAR and select the proper medication from the patient's medication drawer or unit stock.	This is the first check of the label.
8. Compare the label with the MAR. Check expiration dates and perform calculations, if necessary. Scan the bar code on the package, if required.	This is the second check of the label. Verify calculations with another nurse to ensure safety, if necessary.
9. If necessary, withdraw medication from an ampule or vial as described in Skills 5-2 and 5-3.	Allows administration of medication.
10. **Recheck the label with the MAR before taking it to the patient.**	This is a *third* check to ensure accuracy and to prevent errors.
11. Lock the medication cart before leaving it.	Locking the cart or drawer safeguards the patient's medication supply. Hospital accrediting organizations require medication carts to be locked when not in use.
12. Transport medications and equipment to the patient's bedside carefully, and keep the medications in sight at all times.	Careful handling and close observation prevent accidental or deliberate disarrangement of medications. Having equipment available saves time and facilitates performance of the task.
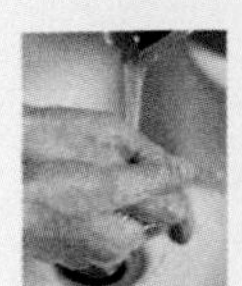 13. Perform hand hygiene.	Hand hygiene deters the spread of microorganisms.
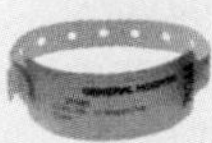 14. **Identify the patient.** Usually, the patient should be identified using two methods. Compare information with the MAR or CMAR.	Identifying the patient ensures the right patient receives the medications and helps prevent errors.
a. Check the name and identification number on the patient's identification band.	This is the most reliable method. Replace the identification band if it is missing or inaccurate in any way.

SKILL 5-14 Introducing Drugs Through a Medication or Drug-Infusion Lock Using the Saline Flush (Intermittent Peripheral Venous Access Device) *(continued)*

ACTION	RATIONALE
b. Ask the patient to state his or her name.	This requires a response from the patient, but illness and strange surroundings often cause patients to be confused.
c. If the patient cannot identify him or herself, verify the patient's identification with a staff member who knows the patient for the second source.	This is another way to double-check identity. Do not use the name on the door or over the bed, because these may be inaccurate.
15. Close the door to the room or pull the bedside curtain.	This provides patient privacy.
16. Complete necessary assessments before administering medications. Check allergy bracelet or ask patient about allergies. Explain the purpose and action of the medication to the patient.	Assessment is a prerequisite to administration of medications. Explanation provides rationale, increases knowledge, and reduces anxiety.
17. Scan the patient's bar code on the identification band, if required.	Scanning provides additional check to ensure that the medication is given to the right patient.
18. **Assess IV site for presence of inflammation or infiltration.**	IV medication must be given directly into a vein for safe administration.
19. Put on clean gloves.	Gloves protect the nurse's hands from contact with the patient's blood.
20. Clean the access port of the medication lock with antimicrobial swab (Figure 1).	Cleaning removes surface contaminants at the lock entry site.

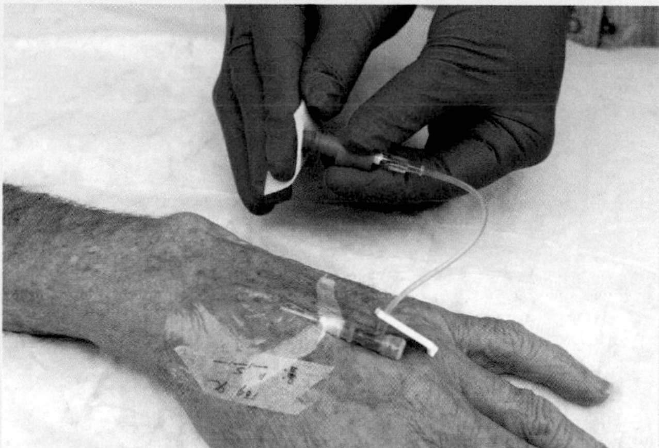

Figure 1. Cleaning port with antimicrobial swab.

ACTION	RATIONALE
21. Stabilize port with your nondominant hand and insert needleless device, syringe, or needle of syringe of normal saline into access port (Figure 2).	This allows for careful insertion into the center circle of the lock.
22. Release the clamp on the extension tubing of the medication lock. Aspirate gently and check for blood return (Figure 3).	This ensures the catheter of the medication lock is in a vein.
23. Gently flush with normal saline by pushing slowly on the syringe plunger. Observe the insertion site while inserting the saline. Remove syringe.	Saline flush ensures that the IV line is patent. Puffiness or swelling as the site is flushed could indicate infiltration of the catheter.

(continued)

SKILL 5-14

Introducing Drugs Through a Medication or Drug-Infusion Lock Using the Saline Flush (Intermittent Peripheral Venous Access Device) *(continued)*

ACTION | RATIONALE

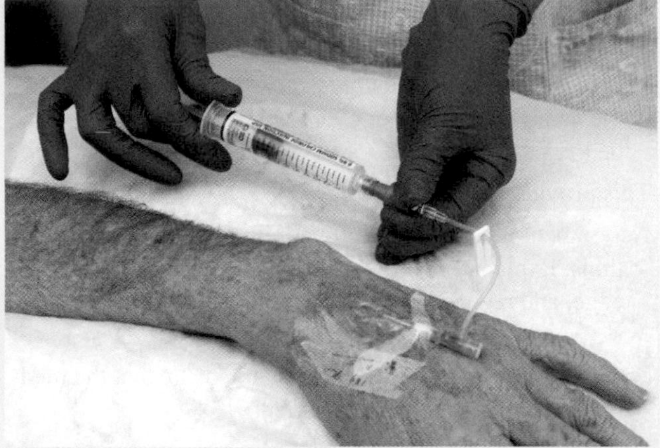

Figure 2. Insert syringe, needle, or needleless device into access port.

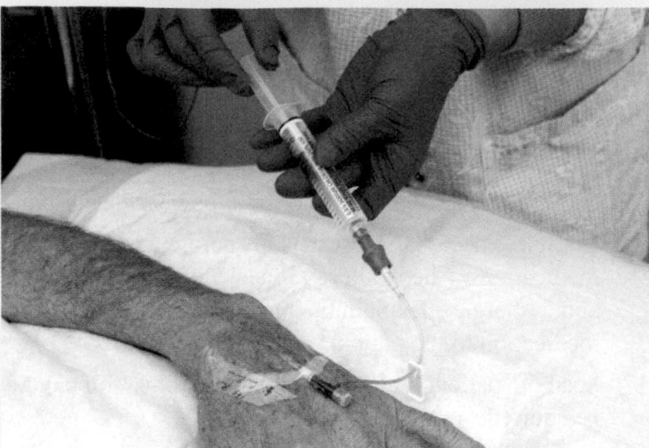

Figure 3. Aspirating for blood return.

24. Insert needleless device or needle of syringe with medication into port and gently inject medication, using a watch to verify correct administration rate. **Do not force the injection if resistance is felt.**

Easy installation of medication usually indicates that the lock is still patent and in the vein. If force is used against resistance, a clot may break away and cause a blockage elsewhere in the body.

25. Remove medication syringe from port. Stabilize port with your nondominant hand and insert needleless device or needle of syringe of normal saline into port. Gently flush with normal saline by pushing slowly on the syringe plunger (Figure 4). To gain positive pressure, clamp the IV tubing as you are still flushing the last of the saline into the medication lock (Figure 5). Remove syringe.

Positive pressure prevents blood from backing into catheter and causing the medication lock to clot off.

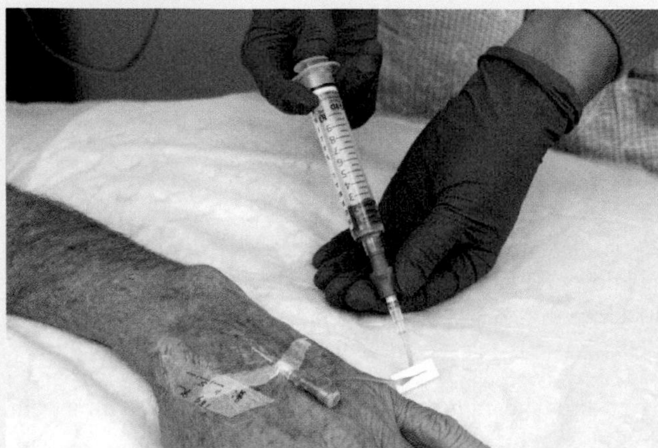

Figure 4. Flushing port with normal saline.

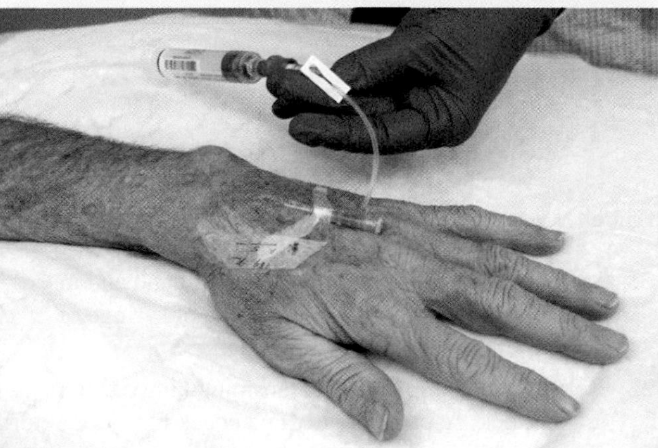

Figure 5. Clamping the access port.

26. Do not recap the used needle. Engage the safety shield or needle guard, if present. Discard the needle and syringe in the appropriate receptacle.

Proper disposal of the needle prevents injury.

SKILL 5-14

Introducing Drugs Through a Medication or Drug-Infusion Lock Using the Saline Flush (Intermittent Peripheral Venous Access Device) *(continued)*

ACTION	RATIONALE
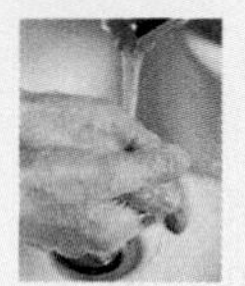 27. Remove gloves and perform hand hygiene.	Hand hygiene deters spread of microorganisms.
28. Evaluate patient's response to medication within appropriate time frame.	Patient requires careful observation because medications given by IV bolus injection may have a rapid effect.
29. Check medication lock site at least every 8 hours or according to facility policy.	This ensures patency of system.

EVALUATION

The expected outcomes are met when the medication is delivered via the parenteral route using sterile technique; the medication is delivered to the patient in a safe manner and at the appropriate infusion rate; patient experiences no adverse effect; the intermittent peripheral venous access device remains patent; and the patient understands and complies with the medication regimen.

DOCUMENTATION

Guidelines

Document the administration of the medication and/or saline flush, including date, time, dose, route of administration, site of administration, and rate of administration on the MAR or record using the required format, immediately after administration. If using a bar-code system, medication administration is automatically recorded when scanned. PRN medications require documentation of the reason for administration. Prompt recording avoids the possibility of accidentally repeating the administration of the drug. If the drug was refused or omitted, record this in the appropriate area on the medication record and notify the physician. This verifies the reason medication was omitted and ensures that the physician is aware of the patient's condition.

Unexpected Situations and Associated Interventions

- *Upon assessing the medication lock site before administering medication, nurse notes that the medication lock has infiltrated:* Remove medication lock from extremity. Restart peripheral venous access in a different location. Continue to monitor new site as medication is administered.
- *While nurse is administering medication, patient begins to complain of pain at the site:* Stop the medication. Assess the medication lock site for signs of infiltration and phlebitis. You may want to flush the medication lock with normal saline again to recheck patency. If the IV site appears within normal limits, resume medication administration at a slower rate. If pain persists, stop, remove medication lock and restart in a different location.
- *As nurse is attempting to access lock, needle or tip of syringe touches patient's arm:* Discard needle and syringe. Prepare new dose for administration.
- *No blood return is noted upon aspiration:* If medication lock appears patent, without signs of infiltration, and normal saline fluid infuses without difficulty, proceed with administration. Observe closely for signs and symptoms of infiltration during and after administration.

(continued)

SKILL 5-14 Introducing Drugs Through a Medication or Drug-Infusion Lock Using the Saline Flush (Intermittent Peripheral Venous Access Device) *(continued)*

Special Considerations

General Considerations

- If medication lock is not used, flush with saline every 8 to 12 hours to maintain patency, according to facility policy.
- Medication lock site is routinely changed every 72 to 96 hours, according to facility policy. This reduces risk of infection and emboli in the bloodstream.
- Intermittent infusions of small-volume IV medications can also be administered through the medication lock. Attach IV medication container to infusion tubing and prime. After flushing the medication lock with saline as outlined above, attach the infusion tubing to the medication lock. Adjust infusion rate with roller clamp on infusion tubing. After infusion is completed, remove tubing from lock and flush with saline as outlined above.
- Ongoing assessment is an important part of nursing care to evaluate patient response to administered medications and early detection of adverse effects. If an adverse effect is suspected, withhold further medication doses and notify the patient's primary healthcare provider. Additional intervention is based on type of reaction and patient assessment.

Infant and Child Considerations

- If the volume of medication being administered is small (<1.0 mL), always include the amount of flush solution as part of the total amount to be injected and take this into account when determining how fast to push a medication. For example, if the medication is to be injected at a rate of 1.0 mL per minute and the total amount of solution to be injected is 2.25 mL (0.25 mL medication volume plus 2.0 mL saline flush solution volume equals 2.25 mL), then the medication would be injected over a period of 2 minutes 15 seconds.

SKILL 5-15 Applying a Transdermal Patch

The transdermal route is being used more frequently to deliver medication. This involves applying to the patient's skin a disk or patch that contains medication intended for daily use or for longer intervals. Transdermal patches are commonly used to deliver hormones, narcotic analgesics, cardiac medications, and nicotine. Medication errors have occurred when patients apply multiple patches at once or fail to remove the overlay on the patch that exposes the skin to the medication. Narcotic analgesic patches are associated with the most adverse drug effects. Clear patches have a cosmetic advantage but can be difficult to find on the patient's skin when they need to be removed or replaced.

Equipment

- Medication patch
- Gloves
- Scissors (optional)
- Washcloth, soap and water
- Medication Administration Record (MAR) or Computer-generated MAR (CMAR)

ASSESSMENT

Assess the patient for any allergies. Check expiration date before administering medication. Assess the appropriateness of the drug for the patient. Review assessment and laboratory data that may influence drug administration. Verify patient name, dose, route, and time of administration. Assess the skin at the location where the patch will be applied. Many patches have different and specific instructions for where the patch is to be placed. Site should be clean, dry, and free of hair. Transdermal patches should not be placed on irritated or broken skin. Check

SKILL 5-15 **Applying a Transdermal Patch** *(continued)*

the manufacturer's instructions for location of the patch. Assess the patient for any old patches. A new transdermal patch should not be placed until old patches have been removed. Assess the patient's knowledge of the medication. If the patient has a knowledge deficit about the medication, this may be the appropriate time to begin education about the medication. If the medication may affect the patient's vital signs, assess them before administration.

NURSING DIAGNOSIS

Determine related factors for the nursing diagnoses based on the patient's current status. Appropriate nursing diagnoses may include:

- Risk for Allergy Response
- Deficient Knowledge
- Risk for Impaired Skin Integrity

OUTCOME IDENTIFICATION AND PLANNING

The expected outcome is that the medication is delivered via the transdermal route. Other outcomes that may be appropriate include the following: patient experiences no adverse effect; the patient's skin remains free from injury; and the patient understands and complies with the medication regimen.

IMPLEMENTATION

ACTION	RATIONALE
1. Gather equipment. Check medication order against the original physician's order according to agency policy. Clarify any inconsistencies. Check the patient's chart for allergies.	This comparison helps to identify errors that may have occurred when orders were transcribed. The physician's order is the legal record of medication orders for each agency.
2. Know the actions, special nursing considerations, safe dose ranges, purpose of administration, and adverse effects of the medications to be administered. Consider the appropriateness of the medication for this patient.	This knowledge aids the nurse in evaluating the therapeutic effect of the medication in relation to the patient's disorder and can also be used to educate the patient about the medication.
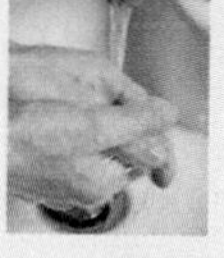 3. Perform hand hygiene.	Hand hygiene prevents the spread of microorganisms.
4. Move the medication cart to the outside of the patient's room or prepare for administration in the medication area.	Organization facilitates error-free administration and saves time.
5. Unlock the medication cart or drawer. Enter pass code and scan employee identification, if required.	Locking of the cart or drawer safeguards each patient's medication supply. Hospital accrediting organizations require medication carts to be locked when not in use. Entering pass code and scanning ID allows only authorized users into the system and identifies user for documentation by the computer.
6. **Prepare medications for one patient at a time.**	This prevents errors in medication administration.
7. Read the MAR and select the proper medication from the patient's medication drawer or unit stock.	This is the first check of the label.
8. Compare the label with the MAR. Check expiration dates and perform calculations, if necessary. Scan the bar code on the package, if required.	This is the second check of the label. Verify calculations with another nurse to ensure safety, if necessary.

(continued)

SKILL 5-15 Applying a Transdermal Patch *(continued)*

ACTION	RATIONALE
9. **When all medications for one patient have been prepared, recheck the label with the MAR before taking them to the patient. Lock the medication cart before leaving it.**	This is a *third* check to ensure accuracy and to prevent errors. Locking the cart or drawer safeguards the patient's medication supply. Hospital accrediting organizations require medication carts to be locked when not in use.
10. Transport medications to the patient's bedside carefully, and keep the medications in sight at all times.	Careful handling and close observation prevent accidental or deliberate disarrangement of medications.
11. **Ensure that the patient receives the medications at the correct time.**	Check agency policy, which may allow for administration within a period of 30 minutes before or 30 minutes after designated time.
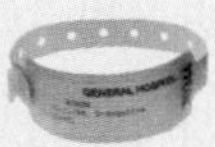 12. **Identify the patient.** Usually, the patient should be identified using two methods. Compare information with the MAR or CMAR.	Identifying the patient ensures the right patient receives the medications and helps prevent errors.
a. Check the name and identification number on the patient's identification band.	This is the most reliable method. Replace the identification band if it is missing or inaccurate in any way.
b. Ask the patient to state his or her name.	This requires a response from the patient, but illness and strange surroundings often cause patients to be confused.
c. If the patient cannot identify him or herself, verify the patient's identification with a staff member who knows the patient for the second source.	This is another way to double-check identity. Do not use the name on the door or over the bed, because these may be inaccurate.
13. **Complete necessary assessments before administering medications. Check allergy bracelet or ask patient about allergies. Explain the purpose and action of each medication to the patient.**	Assessment is a prerequisite to administration of medications.
14. Scan the patient's bar code on the identification band, if required.	This provides an additional check to ensure that the medication is given to the right patient.
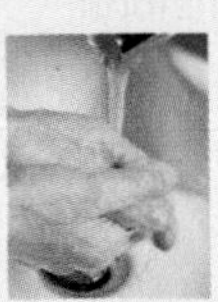 15. Perform hand hygiene and put on gloves.	Hand hygiene deters the spread of microorganisms. Gloves protect the nurse when handling the medication on the transdermal patch.
16. Assess patient's skin where patch is to be placed, looking for any signs of irritation or breakdown. Site should be clean, dry, and free of hair. Rotate application sites.	Transdermal patches should not be placed on skin that is irritated or broken down. Hair can prevent the patch from sticking to the skin. Rotating sites reduces risk for skin irritation.
17. **Remove any old transdermal patches from the patient's skin.** Fold the old patch in half with the adhesive sides sticking together and discard according to facility policy. Gently wash the area where the old patch was with soap and water.	Leaving old patches on patient while applying new ones may lead to delivery of a toxic level of the drug. Folding sides together prevents accidental contact with remaining medication. Washing area with soap and water removes all traces of medication in that area.
18. Remove the patch from its protective covering. Write your initials and the date and time of administration on the label side of the patch.	This allows for easy identification of application date and time.
19. Remove the covering on the patch without touching the medication surface (Figure 1). Apply the patch to the patient's skin (Figure 2). Use the palm of your hand to press firmly for about 10 seconds. Do not massage.	Touching the adhesive side may alter the amount of medication left on the patch. Pressing firmly for 10 seconds ensures that the patch stays on the patient's skin.

SKILL 5-15 **Applying a Transdermal Patch** *(continued)*

ACTION	RATIONALE
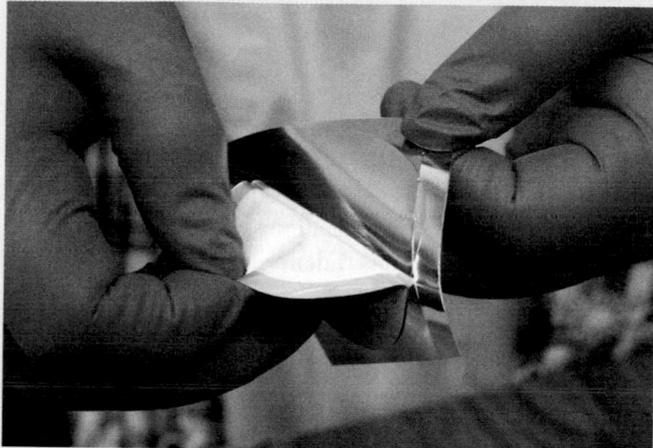 **Figure 1.** Removing covering on the patch.	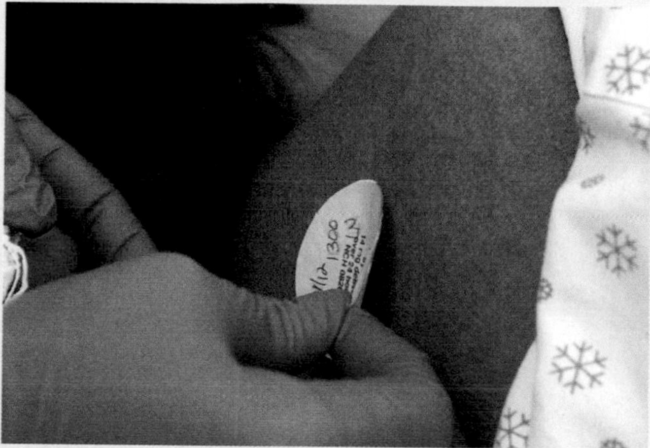 **Figure 2.** Applying patch to patient's skin.
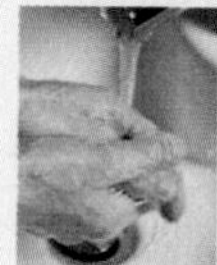 20. Remove gloves and perform hand hygiene.	Hand hygiene deters the spread of microorganisms.
21. Evaluate patient's response to medication within appropriate time frame.	Patient needs to be evaluated to ensure that patch is delivering drug appropriately and that patient is not experiencing any adverse effects.

EVALUATION

The expected outcomes are met when the medication is delivered via the transdermal route; patient experiences no adverse effect; the patient's skin remains intact and free from injury; and the patient understands and complies with the medication regimen.

DOCUMENTATION

Guidelines

Document the administration of the medication immediately after administration, including date, time, dose, route of administration, and site of administration on the MAR or record using the required format. If using a bar-code system, medication administration is automatically recorded when scanned. PRN medications require documentation of the reason for administration. Prompt recording avoids the possibility of accidentally repeating the administration of the drug. If the drug was refused or omitted, record this in the appropriate area on the medication record and notify the physician. This verifies the reason medication was omitted and ensures that the physician is aware of the patient's condition.

Unexpected Situations and Associated Interventions

- *Nurse did not wear gloves while applying transdermal patch:* Immediately perform good hand hygiene using soap and water to remove any medication that may be on the skin. The nurse may feel the effects of the medication if any came into contact with his or her skin.
- *Nurse finds more than one old transdermal patch while applying new transdermal patch:* Remove all old patches of the same kind; remember that more than one medication may be delivered via transdermal patch. Check physician orders to ensure that patient is still receiving medication. Failure to remove old transdermal patches is considered a medication error in some institutions. Notify the physician of potential medication overdose. Follow agency policy regarding paperwork for medication errors.

(continued)

SKILL 5-15 Applying a Transdermal Patch *(continued)*

- *When removing an old transdermal patch, nurse notes skin underneath is erythematous and swollen:* Wash skin with soap and water and assess patient for any latex or adhesive allergies. Discuss with patient whether patch site has been rotated. Notify physician before applying a new patch.

Special Considerations

General Considerations

- Apply the patch at the same time of the day, according to the order and medication specifications.
- Check for dislodgement of the patch if the patient is active. Read information about the patch or consult with the pharmacist to determine reapplication schedule and procedure.
- Aluminum backing on a patch necessitates precautions if defibrillation is required. Burns and smoke may result.
- Assess for any skin irritation at application site. If necessary, remove the patch, wash the area carefully with soap and water, and allow skin to air dry. Apply a new patch at a different site. Assess the potential for adverse reaction.
- Ongoing assessment is an important part of nursing care to evaluate patient response to administered medications and early detection of adverse effects. If an adverse effect is suspected, withhold further medication doses and notify the patient's primary healthcare provider. Additional intervention is based on type of reaction and patient assessment.

SKILL 5-16 Instilling Eye Drops

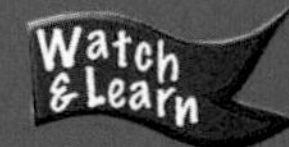

Eye drops are instilled for their local effects, such as for pupil dilation or constriction when examining the eye, for infection treatment, or for controlling intraocular pressure (for patients with glaucoma). The type and amount of solution depend on the purpose of the instillation.

The eye is a delicate organ, highly susceptible to infection and injury. Although the eye is never free of microorganisms, the secretions of the conjunctiva protect against many pathogens. For maximum safety for the patient, the equipment, solutions, and ointments introduced into the conjunctival sac should be sterile. If this is not possible, follow careful guidelines for medical asepsis.

Equipment

- Gloves
- Medication
- Tissues
- Normal saline solution
- Wash cloth, cotton balls, or gauze squares
- Medication Administration Record (MAR) or Computer-generated MAR (CMAR)

ASSESSMENT

Assess the patient for any allergies. Check expiration date before administering medication. Assess the appropriateness of the drug for the patient. Review assessment and laboratory data that may influence drug administration. Verify patient name, dose, route, and time of administration. Assess the affected eye for any drainage, erythema, or swelling. Assess the patient's knowledge of the medication. If the patient has a knowledge deficit about the medication, this may be the appropriate time to begin education about the medication. If the medication may affect the patient's vital signs, assess them before administration.

SKILL 5-16 **Instilling Eye Drops** *(continued)*

NURSING DIAGNOSIS

Determine related factors for the nursing diagnoses based on the patient's current status. Appropriate nursing diagnoses may include:

- Risk for Allergy Response
- Risk for Injury
- Deficient Knowledge

OUTCOME IDENTIFICATION AND PLANNING

The expected outcome to achieve when administering eye drops is that the medication is delivered successfully into the eye. Other outcomes that may be appropriate include the following: patient experiences no allergy response; patient does not exhibit systemic effects of the medication; patient's eye remains free from injury; and patient understands the rationale for medication administration.

IMPLEMENTATION

ACTION	RATIONALE
1. Gather equipment. Check medication order against the original physician's order according to agency policy. Clarify any inconsistencies. Check the patient's chart for allergies.	This comparison helps to identify errors that may have occurred when orders were transcribed. The physician's order is the legal record of medication orders for each agency.
2. Know the actions, special nursing considerations, safe dose ranges, purpose of administration, and adverse effects of the medications to be administered. Consider the appropriateness of the medication for this patient.	This knowledge aids the nurse in evaluating the therapeutic effect of the medication in relation to the patient's disorder and can also be used to educate the patient about the medication.
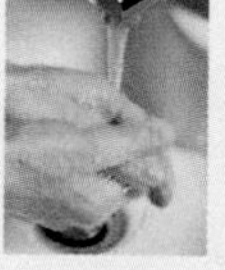 3. Perform hand hygiene.	Hand hygiene prevents the spread of microorganisms.
4. Move the medication cart to the outside of the patient's room or prepare for administration in the medication area.	Organization facilitates error-free administration and saves time.
5. Unlock the medication cart or drawer. Enter pass code and scan employee identification, if required.	Locking of the cart or drawer safeguards each patient's medication supply. Hospital accrediting organizations require medication carts to be locked when not in use. Entering pass code and scanning ID allows only authorized users into the system and identifies user for documentation by the computer.
6. **Prepare medications for one patient at a time.**	This prevents errors in medication administration.
7. Read the MAR and select the proper medication from the patient's medication drawer or unit stock.	This is the first check of the label.
8. Compare the label with the MAR. Check expiration dates and perform calculations, if necessary. Scan the bar code on the package, if required.	This is the second check of the label. Verify calculations with another nurse to ensure safety, if necessary.
9. **When all medications for one patient have been prepared, recheck the label with the MAR before taking them to the patient. Lock the medication cart before leaving it.**	This is a *third* check to ensure accuracy and to prevent errors. Locking the cart or drawer safeguards the patient's medication supply. Hospital accrediting organizations require medication carts to be locked when not in use.

(continued)

SKILL 5-16 Instilling Eye Drops *(continued)*

ACTION	RATIONALE
10. Transport medications to the patient's bedside carefully, and keep the medications in sight at all times.	Careful handling and close observation prevent accidental or deliberate disarrangement of medications.
11. **Ensure that the patient receives the medications at the correct time.**	Check agency policy, which may allow for administration within a period of 30 minutes before or 30 minutes after designated time.
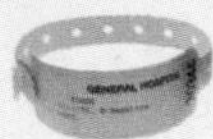 12. **Identify the patient.** Usually, the patient should be identified using two methods. Compare information with the MAR or CMAR.	Identifying the patient ensures the right patient receives the medications and helps prevent errors.
a. Check the name and identification number on the patient's identification band.	This is the most reliable method. Replace the identification band if it is missing or inaccurate in any way.
b. Ask the patient to state his or her name.	This requires a response from the patient, but illness and strange surroundings often cause patients to be confused.
c. If the patient cannot identify him or herself, verify the patient's identification with a staff member who knows the patient for the second source.	This is another way to double-check identity. Do not use the name on the door or over the bed, because these may be inaccurate.
13. **Complete necessary assessments before administering medications. Check allergy bracelet or ask patient about allergies. Explain the purpose and action of each medication to the patient.**	Assessment is a prerequisite to administration of medications.
14. Scan the patient's bar code on the identification band, if required.	Provides additional check to ensure that the medication is given to the right patient.
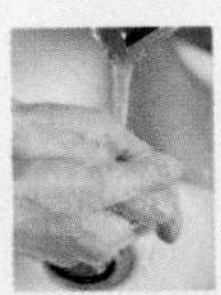 15. Perform hand hygiene and put on gloves.	Hand hygiene deters the spread of microorganisms. Gloves protect the nurse from potential contact with mucous membranes and body fluids.
16. Offer tissue to patient.	Solution and tears may spill from the eye during the procedure.
17. **Cleanse the eyelids and eyelashes of any drainage with a wash cloth, cotton balls, or gauze squares moistened with normal saline solution.** Use each area of the cleaning surface once, moving from the inner toward the outer canthus (Figure 1).	Debris can be carried into the eye when the conjunctival sac is exposed. Using each area of the gauze once and moving from the inner canthus to the outer canthus prevents carrying debris to the lacrimal ducts.

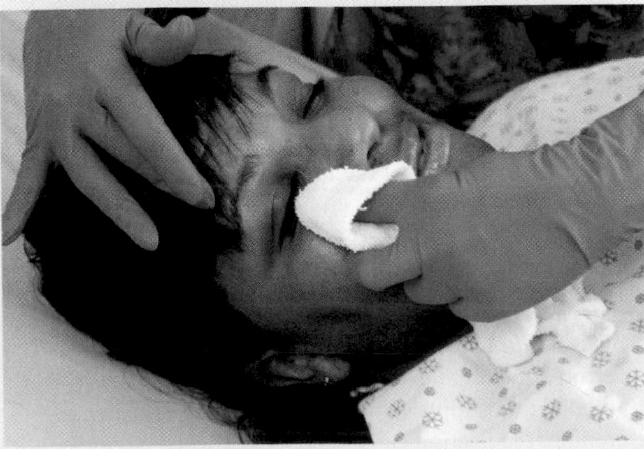

Figure 1. Cleaning lids and lashes from inside of eye to outside.

SKILL 5-16 Instilling Eye Drops *(continued)*

ACTION	RATIONALE
18. Tilt the patient's head back slightly if sitting, or place the patient's head over a pillow if lying down. The head may be turned slightly to the affected side to prevent solution or tears from flowing toward the opposite eye (Figure 2).	Tilting patient's head back slightly makes it easier to reach the conjunctival sac. This should be avoided if the patient has a cervical spine injury. Turning the head to the affected side helps to prevent solution or tears from flowing toward the opposite eye.
19. Remove cap from medication bottle, being careful to not touch the inner side of the cap. (See the accompanying Skill Variation for administering ointment.)	Touching the inner side of the cap may contaminate the bottle of medication.
20. Invert the monodrip plastic container that is commonly used to instill eye drops. Have patient look up and focus on something on the ceiling.	By having the patient look up and focus on something else, the procedure is less traumatic and keeps the eye still.
21. Place thumb or two fingers near margin of lower eyelid immediately below eyelashes, and exert pressure downward over bony prominence of cheek. Lower conjunctival sac is exposed as lower lid is pulled down (Figure 3).	The eye drop should be placed in the conjunctival sac, not directly on the eyeball.

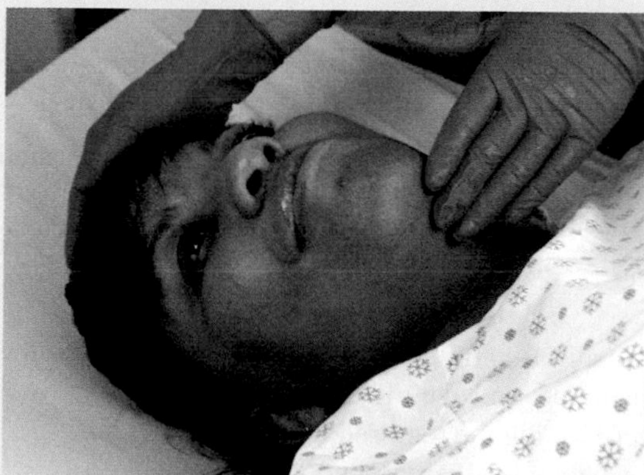

Figure 2. Turning head slightly to affected side.

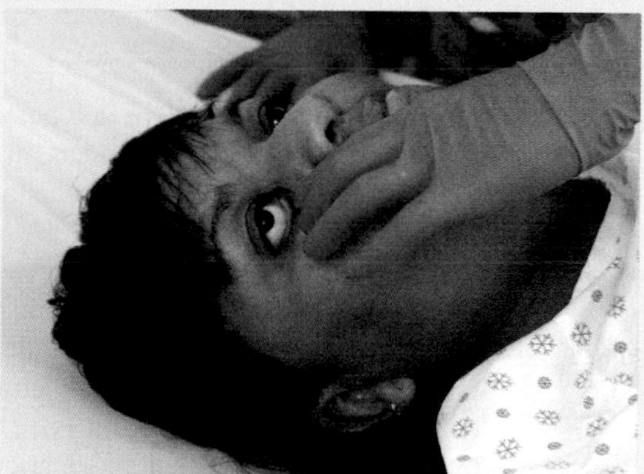

Figure 3. Exerting pressure downward to expose lower conjunctival sac.

ACTION	RATIONALE
22. **Hold dropper close to eye, but avoid touching eyelids or lashes. Squeeze container and allow prescribed number of drops to fall in lower conjunctival sac (Figure 4).**	Touching the eye, eyelids, or lashes can contaminate the medication in the bottle; startle the patient, causing blinking; or injure the eye. Do not allow medication to fall onto cornea. This may injure the cornea or cause the patient to have an unpleasant sensation.
23. Release lower lid after eye drops are instilled. Ask patient to close eyes gently.	This allows the medication to be distributed over the entire eye.
24. Apply gentle pressure over inner canthus to prevent eye drops from flowing into tear duct (Figure 5).	This minimizes the risk of systemic effects from the medication.
25. Instruct patient not to rub affected eye.	This prevents injury and irritation to eye.
26. Remove gloves and perform hand hygiene.	Hand hygiene deters the spread of microorganisms.

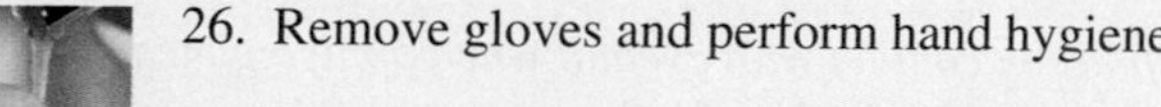

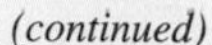

(continued)

SKILL 5-16 Instilling Eye Drops *(continued)*

ACTION	RATIONALE
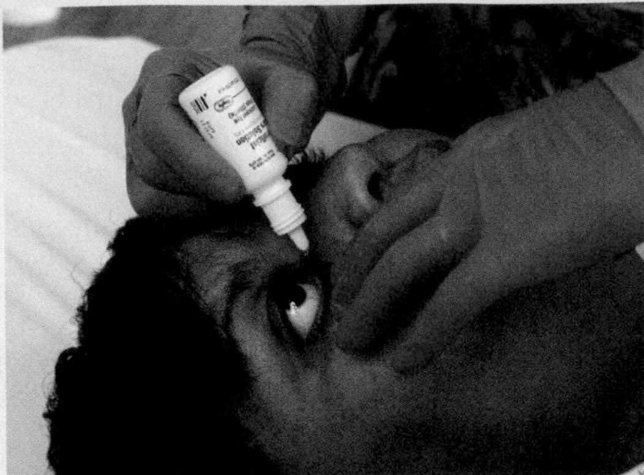 **Figure 4.** Administering drops into conjunctival sac.	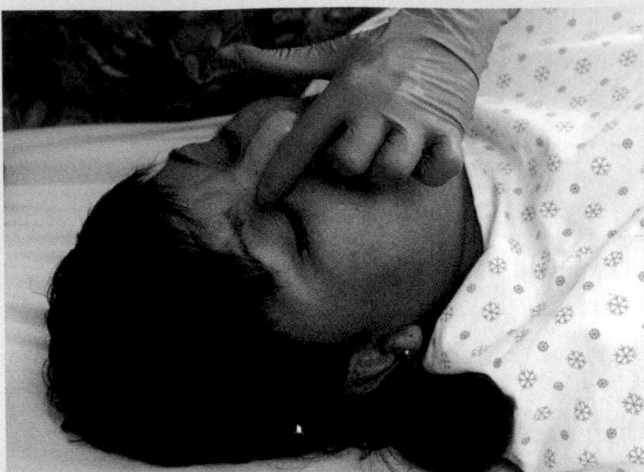 **Figure 5.** Applying gentle pressure over inner canthus.
27. Assist patient to a comfortable position.	This ensures patient comfort.
28. Evaluate patient's response to medication within appropriate time frame.	The patient needs to be evaluated for any adverse affects from the medication.

EVALUATION

The expected outcomes are met when the patient receives the eye drops; experiences no adverse affects, including allergy response, systemic effect, or injury; and understands the rationale for the medication administration.

DOCUMENTATION

Guidelines

Document the administration of the medication immediately after administration, including date, time, dose, route of administration, and site of administration, specifically right, left, or both eyes, on the MAR or record using the required format. If using a bar-code system, medication administration is automatically recorded when scanned. PRN medications require documentation of the reason for administration. Prompt recording avoids the possibility of accidentally repeating the administration of the drug. If the drug was refused or omitted, record this in the appropriate area on the medication record and notify the physician. This verifies the reason medication was omitted and ensures that the physician is aware of the patient's condition.

Unexpected Situations and Associated Interventions

- *Drop is placed on eyelid or outer margin of eyelid due to patient blinking or moving:* Do not count this drop in total number of drops administered. Allow the patient to regain composure and proceed with application of medication. Consider approaching the patient from below their line of sight.
- *Nurse cannot open eyelids due to dried crust and matting of eyelids:* Place a warm wet washcloth over the eye and allow it to remain there for approximately 3 minutes. Cleanse eye as described previously. You may need to repeat this procedure if there is a large amount of matting.
- *Bottle or tube of medication comes in contact with eyeball when applying medication:* Bottle is contaminated; discard appropriately. Notify pharmacy or retrieve new bottle for oncoming shift.

SKILL 5-16 Instilling Eye Drops *(continued)*

Special Considerations

General Considerations

Ongoing assessment is an important part of nursing care to evaluate patient response to administered medications and early detection of adverse effects. If an adverse effect is suspected, withhold further medication doses and notify the patient's primary healthcare provider. Additional intervention is based on type of reaction and patient assessment.

Infant and Child Considerations

- To apply eye drops in a small child, two or more people may be needed to restrain the child. Make sure the child does not reach up to the eye for fear of jabbing the medication bottle into the eye.

SKILL VARIATION Administering Eye Ointment

- Check medication order against the original physician's order according to agency policy. Clarify any inconsistencies. Check the patient's chart for allergies. Know the actions, special nursing considerations, safe dose ranges, purpose of administration, and adverse effects of the medications to be administered. Consider the appropriateness of the medication for this patient.
- Perform hand hygiene.
- Move the medication cart to the outside of the patient's room or prepare for administration in the medication area.
- Unlock the medication cart or drawer. Enter pass code and scan employee identification, if required.
- Read the MAR and select the proper medication from the patient's medication drawer or unit stock.
- Compare the label with the MAR. Check expiration dates. Scan the bar code on the package, if required.
- Recheck the label with the MAR before taking it to the patient.
- Lock the medication cart before leaving it.
- Transport medications and equipment to the patient's bedside carefully, and keep the medications in sight at all times.
- Perform hand hygiene.
- Identify the patient. Usually, the patient should be identified using two methods.
- Close the door to the room or pull the bedside curtain.
- Complete necessary assessments before administering medications. Check allergy bracelet or ask patient about allergies. Explain the purpose and action of the medication to the patient.
- Scan the patient's bar code on the identification band, if required.
- Put on gloves. Offer the patient a tissue.
- Cleanse the eyelids and eyelashes of any drainage with cotton balls or gauze squares moistened with normal saline solution. Use each area of the gauze square once, moving from the inner toward the outer canthus.
- Tilt the patient's head back slightly if sitting, or place the patient's head over a pillow if lying down. The head may be turned slightly to the affected side to prevent solution or tears from flowing toward the opposite eye.
- Have patient look up and focus on something on the ceiling.
- Place thumb or two fingers near margin of lower eyelid immediately below eyelashes and exert pressure downward over bony prominence of cheek. Lower conjunctival sac is exposed as lower lid is pulled down.
- Hold the ointment tube close to eye, but avoid touching eyelids or lashes. Squeeze container and apply about ½″ of ointment from the tube along the exposed sac. Twist tube to break off ribbon of ointment. Do not touch the tip to the eye.
- Release lower lid after ointment is instilled. Ask patient to close eyes gently.
- The warmth helps to liquefy the ointment. Instruct the patient to move the eye, because this helps to spread the ointment under the lids and over the surface of the eyeball.
- Remove gloves and perform hand hygiene.
- Assist the patient to a comfortable position.
- Explain that the ointment may temporarily blur vision; encourage the patient not to rub the eye.
- Evaluate patient's response to medication within appropriate time frame.

SKILL 5-17 Administering an Eye Irrigation

Eye irrigation is performed to remove secretions or foreign bodies or to cleanse and soothe the eye. When irrigating one eye, care should be taken so that the overflowing irrigation fluid does not contaminate the other eye.

Equipment

- Sterile irrigation solution (warmed to 37°C [98.6°F])
- Sterile irrigation set (sterile container and irrigating or bulb syringe)
- Emesis basin or irrigation basin
- Washcloth
- Waterproof pad
- Towel
- Disposable gloves
- Medication Administration Record (MAR) or Computer-generated MAR (CMAR)

ASSESSMENT

Assess the patient's eyes for redness, erythema, edema, drainage or tenderness. Assess the patient for allergies. Verify patient name, dose, route, and time of administration. Assess the patient's knowledge of the procedure. If patient has a knowledge deficit about the procedure, this may be an appropriate time to begin patient education. Assess the patient's ability to cooperate with the procedure.

NURSING DIAGNOSIS

Determine related factors for the nursing diagnoses based on the patient's current status. Appropriate nursing diagnoses may include:

- Deficient Knowledge
- Noncompliance
- Risk for Injury
- Acute Pain

OUTCOME IDENTIFICATION AND PLANNING

The expected outcome to achieve is that the eye is cleansed successfully. Other outcomes that may be appropriate include the following: patient understands the rationale for the procedure and is able to participate; patient's eye remains free from injury; and patient remains free from pain.

IMPLEMENTATION

ACTION	RATIONALE
1. Gather equipment. Check the original physician's order for the irrigation according to agency policy. Clarify any inconsistencies. Check the patient's chart for allergies.	Helps to identify errors that may have occurred when orders were transcribed. The physician's order is the legal record of medication orders for each agency.
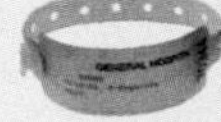 2. **Identify the patient.** Usually, the patient should be identified using two methods. Compare information with the MAR or CMAR.	Identifying the patient ensures the right patient receives the medications and helps prevent errors.
a. Check the name and identification number on the patient's identification band.	This is the most reliable method. Replace the identification band if it is missing or inaccurate in any way.
b. Ask the patient to state his or her name.	This requires a response from the patient, but illness and strange surroundings often cause patients to be confused.
c. If the patient cannot identify him or herself, verify the patient's identification with a staff member who knows the patient for the second source.	This is another way to double-check identity. Do not use the name on the door or over the bed, because these may be inaccurate.
3. Explain procedure to patient.	Explanation facilitates cooperation and reassures patient.

SKILL 5-17 Administering an Eye Irrigation *(continued)*

ACTION	RATIONALE
4. Assemble equipment at patient's bedside.	This provides for an organized approach to the task.
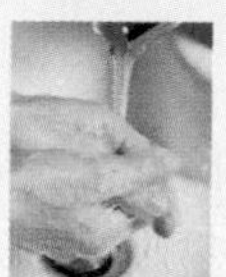 5. Perform hand hygiene.	Hand hygiene deters the spread of microorganisms.
6. Have patient sit or lie with head tilted toward side of affected eye (Figure 1). Protect patient and bed with a waterproof pad.	Gravity aids flow of solution away from unaffected eye and from inner canthus of affected eye toward outer canthus.

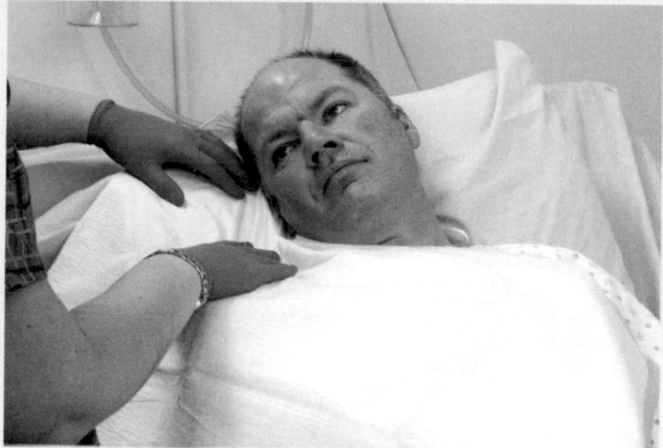

Figure 1. Tilting head toward affected eye.

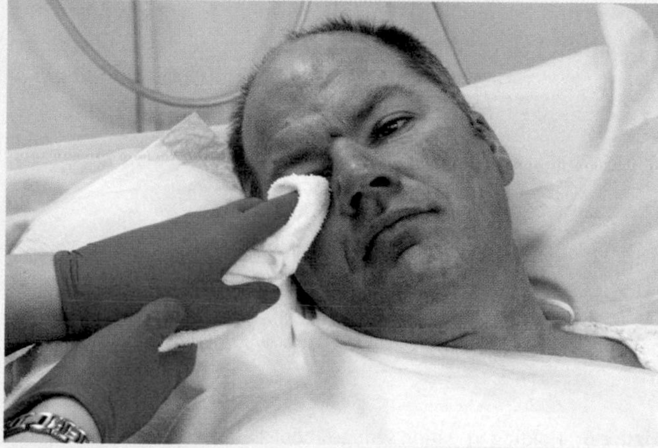

Figure 2. Cleaning lids and lashes from inside of eye to outside.

ACTION	RATIONALE
7. Put on disposable gloves. Clean lids and lashes with washcloth moistened with normal saline or the solution ordered for the irrigation. Wipe from inner canthus to outer canthus (Figure 2). Use a different corner of washcloth with each wipe.	Gloves protect the nurse from contact with mucous membranes, body fluids, and contaminants. Materials lodged on lids or in lashes may be washed into eye. This cleaning motion protects nasolacrimal duct and other eye.
8. Place curved basin at cheek on side of affected eye to receive irrigating solution (Figure 3). If patient is able, ask him or her to support the basin.	Gravity aids flow of solution.

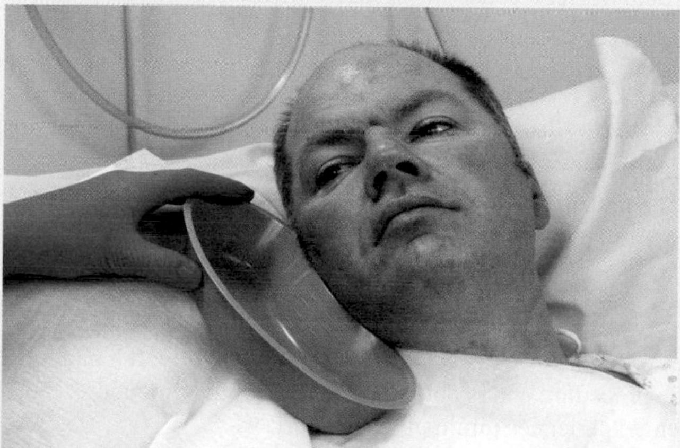

Figure 3. Placing basin to catch irrigating fluid.

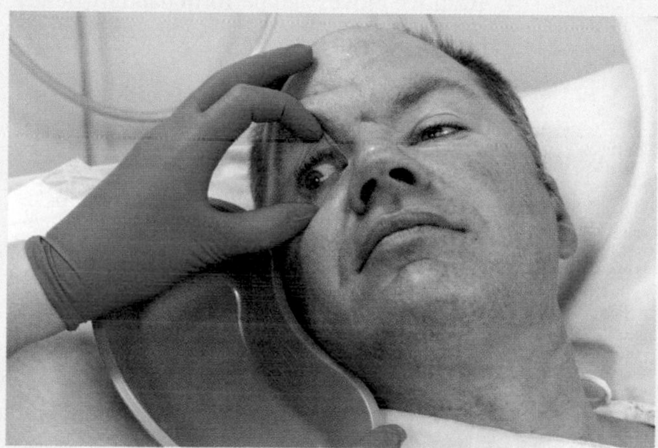

Figure 4. Holding eyelid in position.

(continued)

SKILL 5-17 Administering an Eye Irrigation *(continued)*

ACTION	RATIONALE
9. Expose lower conjunctival sac and hold upper lid open with your nondominant hand (Figure 4).	Solution is directed into lower conjunctival sac because cornea is sensitive and easily injured. This also prevents reflex blinking.
10. Fill the irrigation syringe with the prescribed fluid. **Hold irrigation syringe about 2.5 cm (1″) from eye (Figure 5). Direct flow of solution from inner to outer canthus along conjunctival sac.**	This minimizes the risk for injury to the cornea. Directing solution toward the outer canthus helps to prevent the spread of contamination from the eye to the lacrimal sac, the lacrimal duct, and the nose.

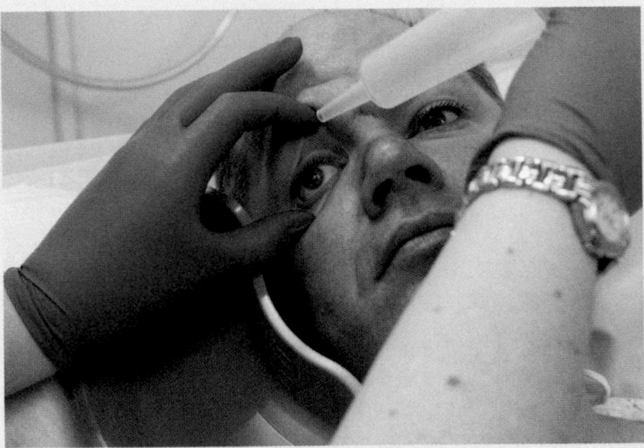

Figure 5. Holding irrigation syringe about 1″ from eye.

ACTION	RATIONALE
11. Irrigate until the solution is clear or all the solution has been used. **Use only enough force to remove secretions gently from the conjunctiva. Avoid touching any part of the eye with the irrigating tip.**	Directing solutions with force may cause injury to the tissues of the eye as well as to the conjunctiva. Touching the eye is uncomfortable for the patient and may cause damage to the cornea.
12. Pause irrigation and have patient close eye periodically during procedure.	Movement of the eye when the lids are closed helps to move secretions from the upper to the lower conjunctival sac.
13. Dry periorbital area after irrigation with gauze sponge. Offer towel to patient if face and neck are wet.	Leaving the skin moist after irrigation is uncomfortable for the patient.
 14. Remove gloves and perform hand hygiene.	Hand hygiene deters the spread of microorganisms.
15. Assist the patient to a comfortable position.	This ensures patient comfort.
16. Evaluate patient's response to medication within appropriate time frame.	The patient needs to be evaluated for any adverse affects from the medication.

EVALUATION

The expected outcomes are met when the eye has been irrigated successfully; the patient understands the rationale for the procedure and is able to comply with the procedure; the eye is not injured; and the patient experiences minimal discomfort.

SKILL 5-17 Administering an Eye Irrigation *(continued)*

DOCUMENTATION

Guidelines

Document the procedure, site, the type of solution and volume used, length of time irrigation performed, pre- and postprocedure assessments, characteristics of any drainage, and the patient's response to the treatment.

Sample Documentation

8/26/08 1820 Sclera of left eye reddened, with periorbital edema and erythema. Thick, yellow liquid draining from left eye. Irrigation of left eye performed using 1000 mL of sterile water. Patient's sclera remains reddened, with slight periorbital edema and erythema. No drainage noted from left eye postirrigation. Patient tolerated procedure with minimal discomfort. Denies need for pain medication at this time. Patient rates pain at present as 1/10.—B. Clapp, RN

Unexpected Situations and Associated Interventions

- *Patient complains of significant pain during procedure:* Stop the procedure and notify the physician. Physician may need to check for any foreign objects such as glass before proceeding with irrigation.
- *Patient cannot keep the eye open during the procedure:* Nurse may need assistance to help patient keep the eye open.

Special Considerations

General Considerations

- Ongoing assessment is an important part of nursing care to evaluate patient response to administered medications and early detection of adverse effects. If an adverse effect is suspected, withhold further medication doses and notify the patient's primary healthcare provider. Additional intervention is based on type of reaction and patient assessment.

SKILL 5-18 Instilling Eardrops

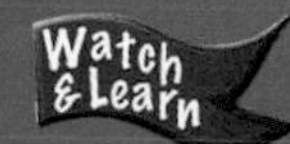

Drugs are instilled into the auditory canal for their local effect. They are used to soften wax, relieve pain, apply local anesthesia, treat infections, or as treatment for an insect lodged in the canal, which can cause great discomfort. If the ear canal has swollen to the point that medication cannot pass, a long piece of cotton material called a wick is inserted into the ear canal. One end of the wick remains external to the ear and the other end is positioned as far as possible into the canal. Medication then may travel along the wick to deliver medication into the canal.

The tympanic membrane separates the external ear from the middle ear. Normally, it is intact and closes the entrance to the middle ear completely. If it is ruptured or has been opened by surgical intervention, the middle ear and the inner ear have a direct passage to the external ear. When this occurs, instillations should be performed with the greatest of care to prevent forcing materials from the outer ear into the middle ear and the inner ear. Sterile technique is used to prevent infection.

Equipment

- Medication (warmed to 37°C [98.6°F])
- Dropper
- Tissue
- Cotton ball (optional)

(continued)

SKILL 5-18

Instilling Eardrops *(continued)*

- Gloves
- Washcloth (optional)
- Normal saline solution
- Medication Administration Record (MAR) or Computer-generated MAR (CMAR)

ASSESSMENT

Assess the affected ear for redness, erythema, edema, drainage or tenderness. Assess the patient for allergies. Verify patient name, dose, route, and time of administration. Assess the patient's knowledge of medication and procedure. If the patient has a knowledge deficit about the medication, this may be an appropriate time to begin education about the medication. Assess the patient's ability to cooperate with the procedure.

NURSING DIAGNOSIS

Determine related factors for the nursing diagnoses based on the patient's current status. Appropriate nursing diagnoses may include:

- Deficient Knowledge
- Anxiety
- Acute Pain
- Risk for Allergy Response
- Risk for Injury

OUTCOME IDENTIFICATION AND PLANNING

The expected outcome to achieve is that drops are administered successfully. Other outcomes that may be appropriate include the following: patient understands the rationale for the eardrop instillation and has decreased anxiety; patient remains free from pain; and patient experiences no allergy response or injury.

IMPLEMENTATION

ACTION	RATIONALE
1. Gather equipment. Check medication order against the original physician's order according to agency policy. Clarify any inconsistencies. Check the patient's chart for allergies.	This comparison helps to identify errors that may have occurred when orders were transcribed. The physician's order is the legal record of medication orders for each agency.
2. Know the actions, special nursing considerations, safe dose ranges, purpose of administration, and adverse effects of the medication to be administered. Consider the appropriateness of the medication for this patient.	This knowledge aids the nurse in evaluating the therapeutic effect of the medication in relation to the patient's disorder and can also be used to educate the patient about the medication.
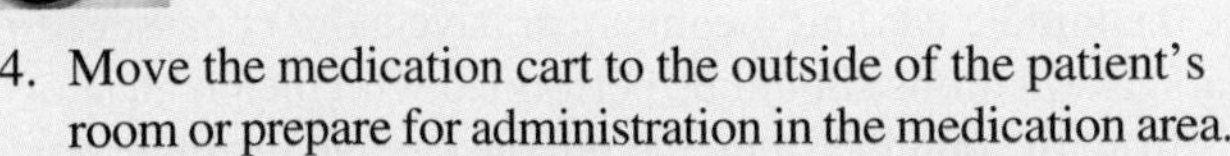 3. Perform hand hygiene.	Hand hygiene prevents the spread of microorganisms.
4. Move the medication cart to the outside of the patient's room or prepare for administration in the medication area.	Organization facilitates error-free administration and saves time.
5. Unlock the medication cart or drawer. Enter pass code and scan employee identification, if required.	Locking of the cart or drawer safeguards each patient's medication supply. Hospital accrediting organizations require medication carts to be locked when not in use. Entering pass code and scanning ID allows only authorized users into the system and identifies user for documentation by the computer.

SKILL 5-18 Instilling Eardrops *(continued)*

ACTION	RATIONALE
6. **Prepare medications for one patient at a time.**	This prevents errors in medication administration.
7. Read the MAR and select the proper medication from the patient's medication drawer or unit stock.	This is the first check of the label.
8. Compare the label with the MAR. Check expiration dates and perform calculations, if necessary. Scan the bar code on the package, if required.	This is the second check of the label. Verify calculations with another nurse to ensure safety, if necessary.
9. **When all medications for one patient have been prepared, recheck the label with the MAR before taking them to the patient. Lock the medication cart before leaving it.**	This is a *third* check to ensure accuracy and to prevent errors. Locking the cart or drawer safeguards the patient's medication supply. Hospital accrediting organizations require medication carts to be locked when not in use.
10. Transport medications to the patient's bedside carefully, and keep the medications in sight at all times.	Careful handling and close observation prevent accidental or deliberate disarrangement of medications.
11. **Ensure that the patient receives the medications at the correct time.**	Check agency policy, which may allow for administration within a period of 30 minutes before or 30 minutes after designated time.
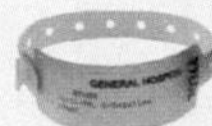 12. **Identify the patient.** Usually, the patient should be identified using two methods. Compare information with the MAR or CMAR.	Identifying the patient ensures the right patient receives the medications and helps prevent errors.
a. Check the name and identification number on the patient's identification band.	This is the most reliable method. Replace the identification band if it is missing or inaccurate in any way.
b. Ask the patient to state his or her name.	This requires a response from the patient, but illness and strange surroundings often cause patients to be confused.
c. If the patient cannot identify him or herself, verify the patient's identification with a staff member who knows the patient for the second source.	This is another way to double-check identity. Do not use the name on the door or over the bed, because these may be inaccurate.
13. **Complete necessary assessments before administering medications. Check allergy bracelet or ask patient about allergies. Explain the purpose and action of each medication to the patient.**	Assessment is a prerequisite to administration of medications.
14. Scan the patient's bar code on the identification band, if required.	Provides additional check to ensure that the medication is given to the right patient.
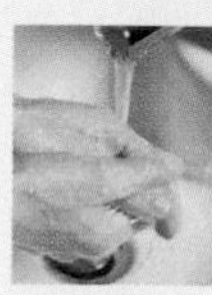 15. Perform hand hygiene and put on gloves.	Hand hygiene deters the spread of microorganisms. Gloves protect the nurse from potential contact with contaminants and body fluids.
16. Cleanse external ear of any drainage with cotton ball or washcloth moistened with normal saline (Figure 1).	Debris and drainage may prevent some of the medication from entering the ear canal.
17. Place patient on his or her unaffected side in bed, or if ambulatory, have patient sit with head well tilted to the side so that affected ear is uppermost (Figure 2).	This positioning prevents the drops from escaping from the ear.

(continued)

SKILL 5-18

Instilling Eardrops *(continued)*

ACTION	RATIONALE
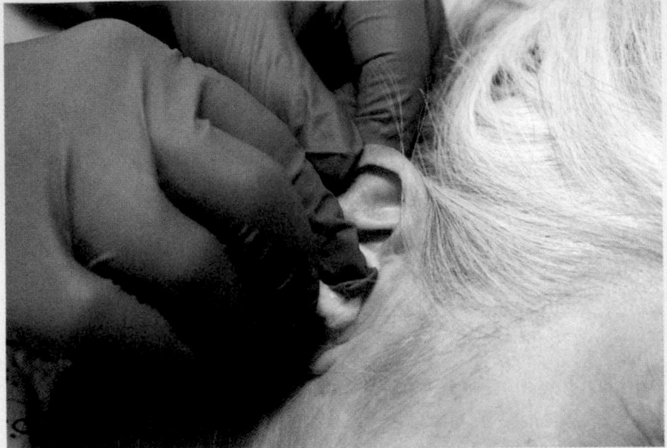 Figure 1. Cleaning external ear.	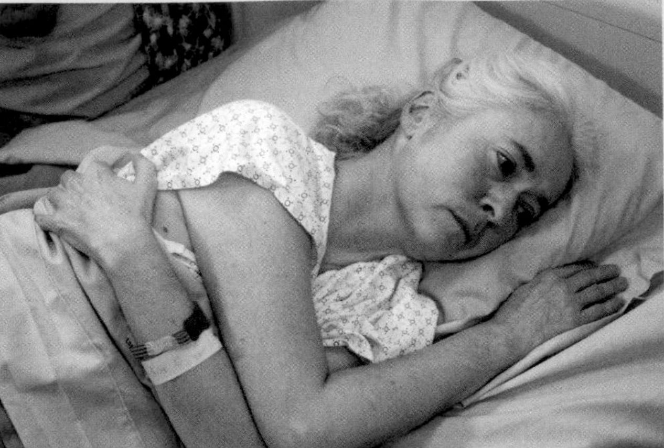 Figure 2. Positioning patient on unaffected side.
18. Draw up the amount of solution needed in dropper. Do not return excess medication to stock bottle. A prepackaged monodrip plastic container may also be used (Figure 3).	Risk for contamination is increased when medication is returned to the stock bottle.
19. Straighten auditory canal by pulling cartilaginous portion of pinna up and back for an adult.	Pulling on the pinna as described helps to straighten the canal properly for eardrop instillation.
20. Hold dropper in ear with its tip above auditory canal (Figure 4). Do not touch dropper to ear. For an infant or an irrational or confused patient, protect dropper with a piece of soft tubing to help prevent injury to ear.	By holding the dropper in the ear, the majority of medication will enter the ear canal. Touching the dropper to the ear contaminates the dropper and medication. The hard tip of the dropper can damage the tympanic membrane if it is jabbed into the ear.
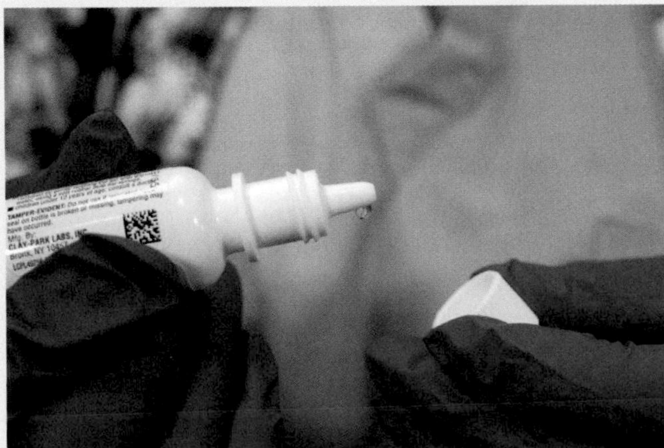 Figure 3. Prepackaged ear drop solution.	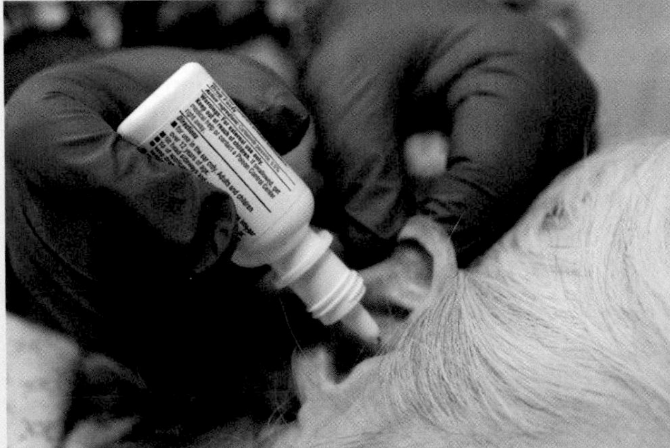 Figure 4. Pulling the pinna up and back and placing the tip of dropper above auditory canal.
21. **Allow drops to fall on side of canal.**	It is uncomfortable for the patient if drops fall directly onto the tympanic membrane.
22. Release pinna after instilling drops, and have patient maintain the position to prevent escape of medication.	Medication should remain in ear canal for at least 5 minutes.

SKILL 5-18 Instilling Eardrops *(continued)*

ACTION	RATIONALE
23. Gently press on tragus a few times (Figure 5).	Pressing on tragus causes medication from canal to move toward tympanic membrane.
24. If ordered, loosely insert a cotton ball into ear canal (Figure 6).	Cotton ball can help prevent medication from leaking out of ear canal.

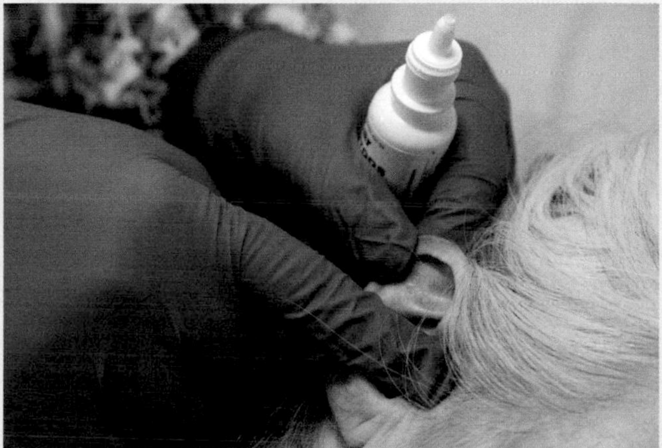

Figure 5. Applying pressure to tragus.

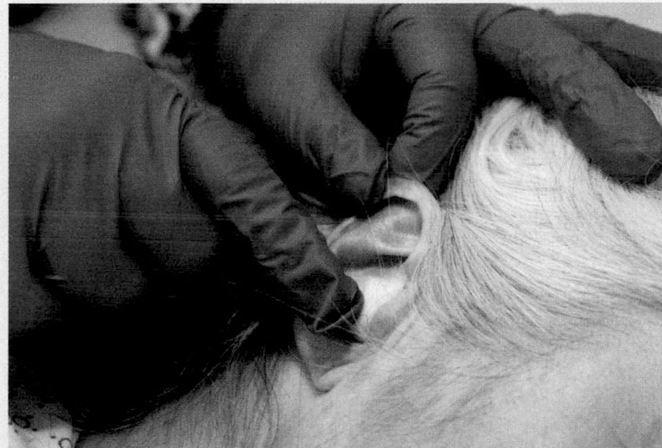

Figure 6. Inserting cotton ball into ear canal.

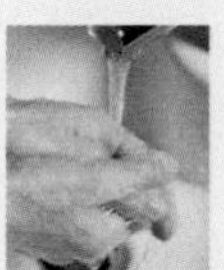

ACTION	RATIONALE
25. Remove gloves and perform hand hygiene.	Hand hygiene deters the spread of microorganisms.
26. Assist the patient to a comfortable position.	This ensures patient comfort.
27. Evaluate patient's response to medication within appropriate time frame.	The patient needs to be evaluated for any adverse affects from the medication.

EVALUATION

The expected outcomes are met when the patient receives the eardrops successfully; understands the rationale for ear drop instillation and exhibits no or decreased anxiety; experiences no or minimal pain; and experiences no allergy response or injury.

DOCUMENTATION

Guidelines

Document the administration of the medication immediately after administration, including date, time, dose, route of administration, and site of administration, specifically right, left, or both eyes, on the MAR or record using the required format. If using a bar-code system, medication administration is automatically recorded when scanned. PRN medications require documentation of the reason for administration. Prompt recording avoids the possibility of accidentally repeating the administration of the drug. If the drug was refused or omitted, record this in the appropriate area on the medication record and notify the physician. This verifies the reason medication was omitted and ensures that the physician is aware of the patient's condition. Document pre- and postadministration assessments, characteristics of any drainage, and the patient's response to the treatment, if appropriate.

(continued)

SKILL 5-18 Instilling Eardrops *(continued)*

Unexpected Situations and Associated Interventions

- *Medication runs from ear into eye:* Notify physician and check with the pharmacy. Eye irrigation may need to be performed.
- *Patient complains of extreme pain when nurse presses on tragus:* Allow patient to press on tragus. If pressure causes too much pain, this part may be deferred.

Special Considerations

General Considerations

- If both ears are to be treated, wait 5 minutes before instilling drops in the second ear.

Infant and Child Considerations

- Pull pinna straight back for a child over 3 years (Figure 7) and down and back for an infant or a child younger than 3 years (Figure 8).
- Distraction techniques, such as TV or a quiet toy, may be helpful when attempting to keep a child quiet for 5 minutes. Reading to the child may not be appropriate because the child's hearing may be compromised during medication administration.
- Ongoing assessment is an important part of nursing care to evaluate patient response to administered medications and early detection of adverse effects. If an adverse effect is suspected, withhold further medication doses and notify the patient's primary healthcare provider. Additional intervention is based on type of reaction and patient assessment.

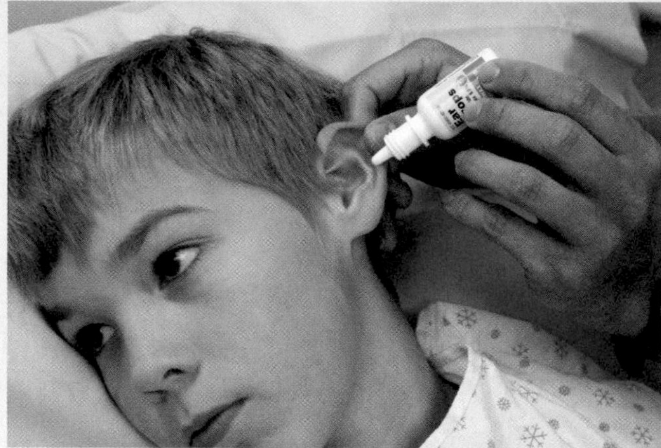

Figure 7. Pulling pinna straight back for child over 3 years.

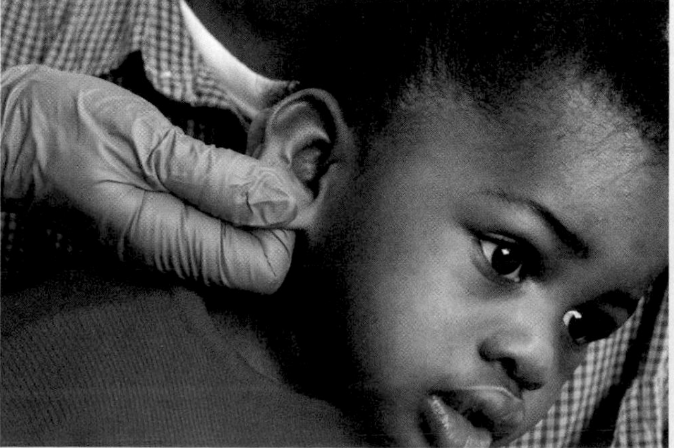

Figure 8. Pulling pinna down and back for an infant or child younger than 3 years.

SKILL
5-19 Administering an Ear Irrigation

Irrigations of the external auditory canal are ordinarily performed for cleaning purposes or for applying heat to the area. Typically, normal saline solution is used, although an antiseptic solution may be indicated for local action. To prevent pain, the irrigation solution should be at least room temperature. Usually, an irrigation syringe is used; however, an irrigating container with tubing and an ear tip may also be used, especially if the purpose of the irrigation is to apply heat to the area.

Equipment

- Prescribed irrigating solution (warmed to 37°C [98.6°F])
- Irrigation set (container and irrigating or bulb syringe)
- Waterproof pad
- Emesis basin
- Cotton-tipped applicators
- Disposable gloves
- Cotton balls
- Medication Administration Record (MAR) or Computer-generated MAR (CMAR)

ASSESSMENT

Assess the affected ear for redness, erythema, edema, drainage or tenderness. Assess the patient's ability to hear. Assess the patient for allergies. Verify patient name, dose, route, and time of administration. Assess the patient's knowledge of medication and procedure. If the patient has a knowledge deficit about the medication, this may be an appropriate time to begin education about the medication. Assess the patient's ability to cooperate with the procedure.

NURSING DIAGNOSIS

Determine related factors for the nursing diagnoses based on the patient's current status. Appropriate nursing diagnoses may include:

- Acute Pain
- Deficient Knowledge
- Risk for Injury

OUTCOME IDENTIFICATION AND PLANNING

The expected outcome to achieve is that the irrigation is administered successfully. Other outcomes that may be appropriate include the following: patient remains free from pain and injury; patient will experience improved hearing; and patient understands the rationale for the procedure.

IMPLEMENTATION

ACTION	RATIONALE
1. Gather equipment. Check the original physician's order for the irrigation according to agency policy. Clarify any inconsistencies. Check the patient's chart for allergies.	Helps to identify errors that may have occurred when orders were transcribed. The physician's order is the legal record of medication orders for each agency.
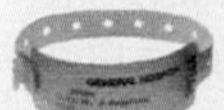 2. **Identify the patient.** Usually, the patient should be identified using two methods. Compare information with the MAR or CMAR.	Identifying the patient ensures the right patient receives the medications and helps prevent errors.
a. Check the name and identification number on the patient's identification band.	This is the most reliable method. Replace the identification band if it is missing or inaccurate in any way.

(continued)

SKILL 5-19 Administering an Ear Irrigation *(continued)*

ACTION	RATIONALE
b. Ask the patient to state his or her name.	This requires a response from the patient, but illness and strange surroundings often cause patients to be confused.
c. If the patient cannot identify him or herself, verify the patient's identification with a staff member who knows the patient for the second source.	This is another way to double-check identity. Do not use the name on the door or over the bed, because these may be inaccurate.
3. Explain procedure to patient.	Explanation facilitates cooperation and reassures patient.
4. Assemble equipment at patient's bedside.	This provides for an organized approach to the task.
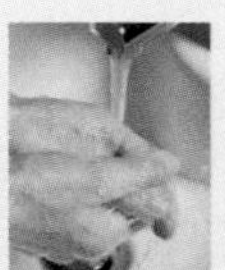 5. Perform hand hygiene and put on gloves.	Hand hygiene deters the spread of microorganisms. Gloves protect the nurse from potential contact with contaminants and body fluids.
6. Have patient sit up or lie with head tilted toward side of affected ear. Protect patient and bed with a waterproof pad. Have patient support basin under the ear to receive the irrigating solution (Figure 1).	Gravity causes the irrigating solution to flow from the ear to the basin.
7. Clean pinna and meatus of auditory canal as necessary with moistened cotton-tipped applicators dipped in warm tap water or the irrigating solution.	Materials lodged on the pinna and at the meatus may be washed into the ear.
8. Fill bulb syringe with warm solution. If an irrigating container is used, prime the tubing.	Priming the tubing allows air to escape from the tubing. Air forced into the ear canal is noisy and therefore unpleasant for the patient.
9. Straighten auditory canal by pulling cartilaginous portion of pinna up and back for an adult (Figure 2).	Straightening the ear canal allows solution to reach all areas of the canal easily.

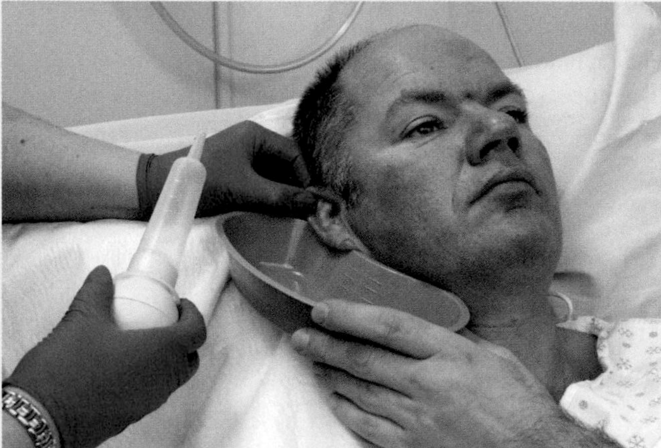

Figure 1. Positioning for ear irrigation.

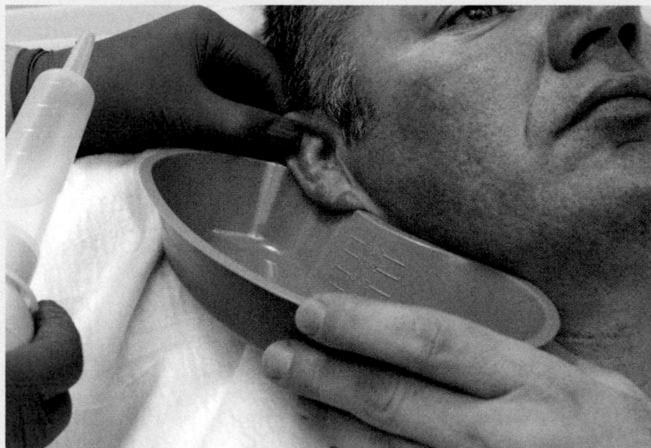

Figure 2. Straightening the ear canal for irrigation.

ACTION	RATIONALE
10. **Direct a steady, slow stream of solution against the roof of the auditory canal, using only enough force to remove secretions. Do not occlude the auditory canal with the irrigating nozzle. Allow solution to flow out unimpeded (Figure 3).**	Directing the solution at the roof of the canal helps prevent injury to the tympanic membrane. Continuous in-and-out flow of the irrigating solution helps to prevent pressure in the canal.
11. When irrigation is complete, place cotton ball loosely in auditory meatus (Figure 4) and have patient lie on side of affected ear on a towel or absorbent pad.	The cotton ball absorbs excess fluid, and gravity allows the remaining solution in the canal to escape from the ear.

SKILL 5-19 **Administering an Ear Irrigation** *(continued)*

ACTION | **RATIONALE**

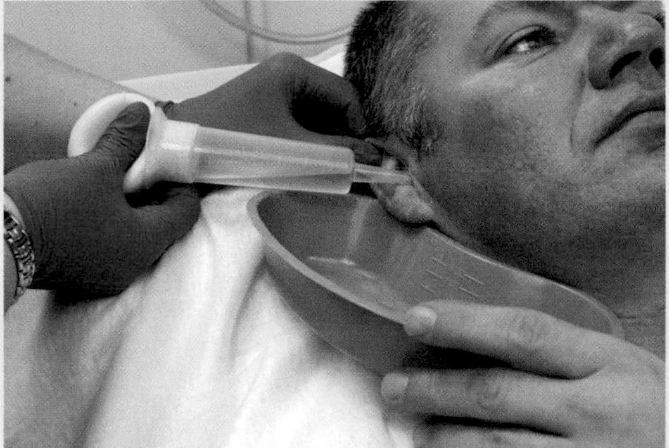

Figure 3. Instilling irrigation fluid.

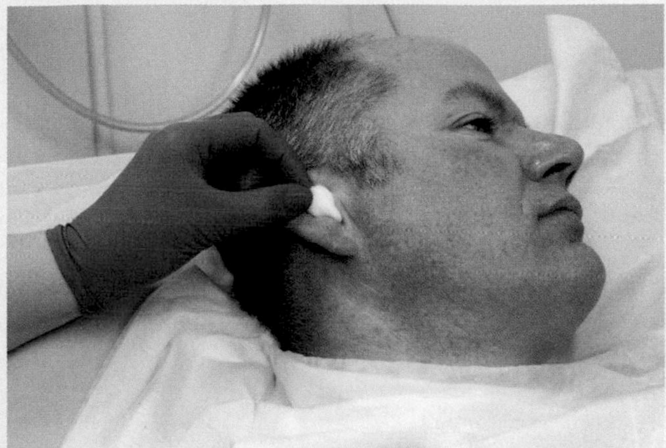

Figure 4. Placing cotton ball in ear.

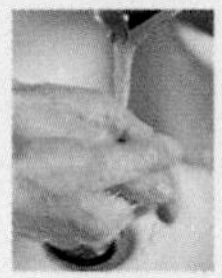

12. Remove gloves and perform hand hygiene.

Hand hygiene deters the spread of microorganisms.

13. Assist the patient to a comfortable position.

This ensures patient comfort.

14. Evaluate patient's response to the procedure. Return in 10 to 15 minutes and remove cotton ball and assess drainage.

The patient needs to be evaluated for any adverse affects from the procedure. Drainage or pain may indicate injury to the tympanic membrane.

EVALUATION

The expected outcomes are met when the ear canal is irrigated successfully; patient experiences no or minimal pain or discomfort; patient's hearing is improved; and patient understands the rationale for the ear irrigation procedure.

DOCUMENTATION

Guidelines

Document the procedure, site, the type of solution and volume used, length of time irrigation performed, pre- and post-procedure assessments, characteristics of any drainage, and the patient's response to the treatment.

Sample Documentation

7/6/09 1830 Right ear noted to be without external edema and redness. No drainage noted. Patient reports slightly decreased hearing in right ear. Slight tenderness noted on palpation. Irrigation of right ear performed using 100 mL of warmed normal saline. Clear return with particles of cerumen noted. Patient tolerated procedure with minimal discomfort. Patient reports no change in hearing in right ear. Denies need for pain medication at this time. Patient rates pain at present as 1/10.—B. Clapp, RN

(continued)

SKILL 5-19 Administering an Ear Irrigation *(continued)*

Unexpected Situations and Associated Interventions

- *Patient complains of significant pain during irrigation:* Stop the irrigation. Check the temperature of the solution. If the solution has cooled, rewarm it and try again. If the patient still complains of pain, stop the irrigation and notify the physician.

Special Considerations

General Considerations

- Ongoing assessment is an important part of nursing care to evaluate patient response to administered medications and early detection of adverse effects. If an adverse effect is suspected, withhold further medication doses and notify the patient's primary healthcare provider. Additional intervention is based on type of reaction and patient assessment.

Infant and Child Considerations

- Pull pinna straight back for a child over 3 years (Figure 5) and down and back for an infant or a child younger than 3 years (Figure 6).

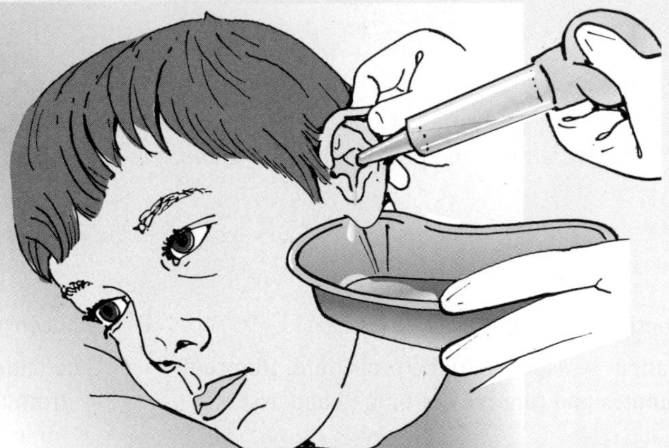

Figure 5. Pulling pinna straight back for child over 3 years.

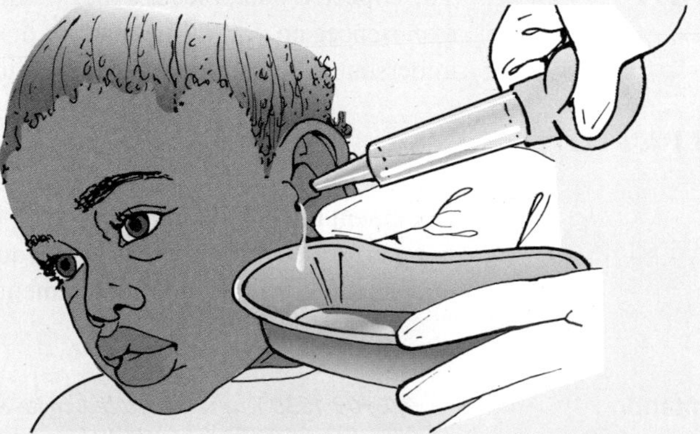

Figure 6. Pulling pinna down and back for an infant or child younger than 3 years.

SKILL
5-20 Instilling Nose Drops

Nasal instillations are used to treat allergies, sinus infections, and nasal congestion. Medications with a systemic effect, such as vasopressin, may also be prepared as a nasal instillation. The nose is normally not a sterile cavity, but because of its connection with the sinuses, medical asepsis should be observed carefully when using nasal instillations.

The following skill describes the steps to administer nasal drops. Refer to the accompanying Skill Variation for guidelines to administer medication via a nasal spray.

Equipment

- Medication
- Dropper, if not part of medication container
- Gloves
- Tissue
- Medication Administration Record (MAR) or Computer-generated MAR (CMAR)

ASSESSMENT

Assess the nares for redness, erythema, edema, drainage, or tenderness. Assess the patient for allergies. Verify patient name, dose, route, and time of administration. Assess the patient's knowledge of medication and procedure. If the patient has a knowledge deficit about the medication, this may be an appropriate time to begin education about the procedure. Assess the patient's ability to cooperate with the procedure

NURSING DIAGNOSIS

Determine related factors for the nursing diagnoses based on the patient's current status. Appropriate nursing diagnoses may include:

- Deficient Knowledge
- Risk for Allergy Response
- Risk for Impaired Skin
- Acute Pain

OUTCOME IDENTIFICATION AND PLANNING

The expected outcome to achieve is that the medication is administered successfully into the nose. Other outcomes that may be appropriate include the following: patient understands the rationale for the nose-drop instillation; patient experiences no allergy response; patient's skin remains intact; patient experiences no, or minimal, pain.

IMPLEMENTATION

ACTION	RATIONALE
1. Gather equipment. Check medication order against the original physician's order according to agency policy. Clarify any inconsistencies. Check the patient's chart for allergies.	This comparison helps to identify errors that may have occurred when orders were transcribed. The physician's order is the legal record of medication orders for each agency.
2. Know the actions, special nursing considerations, safe dose ranges, purpose of administration, and adverse effects of the medication to be administered. Consider the appropriateness of the medication for this patient.	This knowledge aids the nurse in evaluating the therapeutic effect of the medication in relation to the patient's disorder and can also be used to educate the patient about the medication.
3. Perform hand hygiene.	Hand hygiene prevents the spread of microorganisms.
4. Move the medication cart to the outside of the patient's room or prepare for administration in the medication area.	Organization facilitates error-free administration and saves time.

(continued)

SKILL 5-20 Instilling Nose Drops *(continued)*

ACTION	RATIONALE
5. Unlock the medication cart or drawer. Enter pass code and scan employee identification, if required.	Locking of the cart or drawer safeguards each patient's medication supply. Hospital accrediting organizations require medication carts to be locked when not in use. Entering pass code and scanning ID allows only authorized users into the system and identifies user for documentation by the computer.
6. **Prepare medications for one patient at a time.**	This prevents errors in medication administration.
7. Read the MAR and select the proper medication from the patient's medication drawer or unit stock.	This is the first check of the label.
8. Compare the label with the MAR. Check expiration dates and perform calculations, if necessary. Scan the bar code on the package, if required.	This is the second check of the label. Verify calculations with another nurse to ensure safety, if necessary.
9. **When all medications for one patient have been prepared, recheck the label with the MAR before taking them to the patient. Lock the medication cart before leaving it.**	This is a *third* check to ensure accuracy and to prevent errors. Locking the cart or drawer safeguards the patient's medication supply. Hospital accrediting organizations require medication carts to be locked when not in use.
10. Transport medications to the patient's bedside carefully, and keep the medications in sight at all times.	Careful handling and close observation prevent accidental or deliberate disarrangement of medications.
11. **Ensure that the patient receives the medications at the correct time.**	Check agency policy, which may allow for administration within a period of 30 minutes before or 30 minutes after designated time.
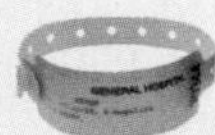 12. **Identify the patient.** Usually, the patient should be identified using two methods. Compare information with the MAR or CMAR.	Identifying the patient ensures the right patient receives the medications and helps prevent errors.
a. Check the name and identification number on the patient's identification band.	This is the most reliable method. Replace the identification band if it is missing or inaccurate in any way.
b. Ask the patient to state his or her name.	This requires a response from the patient, but illness and strange surroundings often cause patients to be confused.
c. If the patient cannot identify him or herself, verify the patient's identification with a staff member who knows the patient for the second source.	This is another way to double-check identity. Do not use the name on the door or over the bed, because these may be inaccurate.
13. **Complete necessary assessments before administering medications. Check allergy bracelet or ask patient about allergies. Explain the purpose and action of each medication to the patient.**	Assessment is a prerequisite to administration of medications.
14. Scan the patient's bar code on the identification band, if required.	Provides additional check to ensure that the medication is given to the right patient.
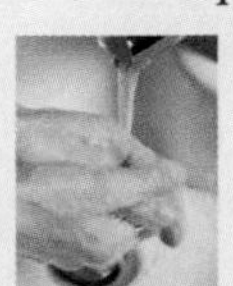 15. Perform hand hygiene and put on gloves.	Hand hygiene deters the spread of microorganisms. Gloves protect the nurse from potential contact with contaminants and body fluids.
16. **Provide patient with paper tissues and ask patient to blow his or her nose.**	Blowing the nose clears the nasal mucosa prior to medication administration.
17. Have patient sit up with head tilted well back. If patient is lying down, tilt head back over a pillow (Figure 1).	These positions allow the solution to flow well back into the nares. Do not tilt head if patient has a cervical spine injury.

SKILL
5-20 Instilling Nose Drops *(continued)*

ACTION | **RATIONALE**

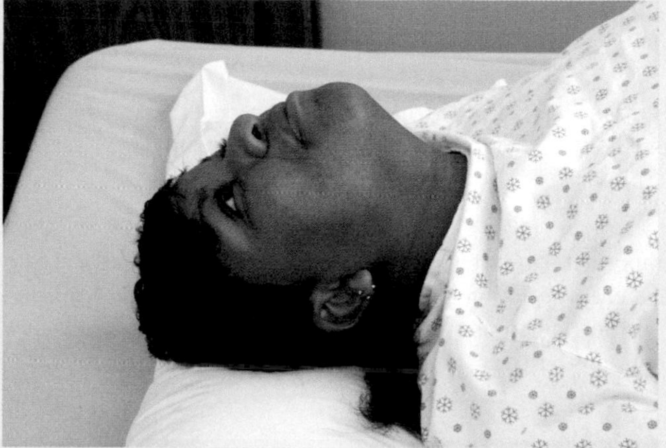

Figure 1. Patient lying down, head tilted back over pillow.

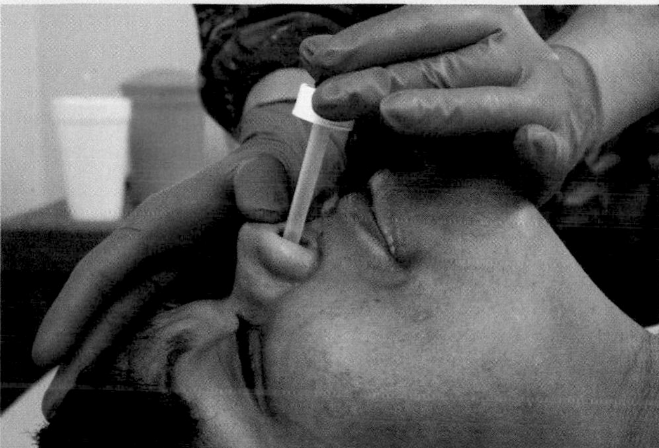

Figure 2. Positioning nose dropper just above naris, about one third of an inch.

18. Draw sufficient solution into dropper for both nares. Do not return excess solution to a stock bottle.

    Returning solution to a stock bottle increases the risk for contamination of the stock bottle.

19. Ask the patient to breathe through the mouth. Hold tip of nose up and place dropper just above naris, about one third of an inch (Figure 2). Instill prescribed number of drops in one naris and then into the other. Protect dropper with a piece of soft tubing if patient is an infant or young child. Avoid touching naris with dropper.

    Breathing through the mouth helps prevent aspiration of solution. The soft tubing will protect the patient's nares from injury during administration of medication. Touching the naris may cause the patient to sneeze and will contaminate the dropper.

20. Have patient remain in position with head tilted back for a few minutes.

    Tilting the head back prevents the escape of the medication.

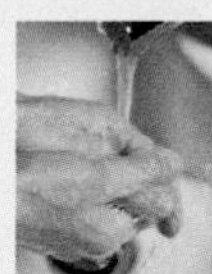

21. Remove gloves and perform hand hygiene.

    Hand hygiene deters the spread of microorganisms.

22. Assist the patient to a comfortable position.

    This ensures patient comfort.

23. Evaluate patient's response to the procedure and medication.

    The patient needs to be evaluated for any adverse affects from the medication or procedure.

EVALUATION

The expected outcomes are met when the patient receives the nose drops successfully; understands the rationale for nose-drop instillation; and experiences no allergy response; patient's skin remains intact; and patient experiences no, or minimal, pain or discomfort.

DOCUMENTATION

Guidelines

Document the administration of the medication, including date, time, dose, route of administration, and site of administration, specifically right, left, or both nares, on the MAR or record using the required format. If using a bar-code system, medication administration is automatically recorded when scanned. PRN medications require documentation of the reason for administration. Prompt recording avoids the possibility of accidentally repeat-

(continued)

SKILL 5-20 Instilling Nose Drops *(continued)*

ing the administration of the drug. If the drug was refused or omitted, record this in the appropriate area on the medication record and notify the physician. This verifies the reason medication was omitted and ensures that the physician is aware of the patient's condition. Document pre- and postadministration assessments, characteristics of any drainage, and the patient's response to the treatment, if appropriate.

Unexpected Situations and Associated Interventions

- *Patient sneezes immediately after receiving nose drops:* Do not repeat the dosage, because you cannot determine how much medication was actually absorbed.

Special Considerations

General Considerations

- Ongoing assessment is an important part of nursing care to evaluate patient response to administered medications and early detection of adverse effects. If an adverse effect is suspected, withhold further medication doses and notify the patient's primary healthcare provider. Additional intervention is based on type of reaction and patient assessment.

SKILL VARIATION Administering Medication via Nasal Spray

- Assist the patient to an upright position with the head tilted back.
- Perform hand hygiene and put on gloves.
- Instruct the patient to inhale gently through the nose as the spray is being administered.
- Have the patient hold one nostril closed. If the spray is indicated for only one naris, close the nostril that will not receive the medication.
- Agitate the medication container, if required, to thoroughly mix the contents.
- Insert the nozzle of the medication container just into the nostril.
- Compress the container, spraying the medication into the nostril, while the patient gently inhales through the nostril.
- Keep the medication container compressed and remove from the nostril. Release the container from the compressed state. Do not allow the container to return to its original position until it is removed from the patient's nose to prevent contamination of the contents of the container.
- Repeat in the other nostril if prescribed.
- Instruct the patient to maintain head position for 1 to 2 minutes.
- Remove gloves and perform hand hygiene.
- Assist the patient to a comfortable position.
- Document medication administration and site, if only one nostril used.

SKILL 5-21 Administering a Vaginal Cream

Creams, foams, and tablets can be applied intravaginally using a narrow, tubular applicator with an attached plunger. Suppositories that melt when exposed to body heat are also administered by vaginal insertion. Suppositories should be refrigerated for storage. Administration should be timed to allow the patient to lie down afterward to retain the medication.

Equipment

- Medication with applicator, if appropriate
- Water-soluble lubricant
- Perineal pad
- Washcloth, skin cleanser, and warm water
- Gloves
- Medication Administration Record (MAR) or Computer-generated MAR (CMAR)

SKILL 5-21 Administering a Vaginal Cream *(continued)*

ASSESSMENT

Assess the external genitalia and vaginal canal for redness, erythema, edema, drainage, or tenderness. Assess the patient for allergies. Verify patient name, dose, route, and time of administration. Assess the patient's knowledge of medication and procedure. If the patient has a knowledge deficit about the medication, this may be an appropriate time to begin education about the medication. Assess the patient's ability to cooperate with the procedure.

NURSING DIAGNOSIS

Determine related factors for the nursing diagnoses based on the patient's current status. Appropriate nursing diagnoses may include:

- Deficient Knowledge
- Risk for Allergy Response
- Risk for Impaired Skin Integrity
- Acute Pain
- Anxiety

OUTCOME IDENTIFICATION AND PLANNING

The expected outcome to achieve is that the medication is administered successfully into the vagina. Other outcomes that may be appropriate include the following: patient understands the rationale for the vaginal instillation; patient experiences no allergy response; patient's skin remains intact; patient experiences no, or minimal, pain; and patient experiences minimal anxiety.

IMPLEMENTATION

ACTION	RATIONALE
1. Gather equipment. Check medication order against the original physician's order according to agency policy. Clarify any inconsistencies. Check the patient's chart for allergies.	This comparison helps to identify errors that may have occurred when orders were transcribed. The physician's order is the legal record of medication orders for each agency.
2. Know the actions, special nursing considerations, safe dose ranges, purpose of administration, and adverse effects of the medication to be administered. Consider the appropriateness of the medication for this patient.	This knowledge aids the nurse in evaluating the therapeutic effect of the medication in relation to the patient's disorder and can also be used to educate the patient about the medication.
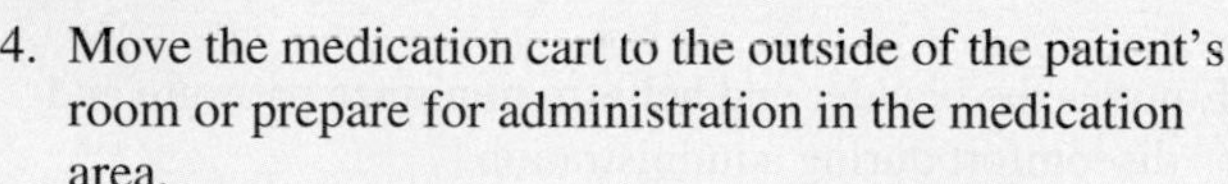 3. Perform hand hygiene.	Hand hygiene prevents the spread of microorganisms.
4. Move the medication cart to the outside of the patient's room or prepare for administration in the medication area.	Organization facilitates error-free administration and saves time.
5. Unlock the medication cart or drawer. Enter pass code and scan employee identification, if required.	Locking of the cart or drawer safeguards each patient's medication supply. Hospital accrediting organizations require medication carts to be locked when not in use. Entering pass code and scanning ID allows only authorized users into the system and identifies user for documentation by the computer.
6. **Prepare medications for one patient at a time.**	This prevents errors in medication administration.

(continued)

SKILL 5-21 Administering a Vaginal Cream *(continued)*

ACTION	RATIONALE
7. Read the MAR and select the proper medication from the patient's medication drawer or unit stock.	This is the first check of the label.
8. Compare the label with the MAR. Check expiration dates and perform calculations, if necessary. Scan the bar code on the package, if required.	This is the second check of the label. Verify calculations with another nurse to ensure safety, if necessary.
9. **When all medications for one patient have been prepared, recheck the label with the MAR before taking them to the patient. Lock the medication cart before leaving it.**	This is a *third* check to ensure accuracy and to prevent errors. Locking the cart or drawer safeguards the patient's medication supply. Hospital accrediting organizations require medication carts to be locked when not in use.
10. Transport medications to the patient's bedside carefully, and keep the medications in sight at all times.	Careful handling and close observation prevent accidental or deliberate disarrangement of medications.
11. **Ensure that the patient receives the medications at the correct time.**	Check agency policy, which may allow for administration within a period of 30 minutes before or 30 minutes after designated time.
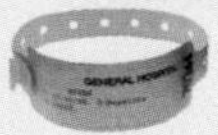 12. **Identify the patient.** Usually, the patient should be identified using two methods. Compare information with the MAR or CMAR.	Identifying the patient ensures the right patient receives the medications and helps prevent errors.
a. Check the name and identification number on the patient's identification band.	This is the most reliable method. Replace the identification band if it is missing or inaccurate in any way.
b. Ask the patient to state his or her name.	This requires a response from the patient, but illness and strange surroundings often cause patients to be confused.
c. If the patient cannot identify herself, verify the patient's identification with a staff member who knows the patient for the second source.	This is another way to double-check identity. Do not use the name on the door or over the bed, because these may be inaccurate.
13. **Complete necessary assessments before administering medications. Check allergy bracelet or ask patient about allergies. Explain the purpose and action of each medication to the patient.**	Assessment is a prerequisite to administration of medications.
14. Scan the patient's bar code on the identification band, if required.	Provides additional check to ensure that the medication is given to the right patient.
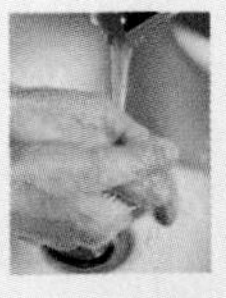 15. Perform hand hygiene and put on gloves.	Hand hygiene deters the spread of microorganisms. Gloves protect the nurse from potential contact with contaminants and body fluids.
16. Ask the patient to void before inserting the medication.	Empties the bladder and helps to minimize pressure and discomfort during administration.
17. Position the patient so that she is lying on her back with the knees flexed. Maintain privacy with draping. Adequate light should be available to visualize the vaginal opening.	Position provides access to vaginal canal and helps to retain medication in the canal. Limits exposure of the patient, promotes warmth and privacy. Adequate light facilitates ease of administration.
18. **Spread labia with fingers, and clean area at vaginal orifice with washcloth and warm water, using a different corner of the washcloth with each stroke. Wipe from above orifice downward toward sacrum (front to back) (Figure 1).**	These techniques prevent contamination of vaginal orifice with debris surrounding anus.

SKILL 5-21

Administering a Vaginal Cream *(continued)*

ACTION	RATIONALE

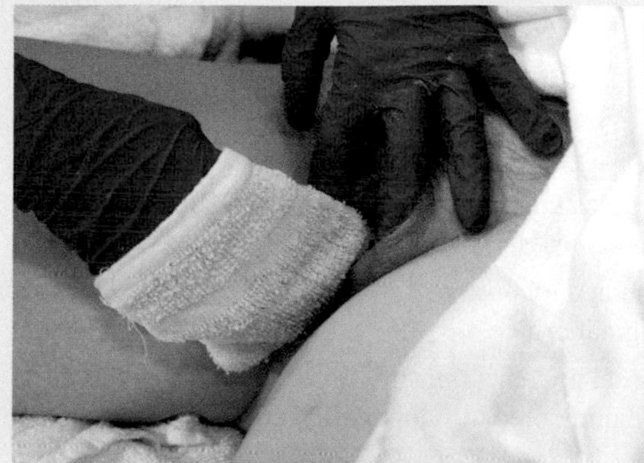

Figure 1. Performing perineal care.

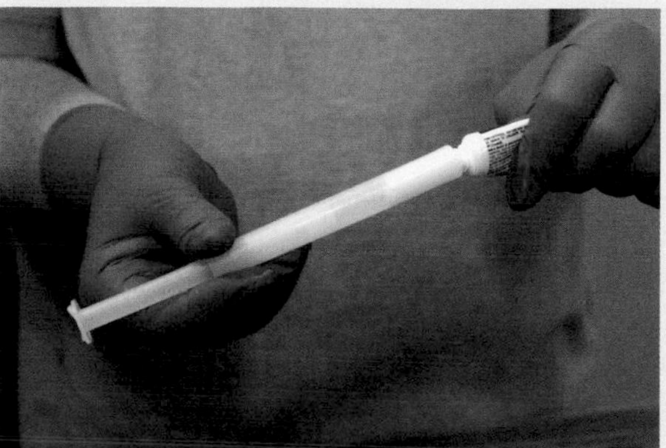

Figure 2. Filling vaginal applicator with cream.

ACTION	RATIONALE
19. Replace your gloves.	Prevents spread of microorganisms.
20. Fill vaginal applicator with prescribed amount of cream (Figure 2). (See the accompanying Skill Variation for administering a vaginal suppository.)	This ensures the correct dosage of medication will be administered.
21. Lubricate applicator with the lubricant, as necessary.	Ordinarily, lubrication is unnecessary, but it may be used to reduce friction while inserting the applicator.
22. Spread the labia with your nondominant hand and introduce applicator with your dominant hand gently, in a rolling manner, while directing it downward and backward.	This follows the normal contour of the vagina for its full length.
23. After applicator is properly positioned (Figure 3), labia may be allowed to fall in place if necessary to free the hand for manipulating plunger. Push plunger to its full length and then gently remove applicator with plunger depressed.	Pushing the plunger will gently deploy the cream into the vaginal orifice.

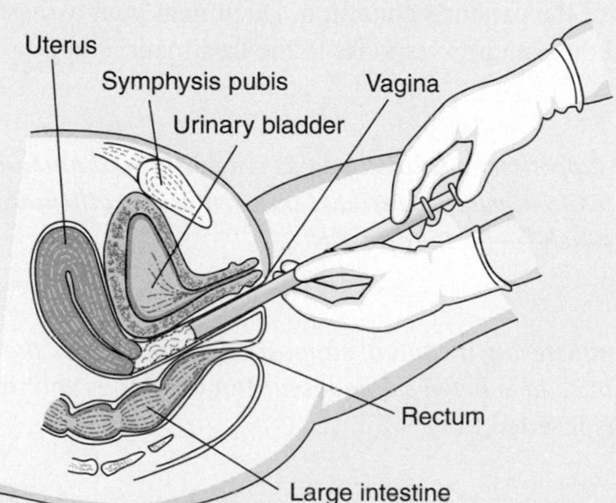

Figure 3. Positioning applicator in the vagina for administration of medication.

(continued)

SKILL 5-21 Administering a Vaginal Cream *(continued)*

ACTION	RATIONALE
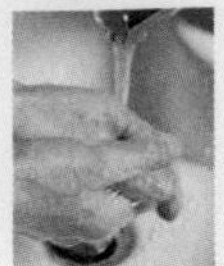 24. Remove gloves and perform hand hygiene.	Hand hygiene deters the spread of microorganisms.
25. **Ask patient to remain in supine position for 5 to 10 minutes after insertion.**	This gives the medication time to be absorbed in the vaginal cavity.
26. Offer patient a perineal pad to collect drainage.	As medication heats up, some medication may leak from vaginal orifice.
27. Dispose of applicator in appropriate receptacle or clean nondisposable applicator according to manufacturer's directions.	Disposal prevents transmission of microorganisms. Cleaning prepares applicator for future use by patient.
28. Evaluate patient's response to the procedure and medication.	The patient needs to be evaluated for any adverse affects from the medication or procedure.

EVALUATION

The expected outcomes are met when the patient receives vaginal medication successfully; patient understands the rationale for the medication administration; patient experiences no allergy response; patient's skin remains intact; patient experiences no or minimal discomfort; and patient experiences no or minimal anxiety.

DOCUMENTATION

Guidelines

Document the administration of the medication immediately after administration, including date, time, dose, and route of administration on the MAR or record using the required format. If using a bar-code system, medication administration is automatically recorded when scanned. PRN medications require documentation of the reason for administration. Prompt recording avoids the possibility of accidentally repeating the administration of the drug. If the drug was refused or omitted, record this in the appropriate area on the medication record and notify the physician. This verifies the reason medication was omitted and ensures that the physician is aware of the patient's condition. Document your assessment, characteristics of any drainage, and the patient's response to the treatment, if appropriate.

Sample Documentation

7/23/08 2300 Monistat vaginal suppository administered as ordered. Small amount of curd-like, white discharge noted from vagina. Perineal skin remains erythematous. Patient states, "It doesn't itch as much."—K. Sanders, RN

Unexpected Situations and Associated Interventions

- *Upon assessing patient after administering a vaginal suppository, nurse notes the suppository is not in the vagina but instead is between the labia:* Put on gloves and reinsert the suppository, ensuring that it is inserted fully.

Special Considerations

General Considerations

- Ongoing assessment is an important part of nursing care to evaluate patient response to administered medications and early detection of adverse effects. If an adverse effect is suspected, withhold further medication doses and notify the patient's primary healthcare provider. Additional intervention is based on type of reaction and patient assessment.

SKILL 5-21 Administering a Vaginal Cream *(continued)*

SKILL VARIATION Administering Vaginal Suppository

- Check medication order against the original physician's order according to agency policy. Clarify any inconsistencies. Check the patient's chart for allergies. Know the actions, special nursing considerations, safe dose ranges, purpose of administration, and adverse effects of the medications to be administered. Consider the appropriateness of the medication for this patient.
- Perform hand hygiene.
- Move the medication cart to the outside of the patient's room or prepare for administration in the medication area.
- Unlock the medication cart or drawer. Enter pass code and scan employee identification, if required.
- Read the MAR and select the proper medication from the patient's medication drawer or unit stock.
- Compare the label with the MAR. Check expiration dates. Scan the bar code on the package, if required.
- Recheck the label with the MAR before taking it to the patient.
- Lock the medication cart before leaving it.
- Transport medications and equipment to the patient's bedside carefully, and keep the medications in sight at all times.
- Perform hand hygiene.
- Identify the patient. Usually, the patient should be identified using two methods.
- Close the door to the room or pull the bedside curtain.
- Complete necessary assessments before administering medications. Check allergy bracelet or ask patient about allergies. Explain the purpose and action of the medication to the patient.
- Scan the patient's bar code on the identification band, if required.
- Perform hand hygiene and put on gloves.
- Ask the patient to void before inserting the medication.
- Position the patient so that she is lying on her back with the knees flexed. Maintain privacy with draping. Adequate light should be available to visualize the vaginal opening.
- **Spread labia with fingers, and clean area at vaginal orifice with washcloth and warm water, using a different corner of the washcloth with each stroke. Wipe from above orifice downward toward sacrum (front to back).**
- Replace your gloves.
- Remove the suppository from its wrapper and lubricate the round end with the water-soluble lubricant (Figure A). Lubricate your gloved index finger on your dominant hand.
- Spread the labia with your nondominant hand.
- Insert the rounded end of the suppository along the posterior wall of the canal (Figure B). Insert to the length of your finger.
- Remove gloves and perform hand hygiene.
- **Ask patient to remain in supine position for 5 to 10 minutes after insertion.**
- Offer patient a perineal pad to collect drainage.
- Evaluate patient's response to the procedure and medication.
- Document the administration of the medication, including date, time, dose, and route of administration on the MAR or record using the required format.

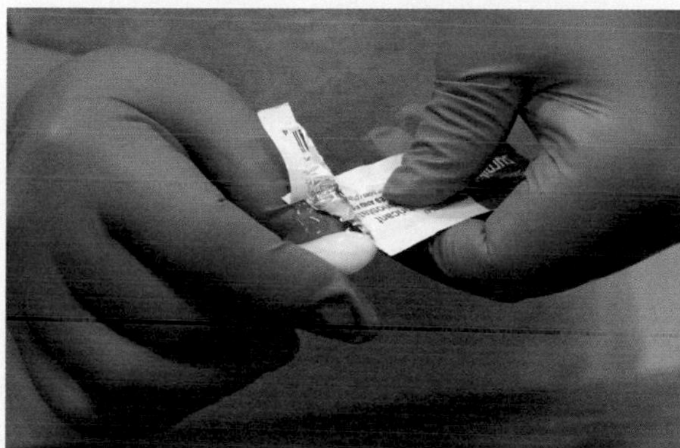

Figure A. Lubricating suppository.

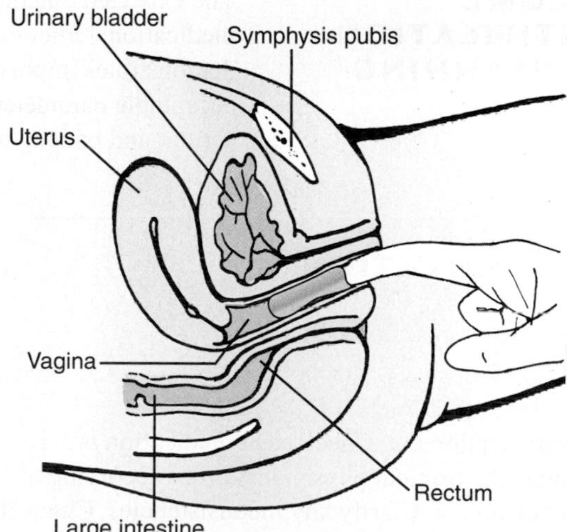

Figure B. Inserting suppository into vagina.

SKILL 5-22 Administering Medication via a Metered-Dose Inhaler (MDI)

Many medications for respiratory problems are delivered via the respiratory system. A metered-dose inhaler (MDI) is a handheld inhaler that uses an aerosol spray or mist to deliver a controlled dose of medication with each compression of the canister. The medication is then absorbed rapidly through the lung tissue, resulting in local and systemic effects.

Equipment

- Stethoscope
- Medication in an MDI
- Spacer or holding chamber (optional)
- Medication Administration Record (MAR) or Computerized-medication Administration Record (CMAR)

ASSESSMENT

Assess lung sounds pre- and post-use to establish a baseline and determine the effectiveness of the medication. Frequently, patients will have wheezes or coarse lung sounds before medication administration. If ordered, assess oxygen saturation level before medication administration. The oxygenation level will usually increase after the medication is administered. Verify patient name, dose, route, and time of administration. Assess patient's ability to manage an MDI; young and older patients may have dexterity problems. Assess the patient's knowledge and understanding of the medication's purpose and action.

NURSING DIAGNOSIS

Determine related factors for the nursing diagnosis based on the patient's current status. Appropriate nursing diagnoses may include:

- Ineffective Airway Clearance
- Ineffective Breathing Pattern
- Impaired Gas Exchange
- Deficient Knowledge
- Risk for Activity Intolerance

OUTCOME IDENTIFICATION AND PLANNING

The expected outcome to achieve when using an MDI is that the patient receives the medication. Other outcomes that may be appropriate include the following: patient demonstrates improved lung expansion and breath sounds; respiratory status is within acceptable parameters; patient verbalizes an understanding of medication purpose and action; and patient demonstrates correct use of MDI.

IMPLEMENTATION

ACTION	RATIONALE
1. Gather equipment. Check each medication order against the original physician's order according to agency policy. Clarify any inconsistencies. Check the patient's chart for allergies.	This comparison helps to identify errors that may have occurred when orders were transcribed. The physician's order is the legal record of medication orders for each agency.
2. Know the actions, special nursing considerations, safe dose ranges, purpose of administration, and adverse effects of the medications to be administered. Consider the appropriateness of the medication for this patient.	This knowledge aids the nurse in evaluating the therapeutic effect of the medication in relation to the patient's disorder and can also be used to educate the patient about the medication.

SKILL 5-22 Administering Medication via a Metered-Dose Inhaler (MDI) *(continued)*

ACTION	RATIONALE
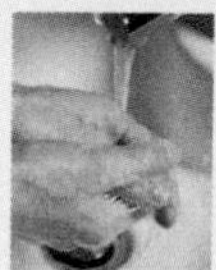 3. Perform hand hygiene.	Hand hygiene prevents the spread of microorganisms.
4. Move the medication cart to the outside of the patient's room or prepare for administration in the medication area.	Organization facilitates error-free administration and saves time.
5. Unlock the medication cart or drawer. Enter pass code and scan employee identification, if required.	Locking of the cart or drawer safeguards each patient's medication supply. Hospital accrediting organizations require medication carts to be locked when not in use. Entering pass code and scanning ID allows only authorized users into the system and identifies user for documentation by the computer.
6. **Prepare medications for one patient at a time.**	This prevents errors in medication administration.
7. Read the MAR and select the proper medication from the patient's medication drawer or unit stock.	This is the first check of the label.
8. Compare the label with the MAR. Check expiration dates and perform calculations, if necessary. Scan the bar code on the package, if required.	This is the second check of the label. Verify calculations with another nurse to ensure safety, if necessary.
9. **When all medications for one patient have been prepared, recheck the label with the MAR before taking them to the patient. Lock the medication cart before leaving it.**	This is a *third* check to ensure accuracy and to prevent errors. Locking the cart or drawer safeguards the patient's medication supply. Hospital accrediting organizations require medication carts to be locked when not in use.
10. Transport medications to the patient's bedside carefully, and keep the medications in sight at all times.	Careful handling and close observation prevent accidental or deliberate disarrangement of medications.
11. **Ensure that the patient receives the medications at the correct time.**	Check agency policy, which may allow for administration within a period of 30 minutes before or 30 minutes after designated time.
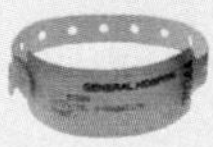 12. **Identify the patient.** Usually, the patient should be identified using two methods. Compare information with the MAR or CMAR.	Identifying the patient ensures the right patient receives the medications and helps prevent errors.
a. Check the name and identification number on the patient's identification band.	This is the most reliable method. Replace the identification band if it is missing or inaccurate in any way.
b. Ask the patient to state his or her name.	This requires a response from the patient, but illness and strange surroundings often cause patients to be confused.
c. If the patient cannot identify him or herself, verify the patient's identification with a staff member who knows the patient for the second source.	This is another way to double-check identity. Do not use the name on the door or over the bed, because these may be inaccurate.
13. **Complete necessary assessments before administering medications. Check allergy bracelet or ask patient about allergies.** Explain what you are going to do and the reason to the patient.	Assessment is a prerequisite to administration of medications. Explanation relieves anxiety and facilitates cooperation.
14. Scan the patient's bar code on the identification band, if required.	Provides additional check to ensure that the medication is given to the right patient.

(continued)

SKILL 5-22

Administering Medication via a Metered-Dose Inhaler (MDI) *(continued)*

ACTION	RATIONALE
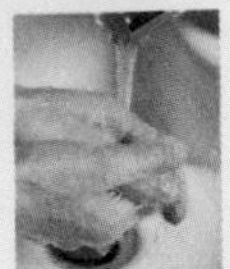 15. Perform hand hygiene.	Hand hygiene deters the spread of microorganisms.
16. **Remove the mouthpiece cover from the MDI and the spacer.** Attach the MDI to the spacer. (See accompanying Skill Variation for using an MDI without a spacer.)	The use of a spacer is preferred because it traps the medication and aids in delivery of the correct dose.
17. Shake the inhaler and spacer well.	The medication and propellant may separate when the canister is not in use. Shaking well ensures that the patient is receiving the correct dosage of medication.
18. Have patient place the spacer's mouthpiece into mouth, grasping securely with teeth and lips (Figure 1). Have patient breathe normally through the spacer.	Medication should not leak out around the mouthpiece.

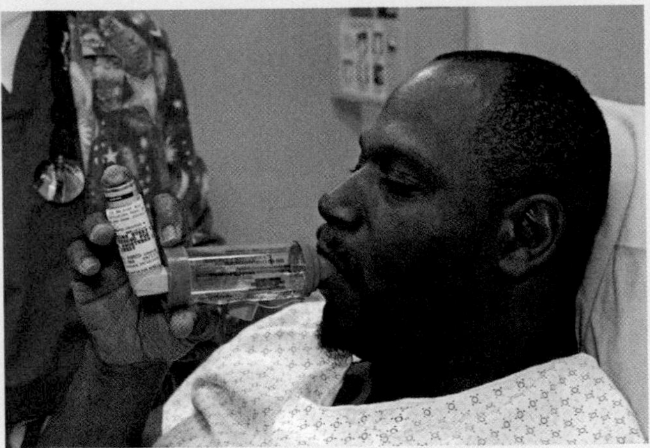

Figure 1. Using an MDI with a spacer.

ACTION	RATIONALE
19. Patient should depress the canister, releasing one puff into the spacer, then inhale slowly and deeply through the mouth.	The spacer will hold the medication in suspension for a short period so that the patient can receive more of the prescribed medication than if it had been projected into the air. Breathing slowly and deeply distributes the medication deep into the airways.
20. **Instruct patient to hold the breath for 5 to 10 seconds, or as long as possible, and then to exhale slowly through pursed lips.**	This allows better distribution and longer absorption time for the medication.
21. **Wait 1 to 5 minutes, as prescribed, before administering the next puff.**	This ensures that both puffs are absorbed as much as possible. Bronchodilation after first puff allows for deeper penetration by subsequent puffs.
22. After the prescribed amount of puffs has been administered, have patient remove the MDI from the spacer and replace the caps on both.	By replacing the cap, the patient is preventing any dust or dirt from entering and being propelled into the bronchioles with later doses.

SKILL 5-22
Administering Medication via a Metered-Dose Inhaler (MDI) *(continued)*

ACTION	RATIONALE
23. **Reassess lung sounds, oxygenation saturation if ordered, and respirations.**	Lung sounds and oxygenation saturation may improve after MDI use. Respirations may decrease after MDI use.
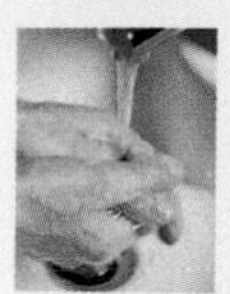 24. Perform hand hygiene.	Hand hygiene deters the spread of microorganisms.

EVALUATION

The expected outcome is met when the patient demonstrates improved lung sounds and ease of breathing. In addition, patient demonstrates correct use of MDI and verbalizes correct information about medication therapy associated with MDI use.

DOCUMENTATION

Guidelines

Document respiratory rate, oxygen saturation, if applicable, and lung assessment. Document medication administration on MAR or CMAR immediately after administration. Document patient teaching and patient response, if appropriate.

Sample Documentation

9/29/08 Wheezes noted in all lobes of lungs before albuterol MDI, O_2 saturation 92%, respiratory rate 24 breaths per minute. After albuterol treatment, lung sounds are clear and equal in all lobes, O_2 saturation 97%, respiratory rate 18 breaths per minute. Patient able to accurately demonstrate use of MDI and spacer and verbalizes understanding of medication purpose and action.—C. Bausler, RN

Unexpected Situations and Associated Interventions

- *Patient uses MDI, but symptoms are not relieved:* Check to make sure that the inhaler still contains medication. The patient may have received only propellant, without medication.
- *Patient is unable to use MDI:* Many companies have adaptive devices that allow patients to use MDI's.
- *Patient reports that relief of symptoms has decreased, even with increased number of puffs:* Have patient demonstrate technique that he or she is using. Many patients develop poor habits over time. Poor administration technique can lead to a decrease in effectiveness and a need for an increased dosage of medication.

Special Considerations

General Considerations

- Spacers and inhalers should be cleaned at least weekly with warm water or soaked in a vinegar solution (1 pint of water to 2 oz vinegar) for 20 minutes. Rinse with clean water and allow to air-dry.
- If the medication being administered is a steroid, the patient should rinse the mouth with water after administration to prevent a thrush infection.
- Ongoing assessment is an important part of nursing care to evaluate patient response to administered medications and early detection of adverse effects. If an adverse effect is suspected, withhold further medication doses and notify the patient's primary healthcare provider. Additional intervention is based on type of reaction and patient assessment.

(continued)

SKILL 5-22 Administering Medication via a Metered-Dose Inhaler (MDI) *(continued)*

Infant and Child Considerations

- Young children usually require a spacer to use an MDI. Spacers with masks are available for young children and should be considered for children less than 5 years of age to aid in the delivery of the medication. Mask must fit securely over both the nose and the mouth to ensure a good seal and prevent medication escaping.
- Children must be able to seal their lips around the mouthpiece in order to use a spacer without a mask.
- Many medications can also be administered as a nebulizer (see Skill 5-23).

Home Care Considerations

- Patients should know how to tell when medication levels are getting low. The most reliable method is to look on the canister and see how many puffs the canister contains. Divide this number by the number of puffs used daily to ascertain how many days the MDI will last. For instance, if the MDI contains 200 puffs and the patient takes 6 puffs per day, the MDI should last for 33 days. The flotation method is also used, but it is not reliable. The patient places the medication canister into a bowl of water. If the canister is full, it will sink to the bottom; if it is empty, it will float horizontally on the top of the water; if it is half full, it will float vertically. To protect the ozone layer, all MDIs are changing the type of propellant used. The flotation method may not work with the new inhalers.

SKILL VARIATION Using an MDI Without a Spacer

- Check medication order against the original physician's order according to agency policy. Clarify any inconsistencies. Check the patient's chart for allergies. Know the actions, special nursing considerations, safe dose ranges, purpose of administration, and adverse effects of the medications to be administered. Consider the appropriateness of the medication for this patient.
- Perform hand hygiene.
- Move the medication cart to the outside of the patient's room or prepare for administration in the medication area.
- Unlock the medication cart or drawer. Enter pass code and scan employee identification, if required.
- Read the MAR and select the proper medication from the patient's medication drawer or unit stock.
- Compare the label with the MAR. Check expiration dates. Confirm the prescribed or appropriate infusion rate. Calculate the drip rate if using gravity system. Scan the bar code on the package, if required.
- Recheck the label with the MAR before taking it to the patient.
- Lock the medication cart before leaving it.
- Transport medications and equipment to the patient's bedside carefully, and keep the medications in sight at all times.
- Perform hand hygiene.
- Identify the patient. Usually, the patient should be identified using two methods.
- Close the door to the room or pull the bedside curtain.
- Complete necessary assessments before administering medications. Check allergy bracelet or ask patient about allergies. Explain the purpose and action of the medication to the patient.
- Scan the patient's bar code on the identification band, if required.
- Perform hand hygiene.
- Remove the cap from the MDI. Shake the inhaler well.
- Have the patient take a deep breath and exhale.
- Have the patient hold the inhaler 1″ to 2″ away from the mouth (Figure A). Begin to inhale slowly and deeply and depress the medication canister. Continue to inhale for a full breath.
- Instruct patient to hold the breath for 5 to 10 seconds, or as long as possible, and then to exhale slowly through pursed lips.
- Wait 1 to 5 minutes, as prescribed, before administering the next puff.
- After the prescribed amount of puffs has been administered, have patient replace the cap on the MDI.
- Reassess lung sounds, oxygenation saturation if ordered, and respirations.
- Perform hand hygiene.

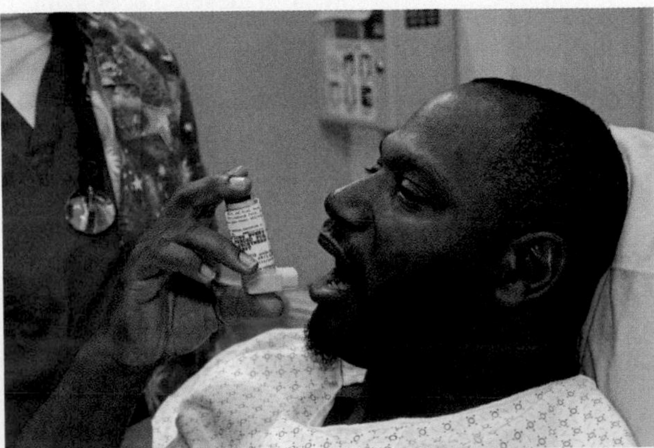

Figure A. Preparing to use an MDI without spacer.

SKILL 5-23 Administering Medication via a Small-Volume Nebulizer

Many medications to help with respiratory problems may be delivered via the respiratory system using a small-volume nebulizer. Nebulizers disperse fine particles of liquid medication into the deeper passages of the respiratory tract, where absorption occurs. The treatment continues until all the medication in the nebulizer cup has been inhaled.

Equipment

- Stethoscope
- Medication
- Nebulizer tubing and chamber
- Air compressor or oxygen hookup
- Sterile saline (if not premeasured)
- Medication Administration Record (MAR) or Computerized-medication Administration Record (CMAR)

ASSESSMENT

Assess lung sounds pre- and postuse to establish a baseline and determine the effectiveness of the medication. Often, patients have wheezes or coarse lung sounds before medication administration. If ordered, assess patient's oxygenation saturation level before medication administration. The oxygenation level will usually increase after the medication has been administered. Verify patient name, dose, route, and time of administration. Assess the patient's knowledge and understanding of the medication's purpose and action.

NURSING DIAGNOSIS

Determine related factors for the nursing diagnosis based on the patient's current status. Appropriate nursing diagnoses may include:

- Deficient Knowledge
- Ineffective Airway Clearance
- Risk for Activity Intolerance
- Ineffective Breathing Pattern
- Impaired Gas Exchange

OUTCOME IDENTIFICATION AND PLANNING

The expected outcome to achieve is that the patient receives the medication. Other outcomes that may be appropriate include the following: patient exhibits improved lung sounds and respiratory effort; patient demonstrates steps for use of nebulizer; and verbalizes understanding of medication purpose and action.

IMPLEMENTATION

ACTION	RATIONALE
1. Gather equipment. Check each medication order against the original physician's order according to agency policy. Clarify any inconsistencies. Check the patient's chart for allergies.	This comparison helps to identify errors that may have occurred when orders were transcribed. The physician's order is the legal record of medication orders for each agency.
2. Know the actions, special nursing considerations, safe dose ranges, purpose of administration, and adverse effects of the medications to be administered. Consider the appropriateness of the medication for this patient.	This knowledge aids the nurse in evaluating the therapeutic effect of the medication in relation to the patient's disorder and can also be used to educate the patient about the medication.

(continued)

SKILL 5-23 Administering Medication via a Small-Volume Nebulizer *(continued)*

ACTION	RATIONALE
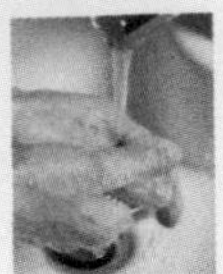 3. Perform hand hygiene.	Hand hygiene prevents the spread of microorganisms.
4. Move the medication cart to the outside of the patient's room or prepare for administration in the medication area.	Organization facilitates error-free administration and saves time.
5. Unlock the medication cart or drawer. Enter pass code and scan employee identification, if required.	Locking of the cart or drawer safeguards each patient's medication supply. Hospital accrediting organizations require medication carts to be locked when not in use. Entering pass code and scanning ID allows only authorized users into the system and identifies user for documentation by the computer.
6. **Prepare medications for one patient at a time.**	This prevents errors in medication administration.
7. Read the MAR and select the proper medication from the patient's medication drawer or unit stock.	This is the first check of the label.
8. Compare the label with the MAR. Check expiration dates and perform calculations, if necessary. Scan the bar code on the package, if required.	This is the second check of the label. Verify calculations with another nurse to ensure safety, if necessary.
9. **When all medications for one patient have been prepared, recheck the label with the MAR before taking them to the patient. Lock the medication cart before leaving it.**	This is a *third* check to ensure accuracy and to prevent errors. Locking the cart or drawer safeguards the patient's medication supply. Hospital accrediting organizations require medication carts to be locked when not in use.
10. Transport medications to the patient's bedside carefully, and keep the medications in sight at all times.	Careful handling and close observation prevent accidental or deliberate disarrangement of medications.
11. **Ensure that the patient receives the medications at the correct time.**	Check agency policy, which may allow for administration within a period of 30 minutes before or 30 minutes after designated time.
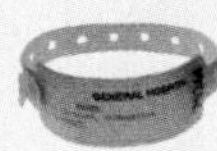 12. **Identify the patient.** Usually, the patient should be identified using two methods. Compare information with the MAR or CMAR.	Identifying the patient ensures the right patient receives the medications and helps prevent errors.
a. Check the name and identification number on the patient's identification band.	This is the most reliable method. Replace the identification band if it is missing or inaccurate in any way.
b. Ask the patient to state his or her name.	This requires a response from the patient, but illness and strange surroundings often cause patients to be confused.
c. If the patient cannot identify him or herself, verify the patient's identification with a staff member who knows the patient for the second source.	This is another way to double-check identity. Do not use the name on the door or over the bed, because these may be inaccurate.
13. **Complete necessary assessments before administering medications. Check allergy bracelet or ask patient about allergies.** Explain what you are going to do and the reason to the patient.	Assessment is a prerequisite to administration of medications. Explanation relieves anxiety and facilitates cooperation.
14. Scan the patient's bar code on the identification band, if required.	Scanning provides additional check to ensure that the medication is given to the right patient.

SKILL 5-23 Administering Medication via a Small-Volume Nebulizer *(continued)*

ACTION	RATIONALE
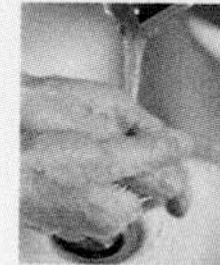 15. Perform hand hygiene.	Hand hygiene deters the spread of microorganisms.
16. Remove the nebulizer cup from the device and open it. Place premeasured unit-dose medication in the bottom section of the cup or use a dropper to place concentrated dose of medication in cup (Figure 1) and add prescribed diluent, if required.	To get enough volume to make a fine mist, normal saline may need to be added to the concentrated medication.
17. Screw the top portion of the nebulizer cup back in place and attach the cup to the nebulizer. Attach one end of tubing to the stem on the bottom of the nebulizer cuff and the other end to the air compressor or oxygen source.	Air or oxygen must be forced through the nebulizer to form a fine mist.
18. Turn on the air compressor or oxygen (Figure 2). Check that a fine medication mist is produced by opening the valve. Have patient place mouthpiece into mouth and grasp securely with teeth and lips.	If there is no fine mist, make sure that medication has been added to the cup and that the tubing is connected to the air compressor or oxygen outlet. Adjust flow meter if necessary.

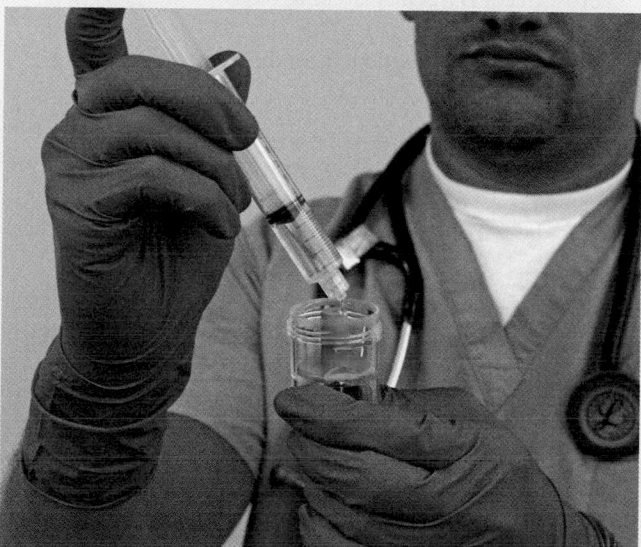

Figure 1. Putting medication into nebulizer chamber.

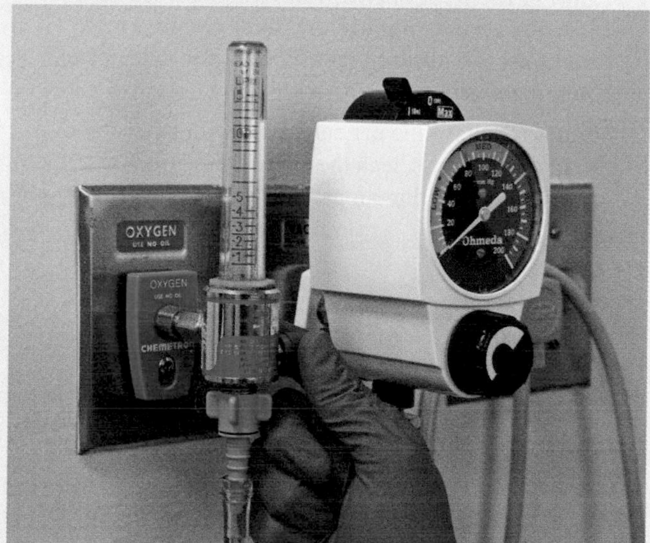

Figure 2. Adjusting flow rate.

ACTION	RATIONALE
19. **Instruct patient to inhale slowly and deeply through the mouth (Figure 3). A nose clip may be necessary if patient is also breathing through nose. Hold each breath for a slight pause, before exhaling.**	While the patient inhales and holds the breath, the medication comes in contact with the respiratory tissue and is absorbed. The longer the breath is held, the more medication can be absorbed.

(continued)

SKILL 5-23 Administering Medication via a Small-Volume Nebulizer *(continued)*

ACTION | **RATIONALE**

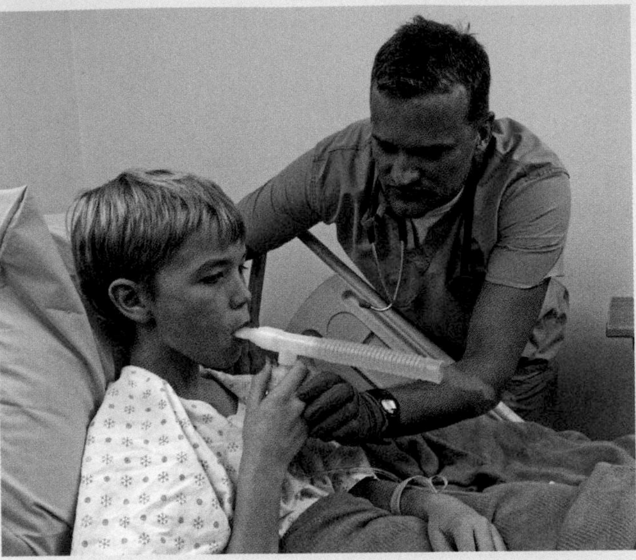

Figure 3. Using nebulizer for treatment.

20. **Continue this inhalation technique until all medication in the nebulizer cup has been aerosolized (usually about 15 minutes). Once the fine mist decreases in amount, gently flick the sides of the nebulizer cup.**

   Once the fine mist stops, the medication is no longer being aerosolized. By gently flicking the cup sides, any medication that is stuck to the sides is knocked into the bottom of the cup, where it can become aerosolized.

21. If desired, have the patient gargle with tap water after using nebulizer. Clean the nebulizer according to the manufacturer's directions.

   Rinsing is necessary when using inhaled steroids, as oral fungal infections can occur. Rinsing removes medication residue from the mouth. The buildup of medication can affect how the medication is delivered, as well as attract bacteria.

22. **Reassess lung sounds, oxygenation saturation if ordered, pulse, and respirations.**

   Lung sounds and oxygenation saturation may improve after nebulizer use. Respirations may decrease after nebulizer use. Checks for adverse effect of medications. Some medications can cause tachycardia.

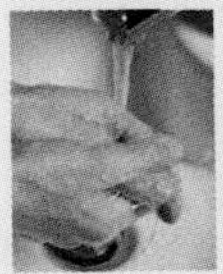

23. Perform hand hygiene.

   Hand hygiene deters the spread of microorganisms.

EVALUATION

The expected outcome is met when the patient receives the medication and exhibits improved lungs sounds and respiratory effort. In addition, the patient demonstrates correct steps for use and verbalizes an understanding of the need for the medication.

DOCUMENTATION

Guidelines

Document respiratory rate, oxygen saturation if appropriate, and lung sounds. Document medication administration on MAR or CMAR immediately after administration. Document patient teaching and patient response, if appropriate.

SKILL 5-23 Administering Medication via a Small-Volume Nebulizer *(continued)*

Sample Documentation

9/29/08 Wheezes noted in all lobes of lungs before albuterol nebulizer, O_2 saturation 92%, respiratory rate 24 breaths per minute, patient reports "feeling like I can't get my breath." After albuterol treatment, lung sounds are clear and equal in all lobes, O_2 saturation 97%, respiratory rate 18 breaths per minute. Patient verbalizes relief of shortness of breath and an understanding of medication purpose and action.—C. Bausler, RN

Unexpected Situations and Associated Interventions

- *Patient reports that nebulizer doesn't smell or taste the way it usually does:* Double-check to make sure that medication was added to nebulizer cup and that it is the appropriate medication.

Special Considerations

General Considerations

- Ongoing assessment is an important part of nursing care to evaluate patient response to administered medications and early detection of adverse effects. If an adverse effect is suspected, withhold further medication doses and notify the patient's primary healthcare provider. Additional intervention is based on type of reaction and patient assessment.

Infant and Child Considerations

- A small child may use a mask instead of a mouthpiece. Mask must fit securely over both the nose and the mouth to ensure a good seal and prevent medication escaping.
- Children must be able to seal their lips around the mouthpiece to use a nebulizer without a mask.

SKILL 5-24 Administering Medication via a Dry Powder Inhaler

Dry powder inhalers (DPI) are another type of delivery method for inhaled medications. The medication is supplied in a powder form, either in a small capsule or disk inserted into the DPI, or in a compartment inside the DPI. DPIs are breath activated. A quick breath by the patient activates the flow of medication, eliminating the need to coordinate activating the inhaler (spraying the medicine) while inhaling the medicine at the same time. Many types of DPIs are available, with distinctive operating instructions. Some have to be loaded with a dose of medication each time they are used and some hold a preloaded number of doses. It is important to understand the particular instructions for the medication and particular delivery device being used.

Equipment

- Stethoscope
- DPI and appropriate medication
- Medication Administration Record (MAR) or Computerized-medication Administration Record (CMAR)

ASSESSMENT

Assess lung sounds pre- and post-use to establish a baseline and determine the effectiveness of the medication. If ordered, assess oxygen saturation level before medication administration. Assess patient's ability to manage the DPI. Verify patient name, dose, route, and time of administration. Assess the patient's knowledge and understanding of the medication's purpose and action.

(continued)

SKILL 5-24 Administering Medication via a Dry Powder Inhaler *(continued)*

NURSING DIAGNOSIS

Determine related factors for the nursing diagnosis based on the patient's current status. Appropriate nursing diagnoses may include:

- Ineffective Airway Clearance
- Ineffective Breathing Pattern
- Impaired Gas Exchange
- Deficient Knowledge
- Risk for Activity Intolerance

OUTCOME IDENTIFICATION AND PLANNING

The expected outcome to achieve is that the patient receives the medication. Other outcomes that may be appropriate include the following: patient demonstrates improved lung expansion and breath sounds; respiratory status is within acceptable parameters; patient verbalizes an understanding of medication purpose and action; and patient demonstrates correct use of the DPI.

IMPLEMENTATION

ACTION	RATIONALE
1. Gather equipment. Check each medication order against the original physician's order according to agency policy. Clarify any inconsistencies. Check the patient's chart for allergies.	This comparison helps to identify errors that may have occurred when orders were transcribed. The physician's order is the legal record of medication orders for each agency.
2. Know the actions, special nursing considerations, safe dose ranges, purpose of administration, and adverse effects of the medications to be administered. Consider the appropriateness of the medication for this patient.	This knowledge aids the nurse in evaluating the therapeutic effect of the medication in relation to the patient's disorder and can also be used to educate the patient about the medication.
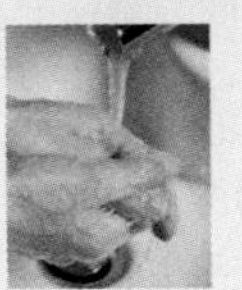 3. Perform hand hygiene.	Hand hygiene prevents the spread of microorganisms.
4. Move the medication cart to the outside of the patient's room or prepare for administration in the medication area.	Organization facilitates error-free administration and saves time.
5. Unlock the medication cart or drawer. Enter pass code and scan employee identification, if required.	Locking of the cart or drawer safeguards each patient's medication supply. Hospital accrediting organizations require medication carts to be locked when not in use. Entering pass code and scanning ID allows only authorized users into the system and identifies user for documentation by the computer.
6. **Prepare medications for one patient at a time.**	This prevents errors in medication administration.
7. Read the MAR and select the proper medication from the patient's medication drawer or unit stock.	This is the first check of the label.
8. Compare the label with the MAR. Check expiration dates and perform calculations, if necessary. Scan the bar code on the package, if required.	This is the second check of the label. Verify calculations with another nurse to ensure safety, if necessary.

SKILL 5-24 Administering Medication via a Dry Powder Inhaler *(continued)*

ACTION	RATIONALE
9. **When all medications for one patient have been prepared, recheck the label with the MAR before taking them to the patient. Lock the medication cart before leaving it.**	This is a *third* check to ensure accuracy and to prevent errors. Locking the cart or drawer safeguards the patient's medication supply. Hospital accrediting organizations require medication carts to be locked when not in use.
10. Transport medications to the patient's bedside carefully, and keep the medications in sight at all times.	Careful handling and close observation prevent accidental or deliberate disarrangement of medications.
11. **Ensure that the patient receives the medications at the correct time.**	Check agency policy, which may allow for administration within a period of 30 minutes before or 30 minutes after designated time.
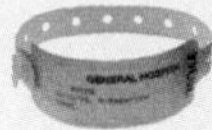 12. **Identify the patient.** Usually, the patient should be identified using two methods. Compare information with the MAR or CMAR.	Identifying the patient ensures the right patient receives the medications and helps prevent errors.
a. Check the name and identification number on the patient's identification band.	This is the most reliable method. Replace the identification band if it is missing or inaccurate in any way.
b. Ask the patient to state his or her name.	This requires a response from the patient, but illness and strange surroundings often cause patients to be confused.
c. If the patient cannot identify him or herself, verify the patient's identification with a staff member who knows the patient for the second source.	This is another way to double-check identity. Do not use the name on the door or over the bed, because these may be inaccurate.
13. **Complete necessary assessments before administering medications. Check allergy bracelet or ask patient about allergies.** Explain what you are going to do and the reason to the patient.	Assessment is a prerequisite to administration of medications. Explanation relieves anxiety and facilitates cooperation.
14. Scan the patient's bar code on the identification band, if required.	Provides additional check to ensure that the medication is given to the right patient.
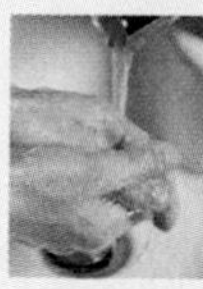 15. Perform hand hygiene.	Hand hygiene deters the spread of microorganisms.
16. **Remove the mouthpiece cover or remove from storage container. Load a dose into the device as directed by the manufacturer, if necessary. Alternately, activate the inhaler if necessary according to manufacturer's directions.**	This is necessary to deliver the medication.
17. Have the patient breathe out slowly and completely, without breathing into the DPI.	This allows for deeper inhalation with the medication dose. Moisture from the patient's breath can clog the inhaler.
18. Patient should place his teeth over and seal his lips around the mouthpiece. Do not block opening with the tongue or teeth (Figure 1).	Prevents medication from escaping and allows for a tight seal, ensuring maximum dosing of medication. Blocking of opening interferes with medication delivery.
19. Breathe in quickly and deeply through the mouth, more than 2 to 3 seconds.	Activates the flow of medication. Deep inhalation allows for maximal distribution of medication to lung tissue.
20. Remove inhaler from mouth. **Instruct patient to hold the breath for 5 to 10 seconds, or as long as possible, and then to exhale slowly through pursed lips.**	This allows better distribution and longer absorption time for the medication.

(continued)

SKILL 5-24 Administering Medication via a Dry Powder Inhaler *(continued)*

ACTION

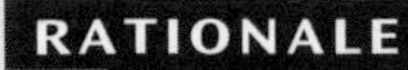

RATIONALE

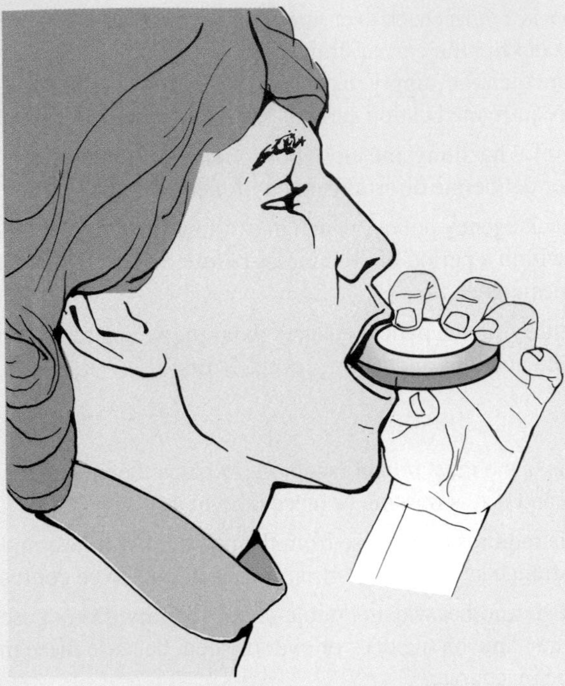

Figure 1. Patient with teeth and lips around mouthpiece of a dry powder inhaler.

ACTION	RATIONALE
21. **Wait 1 to 5 minutes, as prescribed, before administering the next puff.**	This ensures that both puffs are absorbed as much as possible. Bronchodilation after first puff allows for deeper penetration by subsequent puffs.
22. After the prescribed amount of puffs has been administered, have patient replace the cap or storage container.	By replacing the cap, the patient is preventing any dust or dirt from entering and being propelled into the bronchioles with later doses or clogging the inhaler.
23. **Reassess lung sounds, oxygenation saturation if ordered, and respirations.**	Lung sounds and oxygenation saturation may improve after DPI use. Respirations may decrease after DPI use.
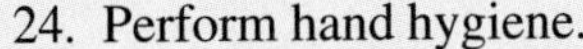 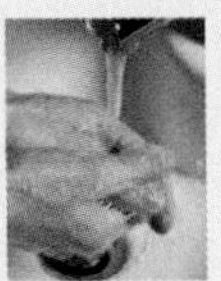 24. Perform hand hygiene.	Hand hygiene deters the spread of microorganisms.

EVALUATION

The expected outcome is met when the patient demonstrates improved lung sounds and ease of breathing. In addition, patient demonstrates correct use of DPI and verbalizes correct information about medication therapy associated with DPI use.

DOCUMENTATION

Guidelines

Document respiratory rate, oxygen saturation, if applicable, and lung assessment. Document medication administration on MAR or CMAR immediately after administration. Document patient teaching and patient response, if appropriate.

SKILL 5-24 Administering Medication via a Dry Powder Inhaler *(continued)*

Sample Documentation

12/22/08 Breath sounds slightly decreased in bases pretreatment. After DPI, lung sounds remain diminished bilaterally in bases, O_2 saturation 97%, respiratory rate 16 breaths per minute. Patient able to accurately demonstrate use of DPI and verbalizes understanding of medication purpose and action.—C. Bausler, RN

Special Considerations

General Considerations

- Instruct the patient to never exhale into the mouthpiece.
- If mist can be seen from the mouth or nose, the DPI is being used incorrectly.
- Follow the manufacturer's directions to clean the DPI.
- Store inhaler, capsules, and discs away from moisture.
- Ongoing assessment is an important part of nursing care to evaluate patient response to administered medications and early detection of adverse effects. If an adverse effect is suspected, withhold further medication doses and notify the patient's primary healthcare provider. Additional intervention is based on type of reaction and patient assessment.

Home Care Considerations

- Patients should know how to tell when medication levels are getting low. The most reliable method is to look on the package and see how many doses the DPI contains. Divide this number by the number of doses used daily to ascertain how many days the DPI will last.
- Some DPIs have dosage counters to keep track of remaining doses.

SKILL 5-25 Administering Medications via a Gastric Tube

Nasogastric and gastrostomy tubes are collectively referred to as gastric tubes. If a patient cannot take medications orally but has a nasogastric tube (NG tube) or gastrostomy tube (G tube) in place, the physician may order the medication to be administered via the tube. Only medications that can be crushed or mixed with other substances such as food or those in liquid form can be given this way.

Equipment

- Irrigation set (60-mL syringe and irrigation container)
- Medications (crushed or in liquid form)
- Water (gastrostomy tubes) or sterile water or saline (nasogastric tubes), according to facility policy

ASSESSMENT

Research each medication to be given, especially for mode of action, side effects, nursing implications, ability to be crushed, and whether medication should be given with or without food. Verify patient name, dose, route, and time of administration. Also assess patient's knowledge of medication and the reason for administration. Auscultate the abdomen for evidence of bowel sounds. Percuss and palpate the abdomen for tenderness and distention. Ascertain the time of the patient's last bowel movement and measure abdominal girth, if appropriate.

(continued)

SKILL 5-25

Administering Medications via a Gastric Tube *(continued)*

NURSING DIAGNOSIS

Determine the related factors for the nursing diagnoses based on the patient's current status. Possible nursing diagnoses may include:

- Deficient Knowledge
- Risk for Injury
- Impaired Swallowing

OUTCOME IDENTIFICATION AND PLANNING

The expected outcome to achieve is that the patient receives the medication via the tube and experiences the intended effect of the medication. In addition, the patient verbalizes knowledge of the medications given; the patient remains free from adverse effect and injury; and the gastric tube remains patent.

IMPLEMENTATION

ACTION	RATIONALE
1. Gather equipment. Check each medication order against the original physician's order according to agency policy. Clarify any inconsistencies. Check the patient's chart for allergies.	This comparison helps to identify errors that may have occurred when orders were transcribed. The physician's order is the legal record of medication orders for each agency.
2. Know the actions, special nursing considerations, safe dose ranges, purpose of administration, and adverse effects of the medications to be administered. Consider the appropriateness of the medication for this patient.	This knowledge aids the nurse in evaluating the therapeutic effect of the medication in relation to the patient's disorder and can also be used to educate the patient about the medication.
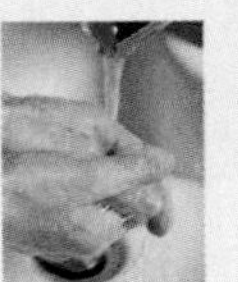 3. Perform hand hygiene.	Hand hygiene prevents the spread of microorganisms.
4. Move the medication cart to the outside of the patient's room or prepare for administration in the medication area.	Organization facilitates error-free administration and saves time.
5. Unlock the medication cart or drawer. Enter pass code and scan employee identification, if required.	Locking of the cart or drawer safeguards each patient's medication supply. Hospital accrediting organizations require medication carts to be locked when not in use. Entering pass code and scanning ID allows only authorized users into the system and identifies user for documentation by the computer.
6. **Prepare medications for one patient at a time.**	This prevents errors in medication administration.
7. Read the MAR and select the proper medication from the patient's medication drawer or unit stock.	This is the first check of the label.
8. Compare the label with the MAR. Check expiration dates and perform calculations, if necessary. Scan the bar code on the package, if required.	This is the second check of the label. Verify calculations with another nurse to ensure safety, if necessary.
9. Check to see if medications to be administered come in a liquid form. **If pills or capsules are to be given, check with pharmacy or drug reference to verify the ability to crush or open capsules.** Ensure that the tube is patent and irrigate as necessary (see Skill 11-4).	To prevent the tube from becoming clogged, all medications should be given in liquid form whenever possible. Medications in extended-release formulations should not be crushed before administration.

SKILL 5-25

Administering Medications via a Gastric Tube *(continued)*

ACTION	RATIONALE
10. Prepare medication.	
Pills: Using a pill crusher, crush each pill one at a time. Dissolve the powder with water or other recommended liquid in a liquid medication cup, keeping each medication separate from the others. Keep the package label with the medication cup, for future comparison of information.	The label is needed for an additional safety check. Some medications require preadministration assessments. Some medications require dissolution in liquid other that water.
Liquid: When pouring liquid medications in a multidose bottle, hold the bottle with the label against the palm. Use the appropriate measuring device when pouring liquids, and read the amount of medication at the bottom of the meniscus at eye level. Wipe the lip of the bottle with a paper towel.	Liquid that may drip onto the label makes the label difficult to read. Accuracy is possible when the appropriate measuring device is used and then read accurately.
11. **When all medications for one patient have been prepared, recheck the label with the MAR before taking them to the patient. Lock the medication cart before leaving it.**	This is a *third* check to ensure accuracy and to prevent errors. Locking the cart or drawer safeguards the patient's medication supply. Hospital accrediting organizations require medication carts to be locked when not in use.
12. Transport medications to the patient's bedside carefully, and keep the medications in sight at all times.	Careful handling and close observation prevent accidental or deliberate disarrangement of medications.
13. **Ensure that the patient receives the medications at the correct time.**	Check agency policy, which may allow for administration within a period of 30 minutes before or 30 minutes after designated time.
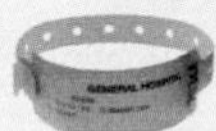 14. **Identify the patient.** Usually, the patient should be identified using two methods. Compare information with the MAR or CMAR.	Identifying the patient ensures the right patient receives the medications and helps prevent errors.
a. Check the name and identification number on the patient's identification band.	This is the most reliable method. Replace the identification band if it is missing or inaccurate in any way.
b. Ask the patient to state his or her name.	This requires a response from the patient, but illness and strange surroundings often cause patients to be confused.
c. If the patient cannot identify him or herself, verify the patient's identification with a staff member who knows the patient for the second source.	This is another way to double-check identity. Do not use the name on the door or over the bed, because these may be inaccurate.
15. **Complete necessary assessments before administering medications. Check allergy bracelet or ask patient about allergies.** Explain what you are going to do and the reason to the patient.	Assessment is a prerequisite to administration of medications. Explanation relieves anxiety and facilitates cooperation.
16. Scan the patient's bar code on the identification band, if required.	This provides an additional check to ensure that the medication is given to the right patient.
17. Assist the patient to the High Fowler's position, unless contraindicated.	This reduces the risk of aspiration.
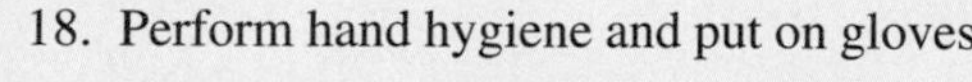 18. Perform hand hygiene and put on gloves.	Hand hygiene deters the spread of microorganisms. Gloves prevent contact with mucous membranes and body fluids.

(continued)

SKILL 5-25 Administering Medications via a Gastric Tube *(continued)*

ACTION	RATIONALE
19. If patient is receiving continuous tube feedings, pause the tube feeding pump (Figure 1).	If the pump is not stopped, tube feeding will flow out of the tube and onto the patient.
20. Pour the water into the irrigation container. Fold the gastric tube over on itself and pinch with fingers (Figure 2). Alternately, open port on gastric tube delegated to medication administration. If necessary, position stopcock to correct direction. Disconnect tubing for feeding or suction from gastric tube. Place cap on end of feeding tubing.	Fluid is ready for flushing of the tube. Folding the tube over and clamping or correct positioning of stopcock prevents any backflow of gastric drainage. Covering end of feeding tubing prevents contamination.

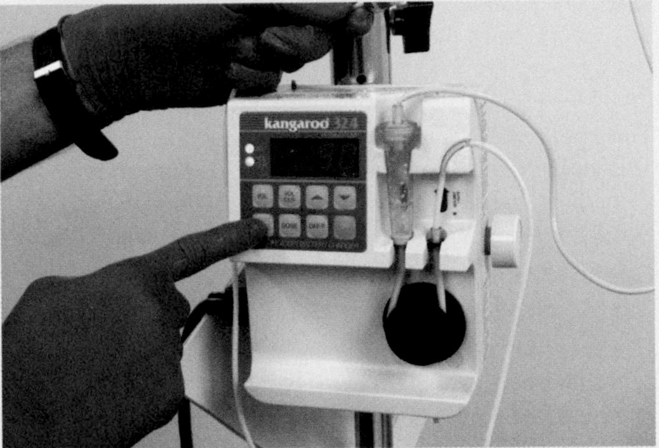

Figure 1. Pausing feeding pump.

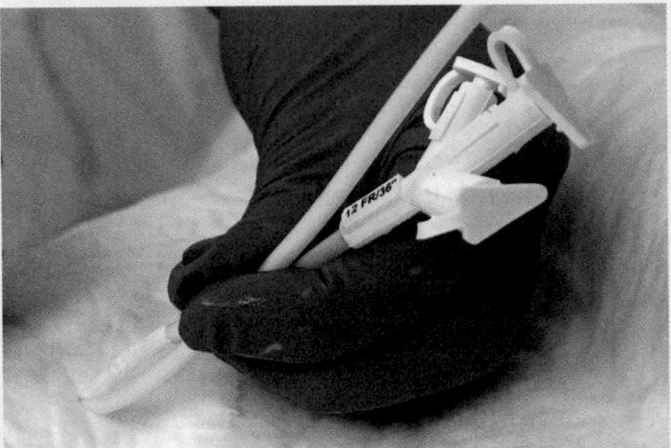

Figure 2. Folding gastric tube over on itself and pinching with fingers.

ACTION	RATIONALE
21. Insert tip of 60-mL syringe into tube. Release gastric tube. Pull plunger back using constant, gentle pressure to check for residual feeding and to check tube placement (Figure 3).	Tube placement must be confirmed before administering anything through the tube to avoid inadvertent instillation in the respiratory tract. Before the medication is administered, assess the stomach for any gastric residual.

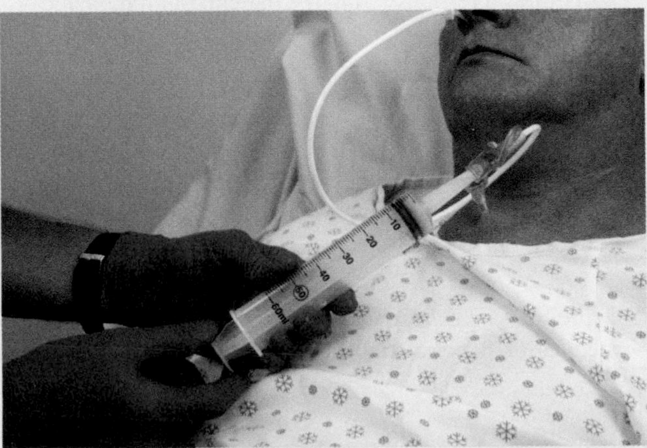

Figure 3. Pulling back on syringe plunger, using constant, gentle pressure.

ACTION	RATIONALE
22. **Note the amount of any residual. Replace residual back into stomach.**	Fluid should be returned to stomach so as not to cause any fluid or electrolyte losses. If residual is a large amount as indicated by above, confer with physician on whether to discard aspirated contents or replace them.

SKILL 5-25 Administering Medications via a Gastric Tube *(continued)*

ACTION	RATIONALE
23. Fold gastric tube over and clamp with fingers. Remove 60-mL syringe. Remove the plunger of the syringe. Reinsert the syringe in the gastric tube without the plunger. Pour 30 mL of water into the syringe. **Unclamp the tube and allow the water to enter the stomach via gravity infusion.**	Folding the tube over and clamping it prevents any backflow of gastric drainage. Flushing the tube ensures all the residual is cleared from tube.
24. Administer the first dose of medication by pouring into the syringe. Follow with a 5- to 10-mL water flush between medication doses. Follow the last dose of medication with 30 to 60 mL of water flush.	Flushing between medications prevents any possible interactions between the medications. Flushing at the end maintains patency of the tube, prevents blockage by medication particles, and ensures all doses enter the stomach.
25. Clamp the tube, remove the syringe, and replace the feeding tubing. If stopcock is used, position stopcock to correct direction. If tube medication port was used, cap port. Unclamp gastric tube and restart tube feeding, if appropriate for medications administered.	Some medications require the holding of the tube feeding for a certain period of time after administration. Consult a drug reference or a pharmacist.
26. Remove gloves and perform hand hygiene.	Hand hygiene deters the spread of microorganisms.
27. Assist the patient to a comfortable position. If receiving a tube feeding, the head of the bed must remain elevated at least 30 degrees.	Ensures patient comfort. Keeping the head of the bed elevated helps prevent aspiration.
28. Evaluate patient's response to medication within appropriate time frame.	The patient needs to be evaluated for any adverse affects from the medication.

EVALUATION

The expected outcome is met when the patient receives the ordered medications and experiences the intended effects of the medications administered. In addition, the patient demonstrates a patent and functioning gastric tube, verbalizes knowledge of the medications given, and remains free from adverse effect and injury.

DOCUMENTATION

Guidelines

Document the administration of the medication immediately after administration, including date, time, dose, and route of administration on the MAR or record using the required format. If using a bar-code system, medication administration is automatically recorded when scanned. PRN medications require documentation of the reason for administration. Prompt recording avoids the possibility of accidentally repeating the administration of the drug. If the drug was refused or omitted, record this in the appropriate area on the medication record and notify the physician. This verifies the reason medication was omitted and ensures that the physician is aware of the patient's condition. Record the amount of gastric residual, if appropriate. Record the amount of liquid given on the intake and output record.

Unexpected Situations and Associated Interventions

- *Medication enters tube and then tube becomes clogged:* Attach a 10-mL syringe onto end of tube. Pull back and then lightly apply pressure to plunger in a repetitive motion. This may dislodge the medication. If the medication does not move through the tube, notify the physician. The tube may have to be replaced.

(continued)

SKILL 5-25 Administering Medications via a Gastric Tube *(continued)*

Special Considerations

General Considerations

- Residual feeding in the stomach is an indicator of gastric emptying. A residual of more than 100 mL from a gastrostomy tube, 200 mL from a nasogastric tube, or more than 10% to 20% above the hourly feeding rate must be reported to the physician, according to policy and physician orders.
- If medications are being administered via a nasogastric tube that is attached to suction, the tube should remain clamped, off suction, for a period of time after medication administration. This allows for medication absorption before returning to suction. Check facility policy and drug reference for specific drug requirements.
- If necessary to use plunger in irrigation syringe to administer medications, instill gently and slowly. Gravity administration is considered best to avoid excess pressure.
- Ongoing assessment is an important part of nursing care to evaluate patient response to administered medications and early detection of adverse effects. If an adverse effect is suspected, withhold further medication doses and notify the patient's primary healthcare provider. Additional intervention is based on type of reaction and patient assessment.

SKILL 5-26 Administering a Rectal Suppository

Rectal suppositories are used primarily for their local action, such as laxatives and fecal softeners. Systemic effects are also achieved with rectal suppositories. It is important to ensure the suppository is placed past the internal anal sphincter and against the rectal mucosa.

Equipment

- Suppository
- Water-soluble lubricant
- Clean gloves
- Medication Administration Record (MAR) or Computer-generated MAR (CMAR)

ASSESSMENT

Assess the rectal area for any alterations in integrity. Suppository should not be administered to patients who have had recent rectal or prostate surgery. Assess recent laboratory values, particularly the patient's white blood cell and platelet counts. Patient who are thrombocytopenic or neutropenic should not receive rectal suppositories. Rectal suppositories should not be administered to patients at risk for cardiac arrhythmias. Assess relevant body systems for the particular medication being administered. Assess the patient for allergies. Verify patient name, dose, route, and time of administration. Assess the patient's knowledge of medication and procedure. If the patient has a knowledge deficit about the medication, this may be an appropriate time to begin education about the medication. Assess the patient's ability to cooperate with the procedure.

NURSING DIAGNOSIS

Determine the related factors for the nursing diagnoses based on the patient's current status. Possible nursing diagnoses may include:

- Deficient Knowledge
- Risk for Injury
- Anxiety

OUTCOME IDENTIFICATION AND PLANNING

The expected outcome is that the medication is administered successfully into the rectum. Other outcomes that may be appropriate include the following: patient understands the rationale for the rectal instillation; patient experiences no allergy response; patient's skin remains intact; patient experiences no, or minimal, pain; and patient experiences minimal anxiety.

SKILL 5-26

Administering a Rectal Suppository *(continued)*

IMPLEMENTATION

ACTION	RATIONALE
1. Gather equipment. Check medication order against the original physician's order according to agency policy. Clarify any inconsistencies. Check the patient's chart for allergies.	This comparison helps to identify errors that may have occurred when orders were transcribed. The physician's order is the legal record of medication orders for each agency.
2. Know the actions, special nursing considerations, safe dose ranges, purpose of administration, and adverse effects of the medication to be administered. Consider the appropriateness of the medication for this patient.	This knowledge aids the nurse in evaluating the therapeutic effect of the medication in relation to the patient's disorder and can also be used to educate the patient about the medication.
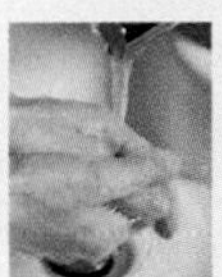 3. Perform hand hygiene.	Hand hygiene prevents the spread of microorganisms.
4. Move the medication cart to the outside of the patient's room or prepare for administration in the medication area.	Organization facilitates error-free administration and saves time.
5. Unlock the medication cart or drawer. Enter pass code and scan employee identification, if required.	Locking of the cart or drawer safeguards each patient's medication supply. Hospital accrediting organizations require medication carts to be locked when not in use. Entering pass code and scanning ID allows only authorized users into the system and identifies user for documentation by the computer.
6. **Prepare medications for one patient at a time.**	This prevents errors in medication administration.
7. Read the MAR and select the proper medication from the patient's medication drawer or unit stock.	This is the first check of the label.
8. Compare the label with the MAR. Check expiration dates and perform calculations, if necessary. Scan the bar code on the package, if required.	This is the second check of the label. Verify calculations with another nurse to ensure safety, if necessary.
9. **When all medications for one patient have been prepared, recheck the label with the MAR before taking them to the patient. Lock the medication cart before leaving it.**	This is a *third* check to ensure accuracy and to prevent errors. Locking the cart or drawer safeguards the patient's medication supply. Hospital accrediting organizations require medication carts to be locked when not in use.
10. Transport medications to the patient's bedside carefully, and keep the medications in sight at all times.	Careful handling and close observation prevent accidental or deliberate disarrangement of medications.
11. **Ensure that the patient receives the medications at the correct time.**	Check agency policy, which may allow for administration within a period of 30 minutes before or 30 minutes after designated time.
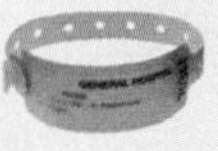 12. **Identify the patient.** Usually, the patient should be identified using two methods. Compare information with the MAR or CMAR.	Identifying the patient ensures the right patient receives the medications and helps prevent errors.
a. Check the name and identification number on the patient's identification band.	This is the most reliable method. Replace the identification band if it is missing or inaccurate in any way.
b. Ask the patient to state his or her name.	This requires a response from the patient, but illness and strange surroundings often cause patients to be confused.

(continued)

SKILL 5-26 Administering a Rectal Suppository *(continued)*

ACTION	RATIONALE
c. If the patient cannot identify him or herself, verify the patient's identification with a staff member who knows the patient for the second source.	This is another way to double-check identity. Do not use the name on the door or over the bed, because these may be inaccurate.
13. **Complete necessary assessments before administering medications. Check allergy bracelet or ask patient about allergies. Explain the purpose and action of each medication to the patient.**	Assessment is a prerequisite to administration of medications.
14. Scan the patient's bar code on the identification band, if required.	Provides additional check to ensure that the medication is given to the right patient.
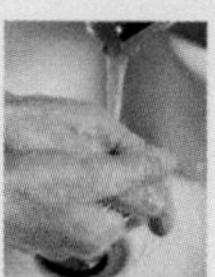 15. Perform hand hygiene and put on gloves.	Hand hygiene deters the spread of microorganisms. Gloves protect the nurse from potential contact with contaminants, mucous membranes, and body fluids.
16. Assist the patient to his or her left side in a Sims' position. Drape accordingly to only expose the buttocks.	Allows for easy access to anal area. Left side decreases chance of expulsion of the suppository. Proper draping maintains privacy.
17. Remove the suppository from its wrapper. Apply lubricant to the rounded end (Figure 1). Lubricate the index finger of your dominant hand.	Lubricant reduces friction on administration and increases patient comfort.
18. Separate the buttocks with your nondominant hand and instruct the patient to breathe slowly and deeply through his or her mouth while the suppository is being inserted.	Slow, deep breaths help to relax the anal sphincter and reduce discomfort.
19. **Using your index finger, insert the suppository, round end first, along the rectal wall. Insert about 3″ to 4″ (Figure 2).**	Suppository must make contact with the rectal mucosa for absorption to occur.

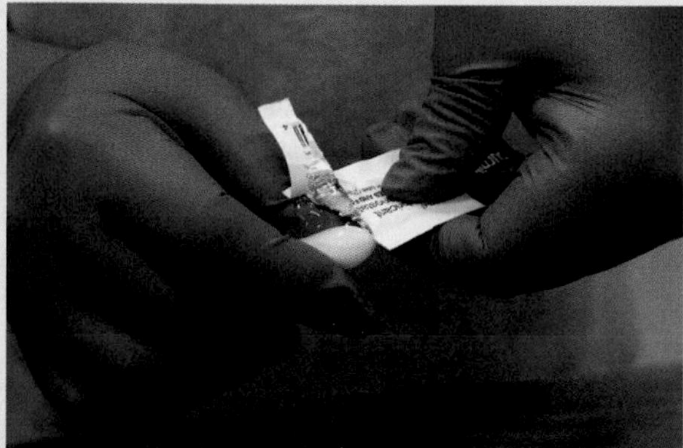

Figure 1. Applying lubricant to the rounded end of the suppository.

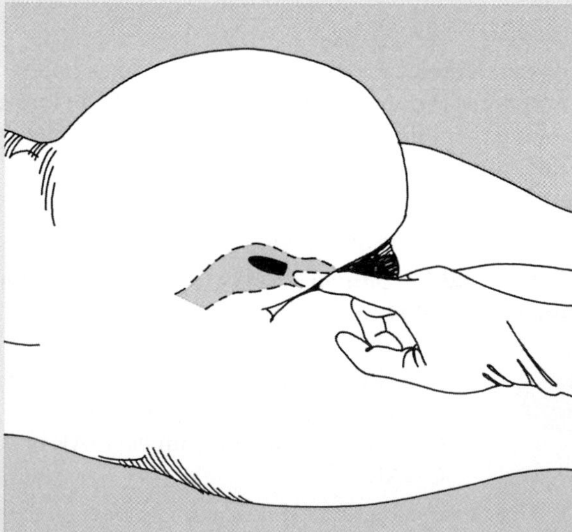

Figure 2. Inserting the suppository round end first along the rectal wall.

SKILL 5-26 **Administering a Rectal Suppository** *(continued)*

ACTION	RATIONALE
20. Use toilet tissue to clean any stool or lubricant from around the anus. Release the buttocks. Encourage the patient to remain on his or her side for at least 5 minutes and retain the suppository for the appropriate amount of time for the specific medication.	Prevents skin irritation. Prevents accidental expulsion of suppository and ensures absorption of medication.
21. Remove gloves and perform hand hygiene.	This prevents spread of microorganisms.
22. Evaluate patient's response to the procedure and medication.	The patient needs to be evaluated for any adverse affects from the medication or procedure.

EVALUATION

The expected outcome is achieved when the medication is administered successfully into the rectum; the patient understood the rationale for the rectal instillation; patient did not experience adverse effect; patient's skin remains intact; and patient experiences minimal anxiety.

DOCUMENTATION

Guidelines

Document the administration of the medication immediately after administration, including date, time, dose, and route of administration on the MAR or record using the required format. If using a bar-code system, medication administration is automatically recorded when scanned. PRN medications require documentation of the reason for administration. Prompt recording avoids the possibility of accidentally repeating the administration of the drug. If the drug was refused or omitted, record this in the appropriate area on the medication record and notify the physician. This verifies the reason medication was omitted and ensures that the physician is aware of the patient's condition. Document your assessments, and the patient's response to the treatment, if appropriate.

Unexpected Situations

- *Patient expels suppository before it is absorbed.* Put on gloves and apply additional lubricant to the suppository. Reinsert past the internal sphincter. If the suppository has warmed and become too soft, discard the suppository and notify the physician. An additional dose may be ordered.

Special Considerations

General Considerations

- If the suppository is for laxative purposes, it must remain in position for 35 to 45 minutes, or until the patient feels the urge to defecate.
- Ongoing assessment is an important part of nursing care to evaluate patient response to administered medications and early detection of adverse effects. If an adverse effect is suspected, withhold further medication doses and notify the patient's primary healthcare provider. Additional intervention is based on type of reaction and patient assessment.

Infant and Child Considerations

- If may be necessary to hold the buttocks closed to relieve pressure on the anal sphincter. Usually, 5 to 10 minutes is sufficient for the urge to defecate to pass.

Older Adult Considerations

- Older adults may have difficulty retaining rectal suppositories, related to decreased muscle tone and loss of sphincter control.

The Taylor Suite offers these additional resources to enhance learning and facilitate understanding:

- thePoint online resource, http://thepoint.lww.com/Lynn2E
- Student CD-ROM included with the book
- Skills Checklist to Accompany Taylor's Clinical Nursing Skills
- Taylor's Interactive Nursing
- Taylor's Video Guide to Clinical Nursing Skills: *Oral and Topical Medications, Injectable Medications* and *Intravenous Medications*

■ Developing Critical Thinking Skills

1. When entering Cooper Jackson's room with the antibiotic, the nurse asks Cooper's mother about any medication allergies that Cooper may have. The mother says, "The only medication that Cooper is allergic to is penicillin. It made it hard for him to breathe the last time he received it." The nurse notes that the ordered medication is a cephalosporin. Should the nurse administer the medication? What is the best technique to administer liquid medication to an uncooperative 2 year old? Thirty minutes after receiving an oral medication, Cooper vomits. Should the nurse readminister the medication?
2. What are some ways that the nurse can make Erika Jenkins feel more relaxed about receiving her injection? What should the nurse do if Erika moves and dislodges the needle during the injection or if Erika tenses her muscles so tightly that the needle does not penetrate the skin?
3. What are some priority points that the nurse needs to discuss with Jonah Dinerman, who has type 1 diabetes, if the education needs to be completed in a short time?

■ Bibliography

Abrams, A. (2001). *Clinical drug therapy* (6th ed.). Philadelphia: Lippincott Williams & Wilkins.

Aschenbrenner, D. & Venable, S. (2006). *Drug therapy in nursing* (2nd ed.). Philadelphia: Lippincott Williams & Wilkins.

Balas, M., Scott, L., & Rogers, A. (2004). The prevalence and nature of errors and near errors reported by hospital staff nurses. *Applied Nursing Research, 17*(4), 224–230.

Burke, K. (2005). Executive summary: The state of the science on safe medication administration symposium. *American Journal of Nursing,* March supplement, 4–7.

Caffrey, R. (2003). Diabetes under control: Are all syringes created equal? *American Journal of Nursing, 103*(6), 46–49.

Carroll, P. (2003). Medication errors: The bigger picture. *RN, 66*(1), 52–58.

Fain, J. (2002). Delivering insulin round the clock. *Nursing, 32*(8), 54–56.

Fain, J. (2003). Pump up your knowledge of insulin pumps. *Nursing, 33*(6), 51–53.

Greenway, K. (2004). Using the ventrogluteal site for intramuscular injection. *Nursing Standard, 18*(25), 39–41.

Haddad, A. (2001). Ethics in action. *RN, 64*(9), 25–28.

Hockenberry, M. (2005). *Wong's essentials of pediatric nursing.* (7th ed.). St. Louis, MO: Elsevier Mosby.

Hughes, R. & Ortiz, E. (2005). Medication errors: Why they happen and how they can be prevented. *American Journal of Nursing,* March supplement, 14–23.

Karch, A., & Karch, F. (2001). Take part in the solution: How to report medication errors. *American Journal of Nursing, 101*(10), 25.

Katsma, D., & Katsma, R. (2000). The myth of the 90°-angle intramuscular injection. *Nurse Educator, 25*(1), 34–37.

Keresztes, P. & Brick, K. (2003). Lantus: A new insulin. *MEDSURG Nursing, 12*(5), 408–410.

King, L. (2003). Subcutaneous insulin injection technique. *Nursing Standard, 17*(34), 45–52.

Koschel, M. (2001). Question of practice: Filter needles. *American Journal of Nursing, 101*(1), 75.

Lee, M., & Phillips, J. (2002). *Transdermal patches: High risk for error? Drug Topics, April 1,* Available at http://fda.gov/dcer/drug/MedErrors/transdermal.pdf. Accessed 6/27/2005.

Lee, S, Im, R., & Magbual, R. (2004). Current perspectives on the use of continuous subcutaneous insulin infusion in the acute care setting and overview of therapy. *Critical Care Nursing Quarterly, 27*(2), 172–184.

McConnell, E. (2001). Clinical do's & don'ts: Instilling eyedrops. *Nursing, 31*(9), 17.

McConnell, E. (2002). Teaching your patient to use a metered-dose inhaler. *Nursing, 32*(2), 73.

McKenry, L., & Salerno, E. (2002). *Pharmacology in nursing* (21st ed.). St. Louis: C. V. Mosby.

McRoberts, S. (2005). The use of bar code technology in medication administration. *Clinical Nurse Specialist, 19*(2), 55–56.

Morris, M. (2002). When a phone order differs from the written one. *RN, 65*(1), 71.

Moshang, J. (2005). Making a point about insulin pens. *Nursing, 35*(2), 46–47.

Nicoll, L., & Hesby, A. (2002). Intramuscular injection: An integrative research review and guideline for evidence-based practice. *Applied Nursing Research, 16*(2), 149–162.

North American Nursing Diagnosis Association. (2005). *Nursing Diagnoses: Definitions and Classification 2005–2006.* Philadelphia: Author.

Olohan, K, & Zappitellli, D. (2003). The insulin pump: Making life with diabetes easier. *American Journal of Nursing, 103*(4), 48–57.

Pape, T. (2003). Applying airline safety practices to medication administration. *Med Surg Nursing, 12*(2), 77–94.

Pope, B. (2002). How to administer subcutaneous and intramuscular injections. *Nursing, 32*(1), 50–51.

Rushing, J. (2004). How to administer a subcutaneous injection. *Nursing, 34*(6), 32.

Small, S. (2004). Preventing sciatic nerve injury from intramuscular injections: Literature review. *Journal of Advanced Nursing, 47*(3), 287–296.

Smeltzer, S., Bare, B., Hinkle, J. H., & Cheever, K.H. (2008). *Brunner and Suddarth's textbook of medical–surgical nursing* (11th ed.). Philadelphia: Lippincott Williams & Wilkins.

Stephens, M. (2003a). Intramuscular injections. *Nursing Times, 99*(26), 27.

Stephens, M. (2003b). Subcutaneous injections. *Nursing Times, 99*(26), 29.

Togger, D., & Brenner, P. (2001). Metered dose inhalers. *American Journal of Nursing, 101*(10), 26–32.

Trooskin, S. (2002). Low-technology, cost-efficient strategies for reducing medication errors. *American Journal of Infection Control, 30*(6), 351–354.

U.S. Food and Drug Administration. (2003). *Strategies to reduce medication errors.* Available at http://www.fda.gov/fdac/features/2003/303_meds.html. Accessed June 27, 2005.

Wentz, J., Karch, A., & Karch, F. (2000). You've caught the error, now how do you fix it? *American Journal of Nursing, 100*(9), 24.

Winland-Brown, J., & Valiante, J. (2000). Effectiveness of different medication management approaches on elders' medication adherence. *Outcomes Management for Nursing Practice, 4*(4), 172–176.

Wolf, Z., Serembus, J., & Beitz, J. (2001). Clinical inference of nursing students concerning harmful outcomes after medication errors. *Nurse Educator, 26*(6), 268–270.

CHAPTER 6

Perioperative Nursing

Focusing on Patient Care

This chapter will help you develop the skills related to safe perioperative nursing care for the following patients:

Josie McKeown, a 2-day-old girl who needs surgery to correct a heart defect

Tatum Kelly, a 28-year-old woman having outpatient surgery for breast reduction

Dorothy Gibbs, an 81-year-old woman having surgery to remove a bowel obstruction

Learning Outcomes

After studying this chapter, you will be able to:

1. Provide safe and effective care for the preoperative patient.
2. Provide safe and effective care for the postoperative patient.
3. Apply a forced-air warming device.

Key Terms

anesthetic: medication that produces such states as narcosis (loss of consciousness), analgesia, relaxation, and loss of reflexes

atelectasis: incomplete expansion or collapse of a part of the lungs

conscious sedation/analgesia: type of anesthesia used for short procedures; the intravenous administration of sedatives and analgesics raises the pain threshold and produces an altered mood and some degree of amnesia, but the patient maintains cardiopulmonary function and can respond to verbal commands

elective surgery: surgery that is recommended but can be omitted or delayed without a negative effect

embolus: foreign body or air in the circulatory system

emergency surgery: surgery that must be performed immediately to save the person's life or a body organ

hemorrhage: excessive blood loss due to the escape of blood from blood vessels

hypovolemic shock: shock due to a decrease in blood volume

perioperative nursing: wide variety of nursing activities carried out before, during, and after surgery

perioperative period: time frame consisting of the preoperative phase (starts with decision that surgery is necessary and lasting until the patient is transferred to the operating room), the intraoperative phase (starts from the arrival in the operating room until transfer to the recovery room), and the postoperative phase (begins with transfer to recovery room and lasts until complete recovery from surgery)

pneumonia: inflammation or infection of the lungs

thrombophlebitis: inflammation in a vein associated with thrombus formation

A wide range of illnesses and injuries may require treatment that includes some type of surgical intervention. Surgery may be planned or unplanned, major or minor, invasive or noninvasive, and may involve any body part or system. A surgical procedure of any extent is a stressor that requires physical and psychosocial adaptations (Fundamentals Review 6-1) for both the patient and the family. The patient's recovery from a surgical procedure requires skillful and knowledgeable nursing care.

Nursing care provided for the patient before, during, and after surgery is called perioperative nursing. Perioperative nursing involves three phases: preoperative phase, beginning with the decision, together with the surgeon, that surgery is necessary and will take place, and lasting until the patient is transferred to the operating room (OR) bed; the intraoperative phase, which begins when the patient is transferred to the OR bed, also called a table, until transfer to the postsurgical recovery area; and the postoperative phase, lasting from admission to the recovery area to complete recovery from surgery. All phases of the nursing process are used in providing nursing care to promote the recovery of health, to prevent further injury or illness, and to facilitate coping with alterations in physical structure and function.

Surgical procedures may be inpatient, performed in a hospital, or ambulatory or outpatient, performed in either a hospital-based surgical center, a freestanding surgical center, or a physician's office. In an ambulatory or outpatient center, the patient goes to the surgical area the day of surgery and returns home on the same day. Whether the surgery is performed in the inpatient or outpatient setting, consistent written policies and procedures for perioperative care grounded in evidence-based practice and agency policy must be followed to ensure patient safety.

In the ambulatory surgery setting, the nurse follows specific criteria and guidelines while conducting the preadmission assessment which includes collecting pertinent physical, emotional, and cultural data (Fundamentals Review 6-2). This preadmission assessment can be accomplished through a telephone call or a face-to face interview. A preoperative teaching plan should include preoperative instructions and patient preparation (Fundamentals Review 6-3 and 6-4). This teaching should include the patient's family members or guardian. For certain types of elective surgery such as joint replacements, patients participate in a group patient teaching session before their admission to the hospital. Nurses may also complete a preoperative checklist (Figure 6-1).

The postoperative care of the patient begins immediately after the surgical procedure is completed. For inpatient surgery, this involves a short stay in the PACU (postanesthesia care unit) for about 1 to 2 hours, depending on the type of surgery and the patient's condition. After this time period and when the patient's condition is stabilized, the patient may be transferred either to the intensive care unit if more in-depth monitoring and nursing care is required, or to the surgical floor in the hospital. In the ambulatory care setting, the patient will be discharged to home. To ensure early identification of complications and address any patient concerns, the patient will receive a telephone call the following day after ambulatory care surgery. Nursing care throughout the postoperative period includes ongoing assessments, monitoring for complications, implementing specific nursing interventions, and patient and family teaching as needed. Before discharge from either the ambulatory care unit or the hospital, all patients will receive both oral and written discharge instructions and information regarding a follow-up appointment with the surgeon.

This chapter will cover the skills to assist the nurse in providing safe perioperative nursing care to the patient.

Fundamentals Review 6-1

Nursing Interventions to Meet Psychological Needs of Patients Having Surgery

- Establish and maintain a therapeutic relationship, allowing the patient to verbalize fears and concerns.
- Use active listening skills to identify and validate verbal and nonverbal messages revealing anxiety and fear.
- Use touch, as appropriate, to demonstrate genuine empathy and caring.
- Be prepared to respond to common patient questions about surgery:
  Will I lose control of my body functions while I'm having surgery?
  How long will I be in the operating room and PACU?
  Where will my family be?
  Will I have pain when I wake up?
  Will the anesthetic make me sick?
  Will I need a blood transfusion?
  How long will it be before I can eat?
  What kind of scar will I have?
  When will I be able to be sexually active?
  When can I go back to work?

Fundamentals Review 6-2

Preadmission Nursing Assessment for Ambulatory Surgery

Preadmission, the nurse assesses for the following:

- Baseline physical status
- Allergies and sensitivities
- Signs of abuse or neglect
- Cultural, emotional, and socioeconomic factors
- Pain (comprehensive assessment)
- Medication history, including nonprescription medications and supplements
- Anesthetic history
- Results of radiologic examinations and other preoperative testing
- Referrals
- Physical alterations that require additional equipment or supplies

The nurse also:

- Provides preoperative patient teaching
- Determines informed consent and/or knowledge of planned procedure
- Asks about advance directive
- Develops a plan of care
- Documents and communicates all information per facility policy

(Source: Association of Operating Room Nurses. [2005]. AORN guidance statement: Preoperative patient care in the ambulatory surgery setting, AORN, 81[4], 871–877)

Fundamentals Review 6-3

Preoperative Information for Ambulatory Surgery

Provide verbal and written instructions for patients having ambulatory surgery as follows:

- List medications routinely taken, and ask the physician which should be taken or omitted the morning of surgery.
- Notify the surgeon's office if a cold or infection develops before surgery.
- List allergies, and be sure the operating staff is aware of these.
- Remove nail polish and do not wear makeup for the procedure.
- Leave all jewelry and valuables at home.
- Wear clothing that buttons in front; short-sleeved garments are better for surgery on the hands.
- Have someone available for transportation home after recovery from anesthesia.

Inform patient of:

- Limitations on eating or drinking before surgery, with a specific time to begin the limitations.
- When and where to arrive for the procedure, as well as the estimated time when the procedure will be performed.

Fundamentals Review 6-4

Sample Preoperative Teaching: Activities and Events for In-Hospital Surgery

Preoperative Phase

- Exercises and physical activities
  - Deep-breathing exercises
  - Coughing
  - Incentive spirometry
  - Turning
  - Leg exercises
  - Pneumatic compression stockings
- Pain management
  - Meaning of PRN orders for medications
  - Timing for best effect of medications
  - Splinting incision
  - Nonpharmacologic pain-management options
- Visit by anesthesiologist
- Physical preparation
  - NPO
  - Sleeping medication the night before
  - Preoperative checklist (review items)
- Visitors and waiting room
- Transported to operating room by stretcher

Intraoperative Phase

- Holding area
  - Skin preparation
  - Intravenous lines and fluids
  - Medications
- Operating room
  - Operating room bed
  - Lights and common equipment (eg, cardiac monitor, pulse oximeter, warming device, etc.)
  - Safety belt
  - Sensations
  - Staff

Postoperative Phase

- Postanesthesia care unit
  - Frequent vital signs, assessments (eg, orientation, movement or extremities, strength of grasp)
  - Dressings/drains/tubes/catheters
  - Intravenous lines
  - Pain medications/comfort measures
  - Family notification
  - Sensations
  - Airway/oxygen therapy/pulse oximetry
  - Staff
- Transfer to unit (on stretcher)
  - Frequent vital signs
  - Sensations
  - Pain medications/nonpharmacologic strategies
  - NPO, diet progression
  - Exercises
  - Early ambulation
  - Family visits

Preoperative Checklist

	YES	NO	N/A	INITIALS
Identification band in place	✓			PL
NPO	✓			PL
Pre-op bath or shower completed	✓			PL
Enema/douche given			✓	PL
Hospital gown	✓			PL
Underwear removed	✓			PL
Voided on call/Foley in place *voided*	✓			PL
Height & weight recorded *68 in* Height *151 lbs.* Weight				AK
Nail polish removed			✓	AK
Make-up removed			✓	AK
Hair ornaments removed			✓	AK
Jewelry removed (earrings, necklaces, bracelets, rings)	✓			AK
Valuables given to family or placed in safe	✓			AK
Dentures removed, placed/given to ________			✓	AK
Prosthesis removed, placed/given to ________			✓	AK
Contact lenses/(glasses) placed/given to *family*	✓			AK
Operative permit signed	✓			PL
Anesthesia permit signed	✓			PL
Hemeprofile, UA (report in chart/in computer)	✓			PL
EKG (report on chart/in computer)	✓			PL
Chest X-ray (report on chart/in computer)	✓			PL
Computer cards, addressograph plate with chart	✓			PL
Medication (record in chart/in computer)	✓			PL
Pre-op teaching completed by *P. LeMone, RN* (see plan)				PL
Side rails up	✓			AK
Allergy sticker on chart front/allergy bracelet on	✓			AK
Correct operative site marked with an X	✓			PL
If no, was the surgeon notified?				
Oxygen ________ liters per nasal cannula ________% per face mask			✓	PL
History and physical updated with last 7 days	✓			PL
Type and cross match done. Number of units of blood set up *2*	✓			PL

Preoperative vital signs: *98.4 - 68 - 16 - 126/78*

Allergies: *none*

Preoperative medications given (time and route) *to be given in preop holding*

Comments: *family will be in surgery waiting room*

Transported to OR per: *cart* Accompanied by *wife*

Date: *10/02/04* Time: *1300* Signed *P. LeMone, RN* (RN or LPN)

Signed *A. Koeplin* (transport personnel)

Figure 6-1. Example of a preoperative checklist.

SKILL 6-1 Providing Preoperative Patient Care: Hospitalized Patient

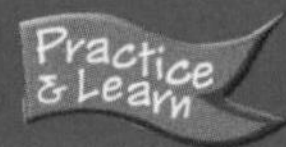

The preoperative phase consists of the time from when it is decided that surgery is needed until the patient arrives in the operating room. This time involves physical, emotional, and cultural assessments of the patient. Patient and family education is conducted at this time. The nurse provides emotional support and allays anxiety as appropriate throughout the preoperative period.

Equipment (will vary depending on the type of surgery)

- Blood pressure cuffs
- Electronic blood pressure machine
- Pulse oximeter sensors
- IV pump
- Antiembolism stockings
- Pneumatic compression stockings
- Tubes, drains, vascular access tubing
- Incentive spirometer
- Small pillow

ASSESSMENT

The preoperative nursing assessment includes a complete baseline health assessment and is completed upon admission. This assessment can begin in various settings, such as the surgeon's office or an inpatient unit. Interview the patient to determine medical and surgical history, including allergies, as well as any emotional, socioeconomic, cultural, and spiritual factors that may influence the patients' care. Ask about/review medications the patient is taking, including nonprescription, herbal medications and supplements, as well as illicit drugs. Any relevant preoperative needs of the patient or family should be explored. If the patient has a preferred speaking language other than English, it is essential to note this in the patient's record. Conduct physical assessments of the skin, respiratory, cardiovascular, abdominal, neurologic, and musculoskeletal function. Take the patient's vital signs. Any assessment abnormalities or areas of concern will need to be communicated to the physician. It is important for the nurse to identify patients who are considered more at risk, such as the very young and very old; obese or malnourished patients; patients with fluid and electrolyte imbalances, patients with chronic disease; patients taking certain medications (such as anticoagulants or analgesics), and patients who are extremely anxious. Depending on the particular at-risk patient, specific assessments and interventions may be warranted.

NURSING DIAGNOSIS

Determine related factors for the nursing diagnosis based on the patient's current status. Appropriate nursing diagnoses may include:

- Anxiety
- Anticipatory Grieving
- Risk for Spiritual Distress
- Fear
- Deficient Knowledge
- Risk for Infection
- Risk for Impaired Physical Mobility
- Risk for Fluid Volume Imbalance
- Risk for Alteration in Nutrition
- Risk for Nausea
- Risk for Aspiration Response
- Risk for Hypothermia
- Risk for Latex Allergy Response

SKILL 6-1 Providing Preoperative Patient Care: Hospitalized Patient *(continued)*

OUTCOME IDENTIFICATION AND PLANNING

The expected outcome to achieve when providing preoperative patient care for the hospitalized patient is that the patient will proceed to surgery. Other outcomes that may be appropriate include the following: the patient will be free from anxiety and fear, and the patient will demonstrate an understanding of the need for surgery and the measures to minimize the postoperative risks associated with surgery.

IMPLEMENTATION

ACTION	RATIONALE
1. Check the patient's chart for the type of surgery and review the physician's orders. Review the nursing database, history, and physical examination. Check that the baseline data are recorded; report those that are abnormal (Figure 1).	Ensures that the care will be provided for the right patient and any specific teaching based on the type of surgery will be addressed. Also, review identifies patients who are surgical risks.

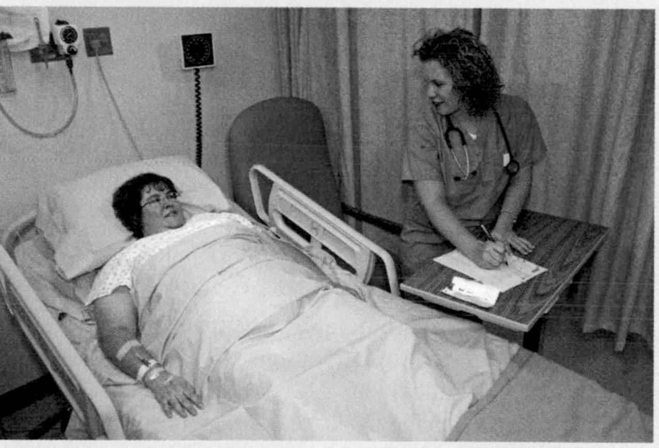

Figure 1. Reviewing baseline data and checking forms.

ACTION	RATIONALE
2. **Check that diagnostic testing has been completed and results are available; identify and report abnormal results.**	This check may influence the type of surgery performed and anesthetic used, as well as the timing of surgery or the need for additional consultation.
3. Gather needed equipment and supplies.	Adequate preparation ensures efficient time management.
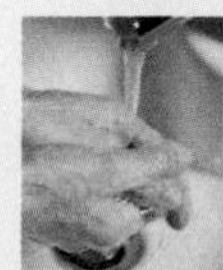 4. Perform hand hygiene.	Hand hygiene deters the spread of microorganisms.
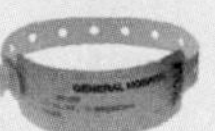 5. Identify the patient.	Identification of the patient ensures that the right patient receives the correct care.
6. Explore the psychological needs of the patient related to the surgery as well as the family.	Meeting the psychological needs of the patient and family before surgery can have a beneficial effect on the postoperative course.
a. Establish the therapeutic relationship, encouraging the patient to verbalize concerns or fears.	
b. Use active learning skills, answering questions and clarifying any misinformation.	

(continued)

SKILL 6-1 Providing Preoperative Patient Care: Hospitalized Patient *(continued)*

ACTION | **RATIONALE**

c. Use touch, as appropriate, to convey genuine empathy.

d. Offer to contact spiritual counselor (priest, minister, rabbi) to meet spiritual needs.

Spiritual beliefs for some patients and family can provide a source of support over the perioperative course.

7. **Identify learning needs of patient and family.** Ensure that the informed consent of the patient for the surgery has been signed, witnessed, and dated. Inquire if the patient has any questions regarding the surgical procedure. Check the patient's record to determine if an advance directive has been completed. If an advance directive has not been completed, discuss with the patient the possibility of completing as appropriate. If patient has had surgery before, ask about this experience.

This enhances surgical recovery and allays anxiety by preparing patient for postoperative convalescence, discharge plans, and self-care. The surgeon is responsible for explaining the details of the surgical procedure and potential risks and complications. The nurse is responsible for clarifying what the surgeon has explained to the patient and contacting the surgeon if the patient does not understand or has further questions. An advance directive provides written communication of the patient's wishes to the healthcare team related to the patient's desire for extraordinary life-sustaining treatments if the patient's condition is deemed unsalvageable. Previous surgical experience may impact preoperative care positively or negatively, depending on this past experience.

8. Provide teaching about deep-breathing exercises.

Deep-breathing exercises improve lung expansion and volume, help expel anesthetic gases and mucus from the airway, and facilitate the oxygenation of body tissues. Coughing helps remove retained mucus from the respiratory tract. Splinting minimizes pain while coughing or moving.

a. Assist or ask the patient to sit up (semi-Fowler's position) and instruct the patient to place the palms of both hands along the lower anterior rib cage (Figure 2).

The upright position promotes chest expansion and lessens exertion of the abdominal muscles. Positioning the hands on the rib cage allows the patient to feel the chest rise and the lungs expand as the diaphragm descends.

b. Instruct the patient to exhale gently and completely.

c. Instruct the patient to breathe in through the nose as deeply as possible and hold breath for 3 seconds.

d. Instruct the patient to exhale through the mouth, pursing the lips like when whistling.

e. Have the patient practice the breathing exercise three times. Instruct the patient that this exercise should be performed every 1 to 2 hours for the first 24 hours after surgery.

Return demonstration ensures that the patient is able to perform the exercises properly.

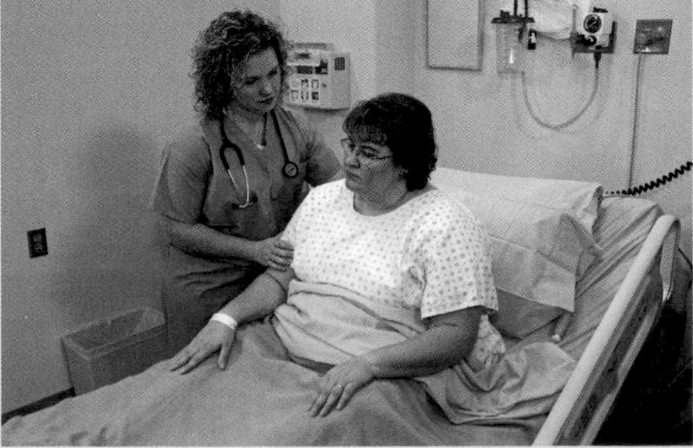

Figure 2. Assisting patient to semi-Fowler's position, leaning forward.

SKILL 6-1

Providing Preoperative Patient Care: Hospitalized Patient *(continued)*

ACTION	RATIONALE
9. Conduct teaching regarding coughing and splinting (providing support to the incision).	Coughing helps remove retained mucus from the respiratory tract. Splinting minimizes pain while coughing or moving.
a. Ask the patient to sit up (semi-Fowler's position) and apply a folded bath blanket or pillow against the part of the body where the incision will be (eg, abdomen or chest) (Figure 3).	These interventions aim to decrease discomfort while coughing.
b. Instruct the patient to inhale and exhale through the nose three times.	
c. Ask the patient to take a deep breath and hold it for 3 seconds and then cough out three short breaths (Figure 4 and Figure 5).	
d. Ask the patient to take a breath through his/her mouth and strongly cough again two times (Figure 6).	
e. Instruct the patient that he/she should perform these actions every 2 hours when awake after surgery.	

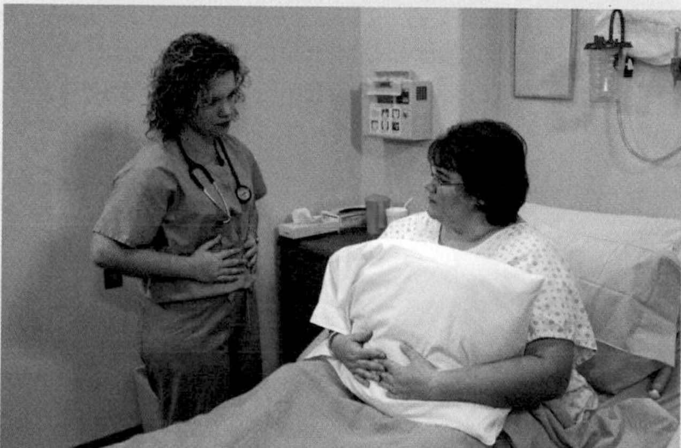

Figure 3. Having patient splint a chest or abdominal incision by holding a folded bath blanket or pillow against the incision.

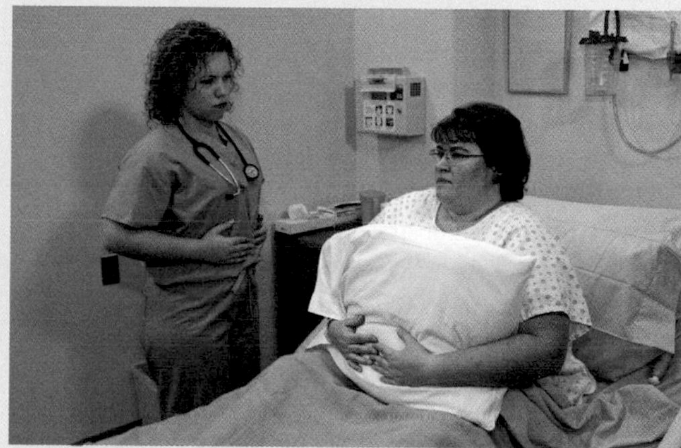

Figure 4. Telling patient to take a deep breath and holds for 3 seconds.

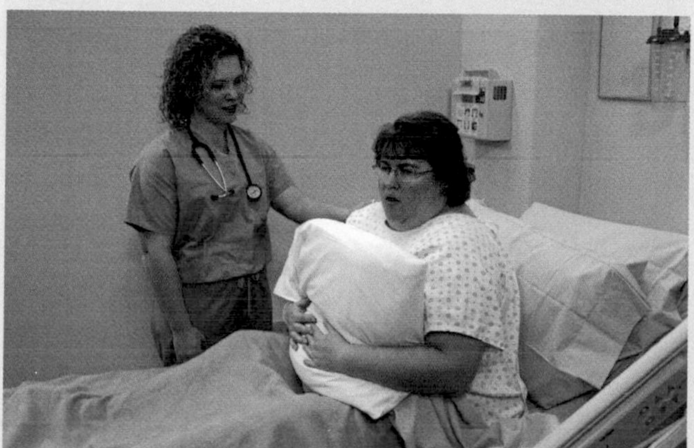

Figure 5. Encouraging patient to "hack" out three short coughs after holding breath.

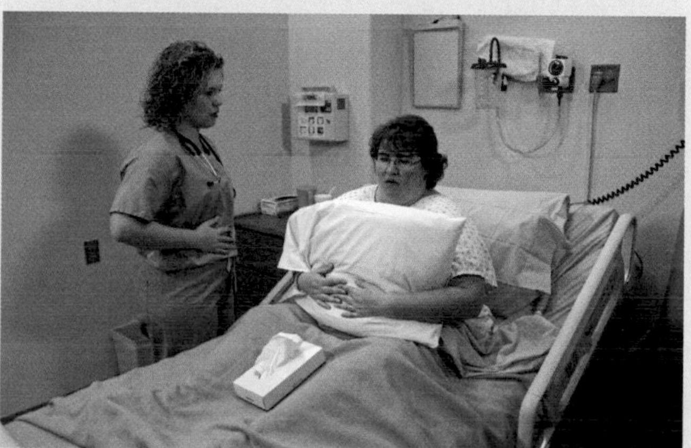

Figure 6. Encouraging patient to cough deeply once or twice and then take another deep breath.

(continued)

SKILL 6-1

Providing Preoperative Patient Care: Hospitalized Patient *(continued)*

ACTION

10. Provide teaching regarding incentive spirometer (Figure 7) (see Chapter 14 for skill practice).

RATIONALE

Incentive spirometry improves lung expansion, helps expel anesthetic gases and mucus from the airway, and facilitates oxygenation of body tissues.

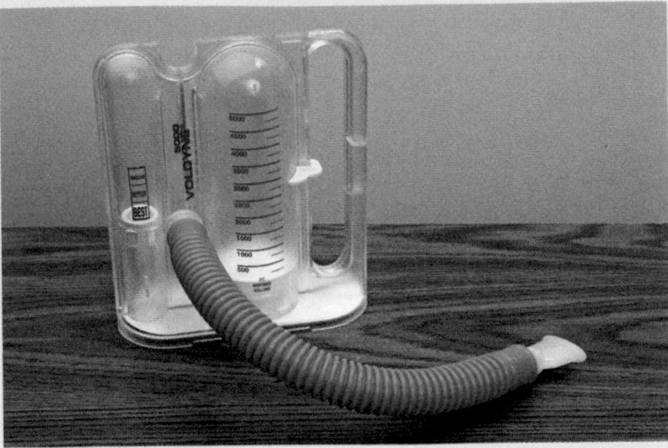

Figure 7. An incentive spirometer helps increase lung volume and promotes inflation of the alveoli.

11. Provide teaching regarding leg exercises.

Leg exercises assist in preventing muscle weakness, promote venous return, and decrease complications related to venous stasis.

a. Assist or ask the patient to sit up (semi-Fowler's position, Figure 8) and explain to patient that you will first demonstrate, and then coach him/her to exercise one leg at a time.
b. Straighten the patient's knee, raise the foot (Figure 9), extend the lower leg and hold this position for a few seconds (Figure 10). Lower the entire leg (Figure 11). Practice this exercise with the other leg.
c. Assist or ask the patient to point the toes of both legs toward the foot of the bed, then relax them (Figure 12). Next, flex or pull the toes toward the chin (Figure 13).
d. Assist or ask the patient to keep legs extended and to make circles with both ankles, first circling to the left and then to the right (Figure 14). Instruct the patient to repeat these exercises three times.

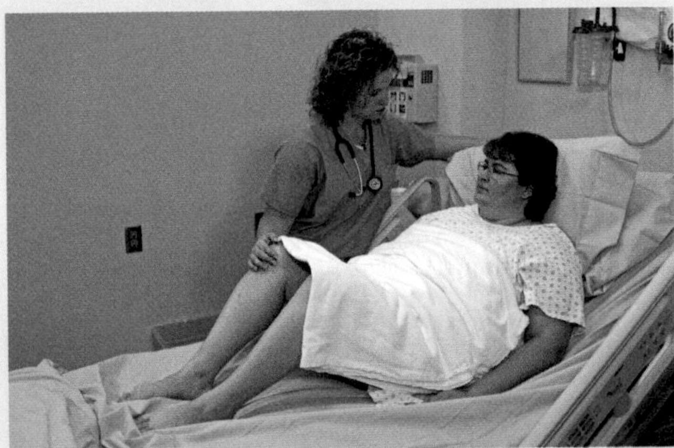

Figure 8. Assisting patient to a semi-Fowler's position.

SKILL 6-1

Providing Preoperative Patient Care: Hospitalized Patient *(continued)*

ACTION

RATIONALE

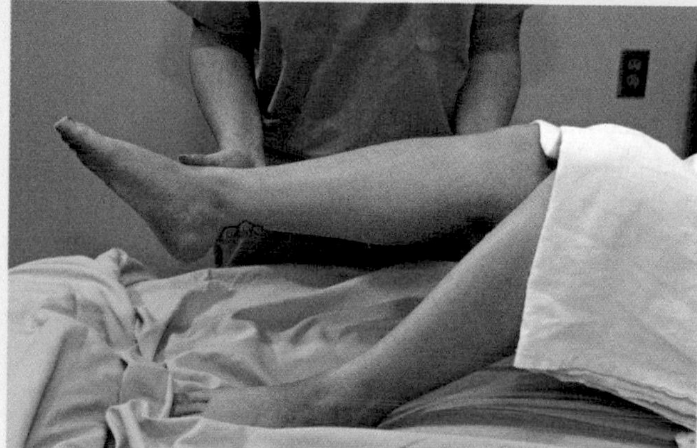
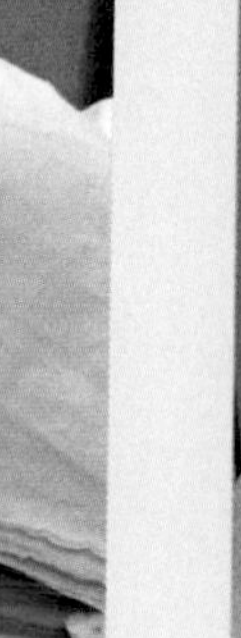

Figure 9. Raising patient's right foot and keeping it elevated for a few seconds.

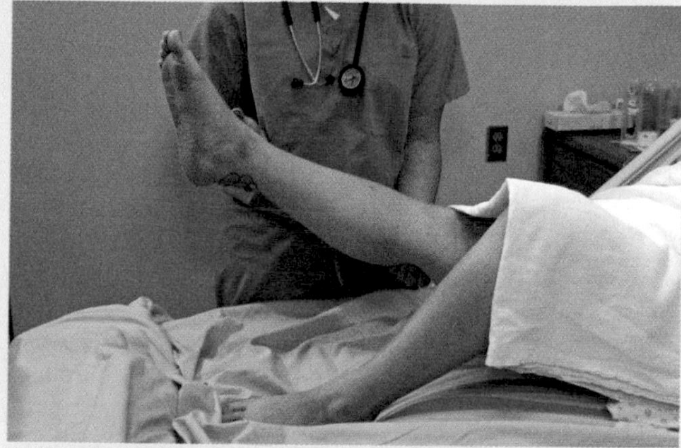

Figure 10. Extending the lower portion of the leg.

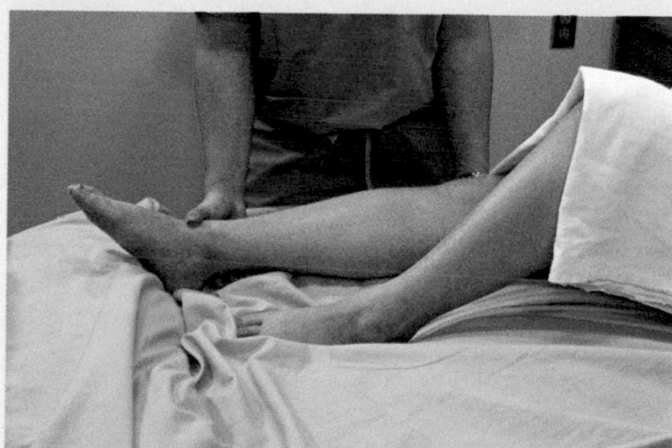

Figure 11. Lowering the entire leg to the bed.

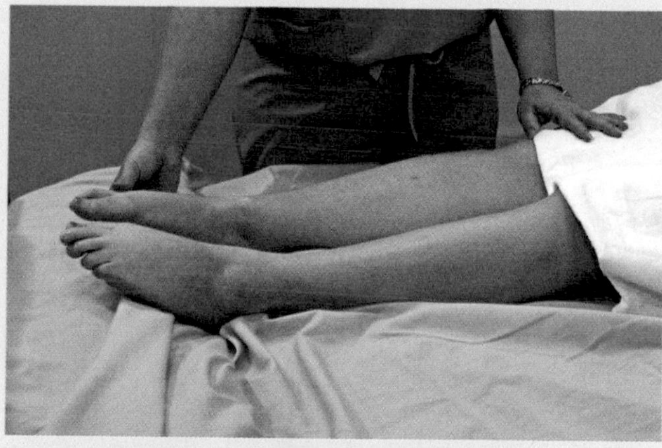

Figure 12. Pointing toes of both feet toward the foot of the bed, with both legs extended.

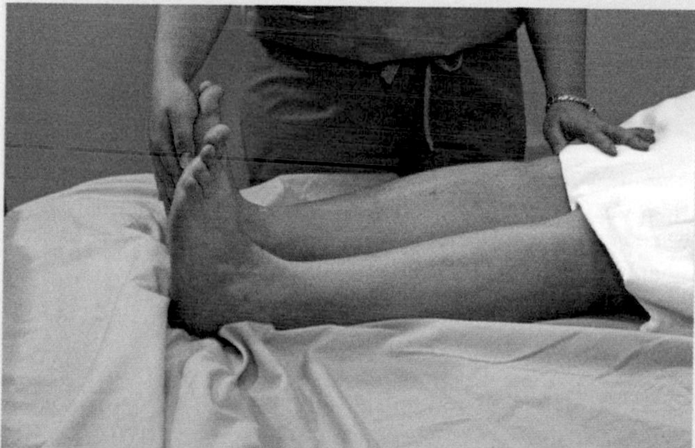

Figure 13. Pulling toes toward chin, as if a string were attached to them.

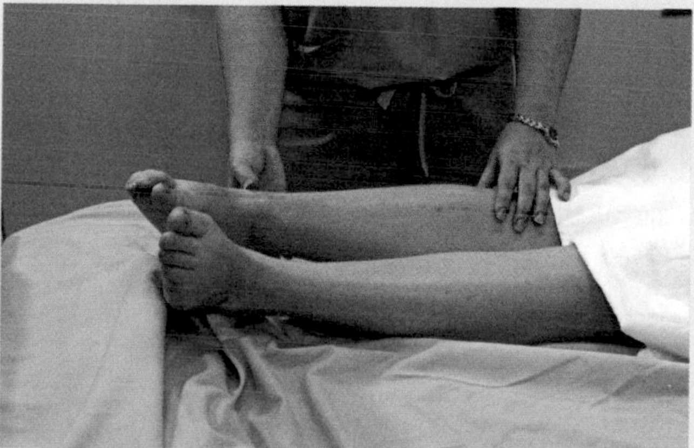

Figure 14. Having patient make circles with both ankles, first one way and then the other.

(continued)

SKILL 6-1 Providing Preoperative Patient Care: Hospitalized Patient *(continued)*

ACTION	RATIONALE
12. Assist the patient in putting on antiembolism stockings (see Chapter 7) and demonstrate how the pneumatic compression device operates (see Chapter 9).	Antiembolism stockings and pneumatic compression devices are used postoperatively for patients who are at risk for a deep-vein thrombosis (DVT) and pulmonary embolism.
13. Provide teaching regarding turning in the bed.	Turning and repositioning of the patient is important for prevention of postoperative complications and for minimizing pain.

a. Instruct the patient to use a pillow or bath blanket to splint where the incision will be. Ask the patient to raise his or her left knee and reach across to grasp the right side rail of the bed when he/she is turning toward his or her right side (Figure 15). If patient is turning to his or her left side, he or she will bend the right knee and grasp the left side rail.

b. When turning the patient onto his or her right side, ask the patient to push with bent left leg and pull on the right side rail (Figure 16). Explain to patient that the nurse will place a pillow behind his/her back to provide support, and that the call bell will be placed within easy reach (Figure 17).

c. Explain to the patient that position change is recommended every 2 hours.

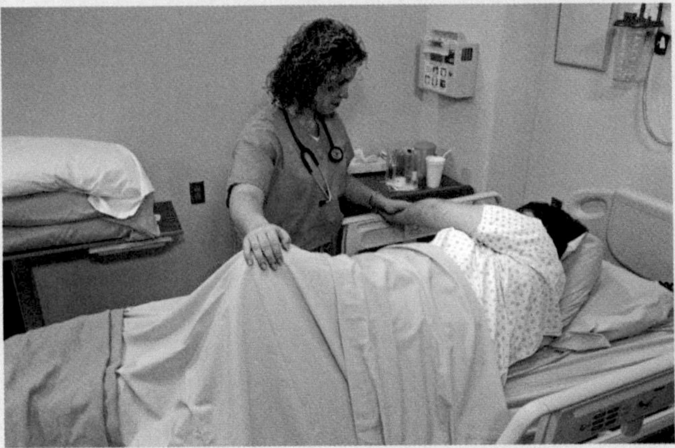

Figure 15. Instructing patient to raise the left knee and reach across to grasp the right side rail toward which she will be turning.

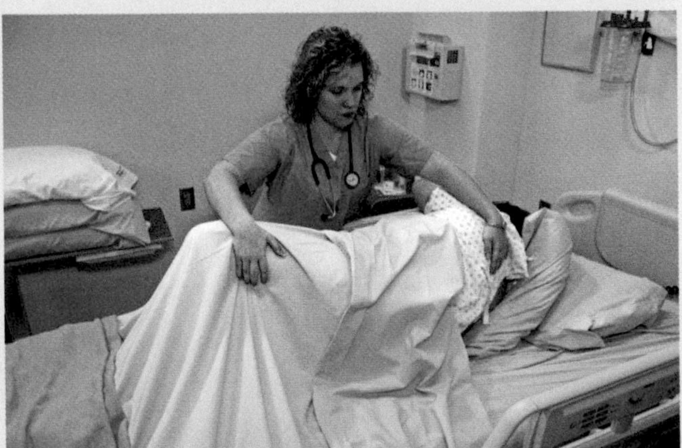

Figure 16. Helping patient to roll over to her right side while she pushes with the left bent leg and pulls on the side rail.

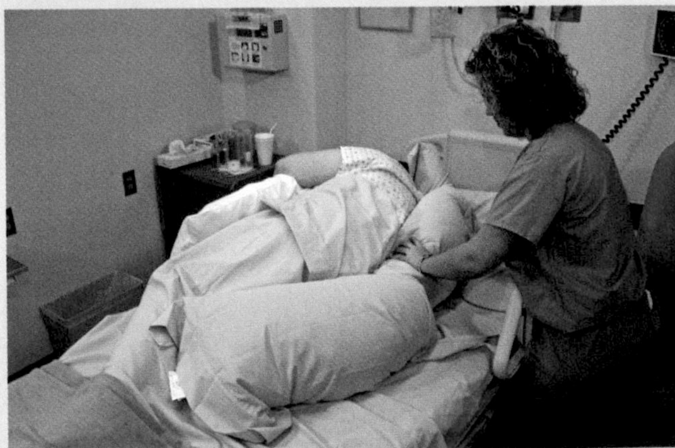

Figure 17. After patient is turned, providing support with pillows behind the patient's back.

ACTION	RATIONALE
14. Provide teaching about pain management.	Using ordered analgesics to minimize pain helps prevent postoperative complications.
a. Discuss past experiences with pain and interventions that the patient has used to reduce pain.	Past experiences with pain can impact patient's ability to manage the pain of surgery. Pain is a subjective experience and individuals vary on what interventions are effective in reducing pain.

SKILL 6-1

Providing Preoperative Patient Care: Hospitalized Patient *(continued)*

ACTION	RATIONALE
b. Discuss the availability of analgesic medication postoperatively.	Depending on the physician's order, the patient may need to request analgesic medication as needed, or a PCA (patient-controlled analgesia) or epidural analgesia may be ordered, for which patient will need specific instruction on how to use. See Chapter 10.
c. Explore the use of other alternative and nonpharmacologic methods to reduce pain, such as position change, massage, relaxation/diversion, guided imagery, and meditation.	These measures may reduce anxiety and may decrease the amount of pain medication that is needed. Analgesic therapy should involve a multimodal approach influenced by age, weight, and comorbidity.
15. Review equipment.	
a. Show the patient various equipment, such as IV pumps, electronic blood pressure cuff, tubes, and surgical drains.	Knowledge can reduce anxiety about equipment. The patient may need a Foley catheter during and after surgery to keep the bladder empty and to monitor urinary output. Drains are frequently used to remove excess fluid around the surgical incision.
16. Provide skin preparation.	An antiseptic shower may be ordered 1 or 2 days before surgery and repeated the morning of surgery to begin the process of preparing the skin before surgery and to prevent infection. Recent research advises against hair removal of the surgical site due to increased potential for infection. The CDC recommends that if shaving is necessary, it should be performed immediately before the surgery, using disposable supplies and aseptic technique. Follow agency policy on skin preparation of the surgical patient. Immediately before the surgical procedure, the skin of the patient's operative site will be cleansed with a product that is compatible with the antiseptic used for showering.
a. **Ask the patient to shower with the antiseptic solution. Remind the patient to carefully clean around the surgical site.**	
b. **For site-specific surgery such as a leg, ask the patient to mark the correct site with a marker.**	This ensures that the correct site is used.
17. Provide teaching about and follow dietary/fluid restrictions.	Common practice in preparation for surgery has included having the patient fast after midnight, nothing by mouth (NPO) the night before surgery. At times, this restriction involved fasting up to 10 to 12 hours when surgery was performed in the later part of the next day. Recent research on both adults and children is challenging this NPO standard or fasting practice before surgery, claiming that a less restricted fluid intake of clear fluids could be safely taken up to 6 hours before surgery for individuals who are considered low risk for aspiration or regurgitation. **Follow agency policy regarding the time period when this restriction will need to be followed.**
a. **Explain to the patient that both food and fluid will be restricted before surgery to ensure that the stomach contains a minimal amount of gastric secretions. This restriction is important to reduce the risk of aspiration. Emphasize to the patient the importance of avoiding food and fluids during the prescribed time period, since failure to adhere may necessitate cancellation of the surgery.**	
18. Provide intestinal preparation. In certain situations, the bowel will need to be prepared through the administering of enemas or laxatives to evacuate the bowel and to reduce the intestinal bacteria.	This preparation will be needed when major abdominal, perineal, perianal, or pelvic surgery is planned.

(continued)

SKILL 6-1 Providing Preoperative Patient Care: Hospitalized Patient *(continued)*

ACTION / **RATIONALE**

a. **As needed, provide explanation of the purpose of enemas or laxatives before surgery. If patient will be administering an enema, clarify the steps as needed.**

Enemas can be stressful, especially when repeated enemas are required to obtain a clear fluid return. Repeated enemas may cause fluid and electrolyte imbalance, orthostatic hypotension, and weakness. Follow safety precautions to guard against patient falls. Anesthetic agents and abdominal surgery can interfere with normal elimination function during the initial postoperative period. Refer to Chapter 13 to review skill for enema administration.

19. **Check administration of regularly scheduled medications.** Review with patient routine medications, OTC, and other herbal supplements that are taken regularly. Check the physician's orders and review with patient which meds he/she will be permitted to take the day of surgery.

Many patients take medications for a variety of chronic medical conditions. Adjustments in taking these medications may be needed before surgery. Certain medications such as aspirin are stopped days before surgery due to its anticoagulant effect. Certain cardiac and respiratory drugs may be taken the day of surgery per physician's order. If the patient is diabetic and takes insulin, the insulin dosage may be reduced.

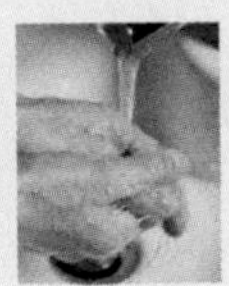

20. Perform hand hygiene.

Hand hygiene reduces transmission of microorganisms.

EVALUATION

The expected outcome is met when the patient prepares for surgery free from excessive anxiety and fear and demonstrates understanding of the importance of perioperative instructions.

DOCUMENTATION

Guidelines

Document that the patient's records were reviewed, including the history, physical assessment, and any laboratory values and diagnostic studies. Record that the surgeon was notified of any abnormal values. Document the components of perioperative teaching that were reviewed with the patient and family if present, such as use of the incentive spirometer, deep-breathing exercises, splinting, leg exercises, antiembolism (T.E.D.®) stockings, and pneumatic compression devices. Record the patient's ability to demonstrate the skills and response to the teaching, and note if any follow-up instruction needs to be performed. Document other preoperative teaching, including pain management, intestinal preparation, medications, and preoperative skin preparation. Record any patient concerns about the surgery and whether the surgeon was contacted to provide any further explanations. Document the emotional support that was offered to the patient and if a spiritual counselor was notified per request of patient.

Sample Documentation

4/2/08 1030 Patient's records were reviewed and no abnormal results were identified. Perioperative teaching points reviewed with patient and his wife, including the rationale for each of these points. Patient demonstrated proper use of incentive spirometry, deep breathing, splinting while coughing, and leg exercises. Reviewed pain management, intestinal preparation, medications, and preoperative skin preparation. Patient stated that he was anxious about the surgery since this will be his first time to the operating room. Emotional support and reassurance was provided.—J. Grabbs, RN

SKILL 6-1 Providing Preoperative Patient Care: Hospitalized Patient *(continued)*

Unexpected Situations and Associated Interventions

- *A patient's laboratory results are noted to be abnormal:* Notify physician. Some abnormalities, such as an elevated INR or abnormalities in the CBC may postpone the surgery.
- *A patient says to you, "I'm not sure I really want this surgery":* Discuss with the patient why he or she feels this way. Notify physician. Patients should not undergo surgery until they are sure that surgery is what they want.

Special Considerations

General Considerations

According to Dunn (2005), obese patients are at greater risk of surgical complications and death compared to optimal-weight patients. In taking the patient's history, the nurse needs to be alert for other medical conditions such as diabetes, hypertension, and sleep apnea.

Infant and Child Considerations

Children have special needs related to their overall health, age, and size. Easing preoperative anxiety of the child is crucial and includes using simple and concrete terms when providing information. Also, the nurse needs to be sensitive to the anxiety level of the parent and provide support, explanations, and patient teaching as needed. Accurate weights are essential for correct medication dosages. Historically, pediatric patients, at times, have been undertreated for pain. Developmentally appropriate pain assessment and therapy needs to be followed. Concerning the older adolescent, ask the patient in private when the parent is not in the room, if he/she uses any substances such as anabolic steroids (Dunn, 2005).

Older Adult Considerations

Age-related changes and preexisting chronic conditions can affect the postoperative course of the geriatric patient. The nurse may encounter resistance from the older patient during the informed consent process, and, thus, a nonjudgmental attitude by the nurse is important if the patient decides not to agree to the surgery. Also, concerning preoperative teaching, it is important to present information slowly with reinforcement, since processing of information can be slower. Due to communication barriers and the comorbidity of many geriatric patients who may respond differently to pain medication, pain assessment and therapy may be suboptimal. Therefore, careful and individualized attention is required in this more vulnerable age group.

SKILL 6-2 Providing Preoperative Patient Care: Hospitalized Patient (Day of Surgery)

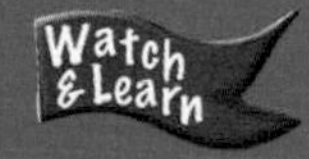

Due to the variety of outpatient and inpatient settings where elective surgery is performed, the day before surgery may be spent at home or in the hospital. If the patient will be arriving the morning of surgery to the surgical setting, he/she will receive a phone call the day before from a healthcare professional reminding the patient of the scheduled surgery, and key points such as showering with an antiseptic cleansing agent, NPO restrictions, and any other pertinent information related to the particular procedure. Additionally, the nurse will clarify any questions that the patient may have. If the patient is a hospitalized patient, the nurse will review the same information, clarify any concerns, and reinforce any perioperative instructions as needed.

Equipment

- Blood pressure cuffs
- Electronic blood pressure machine
- Thermometer
- Pulse oximeter sensors
- IV pump, IV solution vascular access tubing
- Antiembolism stockings
- Incentive spirometer

(continued)

SKILL 6-2 Providing Preoperative Patient Care: Hospitalized Patient (Day of Surgery) *(continued)*

ASSESSMENT

Assessment on the day of surgery involves taking vital signs and reporting any abnormalities in vital signs, as well as any abnormalities in laboratory and diagnostic results to the surgeon. Also, the nurse will review and complete the preoperative checklist (see Figure 6-1 in chapter introduction) and inquire if the patient or family members have any questions. Clarification will be provided as needed.

NURSING DIAGNOSIS

Determine related factors for the nursing diagnosis based on the patient's current status. Appropriate nursing diagnoses may include:

- Anxiety
- Anticipatory Grieving
- Fear
- Deficient Knowledge
- Risk for Infection
- Fatigue
- Risk for Impaired Physical Mobility
- Risk for Fluid Volume Imbalance
- Risk for Alteration in Nutrition
- Risk for Nausea
- Risk for Aspiration Response
- Risk for Hypothermia
- Risk for Latex Allergy Response

OUTCOME IDENTIFICATION AND PLANNING

The expected outcome to achieve when providing preoperative patient care for the hospitalized patient is that the patient will proceed to surgery. Other outcomes that may be appropriate include the following: the patient will be free from anxiety; the patient will be free from fear; and the patient will demonstrate an understanding of the need for surgery and the measures to minimize the postoperative risks associated with surgery.

IMPLEMENTATION

ACTION	RATIONALE
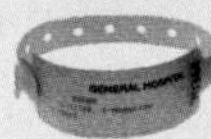 1. Identify the patient.	Identification of the patient ensures that the right patient receives the correct care.
2. Check that preoperative consent forms are signed, witnessed, and correct, that advance directives are in the medical record (as applicable), and that the patient's chart is in order.	This fulfills legal requirements related to informed consent and educates patient regarding advance directives.
3. Gather the needed equipment and supplies.	Adequate preparation ensures efficient time management.
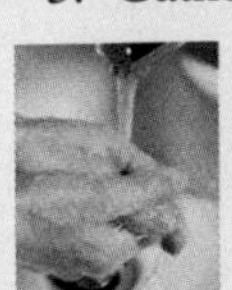 4. Perform hand hygiene.	Hand hygiene helps deter the spread of microorganisms.

SKILL 6-2

Providing Preoperative Patient Care: Hospitalized Patient (Day of Surgery) *(continued)*

ACTION	RATIONALE
5. **Check vital signs.** Notify physician of any pertinent changes (ie, rise or drop in blood pressure, elevated temperature, cough, symptoms of infection) (Figure 1).	This provides baseline data for comparison.

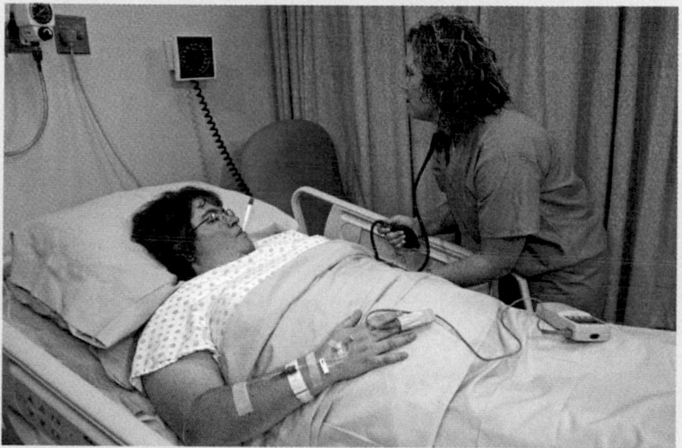

Figure 1. Obtaining preoperative vital signs.

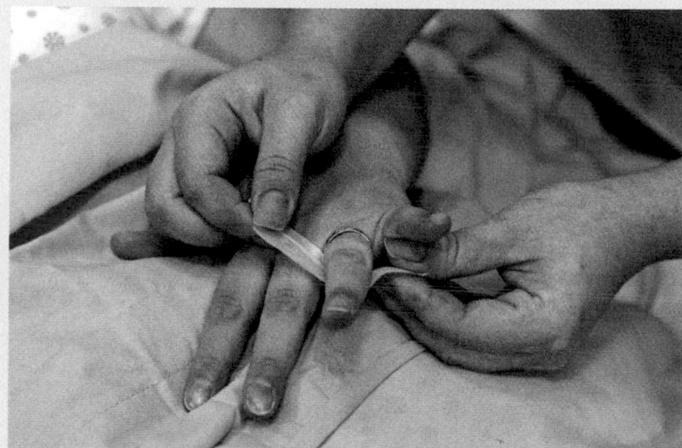

Figure 2. Taping wedding band in place.

ACTION	RATIONALE
6. Provide hygiene and oral care. Assess for loose teeth. **Remind patient of food and fluid restrictions before surgery.**	This promotes comfort and prevents intraoperative complications during anesthesia induction.
7. Instruct the patient to remove all personal clothing including underwear and put on a hospital gown.	Permits access to operative area and ease of assessment during the operative period.
8. Ask patient to remove cosmetics, jewelry including body-piercing, nail polish, and prostheses (eg, contact lenses, false eyelashes, dentures, and so forth). Some facilities allow a wedding band to be left in place depending on the type of surgery, provided it is secured to the finger with tape (Figure 2).	These interfere with assessment during surgery. Some hospital policies advise to have the patient wear eyeglasses and leave hearing aids in place if needed. Notify PACU nurse if patient wears hearing aids.
9. If possible, give valuables to family member or place valuables in appropriate area, such as the hospital safe, if this is not possible. They should not be placed in narcotics drawer.	This ensures safety of valuables and personal possessions. Document where valuables have been secured.
10. **Have patient empty bladder and bowel before surgery.**	An empty bladder and bowel minimize risk for injury or complications during and after surgery.
11. Attend to any special preoperative orders, such as starting an IV line.	This prepares patient for operative procedure.
12. Complete preoperative checklist and record of patient's preoperative preparation.	This ensures accurate documentation and communication with perioperative nurse caring for patient.

(continued)

SKILL 6-2 Providing Preoperative Patient Care: Hospitalized Patient (Day of Surgery) *(continued)*

ACTION	RATIONALE
13. **Administer preoperative medication as prescribed by physician/anesthesia provider.**	Medication reduces anxiety, provides sedation, and diminishes salivary and bronchial secretions. Preoperative medications may be given "on call" (when the OR nurse calls to tell the nurse to give the medication) or at a scheduled time. Certain patients undergoing specific cardiac, colorectal, gynecologic, ophthalmologic, and urinary surgical procedures may be given antibiotic prophylaxis before surgery.
14. Raise side rails of bed; place bed in lowest position. Instruct patient to remain in bed or on stretcher. If necessary, a safety belt may be used.	These actions ensure the patient's safety once the preoperative medication has been given.
15. Help move the patient from the bed to the transport stretcher if necessary. Reconfirm patient identification and ensure that all preoperative events and measures are documented (Figure 3).	Helping the patient move prevents injury. Reconfirming patient identity helps to ensure that the correct patient is being transported to surgery.

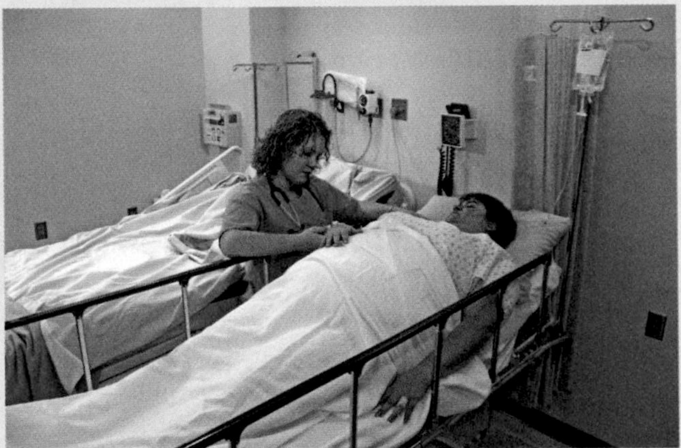

Figure 3. Confirming identification after patient moves from the bed to the stretcher.

ACTION	RATIONALE
16. Tell the family of the patient where the patient will be taken after surgery and the location of the waiting area where the surgeon will come to explain the outcome of the surgery.	If possible, take the family to the waiting area. Informing the family members of what to expect helps allay anxiety and avoid confusion.
17. After the patient leaves for the operating room, prepare the room and make a postoperative bed for the patient. Anticipate any necessary equipment based on the type of surgery and the patient's history.	Preparing for the patient's return helps to promote efficient care in the postoperative period.
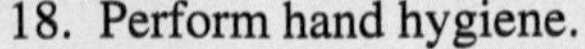 18. Perform hand hygiene.	Hand hygiene reduces the transmission of microorganisms.

SKILL 6-2

Providing Preoperative Patient Care: Hospitalized Patient (Day of Surgery) *(continued)*

EVALUATION

The expected outcome is met when the patient proceeds to surgery, is prepared for surgery so that he or she is free from anxiety and fear, and demonstrates understanding of the importance of pre- and postoperative instructions. Family members exhibit knowledge of what to expect over the remainder of the preoperative course.

DOCUMENTATION

Guidelines

Document that the preoperative checklist was completed and any special interventions that were ordered before sending the patient to the operating room. Record if there were any abnormal results that were communicated to the surgeon or OR nurse. Note if patient valuables were given to a family member. Document that the patient was safely transferred onto the stretcher and escorted to the operating room without incident. Record that the patient's family members were instructed as to where to wait to meet the surgeon after the surgery is performed.

Sample Documentation

4/3/08 0800 Preoperative checklist completed with no abnormalities noted, operative permit signed. Maintained NPO status throughout night. IV started into right forearm, #18-gauge needle inserted without difficulty. IV solution of 1000 cc of D5.45 sodium chloride at 80/cc per hour initiated. Patient verbalized that he will be glad when the surgery is over. Patient assisted onto stretcher for transfer to OR without difficulty. Family instructed to wait in surgical waiting lounge. —D. Irwin, RN

- *A patient admits he ate "just a little bit" this a.m. upon waking from sleep:* Notify the physician. The patient's surgery may have to be postponed for a few hours to prevent aspiration during surgery.
- *Identification band is not in place:* Ensure identity of patient and obtain new identification band. Patient cannot proceed to surgery without identification band. Two patient identifiers are required to meet current patient safety goals.
- *Consent form is not signed:* Notify physician. It is the physician's responsibility to obtain consent for surgery and anesthesia. Preoperative mediations cannot be given until the consent form is signed. The patient should not proceed to surgery without a signed consent form (unless it is an emergency).
- *Patient does not want to remove dentures before surgery, saying, "I never take my dentures out":* Discuss with surgeon or anesthesia provider. Patient may be allowed to go to the preoperative area with dentures and remove the dentures before entering the operating room.
- *Patient refuses to take preoperative medication:* Notify physician before patient goes to operating room. Many medications are necessary to protect the patient pre- or postoperatively.

Special Considerations

General Considerations

Appropriately sized equipment such as blood pressure cuffs, wide stretchers, and lift devices need to be available for obese patients.

(continued)

SKILL 6-2 Providing Preoperative Patient Care: Hospitalized Patient (Day of Surgery) *(continued)*

Infant and Child Considerations

- In many institutions, the parents are allowed to enter the preoperative area with the child. This has been shown to decrease the child's and the parents' anxiety.
- The breastfed infant may be allowed to nurse closer to the time of surgery than a bottle-fed infant would be allowed to have a bottle of formula. Breast milk is easier for the stomach to digest, so the clearance time is shorter than for formula.
- Children have special needs related to their overall health, age, and size. Appropriately sized blood pressure cuffs are essential.

Older Adult Considerations

Due to the prevalence of hearing and vision loss in this age group, the necessity of wearing eyeglasses and hearing aids is essential for processing preoperative teaching and throughout the postoperative course.

SKILL 6-3 Providing Postoperative Care When Patient Returns to Room

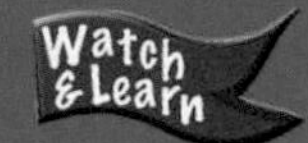

Postoperative care facilitates recovery from surgery and supports the patient in coping with physical changes or alterations. Nursing interventions promote physical and psychological health, prevent complications, and teach self-care skills for the patient to use after the hospital stay. After surgery, patients spend time on the postanesthesia care unit (PACU). From the PACU, they are transferred back to their rooms. At this time, nursing care focuses on accurate assessments and associated interventions. Ongoing assessments are crucial for early identification of postoperative complications.

Equipment (will vary depending upon the surgery)

- Electronic blood pressure machine
- Blood pressure cuff
- Electronic thermometer
- Pulse oximeter sensors
- IV pump, IV solutions
- Antiembolism stockings
- Pneumatic compression boots
- Tubes, drains, vascular access tubing
- Incentive spirometer
- Blankets as needed

ASSESSMENT

A wide variety of factors increase the risk for postoperative complications. Ongoing postoperative assessments and interventions are used to decrease the risk for postoperative complications. Assessment of the patient's and family's learning needs is also important.

NURSING DIAGNOSIS

Determine the related factors for the nursing diagnosis based on the patient's current status. Appropriate nursing diagnoses may include the following:

- Anxiety
- Risk for Spiritual Distress
- Risk for Aspiration
- Disturbed Body Image
- Risk for Imbalanced Body Temperature
- Hypothermia
- Risk for Infection
- Impaired Skin Integrity

SKILL 6-3
Providing Postoperative Care When Patient Returns to Room *(continued)*

- Risk for Perioperative Positioning Injury
- Impaired Physical Mobility
- Acute Pain
- Risk for Fluid Volume Imbalance
- Risk for Latex Allergy Response

Depending on the type and extent of surgery, other nursing diagnoses may apply, such as Ineffective Airway Clearance, Impaired Gas Exchange, Impaired Urinary Elimination, or Deficient Fluid Volume.

OUTCOME IDENTIFICATION AND PLANNING

The expected outcome to achieve when providing postoperative care to a patient is that the patient will recover from the surgery. Other outcomes that may be appropriate include the following: patient is free from anxiety; patient is comfortable with body image; patient's temperature remains between 36.5° and 37.5°C (97.7°–99.5°F); patient will remain free from infection; patient will not experience any skin breakdown; patient will regain mobility; and patient will have pain managed appropriately.

IMPLEMENTATION

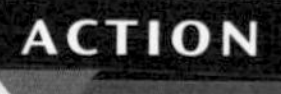

ACTION	RATIONALE
Immediate Care	
1. When patient returns from the PACU, obtain a report from the PACU nurse and review the operating room and PACU data.	Obtaining report ensures accurate communication and promotes continuity of care.
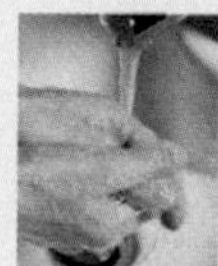 2. Perform hand hygiene.	Hand hygiene deters the spread of microorganisms.
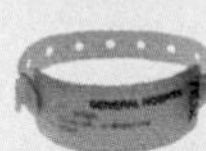 3. Identify the patient.	Identification of the patient ensures that the right patient receives the correct care.
4. Place patient in safe position (semi- or high Fowler's or side-lying) (Figure 1). Note level of consciousness.	A sitting position facilitates deep breathing; the side-lying position with neck slightly extended prevents aspiration and airway obstruction.

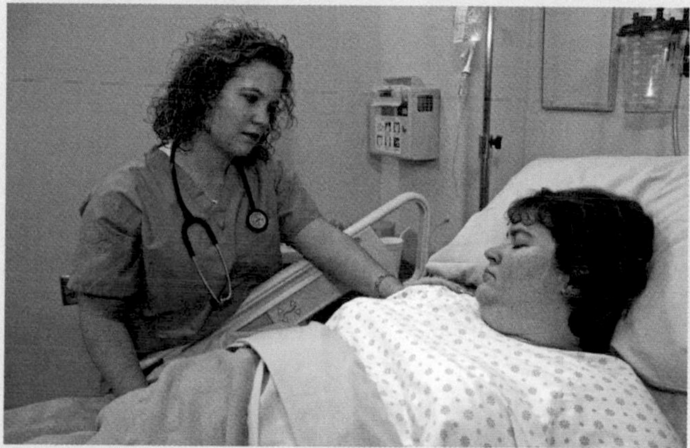

Figure 1. Placing the patient in a safe position (high Fowler's or side-lying).

(continued)

SKILL 6-3 Providing Postoperative Care When Patient Returns to Room *(continued)*

ACTION	RATIONALE
5. **Obtain vital signs (Figure 2). Monitor and record vital signs frequently.** Assessment order may vary, but usual frequency includes taking vital signs every 15 minutes the first hour, every 30 minutes the next 2 hours, every hour for 4 hours, and finally every 4 hours.	Comparison with baseline preoperative vital signs may indicate impending shock or hemorrhage. Some institutions use a paper or computer flow sheet to record initial postoperative data.
6. Provide for warmth, using heated blankets as necessary (Figure 3). Assess skin color and condition.	The operating room is a cold environment. Hypothermia is uncomfortable and may lead to cardiac arrhythmias and impaired wound healing.

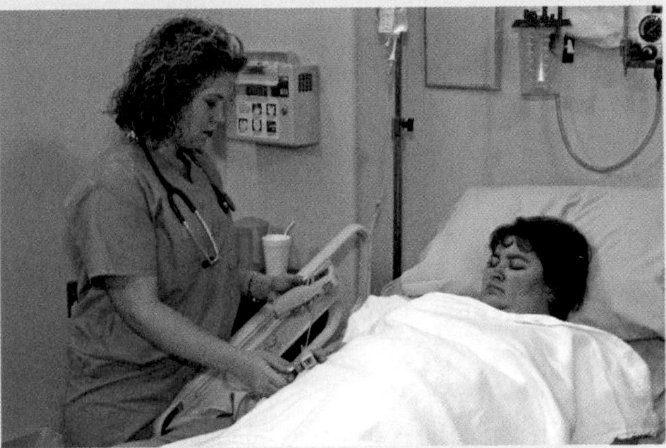

Figure 2. Obtaining postoperative vital signs.

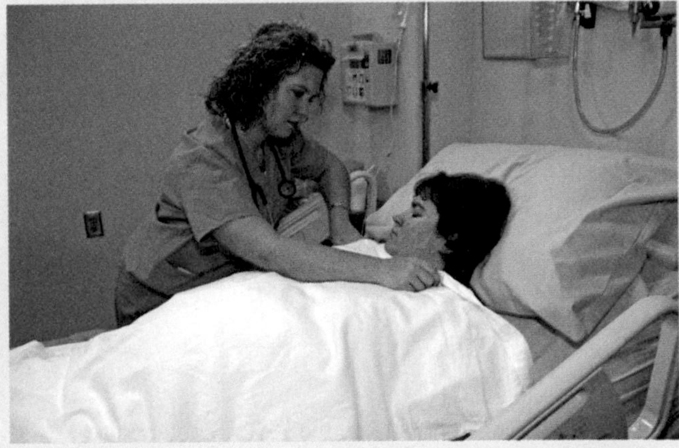

Figure 3. Providing comfort and warmth to the patient.

ACTION	RATIONALE
7. **Check dressings for color, odor, presence of drains, and amount of drainage (Figure 4). Mark the drainage on the dressing by circulating the amount, and include the time. Assess under the patient for bleeding from the surgical site (Figure 5).**	Hemorrhage and shock are life-threatening complications of surgery and early recognition is essential.

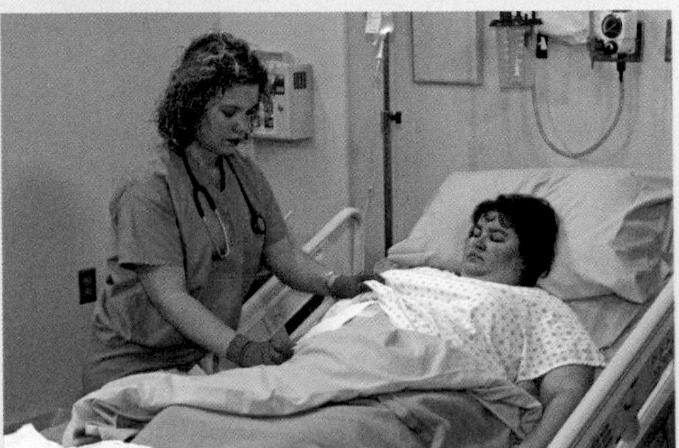

Figure 4. Checking the dressings for color, odor, and amount of drainage.

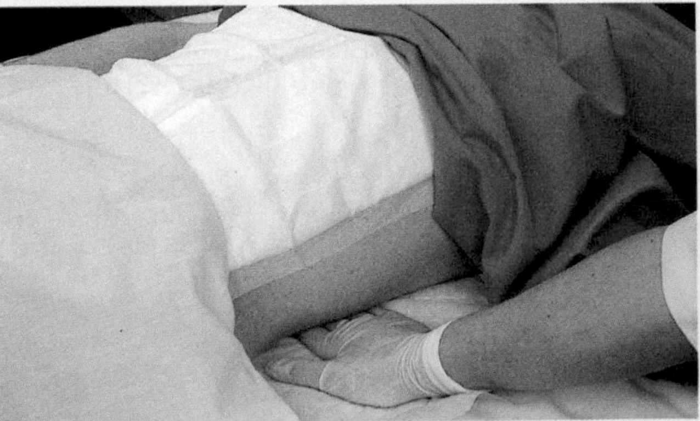

Figure 5. Assessing underneath patient for bleeding.

ACTION	RATIONALE
8. **Verify that all tubes and drains are patent and equipment is operative; note amount of drainage in collection device. If Foley catheter in place, note urinary output.**	This ensures maintenance of vital functions.

SKILL 6-3

Providing Postoperative Care When Patient Returns to Room *(continued)*

ACTION	RATIONALE
9. Maintain IV infusion at correct rate (Figure 6).	This replaces fluid loss and prevents dehydration and electrolyte imbalances.

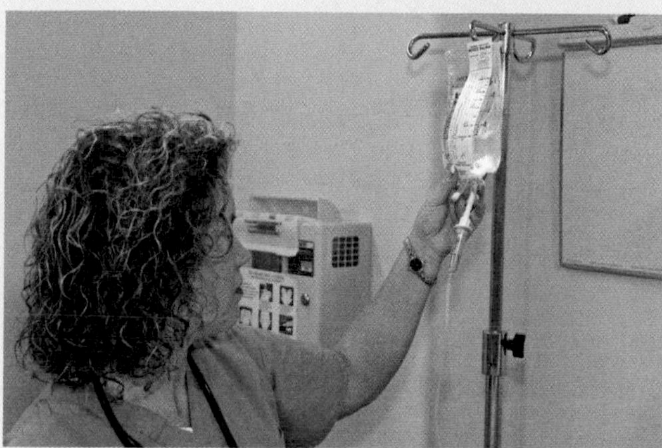

Figure 6. Checking the IV infusion.

ACTION	RATIONALE
10. Provide for a safe environment. Keep bed in low position with side rails up. Have call bell within patient's reach.	This prevents accidental injury. Easy access to call light permits patient to call for nurse when necessary.
11. Assess for and relieve pain by administering medications ordered by physician. If patient has been instructed in use of PCA for pain management, review use. Check record to verify if analgesic medication was administered in the PACU.	Observe for nonverbal behavior that may indicate pain, such as grimacing, crying, and restlessness. Analgesics and other nonpharmacologic pain strategies are used for relief of postoperative pain.
12. Record assessments and interventions on chart.	This provides for accurate documentation.
Ongoing Care	
13. Promote optimal respiratory function.	Anesthetic agents may depress respiratory function. Patients who have existing respiratory or cardiovascular disease, have abdominal or chest incisions, who are obese, elderly, or in a poor state of nutrition are at greater risk for respiratory complications.
a. Assess respiratory rate, depth, quality, color, and capillary refill. Ask if any difficulty breathing.	Postoperative analgesic medication can reduce the rate and quality of the respiratory effort.
b. Assist with coughing and deep-breathing exercises (Figure 7).	
c. Assist with incentive spirometry.	
d. Assist with early ambulation.	
e. Provide frequent position change.	
f. Administer oxygen as ordered.	
g. Monitor pulse oximetry.	

(continued)

SKILL 6-3

Providing Postoperative Care When Patient Returns to Room *(continued)*

ACTION

RATIONALE

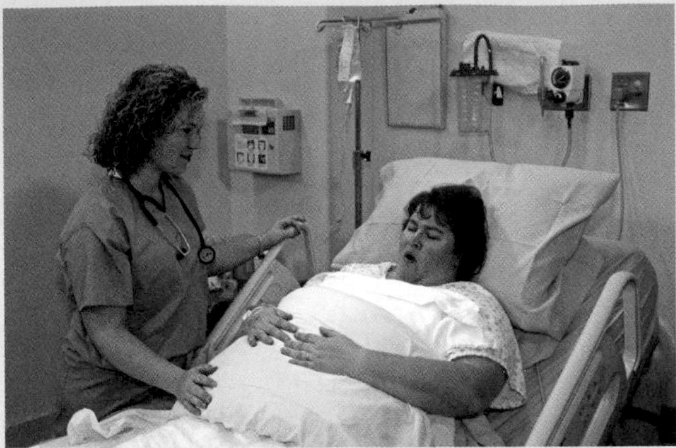

Figure 7. Assisting patient in performing coughing exercises.

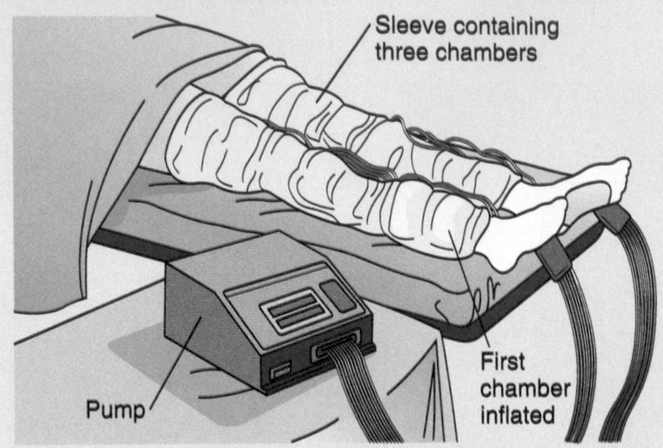

Figure 8. Using pneumatic compression device.

14. Promote optimal cardiovascular function:

Preventive measures can improve venous return and circulatory status.

a. Assess apical rate, rhythm, and quality and compare to peripheral pulses, color, and blood pressure. Ask if the patient has any chest pains or shortness of breath.
b. Provide frequent position changes.
c. Assist with early ambulation.
d. Apply antiembolism stockings or pneumatic compression devices, if ordered by physician (Figure 8).
e. Provide leg and range-of-motion exercises if not contraindicated.

15. Promote optimal neurologic function:

a. Assess level of consciousness, motor, and sensation.
b. Determine the level of orientation to person, place, and time.

Older patients will take longer to return to their level of orientation before surgery. Drug and anesthetics will delay this return.

c. Test motor ability by asking the patient to move each extremity.

Anesthesia alters motor and sensory function.

d. Evaluate sensation by asking the patient if he/she can feel your touch on an extremity.

16. **Promote optimal renal and urinary function and fluid and electrolyte status. Assess intake and output, for urinary retention and serum electrolytes.**

Anesthetic agents and surgical manipulation in the area may temporarily depress bladder tone and response causing urinary retention.

a. Promote voiding by offering bedpan at regular intervals, noting the frequency, amount, and if any burning or urgency symptoms.

Urine output is close to the total intake for a 24-hour period.

b. Monitor urinary catheter drainage if present.

The physician needs to be notified if the urinary output is less than 30 mL/hr or 240 cc/8-hr period.

c. Measure intake and output.

SKILL 6-3

Providing Postoperative Care When Patient Returns to Room *(continued)*

ACTION	RATIONALE
17. Promote optimal gastrointestinal function and meet nutritional needs:	Anesthetic agents and narcotics depress peristalsis and normal functioning of gastrointestinal tract. Flatus indicates return of peristalsis
a. Assess abdomen for distention and firmness. Ask if patient feels nauseated, any vomiting, and if passing flatus.	
b. Auscultate for bowel sounds (Figure 9).	Presence of bowel sounds indicates return of peristalsis.
c. Assist with diet progression.	Patients may experience nausea postsurgery and are encouraged to resume diet slowly, starting with clear liquids and advancing as tolerated. Antiemetics are frequently ordered to alleviate nausea.
d. Encourage fluid intake.	
e. Monitor intake.	
f. Medicate for nausea and vomiting as ordered by physician.	

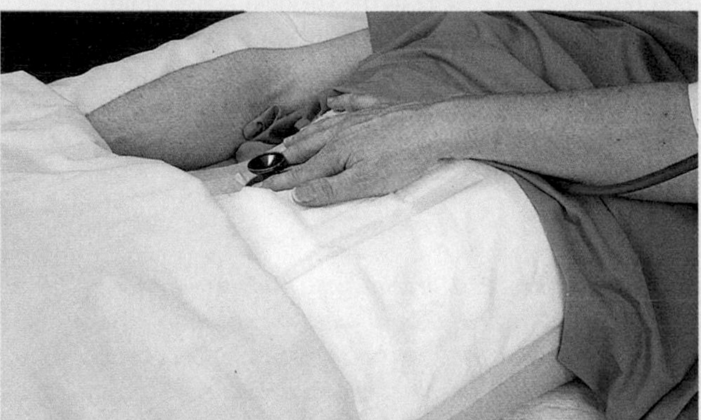

Figure 9. Assessing for bowel sounds.

ACTION	RATIONALE
18. Promote optimal wound healing.	Alterations in nutritional, circulatory, and metabolic status may predispose patient to infection and delayed healing.
a. Assess condition of wound for presence of drains and any drainage.	
b. Use surgical asepsis for dressing changes.	
c. Inspect all skin surfaces for beginning signs of pressure ulcer development and use pressure-relieving supports to minimize potential skin breakdown.	Lying on the operating room table in the same position can predispose some patients to pressure ulcer formation, especially in patients who have undergone surgery lasting more then 4 hours.
19. Promote optimal comfort and relief from pain.	
a. Assess for pain (location and intensity using scale).	
b. Provide for rest and comfort.	This shortens recovery period and facilitates return to normal function. Provide extra blankets as needed for warmth.
c. Administer pain medications as needed or other nonpharmacologic methods.	

(continued)

SKILL 6-3 Providing Postoperative Care When Patient Returns to Room *(continued)*

ACTION	RATIONALE
20. Promote optimal meeting of psychosocial needs: a. Provide emotional support to patient and family as needed. b. Explain procedures and offer explanations regarding postoperative recovery as needed to both patient and family members.	This facilitates individualized care and patient's return to normal health.

EVALUATION

The expected outcome is met when the patient recovers from surgery; is free from anxiety; is comfortable with self-image; has a temperature of 36.5° to 37.5°C (97.7°–99.5°F); remains free from infection; develops no pressure ulcers or areas of skin breakdown; has a dressing that is clean, dry, and intact; can ambulate (if able before surgery); and achieves adequate pain control.

DOCUMENTATION

Guidelines

Document the time that the patient returns from PACU to the surgical hospital unit. Record the patient's level of consciousness, vital signs, and condition of dressing. If patient has oxygen running, an IV, or any other equipment, record this information in the nurses' note. If the patient is experiencing pain, document the interventions that were instituted to alleviate this pain. Document any patient teaching that is reviewed with the patient, such as use of incentive spirometer.

Sample Documentation

4/10/08 1330 Patient returned to room at 11:30, groggy but answers to name. Patient's temperature 38.1° C, pulse 78, BP 122/84. Right lower abdominal dressing dry and intact. Rates pain at a "4" on scale of 1–10, was medicated in PACU with 10-mg morphine sulfate IV at 10:30. Incentive spirometry completed × 10 cycles, 750 mL each. Patient deep breathing and coughing without production and turned to right side with HOB elevated.—J. Grabbs, RN

Unexpected Situations and Associated Interventions

- *Vital signs are progressively increasing or decreasing from baseline:* Notify physician. A continued decrease in blood pressure or an increase in heart rate could indicate internal bleeding.
- *Dressing was clean before but now has large amount of fresh blood:* Do not remove dressing. Reinforce dressing with more bandages. Removing the bandage could dislodge any clot that is forming and lead to further blood loss. Notify physician.
- *Patient reports pain that is not relieved by ordered medication:* After fully assessing pain (location, description, alleviating factors, causal factors), notify physician. Pain can be a clue to other problems, such as hemorrhage.
- *Patient is febrile within 12 hours of surgery:* Assist patient with coughing and deep-breathing. If ordered, begin incentive spirometry. Continue to monitor vital signs and CBC laboratory values.
- *Adult patient has a urine output of less than 30 mL per hour:* Unless this is expected, notify physician. Urine output is a good indicator of tissue perfusion. Patient may need more fluid or may need medication to increase blood pressure if it is low.
- *Family members are anxious and want to be with patient:* Allow family members to visit patient briefly. Stress the need for the patient's continued rest.

SKILL 6-3 Providing Postoperative Care When Patient Returns to Room *(continued)*

Special Considerations

General Considerations

- For patients undergoing throat surgery, such as a tonsillectomy, evaluate swallowing pattern. A patient who has had throat surgery and swallows frequently may be bleeding from the incision site.
- In the obese patient, medications may not perform as expected related to the lack of serum proteins that are needed to bind with drugs to support their effectiveness. Additionally, due to the larger kidney mass of the obese patient, renal elimination rates of certain drugs are increased, reducing the effectiveness of these drugs. Check to make sure that the mattress for the obese patient is of high quality, since this patient is at greater risk for skin breakdown due to the poor vascular supply of adipose tissue.
- Written postoperative instructions specific to the patient and follow-up appointments with the surgeon or other healthcare professionals are provided to each patient upon discharge from the hospital or outpatient center. Patients are required to have a responsible individual accompany them home, and a contact telephone number is to be provided in case of emergency. The patient should be alert and oriented, or mental status should be at the patient's baseline. The vital signs of the patient should be stable. Information such as signs and symptoms to report to the physician as well as restrictions in activity and dietary need to be addressed.

Infant and Child Considerations

According to Dunn (2005), postoperative complications are related to the respiratory system in this age group. After receiving general anesthesia, premature infants are at greater risk for apnea. Infants and children are at great risk for temperature-related complications since their body temperature can change rapidly. It is essential to have warmed blankets and other warming equipment available to avoid this complication.

Older Adult Considerations

In the elderly patient, postoperative pneumonia can be a very serious complication resulting in death. Therefore, it is especially important to encourage and assist the patient in using the incentive spirometer and with deep-breathing exercises.

SKILL 6-4 Applying a Forced-Air Warming Device

Often patients returning from surgery are hypothermic. A more effective way of warming the patient than using warm blankets is application of a forced-air warming device, which circulates warm air around the patient.

Equipment

- Forced-air warming device unit
- Forced-air blanket
- Electronic thermometer

ASSESSMENT

Assess patient's temperature and skin color and perfusion. Patients who are hypothermic are generally pale to dusky and cool to the touch and have decreased peripheral perfusion. In darker skinned individuals, inspect nail beds and mucous membranes for signs of decreased perfusion.

NURSING DIAGNOSIS

Determine the related factors for the nursing diagnosis based on the patient's current status. Appropriate nursing diagnoses may include the following:

- Risk for Imbalanced Body Temperature
- Hypothermia
- Alteration in Comfort

(continued)

SKILL 6-4 Applying a Forced-Air Warming Device *(continued)*

OUTCOME IDENTIFICATION AND PLANNING

The expected outcome to achieve when applying a forced-air warming device is that the patient will return to and maintain a temperature of 36.5° to 37.5°C (97.7°–99.5°F). Other outcomes that may be appropriate include the following: skin will become pink and warm, capillary refill will be less than 2 seconds, and patient will not experience shivering.

IMPLEMENTATION

ACTION	RATIONALE
1. Gather equipment. Check physician's order and explain procedure to patient.	Organization facilitates performance of task. Explanation encourages patient cooperation.
2. Perform hand hygiene.	Hand hygiene deters the spread of microorganisms.
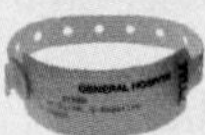 3. Identify the patient.	Identification of the patient ensures that the right patient receives the correct care.
4. **Assess patient's temperature, and document.**	Baseline temperature should be documented before the warming device is used.
5. Plug forced-air warming device into electrical outlet. Place blanket over patient, with plastic side up. Keep air-hose inlet at foot of bed.	Blanket should always be used with device. Do not place air hose under cotton blankets with airflow blanket. "Hosing" is dangerous and can cause burns to the patient.
6. Securely insert air hose into inlet. Place a lightweight fabric blanket over forced-air blanket. Turn machine on and adjust temperature of air to desired effect.	Air hose must be properly inserted to ensure that it will not fall out. Blanket will help keep warmed air near patient. Adjust air temperature depending on desired patient temperature. If blanket is being used to maintain an already stable temperature, it may be turned down lower than if needed to raise patient's temperature.
7. **Monitor patient's temperature at least every 30 minutes while using the forced-air device. If rewarming a patient with hypothermia, do not raise temperature more than 1°C per hour to prevent a rapid vasodilation effect.**	Monitoring the patient's temperature ensures that the patient does not experience too rapid a rise in body temperature, resulting in vasodilation.
8. Discontinue use of forced-air device once patient's temperature is adequate and patient can maintain the temperature without assistance.	Forced-air device is not needed once patient is warm and stable enough to maintain temperature.
9. Remove device and clean according to agency policy and manufacturer's instructions.	Proper care of equipment helps to maintain function of the device.
10. Perform hand hygiene.	Hand hygiene reduces transmission of microorganisms.

SKILL 6-4 Applying a Forced-Air Warming Device *(continued)*

EVALUATION

The expected outcome is met when the patient's temperature returns to the normal range of 36.5° to 37.5°C (97.7°–99.5°F) and the patient can maintain this temperature; skin is pink and warm; and patient is free from shivering.

DOCUMENTATION

Guidelines

Document the patient's temperature and the route. Record that the forced-air warming device was applied to the patient. Document that the patient did not experience any adverse effects from the warming device and the appearance of the skin. Record that the patient's temperature was monitored every 30 minutes, as well as the actual temperature after 30 minutes.

Sample Documentation

4/23/06 1440 Patient's temperature 35.9° C tympanically. Forced-air warming device applied to patient due to decreased temperature. Device temperature set on medium. Patient's temperature after first 30 minutes 36.4° C tympanically. —J. Grabbs, RN

Unexpected Situations and Associated Interventions

- *Patient's temperature is increasing more than 1°C per hour:* Decrease temperature of air. If air is down to lowest setting, turn device off. If patient's temperature increases too rapidly, it can lead to a vasodilation effect that will cause the patient to become hypotensive.

The Taylor Suite offers these additional resources to enhance learning and facilitate understanding of this chapter:

- thePoint online resource, http://thepoint.lww.com/Lynn2E
- Student CD-ROM included with the book
- Skills Checklist to Accompany Taylor's Clinical Nursing Skills
- Taylor's Interactive Nursing: *Perioperative Nursing Care*
- Taylor's Video Guide to Clinical Nursing Skills: *Perioperative Nursing Care*

Developing Critical Thinking Skills

1. Josie has a prophylactic antibiotic ordered to be given "on call to the OR." This means when the preoperative nurses are ready for Josie, they will call and have Josie sent down to this area. When this phone call is received, the nurse is to administer the prescribed medication. However, the phone call comes during a busy period, and the nurse realizes that Josie has been transported down to the preoperative holding area without receiving her dose of prophylactic antibiotics. What should the nurse do?
2. After her surgery, Tatum rates her pain as 8 out of 10. The nurse administers the ordered pain medication. Fifteen minutes later, Tatum is now rating her pain as 9 out of 10 and is beginning to writhe with pain. Tatum has no more ordered pain medications for another hour. What should the nurse do?
3. Dorothy Gibbs returns from surgery with a core temperature of 35.2°C (95.4°F), blood pressure of 128/72 mm Hg, and pulse of 60 beats per minute. Her skin is pale and cool to the touch. A forced-air warming device is placed on Dorothy, and the nurse turns the warmer to the highest heat setting. An hour later, the nurse takes Dorothy's vital signs. Her tympanic temperature is 37.8°C (100.0°F), her blood pressure is 82/48 mm Hg, and her pulse is 100 beats per minute. What should the nurse do?

Bibliography

Allen, G. (2002). Malnutrition and its effect on wound healing. *AORN Journal, 76*(5), 893.

American Association of Nurse Anesthetists. (2003). CRNA. Available at www.aana.com/crna.careerqna.asp.

American Society of Anesthesiologists Task Force on Acute Pain Management. (2004). Practice guidelines for acute pain management in the perioperative setting: An updated report by the

American Society of Anesthesiologists Task Force on Acute Pain Management. *Anesthesiology, 100*(6), 1573–1581.

American Society of Anesthesiologists Task Force on Post-anesthetic Care. (2002). Practice guidelines for postanesthetic care: A report by the American Society of Anesthesiologists Task Force on Postanesthetic Care. *Anesthesiology, 96*(3), 742–752.

American Society of PeriAnesthesia Nurses pain and comfort clinical guideline. (2003). *Journal of PeriAnesthesia Nurses,* Aug. 18(4), 232–236.

Arnstein, P. (2002). Optimizing perioperative pain management. *AORN Journal, 76*(5), 812–818.

Association of Operating Room Nurses. (2002). *AORN standards, recommended practices and guidelines.* Denver, CO: Author.

Association of Operating Room Nurses guidance statement: Postoperative patient care in the ambulatory surgery setting. (2005). *Association of Operating Room Nurses Journal, 81*(4), 881–887.

Association of Operating Room Nurses guidance statement: Preoperative patient care in the ambulatory surgery setting. (2005). *Association of Operating Room Nurses Journal, 81*(4), 871–877.

Beyers, S. (2004). Evidenced-based practice in perioperative nursing. *American Journal of Infection Control, 32*(2), 97–100.

Clinical guideline for the prevention of unplanned perioperative hypothermia. (2001). *Journal of Perianesthesia Nursing,* Oct 16(5), 305–314.

Collins, N. (2003). Obesity and wound healing. *Advances in Skin & Wound Care: The Journal for Prevention and Healing, 16*(1), 45–47.

Crenshaw, J., & Winslow, E. (2002). Original research: Preoperative fasting: Old habits die hard. *American Journal of Nursing, 102*(5), 36–45.

Day, M. (2005). Pulmonary embolism. *Nursing 2005, 35*(9), 88.

Dunn, D. (2004). Preventing perioperative complications in an older adult. *Nursing 2004, 34*(11), 36–41.

Dunn, D. (2005). Preventing perioperative complications in special populations. *Nursing 2005, 35*(11), 36–43.

Golembiewski, J. (2003). Morphine and hydromorphone for postoperative analgesia: Focus on safety. *Journal of PeriAnesthesia Nursing, 18*(2), 120–122.

Ignatavicius, D., & Workman, L. (2006). *Medical–surgical nursing critical thinking for collaborative care* (5th ed.). St. Louis, MO: Elsevier Saunders.

Pasero, C. (2002). The challenge of pain assessment. *Journal of PeriAnesthesia Nursing, 17*(5), 348–350.

Pessagno, J. J. (2002). Recommended practices for managing the patient receiving local anesthesia. *AORN Journal, 75*(4), 849–852.

Plonczynski, D. (2005). Wise use of perioperative antibiotics. *Association of Operating Room Nursing, 81*(6), 1260–1271.

Porth, C. M. (2002). *Pathophysiology: Concepts of altered health states* (5th ed.). Philadelphia: Lippincott.

Rothrock, J., Smith, D., & McEwen, D. (Eds.). (2003). *Alexander's care of the patient in surgery* (12th ed.). St. Louis, MO: Mosby.

Schoonhoven, L., Defloor, T., & Grypdonck, M. (2002). Incidence of pressure due to surgery. *Journal of Clinical Nursing, 11,* 479–487.

Seal, L., & Paul-Cheadle, D. (2004). A systems approach to preoperative surgical patient skin preparation. *American Journal of Infection Control, 32*(2), 57–62.

U • N • I • T

II

Promoting Healthy Physiologic Responses

CHAPTER 7

Hygiene

Focusing on Patient Care

This chapter will help you develop some of the skills related to hygiene necessary to care for the following patients:

Denasia Kerr, a 6-year-old who is on bedrest after surgery and needs her hair washed

Cindy Vortex, age 34, who is in a coma after a car accident and needs her contact lenses removed

Carl Sheen, age 76, who needs help cleaning his dentures

Learning Objectives

After studying this chapter, you will be able to:

1. Give a bed bath.
2. Assist with oral care.
3. Provide oral care for a dependent patient.
4. Provide denture care.
5. Remove contact lenses.
6. Shampoo a patient's hair in bed.
7. Assist with shaving.
8. Apply antiembolism stockings.
9. Make an unoccupied bed.
10. Make an occupied bed.

Key Terms

alopecia: baldness

caries: cavities of the teeth

cerumen: ear wax; consists of a heavy oil and brown pigmentation

dermis: underlying portion of the skin

epidermis: superficial portion of the skin

gingivitis: inflammation of the gingivae (gums)

halitosis: offensive breath

integument: skin

necrosis: death of cells

pediculosis: infestation with lice

plaque: transparent, adhesive coating on teeth consisting of mucin, carbohydrate, and bacteria

podiatrist: one who treats foot disorders; synonym for chiropodist

pyorrhea: extensive inflammation of the gums and alveolar tissues; synonym for periodontitis

sebaceous gland: gland found in the skin that secretes an oily substance called sebum

tartar: hard deposit on the teeth near the gum line formed by plaque buildup and dead bacteria

Measures for personal cleanliness and grooming that promote physical and psychological well-being are called personal hygiene. Personal hygiene practices vary widely among people. The time of day one bathes and how often a person shampoos his or her hair or changes the bed linens and sleeping garments are very individualized choices. It's important that personal care be carried out conveniently and frequently enough to promote personal hygiene and wellness.

People who are well ordinarily are responsible for their own hygiene. In some cases, the nurse may assist a well person through teaching to develop personal hygiene habits the person may lack. Illness, hospitalization, and institutionalization generally require modifications in hygiene practices. In these situations, the nurse helps the patient to continue sound hygiene practices and can teach the patient and family members, when necessary, about hygiene. Nurses assisting patients with basic hygiene should respect individual patient preferences and give only the care that patients cannot or should not provide for themselves.

This chapter will cover skills that the nurse needs to promote hygiene.

SKILL 7-1

Giving a Bed Bath

Some patients must remain in bed as a part of their therapeutic regimen but can still bathe themselves. Other patients are not on bed rest, but require total or partial assistance with bathing in bed due to physical limitations, such as fatigue or limited range of motion. A bed bath may be considered a partial bed bath if the patient is well enough to perform most of the bath, and the nurse needs to assist with washing areas that the patient cannot reach easily. A partial bath may also refer to bathing only those body parts that absolutely have to be cleaned, such as perineal care and soiled body parts. Many of the bedside skin-cleaning products available today do not require rinsing After cleaning body part, just pat dry. See Table 7-1 for a summary of common cleaning products.

Equipment

- Washbasin and warm water
- Personal hygiene supplies (deodorant, lotion, and others)
- Skin-cleaning agent or soap
- Towels (2)
- Washcloths (2)
- Bath blanket
- Gown or pajamas
- Bedpan or urinal
- Laundry bag
- Disposable gloves for anal and perineal care (optional for remainder of bath)

ASSESSMENT

Assess the patient's knowledge of hygiene practices and bathing preferences: frequency, time of day, and type of hygiene products. Assess for any physical-activity limitations. Assess the patient's ability to bathe himself or herself. Allow the patient to do any part of the bath that he or she can do. For example, the patient may be able to wash his face, while the nurse does the rest. Assess the patient's skin for dryness, redness, or areas of breakdown, and gather any other appropriate supplies that may be needed as a result.

NURSING DIAGNOSIS

Determine the related factors for the nursing diagnosis based on the patient's current status. Appropriate nursing diagnoses may include:

- Bathing/Hygiene Self-Care Deficit
- Acute Pain

TABLE 7-1 Bedside Cleaning and Skin-Care Products

PRODUCT	DESCRIPTION
Bathing cloths	Premoistened, pH-balanced, microwaveable, disposable cloths for rinse-free skin cleaning and moisturizing. Each package provides one complete bath using 8–10 cloths.
Bathing wipes	Packaged dry cloths. Adding water to the cloths causes them to foam, providing rinse-free skin pH-balanced cleaning. Cloths are packaged in a resealable package for multiple uses.
No-rinse body wash and shampoo	No-rinse concentrated skin cleanser and moisturizer. Mix with water, apply with a cloth, lather, and dry.
Body foam	Foam cleanser and moisturizer to be used as a body wash, no-rinse shampoo, and perineal cleanser. Pump bottle dispenses foam to be applied with a cloth.

(Adapted from Bauer, J. [2003]. Bedside bathing products. *RN, 66*[6], 65–66.)

(continued)

SKILL 7-1 Giving a Bed Bath *(continued)*

- Ineffective Coping
- Deficient Knowledge
- Risk for Infection
- Disturbed Body Image
- Impaired Skin Integrity
- Risk for Impaired Skin Integrity

OUTCOME IDENTIFICATION AND PLANNING

The expected outcome to achieve when giving a bed bath is that the patient will be clean and fresh. Other outcomes that may be appropriate include the following: patient regains feelings of control by assisting with the bath; patient verbalizes positive body image; and patient demonstrates understanding about the need for cleanliness.

IMPLEMENTATION

ACTION	RATIONALE
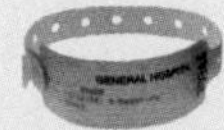 1. Review chart for any limitations in physical activity. Identify the patient. Discuss procedure with patient and assess patient's ability to assist in the bathing process, as well as personal hygiene preferences.	Identifying limitations prevents patient discomfort and injury. Identifying the patient ensures the right patient receives the intervention and helps prevent errors. Discussion promotes reassurance and provides knowledge about the procedure. Dialogue encourages patient participation and allows for individualized nursing care.
2. Bring necessary equipment to the bedside stand or overbed table. Remove sequential compression devices and antiembolism stockings from lower extremities according to agency protocol.	Bringing everything to the bedside conserves time and energy. Arranging items nearby is convenient, saves time, and avoids unnecessary stretching and twisting of muscles on the part of the nurse. Most manufacturers and agencies recommend removal of these devices before the bath to allow for assessment.
3. Close curtains around bed and close door to room if possible. Adjust the room temperature if necessary.	This ensures the patient's privacy and lessens the risk for loss of body heat during the bath.
4. Offer patient bedpan or urinal.	Voiding or defecating before the bath lessens the likelihood that the bath will be interrupted, because warm bath water may stimulate the urge to void.
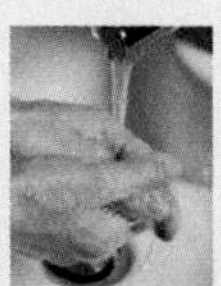 5. Perform hand hygiene.	Hand hygiene deters the spread of microorganisms.
6. Raise bed to a comfortable working height.	Having the bed at a comfortable working height prevents strain on the nurse's back.
7. Lower side rail nearer to you and assist patient to side of bed where you will work. Have patient lie on his or her back.	Having the patient positioned near the nurse and lowering the side rail prevent unnecessary stretching and twisting of muscles on the part of the nurse.
8. Loosen top covers and remove all except the top sheet. Place bath blanket over patient and then remove top sheet while patient holds bath blanket in place. If linen is to be reused, fold it over a chair. Place soiled linen in laundry bag. Take care to prevent linen from coming in contact with your clothing.	The patient is not exposed unnecessarily, and warmth is maintained. If a bath blanket is unavailable, the top sheet may be used in place of the bath blanket.

SKILL 7-1 Giving a Bed Bath *(continued)*

ACTION	RATIONALE
9. Remove patient's gown and keep bath blanket in place. If patient has an IV line and is not wearing a gown with snap sleeves, remove gown from other arm first. **Lower the IV container and pass gown over the tubing and the container. Rehang the container and check the drip rate.**	This provides uncluttered access during the bath and maintains warmth of the patient. IV fluids must be maintained at the prescribed rate.
10. **Raise side rail.** Fill basin with a sufficient amount of comfortably warm water (110°–115°F). Change as necessary throughout the bath. Lower side rail closer to you when you return to the bedside to begin the bath.	Side rails maintain patient safety. Warm water is comfortable and relaxing for the patient. It also stimulates circulation and provides for more effective cleansing.
11. Put on gloves, if necessary. Fold the washcloth like a mitt on your hand so that there are no loose ends (Figure 1, Figure 2, Figure 3).	Gloves are necessary if there is potential contact with blood or body fluids. Having loose ends of cloth drag across the patient's skin is uncomfortable. Loose ends cool quickly and feel cold to the patient.

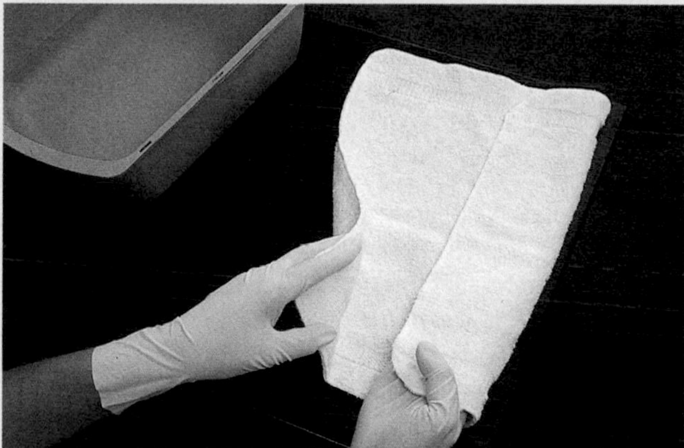

Figure 1. Folding washcloth in thirds around hand to make a bath mitt.

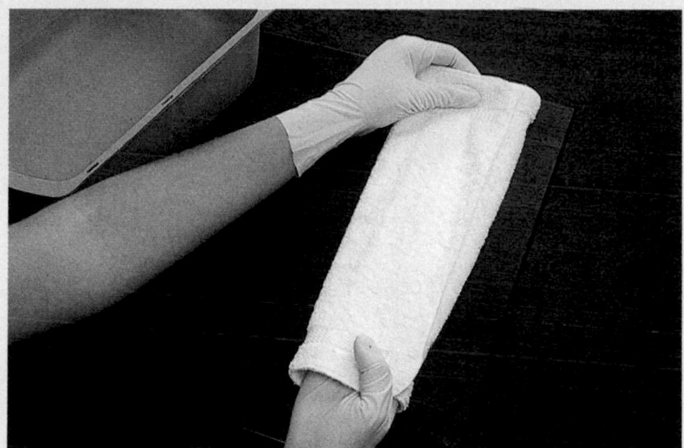

Figure 2. Straightening washcloth before folding into mitt.

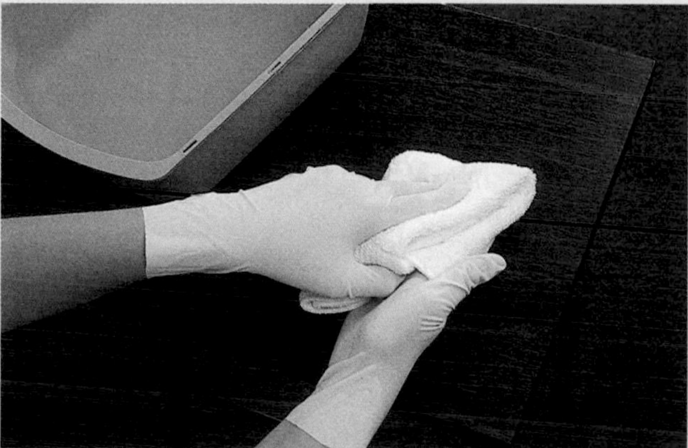

Figure 3. Folding ends over and tucking ends under folded washcloth over palm.

(continued)

SKILL 7-1 Giving a Bed Bath *(continued)*

ACTION	RATIONALE
12. Lay a towel across patient's chest and on top of bath blanket.	This prevents chilling and keeps bath blanket dry.
13. **With no soap on the washcloth, wipe one eye from the inner part of the eye, near the nose, to the outer part (Figure 4). Rinse or turn the cloth before washing the other eye.**	Soap is irritating to the eyes. Moving from the inner to the outer aspect of the eye prevents carrying debris toward the nasolacrimal duct. Rinsing or turning the washcloth prevents spreading organisms from one eye to the other.

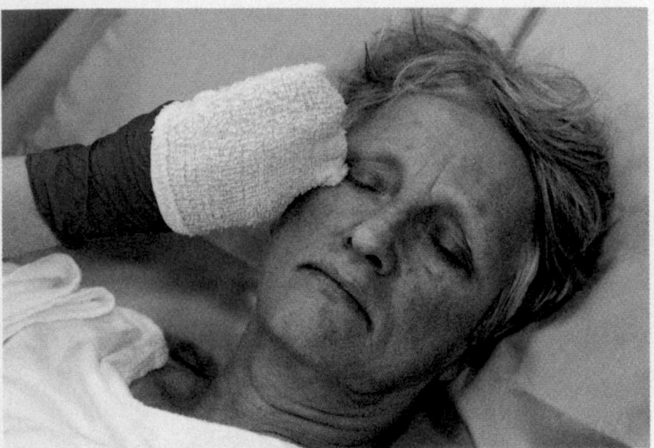

Figure 4. Washing from the inner corner of the eye outward.

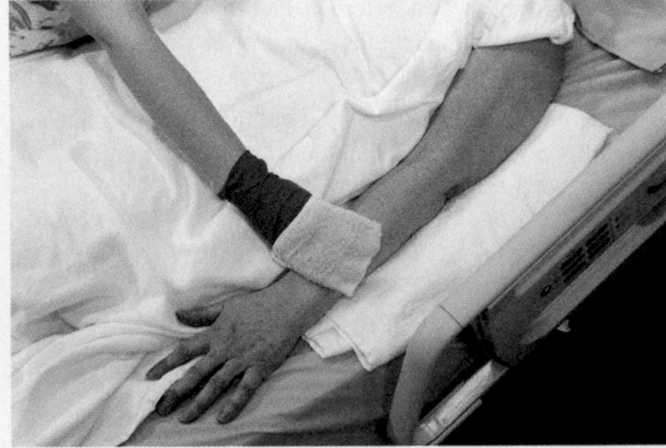

Figure 5. Exposing the far arm and washing it.

ACTION	RATIONALE
14. Bathe patient's face, neck, and ears, avoiding soap on the face if the patient prefers. Apply appropriate emollient.	Soap can be drying and may be avoided as a matter of personal preference.
15. Expose patient's far arm and place towel lengthwise under it. Using firm strokes, wash arm and axilla, lifting the arm as necessary to access axillary region (Figure 5). Rinse, if necessary, and dry. Apply appropriate emollient.	The towel helps to keep the bed dry. Washing the far side first eliminates contaminating a clean area once it is washed. Gentle friction stimulates circulation and muscles and helps remove dirt, oil, and organisms. Long, firm strokes are relaxing and more comfortable than short, uneven strokes.
16. Place a folded towel on the bed next to patient's hand and put basin on it. Soak patient's hand in basin (Figure 6). Wash, rinse, if necessary, and dry hand. Apply appropriate emollient.	Placing the hand in the basin of water is an additional comfort measure for the patient. It facilitates thorough washing of the hands and between the fingers and aids in removing debris from under the nails.
17. Repeat Actions 15 and 16 for the arm nearer you. An option for the shorter nurse or one prone to back strain might be to bathe one side of the patient and move to the other side of the bed to complete the bath.	
18. Spread a towel across patient's chest. Lower bath blanket to patient's umbilical area. Wash, rinse, if necessary, and dry chest. Keep chest covered with towel between the wash and rinse. Pay special attention to skin folds under the breasts.	Exposing, washing, rinsing, and drying one part of the body at a time avoids unnecessary exposure and chilling. Skin-fold areas may be sources of odor and skin breakdown if not cleaned and dried properly.

SKILL 7-1 Giving a Bed Bath *(continued)*

ACTION	RATIONALE
19. Lower bath blanket to perineal area. Place a towel over patient's chest.	Keeping the bath blanket and towel in place avoids exposure and chilling.
20. Wash, rinse, if necessary, and dry abdomen (Figure 7). Carefully inspect and clean umbilical area and any abdominal folds or creases.	Skin-fold areas may be sources of odor and skin breakdown if not cleaned and dried properly.

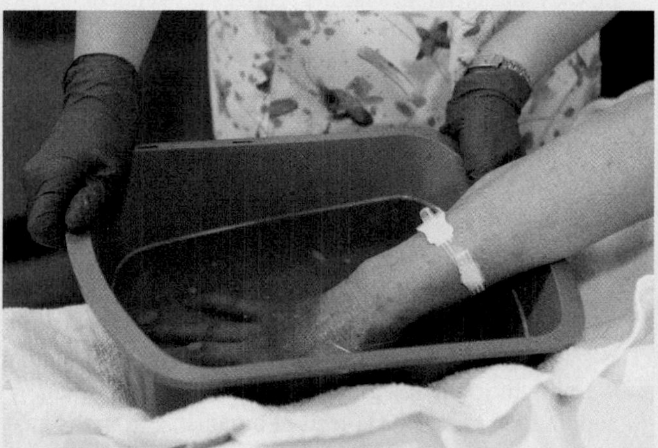

Figure 6. Soaking hand in basin.

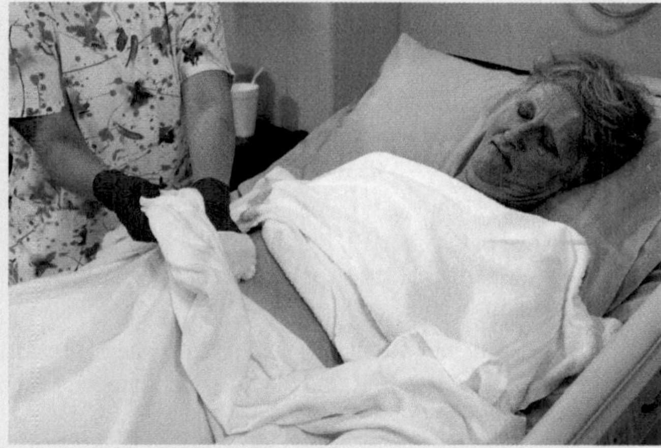

Figure 7. Washing the abdomen, with perineal and chest areas covered.

ACTION	RATIONALE
21. Return bath blanket to original position and expose far leg. Place towel under far leg. Using firm strokes, wash, rinse, if necessary, and dry leg from ankle to knee and knee to groin (Figure 8). Apply appropriate emollient.	The towel protects linens and prevents the patient from feeling uncomfortable from a damp or wet bed. Washing from ankle to groin with firm strokes promotes venous return.
22. Fold a towel near patient's foot area and place basin on it (Figure 9). Place foot in basin while supporting the ankle and heel in your hand and the leg on your arm. Wash, rinse, if necessary, and dry, paying particular attention to area between toes. Apply appropriate emollient.	Supporting the patient's foot and leg helps reduce strain and discomfort for the patient. Placing the foot in a basin of water is comfortable and relaxing and allows for thorough cleaning of the feet and the areas between the toes and under the nails.

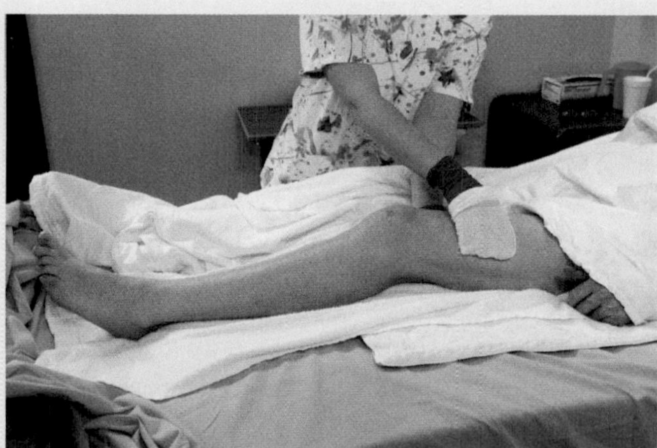

Figure 8. Washing and drying far leg, keeping the other leg covered.

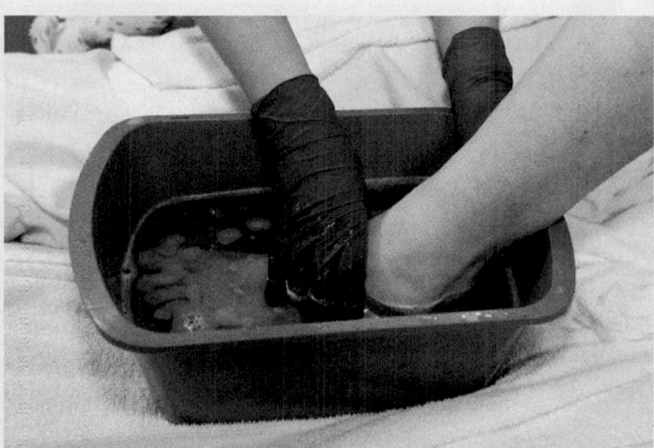

Figure 9. Soaking the foot in basin.

(continued)

SKILL 7-1 Giving a Bed Bath *(continued)*

ACTION	RATIONALE
23. Repeat Actions 21 and 22 for the other leg and foot.	
24. Make sure patient is covered with bath blanket. Change water and washcloth at this point or earlier if necessary.	The bath blanket maintains warmth and privacy. Clean, warm water prevents chilling and maintains patient comfort.
25. Assist patient to prone or side-lying position. Put on gloves, if not applied earlier. Position bath blanket and towel to expose only the back and buttocks.	Positioning the towel and bath blanket protects the patient's privacy and provides warmth. Gloves prevent contact with body fluids.
26. Wash, rinse, if necessary, and dry back and buttocks area (Figure 10). **Pay particular attention to cleansing between gluteal folds, and observe for any redness or skin breakdown in the sacral area.**	Fecal material near the anus may be a source of micro-organisms. Prolonged pressure on the sacral area or other bony prominences may compromise circulation and lead to development of decubitus ulcer.
27. If not contraindicated, give patient a backrub, as described in Chapter 10. Back massage may be given also after perineal care. Apply appropriate emollient and/or skin-barrier product.	A backrub improves circulation to the tissues and is an aid to relaxation. A backrub may be contraindicated in patients with cardiovascular disease or musculoskeletal injuries.
28. Raise the side rail. Refill basin with clean water. Discard washcloth and towel. Remove gloves and put on clean gloves.	The washcloth, towel, and water are contaminated after washing the patient's gluteal area. Changing to clean supplies decreases the spread of organisms from the anal area to the genitals.
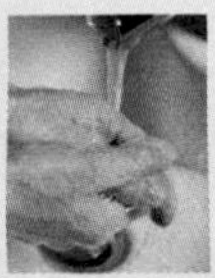 29. Clean perineal area or set up patient so that he or she can complete perineal self-care. If the patient is unable, lower the side rail and complete perineal care, following guidelines in the accompanying Skill Variation. Raise side rail, remove gloves, and perform hand hygiene.	Providing perineal self-care may decrease embarrassment for the patient. Effective perineal care reduces odor and decreases the risk for infection through contamination.
30. Help patient put on a clean gown (Figure 11) and assist with the use of other personal toiletries, such as deodorant or cosmetics.	This provides for the patient's warmth and comfort.

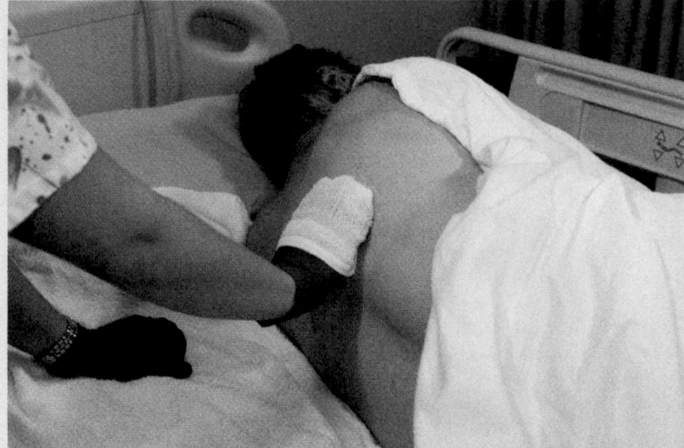

Figure 10. Washing the upper back.

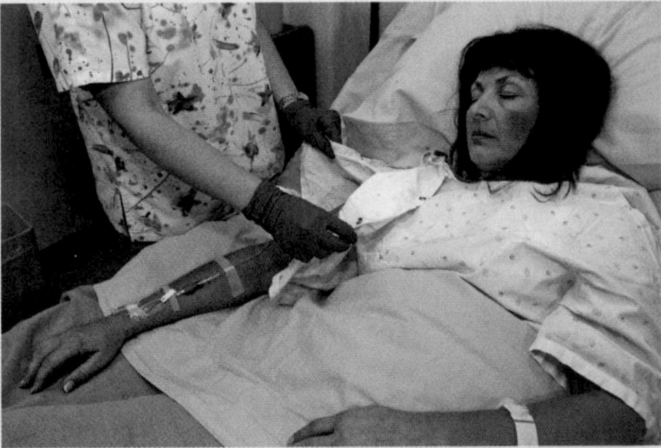

Figure 11. Assisting patient with an IV to put on a new gown.

SKILL 7-1 **Giving a Bed Bath** *(continued)*

ACTION	RATIONALE
31. Protect pillow with towel and groom patient's hair.	
32. Change bed linens, as described in Skills 7-9 and 7-10. Remove gloves and perform hand hygiene. Dispose of soiled linens according to agency policy.	These actions deter the spread of microorganisms.

EVALUATION

The expected outcomes are met when the patient is clean; demonstrates some feeling of control in his or her care; verbalizes an improved body image; and verbalizes the importance of cleanliness.

DOCUMENTATION

Guidelines

Record any significant observations and communication on chart. Document the condition of the patient's skin. Record the procedure, amount of assistance given, and patient participation.

Sample Documentation

7/14/09 2130 Bath provided with complete assistance; reddened area noted on patient's sacral area; skin-care team consultation made.—C. Stone, RN

Unexpected Situations and Associated Interventions

- *Patient becomes chilled during bath:* If the room temperature is adjustable, increase it. Another bath blanket may be needed.
- *The patient becomes unstable during the bath:* Critically ill patients often need to be bathed in stages. For instance, the right arm is bathed, and then the patient is allowed to rest for a short period before the left arm is bathed. The amount of rest time needed depends on how unstable the patient is and which parameter is being monitored. If the blood pressure drops when the patient is stimulated, the nurse may watch the blood pressure while bathing the patient and stop when it begins to decrease. Once the blood pressure returns to the previous level, the nurse can begin to bathe the patient again.

Special Considerations

General Considerations

- To remove the gown from a patient with an IV line, take the gown off the uninvolved arm first and then thread the IV tubing and bottle or bag through the arm of the gown. To replace the gown, place the clean gown on the unaffected arm first and thread the IV tubing and bottle or bag from inside the arm of the gown on the involved side. Never disconnect IV tubing to change a gown, because this causes a break in a sterile system and could introduce infection.
- Lying flat in bed during the bed bath may be contraindicated for certain patients. The position may have to be modified to accommodate their needs.
- Incontinent patients require special attention to perineal care. Patients with urinary or fecal incontinence are at risk for perineal skin damage. This damage is related to moisture, changes in the pH of the skin, overgrowth of bacteria and infection of the skin, and erosion of perineal skin from friction on moist skin. Skin care for these patients should include measures to reduce overhydration (excess exposure to moisture), reduce contact with ammonia and bacteria, and reduce friction. Remove soil and irritants from the skin during routine hygiene, as well as cleansing when the skin becomes exposed to irritants. Avoid using soap and excessive force for cleaning. The use of perineal skin cleansers, moisturizers, and moisture barriers are recommended for skin care for the incontinent patient. These products help promote healing and prevent further skin damage.

(continued)

SKILL 7-1 Giving a Bed Bath *(continued)*

- If the patient has an indwelling catheter and the agency recommends daily care for the catheter, this is usually done after perineal care. Agency policy may recommend use of an antiseptic cleaning agent or plain soap and water on a clean washcloth. Put on clean gloves before cleaning the catheter. Clean 6″ to 8″ of the catheter, moving from the meatus downward. Be careful not to pull or tug on the catheter during the cleaning motion. Also inspect the meatus for drainage and note the characteristics of the urine.

Infant and Child Considerations

- When bathing an infant or young child, have supplies within easy reach, and support or hold the child securely at all times to ensure safety.
- Never leave the child alone.

Older Adult Considerations

- Check the temperature of the water carefully before bathing an older patient, because sensitivity to temperature may be impaired in older persons.
- An older, continent patient may not require a full bed bath with soap and water every day. If dry skin is a problem, water and skin lotion or bath oil may be used on alternate days. If applying lotion, place the lotion dispenser in warm bath water while bathing the patient. This will warm the lotion before it is applied to the patient.
- Refer to Box 7-1 for guidelines to assist in meeting hygiene needs for patients with dementia.

Home Care Considerations

- Evaluate the safety of the bathing area in the home. Tub mats, adhesive strips, grab bars, and shower stools can help prevent falls.
- Use plastic trash bags or a plastic shower-curtain liner to protect the mattress when bathing or shampooing a patient in bed. Disposable washcloths may also be an option to consider. A large plastic container or baby bathtub can effectively serve as a shampoo basin.
- If linens are soiled with blood or body fluids, instruct family members to wear gloves when handling them. They should be rinsed first in cold water and then washed separately from other household wash, using hot water, laundry detergent, and bleach.
- Teach family member or caregiver how to perform comfort measures, such as a backrub.
- Instruct caregivers or patients at home with an indwelling catheter to wash the urinary meatus and perineal area twice daily with soap and water. The anal area should also be cleaned after each bowel movement. Careful hand washing is imperative.

BOX 7-1 Meeting the Bathing Needs of Patients With Dementia

- Shift the focus of the interaction from the "task of bathing" to the needs and abilities of the patient. Focus on comfort, safety, autonomy, and self esteem, in addition to cleanliness.
- Individualize patient care. Consult the patient, the patient's record, family members, and other caregivers to determine patient preferences.
- Consider what can be learned from the behaviors associated with dementia about the needs and preferences of the patient. A patient's behavior may be an expression of unmet needs; flailing and hitting may be a response to uncomfortable water temperatures or levels of sound or light in the room.
- Consider other methods for bathing. Showers and tub baths are not the only options for bathing. Towel baths, washing underclothes, and bathing "body sections" one day at a time are other possible options.
- Maintain a relaxed demeanor. Use calming language. Try to determine phrases and terms the patient understands in relation to bathing and make use of them. Offer frequent reassurance.

(Adapted from Perlmutter, J., & Camberg, L. [2004]. Better bathing for residents with Alzheimer's. *Nursing Homes/Long-Term Care Management, 53*[4], 40, 42–43, and Rasin, J., & Barrick, A. [2004]. Bathing patients with dementia. *American Journal of Nursing, 104*[3], 30–33.)

SKILL 7-1 **Giving a Bed Bath** *(continued)*

SKILL VARIATION Performing Perineal Cleansing

Perineal care may be carried out while the patient remains in bed. When performing perineal care, follow these guidelines:

- Assemble supplies and provide for privacy.
- Explain the procedure to the patient, perform hand hygiene, and put on disposable gloves.
- Wash and rinse the groin area (both male and female patients).
- **For a female patient,** spread the labia and move the washcloth from the pubic area toward the anal area to prevent carrying organisms from the anal area back over the genital area (Figure A). Always proceed from the least contaminated area to the most contaminated area. Use a clean portion of the washcloth for each stroke. Rinse the washed areas well with plain water.
- **For a male patient,** clean the tip of the penis first, moving the washcloth in a circular motion from the meatus outward. Wash the shaft of the penis using downward strokes toward the pubic area (Figure B). Always proceed from the least contaminated area to the most contaminated area. Rinse the washed areas well with plain water. In an *uncircumcised male patient,* retract the foreskin (prepuce) while washing the penis. Pull the *uncircumcised male patient's* foreskin back into place over the glans penis to prevent constriction of the penis, which may result in edema and tissue injury. Wash and rinse the male patient's scrotum. Handle the scrotum, which houses the testicles, with care because the area is sensitive.
- Dry the cleaned areas and apply an emollient as indicated. Avoid the use of powder. Powder may become a medium for the growth of bacteria.
- Turn the patient on his or her side and continue cleansing the anal area. Continue in the direction of least contaminated to most contaminated area. In the female, cleanse from the vagina toward the anus. In both female and male patients, change the washcloth with each stroke until the area is clean. Rinse and dry the area.
- Remove gloves and perform hand hygiene. Continue with additional care as necessary.

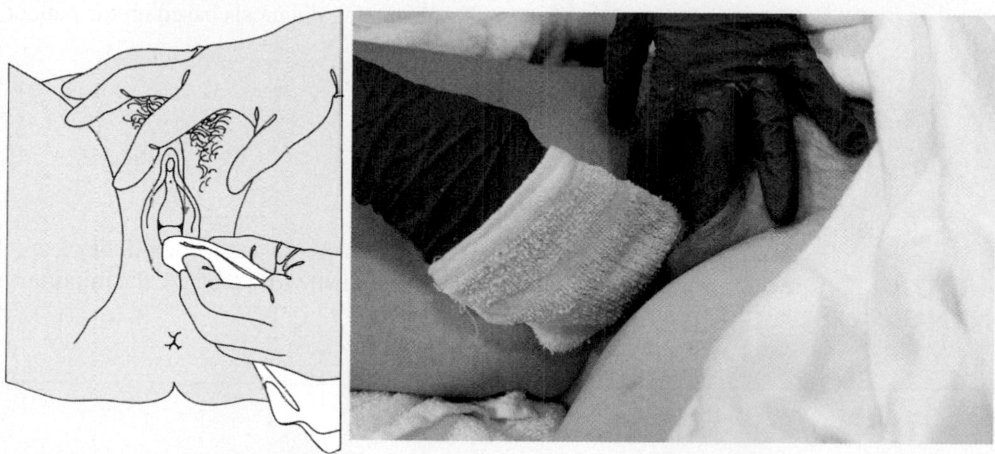

Figure A. Performing female perineal care.

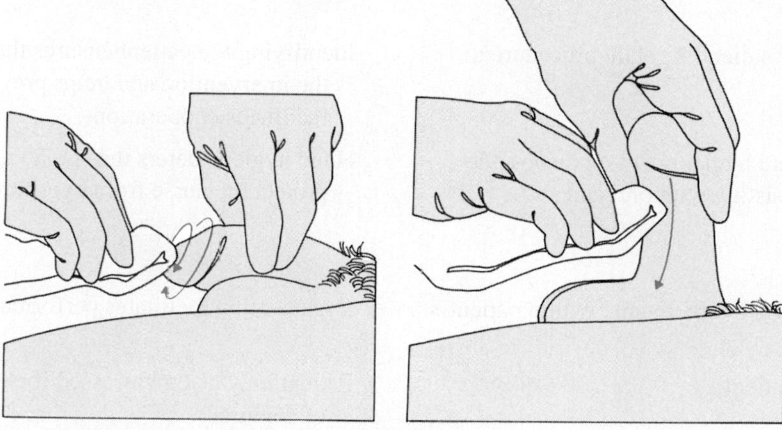

Figure B. Performing male perineal care.

SKILL 7-2 Assisting the Patient With Oral Care

The mouth requires care even during illness, but sometimes care must be modified to meet a patient's needs. If the patient can assist with mouth care, provide the necessary materials. Oral care is important not only to prevent dental caries but also to improve the patient's self-image. Oral care should be done at least twice a day for ambulatory patients.

Equipment

- Toothbrush
- Toothpaste
- Emesis basin
- Glass with cool water
- Disposable gloves
- Towel
- Mouthwash (optional)
- Washcloth or paper towel
- Lip lubricant (optional)
- Dental floss

ASSESSMENT

Assess the patient's oral hygiene preferences: frequency, time of day, and type of hygiene products. Assess for any physical activity limitations. Assess patient's oral cavity and dentition. Look for any caries, sores, or white patches. The white patches may indicate a fungal infection called thrush. Assess patient's ability to perform own care.

NURSING DIAGNOSIS

Determine the related factors for the nursing diagnosis based on the patient's current status. Possible nursing diagnoses may include:

- Ineffective Health Maintenance
- Impaired Oral Mucous Membrane
- Disturbed Body Image
- Deficient Knowledge

OUTCOME IDENTIFICATION AND PLANNING

The expected outcome is that the patient's mouth and teeth will be clean; the patient will exhibit a positive body image; and the patient will verbalize the importance of oral care.

IMPLEMENTATION

ACTION	RATIONALE
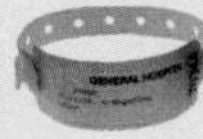 1. Identify the patient. Explain procedure to patient.	Identifying the patient ensures the right patient receives the intervention and helps prevent errors. Explanation facilitates cooperation.
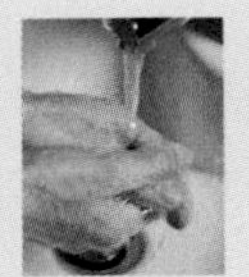 2. Perform hand hygiene. Put on disposable gloves if assisting with oral care.	Hand hygiene deters the spread of microorganisms. Gloves protect the nurse from exposure to blood or body fluids.
3. Assemble equipment on overbed table within patient's reach.	Organization facilitates performance of task.
4. Provide privacy for patient.	Patient may be embarrassed if cleansing involves removal of dentures.
5. Lower side rail and assist patient to sitting position if permitted, or turn patient onto side. Place towel across patient's chest. Raise bed to a comfortable working position.	The sitting or side-lying position prevents aspiration of fluids into the lungs. The towel protects the patient from dampness.

SKILL 7-2 Assisting the Patient With Oral Care *(continued)*

6. Encourage patient to brush own teeth, or assist if necessary.

   a. Moisten toothbrush and apply toothpaste to bristles.

      Water softens the bristles.

   b. Place brush at a 45-degree angle to gum line (Figure 1) and brush from gum line to crown of each tooth (Figure 2). Brush outer and inner surfaces. Brush back and forth across biting surface of each tooth.

      Facilitates removal of plaque and tartar. The 45-degree angle of brushing permits cleansing of all surface areas of the tooth.

   c. Brush tongue gently with toothbrush (Figure 3).

      Removes coating on the tongue. Gentle motion does not stimulate gag reflex.

   d. Have patient rinse vigorously with water and spit into emesis basin (Figure 4). Repeat until clear. Suction may be used as an alternative for removal of fluid and secretions from mouth.

      The vigorous swishing motion helps to remove debris. Suction is appropriate if patient is unable to expectorate well.

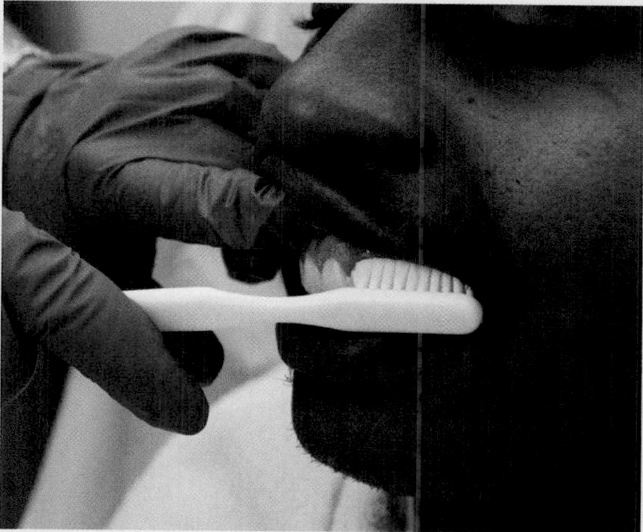

Figure 1. Placing brush at a 45-degree angle to the gum line.

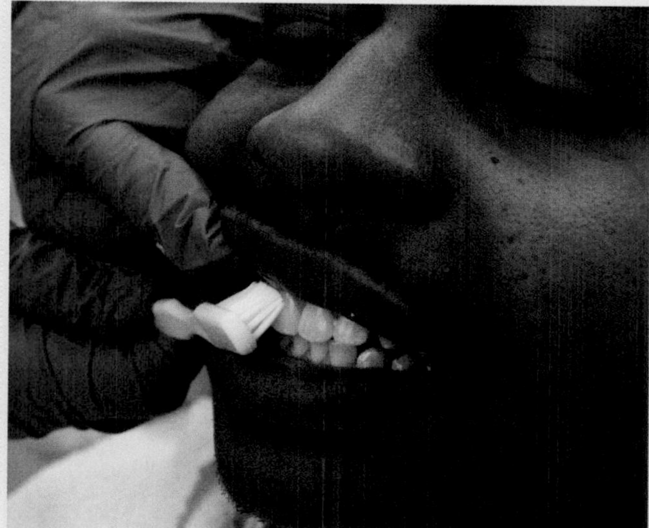

Figure 2. Brushing from the gum line to the crown of each tooth.

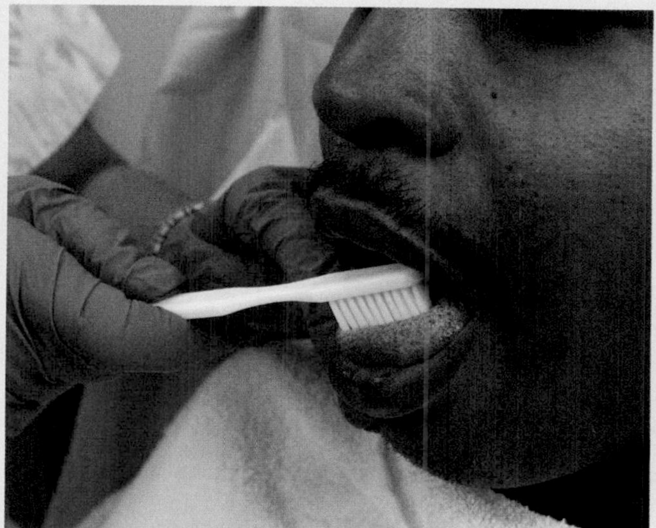

Figure 3. Brushing the tongue.

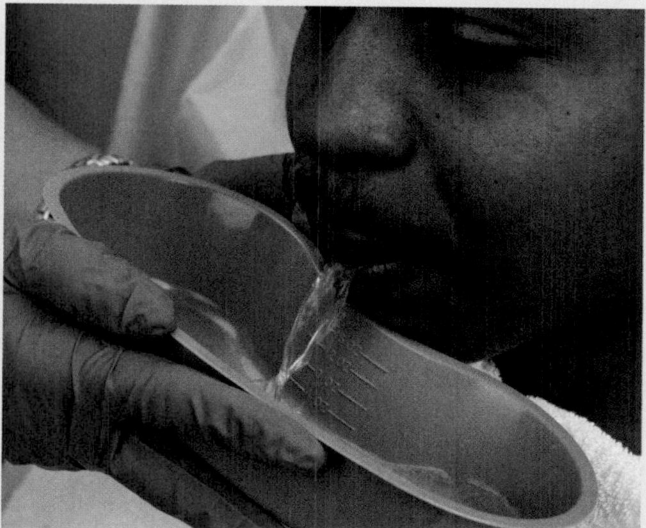

Figure 4. Holding emesis basin for patient to rinse and spit.

(continued)

SKILL 7-2 Assisting the Patient With Oral Care *(continued)*

ACTION	RATIONALE
7. Assist patient to floss teeth, if appropriate:	Flossing aids in removal of plaque and promotes healthy gum tissue.
a. Remove approximately 6″ of dental floss from container or use a plastic floss holder. Wrap the floss around the index fingers, keeping about 1″ to 1.5″ of floss taut between the fingers.	The floss must be held taut to get between the teeth.
b. Insert floss gently between teeth, moving it back and forth downward to the gums.	Trauma to the gums can occur if floss is forced between teeth.
c. Move the floss up and down, first on one side of a tooth and then on the side of the other tooth, until the surfaces are clean (Figure 5). Repeat in the spaces between all teeth.	This ensures that the sides of both teeth are cleaned.
d. Instruct patient to rinse mouth well with water after flossing.	Vigorous rinsing helps to remove food particles and plaque that have been loosened by flossing.

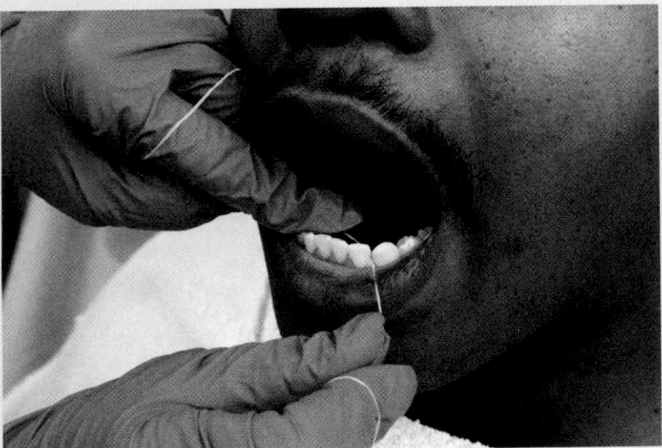

Figure 5. Flossing the teeth.

ACTION	RATIONALE
8. Offer mouthwash if patient prefers.	Mouthwash leaves a pleasant taste in the mouth.
9. Offer lip balm or petroleum jelly.	Lip balm lubricates lips and prevents drying.
10. Remove equipment. Remove gloves and discard. Raise side rail and lower bed. Assist patient to a position of comfort.	These actions promote patient comfort and safety.
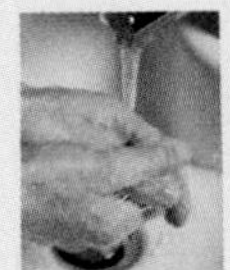 11. Perform hand hygiene.	Hand hygiene deters spread of microorganisms.

EVALUATION

The expected outcomes are met when the patient receives oral care, experiences little to no discomfort, states mouth feels refreshed, and demonstrates understanding of reasons for proper oral care.

SKILL 7-2 Assisting the Patient With Oral Care *(continued)*

DOCUMENTATION

Guidelines

Record oral assessment, significant observations and unusual findings, such as bleeding or inflammation. Document any teaching done. Document procedure and patient response.

Sample Documentation

10/20/09 0930 Patient performed oral care with minimal assistance. Oral-cavity mucosa pink and moist. No evidence of bleeding or ulceration. Lips slightly dry; lip moisturizer applied. Reinforcement provided related to importance of flossing teeth every day. Patient demonstrates appropriate flossing technique.—L. Schneider, RN.

Unexpected Situations and Associated Interventions

- *While cleaning the teeth, you notice a large amount of bleeding from the gum line:* Stop brushing. Allow patient to gently rinse mouth with water and spit into emesis basin. Before brushing again, check most recent platelet level. Consider the use of a toothette to provide oral hygiene.
- *Patient has braces on teeth:* Brush extra thoroughly. Braces collect food particles.

Special Considerations

General Considerations

- Refer to Box 7-2 for guidelines to assist in meeting the oral hygiene needs of patients with cognitive impairments.

Infant and Child Considerations

- When assisting small children with oral care, do not use a toothpaste that contains fluoride if the child cannot spit out excess. Excessive amounts of ingested fluoride can lead to a discoloration of the teeth.
- Oral hygiene should begin as soon as an infant's teeth erupt. Teeth and gums should be cleaned by wiping with a damp cloth. As the infant gets more teeth, a small toothbrush can be introduced. Water should be used to clean an infant's teeth, not toothpaste.

BOX 7-2 Meeting the Oral Hygiene Needs of Patients With Cognitive Impairments

- Choose a time of day when the patient is most calm and accepting of care.
- Enlist the aid of a family member or significant other.
- Break the task into small steps.
- Provide distraction, such as playing favorite music, while providing care.
- Allow the patient to participate. The nurse can put a hand over the patient's to guide the activity.
- The nurse can start the activity, show the patient what to do, then let the patient take over.
- If the patient strongly refuses care, withdraw and reapproach at a later time.
- Effective and ineffective interventions should be documented to provide appropriate information for staff to give consistent, effective care.

(Adapted from Tabloski, R. [2006]. *Gerontological nursing.* Upper Saddle River, NJ: Pearson Prentice Hall, p. 376.)

SKILL 7-3 Providing Oral Care for the Dependent Patient

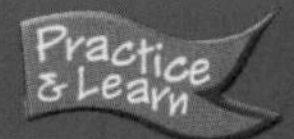

Some patients cannot perform their own oral care. When providing the dependent patient with oral care, the nurse may have to protect the patient's airway. Make certain that the mouth receives care as often as necessary to keep it clean and moist, as often as every 1 or 2 hours, if necessary. This is especially important for patients who cannot drink or are not permitted fluids by mouth.

Equipment

- Toothbrush
- Toothpaste
- Emesis basin
- Glass with cool water
- Disposable gloves
- Towel
- Mouthwash (optional)
- Dental floss (optional)
- Denture-cleaning equipment (if necessary)
- Denture cup
- Denture cleaner
- 4 × 4 gauze
- Washcloth or paper towel
- Lip lubricant (optional)
- Sponge toothette or tongue blades padded with 4 × 4 gauze sponges
- Irrigating syringe with rubber tip (optional)
- Suction catheter with suction apparatus (optional)

ASSESSMENT

Assess the patient's oral hygiene preferences: frequency, time of day, and type of hygiene products. Assess for any physical-activity limitations. Assess the patient's level of consciousness and overall ability to assist with oral care and respond to directions. Assess the patient's risk for oral hygiene problems. Alterations in cognitive function and/or consciousness increase the risk for alterations in oral tissue and structure integrity. Assess the patient's gag reflex. Decreased or absent gag reflex increases the risk for aspiration. Inspect the patient's oral cavity and teeth. Look for any caries, sores, or white patches. The white patches may indicate a fungal infection called thrush.

NURSING DIAGNOSIS

Determine the related factors for the nursing diagnosis based on the patient's current status. Possible nursing diagnoses may include:

- Ineffective Health Maintenance
- Impaired Oral Mucous Membrane
- Disturbed Body Image
- Deficient Knowledge

Other nursing diagnoses also may require the use of this skill.

OUTCOME IDENTIFICATION AND PLANNING

The expected outcome to achieve when performing oral care is that the patient's mouth and teeth will be clean; the patient will not experience impaired oral mucous membranes; the patient will participate as much as possible with oral care; the patient will demonstrate improvement in body image; and the patient will verbalize an understanding about the importance of oral care.

SKILL 7-3

Providing Oral Care for the Dependent Patient *(continued)*

IMPLEMENTATION

ACTION	RATIONALE
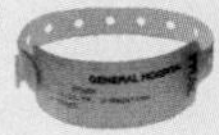 1. Identify the patient. Explain procedure to patient.	Identifying the patient ensures the right patient receives the intervention and helps prevent errors. Explanation facilitates cooperation.
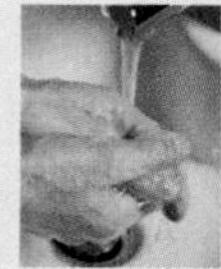 2. Perform hand hygiene and put on disposable gloves.	Hand hygiene and disposable gloves deter the spread of microorganisms.
3. Assemble equipment on overbed table within reach.	Organization facilitates performance of task.
4. Provide privacy for patient. Adjust height of bed to a comfortable position. Lower one side rail and position patient on the side, with head tilted forward. Place towel across patient's chest and emesis basin in position under chin.	The side-lying position with head forward prevents aspiration of fluid into lungs. Towel and emesis basin protects patient from dampness.
5. Open patient's mouth and gently insert a padded tongue blade between back molars if necessary (Figure 1).	A padded tongue blade keeps the mouth open for easier cleaning and prevents the patient from biting the nurse's fingers.
6. If teeth are present, brush carefully with toothbrush and paste (Figure 2). Remove dentures if present and use a toothette or gauze-padded tongue blade moistened with water or dilute mouthwash solution to gently clean gums, mucous membranes, and tongue. Clean the dentures before replacing (see Skill 7-4).	Toothbrush or padded tongue blade provides friction necessary to clean areas where plaque and tartar accumulate. Hydrogen peroxide is considered an irritant and is no longer recommended. The mechanical action of cleansing is more important than the solution used.

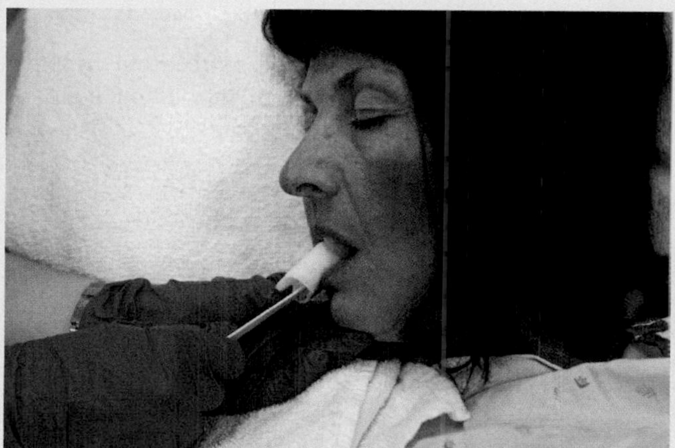

Figure 1. Gently inserting padded tongue blade between back molars.

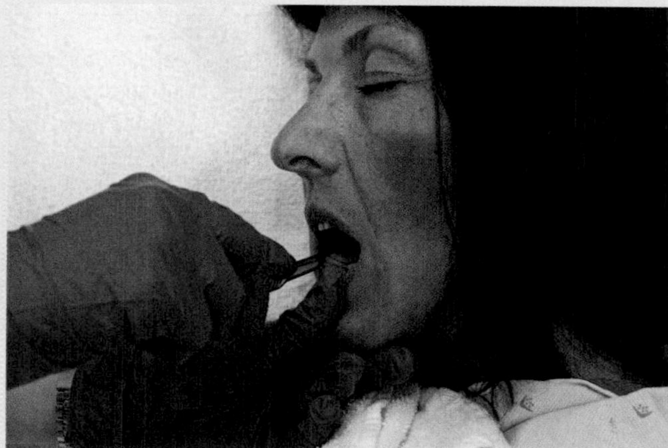

Figure 2. Carefully brushing patient's teeth.

ACTION	RATIONALE
7. Use gauze-padded tongue blade or toothette dipped in mouthwash solution to rinse the oral cavity. If desired, insert the rubber tip of the irrigating syringe into patient's mouth and rinse gently with a small amount of water (Figure 3). Position patient's head to allow for return of water or use suction apparatus to remove the water from oral cavity (Figure 4).	Rinsing helps clean debris from the mouth. Forceful irrigation may cause aspiration.
8. Apply lubricant to patient's lips.	This prevents drying and cracking of lips.

(continued)

SKILL 7-3

Providing Oral Care for the Dependent Patient *(continued)*

ACTION	RATIONALE
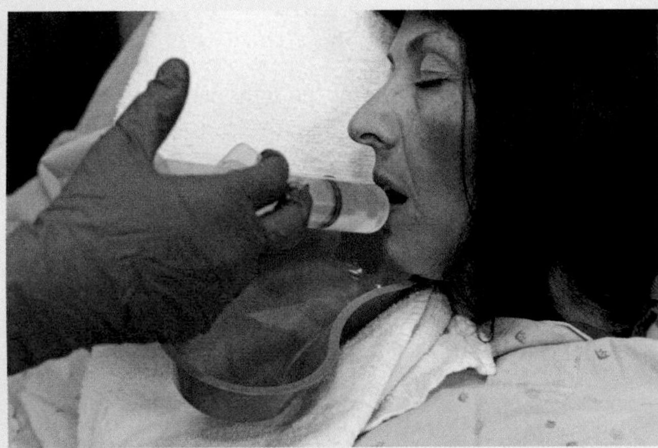 **Figure 3.** Using irrigating syringe and a small amount of water to rinse mouth.	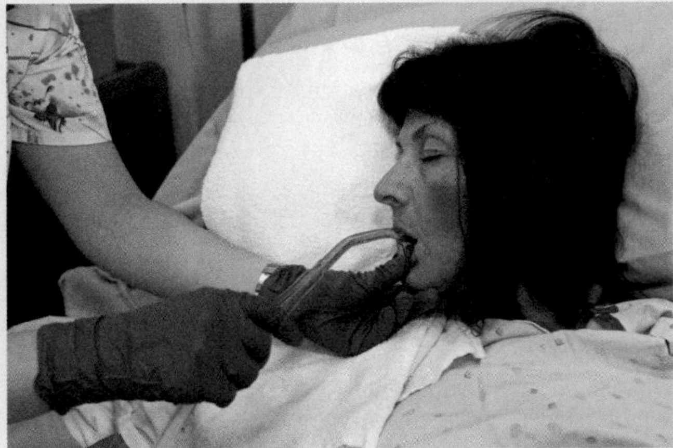 **Figure 4.** Using suction to remove excess fluid.
9. Remove equipment and return patient to a position of comfort. Remove your gloves. Raise side rail and lower bed.	Promotes patient comfort and safety.
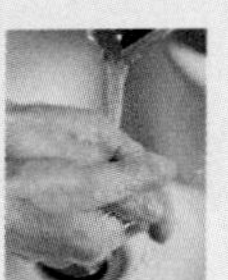 10. Perform hand hygiene.	Hand hygiene deters the spread of microorganisms.

EVALUATION

The expected outcomes are met when the patient's oral cavity is clean, free from complications, and the patient states or demonstrates improved body image. In addition, if the patient is able, verbalizes a basic understanding of the need for oral care.

DOCUMENTATION

Guidelines

Record oral assessment, significant observations, and unusual findings, such as bleeding or inflammation. Document any teaching done. Document procedure and patient response.

Sample Documentation

7/10/09 0945 Oral care performed. Oral cavity mucosa pink and moist. Small amount of bleeding noted from gums after using soft-bristled toothbrush. Resolved spontaneously when brushing completed. No evidence of ulceration. Lips slightly dry; lip moisturizer applied.—C. Stone, RN

Unexpected Situations and Associated Interventions

- *Patient begins to bite on padded tongue blade:* Do not jerk tongue blade out. Wait for patient to relax mouth before removing padded tongue blade.
- *Mouth is extremely dry with crusts that remain after oral care provided:* Increase frequency of oral hygiene. Apply mouth moisturizer to oral mucosa.

Special Considerations

General Considerations

- A patient receiving chemotherapy medication may have bleeding gums and extremely sensitive mucous membranes. Use a soft sponge toothette for cleaning, or substitute a salt water rinse (half teaspoon salt in 1 cup of warm water) for brushing of teeth.

SKILL 7-4

Providing Denture Care

The mouth requires care even during illness, but sometimes care must be modified to meet a patient's needs. If the patient can assist with mouth care, provide the necessary materials. Oral care is important not only to prevent dental caries but also to improve the patient's self-image. Dentures should be cleaned at least daily, to prevent irritation and infection. They may be cleaned more often, based on need and the patient's personal preference. Dentures are often removed at night. Handle dentures with care to prevent breakage.

Equipment

- Soft toothbrush or denture brush
- Toothpaste or denture cleaner
- Denture adhesive (optional)
- Glass of cool water
- Emesis basin
- Denture cup (optional)
- Clean gloves
- Towel
- Mouthwash (optional)
- Washcloth or paper towel
- Lip lubricant (optional)
- Gauze

ASSESSMENT

Assess the patient's oral hygiene preferences: frequency, time of day, and type of hygiene products. Assess for any physical activity limitations. Assess for difficulty chewing, pain, tenderness, and discomfort. Assess patient's oral cavity. Look for inflammation, edema, sores, or white patches. The white patches may indicate a fungal infection called thrush. Assess patient's ability to perform own care.

NURSING DIAGNOSIS

Determine the related factors for the nursing diagnosis based on the patient's current status. Possible nursing diagnoses may include:

- Ineffective Health Maintenance
- Impaired Oral Mucous Membrane
- Disturbed Body Image
- Deficient Knowledge

OUTCOME IDENTIFICATION AND PLANNING

The expected outcome to achieve is that the patient's mouth and dentures will be clean; the patient will exhibit a positive body image; and the patient will verbalize the importance of oral care.

IMPLEMENTATION

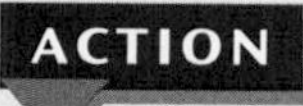

ACTION	RATIONALE
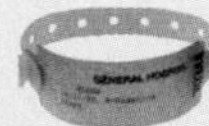 1. Identify patient. Explain procedure to patient.	Identifying the patient ensures the right patient receives the intervention and helps prevent errors. Explanation facilitates cooperation.
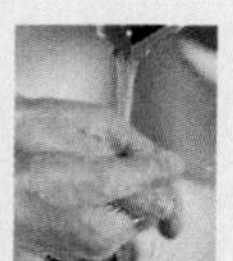 2. Perform hand hygiene. Put on disposable gloves.	Hand hygiene deters the spread of microorganisms. Gloves protect the nurse from exposure to blood or body fluids.
3. Assemble equipment on overbed table within reach.	Organization facilitates performance of task.

(continued)

SKILL 7-4 Providing Denture Care *(continued)*

ACTION	RATIONALE
4. Provide privacy for patient.	Patient may be embarrassed by removal of dentures.
5. Lower side rail and assist patient to sitting position if permitted, or turn patient onto side. Place towel across patient's chest. Raise bed to a comfortable working position.	The sitting or side-lying position prevents aspiration of fluids into the lungs. The towel protects the patient from dampness.
6. Apply gentle pressure with 4 × 4 gauze to grasp upper denture plate and remove (Figure 1). Place it immediately in denture cup. Lift lower dentures with gauze, using slight rocking motion. Remove, and place in denture cup.	Rocking motion breaks suction between denture and gum. Using 4 × 4 gauze prevents slippage and discourages spread of microorganisms.

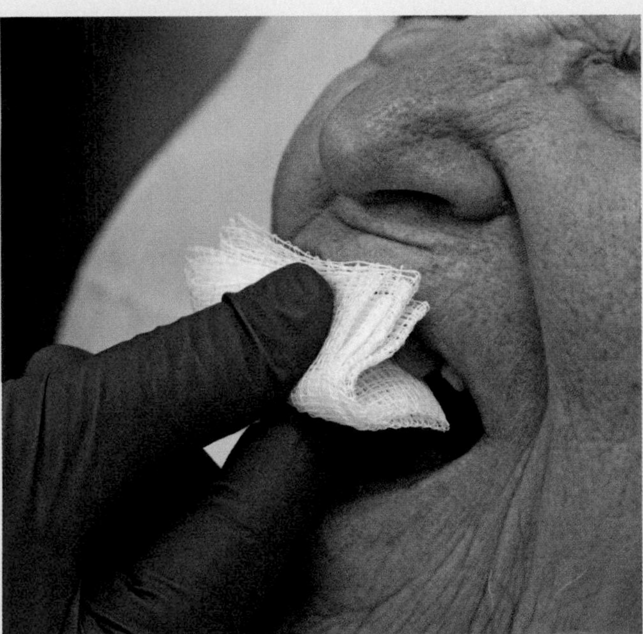

Figure 1. Removing dentures with a gauze sponge.

ACTION	RATIONALE
7. Place paper towels or washcloth in sink while brushing. Using the toothbrush and paste, brush all surfaces gently but thoroughly (Figure 2). If patient prefers, add denture cleaner to cup with water and follow directions on preparation.	Putting paper towels or a washcloth in the sink protects against breakage. Dentures collect food and microorganisms and require daily cleaning.
8. Rinse thoroughly with water. Apply denture adhesive if appropriate.	Water aids in removal of debris and acts as a cleaning agent.
9. Use a toothbrush or toothette moistened with water or dilute mouthwash solution to gently clean gums, mucous membranes, and tongue. Offer mouthwash so patient can rinse mouth before replacing dentures, if desired.	Cleaning removes food particles and plaque, permitting proper fit and preventing infection. Mouthwash leaves a pleasant taste in the mouth.
10. Insert upper denture in mouth and press firmly. Insert lower denture. Check that the dentures are securely in place and comfortable.	This ensures patient comfort.

SKILL 7-4 **Providing Denture Care** *(continued)*

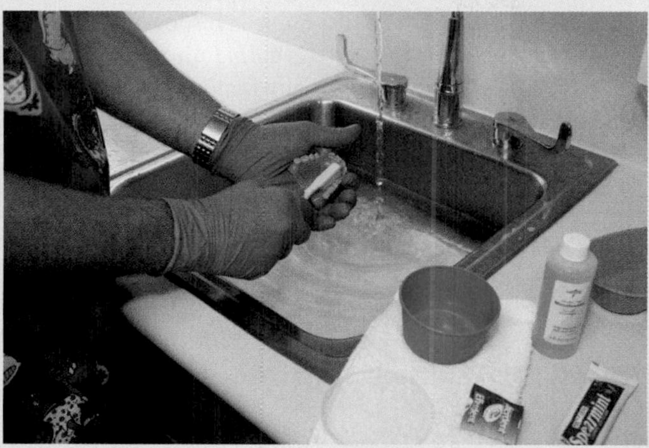

Figure 2. Cleaning dentures at the sink.

11. If the patient desires, dentures can be stored in the denture cup in cold water, instead of returning to the mouth. Label the cup and place in the patient's bedside table.

Storing in water prevents warping of dentures. Proper storage prevents loss and damage.

12. Remove gloves and perform hand hygiene.

Hand hygiene prevents transmission of microorganisms.

EVALUATION

The expected outcomes are met when the patient's oral cavity and dentures are clean, free from complications, and patient states or demonstrates improved body image. In addition, the patient verbalizes a basic understanding of the need for oral care.

DOCUMENTATION

Guidelines

Record oral assessment, significant observations and unusual findings, such as bleeding or inflammation. Document any teaching done. Document procedure and patient response.

Sample Documentation

7/10/09 0945 Oral care performed. Oral cavity mucosa pink and moist. Denture and oral care given. No evidence of bleeding, ulceration, or inflammation.
—C. Stone, RN

Unexpected Situations and Associated Interventions

- *Food or other material doesn't come off denture with brushing:* Place denture in cup with cool water and soak. After soaking, use toothbrush and toothpaste to clean again. If necessary, use commercial denture cleaner added to water in cup to soak, then brush clean.

Special Considerations

General Considerations

- Encourage the patient to wear his dentures, if not contraindicated. Dentures enhance appearance, assist eating, facilitate speech, and maintain the gum line. Denture fit may be altered with long periods of nonuse.
- Encourage the patient to refrain from wrapping the denture in paper towels or napkins because they could be mistaken for trash.
- Encourage the patient to refrain from placing the dentures in the bed clothes because they can be lost in the laundry.

SKILL 7-5 Removing Contact Lenses

If a patient wears contact lenses but cannot remove them, the nurse is responsible for removing them. This may occur, for example, when the nurse is caring for an unconscious patient. Whenever an unconscious patient is admitted without any family present, always assess the patient to determine whether he or she wears contact lenses. Leaving contact lenses in place for long periods could result in permanent eye damage.

Before removing hard or gas-permeable lenses, use gentle pressure to center the lens on the cornea. Once removed, be sure to identify the lenses as being for the right or left eye, because the two lenses are not necessarily identical. If an eye injury is present, do not try to remove lenses because of the danger of causing an additional injury.

Equipment

- Disposable gloves
- Container for contact lenses (if unavailable, two small sterile containers marked "L" and "R" will suffice)
- Sterile normal saline solution
- Rubber pincer, if available (for removal of soft lenses)
- Suction-cup remover, if available (for removal of hard lenses)

ASSESSMENT

Assess both eyes for contact lenses, as some people wear them in only one eye. Assess eyes for any redness or drainage, which may indicate an infection of the eye or an allergic response. Assess for any eye injury. If an injury is present, notify the physician about the presence of the contact lens. Do not try to remove the contact lens in this situation due to the risk for additional eye injury.

NURSING DIAGNOSIS

Determine the related factors for the nursing diagnosis based on the patient's current status. An appropriate nursing diagnosis is Risk for Injury.

OUTCOME IDENTIFICATION AND PLANNING

The expected outcome to achieve when removing contact lenses is that the lenses are removed without trauma to the eye and stored safely.

IMPLEMENTATION

ACTION	RATIONALE
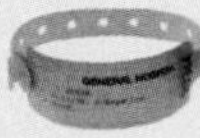 1. Check the patient's identification band and ask the patient to state name, if appropriate.	Positive identification of the patient is essential to ensure the intervention is administered to the correct patient.
2. Explain what you are going to do.	Explanation relieves anxiety and facilitates cooperation.
3. Close curtains around bed and close door to room if possible.	This ensures the patient's privacy.
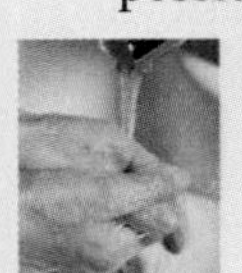 4. Perform hand hygiene and put on clean gloves.	Hand hygiene deters the spread of microorganisms. Gloves prevent exposure to blood and body fluids.
5. Assist patient to supine position. Elevate bed. Lower side rail closest to you.	Supine position with the bed raised and the side rail down is the least stressful position for the nurse to remove the contact lens.
6. If containers are not already labeled, do so now. Place 5 mL of normal saline in each container.	Many patients have different prescription strengths for each eye. The saline will prevent the contact from drying out.

SKILL 7-5 Removing Contact Lenses *(continued)*

ACTION	RATIONALE
7. Remove soft contact lens: a. Have the patient look forward. Retract the lower lid with one hand. Using the pad of the index finger of the other hand, move the lens down to the sclera (Figure 1). b. Using the pads of the thumb and index finger, grasp the lens with a gentle pinching motion and remove (Figure 2). See accompanying Skill Variation display for other techniques for removing both hard and soft lenses.	

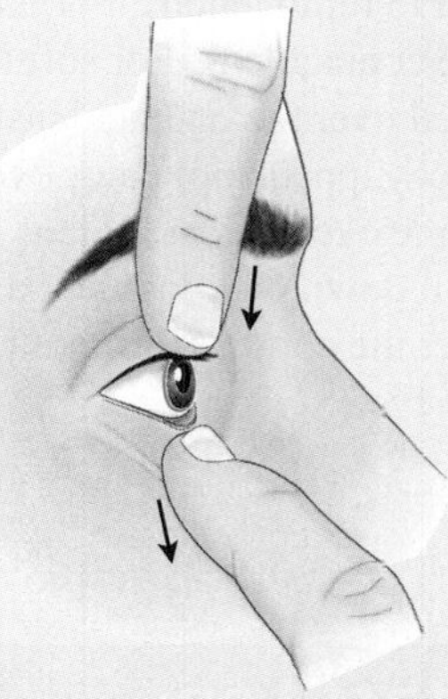

Figure 1. Retracting the lower lid with one hand and using the pad of the index finger of the other hand to move the lens down to the sclera.

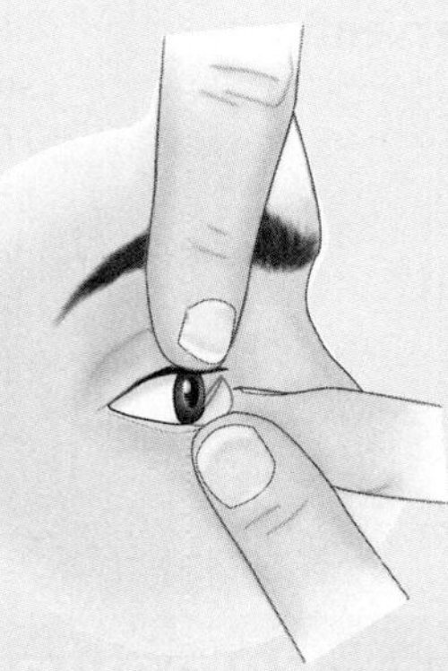

Figure 2. Using the pads of the thumb and index finger to grasp the lens with a gentle pinching motion and remove.

ACTION	RATIONALE
8. Place the first lens in its designated cup in the storage case before removing the second lens (Figure 3).	Lenses may be different for each eye. Avoids mixing them up.

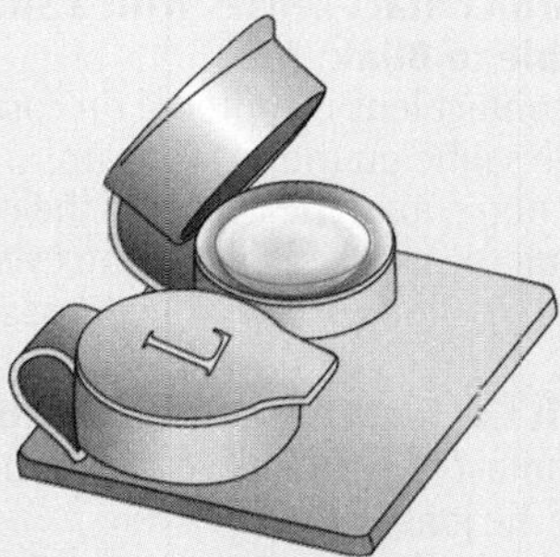

Figure 3. Storage cases are marked L and R, designating left and right lenses. Placing the first lens in its designated cup before removing the second lens avoids mixing them up.

ACTION	RATIONALE
9. Repeat actions to remove other contact lens.	
10. If patient is awake and has glasses at bedside, offer patient glasses.	Not being able to see clearly creates anxiety.
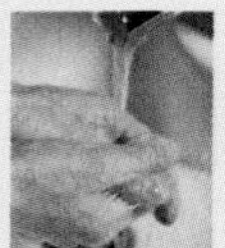 11. Remove gloves. Perform hand hygiene.	Hand hygiene deters the spread of microorganisms.

(continued)

SKILL 7-5 Removing Contact Lenses *(continued)*

EVALUATION

The expected outcome is met when the patient remains free of injury as the contact lenses are removed. Eye exhibits no signs and symptoms of trauma, irritation, or redness.

DOCUMENTATION

Guidelines

Record your assessment, significant observations, and unusual findings, such as drainage or pain. Document any teaching done. Document the removal of the contact lenses and patient response.

Sample Documentation

7/15/09 1045 Soft contacts removed from eyes without trauma. Stored in patient's lens case in normal saline. Sclera white with no drainage from eye. Glasses placed at bedside.—C. Stone, RN

Unexpected Situations and Associated Interventions

- *The contact lens cannot be removed:* Use tool to remove lens. For hard lenses, the tool has a small suction cup that is placed over the contact lens. For soft lenses, the tool is a small pair of rubber grippers that can be placed over the contact lens to aid in removal.
- *Hard contact is not over cornea:* Place a cotton-tipped applicator over upper eyelid and grasp lid, inverting lid over applicator. Examine eye for lens. If lens is not in the upper portion, place finger below eye and gently pull down on lid while having patient look up. When the lens is found, gently slide it over the cornea (Ramponi, 2001). (Soft contacts may be removed from other areas of the eye.)

SKILL VARIATION Removing Different Types of Contact Lens

- Check the patient's identification band and ask the patient to state name, if appropriate.
- Explain what you are going to do.
- Close curtains around bed and close door to room if possible.

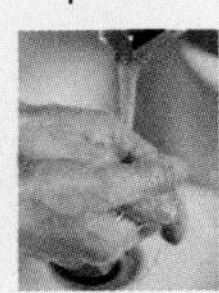

- Perform hand hygiene and put on clean gloves.
- Assist patient to supine position. Elevate bed. Lower side rail closest to you.
- If containers are not already labeled, do so now. Place 5 mL of normal saline in each container.
- **To Remove Hard Contact Lenses—Patient is Able to Blink:**
  - If the lens is not centered over the cornea, apply gentle pressure on the lower eyelid to center the lens (Figure A).
  - Gently pull the outer corner of the eye toward the ear (Figure B).
  - Position the other hand below the lens to catch it and ask patient to blink (Figure C).
- **To Remove Hard Contact Lenses—Patient is Unable to Blink:**
  - Gently spread the eyelids beyond the top and bottom edges of the lens (Figure D).
  - Gently press the lower eyelid up against the bottom of the lens (Figure E).
  - After the lens is tipped slightly, move the eyelids toward one another to cause the lens to slide out between the eyelids (Figure F).
- **To Remove Hard Contact Lenses With a Suction Cup—Patient is Unable to Blink:**
  - Ensure that contact lens is centered on cornea. Place a drop of sterile saline on the suction cup.
  - Place the suction cup in the center of the contact lens and gently pull the contact lens off the eye.
  - To remove the suction cup from the lens, slide the lens off sideways.
- **To Remove Soft Contact Lenses With a Rubber Pincer:**
  - Locate the contact lens and place the rubber pincers in the center of the lens.
  - Gently squeeze the pincers and remove the lens from the eye.
- Place the first lens in its designated cup in the storage case before removing the second lens.
- Repeat actions to remove other contact lens.
- If patient is awake and has glasses at bedside, offer patient glasses.
- Remove gloves. Perform hand hygiene.

SKILL 7-5 Removing Contact Lenses *(continued)*

SKILL VARIATION Removing Different Types of Contact Lens

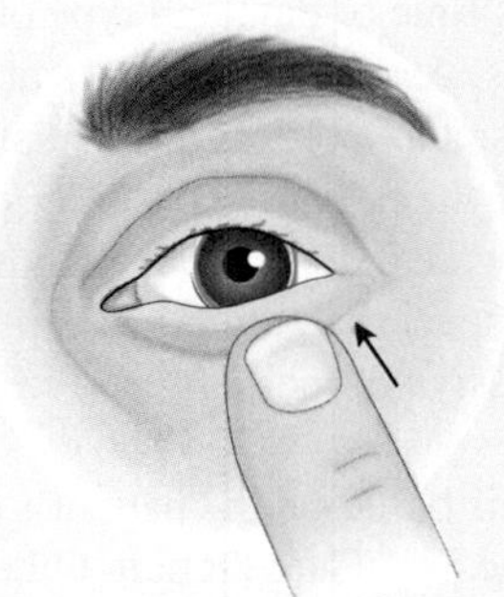

Figure A. Centering the lens.

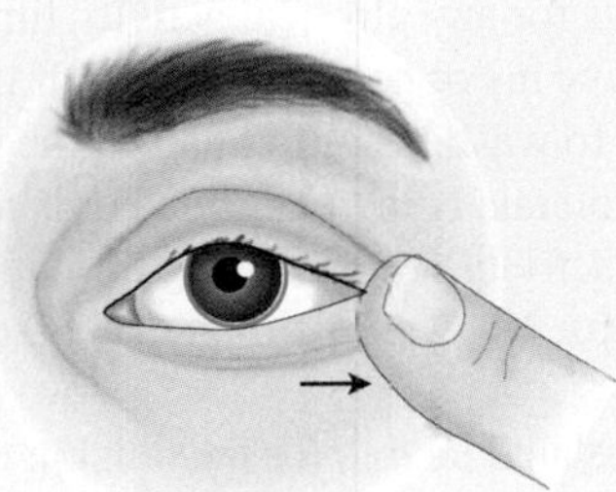

Figure B. Gently pulling outer corner of eye toward ear.

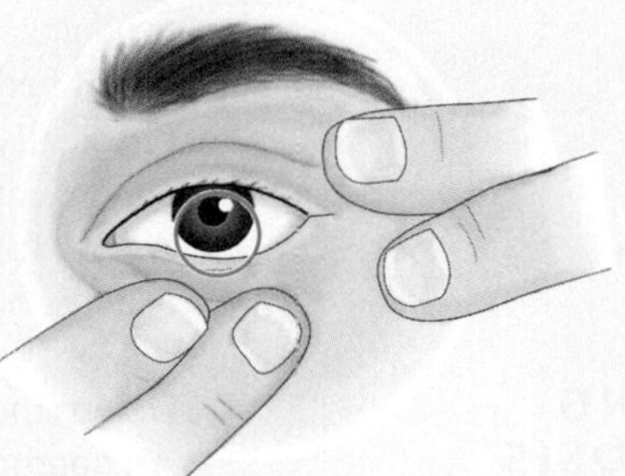

Figure C. Receiving the lens as the patient blinks.

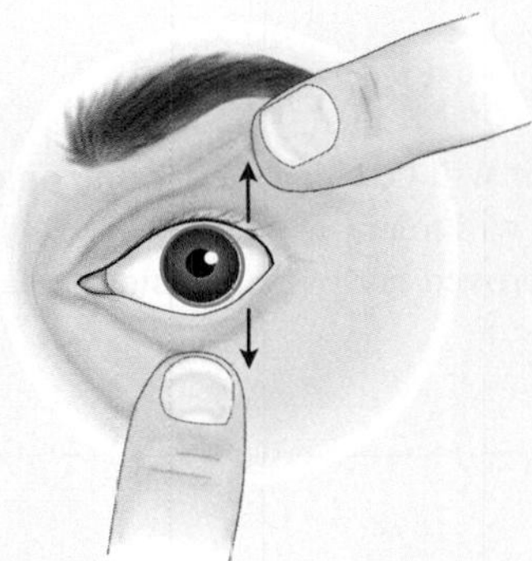

Figure D. Spreading the eyelids.

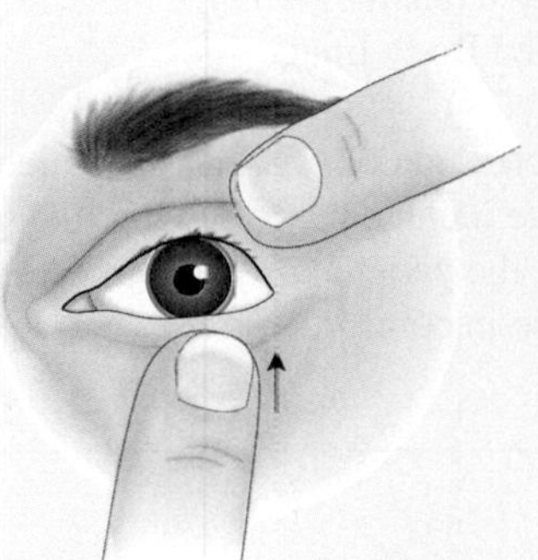

Figure E. Pressing the lower lid up against the bottom of the lens.

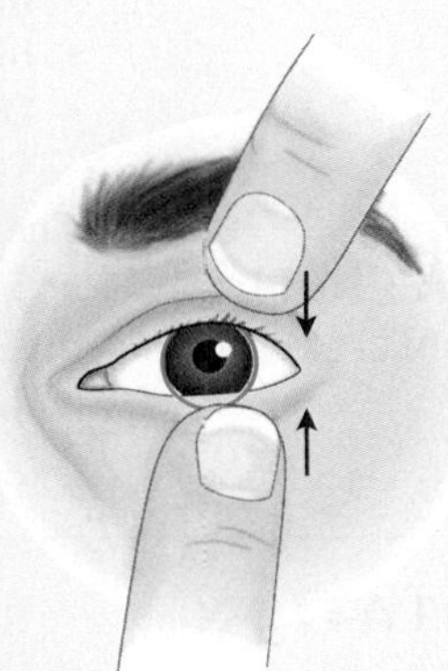

Figure F. Sliding lens out between lids.

SKILL 7-6 Shampooing a Patient's Hair in Bed

The easiest way to wash a patient's hair is to assist him or her in the shower, but not all patients can take showers. If the patient's hair needs to be washed but the patient is unable or not allowed to get out of bed, a bed shampoo can be performed.

Equipment

- Water pitcher
- Warm water
- Shampoo
- Conditioner (optional)
- Disposable gloves (optional)
- Protective pad for bed
- Shampoo board
- Bucket
- Towels
- Gown

(continued)

SKILL 7-6 Shampooing a Patient's Hair in Bed

- Comb or brush
- Blow dryer (optional)

ASSESSMENT

Assess the patient's hygiene preferences: frequency, time of day, and type of hygiene products. Assess for any physical activity limitations. Assess the patient's ability to get out of bed to have his or her hair washed. If the physician's orders allow it and patient is physically able to wash his or her hair in the shower, the patient may prefer to do so. If the patient cannot tolerate being out of bed or is not allowed to do so, perform a bed shampoo. Assess for any activity or positioning limitations. Inspect the patient's scalp for any cuts, lesions, or bumps. Note any flaking, drying, or excessive oiliness.

NURSING DIAGNOSIS

Determine the related factors for the nursing diagnosis based on the patient's current status. An appropriate nursing diagnosis is Bathing/Hygiene Self-Care Deficit. Other nursing diagnosis may include:

- Activity Intolerance
- Impaired Physical Mobility
- Impaired Transfer Ability
- Disturbed Body Image

OUTCOME IDENTIFICATION AND PLANNING

The expected outcome is that the patient's hair will be clean. Other outcomes that may be appropriate include the following: the patient will tolerate the shampoo with little to no difficulty, the patient will demonstrate an improved body image, and the patient will state an increase in comfort.

IMPLEMENTATION

ACTION	RATIONALE
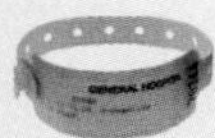 1. Identify the patient. Explain procedure to patient.	Identifying the patient ensures the right patient receives the intervention and helps prevent errors. Explanation facilitates cooperation.
2. Assemble equipment on overbed table within reach.	Organization facilitates performance of task.
3. Close the room door or curtain.	Provides for patient privacy
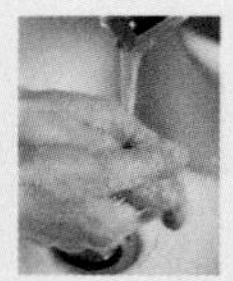 4. Perform hand hygiene. **If you suspect there are any cuts of the scalp or blood in the hair, put on disposable gloves.** Lower head of bed.	Hand hygiene deters the spread of microorganisms. Gloves protect the nurse from contact with blood or body fluids.
5. Remove pillow and place protective pad under patient's head and shoulders (Figure 1).	This protects the sheets from getting wet.
6. **Fill the pitcher with warm water (43°–46°C [110°–115°F]).** Position the patient at the top of the bed, in a supine position. Have the patient lift his head and place shampoo board underneath patient's head (Figure 2). If necessary, pad the edge of the board with a small towel.	Warm water is comfortable and relaxing for the patient. It also stimulates circulation and provides for more effective cleaning. Padding the edge of the shampoo board may help increase patient comfort.
7. Place bucket on floor underneath the drain of the shampoo board (Figure 3).	The bucket will catch the runoff water, preventing a mess on the floor.

SKILL 7-6

Shampooing a Patient's Hair in Bed *(continued)*

ACTION	RATIONALE
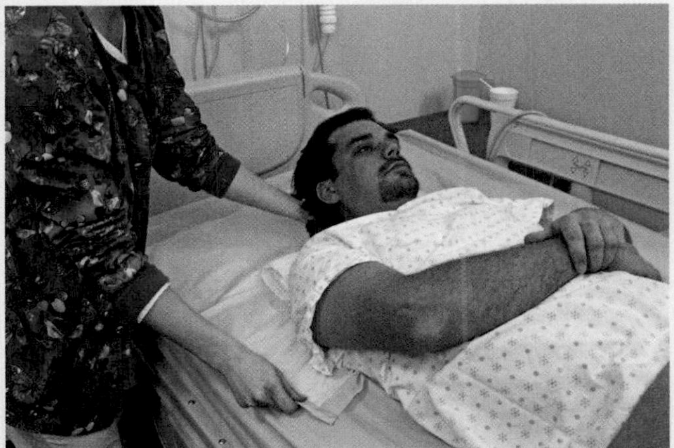 Figure 1. Padding head of bed with protective sheets.	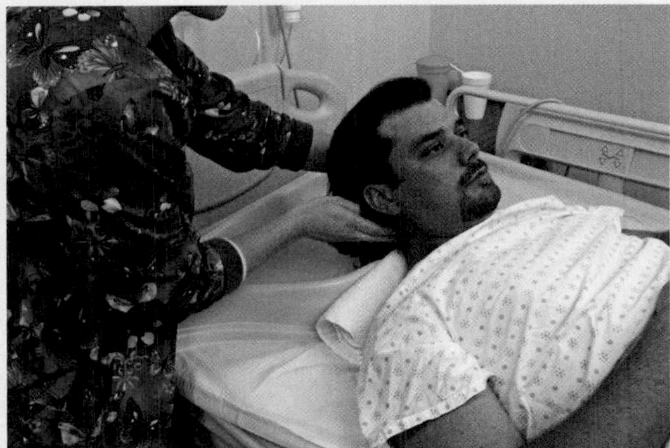 Figure 2. Placing patient's head on shampoo board.
8. If the patient is able, have him or her hold a folded washcloth at the forehead. Pour pitcher of warm water slowly over patient's head, making sure that all hair is saturated (Figure 4). Refill pitcher if needed.	Washcloth prevents water from running into the patient's eyes. By pouring slowly, more hair will become wet, and it is more soothing for the patient.
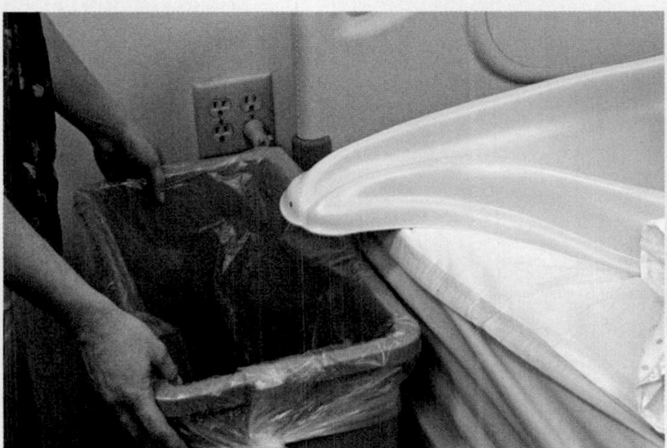 Figure 3. Positioning drain container for shampoo board.	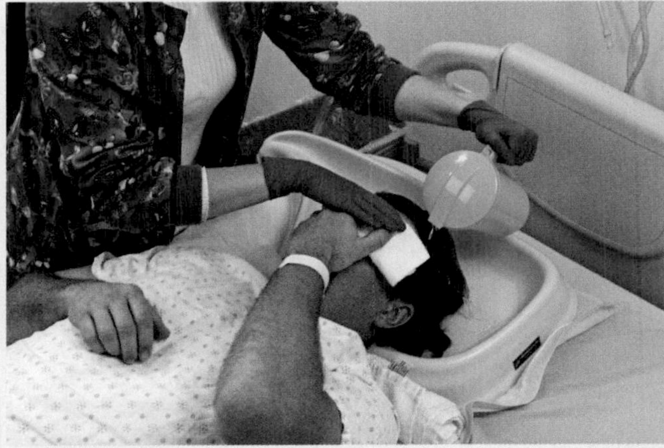 Figure 4. Pouring warm water over patient's head.
9. Apply a small amount of shampoo to patient's hair. **Massage deep into the scalp, avoiding any cuts, lesions, or sore spots (Figure 5).**	Shampoo will help to remove dirt or oil.
10. Rinse with warm water (43°–46°C [110°–115°F]) until all shampoo is out of hair (Figure 6). Repeat shampoo if necessary.	Shampoo left in hair may cause pruritus. If hair is still dirty, another shampoo treatment may be needed.
11. If patient has thick hair or requests it, apply a small amount of conditioner to hair and massage throughout. Avoid any cuts, lesions, or sore spots.	Conditioner eases tangles and moisturizes hair and scalp.

(continued)

SKILL 7-6

Shampooing a Patient's Hair in Bed *(continued)*

ACTION	RATIONALE

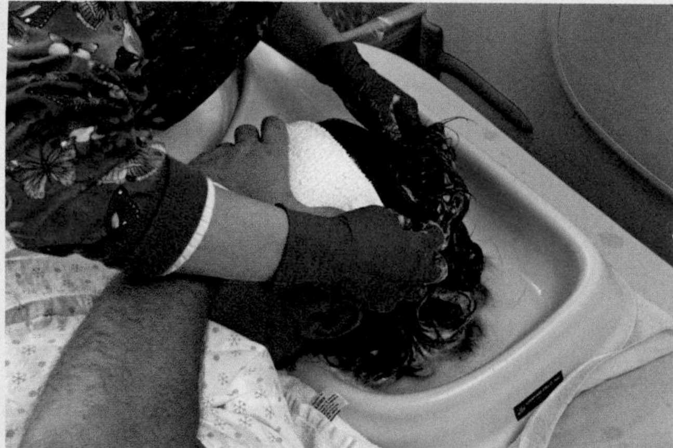

Figure 5. Lathering up shampoo.

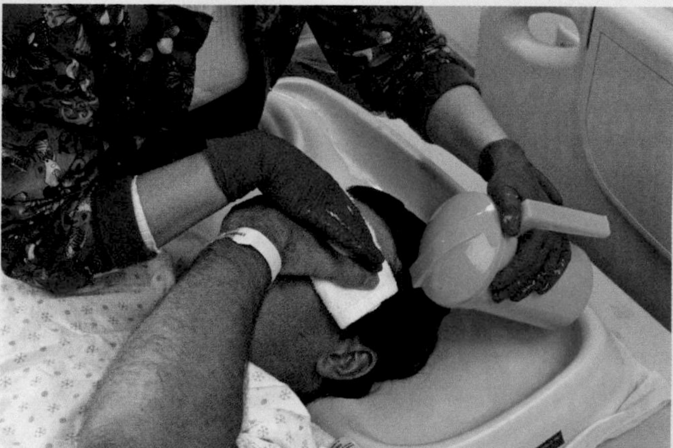

Figure 6. Rinsing shampoo from patient's head.

ACTION	RATIONALE
12. If bucket is small, empty before rinsing hair. Rinse with warm water (43°–46°C [110°–115°F]) until all conditioner is out of hair.	Bucket may overflow if not emptied. Conditioner left in hair may cause pruritus.
13. Remove shampoo board (Figure 7). Place towel around patient's hair.	This prevents the patient from getting cold.

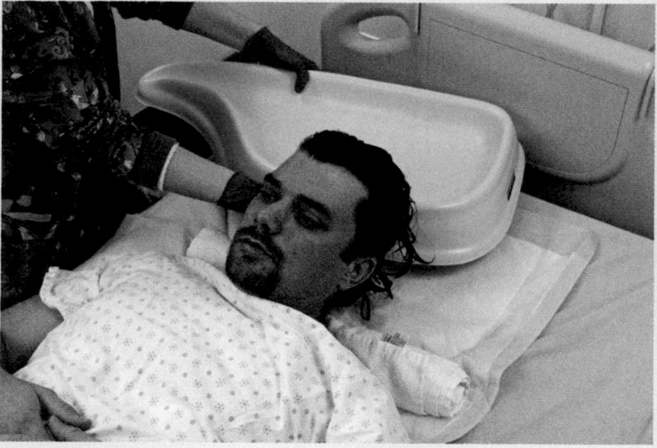

Figure 7. Removing shampoo board from bed.

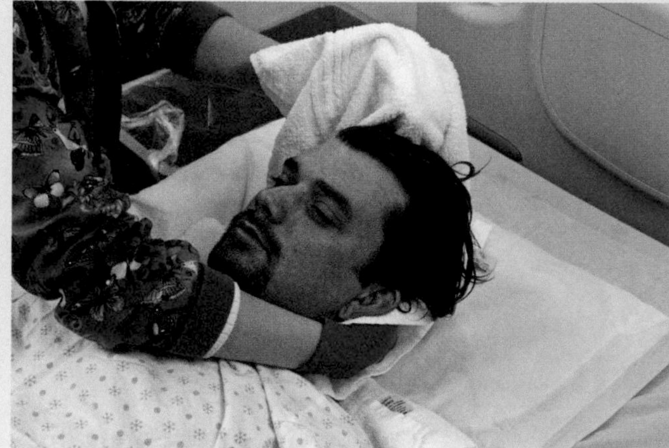

Figure 8. Patting patient's hair dry.

ACTION	RATIONALE
14. Pat hair dry, avoiding any cuts, lesions, or sore spots (Figure 8). Remove protective padding but keep one dry protective pad under patient's hair (Figure 9).	Patting dry removes any excess water without damaging hair or scalp.
15. Gently brush hair, removing tangles as needed.	Removing tangles helps hair to dry faster. Brushing hair improves patient's self-image.
16. Blow-dry hair on a cool setting if allowed and if patient wishes (Figure 10).	Blow-drying hair helps hair to dry faster and prevents patient from becoming chilled.
17. Change patient's gown and remove protective pad. Replace pillow.	If patient's gown is damp, patient will become chilled. Protective pad is no longer needed once hair is dry.

SKILL 7-6 **Shampooing a Patient's Hair in Bed** *(continued)*

ACTION	RATIONALE
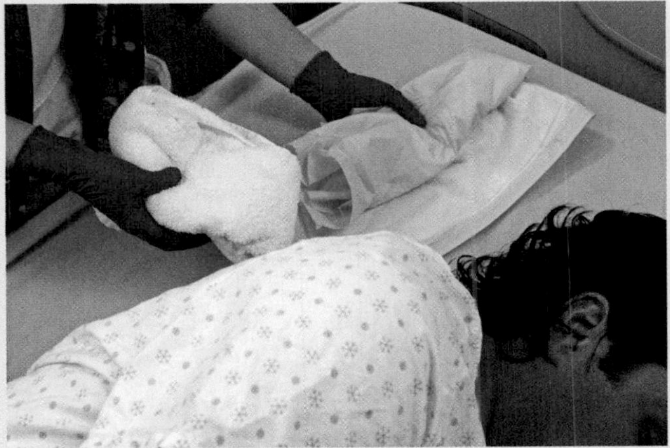 Figure 9. Removing wet protective bedding.	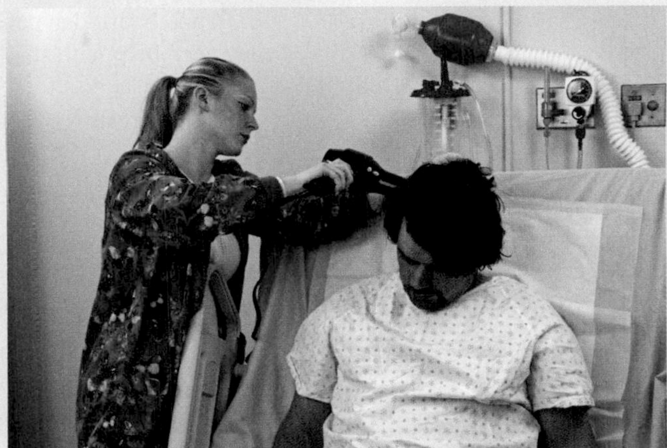 Figure 10. Blow-drying patient's hair.
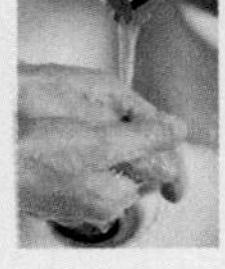 18. Remove gloves. Perform hand hygiene.	Hand hygiene deters spread of microorganisms.

EVALUATION

The expected outcomes are met when the patient's hair is clean, the patient verbalizes a positive body image, and the patient reports an increase in comfort level.

DOCUMENTATION

Guidelines

Record your assessment, significant observations, and unusual findings, such as bleeding or inflammation. Document any teaching done. Document procedure and patient response.

Sample Documentation

7/4/09 1130 Hair washed. Moderate amount of dried blood in hair noted. 3-cm laceration noted over left parietal area. Edges well approximated, sutures intact, and no drainage noted.—C. Stone, RN

Unexpected Situations and Associated Interventions

- *Glass is found in hair:* Carefully comb through hair before washing to remove as much glass as possible. Discard glass in appropriate container. When massaging scalp, be alert to signs of pain from the patient; glass could be cutting the patient's head.

Special Considerations

General Considerations

- If the patient has a spinal cord or neck injury, use of the shampoo board may be contraindicated. In this case, a makeshift protection area can be created to wash the patient's hair without using the board. Place a protective pad underneath the patient's head and shoulders. Roll a towel into the bottom of the protective pad and direct the roll into one area so that water will drain into the container.

SKILL 7-7 Assisting the Patient to Shave

Shaving for many patients is a daily ritual of hygiene. They may feel disheveled and unclean without shaving. Electric shavers are usually recommended when the patient is receiving anticoagulant therapy or has a bleeding disorder, and are especially convenient for ill and bedridden patients, if available and permitted by the facility. Some patients may need help with shaving when using a regular blade.

Equipment

- Shaving cream
- Safety razor
- Towel
- Washcloth
- Bath basin
- Disposable gloves
- Waterproof pad
- Aftershave or lotion (optional)

ASSESSMENT

Assess the patient's shaving preferences: frequency, time of day, and type of shaving products. Assess for any physical activity limitations. Assess patient for any bleeding problems. If patient is receiving any anticoagulant such as heparin or warfarin (Coumadin), has received an antithrombolytic agent, or has a low platelet count, consider using an electric razor. Inspect the area to be shaved for any lesions or weeping areas. Assess the patient's ability to shave himself or assist with the procedure.

NURSING DIAGNOSIS

Determine related factors for the nursing diagnosis based on the patient's current status. Appropriate nursing diagnoses may include:

- Risk for Injury
- Bathing/Hygiene Self-Care Deficit
- Activity Intolerance
- Impaired Physical Mobility

Many other nursing diagnoses may require this skill.

OUTCOME IDENTIFICATION AND PLANNING

The expected outcome to achieve when assisting the patient with shaving is that the patient will be clean, without evidence of hair growth or trauma to the skin. Other outcomes that may be appropriate include the following: the patient tolerates shaving with minimal to no difficulty, and the patient verbalizes feelings of improved self-esteem.

IMPLEMENTATION

ACTION	RATIONALE
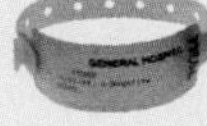 1. Identify patient. Explain procedure to patient.	Identifying the patient ensures the right patient receives the intervention and helps prevent errors. Explanation facilitates cooperation.
2. Assemble equipment on overbed table within reach.	Organization facilitates performance of task.
3. Close the room door or curtain.	Provides for patient privacy.
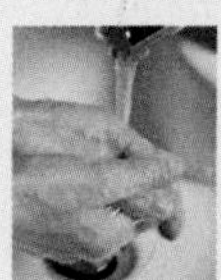 4. Perform hand hygiene and put on disposable gloves.	Hand hygiene deters the spread of microorganisms. Gloves should be worn due to the possibility of contact with blood if the person is cut during shaving.

SKILL 7-7

Assisting the Patient to Shave *(continued)*

ACTION	RATIONALE
5. Cover patient's chest with a towel or waterproof pad. Fill bath basin with warm (43°–46°C [110°–115°F]) water. Moisten the area to be shaved with a washcloth.	Warm water is comfortable and relaxing for the patient.
6. Dispense shaving cream into palm of hand. Rub hands together, then apply to area to be shaved in a layer about 0.5″ thick (Figure 1).	Using shaving cream helps to prevent skin irritation and prevents hair from pulling.

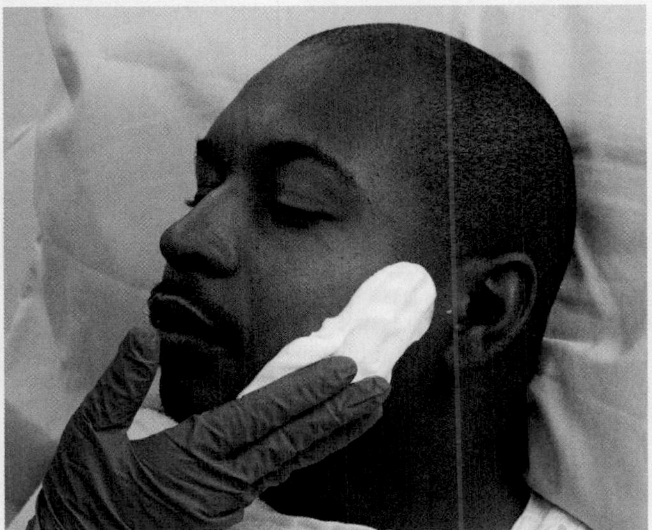

Figure 1. Applying shaving cream to face.

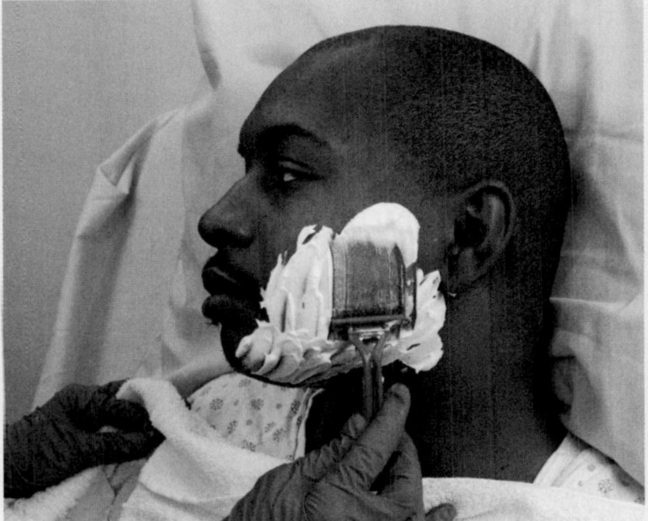

Figure 2. Shaving the face.

ACTION	RATIONALE
7. With one hand, pull the skin taut at the area to be shaved. Using a smooth stroke, begin shaving. *If shaving the face,* shave with the direction of hair growth in downward, short strokes (Figure 2). *If shaving a leg,* shave against the hair in upward, short strokes.	The skin on the face is more sensitive and needs to be shaved with the direction of hair growth to prevent discomfort.
8. Wash off residual shaving cream (Figure 3).	Shaving cream can lead to irritation if left on the skin.

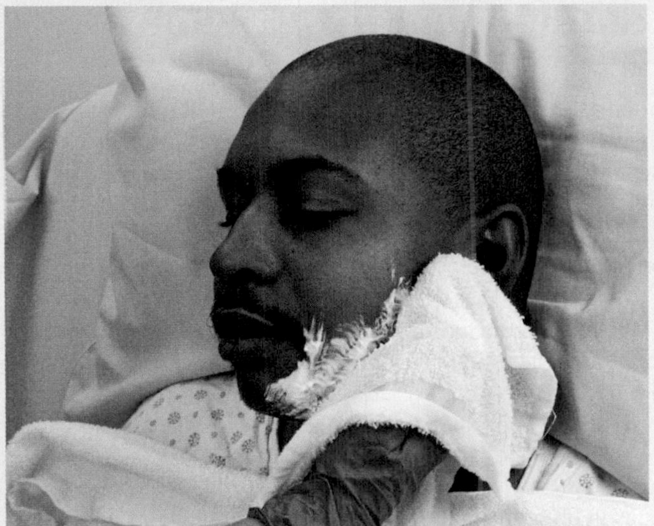

Figure 3. Using a wet washcloth to rinse remaining shaving cream off patient.

(continued)

SKILL 7-7 Assisting the Patient to Shave *(continued)*

ACTION	RATIONALE
9. If patient requests, apply aftershave or lotion to area shaved.	Aftershave and lotion can reduce skin irritation.
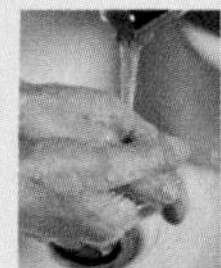 10. Remove and discard gloves and perform hand hygiene.	Proper glove removal and hand hygiene deter the spread of microorganisms.

EVALUATION

The expected outcome is met when the patient exhibits a clean-shaven face without evidence of trauma, irritation, or redness. In addition, the patient verbalizes feeling refreshed and demonstrates improved self-esteem.

DOCUMENTATION

It is not usually necessary to document shaving a patient. However, if your skin assessment reveals any unusual findings, document your assessment and the procedure.

Unexpected Situations and Associated Interventions

- *Patient is cut and bleeding during shave:* Apply pressure with gauze or towel to injured area. Do not release pressure for 2 to 3 minutes. After bleeding has stopped, resume shaving. The water basin may need to be rewarmed before washing the shaving cream off. Document the occurrence and post-shave assessment of area.
- *Patient has large amount of hair to be shaved:* If hair is longer, it may need to be trimmed with scissors before shaving to prevent pulling of hair when shaving.

Special Considerations

General Considerations

- *Patient is brought to hospital with full beard:* Do not shave patient's beard without consent unless it is an emergency situation, such as insertion of an endotracheal tube. For this procedure, shave only the area needed and leave the rest of the beard.

SKILL 7-8 Applying and Removing Antiembolism Stockings

Antiembolism stockings are often used for patients at risk for deep-vein thrombosis, pulmonary embolism, and to help prevent phlebitis (described in Chap. 9, Activity). Manufactured by several companies, they are made of elastic material and are available in either knee-high or thigh-high length. By applying pressure, antiembolism stockings increase the velocity of blood flow in the superficial and deep veins and improve venous valve function in the legs, promoting venous return to the heart. A physician's order is required for their use.

Be prepared to apply the stockings in the morning before the patient is out of bed and while the patient is supine. If the patient is sitting or has been up and about, have the patient lie down with legs and feet elevated for at least 15 minutes before applying the stockings. Otherwise, the leg vessels are congested with blood, reducing the effectiveness of the stockings.

Equipment

- Elastic antiembolism stockings in ordered length in correct size. See Assessment for appropriate measurement procedure.

SKILL 7-8 Applying and Removing Antiembolism Stockings *(continued)*

- Measuring tape
- Talcum powder (optional)

ASSESSMENT

Assess the skin condition and neurovascular status of the legs. Abnormalities should be reported before continuing with the application of the stockings. Assess patient's legs for any redness, swelling, warmth, or tenderness that may indicate a deep-vein thrombosis. If any of these symptoms are noted, notify physician before applying stockings. Measure the patient's legs to obtain the correct size stocking. For knee-high length: Measure around the widest part of the calf and the leg length from the bottom of the heel to the back of the knee, at the bend. For thigh-high length: Measure around the widest part of the calf and the thigh. Measure the length from the bottom of the heel to the gluteal fold. Follow the manufacturer's specifications to select the correct sized stockings.

NURSING DIAGNOSIS

Determine related factors for the nursing diagnosis based on the patient's current status. Appropriate nursing diagnoses may include:

- Ineffective Peripheral Tissue Perfusion
- Risk for Impaired Skin Integrity
- Excess Fluid Volume
- Risk for Injury

OUTCOME IDENTIFICATION AND PLANNING

The expected outcome to achieve when applying and removing antiembolism stockings is that the stockings will be applied and removed with minimal discomfort to patient. Other outcomes that may be appropriate include the following: edema will decrease in the lower extremities; patient will understand the rationale for stocking application; and patient will remain free of deep vein thrombosis.

IMPLEMENTATION

ACTION	RATIONALE
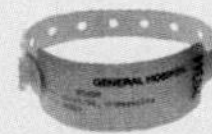 1. Check the patient's identification band and ask the patient to state name, if appropriate.	Positive identification of the patient is essential to ensure the intervention is administered to the correct patient. Ask the patient to state his or her name if possible. It is considered unsafe to call the patient by name because the patient may respond even if the nurse uses the wrong name.
2. Explain what you are going to do and the rationale for use of elastic stockings.	Explanation relieves anxiety and facilitates cooperation
3. Close curtains around bed and close door to room if possible.	This ensures the patient's privacy.
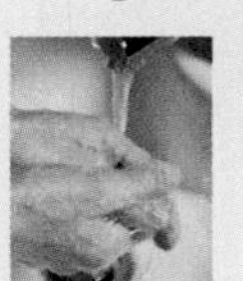 4. Perform hand hygiene.	Hand hygiene deters the spread of microorganisms.
5. Assist patient to supine position. If patient has been sitting or walking, have him or her lie down with legs and feet well elevated for at least 15 minutes before applying stockings.	Dependent position of legs encourages blood to pool in the veins, reducing the effectiveness of the stockings if they are applied to congested blood vessels.

(continued)

SKILL 7-8 Applying and Removing Antiembolism Stockings *(continued)*

ACTION	RATIONALE
6. Expose legs one at a time. Wash and dry legs, if necessary. Powder the leg lightly unless patient has a breathing problem, dry skin, or sensitivity to the powder. If the skin is dry, a lotion may be used. Powders and lotions are not recommended by some manufacturers; check the package material for manufacturer specifications.	Helps maintain patient's privacy. Powder and lotion reduce friction and make application of stockings easier.
7. Stand at the foot of the bed. Place hand inside stocking and grasp heel area securely. Turn stocking inside-out to the heel area, leaving the foot inside the stocking leg (Figure 1).	Inside-out technique provides for easier application; bunched elastic material can compromise extremity circulation.

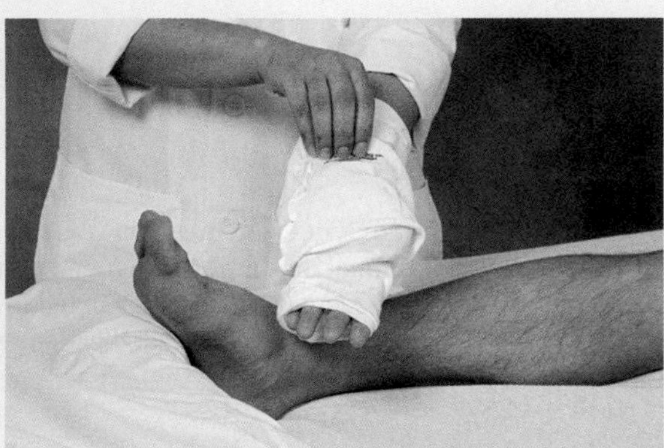

Figure 1. Pulling antiembolism stocking inside-out.

ACTION	RATIONALE
8. With the heel pocket down, ease the foot of stocking over foot and heel (Figure 2). Check that patient's heel is centered in heel pocket of stocking (Figure 3).	Wrinkles and improper fit interfere with circulation.

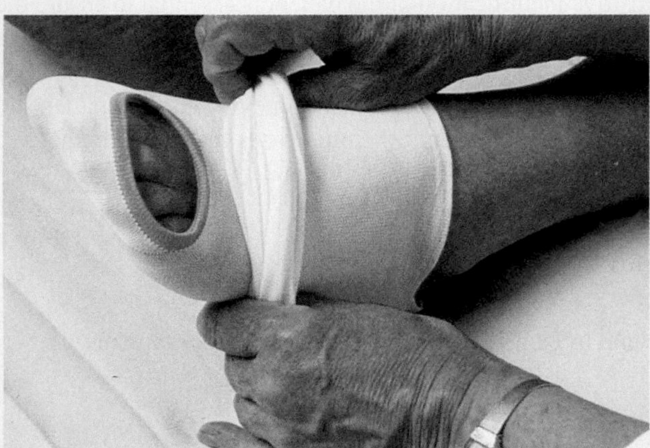

Figure 2. Putting foot of stocking onto patient.

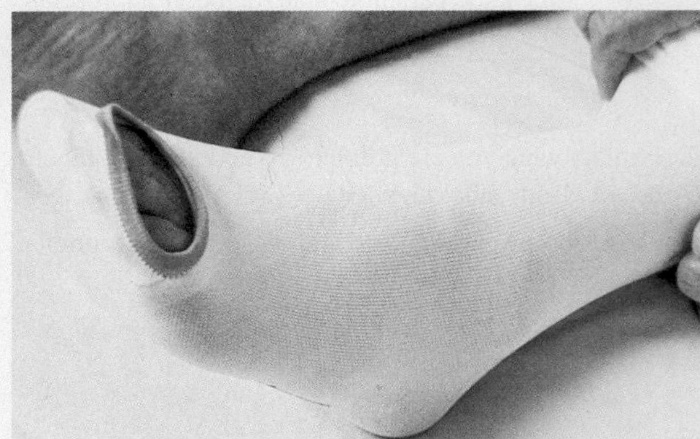

Figure 3. Ensuring heel is centered after stocking is on.

ACTION	RATIONALE
9. Using your fingers and thumbs, carefully grasp edge of stocking and pull it up smoothly over ankle and calf, toward the knee (Figure 4). Make sure it is distributed evenly.	Easing the stocking carefully into position ensures proper fit of the stocking to the contour of the leg. Even distribution prevents interference with circulation.

SKILL 7-8

Applying and Removing Antiembolism Stockings *(continued)*

ACTION	RATIONALE

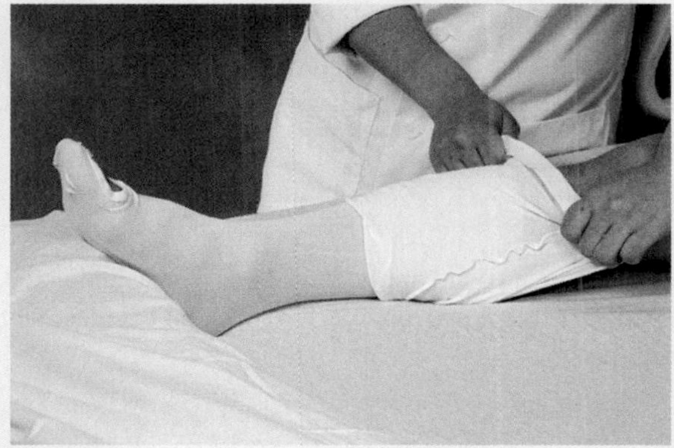

Figure 4. Pulling the stocking up the leg.

ACTION	RATIONALE
10. Pull forward slightly on toe section. If the stocking has a toe window, make sure it is properly positioned. Adjust if necessary to ensure material is smooth.	Ensures toe comfort and prevents interference with circulation.
11. If the stockings are knee-length, make sure each stocking top is 1″–2″ below the patella. Make sure the stocking does not roll down.	Prevents pressure and interference with circulation. Rolling stockings may have a constricting effect on veins.
12. If applying thigh-length stocking, continue the application. Flex the patient's leg. Stretch the stocking over the knee.	This ensures even distribution.
13. Pull the stocking over the thigh until the top is 1-3 inches below the gluteal fold (Figure 5). Adjust the stocking as necessary to distribute the fabric evenly. Make sure the stocking does not roll down.	Prevents excessive pressure and interference with circulation. Rolling stockings may have a constricting effect on veins

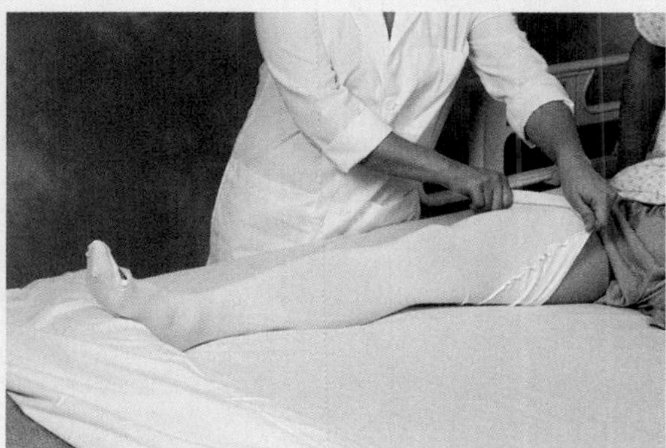

Figure 5. Pulling the stocking up over the thigh.

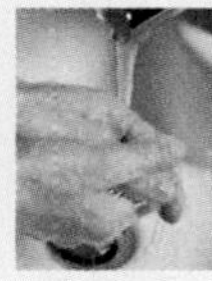

ACTION	RATIONALE
14. Perform hand hygiene.	Hand hygiene deters the spread of microorganisms.

(continued)

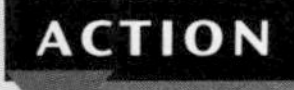

SKILL 7-8 Applying and Removing Antiembolism Stockings *(continued)*

ACTION	RATIONALE
Removing Stockings	
15. To remove stocking, grasp top of stocking with your thumb and fingers and smoothly pull stocking off inside-out to heel. Support foot and ease stocking over it.	This preserves the elasticity and contour of the stocking. It allows assessment of circulatory status and condition of skin on lower extremity and for skin care.

EVALUATION

The expected outcome is met when the stockings are applied and removed as indicated. Other outcomes are met when the patient exhibits a decrease in peripheral edema, and the patient can state the reason for using the stockings.

DOCUMENTATION

Guidelines

Document the patient's leg measurements as a baseline. Document the application of the stockings, size stocking applied, skin and leg assessment, and neurovascular assessment.

Sample Documentation

7/22/09 0945 Leg measurements: calf 14½", length heel to knee 16". Knee-high antiembolism stockings (medium/regular) applied bilaterally. Posterior tibial and dorsalis pedal pulses +2 bilaterally; capillary refill <2 seconds and skin on toes consistent with rest of skin and warm. Skin on lower extremities is intact bilaterally. —C. Stone, RN

Unexpected Situations and Associated Interventions

- *Patient's leg measurements are outside the guidelines for the available sizes:* Notify prescriber. Patient may require custom-fitted stockings.
- *Patient has large amount of pain with application of stockings:* If pain is expected (eg, if the patient has a leg incision), the patient may be premedicated and the stockings applied once the medication has had time to take effect. If the pain is unexpected, a physician may need to be notified because the patient may be developing a deep-vein thrombosis.
- *Patient has an incision on the leg:* When applying and removing stockings, be careful not to hit the incision. If the incision is draining, apply a small bandage to the incision so that it does not drain onto the stockings. If the stockings become soiled by drainage, wash and dry according to instructions.
- *Patient is to ambulate with stockings:* Place skid-resistant socks or slippers on before patient attempts to ambulate.

Special Considerations

General Considerations

- Remove stockings once every shift for 20 to 30 minutes. Wash and air-dry as necessary, according to manufacturer's directions.
- Assess at least every shift for skin color, temperature, sensation, swelling, and the ability to move. If complications are evident, remove the stockings and notify the physician or primary care provider.
- Evaluate stockings to ensure the top or toe opening does not roll with movement. Rolled stocking edges can cause excessive pressure and interfere with circulation.

SKILL 7-8 Applying and Removing Antiembolism Stockings *(continued)*

- Despite the use of elastic stockings, a patient may develop deep-vein thrombosis or phlebitis. A unilateral swelling, redness, tenderness, positive Homans' sign (pain on dorsiflexion), and warmth are possible indicators of these complications. Notify the primary care provider of the presence of any symptoms.

Home Care Considerations

- Make sure that the patient has an extra pair of stockings ordered during hospitalization before discharge (for payment and convenience purposes).
- Stockings may be laundered with other "white" clothing. Avoid excessive bleach. Remove from dryer as soon as "low heat" cycle is complete to avoid shrinkage. Stockings may also be air dried.

SKILL 7-9 Making an Unoccupied Bed

Usually bed linens are changed after the bath, but some agencies change linens only when soiled. If the patient can get out of bed, the bed should be made while it is unoccupied to decrease stress on the patient and the nurse. The following procedure explains how to make the bed using a fitted bottom sheet. Some facilities do not provide fitted bottom sheets, or sometimes a fitted bottom sheet may not be available.

Equipment

- One large flat sheet
- One fitted sheet
- Drawsheet (optional)
- Blankets
- Bedspread
- Pillowcases
- Linen hamper or bag
- Bedside chair
- Waterproof protective pad (optional)
- Disposable gloves (for use if linens are soiled)

ASSESSMENT

Assess the patient's preferences regarding linen changes. Assess for any physical activity limitations before beginning to change linens, inspect the bed for evidence of any body secretions or fluids on the linens. If present, put on disposable gloves before changing linens. Check for any patient belongings that may have accidentally been placed in bed, such as eyeglasses or prayer cloths.

NURSING DIAGNOSIS

Determine the related factors for the nursing diagnosis based on the patient's current status. Many nursing diagnoses may require the use of this skill. Possible nursing diagnoses may include:

- Risk for Impaired Skin Integrity
- Risk for Activity Intolerance
- Impaired Physical Mobility

OUTCOME IDENTIFICATION AND PLANNING

The expected outcome to achieve when making an unoccupied bed is that the bed linens will be changed without injury to the nurse or patient.

(continued)

SKILL 7-9

Making an Unoccupied Bed *(continued)*

IMPLEMENTATION

ACTION	RATIONALE
1. Assemble equipment and arrange on a bedside chair in the order in which items will be used.	Organization facilitates performance of task.
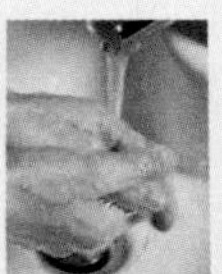 2. Perform hand hygiene.	Hand hygiene deters the spread of microorganisms.
3. Adjust bed to high position and drop side rails.	Having the bed in the high position and the side rails down reduces strain on the nurse while working.
4. Disconnect call bell or any tubes from bed linens.	Disconnecting devices prevents damage to the devices.
5. Put on gloves if linens are soiled. Loosen all linen as you move around the bed, from the head of the bed on the far side to the head of the bed on the near side.	Loosening the linen helps prevent tugging and tearing on linen. Loosening the linen and moving around the bed systematically reduce strain caused by reaching across the bed.
6. Fold reusable linens, such as sheets, blankets, or spread, in place on the bed in fourths and hang them over a clean chair.	Folding saves time and energy when reusable linen is replaced on the bed. Folding linens while they are on the bed reduces strain on the nurse's arms. Some agencies change linens only when soiled.
7. **Snugly roll all the soiled linen inside the bottom sheet and place directly into the laundry hamper (Figure 1). Do not place on floor or furniture. Do not hold soiled linens against your uniform.**	Rolling soiled linens snugly and placing them directly into the hamper helps prevent the spread of microorganisms. The floor is heavily contaminated; soiled linen will further contaminate furniture. Soiled linen contaminates the nurse's uniform, and this may spread organisms to another patient.

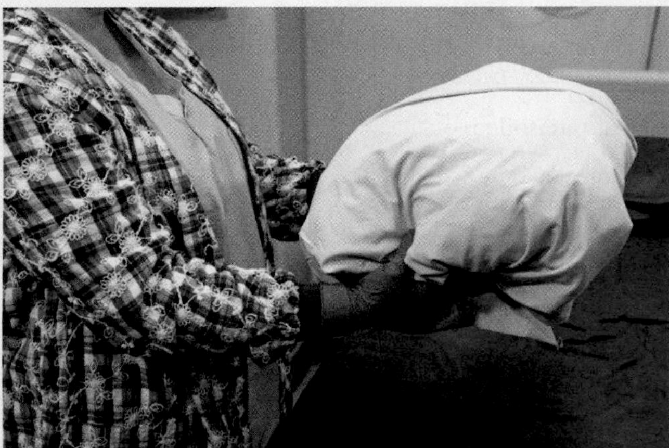

Figure 1. Bundling soiled linens in bottom sheet and holding them away from body.

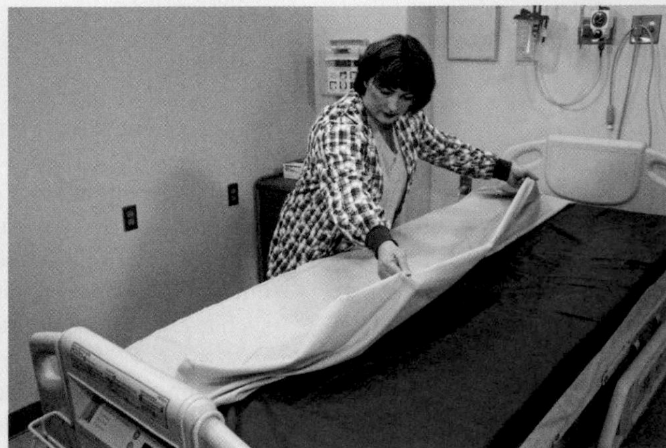

Figure 2. Opening bottom sheet and fan-folding to center of bed.

ACTION	RATIONALE
8. If possible, shift mattress up to head of bed. If mattress is soiled, clean and dry according to facility policy before applying new sheets.	This allows more foot room for the patient.
9. Remove your gloves. Place the bottom sheet with its center fold in the center of the bed. Open the sheet and fan-fold to the center (Figure 2).	Opening linens on the bed reduces strain on the nurse's arms and diminishes the spread of microorganisms. Centering the sheet ensures sufficient coverage for both sides of the mattress.

SKILL 7-9

Making an Unoccupied Bed *(continued)*

ACTION	RATIONALE
10. If using, place the drawsheet with its center fold in the center of the bed and positioned so it will be located under the patient's midsection. Open the drawsheet and fan-fold to the center of the mattress (Figure 3). If a protective pad is used, place it over the drawsheet in the proper area and open to the centerfold. Not all agencies use drawsheets routinely. The nurse may decide to use one.	If the patient soils the bed, drawsheet and pad can be changed without the bottom and top linens on the bed. Having all bottom linens in place before tucking them under the mattress avoids unnecessary moving about the bed. A drawsheet can aid moving the patient in bed.

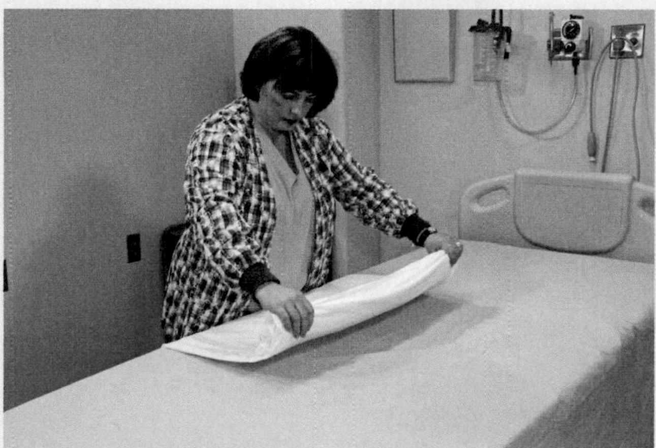

Figure 3. Placing drawsheet on bed.

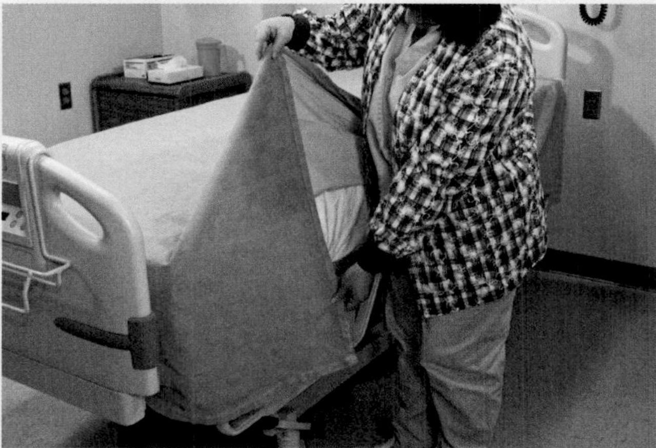

Figure 4. Mitering corner of top sheet and spread.

ACTION	RATIONALE
11. Pull the bottom sheet over the corners at the head and foot of the mattress. (See accompanying Skill Variation for using a flat bottom sheet, instead of a fitted sheet). Tuck the drawsheet securely under the mattress.	Making the bed on one side and then completing the bed on the other side saves time. Having bottom linens free of wrinkles reduces patient discomfort.
12. Move to the other side of the bed to secure bottom linens. Pull the bottom sheet tightly and secure over the corners at the head and foot of the mattress. Pull the drawsheet tightly and tuck it securely under the mattress.	This removes wrinkles from the bottom linens, which can cause patient discomfort and promote skin breakdown.
13. Place the top sheet on the bed with its center fold in the center of the bed and with the hem even with the head of the mattress. Unfold the top sheet. Follow same procedure with top blanket or spread, placing the upper edge about 6″ below the top of the sheet.	Opening linens by shaking them spreads organisms into the air. Holding linens overhead to open them causes strain on the nurse's arms.
14. Tuck the top sheet and blanket under the foot of the bed on the near side. Miter the corners (Figure 4) (also, see accompanying Skill Variation).	This saves time and energy and keeps the top linen in place.
15. Fold the upper 6″ of the top sheet down over the spread and make a cuff.	This makes it easier for the patient to get into bed and pull the covers up.
16. Move to the other side of the bed and follow the same procedure for securing top sheets under the foot of the bed and making a cuff (Figure 5).	Working on one side of the bed at a time saves energy and is more efficient.

(continued)

SKILL 7-9 Making an Unoccupied Bed *(continued)*

ACTION	RATIONALE
17. Place the pillows on the bed. Open each pillowcase in the same manner as you opened other linens. Gather the pillowcase over one hand toward the closed end. Grasp the pillow with the hand inside the pillowcase. Keep a firm hold on the top of the pillow and pull the cover onto the pillow. Place the pillow at the head of the bed (Figure 6).	Opening linens by shaking them causes organisms to be carried on air currents. Covering the pillow while it rests on the bed reduces strain on the nurse's arms and back.

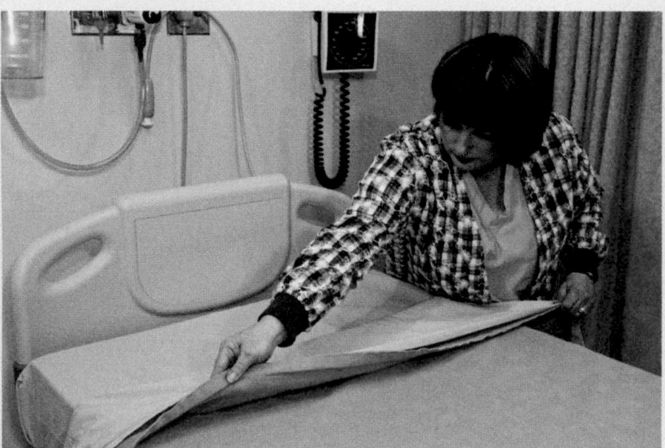

Figure 5. Cuffing top linens.

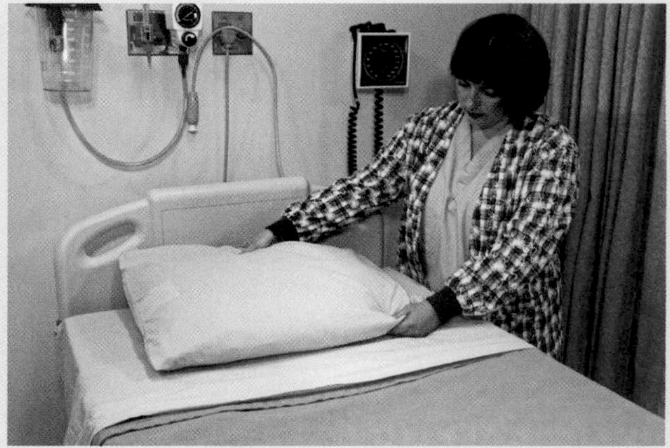

Figure 6. Placing pillow on bed.

ACTION	RATIONALE
18. Fan-fold or pie-fold the top linens.	Having linens opened makes it more convenient for the patient to get into bed.
19. **Secure the signal device on the bed according to agency policy (Figure 7).**	The patient will be able to call for assistance as necessary.

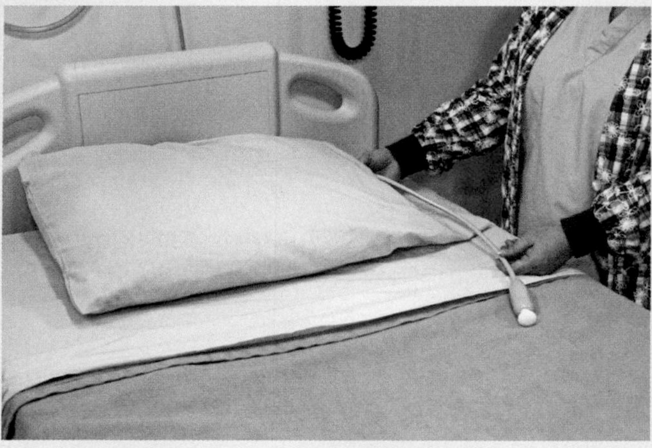

Figure 7. Securing signal device to bed.

ACTION	RATIONALE
20. **Adjust bed to low position.**	Having the bed in the low position makes it easier and safer for the patient to get into bed.
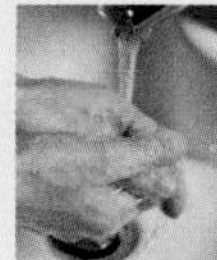 21. Dispose of soiled linen according to agency policy. Perform hand hygiene.	Deters the spread of microorganisms.

SKILL 7-9 Making an Unoccupied Bed *(continued)*

EVALUATION

The expected outcome is met when the bed linens are changed without any injury to the patient or nurse.

DOCUMENTATION

Changing of bed linens does not need to be documented. The use of a specialty bed, or bed equipment, such as Balkan frame or foot cradle, should be documented.

Unexpected Situations and Associated Interventions

- *Drawsheet is not available:* A flat sheet can be folded in half to substitute for a drawsheet, but extra care must be taken to avoid wrinkles in the bed.
- *Patient is frequently incontinent of stool or urine:* More than one protective pad can be placed under the patient to protect the bed, but care must be taken to ensure that the patient is not lying on wrinkles from linens.

SKILL VARIATION Making a Bed With a Flat Bottom Sheet

- Assemble equipment and arrange on a bedside chair in the order in which items will be used. Two large flat sheets are needed.
- Perform hand hygiene.
- Adjust bed to high position and drop side rails.
- Disconnect call bell or any tubes from bed linens.
- Put on gloves if linens are soiled. Loosen all linen as you move around the bed, from the head of the bed on the far side to the head of the bed on the near side.
- Fold reusable linens, such as sheets, blankets, or spread, in place on the bed in fourths and hang them over a clean chair.
- Snugly roll all the soiled linen inside the bottom sheet and place directly into the laundry hamper. Do not place on floor or furniture. Do not hold soiled linens against your uniform.
- If possible, shift mattress up to head of bed.
- Remove your gloves. Place the bottom sheet with its center fold in the center of the bed and high enough to be able to tuck under the head of the mattress. Open the sheet and fan-fold to the center.
- If using, place the drawsheet with its centerfold in the center of the bed and positioned so it will be located under the patient's midsection. Open the drawsheet and fan-fold to the center of the mattress. If a protective pad is used, place it over the drawsheet in the proper area and open to the centerfold.
- Tuck the bottom sheet securely under the head of the mattress on one side of the bed, making a corner. Corners are usually mitered. Grasp the side edge of the sheet about 18″ down from the mattress top (Figure A). Lay the sheet on top of the mattress to form a triangular, flat fold (Figure B). Tuck the portion of the sheet that is hanging loose below the mattress under the mattress without pulling on the triangular fold (Figure C). Pick the top of the triangle fold and place it over the side of the mattress (Figure D). Tuck this loose portion of the sheet under the mattress. Continue tucking the remaining bottom sheet and drawsheet securely under the mattress (Figure E).
- Move to the other side of the bed to secure bottom linens. Pull the sheets across the mattress from the centerfold. Secure the bottom of the sheet under the head of the bed and miter the corner. Pull the remainder of the sheet and the drawsheet tightly and tuck under the mattress, starting at the head and moving toward the foot (Figure F).
- Place the top sheet on the bed with its centerfold in the center of the bed and with the hem even with the head of the mattress. Unfold the top sheet. Follow same procedure with top blanket or spread, placing the upper edge about 6″ below the top of the sheet.
- Tuck the top sheet and blanket under the foot of the bed on the near side. Miter the corners.
- Fold the upper 6″ of the top sheet down over the spread and make a cuff.
- Move to the other side of the bed and follow the same procedure for securing top sheets under the foot of the bed and making a cuff.
- Place the pillows on the bed. Open each pillowcase in the same manner as you opened other linens. Gather the pillowcase over one hand toward the closed end. Grasp the pillow with the hand inside the pillowcase. Keep a firm hold on the top of the pillow and pull the cover onto the pillow. Place the pillow at the head of the bed.
- Fan-fold or pie-fold the top linens.
- Secure the signal device on the bed according to agency policy.
- Adjust bed to low position.
- Dispose of soiled linen according to agency policy. Perform hand hygiene.

(continued)

(continued)

SKILL 7-9 Making an Unoccupied Bed *(continued)*

SKILL VARIATION Making a Bed With a Flat Bottom Sheet *(continued)*

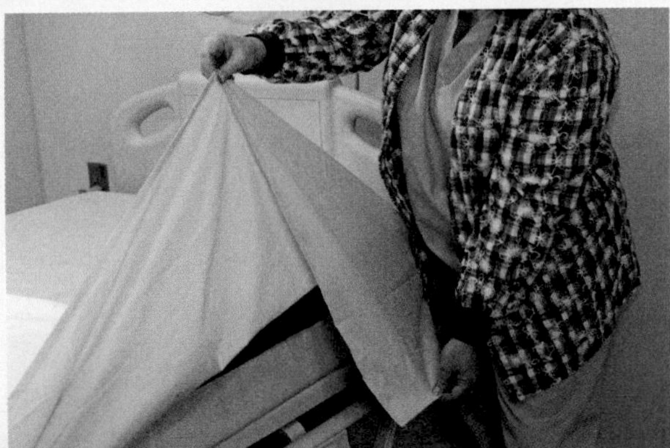

Figure A. Grasping the side edge of the sheet and lifting up to form a triangle.

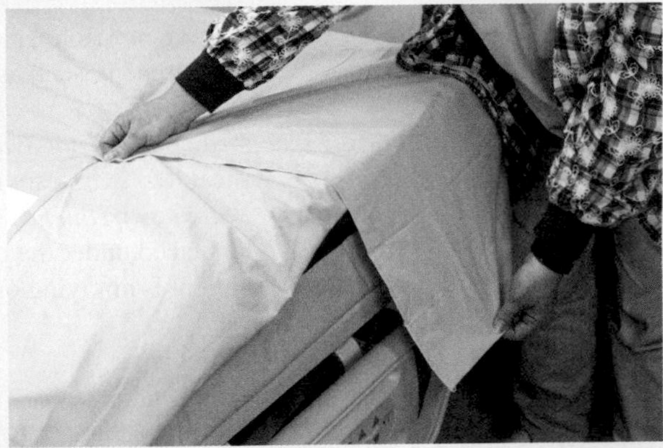

Figure B. Laying sheet on top of the bed to make triangular, flat fold.

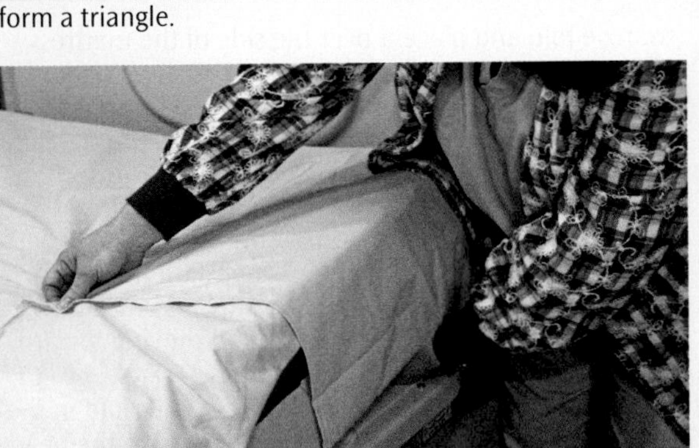

Figure C. Tucking sheet under mattress.

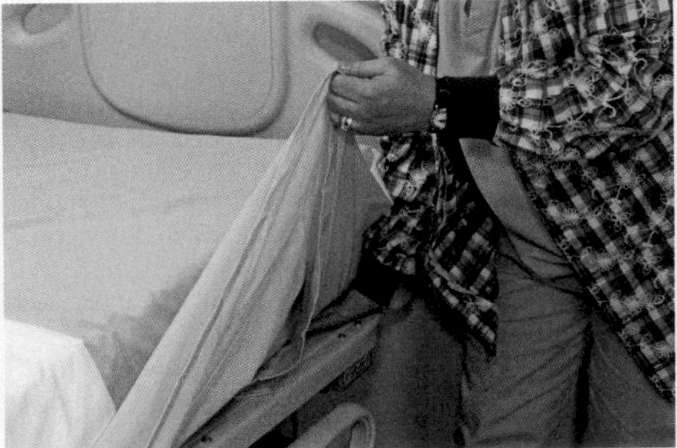

Figure D. Placing top of triangular fold over mattress side.

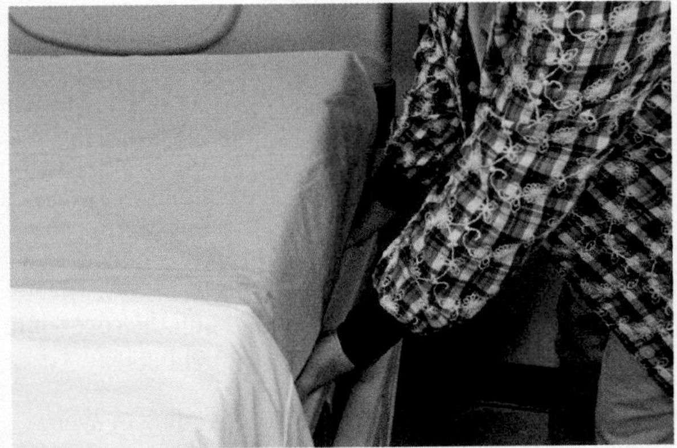

Figure E. Tucking end of triangular linen fold under mattress to complete mitered corner.

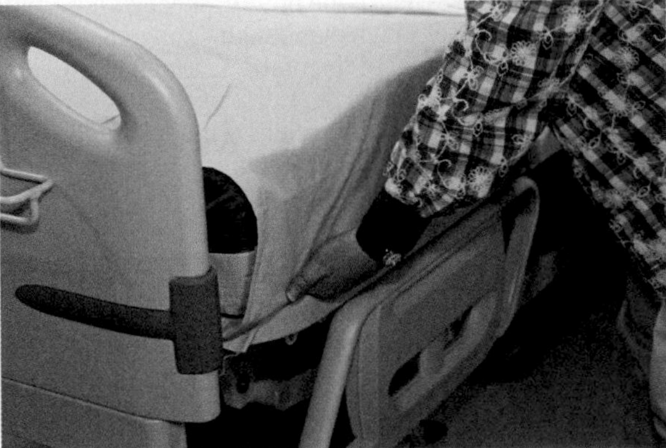

Figure F. Tucking sheet snugly under mattress.

SKILL 7-10

Making an Occupied Bed

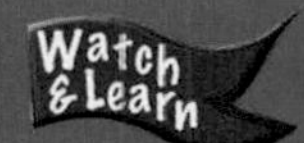

If the patient cannot get out of bed, the linens may need to be changed with the patient still in the bed. This is termed an "occupied" bed.

Equipment

- One large flat sheet
- One fitted sheet
- Drawsheet (optional)
- Blankets
- Bedspread
- Pillowcases
- Linen hamper or bag
- Bedside chair
- Protective pad (optional)
- Disposable gloves (if linens are soiled)

ASSESSMENT

Assess the patient's preferences regarding linen changes. Assess for any precautions or activity restrictions for the patient. Before beginning to change linens, check for evidence of any body secretions or fluids on the linens. If present, put on disposable gloves before changing linens. Check the bed for any patient belongings that may have accidentally been placed or fallen there, such as eyeglasses or prayer cloths. Note the presence and position of any tubes or drains that the patient may have.

NURSING DIAGNOSIS

Determine the related factors for the nursing diagnosis based on the patient's current status. Many nursing diagnoses may require the use of this skill. Possible nursing diagnoses may include:

- Risk for Impaired Skin Integrity
- Risk for Activity Intolerance
- Impaired Physical Mobility
- Impaired Bed Mobility
- Impaired Transfer Ability

OUTCOME IDENTIFICATION AND PLANNING

The expected outcome to achieve when making an occupied bed is that the bed linens are applied without injury to the patient or nurse. Other possible outcomes may include: patient participates in moving from side to side, and patient verbalizes feelings of increased comfort.

IMPLEMENTATION

ACTION	RATIONALE
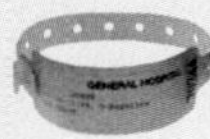 1. Identify patient. Explain procedure to patient. Check chart for limitations on patient's physical activity.	Identifying the patient ensures the right patient receives the intervention and helps prevent errors. This facilitates patient cooperation and determines level of activity.
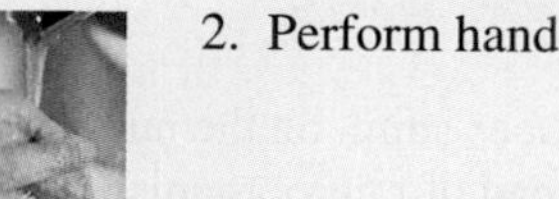 2. Perform hand hygiene.	Hand hygiene deters the spread of microorganisms.
3. Assemble equipment and arrange on bedside chair in the order the items will be used.	Organization facilitates performance of task.

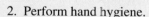

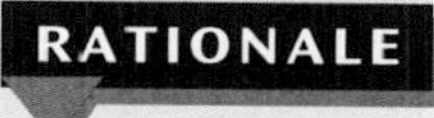

(continued)

SKILL 7-10 Making an Occupied Bed *(continued)*

ACTION	RATIONALE
4. Close door or curtain.	This provides for privacy.
5. Adjust bed to high position. Lower side rail nearest you, leaving the opposite side rail up. Place bed in flat position unless contraindicated.	Having the bed in the high position reduces strain on the nurse while working. Having the mattress flat makes it easier to prepare a wrinkle-free bed.
6. Check bed linens for patient's personal items. **Disconnect the call bell or any tubes/drains from bed linens.**	It is costly and inconvenient when personal items are lost. Disconnecting tubes from linens prevents discomfort and accidental dislodging of the tubes.
7. Put on gloves if linens are soiled. Place a bath blanket over patient. Have patient hold onto bath blanket while you reach under it and remove top linens (Figure 1). Leave top sheet in place if a bath blanket is not used. Fold linen that is to be reused over the back of a chair. Discard soiled linen in laundry bag or hamper. Keep soiled linen away from uniform.	Gloves prevent contact with blood and body fluids. The blanket provides warmth and privacy.

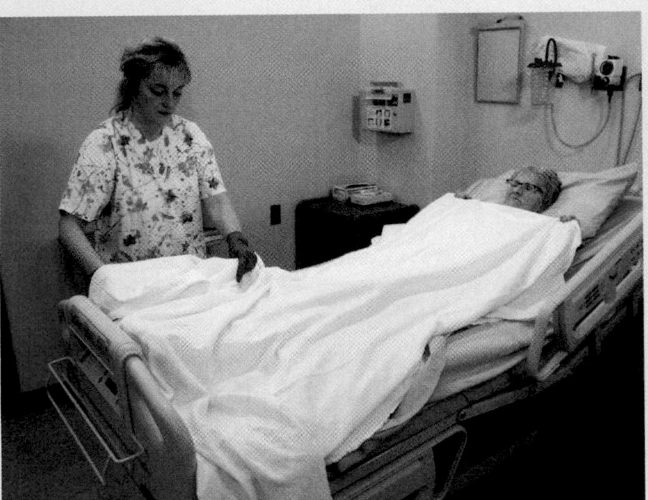

Figure 1. Removing top linens from under bath blanket.

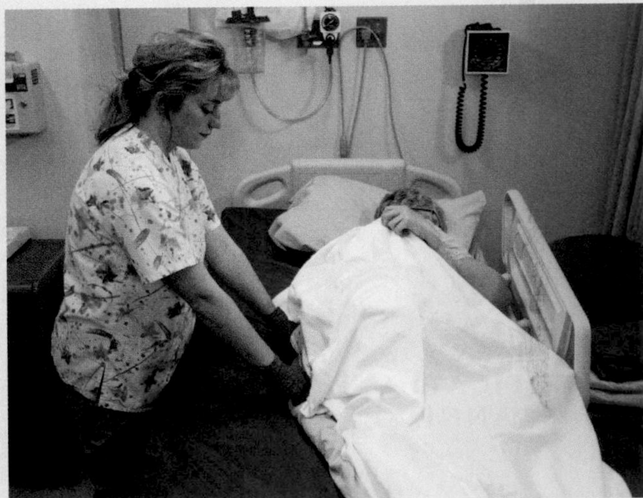

Figure 2. Moving soiled linen as close to patient as possible.

ACTION	RATIONALE
8. If possible and another person is available to assist, grasp mattress securely and shift it up to head of bed.	This allows more foot room for the patient.
9. Assist patient to turn toward opposite side of the bed, and reposition pillow under patient's head.	This allows the bed to be made on the vacant side.
10. Loosen all bottom linens from head, foot, and side of bed.	This facilitates removal of linens.
11. Fan-fold soiled linens as close to patient as possible (Figure 2).	This makes it easier to remove linens when the patient turns to the other side.
12. Remove your gloves, if used. Use clean linen and make the near side of the bed. Place the bottom sheet with its center fold in the center of the bed (Figure 3). Open the sheet and fan-fold to the center, positioning it under the old linens (Figure 4). Pull the bottom sheet over the corners at the head and foot of the mattress.	Opening linens on the bed reduces strain on the nurse's arms and diminishes the spread of microorganisms. Centering the sheet ensures sufficient coverage for both sides of the mattress. Positioning under the old linens makes it easier to remove linens.

SKILL 7-10

Making an Occupied Bed *(continued)*

ACTION | **RATIONALE**

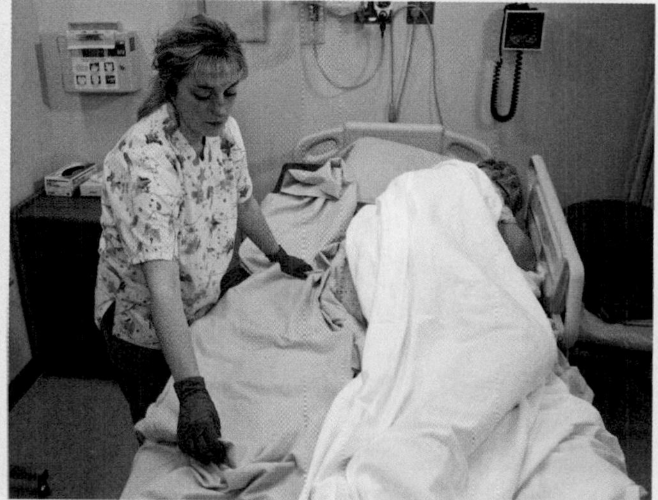

Figure 3. Placing bottom sheet with center fold in center of bed.

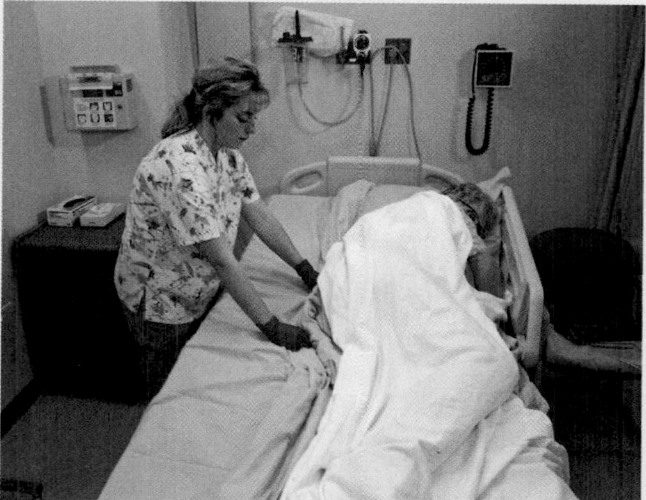

Figure 4. Fan-folding bottom sheet to the center, positioning it under the old linens.

13. If using, place the drawsheet with its center fold in the center of the bed and positioned so it will be located under the patient's midsection. Open the drawsheet and fan-fold to the center of the mattress. Tuck the drawsheet securely under the mattress (Figure 5). If a protective pad is used, place it over the drawsheet in the proper area and open to the centerfold. Not all agencies use drawsheets routinely. The nurse may decide to use one.

    If the patient soils the bed, drawsheet and pad can be changed without the bottom and top linens on the bed. A drawsheet can aid moving the patient in bed.

14. Raise side rail. Assist patient to roll over the folded linen in the middle of the bed toward you. Reposition pillow and bath blanket or top sheet. Move to other side of the bed and lower side rail.

    This ensures patient safety. The movement allows the bed to be made on the other side. The bath blanket provides warmth and privacy.

15. Put on clean gloves, if linen is soiled. Loosen and remove all bottom linen (Figure 6). Place in linen bag or hamper. Hold soiled linen away from your uniform. Remove gloves, if used.

    Proper disposal of soiled linen prevents spread of microorganisms.

16. Ease clean linen from under patient. Pull the bottom sheet taut and secure at the corners at the head and foot of the mattress. Pull the drawsheet tight and smooth. Tuck the drawsheet securely under the mattress.

    This removes wrinkles and creases in the linens, which are uncomfortable to lie on.

17. Assist patient to turn back to the center of bed. If pillowcase is soiled with blood or body fluids, put on unsterile gloves. Remove pillow and change pillowcase. Open each pillowcase in the same manner as you opened other linens. Gather the pillowcase over one hand toward the closed end. Grasp the pillow with the hand inside the pillowcase. Keep a firm hold on the top of the pillow and pull the cover onto the pillow. Place the pillow under the patient's head. Remove gloves, if worn.

    Opening linens by shaking them causes organisms to be carried on air currents.

(continued)

SKILL 7-10 **Making an Occupied Bed** *(continued)*

ACTION | **RATIONALE**

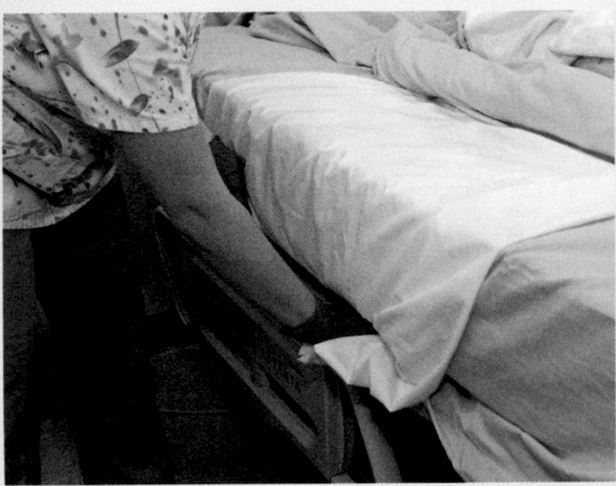

Figure 5. Tucking bottom sheet and drawsheet tightly.

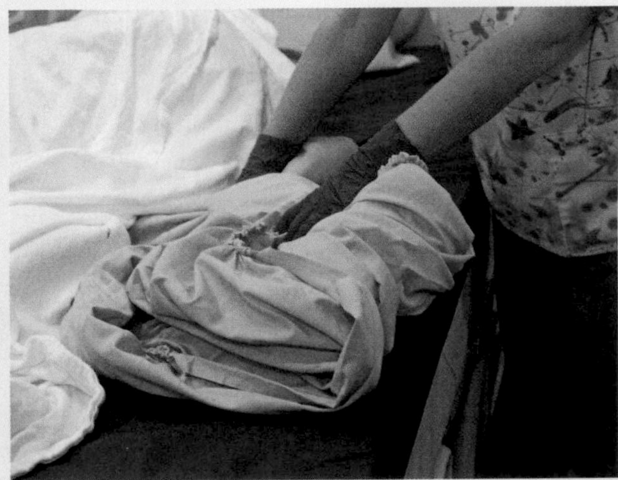

Figure 6. Removing soiled bottom linens from other side of bed.

18. Apply top linen, sheet and blanket if desired, so that it is centered. Fold the top linens over at the patient's shoulders to make a cuff. Have patient hold onto top linen and remove the bath blanket from underneath (Figure 7).

This allows bottom hems to be tucked securely under the mattress and provides for privacy.

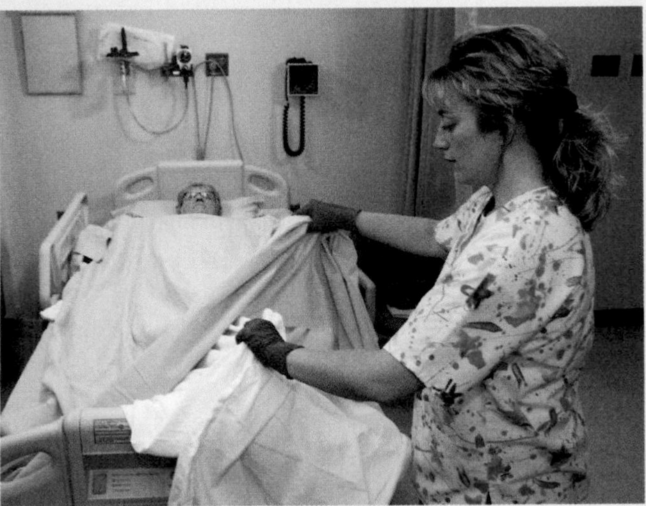

Figure 7. Removing bath blanket from under top linens.

19. Secure top linens under foot of mattress and miter corners (refer to Skill Variation in Skill 7-9). Loosen top linens over patient's feet by grasping them in the area of the feet and pulling gently toward foot of bed.

This provides for a neat appearance. Loosening linens over the patient's feet gives more room for movement.

20. **Raise side rail. Lower bed height and adjust head of bed to a comfortable position. Reattach call bell.**

This provides for the patient's safety.

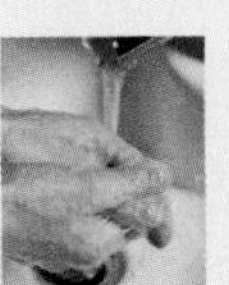

21. Dispose of soiled linens according to agency policy. Perform hand hygiene.

This prevents the spread of microorganisms.

SKILL 7-10 **Making an Occupied Bed** *(continued)*

EVALUATION

The expected outcome is met when the bed linens are changed, and the patient and nurse remain free of injury. In addition, the patient assists in moving from side to side and states feelings of increased comfort after the bed is changed.

DOCUMENTATION

Changing of bed linens does not need to be documented. The use of a specialty bed, or bed equipment, such as Balkan frame or foot cradle, should be documented. Document any significant observations and communication.

Unexpected Situations and Associated Interventions

- *Dirty linens are grossly contaminated with fecal drainage:* Obtain an extra towel or protective pad. Place the pad under and over the soiled linens so that new linens will not be in contact with soiled linens. Clean and dry the mattress according to facility policy before applying new sheets.

Special Considerations

Older Adult Considerations

- Using a soft bath blanket, or a flannelette blanket as a bottom sheet may solve the problem of "coldness" for elderly patients with vascular problems or arthritis.

The Taylor Suite offers these additional resources to enhance learning and facilitate understanding of this chapter:

- thePoint online resource, http://thepoint.lww.com/Lynn2E
- Student CD-ROM included with the book
- Skills Checklist to Accompany Taylor's Clinical Nursing Skills
- Taylor's Interactive Nursing: *Hygiene*
- Taylor's Video Guide to Clinical Nursing Skills: *Hygiene*

Developing Critical Thinking Skills

1. Denasia Kerr, the 6-year-old on bedrest, needs her hair shampooed. It is now several days after surgery. How would you accomplish this task?
2. Cindy Vortex is the 34-year-old woman who is now in a coma after a car accident and who is wearing contact lenses. What information would be important to gather before attempting to remove the contact lenses?
3. Carl Sheen, 76 years old, asks you, "How can I clean my dentures with my right hand all tied up with this IV?" How best could you help Mr. Sheen with this hygiene activity while still fostering his independence?

Bibliography

Applying antiembolism stockings isn't just pulling on socks. (2004). *Nursing, 34*(8), 48–49.

Bailey, R., Gueldner, S., Ledikwe, J., et al. (2005). The oral care of older adults. *Journal of Gerontological Nursing, 31*(7), 11–17.

Bauer, J. (2003). Bedside bathing products. *RN, 66*(6), 65–66.

Brown, A., & Butcher, M. (2005). A guide to emollient therapy. *Nursing Standard, 19*(24), 68–75.

Burr, S., & Penzer, R. (2005). Promoting skin health. *Nursing Standard, 19*(36), 57–65.

Cottrell, B. (2003). Vaginal douching. *Journal of Obstetric, Gynecologic, and Neonatal Nursing, 32*(1), 12–18.

Dougherty, J., & Long, C. (2003). Techniques for bathing without a battle. *Home Healthcare Nurse, 21*(1), 38–39.

Dunn, J., Thiru-Chelvam, B., & Beck, C. (2002). Bathing: Pleasure or pain? *Journal of Gerontological Nursing, 28*(11), 6–13.

Fort, C. (2002). Get pumped to prevent DVT. *Nursing, 32*(9), 50–52.

Gray, M., Ratliff, C., & Donovan, A. (2002). Protecting perineal skin integrity. *Nursing Management,* 33(12), 61–63.

Hayes, J., Lehman, C., & Castonguay, P. (2002). Graduated compression stockings: Updating practice, improving compliance. *MedSurg Nursing, 11*(4), 163–166, 191.

Hess, C. (2003). Managing a diabetic ulcer. *Nursing, 33*(7), 82–83.

Hilgers, J. (2003). Comforting a confused patient. *Nursing, 33*(1), 48–50.

Hockenberry, M. (2005). *Wong's essentials of pediatric nursing.* (7th ed.). St. Louis, MO: Elsevier Mosby.

Holman, C., Roberts, S., & Nicol, M. (2005). Promoting oral hygiene. *Nursing Older People, 16*(10), 37–38.

Larson, E. (2002). The 'hygiene hypothesis': How clean should we be? *American Journal of Nursing, 102*(1), 81–89.

Larson, E., Gomez-Duarte, C., Qureshi, K., & Miranda, D. (2001). How clean is the home environment? A tool to assess home hygiene. *Journal of Community Health Nursing, 18*(3), 139–150.

Larson, E., Ciliberti, T., Chantler, D., Abraham, J., et al. (2004). Comparison of traditional and disposable bed baths in critically ill patients. *American Journal of Critical Care, 13*(3), 235–241.

Lawton, S. (2004). Effective use of emollients in infants and young people. *Nursing Standard, 27*(19), 44–50.

McConnell, E. (2002). Applying antiembolism stockings. *Nursing, 32*(4), 17.

Pauldine, E. (2003). Taking a bite out of Lyme disease. *Nursing, 33*(4), 49–52.

Perlmutter, J., & Camberg, L. (2004). Better bathing for residents with Alzheimer's. *Nursing Homes/Long Term Care Management, 53*(4), 40, 42–43.

Plummer, S. (2001). Chronic complications. *RN, 64*(5), 34–42.

Ramponi, D. (2001). Eye on contact lens removal. *Nursing, 31*(8), 56–57.

Rasin, J., & Barrick, A. (2004). Bathing patients with dementia. *American Journal of Nursing, 104*(3), 30–33.

Smeltzer, S., Bare, B., Hinkle, J. H., & Cheever, K. H. (2008). *Brunner and Suddarth's textbook of medical–surgical nursing.* (11th ed.). Philadelphia: Lippincott Williams & Wilkins.

Tabloski, R. (2006). *Gerontological nursing.* Upper Saddle River, NJ: Pearson Prentice Hall.

CHAPTER 8

Skin Integrity and Wound Care

Focusing on Patient Care

This chapter will help you develop some of the skills related to skin integrity and wound care necessary to care for the following patients:

Lori Downs, a patient with diabetes, is admitted with a chronic ulcer of her left foot.

Tran Nguyen, diagnosed with breast cancer, has had a modified radical mastectomy.

Arthur Lowes has an appointment with his surgeon today for a follow-up examination and removal of surgical staples following a colon resection.

Learning Objectives

After studying this chapter, you will be able to:

1. Clean a wound and apply a sterile dressing.
2. Apply a saline-moistened dressing.
3. Apply a hydrocolloid dressing.
4. Perform a sterile wound irrigation.
5. Collect a wound culture.
6. Apply Montgomery straps.
7. Provide care to a Penrose drain.
8. Provide care to a T-tube drain.
9. Provide care to a Jackson-Pratt drain.
10. Provide care to a Hemovac drain.
11. Apply a wound vacuum-assisted closure (VAC) system.
12. Remove sutures.
13. Remove surgical staples.
14. Apply an external heating device.
15. Apply a warm sterile compress to an open wound.
16. Assist with a sitz bath.
17. Apply a cooling blanket.
18. Apply cold therapy.

Key Terms

approximated wound edges: edges of a wound that are lightly pulled together; epithelialization of wound margins. Edges appear to be touching; wound appears closed.

dehiscence: accidental separation of wound edges, especially a surgical wound

ecchymosis: discoloration of an area resulting from infiltration of blood into the subcutaneous tissue

edema: accumulation of fluid in the interstitial tissues

epithelialization: stage of wound healing in which epithelial cells move across the surface of a wound margin (approximation); tissue color ranges from the color of "ground glass" to pink

erythema: redness or inflammation of an area as a result of dilation and congestion of capillaries

eschar: a thick, leathery scab or dry crust composed of dead cells and dried plasma

granulation tissue: new tissue that is deep pink/red and composed of fibroblasts and small blood vessels that fill an open wound when it starts to heal; characterized by irregular surface like raspberries

hypothermia: condition characterized by a body temperature below 96.8°F

ischemia: insufficient blood supply to a body part due to obstruction of circulation

jaundice: condition characterized by yellowness of the skin, whites of eyes, mucous membranes, and body fluids as a result of deposition of bile pigment resulting from excess bilirubin in the blood

maceration: softening of tissue due to excessive moisture

necrosis: localized tissue death

nosocomial infection: infection acquired while receiving healthcare

pathogens: microorganisms that can harm humans

peripheral neuropathy: abnormal condition characterized by inflammation and degeneration of the peripheral nerves. Sensations reported include burning, tingling, numbness, and pins and needles.

pressure ulcer: lesion caused by unrelieved pressure that results in damage to underlying tissue

sinus tract: cavity or channel underneath a wound that has the potential for infection

sterile technique: surgical asepsis; removing all microorganisms to prevent the introduction or spread of pathogens from the environment into a patient

surgical asepsis: removal of all microorganisms to prevent the introduction or spread of pathogens from the environment into a patient

surgical staples: stainless-steel wire used to close a surgical wound

surgical sutures: thread or wire used to stitch parts of the body together

tachycardia: abnormally rapid heart rate, usually above 100 beats per minute in an adult

tunneling: passageway or opening that may be visible at skin level, but with most of the tunnel under the surface of the skin

undermining: areas of tissue destruction underneath intact skin along the margins of a wound associated with stage 3 or 4 pressure ulcers

vasoconstriction: narrowing of the lumen of a blood vessel

vasodilation: an increase in the diameter of a blood vessel

The skin is the body's first line of defense for protecting it from microbial and foreign-substance invasion. An intact skin surface provides a barrier to harmful microorganisms (see Fundamentals Review 8-1 for the Anatomy and Physiology of Skin and the Integumentary System and Fundamentals Review 8-2 for Factors Affecting the Integumentary System). A disruption in the normal integrity of the skin is called a wound. This disruption creates a potentially dangerous and possibly life-threatening situation. The patient is at risk for wound complications such as infection, hemorrhage, dehiscence, and evisceration (Fundamentals Review 8-3). These complications increase the risk for generalized illness and death, lengthen the time that the patient needs healthcare interventions, and add to healthcare costs. Pressure ulcers, a wound caused by unrelieved pressure that results in damage to underlying tissue, are one of the most common skin and tissue disruptions and are costly in terms of healthcare expenditures (see Fundamentals Review 8-4 for staging of pressure ulcers).

Preventing pressure ulcers (Fundamentals Review 8-5) and caring for wounds are important aspects of nursing care. Nursing responsibilities related to skin integrity involve assessment of the patient and the wound, followed by the development of the nursing plan of care, including the identification of appropriate outcomes, nursing interventions, and evaluation of the nursing care (Fundamentals Review 8-6 describes assessment of the wound). Depending upon the patient's individualized plan of care, specific wound care skills may be needed. Nurses follow Standard Precautions and, if needed, Transmission-Based Precautions in providing wound care. Additionally, ongoing assessment for possible skin or wound complications will be required. Emotional support of the patient will be crucial throughout the provision of physical care. Documentation of all nursing care is essential, as well as the appropriate patient and family education. These interventions facilitate healing, adaptation, and self-care.

This chapter will cover skills to assist the nurse in providing care related to skin integrity and wounds. In addition to the Fundamentals Review boxes in this chapter, please look over those found in Chapter 4 (Asepsis and Infection Control) for a quick review of critical knowledge to assist you in understanding the skills related to skin integrity and wound care.

Fundamentals Review 8-1

Anatomy and Physiology of Skin and the Integumentary System

- Skin is the body's largest organ. It provides protective, sensory, and regulatory functions.
- Changes to or disruptions in skin integrity can interfere with the functions of the integumentary system. The body relies heavily on an intact integumentary system for defense against the environment.
- The skin has two major layers, the epidermis and dermis.
- The epidermis depends on the dermis for nutrition. It forms the hair, nails, and glandular structures of the skin.
- The dermis lies under and is thicker than the epidermis. It produces collagen and elastin. It is home for lymphatic vessels and nerve tissues.
- Skin provides protection from injury, infection, and damage from ultraviolet rays. Secretions produced by the skin inhibit the growth of pathogens present on the skin.
- The dilation and constriction of blood vessels in the skin help to regulate body temperature.
- Nerve endings in the skin are sensitive to pain, itch, vibration, heat, and cold.
- The skin makes vitamin D to aid in the absorption of calcium and phosphorus.
- The skin is a large part of a person's body appearance and attractiveness. It contributes to communication through facial expression and appearance.
- Normal skin tones vary among races of people. Skin is normally warm, dry to the touch, and smooth in texture. Normal skin has good elasticity or turgor. As a person ages, turgor normally decreases.

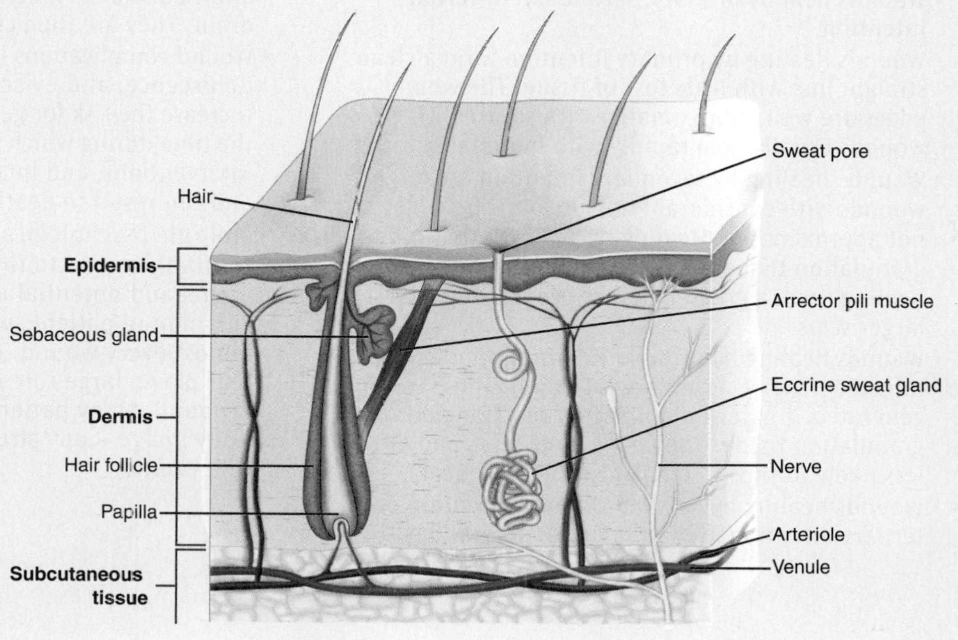

Factors Affecting Integumentary Function

- Healthy, viable skin requires adequate blood flow. Alterations in circulation can lead to skin that has abnormal color, texture, thickness, moisture, or temperature or skin that becomes ulcerated.
- Healthy skin requires a balanced diet. Deficiencies of protein, calories, or multiple vitamins and minerals result in dull, dry hair and dry, flaky skin. Skin that is not healthy becomes more fragile and susceptible to dysfunction.
- Healthy skin requires personal hygiene practices and the avoidance of certain environmental factors. Lack of cleanliness can hinder skin health because bacteria, sweat, and debris are not removed. Overexposure to ultraviolet radiation can lead to wrinkling, changes in texture and elasticity of the skin, and cancer.
- Lack of moisture can lead to breaks in the integrity of the skin, allowing microorganisms to enter the body.
- Allergic reactions, such as those to foods or poison ivy, and resulting skin inflammation can lead to breaks in the integrity of the skin, allowing microorganisms to enter the body.
- An abnormal growth rate of skin cells, such as psoriasis or melanoma, can disrupt the integrity of the skin.
- Many chronic diseases, such as peripheral vascular disease, can lead to disruption in the integrity of the skin due to diminished delivery of blood and oxygen to the underlying tissues.
- Trauma to the skin, such as from surgical or accidental wounds, can disrupt the integrity of the skin.
- Exposure to excessive heat, electricity, chemicals, and radiation results in injuries that can disrupt the integrity of the skin.

Wound Healing and Complications

- Wounds heal by primary, secondary, or tertiary intention.
- Wounds healing by primary intention form a clean, straight line with little loss of tissue. The wound edges are well approximated with sutures. These wounds usually heal rapidly with minimal scarring.
- Wounds healing by secondary intention are large wounds with considerable tissue loss. The edges are not approximated. Healing occurs by formation of granulation tissue. These wounds have a longer healing time, a greater chance of infection, and larger scars.
- Wounds healing by primary intention that become infected heal by secondary intention. These wounds generate a greater inflammatory reaction and more granulation tissue. They have large scars and are less likely to shrink to a flat line as they heal.
- Wounds healing by delayed primary intention or tertiary intention are left open for several days to allow edema or infection to resolve or exudates to drain. They are then closed.
- Wound complications include infection, hemorrhage, dehiscence, and evisceration. These problems increase the risk for generalized illness, lengthen the time during which the patient needs healthcare interventions, and increase the cost of healthcare, and can result in death.
- Multiple psychological effects can occur as a result of trauma to the integumentary system. Actual and potential emotional stressors are common in patients with wounds. Pain is part of almost every wound. In addition, anxiety and fear play a large role in a patient's recovery from a wound. Many patients must deal with changes in body image, body structure, and function related to a wound.

Comparison of Stages of Pressure Ulcers

Stage I

An observable pressure-related alteration of intact skin whose indicators, as compared to the adjacent or opposite area on the body, may include changes in one or more of the following: skin temperature (warmth or coolness), tissue consistency (firm or boggy feel), and sensation (pain, itching). The ulcer appears as a defined area of persistent redness in lightly pigmented skin, whereas in darker skin tones, the ulcer may appear with persistent red, blue, or purple hues.

Pressure-relieving measures:

- Frequent turning
- Pressure-relieving devices
- Positioning

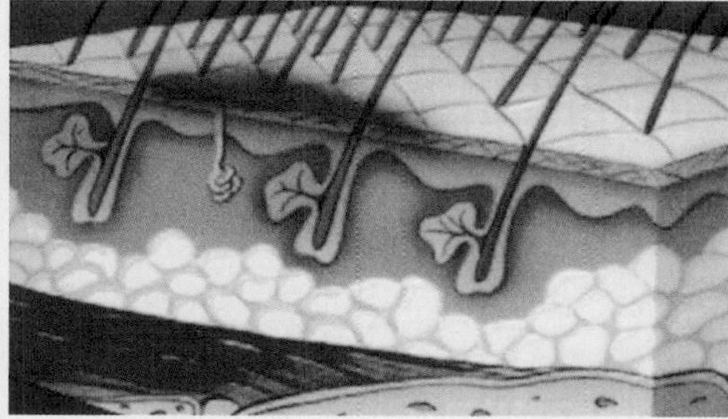
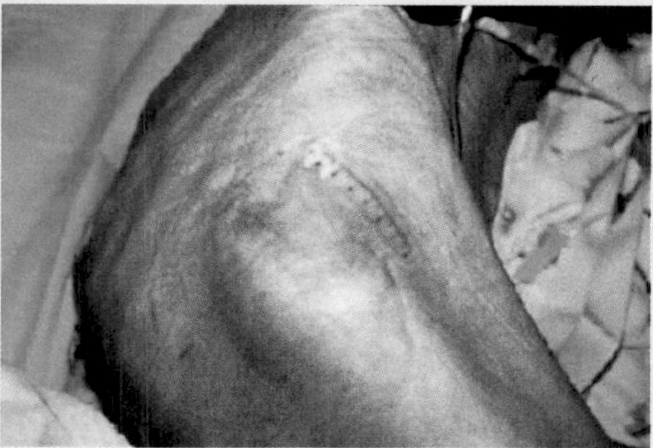

Stage II

Partial-thickness skin loss involving epidermis and/or dermis. The ulcer is superficial and presents clinically as an abrasion, blister, or shallow crater.

Maintenance of a moist healing environment:

- Saline *or*
- Occlusive dressing that promotes natural healing but prevents formation of a scar

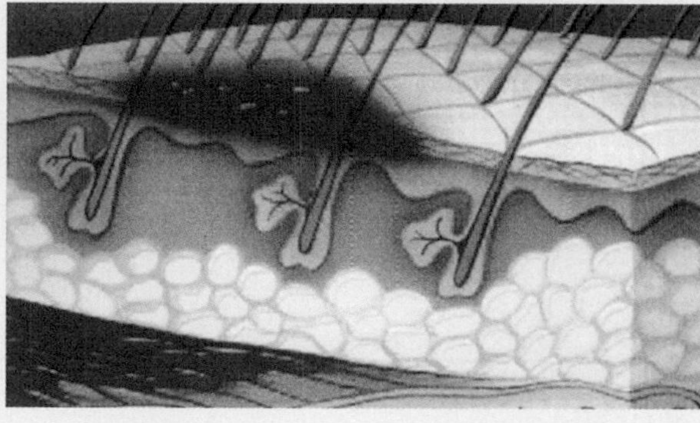
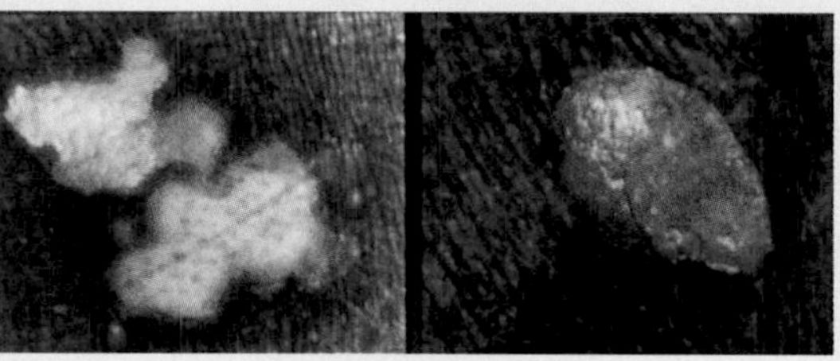

(continued)

Comparison of Stages of Pressure Ulcers *(continued)*

Stage III

Full-thickness skin loss involving damage or necrosis of subcutaneous tissue that may extend down to, but not through, underlying fascia. The ulcer presents clinically as a deep crater with or without undermining of adjacent tissue.

Requires débridement, which can be accomplished by one of the following:

- Wet-to-dry dressings
- Surgical intervention
- Proteolytic enzymes

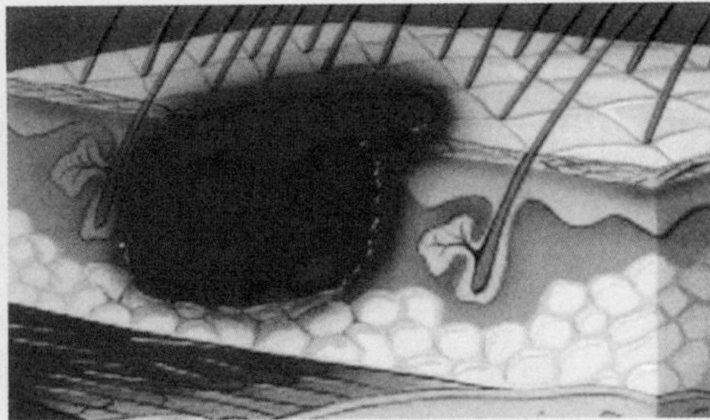

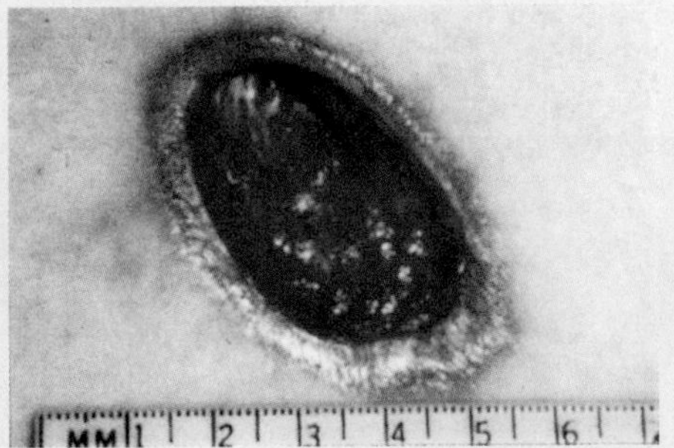

Stage IV

Full-thickness skin loss with extensive destruction, tissue necrosis, or damage to muscle, bone, or supporting structures (eg, tendon or joint capsule). Sinus tracts may also be associated with stage IV ulcers.

Wounds are treated in the following manner:

- Covered with nonadherent dressing
- Changed every 8–12 hours
- May require skin grafts

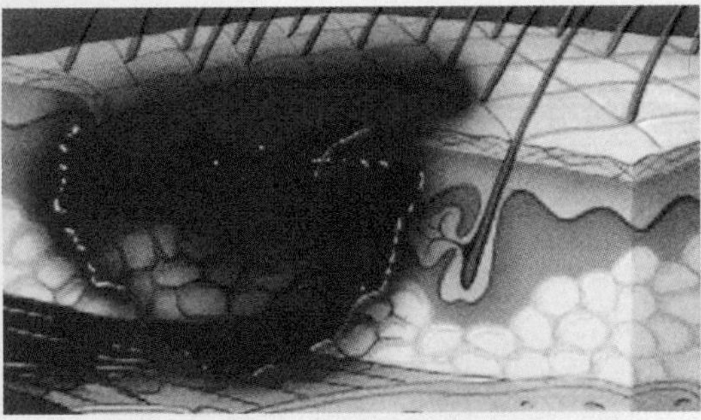

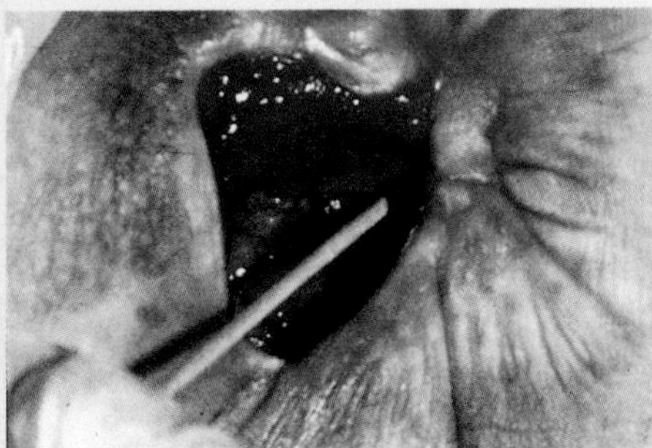

(From U.S. Department of Health and Human Services. Agency for Health Care Policy and Research. [1992]. Pressure ulcers in adults: Prediction and prevention. *Rockville, MD: DHHS; Porth, C. [1994].* Pathophysiology: Concepts of altered health states. *Philadelphia: Lippincott Williams & Wilkins; and National Pressure Ulcer Advisory Panel [NPUAP]. Available at http://www.npuap.org.)*

Fundamentals Review

Preventing Pressure Ulcers

- In patients at risk, assess the skin daily. Pay particular attention to bony prominences.
- Cleanse the skin routinely and whenever soiling occurs. Use mild cleansing agents and minimal friction, and avoid hot water.
- Maintain higher humidity in the environment. Use skin moisturizers for dry skin.
- Avoid massage over bony prominences.
- Protect skin from moisture associated with incontinence or wound drainage.
- Minimize skin injury from friction and shearing forces by using proper positioning, turning, and transfer techniques.
- Monitor dietary intake of protein and calories. Use nutritional supplements and appropriate interventions to ensure adequate intake.
- Initiate interventions to improve mobility and activity.
- Document measures used to prevent pressure ulcers.

Fundamentals Review

Wound Assessment

Wounds are assessed for appearance, size, drainage, pain, presence of sutures, drains, and tubes, and the evidence of complications.

Performing General Wound Assessment

- Assess the wound's appearance by inspecting and palpating. Look for the approximation of the edges and the color of the wound and surrounding area. The edges should be clean and well approximated. Edges may be reddened and slightly swollen for about a week, then closer to normal in appearance. Skin around the wound may be bruised initially. Observe for signs of infection, including increased swelling, redness, and warmth.
- Note the presence of any sutures, drains, and tubes. These areas are assessed in the same manner as the incision. Make sure they are intact and functioning.
- Assess the amount, color, odor, and consistency of any wound drainage.
- Assess the patient's pain, using an objective scale. Incisional pain is usually most severe for the first 2 to 3 days, after which it progressively diminishes. Increased or constant pain, especially an acute change in pain, requires further assessment. It can be a sign of delayed healing, infection, or other complication.
- Assess the patient's general condition for signs and symptoms of infection and hemorrhage.

Measuring Wounds and Pressure Ulcers

Size of the Wound

- Draw the shape and describe it.
- Measure the length, width, and diameter (if circular).

Depth of the Wound

- Perform hand hygiene. Put on gloves.
- Moisten a sterile, flexible applicator with saline and insert it gently into the wound at a 90-degree angle, with the tip down.
- Mark the point on the swab that is even with the surrounding skin surface, or grasp the applicator with the thumb and forefinger at the point corresponding to the wound's margin.
- Remove the swab and measure the depth with a ruler.

Wound Tunneling

- Perform hand hygiene and put on gloves.
- Determine direction: Put on gloves. Gently insert a sterile applicator into the site where tunneling occurs. View the direction of the applicator as if it were the hand of a clock. The direction of the patient's head represents 12 o'clock. Moving in a clockwise direction, document the deepest sites where the wound tunnels.
- Determine the depth: While the applicator is inserted into the tunneling, mark the point on the swab that is even with the wound's edge, or grasp the applicator with the thumb and forefinger at the point corresponding to the wound's margin. Remove the swab and measure the depth with a ruler.
- Document both the direction and depth of tunneling.

(Adapted from Hess, C. [2005]. Wound care *(5th ed., pp. 14–23). Philadelphia: Lippincott Williams & Wilkins.)*

SKILL 8-1 Cleaning a Wound and Applying a Dry, Sterile Dressing

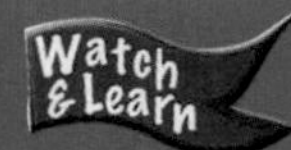

The goal of wound care is to promote tissue repair and regeneration to restore skin integrity. Many times wound care includes cleaning of the wound and the use of a dressing as a protective covering over the wound. Wound cleansing is performed to remove debris, contaminants, and excess exudate. Sterile normal saline is the preferred cleansing solution.

Dressings can rub or stick to the wound, causing superficial injury. They also can create a warm, damp, dark environment, one conducive to the growth of organisms, creating a potential for infection. Dressings are routinely changed to prevent these complications. The frequency of dressing changes depends on the amount of drainage, the physician's order, the nature of the wound, and nursing judgment. One of the most common causes of nosocomial infections is carelessness in practicing asepsis when providing wound care. It is extremely important to use appropriate aseptic technique and follow Standard Precautions. Also, since some patients may experience both physiologic and/or psychological pain related to dressing changes and wound care, nurses must be skilled in assessing for pain and employing strategies to minimize the pain experience of the patient.

Equipment

- Sterile gloves
- Gauze dressings
- Sterile dressing set or suture set (for the sterile scissors and forceps)
- Sterile cleaning solution as ordered (commonly 0.9% normal saline solution)
- Clean disposable gloves
- Sterile basin (may be optional)
- Sterile drape (may be optional)
- Plastic bag or other appropriate waste container for soiled dressings
- Waterproof pad and bath blanket
- Tape or ties
- Surgi-pads or ABD pads
- Additional dressings and supplies needed or required by the physician's order

ASSESSMENT

Assess the situation to determine the need for wound cleaning and a dressing change. Confirm any physician orders relevant to wound care and any wound care included in the nursing plan of care. Assess if the patient experienced any pain in prior dressing changes and what interventions were employed to minimize the patient's pain. Assess the current dressing to determine if it is intact. Assess for excess drainage or bleeding or saturation of the dressing. Inspect the wound and the surrounding tissue. Assess the appearance of the wound for the approximation of wound edges, the color of the wound and surrounding area, and signs of dehiscence. Note the stage of the healing process and characteristics of any drainage. Also assess the surrounding skin for color, temperature, and edema, ecchymosis, or maceration.

NURSING DIAGNOSIS

Determine the related factors for the nursing diagnoses based on the patient's current status. Appropriate nursing diagnoses may include:

- Risk for Infection
- Anxiety
- Disturbed Body Image
- Acute Pain
- Impaired Comfort
- Deficient Knowledge
- Impaired Skin Integrity
- Delayed Surgical Recovery
- Impaired Tissue Integrity

In addition, many other nursing diagnoses may require the use of this skill.

SKILL 8-1 Cleaning a Wound and Applying a Dry, Sterile Dressing *(continued)*

OUTCOME IDENTIFICATION AND PLANNING

The expected outcome to achieve when cleaning a wound and applying a sterile dressing is that the wound is cleaned and protected with a dressing without contaminating the wound area, without causing trauma to the wound, and without causing the patient to experience pain or discomfort. Other outcomes that are appropriate include: the wound continues to show signs of progression of healing, and the patient demonstrates understanding of the need for wound care and dressing change.

IMPLEMENTATION

ACTION	RATIONALE
1. Review the physician's order for wound care or the nursing plan of care related to wound care.	Reviewing the order and plan of care validates the correct patient and correct procedure.
2. Gather the necessary supplies.	Preparation promotes efficient time management and organized approach to the task.
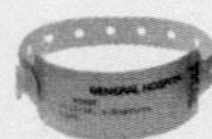 3. Identify the patient.	This ensures the right patient receives the right intervention.
4. Explain the procedure to the patient.	Discussion and explanation help allay anxiety, encourage patient cooperation, and prepare the patient for what to expect.
5. Assess the patient for possible need for nonpharmacologic pain-reducing interventions or analgesic medication before wound care dressing change. Administer appropriate analgesic, consulting physician's orders, and allow enough time for analgesic to achieve its effectiveness.	Pain is a subjective experience influenced by past experience. Wound care and dressing changes may cause pain for some patients.
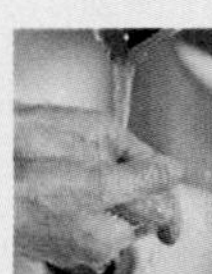 6. Perform hand hygiene.	Hand hygiene prevents the spread of microorganisms.
7. Close the room door or curtains. Place the bed at an appropriate and comfortable working height.	Closing the door or curtain promotes privacy. Proper bed positioning helps reduce back strain while you are performing the procedure.
8. Place a waste receptacle or bag at a convenient location for use during the procedure.	Having a waste container handy means the soiled dressing may be discarded easily, without the spread of microorganisms.
9. Assist the patient to a comfortable position that provides easy access to the wound area. Use the bath blanket to cover any exposed area other than the wound. If necessary, place the waterproof pad under the wound site.	Patient positioning and use of a bath blanket provide for comfort and warmth. Waterproof pad protects underlying surfaces.

(continued)

SKILL 8-1 Cleaning a Wound and Applying a Dry, Sterile Dressing *(continued)*

ACTION | **RATIONALE**

10. Check the position of drains, tubes, or other adjuncts before removing the dressing. Put on clean, disposable gloves and loosen tape on the old dressings (Figure 1). If necessary, use an adhesive remover to help get the tape off.

Checking ensures that a drain is not removed accidentally if one is present. Gloves protect the nurse from contaminated dressings and prevent the spread of microorganisms. Adhesive-tape remover helps reduce patient discomfort during removal of dressing.

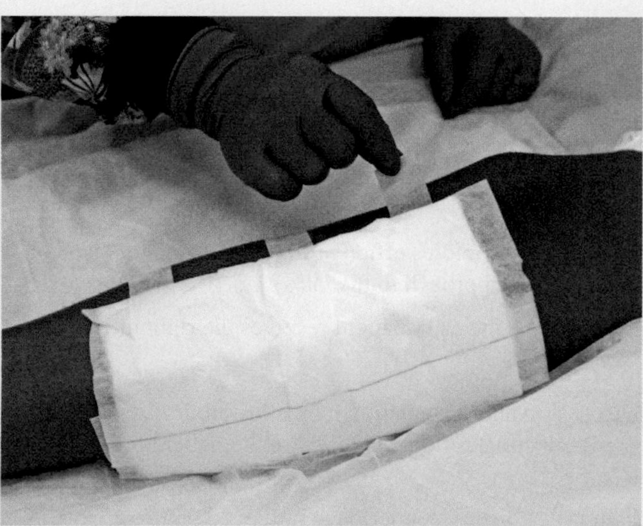

Figure 1. Loosening dressing tape.

11. Carefully remove the soiled dressings (Figure 2). If any part of the dressing sticks to the underlying skin, use small amounts of sterile saline to help loosen and remove (Figure 3). Do not reach over the wound.

Cautious removal of the dressing is more comfortable for the patient and ensures that any drain present is not removed. Sterile saline provides for easier removal of the dressing and prevents tissue damage and minimizes pain.

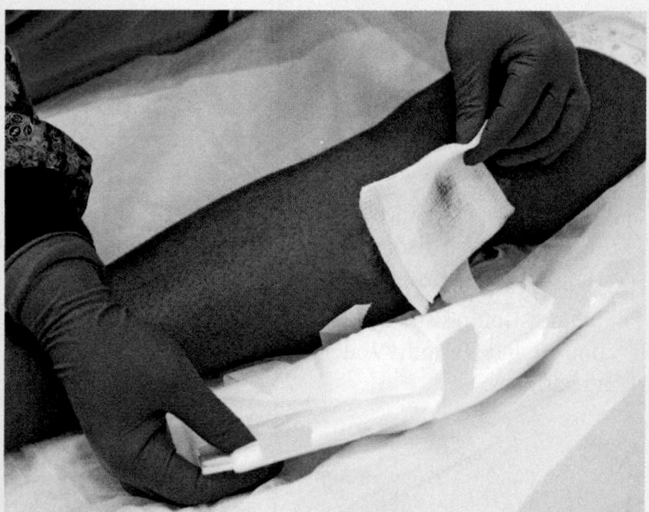

Figure 2. Removing dressing.

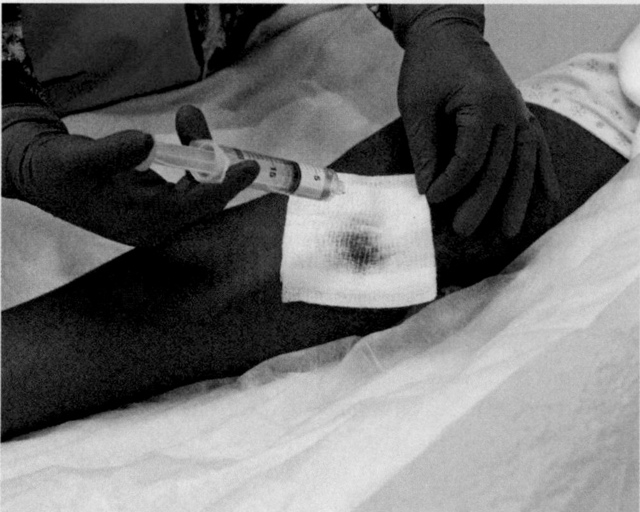

Figure 3. Using saline to aid in removing dressing.

SKILL 8-1

Cleaning a Wound and Applying a Dry, Sterile Dressing *(continued)*

ACTION | **RATIONALE**

12. After removing the dressing, note the presence, amount, type, color, and odor of any drainage on the dressings (Figure 4). Place soiled dressings in the appropriate waste receptacle. Remove your gloves and dispose of them in an appropriate waste receptacle (Figure 5).

The presence of drainage should be documented. Proper disposal of soiled dressings and used gloves prevents spread of microorganisms.

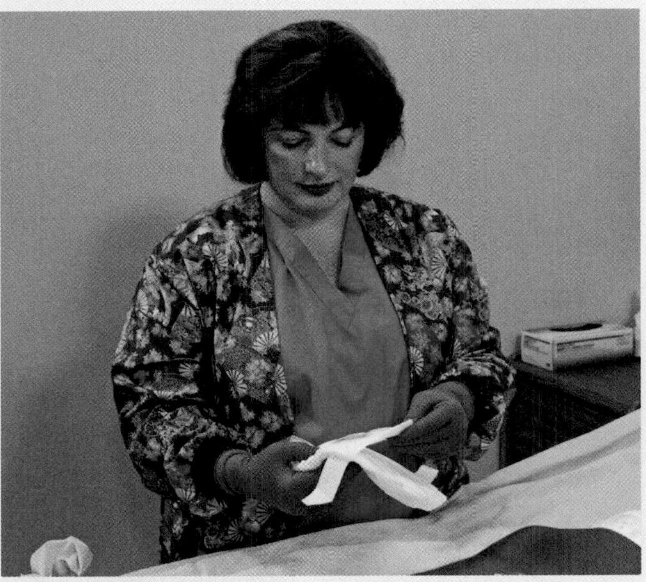

Figure 4. Assessing dressing that has been removed.

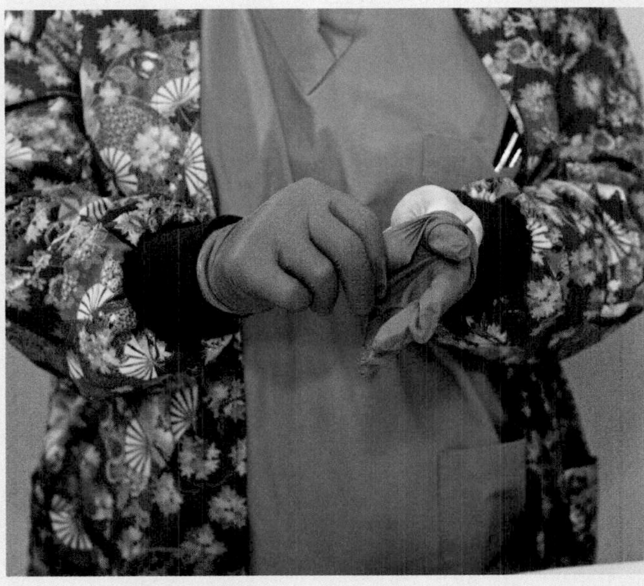

Figure 5. Removing gloves.

13. Inspect the wound site for size, appearance, and drainage. Assess if any pain is present. Check the sutures, Steri-Strips, staples, and drains or tubes. Note any problems to include in your documentation.

Wound healing or the presence of irritation or infection should be documented.

14. **Using sterile technique, prepare a sterile work area and open the needed supplies (Figure 6).**

Supplies are within easy reach and sterility is maintained.

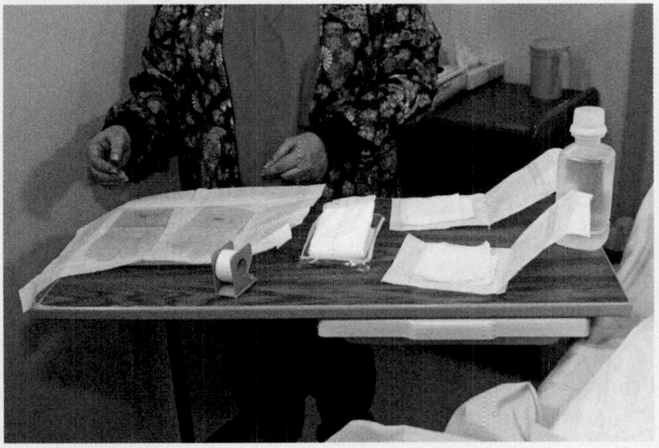

Figure 6. Setting up sterile field.

(continued)

SKILL 8-1 Cleaning a Wound and Applying a Dry, Sterile Dressing *(continued)*

ACTION	RATIONALE
15. Open the sterile cleaning solution. Depending on the amount of cleaning needed, the solution might be poured directly over gauze sponges over a container for small cleaning jobs, or into a basin for more complex or larger cleaning.	Sterility of dressings and solution is maintained.
16. Put on sterile gloves (Figure 7).	Use of sterile gloves maintains surgical asepsis and sterile technique and reduces the risk for spreading microorganisms.
17. Clean the wound. If needed, use sterile forceps to clean the area. **Clean the wound from top to bottom and from the center to the outside (Figure 8). Following this pattern, use a new gauze for each wipe, placing the used gauze in the waste receptacle. Do not touch any surface with the gloves or forceps.**	Cleaning occurs from the least to most contaminated area. Using a single gauze for each wipe ensures that the previously cleaned area is not contaminated again.

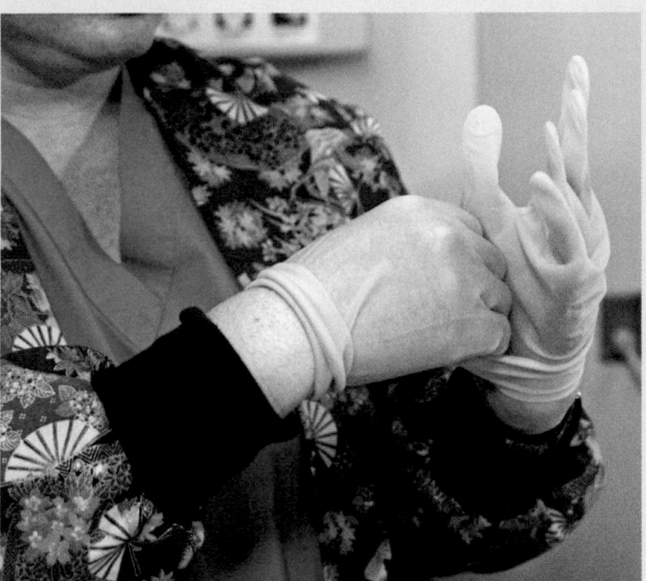

Figure 7. Putting on sterile gloves.

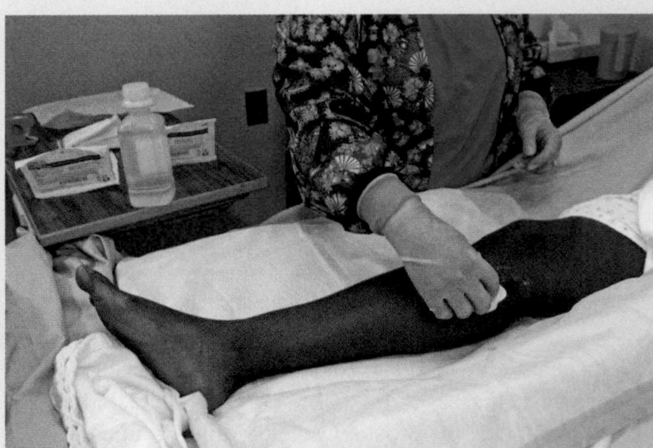

Figure 8. Cleaning wound with dampened gauze.

ACTION	RATIONALE
18. **If a drain is in use, clean around the drain using a circular motion. Wipe from the center toward the outside. Use the gauze a single time and then dispose of it.**	Cleaning occurs from least to most contaminated area.
19. Once the wound is cleaned, dry the area using a gauze sponge in the same manner. Apply ointment or any other treatments if ordered (Figure 9).	Moisture provides a medium for growth of microorganisms. The growth of microorganisms may be retarded and the healing process improved with the use of ordered ointments or other applications.
20. Apply a layer of dry sterile dressing over the wound (Figure 10). Forceps may be used to apply the dressing.	Primary dressing serves as a wick for drainage. Use of forceps helps ensure that sterile technique is maintained.
21. Place a second layer of gauze over the wound site.	A second layer provides for increased absorption of drainage.

SKILL 8-1

Cleaning a Wound and Applying a Dry, Sterile Dressing *(continued)*

ACTION

RATIONALE

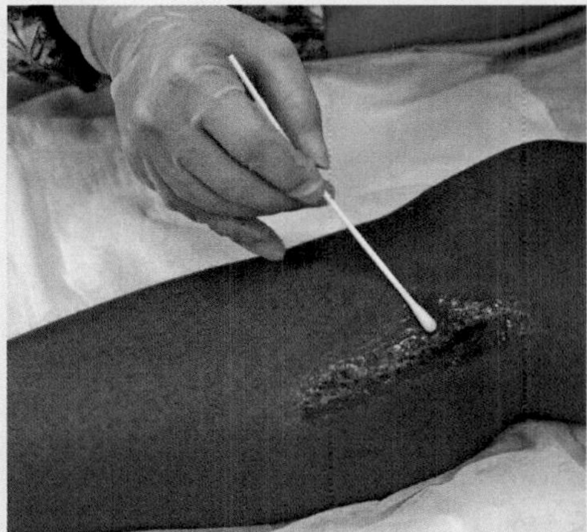

Figure 9. Applying antimicrobial ointment to wound with cotton applicator.

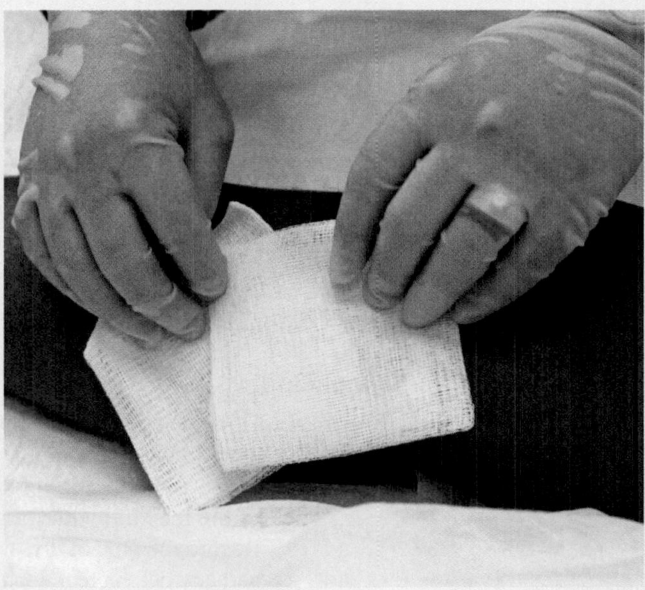

Figure 10. Applying dry dressing to site.

22. Apply a Surgi-pad or ABD dressing over the gauze at the site as the outermost layer of the dressing (Figure 11).

The dressing acts as additional protection for the wound against microorganisms in the environment.

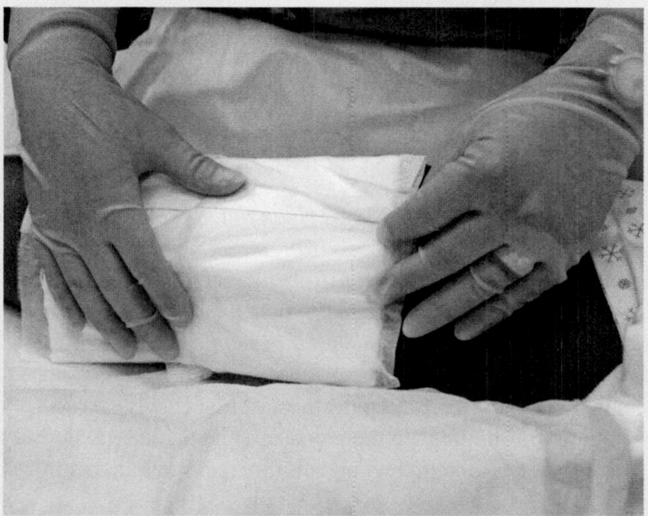

Figure 11. Applying a Surgi-pad (ABD) over dressing and securing with tape.

23. Remove and discard sterile gloves. Apply tape or tie tapes to secure the dressings.

Tape is easier to apply after gloves have been removed. Proper disposal of gloves prevents the spread of microorganisms.

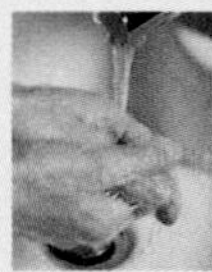

24. After securing the dressing, label dressing with date and time. Remove all remaining equipment, place the patient in a comfortable position. with side rails up and bed in the lowest position. Perform hand hygiene.

Recording date and time provides communication and demonstrates adherence to plan of care. Proper patient and bed positioning promotes safety. Hand hygiene prevents spread of microorganisms.

(continued)

SKILL 8-1 Cleaning a Wound and Applying a Dry, Sterile Dressing *(continued)*

ACTION	RATIONALE
25. Check all wound dressings every shift. More frequent checks may be needed if the wound is more complex or dressings become saturated quickly.	Checking dressings ensures the assessment of changes in patient condition and timely intervention to prevent complications.

EVALUATION

The expected outcome is met when the patient exhibits a clean, intact wound with a clean sterile dressing in place; the wound is free of contamination and trauma; the patient reports little to no pain or discomfort during care; and the patient demonstrates signs and symptoms of progressive wound healing.

DOCUMENTATION

Guidelines

Document the location of the incision and that the dressing was removed. Record your assessment of the incision including the approximation of the sutures and the condition of the surrounding skin. Note if redness, edema or drainage is observed. Document cleansing of the incision with normal saline and any application of antibiotic ointment as ordered. Record the type of dressing that was reapplied. Note pertinent patient and family education and any patient reaction from this procedure. including patient's pain level and effectiveness of nonpharmacologic interventions or analgesia if administered.

Sample Documentation

9/8/09 0600 Dressing removed from leg incision. Scant purulent secretions noted on dressing. Incision edges approximately 1 mm apart, red, with ecchymosis and edema present. Small amount of purulent drainage from wound noted. Area cleansed with normal saline, dried, antibiotic ointment applied per order. Surrounding tissue red and ecchymotic. Redressed with nonadhering dressing, gauze, and wrapped with stretch gauze. Patient reports adequate pain control after preprocedure analgesic. —N. Joiner, RN

Unexpected Situations and Associated Interventions

- *The previous wound assessment states that the incision was clean and dry and the wound edges were approximated, with the staples and surgical drain intact. The surrounding tissue was without inflammation, edema, or erythema. After the dressing is removed, you note the incision edges are not approximated at the distal end, multiple staples are evident in the old dressing, the surrounding skin tissue is red and swollen, and purulent drainage is on the dressing and leaking from the wound:* Assess the patient for any other signs and symptoms, such as pain, malaise, fever, and paresthesias. Place a dry sterile dressing over the wound site. Report your findings to the physician and document the event in the patient's record. Be prepared to obtain a wound culture and implement any changes in wound care as ordered.
- *After you have put on sterile gloves, the patient moves too close to the edge of the bed and you support her with your hands to prevent her from falling:* If nothing else in the sterile field was touched, remove the contaminated gloves and put on new sterile gloves. If you did not bring a second pair, use the call light to summon a coworker to provide a new pair of gloves.
- *You have set up your supplies, removed the old dressing, and put on sterile gloves to clean the wound. You realize you have forgotten a necessary piece of dressing material:* Ask the patient to press the call bell to summon a coworker to provide the missing supplies.

SKILL 8-1 Cleaning a Wound and Applying a Dry, Sterile Dressing *(continued)*

Special Considerations

General Considerations

- Instruct the patient, if appropriate, and ancillary staff members to observe for excessive drainage that may overwhelm the dressing. They should also report when dressings become soiled or loosened from the skin.
- Lloyd-Jones (2004) suggests warm saline solution to minimize discomfort for patients who experience discomfort from cold saline wound cleansing.

Older Adult Considerations

- The skin of older adults is less elastic and more sensitive, so use paper tape or Montgomery straps to prevent tearing of the skin.

SKILL 8-2 Applying a Saline-Moistened Dressing

A dressing is a protective covering placed on a wound. Gauze dressings are easy to use and adapt to many applications. Gauze can be moistened with saline to keep the surface of open wounds moist. This type of dressing promotes moist wound healing and protects the wound from contamination and trauma. A moist wound surface enhances the cellular migration necessary for tissue repair and healing. This dressing is often used with chronic wounds and pressure wounds. It is important that the dressing material be moist, not wet, when placed in open wounds. Dressing materials are soaked in normal saline solution and squeezed to remove excess saline so that the dressing is only slightly moist. The dressing can be loosely packed in the wound bed if appropriate, then covered with a secondary dressing to absorb drainage.

At times, wet-to-dry dressings are applied for débridement. These dressings are used to soften debris and facilitate removal of necrotic tissue. The accompanying Skill Variation discusses technique.

Equipment

- Clean disposable gloves
- Sterile gloves
- Sterile dressing set or suture set (for the sterile scissors and forceps)
- Sterile thin-mesh gauze dressing for packing, if ordered
- Sterile gauze dressings
- Surgi-pads or ABD pads
- Skin-protectant wipes
- Sterile basin
- Sterile cleaning solution as ordered (commonly 0.9% normal saline solution)
- Sterile saline
- Tape or ties
- Plastic bag or other appropriate waste container for soiled dressings
- Sterile cotton-tipped applicators
- Supplies for wound cleansing or irrigation, as necessary
- Waterproof pad and bath blanket
- Personal protective equipment, such as a gown, mask, and eye protection
- Bath blanket

ASSESSMENT

Assess the situation to determine the need for a dressing change. Confirm any physician orders relevant to wound care and any wound care included in the nursing plan of care.

(continued)

SKILL 8-2 Applying a Saline-Moistened Dressing

Assess the current dressing, if there is one, to see if it is intact and if there is excess drainage or bleeding or saturation of the dressing. Assess the patient's level of comfort and the need for analgesics before wound care. Assess the location, stage, drainage, and types of tissue present in the wound. Measure the wound. Assess the surrounding skin for color, temperature, edema, ecchymosis, or maceration.

NURSING DIAGNOSIS

Determine the related factors for the nursing diagnoses based on the patient's current status. An appropriate nursing diagnosis is Impaired Skin Integrity. Other nursing diagnoses that may be appropriate include:

- Anxiety
- Disturbed Body Image
- Impaired Comfort
- Risk for Infection
- Acute Pain
- Chronic Pain
- Impaired Tissue Integrity

OUTCOME IDENTIFICATION AND PLANNING

The expected outcome to achieve when applying a saline-moistened dressing is that the procedure is accomplished without contaminating the wound area, without causing trauma to the wound, and without causing the patient to experience pain or discomfort. Other outcomes that are appropriate include sterile technique is maintained (if appropriate); wound healing is promoted; the surrounding skin is without signs of irritation, infection, and maceration; and the wound continues to show signs of progression of healing.

IMPLEMENTATION

ACTION	RATIONALE
1. Review the physician's order and/or nursing plan of care for the application of a saline-moistened dressing.	This action validates the correct patient and correct procedure.
2. Gather the necessary supplies.	This action promotes efficient time management and provides an organized approach to the task.
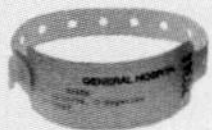 3. Identify the patient.	This ensures that the right patient receives the right intervention.
4. Explain the procedure to the patient.	Discussion and explanation help allay anxiety, encourage patient cooperation, and prepare the patient for what to expect.
5. Assess the patient for possible need for nonpharmacologic pain-reducing interventions or analgesic medication before wound care dressing change. Administer appropriate analgesic, consulting physician's orders, and allow enough time for analgesic to achieve its effectiveness before beginning procedure.	Pain is a subjective experience influenced by past experience. Wound care and dressing changes may cause pain for some patients.
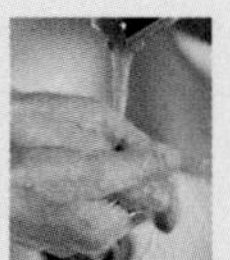 6. Perform hand hygiene.	Hand hygiene prevents the spread of microorganisms.
7. Close the room door or curtains. Place the bed at a comfortable working height.	Closing the door or curtains provides privacy. Having the bed at a comfortable height helps reduce back strain while you are performing the procedure.

SKILL 8-2 Applying a Saline-Moistened Dressing *(continued)*

ACTION	RATIONALE
8. Place a waste receptacle or bag at a convenient location for use during procedure.	Having the waste receptacle handy means that soiled dressings and supplies may be discarded easily, without the spread of microorganisms.
9. Assist the patient to a comfortable position that provides easy access to the wound area. Position the patient so the irrigation solution will flow from the clean end of the wound toward the dirtier end, if wound irrigation is necessary (See Skill 8-4 for irrigation techniques). Expose the area and drape the patient with the bath blanket if needed. Put the waterproof pad under the wound area to protect the bed.	A comfortable position and bath blanket provide comfort and warmth for the patient. Gravity directs the flow of liquid from the least contaminated to the most contaminated area. The waterproof pad protects the patient and the bed linens.
10. Put on personal protective equipment as appropriate.	Using personal protective equipment prevents contamination from microorganisms and the spread of infection. The nurse uses standard and transmission-based precautions as needed.
11. Put on clean disposable gloves and gently remove the soiled dressings. If the dressing adheres to the underlying tissues, moisten it with saline to loosen it.	Gloves protect the nurse from handling contaminated dressings. Moistening the dressing prevents disruption of healing tissue.
12. After removing the dressing, note the presence, amount, type, color, and odor of any drainage on the dressings. Place soiled dressings in the appropriate waste receptacle.	The presence of drainage should be documented. Discarding dressings appropriately prevents the spread of microorganisms.
13. Assess the wound for appearance, stage, the presence of eschar, granulation tissue, epithelialization, undermining, tunneling, necrosis, sinus tract, and drainage. Assess the appearance of the surrounding tissue. Measure the wound.	This information provides evidence about the wound healing process and/or the presence of infection.
14. Remove your gloves and put them in the receptacle.	Discarding gloves prevents the spread of microorganisms.
15. Using sterile technique, open the supplies and dressings. Place the fine-mesh gauze into the basin and pour the ordered solution over the mesh to saturate it.	Gauze touching the wound surface must be moistened to increase the absorptive ability and promote healing.
16. Put on the sterile gloves.	Sterile gloves maintain surgical asepsis.
17. Clean the wound. If needed, use sterile forceps to clean the area. **Clean the wound from top to bottom and from the center to the outside. Following this pattern, use a new gauze for each wipe, placing the used gauze in the waste receptacle. Do not touch any surface with the gloves or forceps.** Irrigate the wound, if needed (see Skill 8-4).	Using a single gauze for each wipe ensures that previously cleaned areas are not contaminated again.
18. Dry the surrounding skin with sterile gauze dressings.	Moisture provides a medium for growth of microorganisms.
19. Squeeze excess fluid from the gauze dressing. Unfold and fluff the dressing.	The gauze provides a thin, moist layer to contact all the wound surfaces.
20. Gently press to loosely pack the moistened gauze into the wound (Figure 1). If necessary, use the forceps or cotton-tipped applicators to press the gauze into all wound surfaces (Figure 2).	The dressing provides a moist environment for all wound surfaces. Avoid overpacking the gauze and loosely pack to prevent too much pressure in the wound bed, which could impede wound healing.

(continued)

SKILL 8-2 Applying a Saline-Moistened Dressing *(continued)*

ACTION | **RATIONALE**

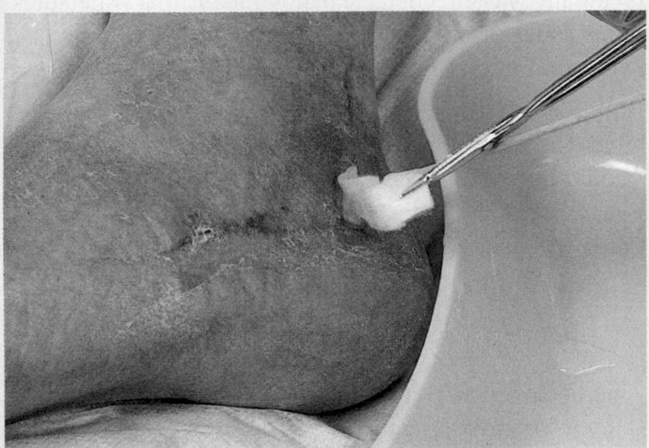

Figure 1. Gently pressing gauze into wound.

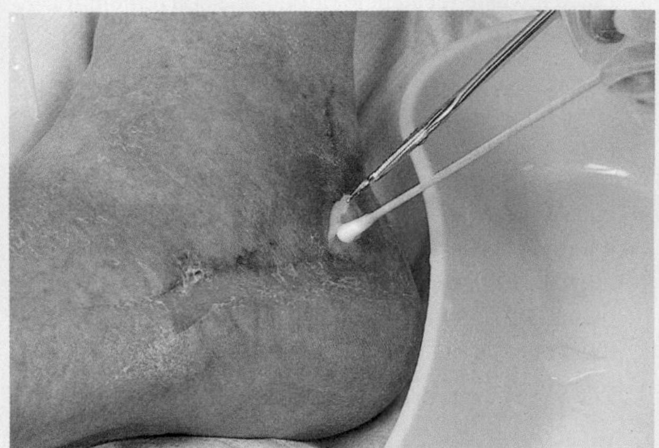

Figure 2. Using a cotton-tipped applicator to press gauze into all wound surfaces.

21. Apply several dry, sterile gauze pads over the wet gauze.

    Dry gauze absorbs excess moisture and drainage.

22. Place the ABD pad over the gauze.

    The ABD pad prevents contamination.

23. Remove and discard your sterile gloves. Apply a skin protectant to the surrounding skin if needed Apply tape or tie tapes to secure the dressings.

    Discarding gloves prevents the spread of microorganisms. A skin protectant prevents skin irritation and breakdown. Tape is easier to apply after gloves have been removed.

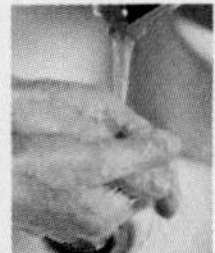

24. After securing the dressing, remove all remaining equipment, place the patient in a position of comfort, with side rails up and the bed in the lowest position, and perform hand hygiene.

    These actions ensure safety. Hand hygiene prevents the spread of microorganisms.

25. Check all wound dressings every shift. You might need to check more frequently if a wound is more complex or dressings become saturated more frequently.

    Frequent checks ensure that changes in patient condition are noted and timely intervention is performed to prevent complications.

EVALUATION

The expected outcome when applying a saline-moistened dressing is met when the procedure is accomplished without contaminating the wound area, without causing trauma to the wound, and without causing the patient to experience pain or discomfort. Other outcomes are met when sterile technique is maintained (if appropriate); wound healing is promoted; the surrounding skin is without signs of irritation, infection, and maceration; and the wound continues to show signs of progression of healing.

DOCUMENTATION

Guidelines

Document the procedure, your wound assessment, and the patient's reaction to the procedure. Record the condition of the wound, such as evidence of granulation tissue, presence of necrotic tissue, and characteristics of drainage. Include the appearance of the surrounding skin. Include if an irrigation of the wound was needed. Record the patient's response to the treatment including a pain assessment. Document pertinent patient and family education.

SKILL 8-2 Applying a Saline-Moistened Dressing *(continued)*

Sample Documentation

11/20/09 1645 Healing abdominal incision with granulating tissue noted. No evidence of necrosis or tunneling. Scant amount of serous drainage from upper aspect of incision. Saline-moistened dressing applied; covered loosely with ABD dressing. Patient denies pain from incision. Instructed patient that moist saline gauze will facilitate the healing process and to notify nurse for any discomfort related to incision.—R. Dobbins, RN

Unexpected Situations and Related Interventions

- *When removing a patient's dressing, you note eschar in the wound:* The presence of eschar in a wound precludes the staging of the wound. The eschar must be removed for adequate pressure ulcer staging to be done.
- *You note several depressions or crater-like areas on inspection of a wound:* Notify the physician, who may order the wound to be packed. Pack wound cavities loosely with dressing material. Overpacking may increase pressure and interfere with tissue healing.
- *You note that the wound dressing is dry upon removal:* Reduce the time interval between changes to prevent drying of the materials, which may disrupt healing tissue.

Special Considerations

General Considerations

- Make sure ancillary staff understand the importance of reporting excessive drainage from the dressing, and any soiled or loose dressings.
- Many products are available to treat chronic and pressure ulcers. Treatment varies based on facility policy, nursing protocol, clinical specialist referrals, and physician orders.

SKILL VARIATION Wet-to-Dry or Wet-to-Moist Dressings for Débridement

Wet-to-dry dressings may be used for débridement. These dressings soften debris and facilitate removal of necrotic tissue. Gauze is moistened with an appropriate solution, such as normal saline and applied to the wound. The dressing is covered with dry gauze and the dressings are allowed to dry. Debris and necrotic tissue adhere to the gauze and are removed from the wound when the dressing is changed. However, when the dressing dries completely, new granulation can be removed, which slows wound healing. Other research recommends that to preserve the newly forming granulation tissue, remove the dressing when it is moist rather then completely dry. This dressing is referred to as a wet-to-moist dressing.

- Gather equipment and verify the physician's order.
- Identify the patient and explain the procedure.
- Assess the patient for pain and need for analgesic before procedure.
- Administer analgesic if needed and wait appropriate time for effectiveness to be reached.
- Perform hand hygiene and put on clean gloves.
- Remove dressing and inspect the wound for color, presence of drainage, and granulation tissue.
- Remove gloves.
- If needed, prepare sterile field. Pour prescribed cleaning solution into sterile basin and open sterile gauze dressings and forceps wrapper.
- Put on sterile gloves.
- Place sterile gauze dressings into sterile basin and place forceps onto sterile field.
- Clean wound with sterile gauze as needed.
- Apply wet, sterile, saline gauze dressings directly into wound, loosely filling all spaces of the wound. Use forceps if needed to loosely place gauze into deeper areas.
- Place dry, sterile gauze dressing over the wet gauze and cover with ABD dressing.
- Dispose of supplies as needed and remove sterile gloves. Perform hand hygiene. Ensure patient comfort.
- When the dressings have dried, carefully remove the dry dressings. This procedure may cause discomfort to the patient, so, if needed, analgesic medication may be prescribed.

SKILL 8-3 Applying a Hydrocolloid Dressing

Hydrocolloid dressings are wafer-shaped dressings that come in many shapes, sizes, and thicknesses. An adhesive backing provides adherence to the wound and surrounding skin. They absorb drainage, maintain a moist wound surface, and decrease the risk for infection by covering the wound surface (Table 8-1 provides example of moisture-retentive dressings).

They are used for shallow to moderate-depth wounds with minimal drainage and stay in place for 3 to 7 days. Polyurethane dressings are nonadhesive hydrocolloid dressings that must be secured to prevent wound contamination, as they do not adhere to the wound or surrounding skin. Application can be done using clean or sterile technique, depending on facility policy (see Special Considerations).

Equipment

- Hydrocolloid dressing
- Clean disposable gloves
- Sterile gloves
- Sterile dressing instrument set or suture set (for the scissors and forceps)
- Sterile cleaning solution as ordered (commonly 0.9% normal saline solution)

TABLE 8-1 Examples of Moisture-Retentive Dressings

TYPE	PURPOSES	USE
Transparent films Acu-derm Bioclusive BlisterFilm Mefilm Polyskin Uniflex Op-Site Tegaderm	• Allow exchange of oxygen between wound and environment • Are self-adhesive • Protect against contamination • Prevent loss of wound fluid • Maintain a moist wound environment • Allow visualization of wound • May remain in place for 24 to 72 hours, resulting in less interference with healing	• Wounds with minimal drainage • Wounds that are small and superficial, such as stage I and II pressure ulcers and superficial burns
Hydrocolloid dressings DuoDerm Intact Comfeel IntraSite Tegasorb Ultec	• Are occlusive • Absorb drainage • Provide cushioning • Do not allow entry of contaminants • May be left in place for 3 to 5 days, resulting in less interference with healing	• Shallow to moderate-depth skin ulcers • Wounds with drainage • In conjunction with packing for open, deep wounds
Hydrogels Vigilon IntraSite Gel Aquasorb ClearSite Nu-Gel Hypergel	• Maintain a moist wound environment • Do not adhere to wound • Reduce pain	• Partial- and full-thickness wounds • Necrotic wounds • Burns
Alginates Sorban AlgiDerm Curasorb Dermacea Melgisorb	• Absorb some exudate • Are compatible with topical medication • Absorb exudate • Maintain moisture	• Infected wounds
Foams LYOfoam Allevyn	• Maintain moist wound surface • Do not adhere to wound • Insulate wound	• Chronic wounds

SKILL 8-3 Applying a Hydrocolloid Dressing *(continued)*

- Skin-protectant wipes
- Additional supplies needed for wound cleansing
- Sterile cotton-tipped applicators
- Waterproof waste receptacle
- Waterproof pad or bath blanket as needed
- Personal protective equipment such as gown, mask, and eye protection, as needed
- Measuring tape or other supplies, such as sterile flexible applicator (if needed for assessing wound measurements)

ASSESSMENT

Assess the situation to determine the need for a dressing change. Check the date when the current dressing (if present) was placed. Confirm any physician orders relevant to wound care and any wound care included in the nursing plan of care. Assess the current dressing, if there is one, to determine if it is intact. Assess the patient's level of comfort and the need for analgesics before wound care. Assess the location, stage, drainage, and types of tissue present in the wound. Measure the wound. Assess the surrounding skin for color, temperature, edema, ecchymosis, or maceration.

NURSING DIAGNOSES

Determine the related factors for the nursing diagnoses based on the patient's current status. An appropriate nursing diagnosis is Impaired Skin Integrity. Other nursing diagnoses that may be appropriate include:

- Anxiety
- Disturbed Body Image
- Impaired Comfort
- Risk for Infection
- Acute Pain
- Chronic Pain
- Impaired Tissue Integrity

OUTCOME IDENTIFICATION AND PLANNING

The expected outcome to achieve when applying a hydrocolloid dressing is that the procedure is accomplished without contaminating the wound area, without causing trauma to the wound, and without causing the patient to experience pain or discomfort. Other outcomes that are appropriate include sterile technique is maintained (if appropriate); wound healing is promoted; the surrounding skin is without signs of irritation, infection, and maceration; and the wound continues to show signs of progression of healing.

IMPLEMENTATION

ACTION	RATIONALE
1. Review the physician's order and/or nursing plan of care for the application of a hydrocolloid dressing.	Checking the order validates the correct patient and correct procedure.
2. Gather the necessary supplies.	Having supplies at hand promotes efficient time management and provides an organized approach to the task.
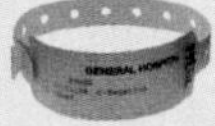 3. Identify the patient.	This ensures the right patient receives the right intervention.
4. Explain the procedure to the patient.	Discussion and explanation help allay anxiety, encourage patient cooperation, and prepare the patient for what to expect.

(continued)

SKILL 8-3 Applying a Hydrocolloid Dressing *(continued)*

ACTION	RATIONALE
5. Assess the patient for possible need for nonpharmacologic pain-reducing interventions or analgesic medication before wound care dressing change. Administer appropriate analgesic, consulting physician's orders, and allow enough time for analgesic to achieve its effectiveness before beginning procedure.	Pain is a subjective experience influenced by past experience. Wound care and dressing changes may cause pain for some patients
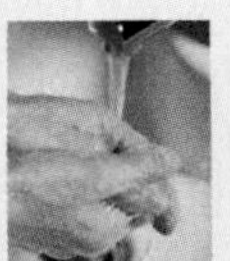 6. Perform hand hygiene.	Hand hygiene prevents the spread of microorganisms.
7. Close the room door or curtains. Place the bed at a comfortable working height.	Closing the door or curtains provides privacy. Having the bed at a comfortable height helps reduce back strain while you are performing the procedure.
8. Have the disposal bag or waste receptacle within easy reach.	Having the waste receptacle handy means that dressings and supplies may be discarded easily, without the spread of microorganisms.
9. Assist the patient to a comfortable position that provides easy access to the wound area. Position the patient so the irrigation solution will flow from the cleanest to the dirtiest end of the wound, if necessary. Expose the area and drape the patient with the bath blanket if needed. Put the waterproof pad under the wound area to protect the bed.	A comfortable position and the bath blanket provide for comfort and warmth. Gravity directs the flow of liquid from the least contaminated to the most contaminated area. The waterproof pad protects the patient and the bed linens.
10. Put on personal protective equipment as appropriate.	Using personal protective equipment prevents contamination from microorganisms and the spread of infection.
11. Put on clean disposable gloves and gently remove the soiled dressing. Discard it in the receptacle.	The nurse is protected from handling a contaminated dressing.
12. Assess the wound for appearance, stage, granulation tissue, epithelialization, undermining, tunneling, necrosis, sinus tract, and drainage. Assess the appearance of the surrounding tissue. Measure the wound if needed.	This information provides evidence about the wound healing process and/or the presence of infection.
13. Remove your gloves and put them in the receptacle.	Discarding gloves prevents the spread of microorganisms.
14. Set up a sterile field and put on the sterile gloves if indicated.	Using sterile gloves prevents contamination of the wound or supplies and prevents the spread of microorganisms.
15. Clean the wound. If needed, use sterile forceps to clean the area. **Clean the wound from top to bottom and from the center to the outside. Following this pattern, use a new gauze for each wipe, placing the used gauze in the waste receptacle. Do not touch any surface with the gloves or forceps.** Irrigate the wound, if appropriate (see Skill 8-4).	Cleaning removes debris, contaminants, and excess exudate. Using a single gauze for each wipe ensures that previously cleaned areas are not contaminated again.
16. Dry the surrounding skin with sterile gauze dressings.	Moisture provides a medium for growth of microorganisms.
17. Choose a clean, dry, presized dressing or cut one to size using sterile scissors. The dressing must be sized generously, allowing at least a 1″ margin of healthy skin around the wound to be covered with the dressing.	These actions ensure proper adherence, coverage of the wound, and wear of the dressing.

SKILL 8-3

Applying a Hydrocolloid Dressing *(continued)*

ACTION	RATIONALE
18. Remove the release paper from the adherent side of the dressing. Apply the dressing to the wound without stretching the dressing. Smooth wrinkles as it is applied.	Proper application prevents shearing force on the wound and minimizes irritation.
19. Apply a skin protectant to the skin surrounding the wound if needed. If necessary, secure the dressing edges with tape. Dressings that are near the anus need to have the edges taped. Apply additional skin barrier to the areas to be covered with tape, if necessary.	Taping helps keep the dressing intact. Taping the edges of dressings near the anus prevents wound contamination from fecal material. Skin protectant prevents surrounding skin irritation and breakdown.
20. Remove and discard your sterile gloves.	Discarding gloves prevents the spread of microorganisms.
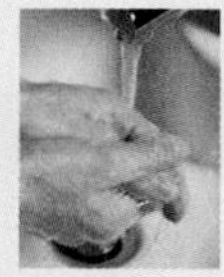 21. Remove all remaining equipment, place the patient in a position of comfort with side rails up and the bed in the lowest position, and perform hand hygiene.	These actions ensure safety. Hand hygiene prevents the spread of microorganisms.
22. Check all wound dressings every shift to validate that they are intact.	Frequent checks ensure that changes in patient condition are noted and timely intervention is performed to prevent complications.

EVALUATION

The expected outcome when applying a hydrocolloid dressing is met when the procedure is accomplished without contaminating the wound area, without causing trauma to the wound, and without causing the patient to experience pain or discomfort. Other outcomes are met when sterile technique is maintained (if appropriate); wound healing is promoted; surrounding skin is without signs of irritation, infection, and maceration; and the wound continues to show signs of progression of healing.

DOCUMENTATION

Guidelines

Record the procedure, your wound assessment, and the patient's reaction to the procedure. Describe the stage of the wound, including length, width, and depth. Note the presence of granulating tissue, necrotic tissue, and undermining and tunneling of the wound. Include a description of the drainage and its characteristics. Also document the appearance of the surrounding tissue and whether a skin barrier was applied. Record the type of hydrocolloid dressing that was applied. Note the date for the next dressing change, based on facility policy (normally 3–7 days).

Sample Documentation

11/4/08 0930 Stage 3 wound on right hip area (3 × 2 × 2 cm) assessed. Granulation tissue about 50%, no necrosis, undermining, or tunneling present. Minimal serous drainage on old dressing. Wound cleansed with normal saline. Hydrocolloid dressing applied. Due to be changed in 5 days. Skin barrier applied to surrounding intact skin. Prior to dressing change, patient was medicated with Tylenol 650 mg PO for anticipated pain. Patient tolerated dressing change. Stated "pain not so bad," about a "3." Instructed patient to call for nurse for any discomfort related to dressing.
—M. Semet, RN

(continued)

SKILL 8-3 Applying a Hydrocolloid Dressing *(continued)*

Unexpected Situations and Related Intervention

- *When performing wound care, you observe adherent necrotic material in the wound:* Notify the wound care specialist and/or the physician, as further débridement may be necessary.

Special Considerations

- Guidelines from the Agency for Health Care Policy and Research state that clean gloves and clean dressings may be used to treat pressure ulcers as long as the agency infection-control procedures are followed. The *no-touch technique* may be used within these guidelines. Clean gloves are used to handle dressing material. Irrigants and dressings are sterile. The wound is redressed by picking up dressing materials by the corner and placing the untouched side over the pressure ulcer.
- Many products are available to treat chronic and pressure ulcers. Treatment varies based on facility policy, nursing protocol, clinical specialist referrals, and physician orders.

SKILL 8-4 Performing a Sterile Irrigation of a Wound

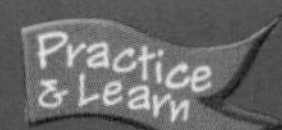

Irrigation is a directed flow of solution over tissues. Physicians may order wound irrigations to clean the area of pathogens and other debris and to promote wound healing. Irrigation procedures may also be ordered to apply heat or antiseptics locally. If the wound is closed, clean technique may be used; if the wound is open, sterile equipment and solutions are used for irrigation. Normal saline is often the solution of choice when irrigating wounds.

Equipment

- A sterile irrigation set, including a basin, irrigant container, and irrigation syringe
- Sterile irrigation solution as ordered by the physician, warmed to body temperature, commonly 0.9% normal saline solution
- Plastic bag or other waste container to dispose of soiled dressings
- Sterile gloves
- Sterile drape (may be optional)
- Clean disposable gloves
- Sterile dressing set or suture set (for the sterile scissors and forceps)
- Waterproof pad and bath blanket as needed
- Sterile gauze dressings
- Sterile packing gauze as needed
- Tape or ties
- Skin-protectant wipes
- Personal protective equipment, such as a gown, mask, and eye protection

ASSESSMENT

Assess the situation to determine the need for wound irrigation. Confirm any physician orders relevant to wound care and any wound care included in the nursing plan of care. Assess the current dressing to determine if it is intact. Assess for excess drainage or bleeding or saturation of the dressing. Inspect the wound and the surrounding tissue. Assess the wound for the approximation of wound edges, the color of the wound and surrounding area, and signs of dehiscence. Note the stage of the healing process and characteristics of any drainage. Assess the surrounding skin for color, temperature, and edema, ecchymosis, or maceration. Determine the patient's level of pain and administer analgesics as ordered.

NURSING DIAGNOSIS

Determine the related factors for the nursing diagnoses based on the patient's current status. An appropriate nursing diagnosis would be Risk for Infection. Other nursing diagnoses may include:

- Anxiety
- Acute Pain

SKILL 8-4 Performing a Sterile Irrigation of a Wound *(continued)*

- Disturbed Body Image
- Deficient Knowledge
- Impaired Skin Integrity
- Delayed Surgical Recovery
- Impaired Tissue Integrity
- Risk for Trauma

OUTCOME IDENTIFICATION AND PLANNING

The expected outcome to achieve when irrigating a wound is that the wound is cleaned without contamination or trauma and without causing the patient to experience pain or discomfort. Other outcomes that might be appropriate include: the wound continues to show signs of progression of healing, and the patient demonstrates understanding about the need for wound irrigation.

IMPLEMENTATION

ACTION	RATIONALE
1. Review the physician's order for wound care or the nursing plan of care related to wound care.	Reviewing the order and nursing plan of care validates the correct patient and correct procedure.
2. Gather the necessary supplies.	Preparation promotes efficient time management and provides an organized approach to the task.
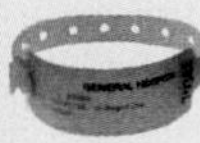 3. Identify the patient.	This ensures that the right patient receives the right intervention.
4. Explain the procedure to the patient.	Discussion and explanation help allay anxiety, encourage patient cooperation, and prepare the patient for what to expect.
5. Assess the patient for possible need for nonpharmacologic pain-reducing interventions or analgesic medication before wound care dressing change. Administer appropriate analgesic, consulting physician's orders, and allow enough time for analgesic to achieve its effectiveness.	Pain is a subjective experience influenced by past experience. Wound care and dressing changes may cause pain for some patients.
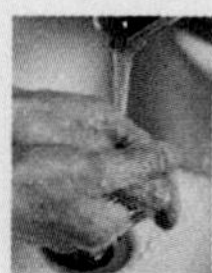 6. Perform hand hygiene.	Hand hygiene prevents the spread of microorganisms.
7. Close the room door or curtains. Place the bed at a comfortable working height.	Closing the door or curtains provides privacy. Proper bed positioning helps reduce back strain while you are performing the procedure.
8. Have the disposal bag or waste receptacle within easy reach prior to the irrigation for soiled dressing disposal.	Having the waste container handy means that soiled dressings and supplies may be discarded easily, without the spread of microorganisms.
9. Assist the patient to a comfortable position that provides easy access to the wound area. **Position the patient so that the irrigation solution will flow from the clean to dirty end of the wound.** Expose the area and drape the patient with a bath blanket if needed. Put the waterproof pad under the wound area.	Patient positioning and use of a bath blanket provide for comfort and warmth. Gravity directs the flow of liquid from the least contaminated to the most contaminated area. Waterproof pad protects the patient and the bed linens.

(continued)

SKILL 8-4 Performing a Sterile Irrigation of a Wound *(continued)*

ACTION	RATIONALE
10. Put on a gown, mask, and eye protection.	Using personal protective equipment such as gowns, masks, and eye protection is part of Standard Precautions. A gown protects clothes from contamination should splashing occur. Goggles protect mucous membranes of eyes from contact with irrigant fluid or wound drainage.
11. Put on clean disposable gloves and remove the soiled dressings.	The nurse is protected from handling contaminated dressings.
12. Assess the wound for size, appearance, and drainage on the dressing. Assess the appearance of the surrounding tissue.	Assessment provides information about the wound healing process or the presence of infection.
13. Discard the dressings in the receptacle. Remove gloves and put them in the receptacle.	Proper disposal of dressings and gloves prevents the spread of microorganisms.
14. **Using sterile technique, prepare a sterile field and add all the sterile supplies needed for the procedure to the field. Pour warmed sterile irrigating solution into the sterile container.**	Supplies are within easy reach and sterile technique is maintained. Using warmed solution prevents chilling of the patient and may minimize patient discomfort.
15. Put on sterile gloves.	Using sterile gloves maintains surgical asepsis.
16. Position the sterile basin below the wound to collect the irrigation fluid.	Patient and bed linens are protected from contaminated fluid.
17. Fill the irrigation syringe with solution (Figure 1). **Using your nondominant hand, gently apply pressure to the basin against the skin below the wound to form a seal with the skin (Figure 2).**	The solution will collect in the basin and prevent the irrigant from running down the skin. Patient and bed linens are protected from contaminated fluid.

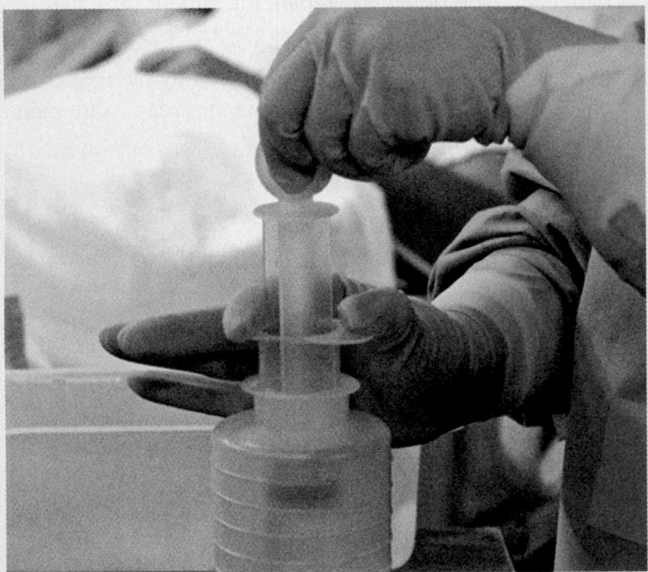

Figure 1. Drawing up sterile solution from sterile container into irrigation syringe.

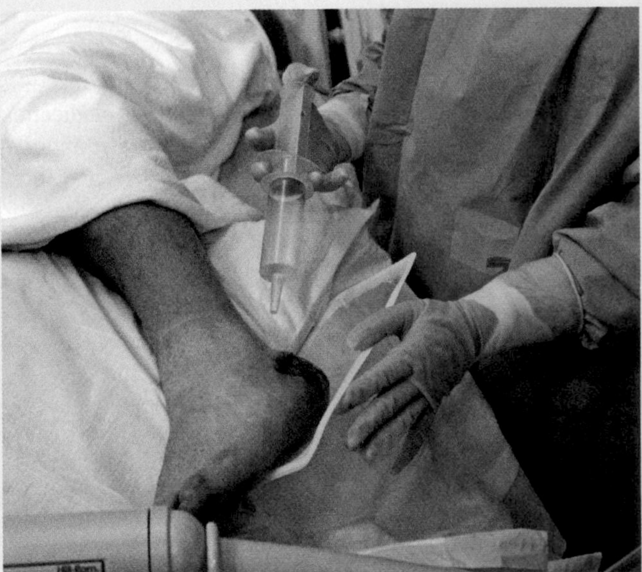

Figure 2. Patient lying on side with wound exposed, sterile collection container placed against skin, bed protected with waterproof pad.

ACTION	RATIONALE
18. **Gently direct a stream of solution into the wound (Figure 3). Keep the tip of the syringe at least 1″ above the upper tip of the wound. When using a catheter tip, insert it gently into the wound until it meets resistance. Gently flush all wound areas.**	Debris and contaminated solution flow from the least contaminated to most contaminated area. High-pressure irrigation flow may cause patient discomfort as well as damage granulation tissue. A catheter tip allows the introduction of irrigant into a wound with a small opening or one that is deep.

SKILL 8-4

Performing a Sterile Irrigation of a Wound *(continued)*

ACTION	RATIONALE
19. Watch for the solution to flow smoothly and evenly. When the solution from the wound flows out clear, discontinue irrigation.	Irrigation removes exudate and debris.
20. Dry the surrounding skin with a sterile gauze sponge. (Figure 4).	Moisture provides a medium for growth of microorganisms.

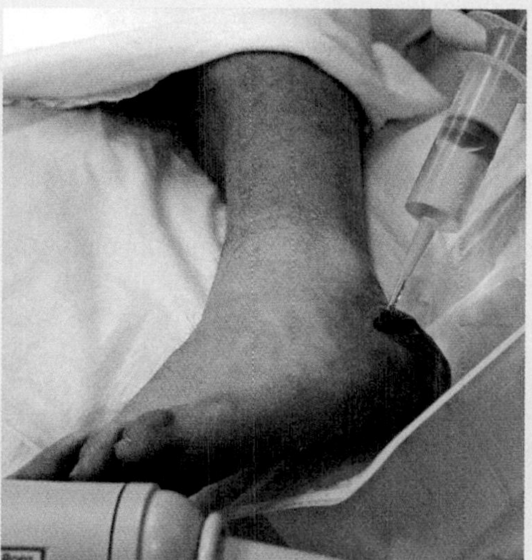

Figure 3. Irrigating wound with a gentle stream of solution. Solution drains into collection container.

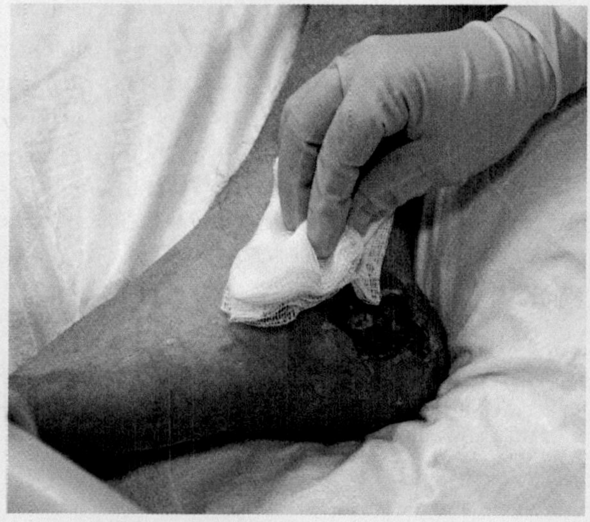

Figure 4. Drying around wound, not in wound, with sterile gauze pad.

ACTION	RATIONALE
21. Apply a new sterile dressing to the wound (see Skill 8-1) (Figure 5).	Dressings absorb drainage and protect the surrounding skin.

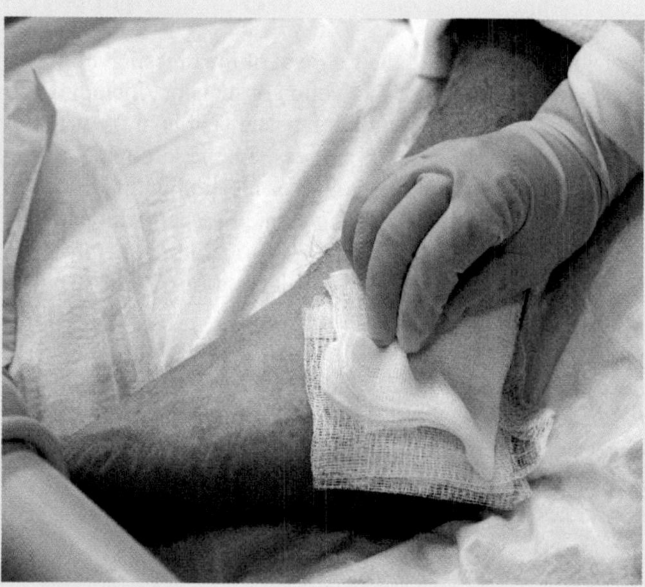

Figure 5. Applying sterile dressing to wound.

(continued)

SKILL 8-4 Performing a Sterile Irrigation of a Wound *(continued)*

ACTION	RATIONALE
22. Remove gloves and dispose of them properly. Apply a skin protectant to the surrounding skin if needed. Apply tie straps or tape as needed to secure the dressing. Remove other protective equipment and dispose in bedside waste receptacle container or bag.	Tape is easier to apply after gloves have been removed. A skin protectant prevents skin irritation and breakdown.
23. Return the bed to the lowest position while making the patient comfortable and raising the side rails as needed.	Repositioning the bed promotes patient safety.
24. Remove any remaining personal protective equipment and the waste receptacle out of the patient's room and dispose of it properly. If any irrigating solution remains in the bottle, recap the bottle and note on the bottle the date and time it was opened.	Open bottles of solution for wound care are usually good for 24 hours and can be reused. Always follow your facility's guidelines regarding solution storage and disposal.
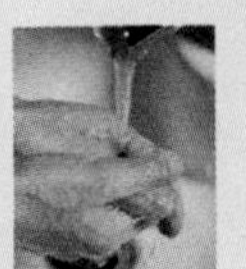 25. Perform hand hygiene.	Hand hygiene prevents spread of microorganisms.
26. Check all wound dressings every shift. You might need to check more frequently if a wound is more complex or dressings become saturated more frequently.	Frequent assessment ensures identification of changes in patient condition and timely intervention to prevent complications.

EVALUATION

The expected outcome is met when the patient exhibits a wound that is clean and dry after being irrigated; the wound is free of contamination and trauma; the patient verbalizes little to no pain or discomfort; the patient verbalizes understanding of the need for irrigation; and the wound exhibits signs and symptoms of progressive healing.

DOCUMENTATION

Guidelines

Document the location of the incision or wound and the removal of the dressing, noting any drainage on dressing. Record your assessment of the wound or incision, including the approximation of the sutures and evidence of any granulation tissue visible in the wound. Describe the condition of the surrounding skin. Note if redness, edema, drainage, or maceration is observed. Document the irrigation of the wound or incision with normal saline. Record if any skin barrier was applied to surrounding skin. Note pertinent patient and family education and any patient reaction from this procedure, including the presence of pain and effectiveness or ineffectiveness of pain-reducing interventions.

Sample Documentation

3/5/08 1700 Dressing removed from left outer heel area. Minimal serosanguineous drainage noted on dressings. Wound 4 × 5 × 2 cm, pink, with granulation tissue evident. Surrounding skin tone consistent with patient's skin, no edema or redness noted. Irrigated with normal saline, lightly packed with moist saline gauze, and redressed with gauze.—J. Lark, RN

Unexpected Situations and Associated Interventions

- *The patient experiences pain when you begin the wound irrigation:* Stop the procedure and administer an analgesic as ordered. Obtain new sterile supplies and begin the proce-

SKILL 8-4 Performing a Sterile Irrigation of a Wound *(continued)*

dure after an appropriate amount of time has elapsed to allow the analgesic to begin working. Note the patient's pain on the nursing plan of care so that pain medication can be given before future wound treatments.

- *During the wound irrigation, you note bleeding from the wound. This has not happened in the past:* Stop the procedure. Assess the patient for other symptoms. Obtain vital signs. Report your findings to the physician and document the event in the patient's record.

SKILL 8-5 Collecting a Wound Culture

If your assessment of a patient and the patient's wound suggests infection, a wound culture may be ordered to identify the causative organism. Identifying the invading microorganism will provide useful information to select the most appropriate therapy. A nurse or physician can perform a wound culture. Maintaining strict asepsis is crucial so that only the pathogen present in the wound is isolated. Also, using the correct Culturette kit for collection of an aerobic or anaerobic organism is essential.

Equipment

- A sterile Culturette kit (aerobic or anaerobic) with swab, or a culture tube with individual sterile swabs
- Sterile gloves
- Clean disposable gloves
- Plastic bag or appropriate waste receptacle
- Patient label for the sample tube
- Biohazard specimen bag
- Bath blanket (if necessary to drape the patient)
- Supplies to clean the wound and reapply a sterile dressing after obtaining the culture

ASSESSMENT

Assess the situation to determine the need for a wound culture. Confirm any physician orders relevant to obtaining a wound culture. Complete an assessment of the wound and the surrounding tissue. Inspect the wound for the approximation of wound edges, the color of the wound and surrounding area, and signs of dehiscence. Note the stage of the healing process and characteristics of any drainage. Assess the surrounding skin for color, temperature, and edema, ecchymosis, or maceration.

NURSING DIAGNOSIS

Determine the related factors for the nursing diagnoses based on the patient's current status. An appropriate nursing diagnosis would be Risk for Infection. Other appropriate diagnoses may include:

- Acute Pain
- Impaired Skin Integrity
- Impaired Tissue Integrity
- Delayed Surgical Recovery
- Disturbed Body Image
- Hyperthermia

OUTCOME IDENTIFICATION AND PLANNING

The expected outcome to achieve when collecting a wound culture is that the culture is obtained without evidence of contamination, without exposing the patient to additional pathogens, and without causing discomfort for the patient.

(continued)

SKILL 8-5

Collecting a Wound Culture

IMPLEMENTATION

ACTION	RATIONALE
1. Review the physician's order for obtaining a wound culture.	Review of the order validates the correct patient and correct procedure.
2. Gather the necessary supplies.	Preparation promotes efficient time management and provides for organized approach to task.
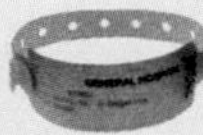 3. Identify the patient.	This ensures the right patient receives the right intervention.
4. Explain the procedure to the patient.	Discussion and explanation help allay anxiety and prepare the patient for what to expect.
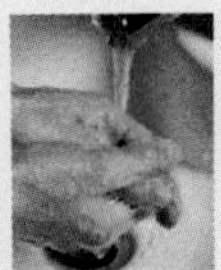 5. Perform hand hygiene.	Hand hygiene prevents the spread of microorganisms.
6. Close the room door or curtains. Place the bed at an appropriate and comfortable working height.	Closing the door or curtain promotes privacy. Proper bed positioning helps reduce back strain while you are performing the procedure.
7. Place an appropriate waste receptacle within easy reach for use during the procedure.	Having the waste container handy means that soiled materials may be discarded easily, without the spread of microorganisms.
8. Assist the patient to a comfortable position that provides easy access to the wound. If necessary, drape the patient with the bath blanket to expose only the wound area. Check the culture label again against the patient's identification bracelet (Figure 1).	Patient positioning and use of a bath blanket provide for comfort and warmth. Checking the culture label with the patient's identification ensures the correct patient and the correct procedure.

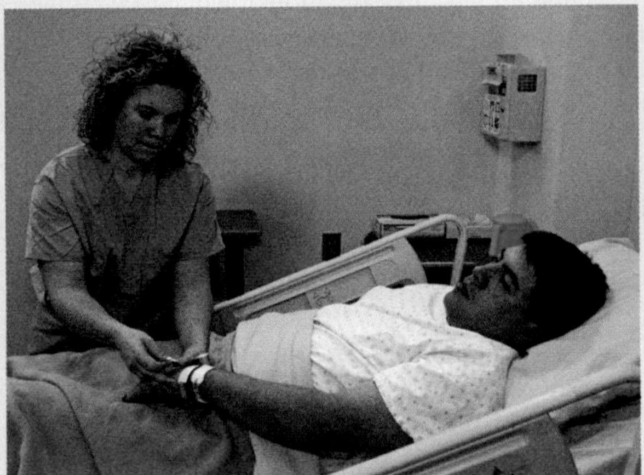

Figure 1. Checking culture label with the patient's identification band.

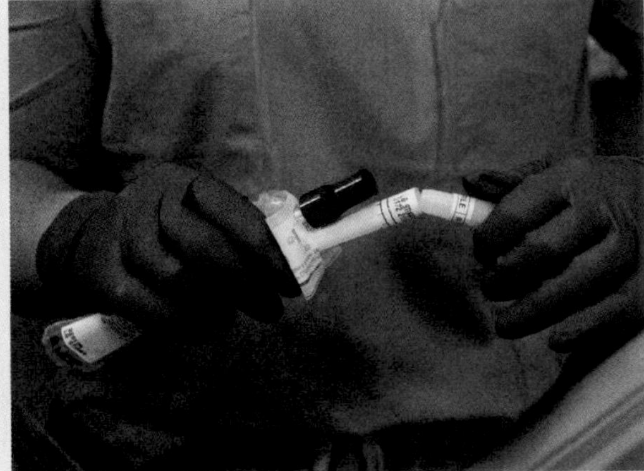

Figure 2. Twisting cap on Culturette, keeping swab in the tube.

ACTION	RATIONALE
9. Put on the clean, disposable gloves to remove any dressings. Loosen the tape and old dressings. Do not reach over the wound. Remove the dressing and dispose of it in the receptacle. Assess the wound and the characteristics of any drainage. Remove gloves and dispose of them.	Gloves protect the nurse from handling contaminated dressings. Assessment provides information about wound healing or the presence of irritation or infection that should be documented.

SKILL 8-5 Collecting a Wound Culture *(continued)*

ACTION	RATIONALE
10. Set up sterile field with supplies if necessary. Put on sterile gloves and clean the wound according to facility policies and procedures. Remove the sterile gloves.	A sterile field prevents contamination of the wound. Previous drainage and skin flora, which could contaminate the culture, are removed.
11. Put on clean gloves. Twist the cap to loosen the swab on the Culturette tube, or open the separate swab and remove the cap from the culture tube. **Keep the swab and inside of the culture tube sterile (Figure 2).**	Supplies are ready to use and within easy reach, and aseptic technique is maintained.
12. Put on a clean glove or new sterile glove, if necessary.	The use of a Culturette or swab does not require immediate contact with the skin or wound. If contact with the wound is necessary to collect the specimen, wear a sterile glove on that hand.
13. **Carefully insert the swab into the wound and gently roll the swab to obtain a sample (Figure 3). Use another swab if collecting a specimen from another site.**	Cotton tip absorbs wound drainage. Using another swab at a different site prevents cross-contamination of the wound.
14. Place the swab back in the culture tube (Figure 4). **Do not touch the outside of the tube with the swab.** Secure the cap. Some Culturette tubes have an ampule of medium at the bottom of the tube. It might be necessary to crush this ampule to activate. Follow the manufacturer's instructions for use.	The outside of the container is protected from contamination with microorganisms, and the sample is not contaminated with organisms not in the wound. Surrounding the swab with culture medium is necessary for accurate culture results.

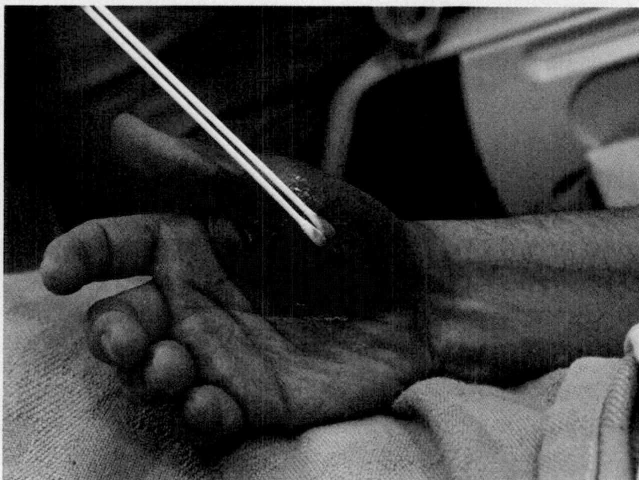

Figure 3. Swabbing the wound with cotton applicator from Culturette.

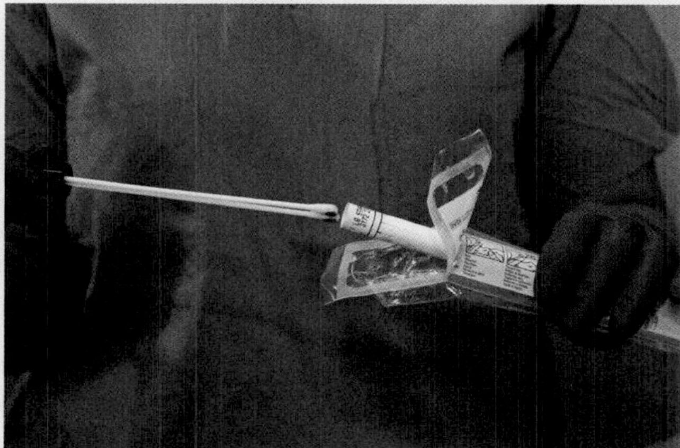

Figure 4. Placing applicator swab back in the Culturette.

ACTION	RATIONALE
15. Remove gloves and discard them accordingly.	Follow Standard Precautions for disposal of gloves.
16. Put on sterile gloves and replace the dressing as needed following the appropriate procedure.	Gloving maintains aseptic technique. Dressings provide for drainage absorption and protect the wound.
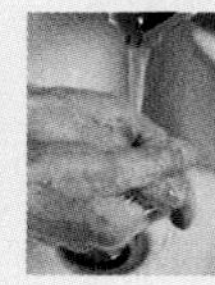 17. Remove gloves and perform hand hygiene. Remove any equipment and leave the patient comfortable, with the side rails up and the bed in the lowest position.	Removing gloves and performing hand hygiene prevent the spread of microorganisms. Proper bed positioning promotes patient safety.

(continued)

SKILL 8-5

Collecting a Wound Culture *(continued)*

ACTION	RATIONALE
18. Label the specimen according to your institution's guidelines and send it to the laboratory in a biohazard bag (Figure 5).	Proper labeling ensures proper identification of the specimen.

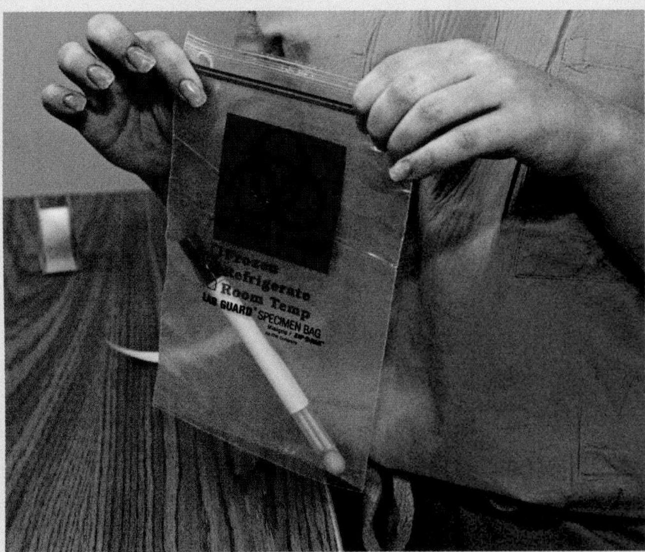

Figure 5. Culturette/specimen container in biohazard bag.

EVALUATION

The expected outcome is met when the patient's wound is cultured without evidence of contamination, and the patient remains free of exposure to additional pathogens.

DOCUMENTATION

Guidelines

Document the location of the incision or wound, including length, width, and depth. Record your assessment of the wound or incision, including the approximation of the sutures and the condition of the surrounding skin. Note if redness, edema, drainage, or maceration is observed. Document cleansing of the wound or incision with normal saline and the obtaining of the culture. Record if any skin barriers were applied to surrounding skin. Note pertinent patient and family education and any patient reaction from this procedure, including the presence of tenderness of the wound or incision site.

Sample Documentation

6/22/08 2100 Wound noted on patient's left ankle; 2 cm × 3 cm × 1 cm, red, tender, with purulent drainage present. Edges macerated, without erythema and tenderness. Wound cleaned with normal saline, culture obtained. Skin barrier applied to surrounding area, wound packed with moist saline gauze, dressed with dry gauze and Kling. Left-lower extremity elevated. Culture labeled and sent to lab.—J. Wentz, RN

Unexpected Situations and Associated Interventions

- *You have the culture swab in the patient's wound to obtain the specimen. You realize that you did not clean the wound first:* Discard this swab. Obtain the additional supplies needed to clean the wound according to facility policy and a new culture swab. Clean the wound, then proceed to obtain the culture specimen.
- *As you prepare to insert the culture swab into the wound, you inadvertently touch the swab to the patient's bedclothes:* Discard this swab, obtain a new culture swab, and collect the specimen.

SKILL 8-6 Applying Montgomery Straps

Montgomery straps are recommended to secure dressings on wounds that require frequent dressing changes, such as wounds with increased drainage. These straps allow the nurse to perform wound care without the need to remove adhesive strips, such as tape, with each dressing change, thus decreasing the risk of skin irritation and injury.

Montgomery straps are prepared strips of nonallergenic tape with ties inserted through holes at one end. One set of straps is placed on either side of a wound, and the straps are tied like shoelaces to secure the dressings. When it is time to change the dressing, the straps are untied, the wound is cared for, and then the straps are retied to hold the new dressing. Often a skin barrier is applied before the straps to protect the skin. The straps or ties need to be changed only if they become loose or soiled.

Equipment

- Clean disposable gloves
- Dressings for wound care as ordered
- Commercially available Montgomery straps or 2″ to 3″ hypoallergenic tape and strings for ties
- Cleansing solution, usually normal saline
- Gauze pads
- Skin-protectant wipe
- Skin-barrier sheet (hydrocolloidal or nonhydrocolloidal)

ASSESSMENT

Assess the wound for amount of drainage and the frequency of dressing changes. Assess the integrity of any straps currently in use. Loose or soiled straps or ties should be replaced. Assess the wound and surrounding skin.

NURSING DIAGNOSIS

Determine the related factors for the nursing diagnoses based on the patient's current status. An appropriate nursing diagnosis is Risk for Impaired Skin Integrity. Other nursing diagnoses that may be appropriate include:

- Impaired Tissue Integrity
- Risk for Infection
- Risk for Injury
- Anxiety
- Acute Pain
- Disturbed Body Image
- Deficient Knowledge
- Impaired Skin Integrity
- Delayed Surgical Recovery

OUTCOME IDENTIFICATION AND PLANNING

The expected outcome to achieve when applying Montgomery straps is that the patient's skin is free from irritation and injury. Other outcomes that may be appropriate include that the care is accomplished without contaminating the wound area, without causing trauma to the wound, and without causing the patient to experience pain or discomfort, and the wound continues to show signs of progression of healing.

IMPLEMENTATION

ACTION	RATIONALE
1. Review the physician's order for wound care or the nursing plan of care related to wound care.	Reviewing the order validates the correct patient and correct procedure.
2. Gather the necessary supplies.	Preparation promotes efficient time management and an organized approach to the task.

(continued)

SKILL 8-6 Applying Montgomery Straps *(continued)*

ACTION	RATIONALE
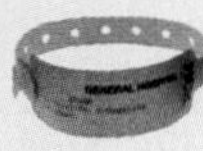 3. Identify the patient.	This ensures the right patient received the right intervention.
4. Explain the procedure to the patient.	Discussion and explanation help allay anxiety, encourage patient cooperation, and prepare the patient for what to expect.
5. Assess the patient for possible need for nonpharmacologic pain-reducing interventions or analgesic medication before wound care dressing change. Administer appropriate analgesic, consulting physician's orders, and allow enough time for analgesic to achieve its effectiveness before beginning procedure.	Pain is a subjective experience influenced by past experience. Wound care and dressing changes may cause pain for some patients.
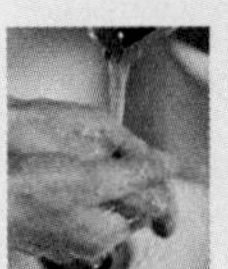 6. Perform hand hygiene.	Hand hygiene prevents the spread of microorganisms.
7. Close the room door or curtains. Place the bed at an appropriate and comfortable working height.	Closing the door or curtains provides privacy. Proper bed positioning helps reduce back strain while you are performing the procedure.
8. Place a waste receptacle at a convenient location for use during the procedure.	Having a waste container handy means that the soiled dressing may be discarded easily, without the spread of microorganisms.
9. Assist the patient to a comfortable position that provides easy access to the wound area. Use a bath blanket to cover any exposed area other than the wound. If necessary, place a waterproof pad under the wound site.	Patient positioning and use of a bath blanket provide for comfort and warmth. Waterproof pad protects underlying surfaces.
10. Perform wound care and a dressing change as outlined in Skill 8-1, as ordered.	Wound care aids in healing and provides protection for the wound.
11. If ready-made straps are not available, cut four to six strips of tape long enough to extend about 6″ beyond the wound. The number of strips will depend on the size of the wound and dressing.	Proper sizing is necessary to allow enough tape to secure to the patient's skin and hold the dressing in place.
12. Fold one end of each strip 2″ to 3″ back on itself, sticky sides together, to form a nonadhesive tab. Cut a small hole in the folded tab's center, close to the top edge. Make as many pairs of straps as necessary to secure the dressing.	Straps should be long enough to allow removal and replacement of the dressing multiple times.
13. Put on clean gloves. Clean the skin on either side of the wound with the gauze, moistened with normal saline. Dry the skin.	Gloves prevent the spread of microorganisms. Cleaning and drying the skin prevents irritation and injury.
14. **Apply a skin protectant to the skin where the straps will be placed.**	Skin protectant minimizes the risk for skin breakdown and irritation.
15. Remove gloves.	Tape is easier to handle without gloves. Wound is covered with the dressing.
16. Apply the sticky side of each tape or strap to a skin barrier sheet (Figure 1). Apply the sheet directly to the skin near the dressing. Repeat for the other side.	Skin barrier prevents skin irritation and breakdown.

SKILL
8-6

Applying Montgomery Straps *(continued)*

ACTION | **RATIONALE**

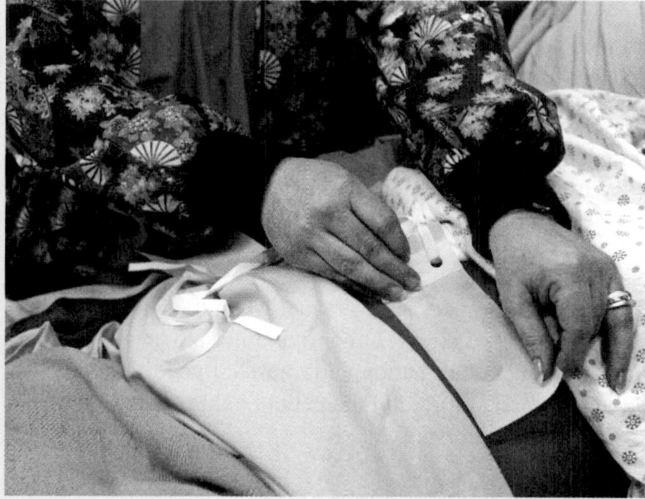

Figure 1. Applying Montgomery straps and skin barrier sheet to the patient's abdomen.

17. Thread a separate string through each pair of holes in the straps. Tie one end of the string in the hole. Fasten the other end with the opposing tie, like a shoelace (Figure 2). **Do not secure too tightly.** Repeat according to the number of straps needed. If commercially prepared straps are used, tie strings like a shoelace. Note date and time of application on strap (Figure 3).

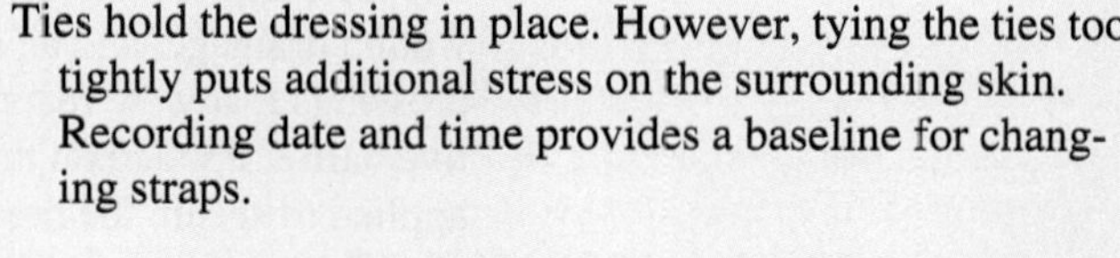

Ties hold the dressing in place. However, tying the ties too tightly puts additional stress on the surrounding skin. Recording date and time provides a baseline for changing straps.

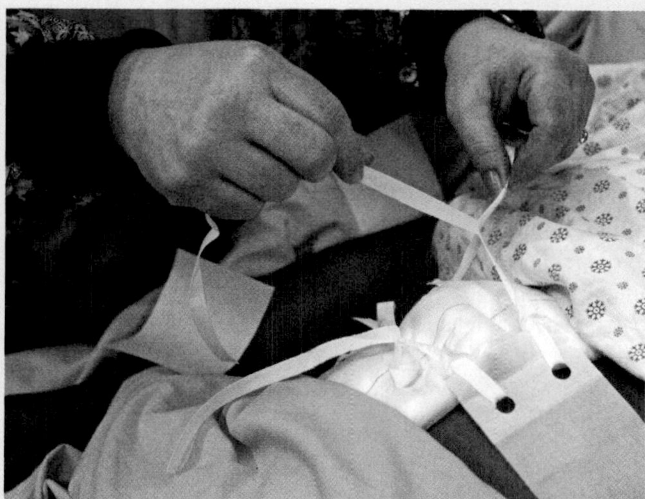

Figure 2. Tying Montgomery straps.

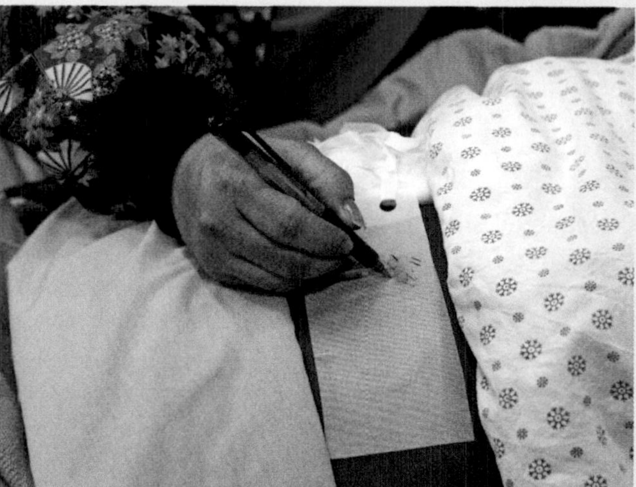

Figure 3. Labeling Montgomery straps.

18. Return the bed to the lowest position while making the patient comfortable and raising the side rails as needed.

Repositioning the bed and patient promotes safety.

(continued)

SKILL 8-6 Applying Montgomery Straps *(continued)*

ACTION	RATIONALE
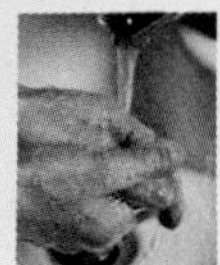 19. Perform hand hygiene.	Hand hygiene prevents spread of microorganisms.
20. Replace the ties and straps whenever they are soiled, or every 2 to 3 days.	Replacing soiled ties and straps prevents growth of pathogens.

EVALUATION

The expected outcome when applying Montgomery straps is met when the patient's skin is clean, dry, intact, and free from irritation and injury. Other outcomes are met when the patient exhibits a clean wound area free of contamination and trauma. In addition, the patient verbalizes minimal to no pain or discomfort, and the patient exhibits signs and symptoms indicative of progressive wound healing.

DOCUMENTATION

Guidelines

Document the procedure, the patient's response, and your assessment of the area before and after application. Record a description of the wound, amount and character of the wound drainage, and an assessment of the surrounding skin. Note the amount and type of dressings that were reapplied and the frequency, as well as if there was any skin protective barrier applied on the surrounding skin. Document that Montgomery straps were applied to secure the dressings.

Record the patient's response to the dressing care and associated pain assessment. Include any pertinent patient and family education.

Sample Documentation

10/20/08 1930 Patient's abdominal wound has large amounts of serosanguineous drainage, saturating multiple layers of gauze and ABDs, requiring dressing changes at least q 3 hours. Surrounding skin cleansed, skin protectant applied, and Montgomery straps applied to secure wound dressings.—D. Rightner, RN

Unexpected Situation and Associated Intervention

- *Your patient has had an abdominal wound for several weeks. Despite careful wound and skin care, you observe signs of redness and irritation where the tape for the dressings has been repeatedly placed:* Obtain the supplies listed in this skill. Apply Montgomery straps, being sure to move the skin barrier sheet at least 1″ away from the area of irritation.

SKILL 8-7 Caring for a Penrose Drain

Drains are inserted into or near a wound when it is anticipated that a collection of fluid in a closed area would delay healing. A Penrose drain is a hollow, open-ended rubber tube. It allows fluid to drain via capillary action into absorbent dressings. Penrose drains are commonly used after a surgical procedure or for drainage of an abscess. After a surgical

SKILL 8-7

Caring for a Penrose Drain *(continued)*

procedure, the surgeon places one end of the drain in or near the area to be drained. The other end passes through the skin, directly through the incision or through a separate opening referred to as a stab wound. A Penrose drain is not sutured. A large safety pin is usually placed in the part outside the wound to prevent the drain from slipping back into the incised area. This type of drain can be advanced or shortened to drain different areas. The patency and placement of the drain are included in the wound assessment.

Equipment

- Sterile cleansing solution and sterile container
- Sterile gloves
- Gauze dressings
- Sterile cotton-tipped applicators, if appropriate
- Sterile drain sponges
- Surgi-pads or ABD pads
- Sterile dressing set or suture set (for the sterile scissors and forceps)
- Sterile cleaning solution as ordered (commonly 0.9% normal saline solution)
- Clean disposable gloves
- Sterile basin (optional)
- Sterile drape (optional)
- Plastic bag or other appropriate waste container for soiled dressings
- Waterproof pad and bath blanket
- Tape or ties
- Skin-protectant wipes if needed
- Additional dressings and supplies needed or as required by the physician's order

ASSESSMENT

Assess the situation to determine the necessity for wound cleaning and a dressing change. Confirm any physician orders relevant to drain care and any drain care included in the nursing plan of care. Assess the current dressing to determine if it is intact, and assess for the presence of excess drainage, bleeding, or saturation of the dressing. Assess the patency of the Penrose drain.

Inspect the wound and the surrounding tissue. Assess the appearance of the wound for the approximation of wound edges, the color of the wound and surrounding area, and signs of dehiscence. Note the stage of the healing process and the characteristics of any drainage. Assess the surrounding skin for color, temperature, and the presence of edema, ecchymosis, or maceration.

NURSING DIAGNOSIS

Determine the related factors for the nursing diagnosis based on the patient's current status. An appropriate nursing diagnosis is Risk for Infection. Other nursing diagnoses may also be appropriate, including:

- Anxiety
- Disturbed Body Image
- Acute Pain
- Deficient Knowledge
- Impaired Skin Integrity
- Delayed Surgical Recovery
- Impaired Tissue Integrity

OUTCOME IDENTIFICATION AND PLANNING

The expected outcome to achieve when performing care for a Penrose drain is that the Penrose drain remains patent and intact. Care is accomplished without contaminating the wound area, without causing trauma to the wound, and without causing the patient to experience pain or discomfort. Other outcomes that are appropriate may include: the wound shows signs of progressive healing without evidence of complications, and the patient demonstrates understanding about the need for drain care.

(continued)

SKILL 8-7

Caring for a Penrose Drain *(continued)*

IMPLEMENTATION

ACTION	RATIONALE
1. Review the physician's order for drain and site care or the nursing plan of care related to drain care.	Review of the order or plan of care validates the correct patient and correct procedure.
2. Gather the necessary supplies.	Preparation promotes efficient time management and organized approach to the task.
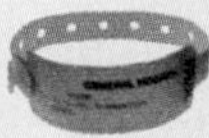 3. Identify the patient.	This ensures the right patient receives the right intervention.
4. Explain the procedure to the patient.	Discussion and explanation help allay anxiety, encourage patient cooperation, and prepare the patient for what to expect.
5. Assess the patient for possible need for nonpharmacologic pain-reducing interventions or analgesic medication before wound care dressing change. Administer appropriate analgesic, consulting physician's orders, and allow enough time for analgesic to achieve its effectiveness.	Pain is a subjective experience influenced by past experience. Wound care and dressing changes may cause pain for some patients.
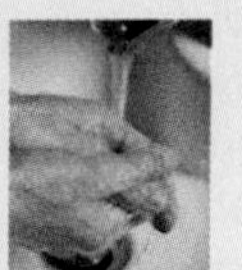 6. Perform hand hygiene.	Hand hygiene prevents the spread of microorganisms.
7. Close the room door or curtains. Place the bed at an appropriate and comfortable working height.	Closing the door or curtain provides privacy. Placing the bed at an appropriate height helps reduce back strain when providing drain care.
8. Place a waste receptacle at a convenient location for use during the procedure.	Soiled dressing may be discarded easily, without the spread of microorganisms.
9. Assist the patient to a comfortable position that provides easy access to the drain area. Use the bath blanket to cover any exposed area other than the drain. If necessary, place the waterproof pad under the drain site.	Proper patient positioning and use of bath blankets provide for comfort and warmth. Waterproof pad protects underlying surfaces.
10. Check the position of the drain or drains before removing the dressing. Put on clean, disposable gloves and loosen tape on the old dressings. Use an adhesive remover to help get the tape off, if necessary.	Checking the position ensures that a drain is not removed accidentally if one is present. Use of gloves protects the nurse from contaminated dressings and prevents the spread of microorganisms. Using adhesive remover helps to reduce patient discomfort during removal of dressing.
11. **Carefully remove the soiled dressings.** If any part of the dressing sticks to the underlying skin, use small amounts of sterile saline to help loosen and remove it. Do not reach over the drain site.	Cautious removal of the dressing is more comfortable for the patient and ensures that any drain present is not inadvertently removed. Sterile saline provides for easier removal of the dressing and prevents tissue damage.
12. After removing the dressing, note the presence, amount, type, color, and odor of any drainage on the dressings. Place soiled dressings in the appropriate waste receptacle. Remove gloves and dispose of them in the appropriate waste receptacle.	The presence of drainage should be documented. Proper use and disposal of gloves prevent the spread of microorganisms.

SKILL 8-7

Caring for a Penrose Drain *(continued)*

ACTION	RATIONALE
13. Inspect the drain site for appearance and drainage. Assess if any pain is present. **Closely observe the safety pin in the drain** (Figure 1). Include any problems noted in documentation.	The wound healing process and/or the presence of irritation or infection must be documented.
14. If the pin or drain is crusted, replace the pin with a new sterile pin. Take care not to dislodge the drain.	Microorganisms grow more easily in a soiled environment. The safety pin ensures proper placement because the drain is not sutured in place.
15. Using sterile technique, prepare a sterile work area and open the needed supplies.	Supplies are within easy reach and sterility is maintained.
16. Open the sterile cleaning solution. Pour the cleansing solution into the basin. Add the gauze sponges.	Sterility of dressings and solution is maintained.
17. Put on sterile gloves.	Sterile gloves help to maintain surgical asepsis and sterile technique and prevent the spread of microorganisms.
18. Cleanse the drain site with the cleaning solution. Use the forceps and the moistened gauze or cotton-tipped applicators. **Start at the drain insertion site, moving in a circular motion toward the periphery (Figure 2). Use each gauze sponge or applicator only once. Discard and use new gauze if additional cleansing is needed.**	Using a circular motion ensures that cleaning occurs from the least to most contaminated area and a previously cleaned area is not contaminated again.

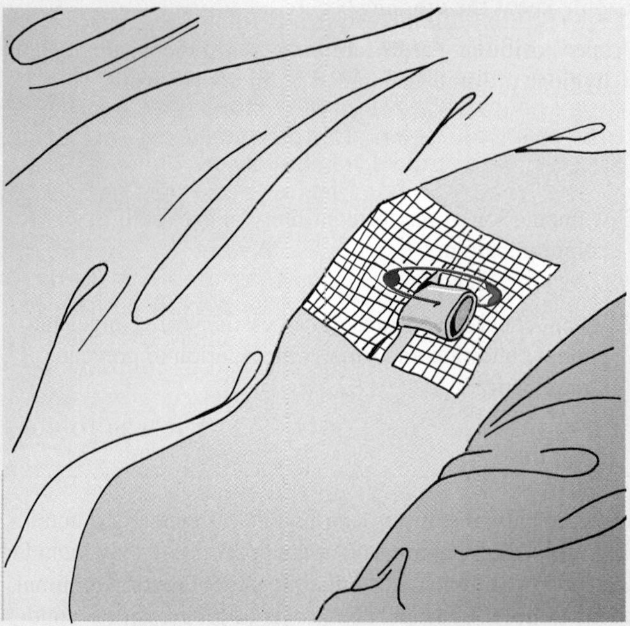

Figure 1. Penrose drain in place.

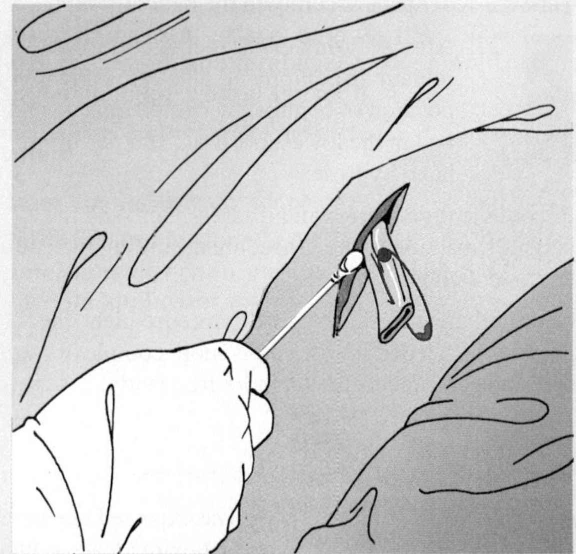

Figure 2. Using gloved hands to clean around a Penrose drain with saline-soaked gauze sponge.

ACTION	RATIONALE
19. Dry the skin with a new gauze pad. Place the presplit drain sponge under the drain. Place several gauze pads around the drain site. Apply gauze pads over the drain (Figure 3).	Drying prevents skin irritation. The gauze absorbs drainage and prevents the drainage from accumulating on the patient's skin.
20. Apply ABD pads over the gauze. Remove gloves and dispose of them.	Pads provide extra absorption for excess drainage and provide a moisture barrier. It is easier to handle the tape without gloves.

(continued)

SKILL 8-7 Caring for a Penrose Drain *(continued)*

ACTION	RATIONALE
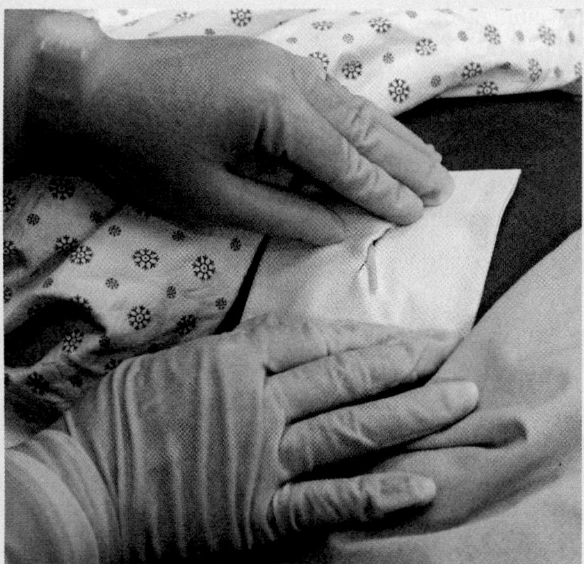 Figure 3. Placing the presplit drainage sponge around Penrose drain with gloved hands.	
21. Tape the ABD pads securely to the patient's skin.	Taping keeps the dressing secure.
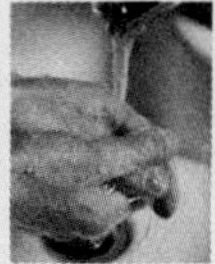 22. After securing the dressing, remove all remaining equipment, place the patient in a position of comfort, with side rails up and bed in the lowest position, and perform hand hygiene.	Proper positioning after care maintains patient safety. Hand hygiene prevents the spread of microorganisms.
23. Record the procedure, wound assessment, and the patient's reaction to the procedure according to institution's guidelines.	Documentation promotes continuity of care and communication.
24. Check all dressings every shift. More frequent checking may be needed if a wound is more complex or dressings become saturated more frequently.	Frequent checking ensures the assessment of changes in patient condition and timely intervention to prevent complications.

EVALUATION

The expected outcome is met when the patient exhibits a wound that is clean, dry, and intact, with a patent, intact Penrose drain. Other outcomes that are appropriate may include: the patient remains free of wound contamination and trauma; the patient reports minimal to no pain or discomfort; the patient exhibits signs and symptoms of progressive wound healing; and the patient states the reason for drain care.

DOCUMENTATION

Guidelines

Document whether the patient received any pain/analgesic medication before the dressing care procedure, recording type, dosage, and route. Comment on the presence of drainage on the old dressing upon removal. Document the appearance of the wound or incision, including the presence of erythema, edema, approximation of sutures or staples, and intactness of Penrose drain. Describe the care provided to the area, including any solution

SKILL 8-7 Caring for a Penrose Drain *(continued)*

used in cleaning the area, such as normal saline, and the dressings that were used for this care. Document the patient's reaction to the care, the effectiveness of the pain medication, and any patient-teaching information that was provided.

Sample Documentation

3/13/08 1400 Patient medicated with morphine 3 mg IV as ordered prior to dressing change. Dressing to right forearm removed. Dressings noted with small amount of serosanguineous drainage. Forearm with gross edema and erythema. Penrose drain intact. Incision edges approximated, staples intact. Area irrigated with normal saline, dried, and redressed with gauze, ABD pads, and stretch gauze. Reinforced the importance of keeping arm elevated on pillows, with patient verbalizing understanding.—P. Towns, RN

Unexpected Situations and Associated Interventions

- *Assessment of the drain site reveals significantly increased edema, erythema, and drainage from the site, in addition to drainage via the drain:* Cleanse the site as ordered or per the nursing plan of care. Obtain vital signs, including the patient's temperature. Document care and assessments. Notify the physician of your findings.
- *Assessment of the drain site reveals that the drain has slipped back into the incision:* Follow facility policy and the physician's orders related to advancing Penrose drains. Document assessments and interventions. Notify the physician of your findings and interventions.
- *When preparing to change a dressing on a Penrose drain site, you remove the old dressing and note that the drain is completely out, lying in the dressing when you remove it:* Assess the site and the patient for other symptoms. Provide site care as ordered. Notify the physician. Often, depending on the patient's stage of recovery, the drain is left out. Document your findings and interventions.

Special Considerations

General Considerations

- A sudden increase in the amount of drainage or bright red drainage should be evaluated and the physician notified of these findings.
- Wound care is often uncomfortable, and patients may experience significant pain. Assess the patient's comfort level and past experiences with wound care. Offer analgesics as ordered to maintain the patient's level of comfort.

SKILL 8-8 Caring for a T-Tube Drain

A biliary drain or T-tube (Figure 1) is sometimes placed in the common bile duct after removal of the gallbladder (cholecystectomy) or a portion of the bile duct (choledochostomy). The tube drains bile while the surgical site is healing. A portion of the tube is inserted into the common bile duct and the remaining portion is anchored to the abdominal wall, passed through the skin, and connected to a closed drainage system. Often, a three-way valve is inserted between the drain tube and the drainage system to allow for clamping and flushing of the tube if necessary. The drainage amount is measured every shift, recorded, and included in output totals.

(continued)

SKILL 8-8 Caring for a T-Tube Drain *(continued)*

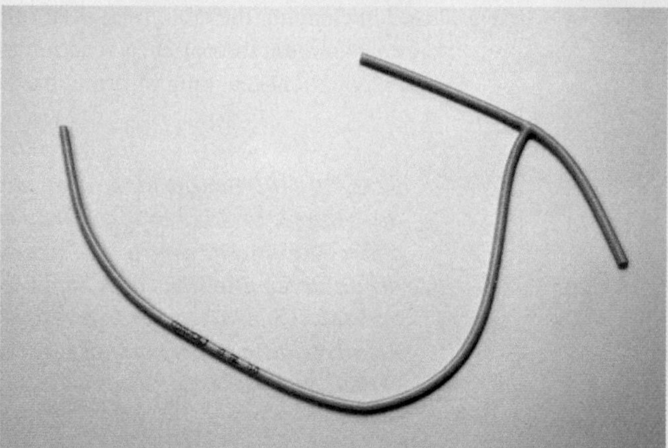

Figure 1. T-tube.

Equipment

- Sterile gloves
- Clean disposable gloves
- Sterile gauze pads
- Sterile drain sponges
- Cleansing solution, usually sterile normal saline
- Sterile cotton-tipped applicators (if appropriate)
- Transparent dressing
- Graduated collection container
- Waste receptacle
- Sterile basin
- Sterile forceps
- Tape
- Skin-protectant wipes
- Waterproof pad and bath blanket, if needed

ASSESSMENT

Assess the situation to determine the need for wound cleaning, a dressing change, or emptying of the drain. Confirm any physician orders relevant to drain care and any drain care included in the nursing plan of care. Assess the current dressing to determine if it is intact, and assess for evidence of excessive drainage or bleeding or saturation of the dressing. Assess the patency of the T-tube and the drain site.

Inspect the wound and the surrounding tissue. Assess the appearance of the incision for the approximation of wound edges, the color of the wound and surrounding area, and signs of dehiscence. Note the stage of the healing process and characteristics of any drainage. Assess the surrounding skin for color, temperature, and edema, ecchymosis, or maceration.

NURSING DIAGNOSIS

Determine the related factors for the nursing diagnoses based on the patient's current status. An appropriate nursing diagnosis is Risk for Infection. Other nursing diagnoses may also be appropriate, including:

- Acute Pain
- Anxiety
- Disturbed Body Image
- Deficient Knowledge
- Impaired Skin Integrity
- Delayed Surgical Recovery
- Impaired Tissue Integrity

OUTCOME IDENTIFICATION AND PLANNING

The expected outcome to achieve when performing care for a T-tube drain is that the drain remains patent and intact. Care is accomplished without contaminating the wound area, without causing trauma to the wound, and without causing the patient to experience pain or

SKILL 8-8 Caring for a T-Tube Drain *(continued)*

discomfort. Other outcomes that are appropriate may include: the wound continues to show signs of progression of healing, and the drainage amounts are measured accurately at the frequency required by facility policy and recorded as part of the intake and output record.

IMPLEMENTATION

ACTION	RATIONALE
1. Review the physician's order for drain and site care or the nursing plan of care related to drain care.	Review validates the correct patient and correct procedure.
2. Gather the necessary supplies.	Preparation promotes efficient time management and organized approach to the task.
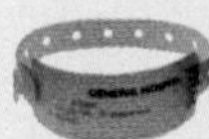 3. Identify the patient.	This ensures the right patient receives the right intervention.
4. Explain the procedure to the patient.	Discussion and explanation help allay anxiety, encourage patient cooperation, and prepare the patient for what to expect.
5. Assess the patient for possible need for nonpharmacologic pain-reducing interventions or analgesic medication before wound care dressing change. Administer appropriate analgesic, consulting physician's orders, and allow enough time for analgesic to achieve its effectiveness.	Pain is a subjective experience influenced by past experience. Wound care and dressing changes may cause pain for some patients.
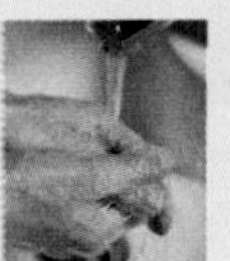 6. Perform hand hygiene.	Hand hygiene prevents the spread of microorganisms.
7. Close the room door or curtains. Place the bed at an appropriate and comfortable working height.	Closing the door or curtain provides privacy. Proper bed positioning helps reduce back strain when providing care.
8. Place a waste receptacle at a convenient location for use during the procedure.	Having a waste receptacle handy means that the soiled dressing may be discarded easily, without the spread of microorganisms.
9. Assist the patient to a comfortable position that provides easy access to the drain area. Use the bath blanket to cover any exposed area other than the drain. Place the waterproof pad under the drain site.	Patient positioning and use of a bath blanket provide for comfort and warmth. Waterproof pad protects underlying surfaces.
Emptying Drainage	
10. Put on clean gloves.	Gloves help prevent the spread of microorganisms.
11. Using sterile technique, open a gauze pad, making a sterile field with the outer wrapper.	Using sterile technique deters the spread of microorganisms.
12. Place the graduated collection container under the outlet valve of the drainage bag **Without contaminating the outlet valve, pull the cap off and empty the bag's contents completely into the container (Figure 2); use the gauze to wipe the valve, and reseal the outlet valve (Figure 3).**	Draining contents into container allows for accurate measurement of the drainage. Wiping the valve with gauze prevents contamination of the valve. Wiping the valve and resealing it prevents the spread of microorganisms.

(continued)

SKILL 8-8 **Caring for a T-Tube Drain** *(continued)*

ACTION	RATIONALE
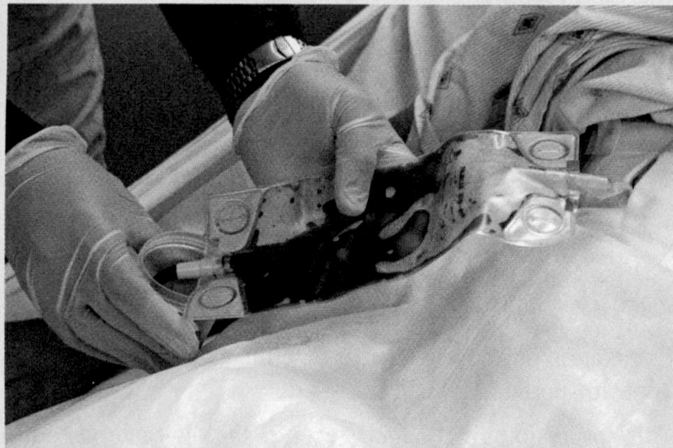 **Figure 2.** Holding the collection container at the outlet valve.	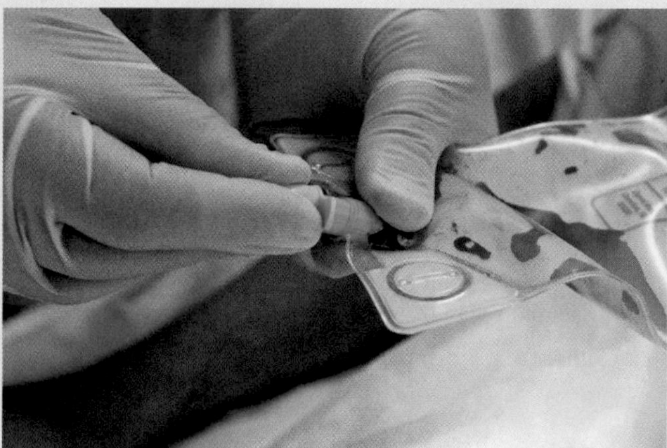 **Figure 3.** Resealing the outlet valve.
13. Carefully measure and record the character, color, and amount of the drainage. Discard the drainage according to facility policy.	Documentation promotes continuity of care and communication. Appropriate disposal of biohazard material reduces the risk for microorganism transmission.
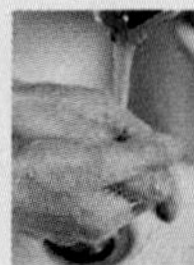 14. Remove gloves and perform hand hygiene.	Proper glove removal and performing hand hygiene prevent spread of microorganisms.
Cleaning the Drain Site	
15. Put on clean gloves. Check the position of the drain or drains before removing the dressing. Loosen the tape on the old dressings. If necessary, use an adhesive remover to help get the tape off.	Checking position ensures that a drain is not removed accidentally. Gloves protect the nurse from contaminated dressings and prevent the spread of microorganisms. Adhesive-tape remover helps to reduce patient discomfort during dressing removal.
16. Carefully remove the soiled dressings. If any part of the dressing sticks to the underlying skin, use small amounts of sterile saline to help loosen and remove. Do not reach over the drain site.	Cautious removal of the dressing is more comfortable for the patient and ensures that any drain present is not removed. Sterile saline provides for easier removal of the dressing and prevents tissue damage. Not reaching over the drain site reduces the risk for contamination.
17. After removing the dressing, note the presence, amount, type, color, and odor of any drainage on the dressings. Place soiled dressings in the appropriate waste receptacle. Remove gloves and dispose of in appropriate waste receptacle.	The presence of drainage should be documented. Proper disposal of gloves prevents spread of microorganisms.
18. Inspect the drain site for appearance and drainage. Assess if any pain is present. Note any problems to include in your documentation.	Wound healing process and/or the presence of irritation or infection should be documented.
19. Using sterile technique, prepare a sterile work area and open the needed supplies.	Preparing a sterile work area ensures that supplies are within easy reach and sterility is maintained.
20. Open the sterile cleaning solution. Pour the cleansing solution into the basin. Add the gauze sponges.	Sterility of dressings and solution is maintained.
21. Put on sterile gloves.	Use of sterile gloves maintains surgical asepsis and sterile technique and reduces the risk of microorganism transmission.

SKILL 8-8

Caring for a T-Tube Drain *(continued)*

ACTION	RATIONALE
22. Cleanse the drain site with the cleaning solution. Use the forceps and the moistened gauze or cotton-tipped applicators. **Start at the drain insertion site, moving in a circular motion toward the periphery. Use each gauze sponge only once. Discard and use new gauze if additional cleansing is needed.**	Cleaning is done from the least to most contaminated area so that a previously cleaned area is not contaminated again.
23. Allow the area to dry or dry with a new sterile gauze.	Drying deters the growth of microorganisms, which occurs in moist environments.
24. Place the drain sponge under the drain. Place several gauze pads around the drain site. Apply gauze pads over the drain. Alternatively, place the transparent dressing over the tube and dressings.	Dressings absorbs any drainage from the site.
25. Secure the dressings with tape as needed. **Be careful not to kink the tubing.**	Kinked tubing could block drainage.
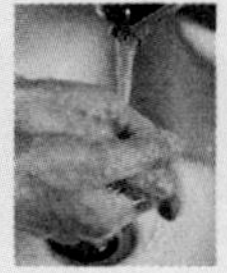 26. After securing the dressing, remove all remaining equipment. Apply skin protectant to the surrounding skin if needed. Place the patient in a position of comfort, with side rails up and bed in the lowest position, and perform hand hygiene.	Proper patient positioning promotes safety. Skin protectant prevents skin breakdown and irritation. Hand hygiene prevents spread of microorganisms.
27. Check all dressings every shift. More frequent checking may be needed if a wound is more complex or dressings become saturated quickly.	Follow-up assessment ensures identification of changes in patient condition and timely intervention to prevent complications.

EVALUATION

The expected outcome is met when the patient exhibits a patent and intact T-tube drain with a wound area that is free of contamination and trauma. The patient verbalizes minimal to no pain or discomfort. Other outcomes that are appropriate may include: the patient exhibits signs and symptoms of progressive wound healing, with drainage being measured accurately at the frequency required by facility policy, and amounts recorded as part of the intake and output record; and the patient states the reason for T-tube care.

DOCUMENTATION

Guidelines

Document the appearance of the T-tube dressing that was removed, noting color, odor, and amount of drainage if present. Include documentation of the condition of the drain site, noting if any redness, edema, drainage, or ecchymosis. Document the care that was provided to the drain site, such as cleaned with normal saline, and the redressing of the site. Note if sutures are intact. Document the amount of bile drainage obtained from the drainage bag on the appropriate intake and output record. Include in the documentation note whether patient was medicated for pain before the procedure, identifying the medication, dosage, and route of the medication. Document the patient's reaction to the procedure and note whether the patient experienced any pain. Include patient and family education concerning this procedure.

Sample Documentation

8/9/09 1500 Dressing removed from T-tube site. No drainage noted on dressings. Drain site without redness, edema, drainage, or ecchymosis. Suture intact. Exit site cleaned with normal saline, dried, and redressed with dry dressing. Patient denies pain. Emptied collection bag of 20 cc bile-colored drainage.—L. Saunders, RN

(continued)

SKILL 8-8 Caring for a T-Tube Drain *(continued)*

Unexpected Situations and Associated Interventions

- *A patient's T-tube has been consistently draining 30 to 50 mL a shift, but now there is no output for the current shift. You check the tubing and site and do not observe kinks or other exterior obstructions:* Assess for signs of obstructed bile flow, including chills, fever, tachycardia, nausea, right upper quadrant fullness and pain, jaundice, dark foamy urine, and clay-colored stools. Obtain vital signs. Notify the physician of the situation and your findings and document the event in the patient's record. Flushing of the tube with sterile saline may be ordered as part of the patient's care.
- *Patient had a T-tube placed after surgery. The surgeon has asked that the tube be clamped for 1 hour before and after meals:* This diverts bile into the duodenum to aid in digestion and is accomplished by occluding the tube with a clamp or rubber band. Monitor the patient's response to clamping the tube. If the patient reports new symptoms, such as right upper quadrant pain, nausea, or vomiting, unclamp the tube. Assess for other symptoms and obtain vital signs. Report your findings to the surgeon and document the event in the patient's record.

SKILL 8-9 Caring for a Jackson-Pratt Drain

A Jackson-Pratt (J-P) or grenade drain collects wound drainage in a bulblike device that is compressed to create gentle suction (Figure 1). It consists of perforated tubing connected to a portable vacuum unit. After a surgical procedure, the surgeon places one end of the drain in or near the area to be drained. The other end passes through the skin via a separate incision. These drains are usually sutured in place. The site may be treated as an additional surgical wound, but often these sites are left open to air after the first 24 hours after surgery. They are typically used with breast and abdominal surgery.

As the drainage accumulates in the bulb, the bulb expands and suction is lost, requiring recompression. Typically, these drains are emptied every 4 to 8 hours, and when they are half full of drainage or air. However, based on nursing assessment and judgment, the drain could be emptied and recompressed more frequently. The patency, placement of the drain, and the amount and characteristics of the drainage are included in the wound assessment.

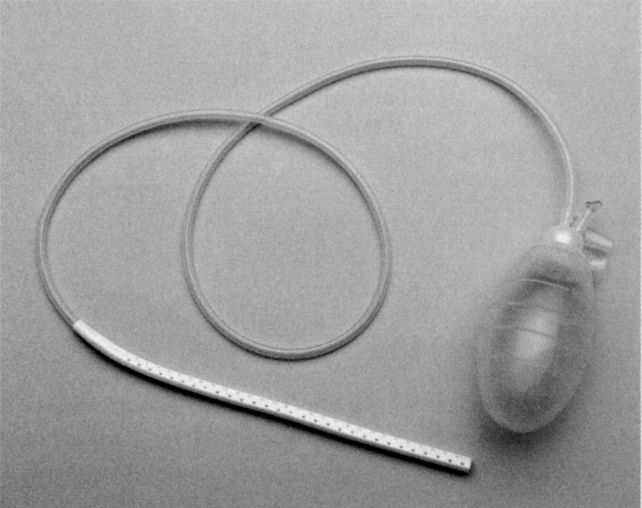

Figure 1. Jackson-Pratt drain.

SKILL 8-9 Caring for a Jackson-Pratt Drain *(continued)*

Equipment

- Graduated container for measuring drainage
- Clean disposable gloves
- Alcohol pad
- Cleansing solution, usually sterile normal saline
- Sterile gauze pads
- Skin-protectant wipes
- Personal protective equipment, such as mask or face shield, if indicated

ASSESSMENT

Assess the patency of the Jackson-Pratt drain and the drain site. Confirm any physician orders relevant to drain care and any drain care included in the nursing plan of care.

Assess the situation to determine the need for wound cleaning, a dressing change, or emptying of the drain. Assess the current dressing, if there is one, to determine whether it is intact. Assess for the presence of excess drainage or bleeding or saturation of the dressing.

Inspect the wound and the surrounding tissue. Assess the appearance of the incision for the approximation of wound edges, the color of the wound and surrounding area, and signs of dehiscence. Note the stage of the healing process and characteristics of any drainage. Also assess the surrounding skin for color, temperature, and edema, ecchymosis, or maceration.

NURSING DIAGNOSIS

Determine the related factors for the nursing diagnoses based on the patient's current status. An appropriate nursing diagnosis is Risk for Infection. Many other nursing diagnoses may also be appropriate, including:

- Anxiety
- Disturbed Body Image
- Acute Pain
- Deficient Knowledge
- Impaired Skin Integrity
- Delayed Surgical Recovery
- Impaired Tissue Integrity

OUTCOME IDENTIFICATION AND PLANNING

The expected outcome to achieve when performing care for a Jackson-Pratt drain is that the drain is patent and intact. Care is accomplished without contaminating the wound area, without causing trauma to the wound, and without causing the patient to experience pain or discomfort. Other outcomes that are appropriate may include: drainage amounts are measured accurately at the frequency required by facility policy and amounts are recorded as part of the intake and output record; and the patient states positive aspects about self and verbalizes an understanding of the need for drain care.

IMPLEMENTATION

ACTION	RATIONALE
1. Review the physician's order for drain and site care or the nursing plan of care related to drain care.	Reviewing the order and plan of care validates the correct patient and correct procedure.
2. Gather the necessary supplies.	Preparation promotes efficient time management and organized approach to the task.
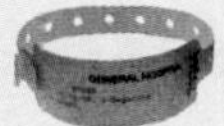 3. Identify the patient.	This ensures the right patient receives the right intervention.

(continued)

SKILL 8-9 Caring for a Jackson-Pratt Drain *(continued)*

ACTION	RATIONALE
4. Assess the patient for possible need for nonpharmacologic pain-reducing interventions or analgesic medication before wound care dressing change. Administer appropriate analgesic, consulting physician's orders, and allow enough time for analgesic to achieve its effectiveness.	Pain is a subjective experience influenced by past experience. Wound care and dressing changes may cause pain for some patients.
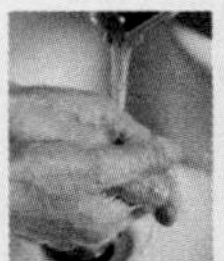 5. Perform hand hygiene.	Hand hygiene prevents the spread of microorganisms.
6. Close the room door or curtains. Place the bed at an appropriate and comfortable working height.	Closing the door or curtain provides privacy. Placing the bed at the appropriate height helps reduce back strain when providing care.
7. Assist the patient to a comfortable position that provides easy access to the drain area. Use the bath blanket to cover any exposed area other than the drain. Place the waterproof pad under the drain site.	Patient positioning and use of a bath blanket promote comfort and warmth. Waterproof pad protects underlying surfaces.
8. Put on clean gloves; put on mask or face shield if indicated.	Gloves prevent the spread of microorganisms; mask reduces the risk of transmission should splashing occur.
9. Place the graduated collection container under the outlet valve of the drain. Without contaminating the outlet valve, pull the cap off. The chamber will expand completely as it draws in air. **Empty the chamber's contents completely into the container (Figure 2). Use the alcohol pad to clean the chamber's spout and cap. Fully compress the chamber with one hand and replace the plug with your other hand (Figure 3).**	Emptying the drainage allows for accurate measurement. Cleaning the spout and cap reduces the risk of contamination and helps prevent the spread of microorganisms. Compressing the chamber reestablishes the vacuum.

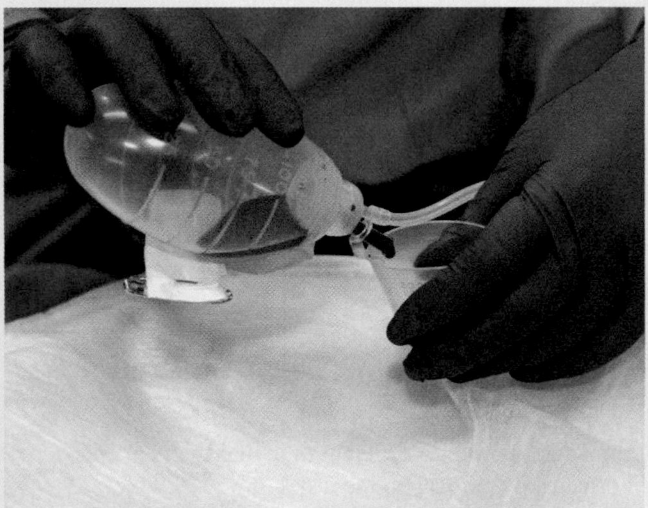

Figure 2. Emptying contents of Jackson-Pratt drain into collection device.

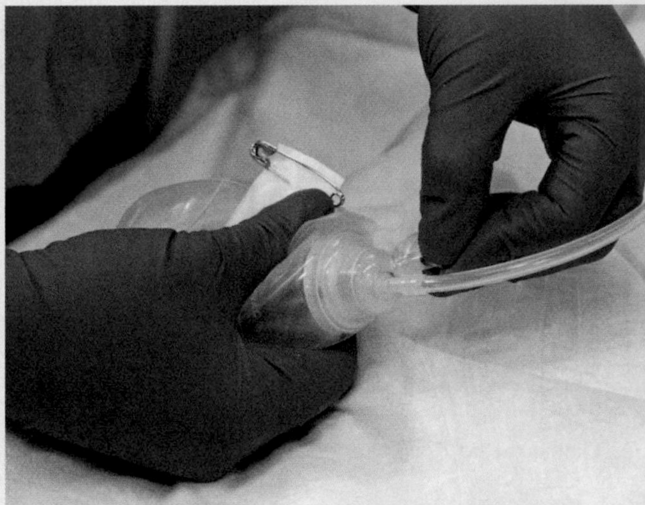

Figure 3. With gloved hand, compressing a Jackson-Pratt drain and replacing plug.

SKILL 8-9 Caring for a Jackson-Pratt Drain *(continued)*

10. Check the patency of the equipment. Make sure the tubing is free from twists and kinks.

    Patent, untwisted, or unkinked tubing promotes appropriate drainage from wound.

11. Secure the Jackson-Pratt drain to the patient's gown below the wound with a safety pin, making sure that there is no tension on the tubing.

    Securing the drain prevents injury to the patient and accidental removal of the drain.

12. Carefully measure and record the character, color, and amount of the drainage. Discard the drainage according to facility policy.

    Documentation promotes continuity of care and communication. Appropriate disposal of biohazard material reduces the risk for microorganism transmission.

13. If the drain site has a dressing, redress the site as outlined in Skill 8-3.

    Dressing protects the site.

14. If the drain site is open to air, observe the sutures that secure the drain to the skin. Look for signs of pulling, tearing, swelling, or infection of the surrounding skin.

    Early detection of problems leads to prompt intervention and prevents complications.

15. Gently clean the sutures with the gauze pad soaked in normal saline. Dry with a new gauze pad. Apply skin protectant to the surrounding skin if needed.

    Gentle cleaning and drying prevent the growth of microorganisms. Skin protectant prevents skin irritation and breakdown.

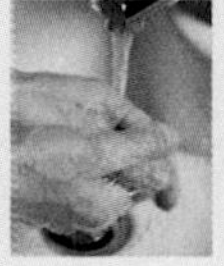

16. Remove gloves and all remaining equipment, place the patient in a position of comfort, with side rails up and bed in the lowest position, and perform hand hygiene.

    Proper patient positioning promotes safety. Proper removal of gloves and hand hygiene prevent spread of microorganisms.

EVALUATION

The expected outcome is met when the patient exhibits a patent and intact Jackson-Pratt drain, with a wound that is free of contamination and trauma. The patient reports minimal to no pain or discomfort with the care. Other outcomes are met when the patient exhibits signs and symptoms of progressive healing without evidence of complications, with wound drainage being measured accurately at the frequency required by facility policy and recorded as part of the intake and output record.

DOCUMENTATION

Guidelines

Document the location of the incision as well as the appearance of the incision noting the approximation of the wound edges and presence or absence of edema, redness, or drainage. Note if Steri-Strips are present or other dressings. Document the patency of the drain and if sutures are in place. Note that the drain was emptied, recompressed, and the amount and type of drainage that was obtained. Document the patient's reaction to the procedure, including if the patient received any analgesic medication, noting type, dosage, and route prior to the procedure and its effectiveness. Include pertinent patient and family teaching as well as any patient concerns.

Sample Documentation

2/7/09 2400 Right chest incision and drain open to air. Wound edges approximated, slight ecchymosis, no edema, redness, or drainage. Steri-Strips intact. Drain patent and secured with suture. Exit site without edema, drainage, or redness. Drain emptied and recompressed. 40 cc sanguineous drainage recorded.
—Carol White, RN

(continued)

SKILL 8-9 Caring for a Jackson-Pratt Drain *(continued)*

Unexpected Situations and Associated Interventions

- *A patient has a Jackson-Pratt drain in the right lower quadrant following abdominal surgery. The record indicates it has been draining serosanguineous fluid, 40 to 50 mL every shift. While performing your initial assessment, you note that the dressing around the drain site is saturated with serosanguineous secretions and there is minimal drainage in the collection chamber:* Inspect the tubing for kinks or obstruction. Assess the patient for changes in condition. Remove the dressing and assess the site. Often, if the tubing becomes blocked with a blood clot or drainage particles, the wound drainage will leak around the exit site of the drain. Cleanse the area and redress the site. Notify the physician of your findings and document the event in the patient's record.
- *Your patient calls you to the room and says, "I found this in the bed when I went to get up." He has his Jackson-Pratt drain in his hand. It is completely removed from the patient:* Assess the patient for any new and abnormal signs or symptoms, and assess the surgical site and drain site. Apply a sterile dressing with gauze and tape to the drain site. Notify the physician of your findings and document the event in the patient's record.

Special Considerations

General Considerations

- Often patients have more than one Jackson-Pratt drain. Number or letter the drains for easy identification. Record the drainage from each drain separately, identified by the number or letter, on the intake and output record.

SKILL 8-10 Caring for a Hemovac Drain

A Hemovac drain is placed into a vascular cavity where blood drainage is expected after surgery, such as with abdominal and orthopedic surgery. The drain consists of perforated tubing connected to a portable vacuum unit (Figure 1). Suction is maintained by compressing a springlike device in the collection unit. After a surgical procedure, the surgeon places one end of the drain in or near the area to be drained. The other end passes through the skin via a separate incision. These drains are usually sutured in place. The site may be treated as an additional surgical wound, but often these sites are left open to air after the first 24 hours after surgery.

As the drainage accumulates in the collection unit, it expands and suction is lost, requiring recompression. Typically, the drain is emptied every 4 or 8 hours and when it is half full of drainage or air. However, based on the physician's orders and nursing assessment and judgment, it could be emptied and recompressed more frequently. The patency, placement of the drain, and the amount and characteristics of the drainage are included in the wound assessment.

Equipment

- Graduated container for measuring drainage
- Clean gloves
- Alcohol pad
- Cleansing solution, usually sterile normal saline
- Sterile gauze pads
- Skin protectant as needed
- Personal protective equipment, such as mask or face shield, if indicated

SKILL 8-10 Caring for a Hemovac Drain *(continued)*

ASSESSMENT

Assess the patency of the Hemovac drain and the drain site. Confirm any physician orders relevant to drain care and any drain care included in the nursing plan of care. Also assess the situation to determine the need for wound cleaning, a dressing change, or emptying of the drain. Assess the current dressing, if there is one, to determine if it is intact. Assess for the presence of excess drainage or bleeding or saturation of the dressing. Inspect the wound and the surrounding tissue. Assess the appearance of the incision for the approximation of wound edges, the color of the wound and surrounding area, and signs of dehiscence. Note the stage of the healing process and characteristics of any drainage. Assess the surrounding skin for color, temperature, and edema, ecchymosis, or maceration.

NURSING DIAGNOSIS

Determine the related factors for the nursing diagnoses based on the patient's current status. An appropriate nursing diagnosis is Risk for Infection. Many other nursing diagnoses may also be appropriate, including:

- Anxiety
- Disturbed Body Image
- Acute Pain
- Deficient Knowledge
- Impaired Skin Integrity
- Delayed Surgical Recovery
- Impaired Tissue Integrity

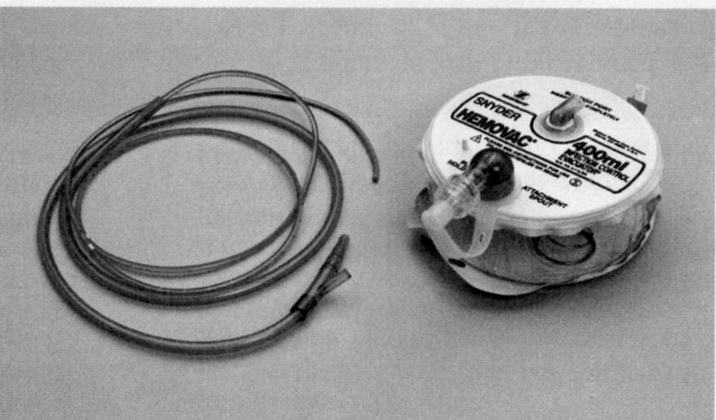

Figure 1. Hemovac drain.

OUTCOME IDENTIFICATION AND PLANNING IMPLEMENTATION

The expected outcome to achieve when performing care for a Hemovac drain is that the drain is patent and intact. Care is performed without contaminating the wound area, without causing trauma to the wound, and without causing the patient to experience pain or discomfort. Other outcomes that are appropriate may include: drainage amounts are measured accurately at the frequency required by facility policy and recorded as part of the intake and output record; and the patient demonstrates understanding of the need for drain care.

ACTION	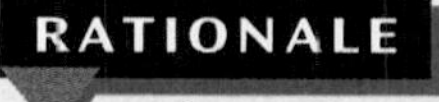 RATIONALE
1. Review the physician's order for drain and site care or the nursing plan of care related to drain care.	Review of the order and plan of care validates the correct patient and correct procedure.

(continued)

SKILL 8-10 Caring for a Hemovac Drain *(continued)*

ACTION	RATIONALE
2. Gather the necessary supplies.	Preparation promotes efficient time management and organized approach to the task.
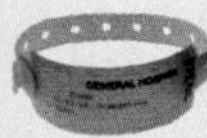 3. Identify the patient.	This ensures the right patient receives the right intervention.
4. Explain the procedure to the patient.	Discussion and explanation help allay anxiety, encourage patient cooperation, and prepare the patient for what to expect.
5. Assess the patient for possible need for nonpharmacologic pain-reducing interventions or analgesic medication before wound care dressing change. Administer appropriate analgesic, consulting physician's orders, and allow enough time for analgesic to achieve its effectiveness.	Pain is a subjective experience influenced by past experience. Wound care and dressing changes may cause pain for some patients.
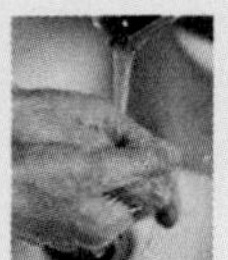 6. Perform hand hygiene.	Hand hygiene prevents the spread of microorganisms.
7. Close the room door or curtains. Place the bed at an appropriate and comfortable working height.	Closing the door or curtain provides privacy. Positioning the bed at the proper height helps reduce back strain when providing care.
8. Assist the patient to a comfortable position that provides easy access to the drain area. Use the bath blanket to cover any exposed area other than the drain. Place the waterproof pad under the drain site.	Patient positioning and use of a bath blanket provide for comfort and warmth. Waterproof pad protects underlying surfaces.
9. Put on clean gloves and other personal protective equipment, such as mask or face shield, as necessary.	Gloves prevent the spread of microorganisms. Personal protective equipment such as a face shield prevents transmission should splashing occur.
10. Place the graduated collection container under the pouring spout of the drain. Without contaminating the outlet valve, uncap the valve. The chamber will expand completely as it draws in air. Empty the chamber's contents completely into the container (Figure 2). Use the alcohol pad to clean the chamber's spout and cap. **Fully compress the chamber by pushing the top and bottom together with your hands. Keep the device tightly compressed while you reinsert the plug (Figure 3).**	Uncapping allows for accurate measurement of the drainage. Cleaning with alcohol prevents contamination of the valve and reduces the risk for microorganism transmission. Compression with both hands helps to reestablish the vacuum.
11. Check the patency of the equipment. Make sure the tubing is free from twists and kinks.	Free, untwisted, and unkinked tubing promotes drainage from wound.
12. Secure the Hemovac drain to the patient's gown below the wound with pins, making sure that there is no tension on the tubing.	Securing the drain prevents injury to the patient or accidental removal of the drain.
13. Carefully measure and record the character, color, and amount of the drainage. Discard the drainage according to facility policy.	Documentation promotes continuity of care and communication. Appropriate disposal of biohazard material prevents transmission of microorganisms.

SKILL 8-10

Caring for a Hemovac Drain *(continued)*

ACTION | RATIONALE

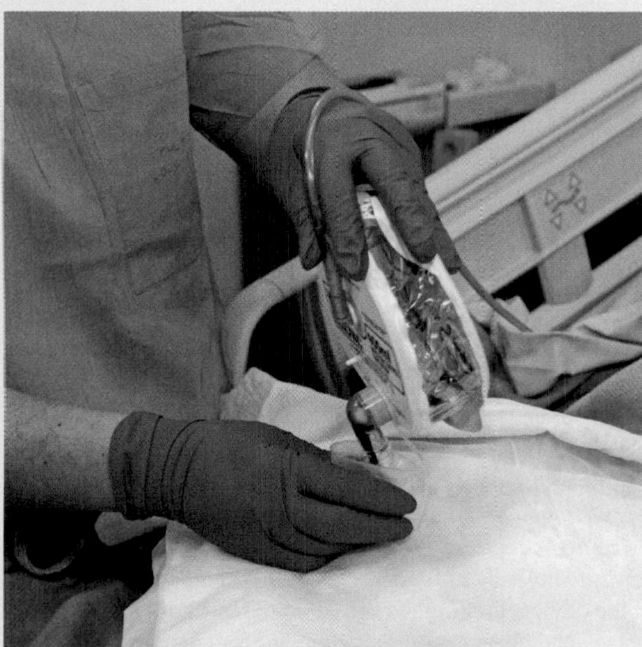
Figure 2. Emptying Hemovac drain into collection device.

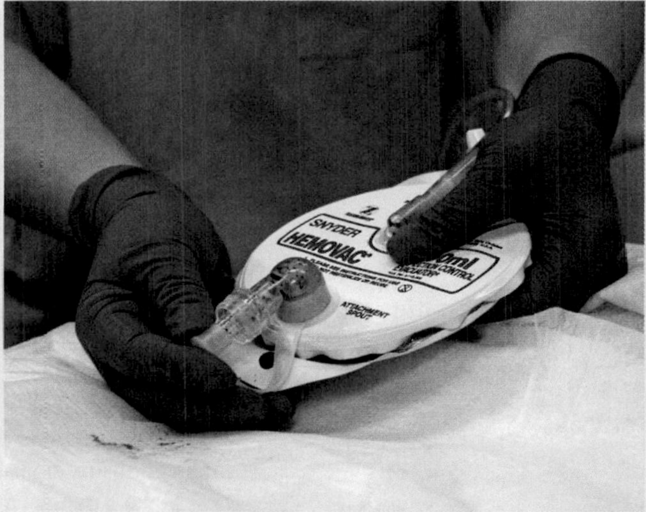

Figure 3. Compressing the Hemovac and securing the cap.

14. If the drain site has a dressing, redress the site as outlined in Skill 8-3. Assess the patient for possible need for pain/analgesic medication prior to dressing change

Dressing protects the site. Dressing changes may be painful and pain is a subjective experience.

15. If the drain site is open to air, observe the sutures that secure the drain to the skin. Look for signs of pulling, tearing, swelling, or infection of the surrounding skin.

Early detection of problems leads to prompt intervention and prevents complications.

16. Gently clean the sutures with the gauze pad soaked in normal saline. Dry with a new gauze pad.

Cleaning prevents the growth of microorganisms.

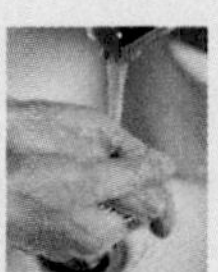

17. Remove gloves and all remaining equipment, place the patient in a position of comfort, with side rails up and bed in the lowest position, and perform hand hygiene.

Patient positioning promotes safety. Proper glove removal and hand hygiene prevent spread of microorganisms.

EVALUATION

The expected outcome is met when the patient demonstrates a patent, intact Hemovac drain with a wound that is free of contamination and trauma. The patient verbalizes little to no pain or discomfort. Other outcomes are met when the patient exhibits signs and symptoms of progressive healing without evidence of complications, with wound drainage being measured accurately at the frequency required by facility policy and recorded as part of the intake and output record.

(continued)

SKILL 8-10 Caring for a Hemovac Drain *(continued)*

DOCUMENTATION

Guidelines

Document the location of the Hemovac drain. Note the presence of sutures and the condition of the drain site and surrounding skin. Record if redness, edema or drainage is observed. Document cleansing of exit site with normal saline. Record the amount and type of drainage emptied from the Hemovac drain and that it was recompressed to maintain the negative suction of the drainage system. Note pertinent patient and family education and any patient reaction from this procedure.

Sample Documentation

1/18/09 1000 Hemovac drain in place in left lower extremity, site open to air. Suture intact; exit site slightly pink, without redness, edema, or drainage. Surrounding skin without edema, ecchymosis, or redness. Exit site and suture cleansed with normal saline. Hemovac emptied of 90 cc sanguineous secretions and recompressed. —A. Smith, RN

Unexpected Situations and Associated Interventions

- *A patient has a Hemovac drain placed in the left knee following surgery. The record indicates it has been draining serosanguineous secretions, 40 to 50 mL every shift. While performing your initial assessment, you note that the collection chamber is completely expanded. You empty the device and compress to resume suction. A short time later, you observe that the chamber is completely expanded again:* Inspect the tubing for kinks or obstruction. Inspect the device, looking for breaks in the integrity of the chamber. Make sure the cap is in place and closed. Assess the patient for changes in condition. Remove the dressing and assess the site. Make sure the drainage tubing has not advanced out of the wound, exposing any of the perforations in the tubing. If you are not successful in maintaining the vacuum, notify the physician of your findings and interventions and document the event in the patient's record.

Special Considerations

General Considerations

- When the patient with a drain is ready to ambulate, empty and compress the drain before activity. Secure the drain to the patient's gown below the wound, making sure there is no tension on the drainage tubing. This removes excess drainage, maintains maximum suction, and avoids strain on the drain's suture line.

SKILL 8-11 Applying a Wound Vacuum-Assisted Closure

Vacuum-assisted closure (VAC) is a therapy that assists in wound closure by applying localized negative pressure to the wound bed. It is also known as topical negative pressure (TNP) or negative-pressure wound therapy (NPWT). An open-cell foam dressing is applied in the wound. A fenestrated tube is embedded in the foam, allowing the application of the negative pressure. The dressing and distal tubing are covered by a transparent, occlusive, air-permeable dressing that provides a seal, allowing the application of the negative pressure. Excess wound fluid is removed through tubing, and it also acts to pull the wound edges together.

This wound treatment increases blood flow to the wound, promotes granulation tissue formation, removes excess exudate, and reduces wound bacterial counts. Wound VAC dressings are changed every 48 to 72 hours, depending on the manufacturer's specifications and physician's orders.

SKILL 8-11 Applying a Wound Vacuum-Assisted Closure *(continued)*

Vacuum-assisted therapy is indicated for acute and traumatic wounds, pressure ulcers, and chronic open wounds. It should be used cautiously in patients with active bleeding and those taking anticoagulants. It is contraindicated in malignant wounds, untreated osteomyelitis (bone infection), exposed arteries or veins, and when there are fistulas to body cavities or organs. Additionally, this therapy is not indicated when necrotic tissue cannot be removed.

Equipment

- Vacuum unit
- Evacuation/collection canister
- Reticulated foam
- Fenestrated tubing
- Evacuation tubing
- Transparent occlusive air-permeable dressing
- Skin-protectant wipes
- Sterile gauze sponge
- A sterile irrigation set, including a basin, irrigant container, and irrigation syringe
- Sterile irrigation solution as ordered by the physician, warmed to body temperature
- Waste receptacle to dispose of contaminated materials
- Sterile gloves (2 pairs) and a set of clean disposable gloves
- Sterile scissors
- Waterproof pad and bath blanket
- Personal protective equipment, such as a gown, mask, and eye protection

ASSESSMENT

Confirm the physician's order for the application of wound VAC therapy. Check the patient's chart and question the patient about current treatments and medications that may make the application contraindicated, such as current or recent past anticoagulation therapy, bleeding from the wound, malignant wound, unstable diabetes, untreated osteomyelitis, or the presence of large amounts of necrosis. Assess the patient for pain. Assess the equipment to be used, including the condition of cords and plugs.

Complete a wound assessment. Inspect the wound and the surrounding tissue. Assess the wound for the approximation of wound edges, the color of the wound and surrounding area, and signs of dehiscence. Note the stage of the healing process and characteristics of any drainage. Assess the surrounding skin for color, temperature, and edema, ecchymosis, or maceration.

NURSING DIAGNOSIS

Determine the related factors for the nursing diagnoses based on the patient's current status. An appropriate nursing diagnosis is Impaired Skin Integrity. Other nursing diagnoses that may be appropriate or require the use of this skill include:

- Anxiety
- Disturbed Body Image
- Acute Pain
- Risk for Infection
- Risk for Injury
- Deficient Knowledge
- Acute Pain
- Impaired Tissue Integrity

OUTCOME IDENTIFICATION AND PLANNING

The expected outcome to achieve when applying a wound VAC is that the therapy is accomplished without contaminating the wound area, without causing trauma to the wound, and without causing the patient to experience pain or discomfort. Other outcomes that may be appropriate include: the vacuum device functions correctly; the appropriate and ordered pressure is maintained throughout therapy; and the wound exhibits healing.

(continued)

SKILL 8-11 Applying a Wound Vacuum-Assisted Closure *(continued)*

IMPLEMENTATION

ACTION	RATIONALE
1. Review the physician's order for the application of wound VAC therapy, including the ordered setting for the negative pressure.	Reviewing the order validates the correct patient and correct procedure.
2. Gather the necessary supplies.	Preparation promotes efficient time management and provides an organized approach to the task.
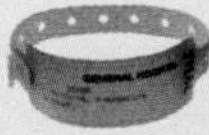 3. Identify the patient.	This ensures the right patient receives the right intervention.
4. Explain the procedure.	Discussion and explanation help allay anxiety, encourage patient cooperation, and prepare the patient for what to expect.
5. Assess the patient for possible need for nonpharmacologic pain-reducing interventions or analgesic medication before wound care dressing change. Administer appropriate analgesic, consulting physician's orders, and allow enough time for analgesic to achieve its effectiveness before beginning procedure.	Pain is a subjective experience influenced by past experience. Wound care and dressing changes may cause pain for some patients.
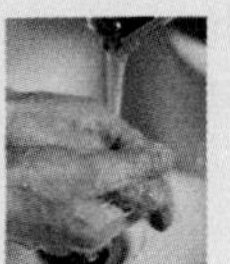 6. Perform hand hygiene.	Hand hygiene prevents the spread of microorganisms.
7. Close the room door or curtains. Place the bed in a comfortable working height.	Closing the door or curtains provides privacy. Proper bed positioning helps reduce back strain while you are performing the procedure.
8. Assist the patient to a comfortable position that provides easy access to the wound area. Position the patient so the irrigation solution will flow from the clean end of the wound toward the dirty end. Expose the area and drape the patient with a bath blanket if needed. Put a waterproof pad under the wound area.	Patient positioning and draping provide for comfort and warmth. Gravity directs the flow of liquid from the least contaminated to the most contaminated area. Waterproof pad protects the patient and the bed linens.
9. Have the disposal bag or waste receptacle within easy reach for use during the procedure.	Having the waste container handy means that soiled dressings and supplies may be discarded easily, without the spread of microorganisms.
10. Assemble the VAC device according to the manufacturer's instructions. Set the negative pressure according to the physician's order (25–200 mm Hg).	Assembling the equipment promotes efficient time management and provides an organized approach to the task. Setting the pressure ensures appropriate pressure is applied to the wound.
11. Using sterile technique, prepare a sterile field and add all the sterile supplies needed for the procedure to the field. Pour warmed, sterile irrigating solution into the sterile container.	Proper preparation ensures that supplies are within easy reach and sterility is maintained. Warmed solution may result in less discomfort.

SKILL
8-11 Applying a Wound Vacuum-Assisted Closure *(continued)*

ACTION	RATIONALE
12. Put on a gown, mask, and eye protection.	Use of personal protective equipment is part of Standard Precautions. A gown protects your clothes from contamination if splashing should occur. Goggles protect mucous membranes of your eyes from contact with irrigant fluid.
13. Put on clean disposable gloves and remove the soiled dressings.	Gloves provide protection from contaminated dressings.
14. Assess the wound for appearance and drainage. Assess the appearance of the surrounding tissue.	Assessment provides information about the wound healing process or the presence of infection.
15. Discard the dressings in the receptacle. Remove your gloves and put them in the receptacle.	Proper disposal of dressings and used gloves prevents the spread of microorganisms.
16. Put on sterile gloves. Using sterile technique, irrigate the wound (see Skill 8-4).	Irrigation removes exudate and debris.
17. Clean the area around the skin with normal saline. Dry the surrounding skin with a sterile gauze sponge.	Moisture provides a medium for growth of microorganisms.
18. **Wipe intact skin around the wound with a skin-protectant wipe and allow it to dry well.**	Skin protectant provides a barrier against irritation and breakdown.
19. Remove gloves if they become contaminated and discard them into the receptacle.	Proper disposal of gloves prevents spread of microorganisms.
20. Put on a new pair of sterile gloves. **Using sterile scissors, cut the foam to the shape and measurement of the wound.** More than one piece of foam may be necessary if the first piece is cut too small. **Carefully place the foam in the wound.**	Aseptic technique maintains sterility of items to come in contact with wound. Foam should fill the wound but not cover intact surrounding skin. Black polyurethane foam has larger pores, thus requires lower negative pressure. White polyurethane foam requires higher negative pressure and is used when tissue granulation stimulation needs to be limited.
21. **Place the fenestrated tubing into the center of the foam (Figure 1). There should be foam between the tubing and the base of the wound and foam over top of the tubing.**	The fenestrated tubing embedded into the foam delivers negative pressure to the wound.
22. **Cover the foam and tubing with the transparent occlusive air-permeable dressing, leaving at least a 2″ margin on the intact skin around the wound.**	The occlusive air-permeable dressing provides a seal, allowing the application of the negative pressure.
23. Connect the free end of the fenestrated tubing to the tubing that is connected to the evacuation canister (Figure 2).	Connection to canister provides a collection chamber for wound drainage and allows measurement of drainage.
24. Remove and discard gloves. Turn on the vacuum unit (Figure 3). **Observe the shrinking of the transparent dressing to the foam and skin.**	Shrinkage confirms good seal, allowing for accurate application of pressure and treatment.
25. Lower the bed and make sure the patient is comfortable.	Repositioning the bed and the patient promotes safety and comfort.

(continued)

SKILL 8-11 Applying a Wound Vacuum-Assisted Closure *(continued)*

ACTION	RATIONALE

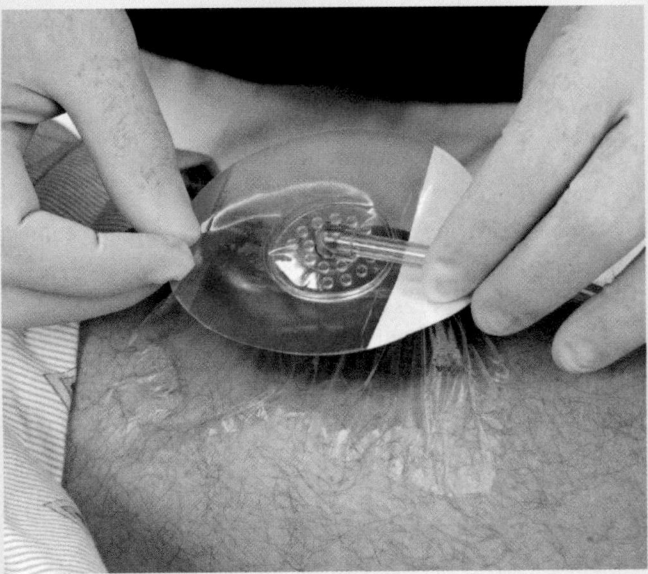

Figure 1. Applying fenestrated tubing.

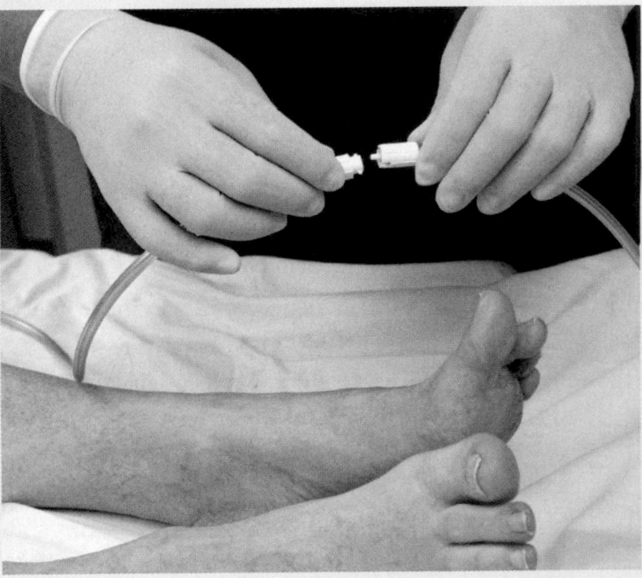

Figure 2. Connecting tubing to collection canister.

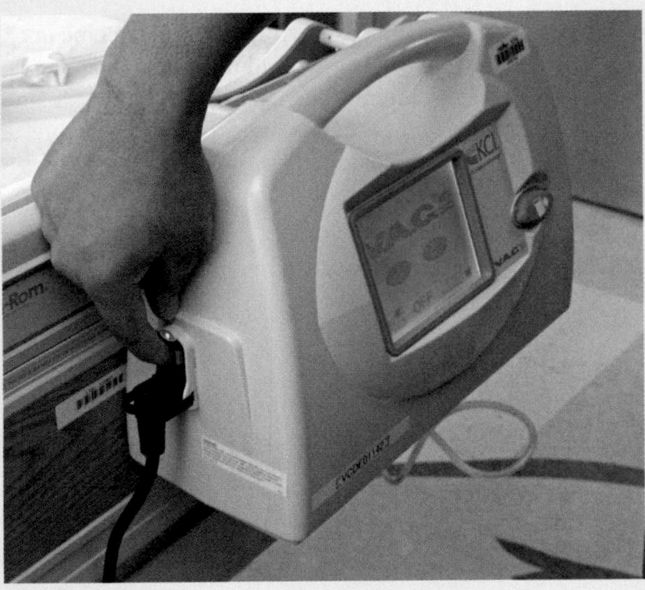

Figure 3. Turning on wound VAC.

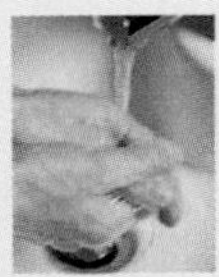

ACTION	RATIONALE
26. Perform hand hygiene.	Hand hygiene prevents spread of microorganisms.
27. Dispose of used supplies and equipment according to facility policy.	Proper disposal of supplies and equipment prevents spread of microorganisms.
28. Check all wound dressings every shift.	Assessment ensures identification of changes in patient condition and timely intervention to prevent complications.

SKILL
8-11 Applying a Wound Vacuum-Assisted Closure *(continued)*

EVALUATION

The expected outcome is met when the patient exhibits a wound VAC applied without contamination or trauma to the wound. The patient verbalizes little to no pain or discomfort. Other outcomes that may be appropriate include: the patient demonstrates a wound with the appropriate and ordered pressure being maintained; the device functions properly; and the wound shows signs of progressive healing.

DOCUMENTATION

Guidelines

Document the location of the wound VAC dressing application, noting the pressure setting, patency, and seal of the VAC dressing. Describe the color and characteristics of the drainage in the collection chamber. Document the condition of the surrounding tissue, noting the presence of any edema, redness, or ecchymosis. Record pertinent patient and family education and any patient reaction from this procedure, including the presence of pain and effectiveness or ineffectiveness of pain reducing interventions.

Sample Documentation

4/5/09 0800 Wound VAC dressing intact with good seal maintained, VAC system patent, pressure setting 50 mm Hg. Purulent, sanguineous drainage noted in collection chamber and tubing. Surrounding tissue without edema, redness, ecchymosis, or signs of irritation. Patient verbalizes an understanding of movement limitations related to the system.—B. Clark, RN

Unexpected Situations and Associated Interventions

- *While assessing the patient, you note that the seal between the transparent dressing and the foam and skin is not tight:* If the seal is broken, the appropriate pressure is not being applied to the wound. Change the dressing, regardless of the length of time it is has been in place.
- *The patient complains of acute pain while the wound VAC is operating:* Assess the patient for other symptoms, obtain vital signs, assess the wound, and assess the vacuum device for proper functioning. Report your findings to the physician and document the event in the patient's record. Administer analgesics as ordered. Continue or change the wound therapy as ordered.

Special Considerations

General Considerations

- Change the wound dressing every 48 to 72 hours, as ordered. Time dressing changes to allow for wound assessment by the other members of the healthcare team.
- Measure and record the amount of drainage each shift as part of the intake and output record.
- Be alert for audible and visual alarms on the vacuum device to alert you to problems, such as tipping of the device greater than 45 degrees, a full collection canister, an air leak in the dressing, or dislodgment of the canister.
- The VAC therapy should be operating for 24 hours. It should not be shut off for more than 2 hours at a time because this will lead to stagnation of wound fluid in the injury site (Kaufman & Pahl, 2003).
- When maceration of the surrounding skin beneath the occlusive dressing occurs, this may be treated by placing a calcium alginate dressing beneath the transparent dressing to absorb drainage. Verify with hospital policy as needed.

SKILL 8-12 Removing Sutures

Skin sutures are used to hold tissue and skin together. Sutures may be black silk, synthetic material, or fine wire. Sutures are removed when enough tensile strength has developed to hold the wound edges together during healing. The time frame varies depending on the patient's age, nutritional status, and wound location. Frequently, after skin sutures are removed, Steri-Strips (small wound-closure strips of adhesive) are applied across the wound to give additional support as it continues to heal. The removal of sutures may be done by the physician or by the nurse with a physician's order.

Equipment

- Sterile suture removal kit or sterile forceps and scissors
- Gauze
- Wound cleansing agent, according to facility policy
- Clean disposable gloves
- Sterile gloves
- Steri-Strips
- Tincture of benzoin, if indicated

ASSESSMENT

Inspect the surgical incision and the surrounding tissue. Assess the appearance of the wound for the approximation of wound edges, the color of the wound and surrounding area, presence of wound drainage, noting color, volume, and odor, and for signs of dehiscence. Note the stage of the healing process and characteristics of any drainage. Assess the surrounding skin for color, temperature, and the presence of edema, maceration, or ecchymosis.

NURSING DIAGNOSIS

Determine the related factors for the nursing diagnoses based on the patient's current status. An appropriate nursing diagnosis is Risk for Infection. Other nursing diagnoses that may be appropriate include:

- Anxiety
- Pain
- Acute Pain
- Impaired Skin Integrity
- Delayed Surgical Recovery
- Risk for Situational Low Self-Esteem

OUTCOME IDENTIFICATION AND PLANNING

The expected outcome to achieve when removing surgical sutures is that the sutures are removed without contaminating the incisional area by maintaining sterile technique, without causing trauma to the wound, and without causing the patient to experience pain or discomfort. In addition, other outcomes that are appropriate include: the patient remains free from exposure to infectious microorganisms; the patient remains free of complications that would delay recovery; and the patient verbalizes positive aspects about self.

IMPLEMENTATION

ACTION	RATIONALE
1. Review the physician's order for suture removal.	Reviewing the order validates the correct patient and correct procedure.
2. Gather the necessary supplies.	Adequate preparation ensures efficient time management.
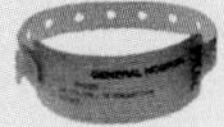 3. Identify the patient.	This ensures the right patient receives the right intervention.

SKILL 8-12 **Removing Sutures** *(continued)*

ACTION	RATIONALE
4. Explain the procedure to the patient. Describe the sensation as a pulling or slightly uncomfortable experience.	Discussion and explanation help allay anxiety and prepare the patient for what to expect.
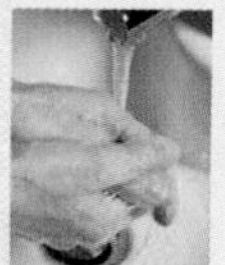 5. Perform hand hygiene.	Hand hygiene prevents the spread of microorganisms.
6. Close the room door or curtains. Place the bed at an appropriate and comfortable working height.	Closing the door or curtains provides privacy. Placing the bed at an appropriate height helps reduce back strain when performing the procedure.
7. Assist the patient to a comfortable position that provides easy access to the wound area. Use the bath blanket to cover any exposed area other than the wound.	A comfortable patient position helps reduce anxiety. Bath blanket provides for comfort and warmth.
8. Put on clean gloves. Remove and dispose of any dressings on the surgical incision. Remove gloves and put on sterile gloves. Inspect the incision area (Figure 1).	Use of gloves and proper removal of dressings help prevent spread of microorganisms. Removal of dressings allows access to the incision.

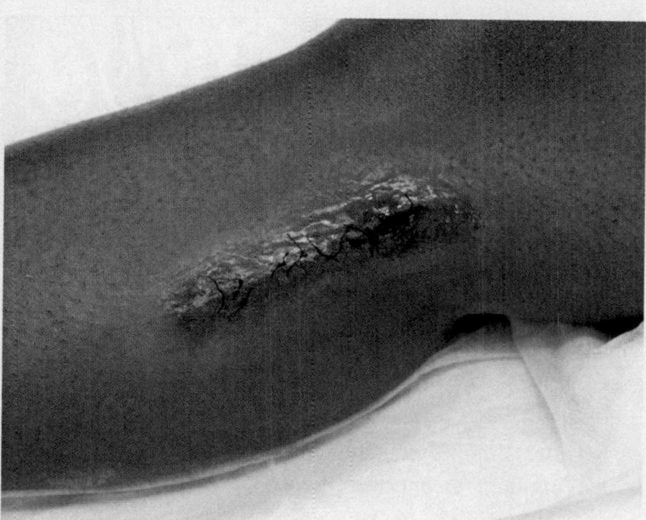

Figure 1. Incision with sutures.

ACTION	RATIONALE
9. Clean the incision using the wound cleanser and gauze, according to facility policies and procedures.	Incision cleaning prevents the spread of microorganisms and contamination of the wound.
10. **Using the sterile forceps, grasp the knot of the first suture and gently lift the knot up off the skin.**	Raising the suture knot prevents accidental injury to the wound or skin when cutting.

(continued)

SKILL 8-12 Removing Sutures *(continued)*

ACTION | **RATIONALE**

11. Using the sterile scissors, cut one side of the suture below the knot, close to the skin. **Grasp the knot with the forceps and pull the cut suture through the skin (Figure 2). Avoid pulling the visible portion of the suture through the underlying tissue.**

Pulling the cut suture through the skin helps reduce the risk for contamination of the incision area and resulting infection.

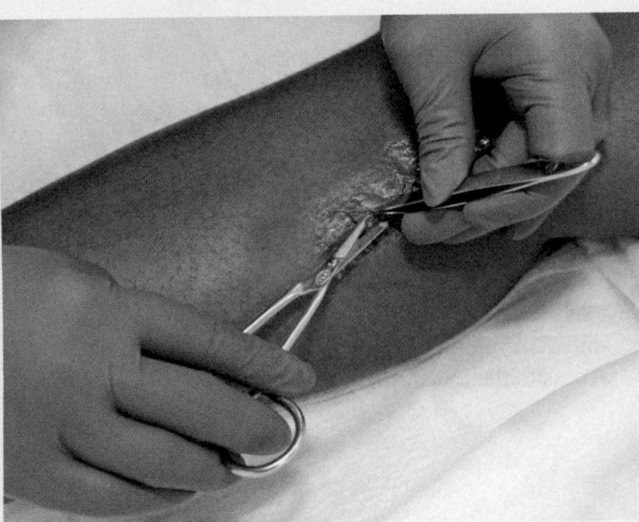

Figure 2. Using gloved hands to pull up on a suture with forceps and cutting the suture with sterile scissors.

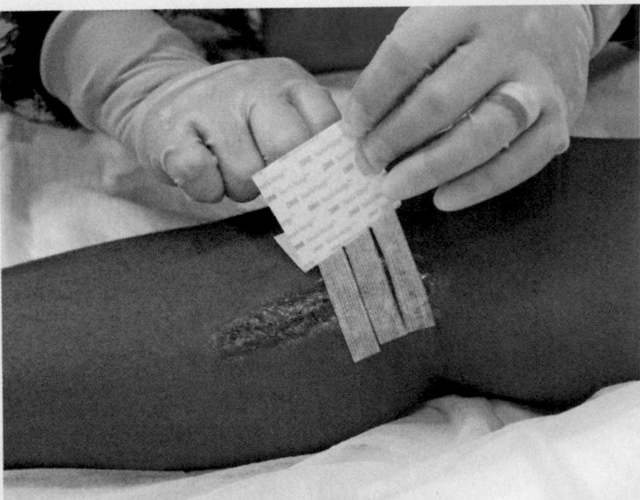

Figure 3. Applying Steri-Strips on incision.

12. Remove every other suture to be sure the wound edges are healed. If they are, remove the remaining sutures as ordered. Dispose of sutures in a biohazard bag.

Removing every other suture allows for inspection of the wound, while leaving adequate suture in place to promote continued healing if the edges are not totally approximated. Follow Standard Precautions in disposing of sutures.

13. Apply Steri-Strips if ordered. If necessary, prepare skin with tincture of benzoin before applying Steri-Strips (Figure 3).

Steri-Strips provide additional support to the wound as it continues to heal. Applying benzoin aids in adherence of Steri-Strips.

14. Reapply the dressing, depending on the physician's orders and facility policy.

A new dressing protects the wound. Some policies advise leaving the area uncovered.

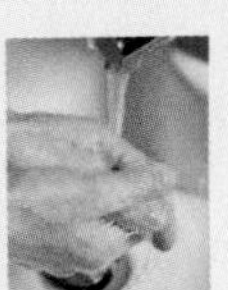

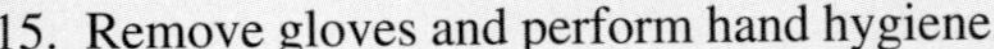

15. Remove gloves and perform hand hygiene.

Removing gloves and performing hand hygiene prevent the spread of microorganisms.

EVALUATION

The expected outcome is met when the patient exhibits an incision area that is clean, dry, and intact without sutures. The incision area is free of trauma and infection, and the patient verbalizes minimal to no complaints of pain or discomfort and positive aspects about self.

SKILL 8-12 Removing Sutures *(continued)*

DOCUMENTATION

Guidelines

Document the location of the wound and the suture removal. Comment on whether the wound appears healed, including if the incision edges are approximated and if Steri-Strips or a dressing was applied. Document presence or absence of erythema, edema, ecchymosis, or drainage, as well as temperature and color of the skin. Include a statement related to how the patient tolerated the suture removal and the patient care education that was provided to both the patient and family member, if available.

Sample Documentation

3/4/08 1800 Right leg surgical wound appears healed. Incision edges are approximated, without erythema, edema, ecchymosis, or drainage. Skin warm and pink. Sutures removed without difficulty, Steri-Strips applied. Patient instructed in how to care for wound and expectations regarding Steri-Strips; patient and wife verbalized an understanding of information and asked appropriate questions.—R. Downs, RN

Unexpected Situations and Associated Interventions

- *Sutures are crusted with dried blood or secretions, making them difficult to remove:* Moisten sterile gauze with sterile saline and gently loosen crusts before removing sutures.
- *Resistance is met when attempting to pull suture through the tissue:* Use a gentle, continuous pulling motion to remove the suture. If the suture still does not come out, do not use excessive force. Report your findings to the physician and document the event in the patient's record.

Special Considerations

General Considerations

- Encourage the patient to splint chest and abdominal wounds during activity, such as changing position, ambulation, coughing, and sneezing. This provides increased support for the underlying tissues and can decrease discomfort.

SKILL 8-13 Removing Surgical Staples *(continued)*

Surgical skin staples are made of stainless steel and are used to hold tissue and skin together. Staples decrease the risk of infection and allow faster wound closure. Surgical staples are removed when enough tensile strength has developed to hold the wound edges together during healing. The time frame varies depending on the patient's age, nutritional status, and wound location. After skin staples are removed, Steri-Strips (small wound-closure strips of adhesive) are applied across the wound to keep the skin edges approximated as it continues to heal. The removal of surgical staples may be done by the physician or by the nurse with a physician's order.

Equipment

- Sterile staple remover
- Gauze
- Wound cleansing agent, according to facility policy
- Gloves
- Steri-Strips
- Tincture of benzoin if indicated

(continued)

SKILL 8-13 Removing Surgical Staples *(continued)*

ASSESSMENT

Inspect the surgical incision and the surrounding tissue. Assess the appearance of the wound for the approximation of wound edges, the color of the wound and surrounding area, and signs of dehiscence. Note the stage of the healing process and the characteristics of any drainage. Assess the surrounding skin for color, temperature, and the presence of edema or ecchymosis.

NURSING DIAGNOSIS

Determine the related factors for the nursing diagnoses based on the patient's current status. An appropriate nursing diagnosis is Risk for Infection. Other nursing diagnoses that may be appropriate include:

- Anxiety
- Impaired Comfort
- Acute Pain
- Impaired Skin Integrity
- Delayed Surgical Recovery
- Risk for Situational Low Self-Esteem

OUTCOME IDENTIFICATION AND PLANNING

The expected outcome to achieve when removing surgical staples is that the staples are removed without contaminating the incision area, without causing trauma to the wound, and without causing the patient to experience pain or discomfort. Other outcomes that are appropriate include: the patient remains free from exposure to infectious microorganisms; the patient remains free of complications that would delay recovery; and the patient verbalizes positive aspects about self.

IMPLEMENTATION

ACTION	RATIONALE
1. Review the physician's order for staple removal.	Reviewing the order validates the correct patient and correct procedure.
2. Gather the necessary supplies.	Preparation promotes efficient time management.
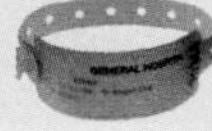 3. Identify the patient. Explain the procedure to the patient. Describe the sensation as a pulling or slightly uncomfortable experience.	Patient identification validates the correct patient and correct procedure. Discussion and explanation help allay anxiety and prepare the patient for what to expect.
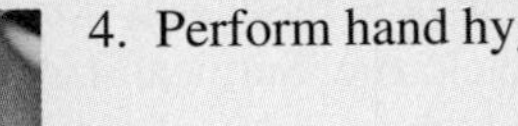 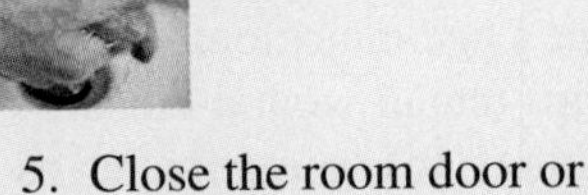 4. Perform hand hygiene.	Hand hygiene prevents the spread of microorganisms.
5. Close the room door or curtains. Place the bed at an appropriate and comfortable working height.	Closing the door or curtain provides privacy. Raising the bed to an appropriate height helps reduce back strain when performing the procedure.
6. Assist the patient to a comfortable position that provides easy access to the wound area. Use the bath blanket to cover any exposed area other than the wound.	A comfortable position helps reduce the patient's anxiety. Bath blankets provide for comfort and warmth.
7. Put on gloves. Remove and dispose of any dressings on the surgical incision using proper technique. Remove gloves and put on a new pair.	Use of gloves and proper dressing removal prevent the spread of microorganisms. Dressing removal also allows access to the incision.

SKILL 8-13 Removing Surgical Staples *(continued)*

ACTION	RATIONALE
8. Clean the incision using the wound cleanser and gauze, according to facility policies and procedures.	Wound cleaning prevents the spread of microorganisms and contamination of the wound.
9. **Position the sterile staple remover under the staple to be removed. Firmly close the staple remover. The staple will bend in the middle and the edges will pull up out of the skin.**	Correct use of staple remover prevents accidental injury to the wound and contamination of the incision area and resulting infection.
10. Remove every other staple to be sure the wound edges are healed. If they are, remove the remaining staples as ordered. Dispose of staples in the sharps container.	Removing every other staple allows for inspection of the wound, while leaving an adequate number of staples in place to promote continued healing if the edges are not totally approximated.
11. Apply Steri-Strips according to facility policy or physician's order. Prepare skin with tincture of benzoin if indicated.	Steri-Strips provide additional support to the wound as it continues to heal. Applying benzoin helps to ensure adherence of Steri-Strips.
12. Reapply the dressing, depending on the physician's orders and facility policy.	A dressing protects the wound.
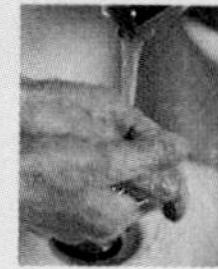 13. Remove gloves and perform hand hygiene.	Removing gloves and performing hand hygiene prevent the spread of microorganisms.

EVALUATION

The expected outcome is met when the patient exhibits a wound that is clean, dry, and intact with the staples removed. Additionally, the patient's wound is free of contamination and trauma. Other outcomes are met when the patient verbalizes little to no pain or discomfort during the removal and states positive aspects about self.

DOCUMENTATION

Guidelines

Document a description of the condition of the incision and the staples, noting whether the edges are approximated or there is any presence of erythema. Also note if there is any drainage and the color and amount of the drainage. Include any subjective comments offered by the patient, such as pain or itchiness. Include in the documentation note the name of the individual who removed the staples. Describe any interventions that were performed related to the incision, such as cleansing with normal saline or application of Steri-Strips or gauze dressings. Document the patient's reaction to the procedure and patient-teaching information.

Sample Documentation

10/3/09 0930 Patient reports itching and "new stuff coming from my incision." Leg incision examined. Noted to have serosanguineous drainage from proximal 6 cm of the incision. Proximal 6 to 8 cm with erythema and slight opening of wound edges, rest of incision with approximated edges, no erythema or drainage. Staples removed 10/1/09. Dr. Coles notified. Incision cleansed with normal saline solution, dried, Steri-Strips applied to proximal 6 cm of incision, dressed with dry gauze and wrapped with stretch gauze per order.—S. Hoffman, RN

(continued)

SKILL 8-13 Removing Surgical Staples *(continued)*

Unexpected Situations and Associated Interventions

- *The wound edges appear approximated before staple removal but pull apart afterward:* Report your findings to the physician and document the event in the patient's record. Apply Steri-Strips according to facility policy or physician's order.
- *The staples are stuck to the wound because of dried blood or secretions:* Per facility policy or physician's order, apply moist saline compresses to loosen crusts before attempting to remove the staples.

Special Considerations

General Considerations

- Encourage the patient to splint chest and abdominal wounds during activity, such as changing position, ambulation, coughing, and sneezing. This provides increased support for the underlying tissues and can help decrease patient discomfort.

SKILL 8-14 Applying an External Heating Device: Aquathermia Pad and Hot Water Bag

Heat dilates peripheral blood vessels, helping to dissipate heat from the body and increasing blood flow to the area. This increases the supply of oxygen and nutrients to the area and reduces venous congestion. Heat applications accelerate the inflammatory response, promoting healing. Heat is also used to reduce muscle tension, relieve muscle spasm, and relieve joint stiffness. Heat also helps relieve pain. It is used to treat infections, surgical wounds, inflammation, arthritis, joint pain, muscle pain, and chronic pain.

Heat is applied by moist and dry methods. The physician's order should include the type of application, the body area to be treated, the frequency of application, and the length of time for the applications. Water used for heat applications needs to be at the appropriate temperature to avoid skin damage: 115° to 125°F for older children and adults and 105° to 110°F for infants, young children, older adults, and patients with diabetes or those who are unconscious.

Three common types of external heating devices are Aquathermia pads, hot water bags and the newer crushable, microwaveable hot pack. Aquathermia pads are used in healthcare agencies and are safer to use than heating pads. The temperature setting for an Aquathermia pad should not exceed 105° to 109.4°F, depending on facility policy.

Hot water bags and microwaveable packs are easy and inexpensive to use but have several disadvantages. They may leak and pose a danger from burns related to improper use. They are used most often in the home setting.

Equipment

- Hot water bag with cover
- Commercially prepared hot pack with cover
- Water at the appropriate temperature
- Bath thermometer
- Aquathermia pad with electronic unit
- Distilled water
- Cover for the pad, if not part of pad
- Gauze bandage or tape to secure the pad
- Waterproof pad for under the hot water bag or commercially prepared hot pack
- Bath blanket

SKILL 8-14

Applying an External Heating Device: Aquathermia Pad and Hot Water Bag *(continued)*

ASSESSMENT

Assess the situation to determine the appropriateness for the application of heat. Assess the patient's physical and mental status and the condition of the body area to be treated with heat. Confirm the physician's order for heat therapy, including frequency, type of therapy, body area to be treated, and length of time for the application. Check the equipment to be used, including the condition of cords, plugs, and heating elements. Look for fluid leaks. Once the equipment is turned on, make sure there is a consistent distribution of heat and the temperature is within safe limits.

NURSING DIAGNOSIS

Determine the related factors for the nursing diagnoses based on the patient's current status. Nursing diagnoses that may be appropriate or require the use of this skill include:

- Chronic Pain
- Acute Pain
- Impaired Skin Integrity
- Risk for Impaired Skin Integrity
- Delayed Surgical Recovery
- Impaired Tissue Integrity
- Risk for Injury

Many other nursing diagnoses may require the use of this skill.

OUTCOME IDENTIFICATION AND PLANNING

The expected outcome to achieve when applying an external heat source depends on the patient's nursing diagnosis. Outcomes that may be appropriate include the following: the patient experiences increased comfort; the patient experiences decreased muscle spasms; the patient exhibits improved wound healing; the patient demonstrates a reduction in inflammation; and the patient remains free of injury.

IMPLEMENTATION

ACTION	RATIONALE
1. Review the physician's order for the application of heat therapy, including frequency, type of therapy, body area to be treated, and length of time for the application.	Reviewing the order validates the correct patient and correct procedure.
2. Gather the necessary supplies.	Preparation promotes efficient time management and provides an organized approach to the task.
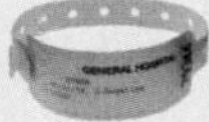 3. Identify the patient.	This ensures the right patient receives the right intervention.
4. Explain the procedure.	Discussion and explanation help allay anxiety, encourage patient cooperation, and prepare the patient for what to expect.
5. Assess the condition of the skin where the heat is to be applied.	Assessment supplies baseline data for posttreatment comparison and identifies conditions that may contraindicate the application.
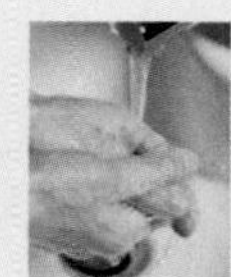 6. Perform hand hygiene.	Hand hygiene prevents the spread of microorganisms.

(continued)

SKILL 8-14

Applying an External Heating Device: Aquathermia Pad and Hot Water Bag *(continued)*

ACTION	RATIONALE
7. Close the room door or curtains. Place the bed at a comfortable working height.	Closing door or curtains provides privacy. Proper bed positioning helps reduce back strain while you are performing the procedure.
8. Assist the patient to a comfortable position that provides easy access to the area to be treated. Expose the area and drape the patient with a bath blanket if needed. Put a waterproof pad under the wound area to protect the bed, if necessary.	Patient positioning and use of a bath blanket provide for comfort and warmth. Waterproof pad protects the patient and the bed linens.
9. Check that the water is at the appropriate level. Fill the control unit two-thirds full with distilled water, or to the fill mark, if necessary. Check the temperature setting on the unit to ensure it is within the safe range	Tap water leaves mineral deposits in the unit. Checking the temperature setting helps to prevent skin or tissue damage.
10. Check for leaks and tilt the unit in several directions.	This action clears the pad's tubing of air.
11. Plug in the unit and warm the pad before use. Cover the pad with an absorbent cloth. Apply the heat source to the prescribed area. Secure with gauze bandage or tape.	Plugging in the pad readies it for use. Cover protects the skin from direct contact with the bag. Heat travels by conduction from one object to another. Gauze bandage or tape holds the pad in position; do not use pins, as they may puncture and damage the pad.
12. **Assess the condition of the skin and the patient's response to the heat at frequent intervals, according to facility policy. Do not exceed the prescribed length of time for the application of heat.**	Maximum vasodilatory therapeutic effects from the application of heat occur within 20 to 30 minutes. Using heat for more than 45 minutes results in tissue congestion and vasoconstriction, known as the rebound phenomenon. Also, prolonged heat application may result in an increased risk of burns.
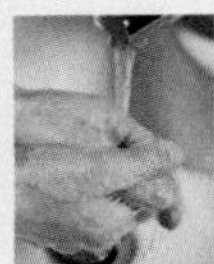 13. Remove after the prescribed amount of time. Perform hand hygiene.	Removal reduces risk of injury. Hand hygiene prevents spread of microorganisms.

EVALUATION

The expected outcome is met when the patient exhibits increased comfort, decreased muscle spasm, less pain, improved wound healing, or decreased inflammation. In addition, the patient remains free of injury.

DOCUMENTATION

Guidelines

Document the rationale for application of heat therapy. If patient is receiving heat therapy for pain, ask the patient to rate the pain on a scale of 1 to 10, with 10 being the greatest pain. Specify the type of heat therapy and location where it is being applied, as well as length of time. Record the condition of the skin, noting any redness or irritation before the heat application and after the application. Document the patient's reaction to the heat therapy. Include an assessment of pain if heat provided for the purpose of decreasing pain. Record any appropriate patient or family education.

SKILL 8-14 Applying an External Heating Device: Aquathermia Pad and Hot Water Bag *(continued)*

Sample Documentation

9/13/09 2300 Patient complaining of pain, rating it 5 out of 10. Aquathermia pad applied to patient's lower back for 30 minutes; now rating pain as 2 out of 10. Skin without signs of redness or irritation before and after application.—M. Martinez, RN

Unexpected Situations and Associated Interventions

- *When performing your periodic assessment of the site during the application of heat, you note excessive swelling and redness at the site and the patient complains of pain that was not present before applying the heat:* Remove the hot water bag or Aquathermia pad. Assess the patient for other symptoms and obtain vital signs. Report your findings to the physician and document your interventions in the patient's record.
- *When performing your periodic assessment of the site during the application of heat, you note that the hot water bag seems to be significantly cooler:* Refill the hot water bag as necessary to maintain the correct temperature.

Special Considerations

General Considerations

- Direct heat treatment is contraindicated for patients at risk for bleeding, patients with a sprained limb in the acute stage, or patients with a condition associated with acute inflammation. Use cautiously with children and older adults. Patients with diabetes, stroke, spinal cord injury, and peripheral neuropathy are at risk for thermal injury, as are patients with very thin or damaged skin. Be extremely careful when applying to heat-sensitive areas, such as scar tissue and stomas.
- Instruct the patient not to lean or lie directly on the heating device, as this reduces air space and increases the risk of burns.
- Check the water level in the Aquathermia unit periodically. Evaporation may occur. If the unit runs dry, it could become damaged. Refill with distilled water periodically.

Home Care Considerations

- A hot water bag or commercially prepared hot pack may be used in the home to apply heat. If using a hot water bag, fill with hot tap water to warm the bag, then empty it to detect any leaks. Check the temperature of the water with the bath thermometer or test on your inner wrist, adjusting the temperature as ordered (usually 115°–125°F for adults). Checking the temperature ensures that the heat applied is within the acceptable range of temperatures. Fill the bag one-half to two-thirds full. Partial filling keeps the bag lightweight and flexible so that it can be molded to the treatment area. Squeeze the bag until the water reaches the neck; this expels air, which would make the bag inflexible and would reduce heat conduction. Fasten the top, and cover the bag with an absorbent cloth. The covering protects the skin from direct contact with the bag. If using a commercially prepared hot pack, follow manufacturer's directions and carefully assess skin before and after heat application.

SKILL 8-15 Applying a Warm Sterile Compress to an Open Wound

Sterile warm moist compresses are used on wounds to help promote circulation to the wound, encourage wound healing, decrease edema, promote consolidation of wound exudate, and decrease pain and discomfort at the wound site. Moist heat softens crusted material and is less drying to the skin. Moist heat also penetrates tissues more deeply than dry heat.

(continued)

SKILL 8-15 Applying a Warm Sterile Compress to an Open Wound *(continued)*

The heat of a warm compress dissipates quickly, so the compresses must be changed frequently. Applying a layer of plastic over the compress can help retain the heat longer. If a constant warm temperature is required, a heating device such as an Aquathermia pad (refer to Skill 8-14) is applied over the compress. However, because moisture conducts heat, a low temperature setting is needed on the heating device. Many facilities have warming devices to heat the dressing package to an appropriate temperature for the compress. These devices help reduce the risk of burning or skin damage.

Equipment

- Prescribed solution to moisten the compress material, warmed to 105° to 110°F
- Sterile container for solution
- Sterile gauze dressings or compresses
- Sterile gloves
- Clean disposable gloves
- Waterproof pad and bath blanket
- Dry bath towel
- Tape or ties
- Aquathermia or other external heating device, if ordered or required to maintain the temperature of the compress
- Sterile bath thermometer (if available) to check the solution's temperature
- Sterile supplies to replace the wound dressing after the procedure is completed

ASSESSMENT

Assess for circulatory compromise in the area where compress will be applied, including skin color, pulses distal to the site, evidence of edema, and the presence of sensation. Assess the situation to determine the appropriateness for the application of heat. Confirm the physician's order for the compresses, including the solution to be used, frequency, body area to be treated, and length of time for the application. Assess the equipment to be used, if necessary, including the condition of cords, plugs, and heating elements. Look for fluid leaks. Once the equipment is turned on, make sure there is a consistent distribution of heat and the temperature is within safe limits. Assess the application site frequently during the treatment, as tissue damage can occur.

NURSING DIAGNOSIS

Determine the related factors for the nursing diagnoses based on the patient's current status. An appropriate nursing diagnosis is Risk for Injury. Many other nursing diagnoses may be appropriate, including:

- Anxiety
- Disturbed Body Image
- Acute Pain
- Chronic Pain
- Impaired Skin Integrity
- Risk for Impaired Skin Integrity
- Impaired Tissue Integrity
- Deficient Knowledge

OUTCOME IDENTIFICATION AND PLANNING

The expected outcome to achieve when applying warm sterile compresses is that the patient shows signs such as decreased inflammation, decreased muscle spasms, or decreased pain that indicate problems have been relieved. Other outcomes that may be appropriate include: the patient experiences improved wound healing, and the patient remains free from injury.

SKILL 8-15 Applying a Warm Sterile Compress to an Open Wound *(continued)*

IMPLEMENTATION

ACTION	RATIONALE
1. Review the physician's order.	Reviewing the order validates the correct patient and correct procedure.
2. Gather the necessary supplies.	Preparation promotes efficient time management and provides an organized approach to the task.
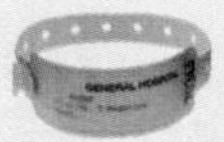 3. Identify the patient.	This ensures the right patient receives the right intervention.
4. Explain the procedure.	Discussion and explanation help allay anxiety, encourage patient cooperation, and prepare the patient for what to expect.
5. Assess the patient for possible need for nonpharmacologic pain-reducing interventions or analgesic medication before wound care dressing change. Administer appropriate analgesic, consulting physician's orders, and allow enough time for analgesic to achieve its effectiveness before beginning procedure.	Pain is a subjective experience influenced by past experience. Wound care and dressing changes may cause pain for some patients.
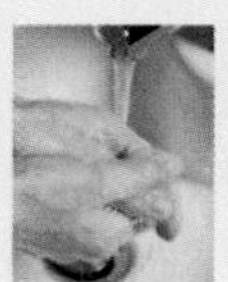 6. Perform hand hygiene.	Hand hygiene prevents the spread of microorganisms.
7. Close the room door or curtains. Place the bed at a comfortable working height.	Closing the door or curtain provides privacy. Proper bed positioning helps reduce back strain while you are providing care.
8. Assist the patient to a comfortable position that provides easy access to the wound area. Expose the area and drape the patient with a bath blanket if needed. Put the waterproof pad under the wound area.	Patient positioning and use of a bath blanket provide for comfort and warmth. Waterproof pad protects the patient and the bed linens.
9. Have the disposal bag or waste receptacle within easy reach for use during the procedure.	Having a waste container handy means that soiled dressings and supplies may be discarded easily, without the spread of microorganisms.
10. Prepare the external heating pad or Aquathermia pad if one is being used.	Having equipment ready provides for an organized approach to the task. The external heating device (Figure 1) allows the compress to retain heat for a longer interval.
11. Using sterile technique, prepare a working field and open all sterile packaging, dressings, and the warmed solution. Pour the solution into the sterile container and drop the sterile gauze for the compress into the solution.	Sterile technique is used for warm moist compresses to an open wound to prevent contamination with microorganisms.
12. Put on clean disposable gloves and remove any old dressing in place. Discard the old dressing in the appropriate receptacle. Remove your gloves and discard them.	Adherence to medical aseptic practices and proper disposal of soiled dressings and supplies prevent the spread of microorganisms.
13. Assess wound site and surrounding tissues. Look for inflammation, drainage, skin color, ecchymosis, and odor.	Assessment provides information about the wound healing process and about the presence of infection and allows for documentation of the condition of the wound before the compress is applied.

(continued)

SKILL 8-15 Applying a Warm Sterile Compress to an Open Wound *(continued)*

ACTION	RATIONALE
	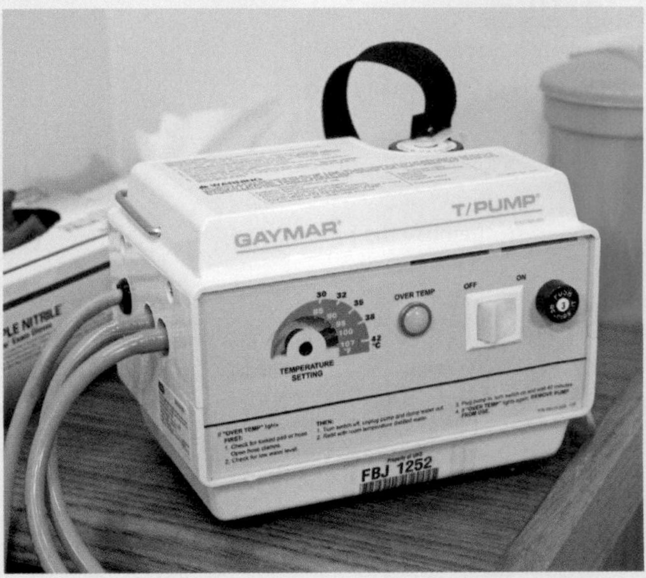 **Figure 1.** External heating device.
14. Put on sterile gloves, following proper procedure.	Use of sterile gloves maintains sterile technique.
15. **Retrieve the sterile compress from the warmed solution, squeezing out any excess moisture (Figure 2). Apply the compress by gently and carefully molding it around the wound site (Figure 3). Ask patient if the application feels too hot.**	Excess moisture may contaminate the surrounding area and is uncomfortable for the patient. Molding the compress to the skin promotes retention of warmth around the site.
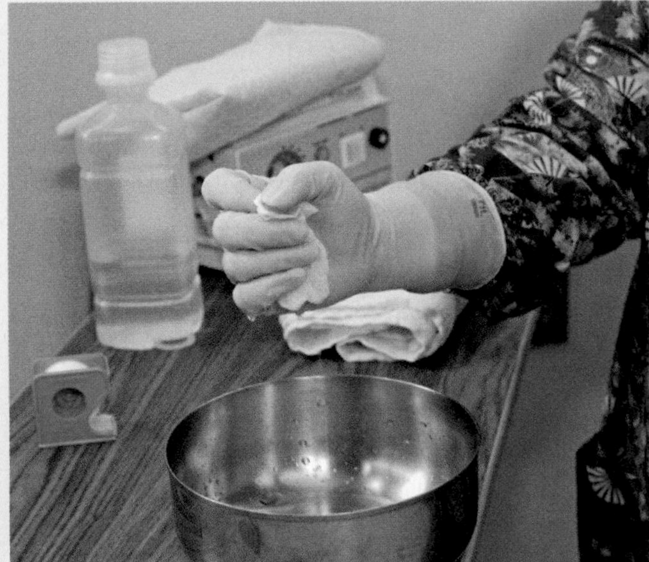 **Figure 2.** Squeezing excess solution out of a dressing.	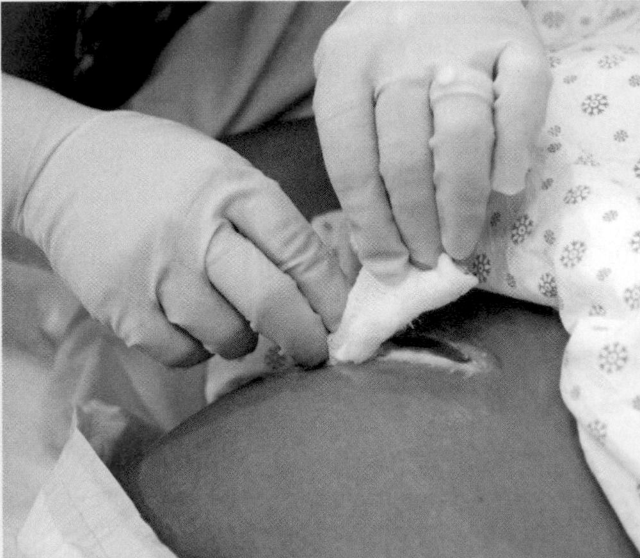 **Figure 3.** Molding moist gauze around the wound.
16. **Cover the site with a single layer of gauze and with a clean dry bath towel;** secure in place if necessary (Figure 4).	Towel provides extra insulation.

SKILL 8-15 Applying a Warm Sterile Compress to an Open Wound *(continued)*

ACTION	RATIONALE
17. Place the Aquathermia or heating device, if used, over the towel (Figure 5).	Use of heating device maintains the temperature of the compress and extends the therapeutic effect.

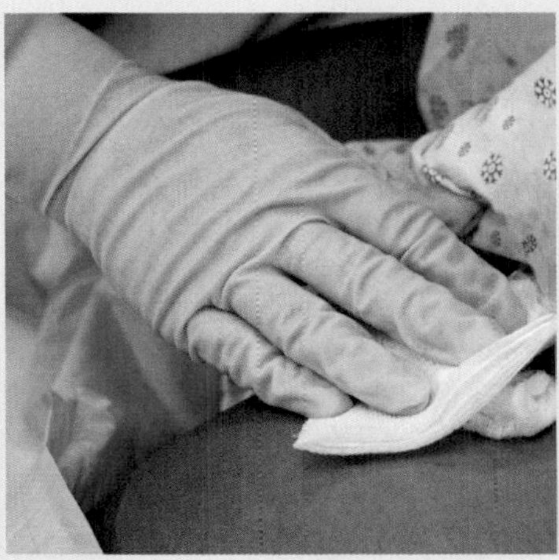

Figure 4. Applying single layer of gauze.

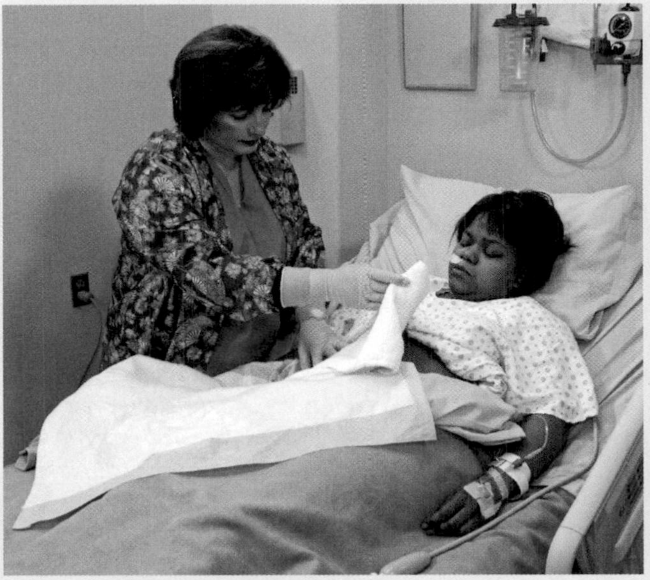

Figure 5. Applying external heating device.

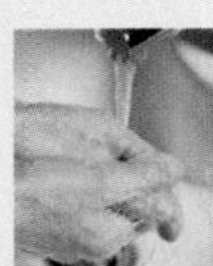

ACTION	RATIONALE
18. Remove sterile gloves and discard them appropriately. Perform hand hygiene.	Hand hygiene prevents the spread of microorganisms.
19. **Monitor the time the compress is in place to prevent burns or skin damage. Monitor the condition of the patient's skin and the patient's response at frequent intervals.**	Extended use of heat results in an increased risk for burns from the heat. Impaired circulation may affect the patient's sensitivity to heat.
20. After the prescribed time for the treatment (up to 30 minutes), remove the external heating device (if used) and put on sterile gloves.	Use of sterile gloves helps to maintain sterile technique.
21. Carefully remove the compress while assessing the skin condition around the wound site and observing the patient's response to the heat application. Note any wound changes.	Assessment provides information about the wound healing process; the presence of irritation or infection should be documented.
22. Apply a new dry sterile dressing to the wound, following proper procedure.	Dressing provides protection for the wound.
23. Remove gloves. Place the patient in a comfortable position. Lower the bed. Dispose of any other supplies appropriately.	Repositioning promotes patient comfort and safety.
24. Perform hand hygiene.	Hand hygiene prevents spread of microorganisms.

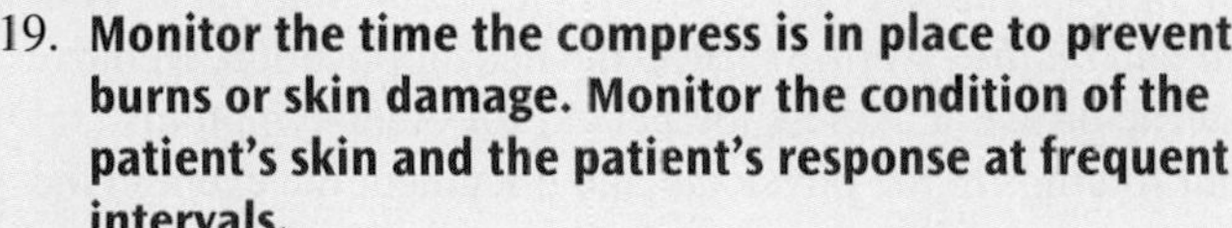

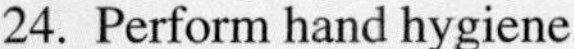

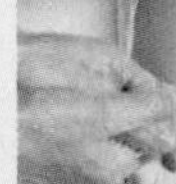

(continued)

SKILL 8-15 Applying a Warm Sterile Compress to an Open Wound *(continued)*

EVALUATION

The expected outcome is met when the patient reports relief of symptoms, such as decreased inflammation, pain, or muscle spasms. In addition, the patient remains free of signs and symptoms of injury.

DOCUMENTATION

Guidelines

Document the procedure, the length of time the compress was applied, including use of an Aquathermia pad. Record the temperature of the Aquathermia pad and length of application time. Include a description of the wound, noting any edema, redness, or drainage, as well as the surrounding skin. Record that the wound was redressed. Document the patient's reaction to the procedure including pain assessment. Record any patient and family education that was provided.

Sample Documentation

7/6/08 0900 Left forearm with positive radial pulse, sensation and movement within normal limits, skin pale with brisk capillary refill. Wound dressing removed from left forearm. Wound 2 × 2 × 2 cm on dorsal aspect, red, scant purulent drainage, surrounding area red, with edema, no evidence of maceration. Moist saline compress applied with Aquathermia pad set at 100° F for 30 min. Site assessed every 10 min; no evidence of injury noted. Wound redressed and wrapped with stretch gauze. Left arm elevated on pillows.—S. Tran, RN

Unexpected Situations and Associated Interventions

- *You are monitoring a patient with a warm compress applied to a wound. Procedure requires that you check the area of application every 5 minutes for tissue tolerance. You note excessive redness and slight maceration of the surrounding skin, and the patient verbalizes increased discomfort:* Stop the heat application. Remove the compress. Apply a new sterile dressing. Assess the patient for other symptoms. Obtain vital signs. Report your findings to the physician and document the event in the patient's record.
- *You are monitoring a patient with a warm compress applied to a wound. Procedure requires that you check the area of application every 5 minutes for tissue tolerance. You note bleeding from the wound and on the compress:* Stop the heat application. Remove the compress. Apply a new sterile dressing. Assess the patient for other symptoms. Obtain vital signs. Report your findings to the physician and document the event in the patient's record.

Special Considerations

General Considerations

- Patients with diabetes, stroke, spinal cord injury, and peripheral neuropathy are at risk for thermal injury, as are patients with very thin or damaged skin.
- Be extremely careful when applying to heat-sensitive areas, such as scar tissue and stomas.

SKILL 8-16 Assisting With a Sitz Bath

A sitz bath can help relieve pain and discomfort in the perineal area, such as after child-birth or surgery and can increase circulation to the tissues, promoting healing.

Equipment

- Clean disposable gloves
- Towel
- Disposable sitz bath bowl with water bag

ASSESSMENT

Review any orders related to the sitz bath. Determine patient's ability to ambulate to the bathroom and maintain sitting position for 15 to 20 minutes. Prior to the sitz bath, inspect perineal/rectal area for swelling, drainage, redness, warmth, and tenderness. Assess bladder fullness and encourage patient to void before sitz bath.

NURSING DIAGNOSIS

Determine related factors for the nursing diagnosis based on the patient's current status. Possible nursing diagnoses may include:

- Acute Pain
- Risk for Hypothermia
- Risk for Infection
- Impaired Tissue Integrity

OUTCOME IDENTIFICATION AND PLANNING

The expected outcome to achieve when administering a sitz bath is that the patient states an increase in comfort. Other outcomes that may be appropriate include the following: the patient experiences a decrease in healing time, maintains normal body temperature, remains free of any signs and symptoms of infection, and exhibits signs and symptoms of healing.

IMPLEMENTATION

ACTION	RATIONALE
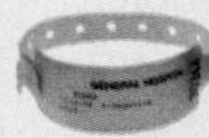 1. Identify the patient.	Positive identification of the patient is essential to ensure the intervention is administered to the correct patient.
2. Explain what you are going to do.	Explanation relieves anxiety and facilitates cooperation.
3. Close curtains around bed and close door to room if possible.	This ensures the patient's privacy.
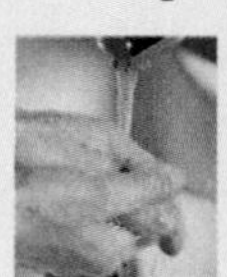 4. Perform hand hygiene and put on clean gloves.	Hand hygiene deters the spread of microorganisms. Gloves prevent exposure to blood and body fluids.
5. Assemble equipment in bathroom.	Organization facilitates performance of task.

(continued)

SKILL 8-16 Assisting With a Sitz Bath *(continued)*

ACTION	RATIONALE
6. Raise lid of toilet. Place bowl of sitz bath, with drainage ports to rear and infusion port in front, in the toilet (Figure 1). Fill bowl of sitz bath about halfway full with tepid to warm water (37°–46°C [98°–115°F]).	Sitz bath will not drain appropriately if placed in toilet backwards. Tepid water can promote relaxation and help with edema; warm water can help with circulation.

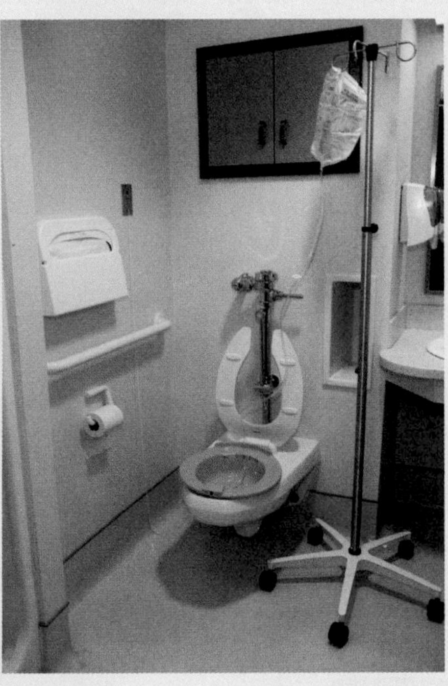

Figure 1. Disposable sitz bath.

ACTION	RATIONALE
7. Clamp tubing on bag. Fill bag with same temperature water as mentioned above. Hang bag above patient's shoulder height on hook or IV pole.	If bag is hung lower, the rate of flow will not be sufficient and water may cool too quickly.
8. Assist patient to sit on toilet and provide any extra draping if needed. Insert tubing into infusion port of sitz bath. Slowly unclamp tubing and allow sitz bath to fill.	If tubing is placed into sitz bath before patient sits on toilet, patient may trip over tubing. Filling the sitz bath ensures that the tissue is submerged in water.
9. Clamp tubing once sitz bath is full. Instruct patient to open clamp when water in bowl becomes cool. **Ensure that call bell is within reach. Instruct patient to call if she feels light-headed or dizzy or has any problems. Instruct patient not to try standing without assistance.**	Cool water may produce hypothermia. Patient may become light-headed due to vasodilation, so call bell should be within reach.
10. When patient is finished (in about 15–20 minutes), help patient stand and gently pat perineal area dry. Assist patient to bed or chair. Ensure that call bell is within reach.	Patient may be light-headed and dizzy due to vasodilation. Patient should not stand alone, and bending over to dry self may cause patient to fall.
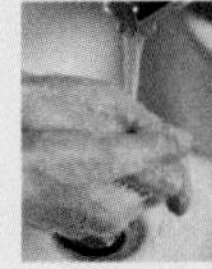 11. Empty and disinfect sitz bath bowl according to agency policy. Remove gloves and perform hand hygiene.	Proper equipment cleaning and hand hygiene deter the spread of microorganisms.

SKILL 8-16 Assisting With a Sitz Bath *(continued)*

EVALUATION

The expected outcomes are met when the patient verbalizes a decrease in pain or discomfort, patient tolerates sitz bath without incident, area remains clean and dry, and patient demonstrates signs of healing.

DOCUMENTATION

Guidelines

Document administration of the sitz bath, including water temperature and duration. Document patient response, and assessment of perineum before and after administration.

Sample Documentation

7/30/09 1620 Perineum assessed. Episiotomy mediolateral; edges well approximated, no drainage noted. Patient assisted to sitz bath. Patient took warm water sitz bath (temperature 99° F) for 20 minutes. Denies feeling light-headed or dizzy. Assisted back to bed after bath. Patient states pain level has dropped "from a 5 to a 2."
—C. Stone, RN

Unexpected Situations and Associated Interventions

- *Patient complains of feeling light-headed or dizzy during sitz bath:* Stop sitz bath. Do not attempt to ambulate patient by self. Use call light to summon help. Let patient sit on toilet with face up until feeling subsides or help has arrived to assist patient back to bed.
- *Temperature of water is uncomfortable:* The water may be too warm or cold, depending on the patient's preference. If this happens, clamp the tubing, disconnect the water bag, and refill it with water that is comfortable for the patient, but no warmer than 115°F (46°C).

SKILL 8-17 Using a Cooling Blanket

A cooling blanket, or hypothermia pad, is a blanket-sized Aquathermia pad that conducts a cooled solution, usually distilled water, through coils in a rubber or plastic blanket or pad (Figure 1). Placing a patient on a hypothermia blanket or pad helps to lower body temperature. The nurse monitors the patient's body temperature and can reset the blanket setting accordingly. The blanket also may be preset to maintain a specific body temperature; the

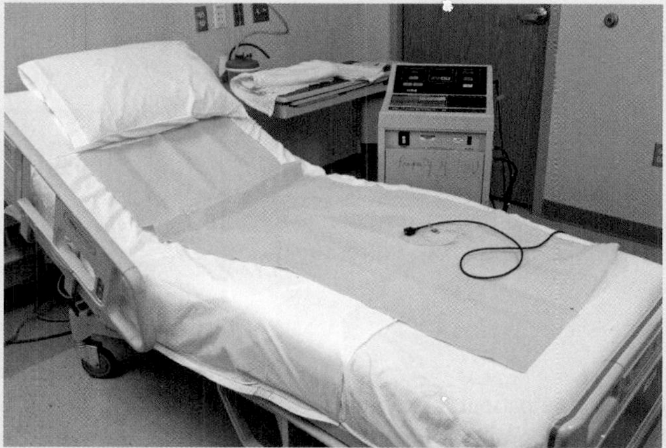

Figure 1. Hypothermia blanket.

(continued)

SKILL 8-17 Using a Cooling Blanket *(continued)*

device continually monitors the patient's body temperature using a temperature probe (which is inserted rectally or in the esophagus, or placed on the skin) and adjusts the temperature of the circulating liquid accordingly.

Equipment

- Disposable cooling blanket or pad
- Control panel
- Distilled water to fill the device, if necessary
- Thermometer, if needed to monitor the patient's temperature
- Sphygmomanometer
- Stethoscope
- Temperature probe, if needed
- Thin blanket or sheet
- Towels
- Disposable clean gloves

ASSESSMENT

Assess the patient's condition, including current body temperature, to determine the need for the cooling blanket. Consider alternative measures to help lower the patient's body temperature before implementing the blanket. Also verify the physician's order for the application of a hypothermia blanket. Assess the patient's vital signs, neurologic status, peripheral circulation, and skin integrity. Assess the equipment to be used, including the condition of cords, plugs, and cooling elements. Look for fluid leaks. Once the equipment is turned on, make sure there is a consistent distribution of cooling.

NURSING DIAGNOSIS

Determine the related factors for the nursing diagnoses based on the patient's current status. Appropriated nursing diagnoses may include:

- Hyperthermia
- Risk for Injury
- Deficient Knowledge
- Risk for Impaired Skin Integrity
- Ineffective Thermoregulation
- Acute Pain

OUTCOME IDENTIFICATION AND PLANNING

The expected outcome to achieve when using a hypothermia blanket is that the patient maintains a normal body temperature. Other outcomes that may be appropriate include: the patient does not experience shivering; the patient's vital signs are within normal limits; and the patient does not experience alterations in skin integrity.

IMPLEMENTATION

ACTION	RATIONALE
1. Review the physician's order for the application of the hypothermia blanket. Obtain consent for the therapy per facility policy.	Reviewing the order validates the correct patient and correct procedure.
2. Gather the necessary supplies.	Preparation promotes efficient time management and provides an organized approach to the task.
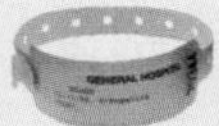 3. Identify the patient. Determine if the patient has had any previous adverse reaction to hypothermia therapy.	This ensures the right patient receives the right intervention. Individual differences exist in tolerating specific therapies.

SKILL 8-17 Using a Cooling Blanket *(continued)*

ACTION	RATIONALE
4. Explain the procedure.	Discussion and explanation help allay anxiety, encourage cooperation, and prepare the patient for what to expect.
5. Assess the patient's vital signs, neurologic status, peripheral circulation, and skin integrity.	Assessment supplies baseline data for comparison during therapy and identifies conditions that may contraindicate the application.
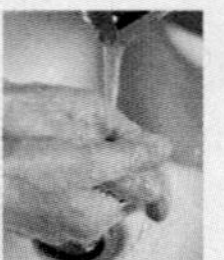 6. Perform hand hygiene.	Hand hygiene prevents the spread of microorganisms.
7. Close the room door or curtains. Place the bed at a comfortable working height.	Closing the room or curtains provides privacy. Proper bed positioning helps reduce back strain while you are performing the procedure.
8. Make sure the patient's gown has cloth ties, not snaps or pins.	Cloth ties minimize the risk of cold injury.
9. Apply lanolin or a mixture of lanolin and cold cream to the patient's skin where it will be in contact with the blanket.	These agents help protect the skin from cold.
10. Turn on the blanket and make sure the cooling light is on. Verify that the temperature limits are set within the desired safety range (Figure 2).	Turning on the blanket prepares it for use. Keeping temperature within the safety range prevents excessive cooling.
11. Cover the hypothermia blanket with a thin sheet or bath blanket.	A sheet or blanket protects the patient's skin from direct contact with the cooling surface, reducing the risk for injury.
12. Position the blanket under the patient so that the top edge of the pad is aligned with the patient's neck (Figure 3).	The blanket's rigid surface may be uncomfortable. The cold may lead to tissue breakdown.

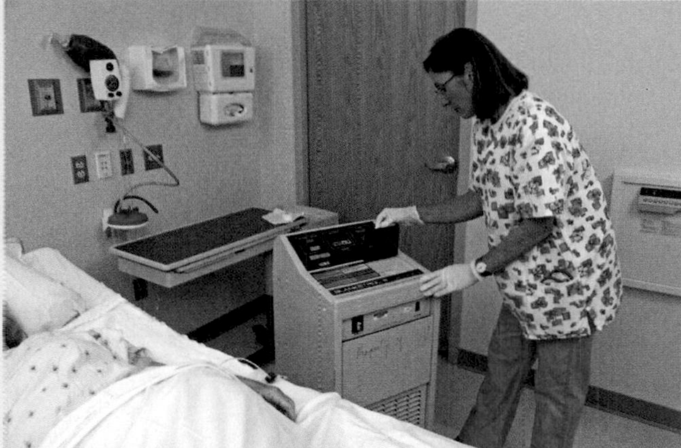

Figure 2. Checking the settings on the cooling blanket control unit and turning it on.

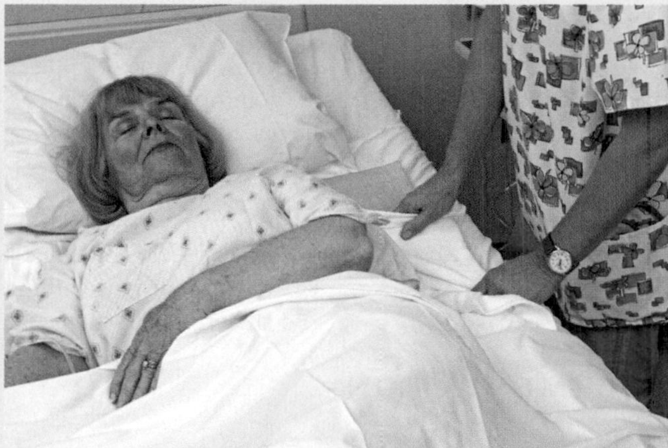

Figure 3. Aligning cooling blanket on bed.

(continued)

SKILL 8-17 Using a Cooling Blanket *(continued)*

ACTION	RATIONALE
13. Put on gloves. Lubricate the rectal probe and insert it into the patient's rectum unless contraindicated. Or tuck the skin probe deep into the patient's axilla and tape it in place. For patients who are comatose or anesthetized, use an esophageal probe. Attach the probe to the control panel for the blanket.	The probe allows continuous monitoring of the patient's core body temperature. Rectal insertion may be contraindicated in patients with a low white blood cell count or platelet count.
14. Wrap the patient's hands and feet in gauze if ordered, or if the patient desires. **For male patients, elevate the scrotum off the cooling blanket with towels.**	These actions minimize chilling, promote comfort, and protect sensitive tissues from direct contact with cold.
15. Recheck the thermometer and settings on the control panel.	Rechecking verifies that the blanket temperature is maintained at a safe level.
16. Remove gloves and perform hand hygiene.	Hand hygiene prevents spread of microorganisms.
17. **Turn and position the patient regularly (every 30 minutes to 1 hour).** Keep linens free from condensation. Reapply cream as needed. Observe the patient's skin for change in color, changes in lips and nail beds, edema, pain, and sensory impairment.	Turning and repositioning prevent alterations in skin integrity and provide for assessment of potential skin injuries.
18. **Monitor vital signs and perform a neurologic assessment per facility policy, usually every 15 minutes, until the body temperature is stable.**	Continuous monitoring provides evaluation of the patient's response to the therapy and permits early identification and intervention if adverse effects occur.
19. Observe for signs of shivering, including verbalized sensations, facial muscle twitching, hyperventilation, or twitching of extremities.	Shivering increases heat production.
20. Assess the patient's level of comfort.	Hypothermia therapy can cause discomfort. Prompt assessment and action can prevent injuries.
21. Turn off blanket according to facility policy, usually when the patient's body temperature reaches 1° above the desired temperature. Continue to monitor the patient's temperature until it stabilizes.	Body temperature can continue to fall after this therapy.
22. Document assessments, vital signs, and time of initiation of therapy. Document the control settings, the duration of treatment, and the patient's response.	Documentation promotes continuity of care and communication.

EVALUATION

The expected outcome is met when the patient exhibits a stable body temperature and other vital signs within acceptable parameters. In addition, the patient remains free from shivering, and the patient's skin is pink, clean, warm, and dry, without evidence of injury.

DOCUMENTATION

Guidelines

Document assessments such as vital signs, neurologic, peripheral circulation, and skin integrity status before use of hypothermia blanket. Record verification of physician's order and that the procedure was explained to the patient. Document the control settings, the length of the treatment, and the route of the temperature monitoring. Include the application of lanolin cream to skin as well as the frequency of position changes. Document the patient's response to the therapy using agency flow sheet, especially noting decrease in

SKILL 8-17 Using a Cooling Blanket *(continued)*

temperature and discomfort assessment. Record the possible use of medication to reduce shivering or other discomforts. Include any pertinent patient and family teaching.

Sample Documentation

11/10/08 1800 Patient's temp 106° F, pulse 122, respirations 24, BP 118/72. Dr. Fenter notified. Order received for application of cooling blanket. Procedure explained to patient. Lanolin applied to skin, bath sheet applied between blanket and patient, axillary probe applied, cooling blanket setting 99° F per order. Vital signs and skin assessment every 30 min; see flow sheet.—J. Lee, RN

11/10/08 1930 Patient reports chills and shivering. Temp 100° F, pulse 104, respirations 20, BP 114/68. Dr. Fenter notified. Cooling blanket discontinued per order.—J. Lee, RN

Unexpected Situations and Associated Interventions

- *The patient states he is cold and has chills. You observe shivering of his extremities:* Obtain vital signs. Assess for other symptoms. Increase the blanket temperature to a more comfortable range. Administer tranquilizers as ordered. If shivering persists or is excessive, discontinue the therapy. Notify the physician of your findings and document the event in the patient's record.
- *When performing a skin assessment during therapy, you note increased pallor on pressure points and sluggish capillary refill. The patient reports alterations in sensation on these points:* Discontinue therapy, obtain vital signs, assess for other symptoms, notify the physician, and document the event in the patient's record.

Special Considerations

- The patient may experience a secondary defense reaction, vasodilation, that causes body temperature to rebound, defeating the purpose of the therapy.

Older Adult Considerations

- Older adults are more at risk for skin and tissue damage because of their thin skin, loss of cold sensation, decreased subcutaneous tissue, and changes in the body's ability to regulate temperature. Check these patients more frequently during therapy.

SKILL 8-18 Applying Cold Therapy

Cold constricts the peripheral blood vessels, reducing blood flow to the tissues and decreasing the local release of pain-producing substances. Cold reduces the formation of edema and inflammation, reduces muscle spasm, and promotes comfort by slowing the transmission of pain stimuli. The application of cold therapy reduces bleeding and hematoma formation. The application of cold, using ice, is appropriate after direct trauma, for dental pain, for muscle spasms, after muscle sprains, and for the treatment of chronic pain. Ice can be used to apply cold therapy, usually in the form of an ice bag or ice collar, or in a glove. Commercially prepared cold packs are also available. For electronically-controlled cooling devices, see the accompanying Skill Variation.

Equipment

- Ice
- Ice bag, ice collar, glove
- Commercially prepared cold packs
- Small towel or washcloth
- Clean disposable gloves
- Disposable waterproof pad

(continued)

SKILL 8-18 Applying Cold Therapy *(continued)*

- Gauze wrap or tape
- Bath blanket

ASSESSMENT

Assess the situation to determine the appropriateness for the application of cold therapy. Assess the patient's physical and mental status and the condition of the body area to be treated with the cold therapy. Confirm the physician's order, including frequency, type of therapy, body area to be treated, and length of time for the application. Assess the equipment to be used to make sure it will function properly.

NURSING DIAGNOSIS

Determine the related factors for the nursing diagnoses based on the patient's current status. An appropriate nursing diagnosis is Acute Pain. Other nursing diagnoses that may be appropriate or require the use of this skill include:

- Impaired Skin Integrity
- Chronic Pain
- Ineffective Tissue Perfusion
- Delayed Surgical Recovery

OUTCOME IDENTIFICATION AND PLANNING

The expected outcome to achieve when applying an external cold source depends on the patient's nursing diagnosis. Outcomes that may be appropriate include the following: the patient experiences increased comfort; the patient experiences decreased muscle spasms; the patient experiences decreased inflammation; and the patient does not show signs of bleeding or hematoma at the treatment site.

IMPLEMENTATION

ACTION	RATIONALE
1. Review the physician's order for the application of cold therapy, including frequency, type of therapy, body area to be treated, and length of time for the application.	Reviewing the order validates the correct patient and correct procedure.
2. Gather the necessary supplies.	Preparation promotes efficient time management and provides an organized approach to the task.
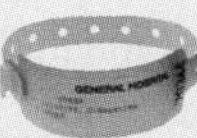 3. Identify the patient. Determine if the patient has had any previous adverse reaction to cold therapy.	This ensures the right patient receives the right intervention. Individual differences exist in tolerating specific therapies.
4. Explain the procedure.	Discussion and explanation help allay anxiety, encourage cooperation, and prepare the patient for what to expect.
5. Assess the condition of the skin where the ice is to be applied.	Assessment supplies baseline data for posttreatment comparison and identifies any conditions that may contraindicate the application.
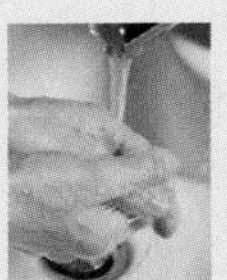 6. Perform hand hygiene.	Hand hygiene prevents the spread of microorganisms.
7. Close the room door or curtains. Place the bed at a comfortable working height.	Closing the door or curtain provides privacy. Proper bed positioning helps reduce back strain while you perform the procedure.

SKILL 8-18 Applying Cold Therapy *(continued)*

ACTION	RATIONALE
8. Assist the patient to a comfortable position that provides easy access to the area to be treated. Expose the area and drape the patient with a bath blanket if needed. Put the waterproof pad under the wound area, if necessary.	Patient positioning and use of a bath blanket provide for comfort and warmth. Waterproof pad protects the patient and the bed linens.
9. Prepare device:	
Fill the bag, collar, or glove about three-fourths full with ice (Figure 1). **Remove any excess air from the device.** Securely fasten the end of the bag or collar; tie the glove closed, checking for holes and leakage of water.	Ice provides a cold surface. Excess air interferes with cold conduction. Fastening the end prevents leaks.
Prepare commercially prepared ice pack if appropriate.	

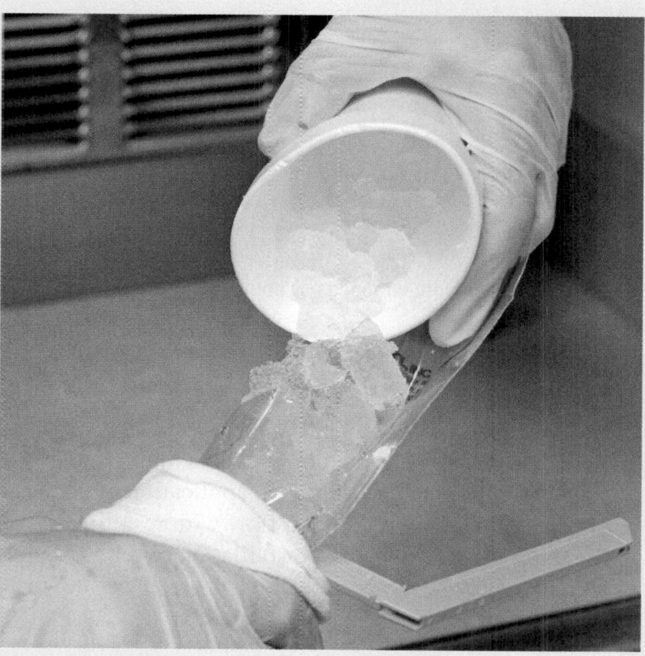

Figure 1. Filling ice bag with ice.

ACTION	RATIONALE
10. **Cover the device with a towel or washcloth (Figure 2).** (If the device has a cloth exterior, this is not necessary.)	The cover protects the skin and absorbs condensation.
11. Put on gloves. Position cooling device on top of dressing and lightly secure in place as needed.	Use of gloves and leaving the dressing in place prevents the spread of microorganisms. Proper positioning ensures the cold therapy to the specific area of the body.
12. **Remove the ice and assess the site for redness after 30 seconds. Ask the patient about the presence of burning sensations.**	These actions prevent burn injury.
13. Replace the device snugly against the site if no problems are evident. Secure it in place with gauze wrap or tape (Figure 3).	Wrapping or taping stabilizes the device in the proper location.

(continued)

SKILL 8-18 Applying Cold Therapy *(continued)*

ACTION	RATIONALE
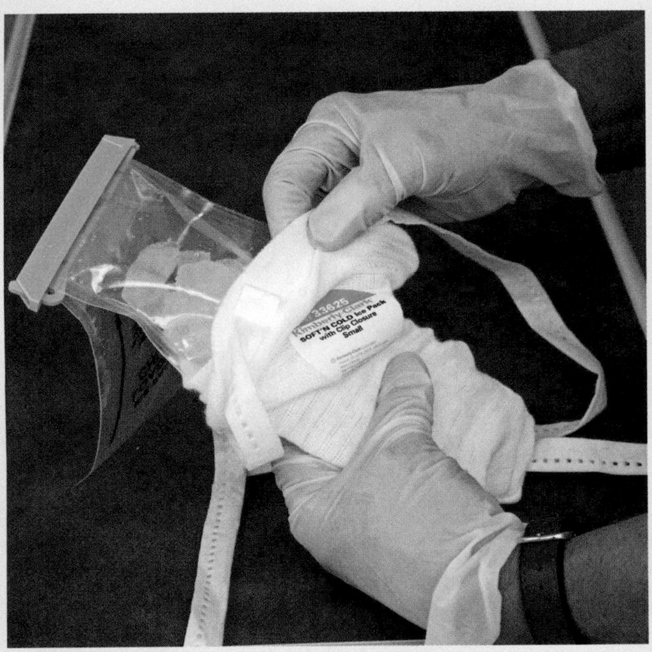 **Figure 2.** Wrapping ice bag with cloth.	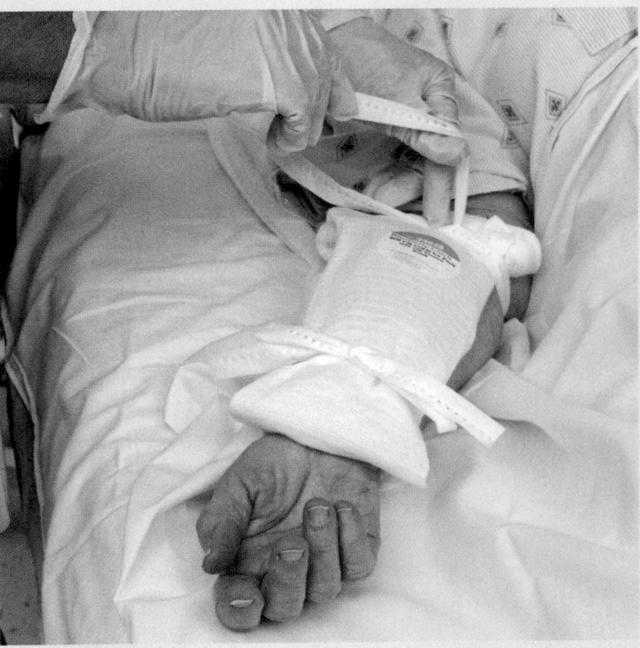 **Figure 3.** Applying cloth-wrapped bag and securing with gauze.
14. Reassess the treatment area every 5 minutes or according to facility policy.	Assessment of the patient's skin is necessary for early detection of adverse effects, thereby allowing prompt intervention to avoid complications.
15. **After 20 minutes or the prescribed amount of time, remove the ice and dry the skin.**	Limiting the time of application prevents injury due to overexposure to cold. Prolonged application of cold may result in decreased blood flow with resulting tissue ischemia. A compensatory vasodilation or rebound phenomenon may occur as a means to provide warmth to the area.
16. Apply a new dressing to site, if necessary.	Dressing provides protection to the skin.
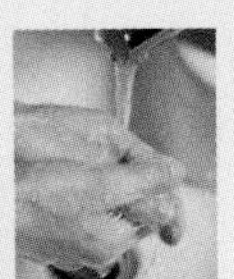 17. Perform hand hygiene.	Hand hygiene prevents spread of microorganisms.

EVALUATION

The expected outcome is met when the patient reports a relief of pain and increased comfort. Other outcomes that may be appropriate include: the patient verbalizes a decrease in muscle spasms; the patient exhibits a reduction in inflammation; and the patient remains free of any injury, including signs of bleeding or hematoma at the treatment site.

DOCUMENTATION

Guidelines

Document the procedure, the patient's response, and your assessment of the area before and after the cold application. Record the assessment of the area where the cold therapy was applied, noting the patient's mobility, sensation, color, temperature, and any presence

SKILL 8-18 **Applying Cold Therapy** *(continued)*

of numbness, tingling, or pain. Include that the cold pack was covered with cloth and the duration of the treatment. Document the patient's response, such as any decrease in pain or change in sensation. Include any pertinent patient and family education.

Sample Documentation

11/1/08 1430 Swelling noted on right lower extremity from mid-calf to foot. Toes warm, pink, positive sensation and movement, negative for numbness, tingling, and pain. Ice bags wrapped in cloth applied to right ankle and lower calf. Patient instructed to communicate any changes in sensation or pain; verbalizes an understanding of information.—L. Semet, RN

Unexpected Situations and Associated Interventions

- *When performing a skin assessment during therapy, you note increased pallor at the treatment site and sluggish capillary refill, and the patient reports alterations in sensation at the application site:* Discontinue therapy, obtain vital signs, assess for other symptoms, notify the physician, and document the event in the patient's record.

Special Considerations

General Considerations

- The patient may experience a secondary defense reaction, vasodilation, that causes body temperature to rebound, defeating the purpose of the therapy.

Older Adult Considerations

- Older adults are more at risk for skin and tissue damage because of their thin skin, loss of cold sensation, decreased subcutaneous tissue, and changes in the body's ability to regulate temperature. Check these patients more frequently during therapy.

SKILL VARIATION Applying an Electronically-Controlled Cooling Device

Electronically controlled cooling devices are used in situations to deliver a constant cooling effect. Postoperative orthopedic patients as well as other patients with acute musculoskeletal injuries may benefit from this therapy. A physician's order is required for use of this device. Initial assessment of the extremity is involved, as well as ongoing assessment throughout the period of use. As with application of any electronic device, ongoing monitoring for proper functioning and temperature regulation is necessary.

- Gather equipment and verify the physician's order.
- Identify the patient and explain the procedure.
- Perform hand hygiene.
- Assess the involved extremity or body part.
- Set the correct temperature on the device.
- Wrap the cooling water-flow pad around the involved body part.
- Wrap Ace bandage or gauze pads around the water-flow pads.
- Assess to ensure that the cooling pads are functioning properly.
- Recheck frequently to ensure proper functioning of equipment.
- Unwrap at intervals to assess skin integrity of the body part.

The Taylor Suite offers these additional resources to enhance learning and facilitate understanding of this chapter:

- thePoint online resource, http://thepoint.lww.com/Lynn2E
- Student CD-ROM included with the book
- Skills Checklist to Accompany Taylor's Clinical Nursing Skills
- Taylor's Interactive Nursing: *Skin Integrity and Wound Care*
- Taylor's Video Guide to Clinical Nursing Skills: *Skin Integrity and Wound Care*

Developing Critical Thinking Skills

1. While providing wound care for Lori Downs' foot ulcer, you note that the drainage, which was scant and yellow

yesterday, is now green and has saturated the old dressing. Should you continue with the prescribed wound care?

2. Three days ago Tran Nguyen underwent a modified radical mastectomy. She has three Jackson-Pratt drains at her surgical site. She has started asking questions about her surgery and anticipated discharge home. Until this morning, she has avoided looking at her surgical site. You are helping her with her bathing and dressing. As you help her remove her gown, she becomes visibly upset and anxious and exclaims, "Oh no! What's wrong? I'm bleeding from the cuts!" You realize she is looking at her drains. How should you respond?

3. Arthur Lowes has come to his surgeon's office today for a follow-up examination after a colon resection. After he sees the physician, you, the treatment nurse, will remove the surgical staples from the incision. As you prepare to remove the staples, Mr. Lowes comments, "I hope my stomach doesn't pop out now!" What should you tell him?

Bibliography

Agency for Health Care Policy & Research (AHCPR). (1994). *Treatment of pressure ulcers: Clinical practice guideline.* Number 15. Publication Number 95-0652. Rockville, MD: U.S. Department of Health and Human Services.

Agency for Health Care Policy & Research (AHCPR). (1992). *Pressure ulcers in adults: Prediction and prevention.* Number 3. Publication Number 92-0047. Rockville, MD: U.S. Department of Health and Human Services

Atkinson, A. (2002). Body image considerations in patients with wounds. *Journal of Community Nursing, 16*(10), 32–36.

Braden, B., & Maklebust, J. (2005). Preventing pressure ulcers with the Braden Scale. *American Journal of Nursing, 105*(6), 70–72.

Braden, B., & Ayello, E. (2002). How and why to do pressure ulcer risk assessment. *Advances in Skin & Wound Care: The Journal for Prevention and Healing, 15*(3), 125–131

Carpenito, L. (2002). *Nursing diagnosis: Application to clinical practice* (9th ed.). Philadelphia: Lippincott Williams & Wilkins.

Clinical Skills. (Jan. 21–27, 2003). Wound VACs. *Nursing Times, 99*(3), 29.

Craven, R., & Hirnle, C. (2007). *Fundamentals of nursing. Human health and function* (5th ed.). Philadelphia: Lippincott Williams & Wilkins.

Davidson, M. (2002). Sharpen your wound assessment skills. *Nursing, 32*(10), 32hn1.

Doughty, D. (2004). Wound assessment: Tips and techniques. *Home Healthcare Nurse, 22*(3), 192–195.

Ellis, J., & Bentz, P. (2007). *Modules for basic nursing care* (7th ed). Philadelphia: Lippincott Williams & Wilkins.

Franz, R., Gardner, S., Specht, J., et al. (2001). Integration of pressure ulcer treatment protocol into practice: Clinical outcomes and care environment attributes. *Outcomes Management for Nursing Practice, 5*(3), 112–120.

Harvey, C. (2005). Wound healing. *Orthopaedic Nursing, 24*(2), 143–157.

Hess, C. (2005). *Wound care.* (5th ed.). Philadelphia: Lippincott Williams & Wilkins.

Hess, C., & Kirsner, R. (2003). Uncover the latest techniques in wound bed preparation. *Nursing Management, 34*(12), 54–56.

Kaufman, M., & Pahl, D. (2003). Vacuum-assisted closure therapy: Wound care and nursing implications. *Dermatology Nursing, 15*(4), 317–325.

Lloyd-Jones, M. (2004). Minimising pain at dressing changes. *Nursing Standards, 18* (24), 65–70.

Mayo Clinic Geriatric Medicine. (2001). *Pressure ulcers: Prevention and management.* Available at http://www.mayo.edu/geriatrics-rst/PU.

McCloskey, J. C., & Bulechek, G. M. (2000). *Iowa Intervention Project: Nursing Interventions Classification (NIC)* (3rd ed.). St. Louis, MO: C. V. Mosby.

McConnell, E. A. (July 2001). Clinical do's & don'ts: Emptying a closed wound drainage device. *Nursing, 31*(7), 17.

Mendez-Eastman, S. (2005). Using negative-pressure for positive results. *Nursing, 35*(5), 48–50.

Nelson, D., & Dilloway, M. (2002). Principles, products, and practical aspects of wound care. *Critical Care Nursing Quarterly, 25*(1), 33–54.

North American Nursing Diagnosis Association. (2002). *NANDA nursing diagnoses: Definitions and classification 2002–2003.* Philadelphia: Author.

Pieper, B., Templin, T., et al. (2002). Home care nurses' ratings of appropriateness of wound treatments and wound healing. *Journal of WOCN, 29*(1), 20–28.

Pullen, R. L., Jr. (October 2003). Clinical do's & don'ts: Removing sutures and staples. *Nursing, 33*(10), 18.

Sarvis, C. (2004). The role of bacterial toxins in wounds. *Nursing, 34*(7), 68.

Taylor, C., Lillis, C., LeMone, P., & Lynn, P. (2008). *Fundamentals of nursing. The art & science of nursing care* (6th ed.). Philadelphia: Lippincott Williams & Wilkins.

Weber, J., & Kelley, J. (2007). *Health assessment in nursing.* (3rd ed.). Philadelphia: Lippincott Williams & Wilkins.

Worley, C. (2004). Assessment and terminology: Critical issues in wound care. *Dermatology Nursing, 16*(5), 451, 457.

Worley, C. (2004). Quality of life—Part I: Using the holistic caring praxis in skin and wound care. *Dermatology Nursing, 16*(6), 527–528.

Worley, C. (2004). Why won't this wound heal? Factors affecting wound repair. *Dermatology Nursing, 16*(4), 360–361.

Worley, C. (2005). So, what do I put on this wound? The wound dressing puzzle: Part I. *Dermatology Nursing, 17*(2), 143–144.

Worley, C. (2005). So, what do I put on this wound? The wound dressing puzzle: Part II. *Dermatology Nursing, 17*(3), 204–205.

Worley, C. (2005). So, what do I put on this wound? The wound dressing puzzle: Part III. *Dermatology Nursing, 17*(4), 299–300.

CHAPTER 9

Activity

Focusing on Patient Care

This chapter will help you develop some of the skills related to activity necessary to care for the following patients:

Bobby Rowden was knocked down during soccer practice and has come to the emergency room with pain, swelling, and deformity of his right forearm. He is diagnosed with a fracture.

Esther Levitz has been admitted to the hospital with nausea, anorexia, debilitating fatigue, and weight loss. Her underlying diagnosis of lymphoma and inactivity put her at risk for thrombus formation.

Manuel Esposito is scheduled for surgery tomorrow to repair a fractured hip. His physician has ordered skin traction to immobilize the injury before surgery.

Learning Objectives

After studying this chapter, you will be able to:

1. Assist a patient with turning in bed.
2. Provide range-of-motion exercises.
3. Move a patient up in bed with the assistance of another nurse.
4. Transfer a patient from the bed to a stretcher.
5. Transfer a patient from the bed to a chair.
6. Transfer a patient using a full-powered body sling lift.
7. Assist a patient with ambulation.
8. Assist a patient with ambulation using a walker.
9. Assist a patient with ambulation using crutches.
10. Assist a patient with ambulation using a cane.
11. Apply pneumatic compression devices.
12. Apply a continuous passive motion device.
13. Apply a sling.
14. Apply a figure-eight bandage.
15. Assist with a cast application.
16. Care for a patient with a cast.
17. Apply and care for a patient in skin traction.
18. Care for patient in skeletal traction.
19. Care for a patient with an external fixation device.

Key Terms

abduction: movement away from the center or median line of the body

adduction: movement toward the center or median line of the body

arthroplasty: surgical formation or reformation of a joint

compartment syndrome: occurs when there is increased tissue pressure within a limited space; leads to compromises in the circulation and the function of the involved tissue

contracture: permanent shortening or tightening of a muscle due to spasm or paralysis

contusion: an injury in which the skin is not broken; a bruise

deep-vein thrombosis: a blood clot in a blood vessel originating in the large veins of the legs

extension: the return movement from flexion; the joint angle is increased

flexion: bending of a joint so that the angle of the joint diminishes

fracture: a break in the continuity of the bone

goniometer: an apparatus to measure joint movement and angles

Homans' sign: pain in the calf when the toe is passively dorsiflexed; can be an early sign in venous thrombosis of the deep veins of the calf

hyperextension: extreme or abnormal extension

orthostatic hypotension: an abnormal drop in blood pressure that occurs as a person changes from a supine to a standing position

peripheral vascular disease: pathologic conditions of the vascular system characterized by reduced blood flow through the peripheral blood vessels

pronation: the act of lying face downward; the act of turning the hand so the palm faces downward or backward

rotation: process of turning on an axis; twisting or revolving

shearing force: force created by the interplay of gravity and friction on the skin and underlying tissues; shear causes tissue layers to slide over one another and blood vessels to stretch and twist and disrupts the microcirculation of the skin and subcutaneous tissue

supination: turning of the palm or foot upward

thrombophlebitis: a blood clot that accompanies vein inflammation

thrombosis: the formation or development of a blood clot

venous stasis: decrease in blood flow in the venous system related to dysfunctional valves or inactivity of the muscles of the affected extremity

The ability to move is closely related to the fulfillment of other basic human needs. Regular exercise contributes to the healthy functioning of each body system. Conversely, lack of exercise and immobility negatively affect each body system. A summary of the effects of immobility on the body is outlined in Fundamentals Review 9-1. Nurses should encourage activity and exercise to promote wellness, prevent illness, and restore health.

Nurses must recognize cues that indicate both potential and actual problems related to a patient's activity and mobility status. Nursing interventions are directed to preventing these problems whenever possible. Strategies designed to promote correct body alignment, mobility, and fitness are important parts of nursing care. Nurses use knowledge of body mechanics and mobility and knowledge of safe patient-handling techniques along with specific nursing interventions to promote fitness and to resolve mobility problems. See Fundamentals Review 9-2: Principles of Body Mechanics.

When promoting activity for a patient, the safety of the patient and the nurse is key. Research conducted at the VISN 8 Patient Safety Center of Inquiry at the James A. Haley Veterans Hospital/Veterans Administration medical center supports the consistent use of standardized protocols and mechanical lifting devices as a more effective approach to decrease the risk of injury for healthcare workers, rather than just using proper body mechanics (Nelson, Fragala, & Menzel, 2003; Nelson, et al, 2003). The Occupational Safety &

Health Administration (OSHA) recommends minimizing manual lifting of patients/residents in all cases and eliminating lifting when possible (U.S. Department of Labor, 2003). Even routine repetitive care activities such as changing bed linens and bathing patients have the potential to cause back injury. Therefore, preventive measures should focus on careful assessment of the patient care environment so that patients can be moved safely and effectively. In some institutions, specially trained staff members who function as "back injury resource nurses" are responsible for assisting nurses to assess patients. Step-by-step protocols or algorithms are available to aid decision making to prevent injury to staff and patients.

Samples are provided in the skills related to patient movement and handling. Always check institution practices and guidelines and available equipment related to safe patient handling and movement. When using any equipment, check for proper functioning before using with the patient. Fundamentals Review 9-3 presents guidelines for safe patient handling and movement. Fundamentals Review 9-4 discusses examples of equipment and assistive devices that are available to aid with safe patient movement and handling.

This chapter will cover skills to assist the nurse in providing care related to activity, inactivity, and healthcare problems related to the musculoskeletal system.

Fundamentals Review 9-1

Effects of Immobility on the Body

- Decreased muscle strength and tone, decreased muscle size
- Decreased joint mobility and flexibility
- Limited endurance and activity intolerance
- Bone demineralization
- Lack of coordination and altered gait
- Decreased ventilatory effort and increased respiratory secretions, atelectasis, respiratory congestion
- Increased cardiac workload, orthostatic hypotension, venous thrombosis
- Impaired circulation and skin breakdown
- Decreased appetite, constipation
- Urinary stasis, infection
- Altered sleep patterns, pain, depression, anger, anxiety

Fundamentals Review 9-2

Principles of Body Mechanics

- Correct body alignment is important to prevent undue strain on joints, muscles, tendons, and ligaments while maintaining balance.
- Maintaining balance involves keeping the spine in vertical alignment, body weight close to the center of gravity, and feet spread for a broad base of support.
- Using the body's major muscle groups and natural levers and fulcrums allows for coordinated movement to avoid musculoskeletal strain and injury.
- Assess the situation before acting so that you can plan to use good body mechanics.
- Use the large muscle groups in the legs to provide force for movement. Keep the back straight, with hips and knees bent. Slide, roll, push, or pull rather than lift an object.
- Perform work at the appropriate height for your body position, close to your center of gravity.
- Use mechanical lifts and/or assistance to ease the movement.

Guidelines for Safe Patient Handling and Movement

Keep the patient in good alignment and protect from injury while being moved. Follow these recommended guidelines when moving and lifting patients:

- Assess the patient. Know the patient's medical diagnosis, capabilities, and any movement not allowed. Put in place braces or any device the patient wears before helping from bed.
- Assess the patient's ability to assist with the planned movement. Patients should be encouraged to assist in their own transfers. Encouraging the patient to perform tasks that are within his or her capabilities promotes independence. Eliminating or reducing unnecessary tasks by the nurse reduces the risk of injury.
- Assess the patient's ability to understand instructions and cooperate with the staff to achieve the movement.
- Ensure enough staff is available and present to safely move the patient.
- Assess the area for clutter, accessibility to the patient and availability of devices. Remove any obstacles that may make moving and lifting inconvenient.
- Decide which equipment to use. Handling aids should be used whenever possible to help reduce risk of injury to the nurse and patient.
- Plan carefully what you will do before moving or lifting a patient. Assess the mobility of attached equipment. You may injure the patient or yourself if you have not planned well. If necessary, enlist the support of another nurse. This reduces the strain on everyone involved. Communicate the plan with staff and the patient, to ensure coordinated movement.
- Explain to the patient what you plan to do. Then use what abilities the patient has to assist you. This technique often decreases the effort required and the possibility of injury to you.
- If the patient is in pain, administer the prescribed analgesic sufficiently in advance of the transfer to allow the patient to participate in the move comfortably.
- Elevate the bed as necessary so that you are working at a height that is comfortable and safe for you.
- Lock the wheels of the bed, wheelchair, or stretcher so that they do not slide while you are moving the patient.
- Observe the principles of body mechanics to prevent injuring yourself while you work.
- Be sure the patient is in good body alignment while being moved and lifted to protect the patient from strain and muscle injury.
- Support the patient's body well. Avoid grabbing and holding an extremity by its muscles.
- Avoid friction on the patient's skin during moving. Use friction-reducing sheets, if available, or positioning linens, such as a drawsheet, as well as sprinkling powder or cornstarch between the surface linens and positioning linens.
- Move your body and the patient in a smooth, rhythmic motion. Jerky movements tend to put extra strain on muscles and joints and are uncomfortable for the patient.
- Use mechanical devices such as lifts, slides, transfer chairs, or gait belts for moving patients. Be sure that you understand how the device operates and that the patient is properly secured and informed of what will occur. Patients who do not understand or are afraid may be unable to cooperate and may suffer injury as a result.
- Assure equipment used meets weight requirements. Bariatric patients (BMI greater than 50) require bariatric transfer aids and equipment.

Fundamentals Review 9-4

Equipment and Assistive Devices

Many devices and equipment are available to aid in transferring, repositioning, and lifting patients. It is important to use the right equipment and appropriate device based on patient assessment and desired movement.

Gait Belts

A gait belt is a belt with handles. It is placed around the patient's waist and secured by Velcro fasteners. The handles can be placed in a variety of configurations so the caregiver can have better access to, improved grasp, and control of the patient (Nelson, Fragala, & Menzel, 2003). Some belts are hand-held slings that go around the patient, providing a firm grasp for the caregiver and facilitating the transfer (Nelson, Owen, Lloyd et al, 2003). Gait belts should not be used on patients with abdominal or thoracic incisions (Blocks, 2005). (See Figure A for a gait belt.)

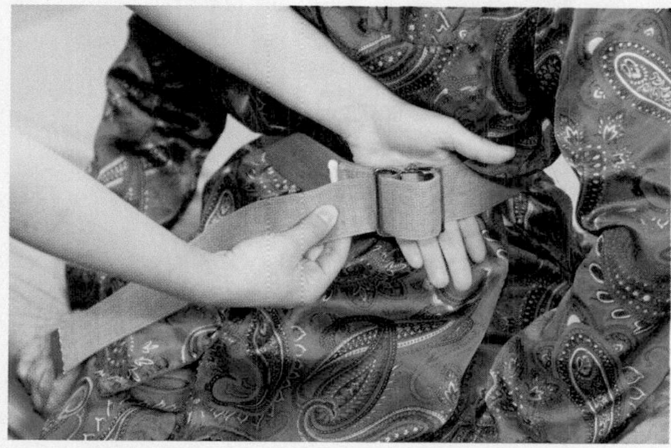

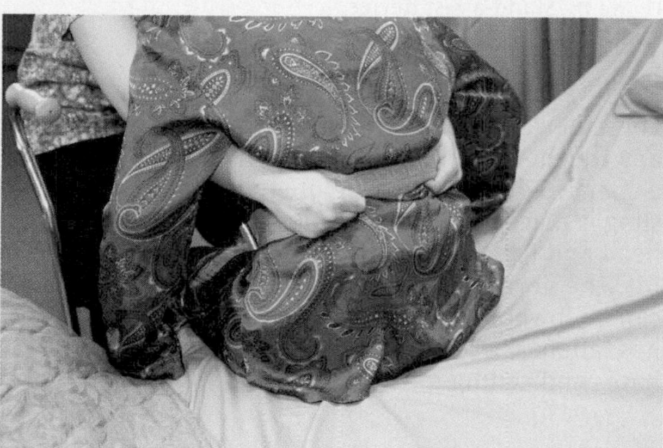

Figure A. Using gait belt.

Stand-assist and Repositioning Aids

Some patients need minimal assistance to stand up. With an appropriate support to grasp, they can lift themselves. Many types of secure devices can help a patient to stand. These devices are freestanding or attach to the bed or wheelchair. One type of stand-assist aid attaches to the bed. Other aids have a pull bar to assist the patient to stand, and then a seat unfolds under the patient. After sitting on the seat, the device can be wheeled to the toilet, chair, shower, or bed.

Lateral-assist Devices

Lateral-assist devices reduce patient-surface friction during lateral transfers. Roller boards, slide boards, transfer boards, inflatable mattresses, and friction-reducing, lateral-assist devices are examples of these devices that make transfers safer and more comfortable for the patient. An inflatable lateral-assist device is a flexible mattress that is placed under the patient. An attached, portable air supply inflates the mattress, which provides a layer of air under the patient. This air cushion allows nursing staff to perform the move with much less effort (Nelson, Owen, Lloyd et al., 2003). Transfer boards are placed under the patient. They provide a slick surface for the patient during transfers, reducing friction and the force required to move the patient. Transfer boards are made of smooth, rigid, low-friction material such as coated wood or plastic. Another lateral sliding aid is made of special fabric that reduces friction. Some devices have long handles that reduce reaching by staff, to improve safety and make the transfer easier (Figure B).

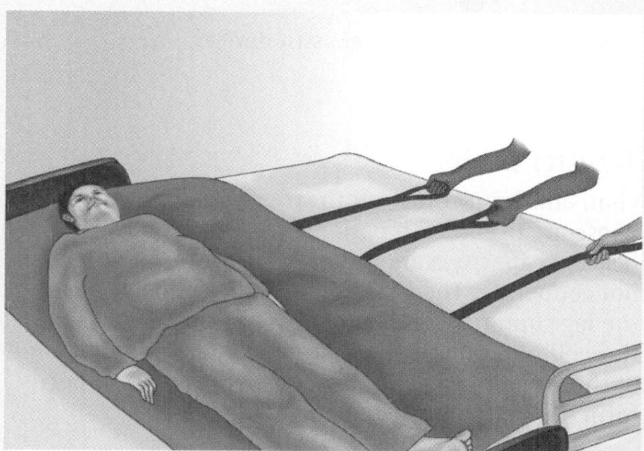

Figure B. Lateral-assist device with long handles to reduce reaching by the staff.

(continued)

Fundamentals Review 9-4

Equipment and Assistive Devices *(continued)*

Friction-reducing Sheets

Friction-reducing sheets can be used under patients to prevent skin shearing when moving a patient in the bed and to assist with lateral transfers. The use of these sheets when moving the patient up in bed, turning, and repositioning reduces friction and the force required to move the patient.

Mechanical Lateral-assist Devices

These stretchers and devices eliminate the need to slide the patient manually. Some devices are motorized and some use a hand crank (Figure C). A portion of the device moves from the stretcher to the bed, sliding under the patient, bridging the bed and stretcher. The device is then returned to the stretcher, effectively moving the patient without pulling by staff members.

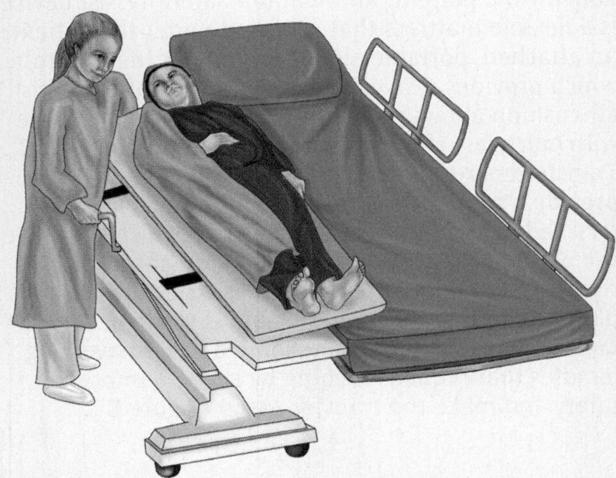

Figure C. Mechanical lateral-assist device.

Transfer Chairs

Chairs that can convert into stretchers are available. These are useful with patients who have no weight-bearing capacity, cannot follow directions, and/or cannot cooperate. The back of the chair bends back and the leg supports elevate to form a stretcher configuration, eliminating the need for lifting the patient. Some of these chairs have built-in mechanical aids to perform the patient transfer, as detailed above.

Powered Stand-assist and Repositioning Lifts

These devices can be used with patients who have weight-bearing ability in at least one leg, who can follow directions, and are cooperative. A simple sling is placed around the patient's back and under the arms (Figure D). The patient rests his feet on the device's footrest and places his hands on the handle. The device mechanically assists the patient to stand, without any lifting by the nurse. Once the patient is standing, the device can be wheeled to a chair, the toilet, or bed. Some devices have removable foot rests and can be used as a walker. Some have scales incorporated into the device that can be used to weigh the patient.

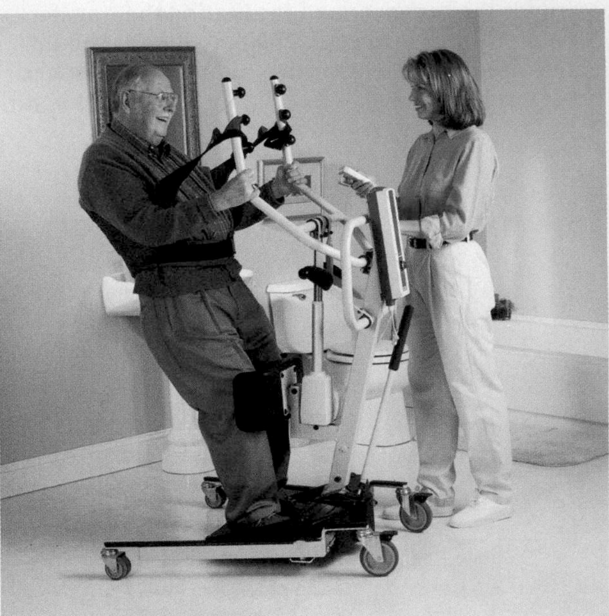

Figure D. Stand-assist device.

Powered Full-body Lifts

These devices are used with patients who cannot bear any weight to move them out of bed, into and out of a chair, and to a commode or stretcher. A full-body sling is placed under the patient's body, including head and torso, and then the sling is attached to the lift. The device slowly lifts the patient. Some devices can be lowered to the floor to pick up a patient who has fallen. These devices are available on portable bases and ceiling-mounted tracks.

SKILL 9-1 Assisting a Patient With Turning in Bed

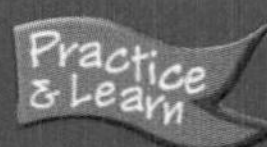

Individuals who are forced into inactivity by illness or injury are at high risk for serious health complications. One of the most common skills that you may use involves helping patients who cannot turn themselves in bed without assistance. You need to use your knowledge of body mechanics, correct body alignment, and assistive devices to turn the patient in bed. Figure 1, Safe Patient Handling Algorithm 4, can help you make decisions about safe patient handling and movement. Mastering and using these techniques will help you maintain a turn schedule to prevent complications for a patient who is immobile. If a patient requires logrolling, please refer to Skill 17-4.

Equipment

- Friction-reducing sheet or draw sheet
- Bed surface that inflates to aid in turning
- Pillows or other supports to help the patient maintain the desired position after turning and to maintain correct body alignment for the patient
- Nonsterile gloves, if indicated

ASSESSMENT

Before moving a patient, check the medical record for any conditions or orders that will limit mobility. Perform a pain assessment before the time for the activity. If the patient reports pain, administer the prescribed medication in sufficient time to allow for the full effect of the analgesic. Assess the patient's ability to assist with moving and the need for a second or third individual to assist with the activity. Assess the patient's skin for signs of irritation, redness, edema, or blanching.

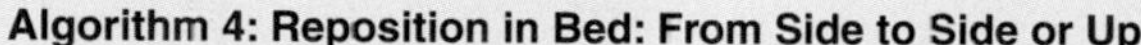

Algorithm 4: Reposition in Bed: From Side to Side or Up

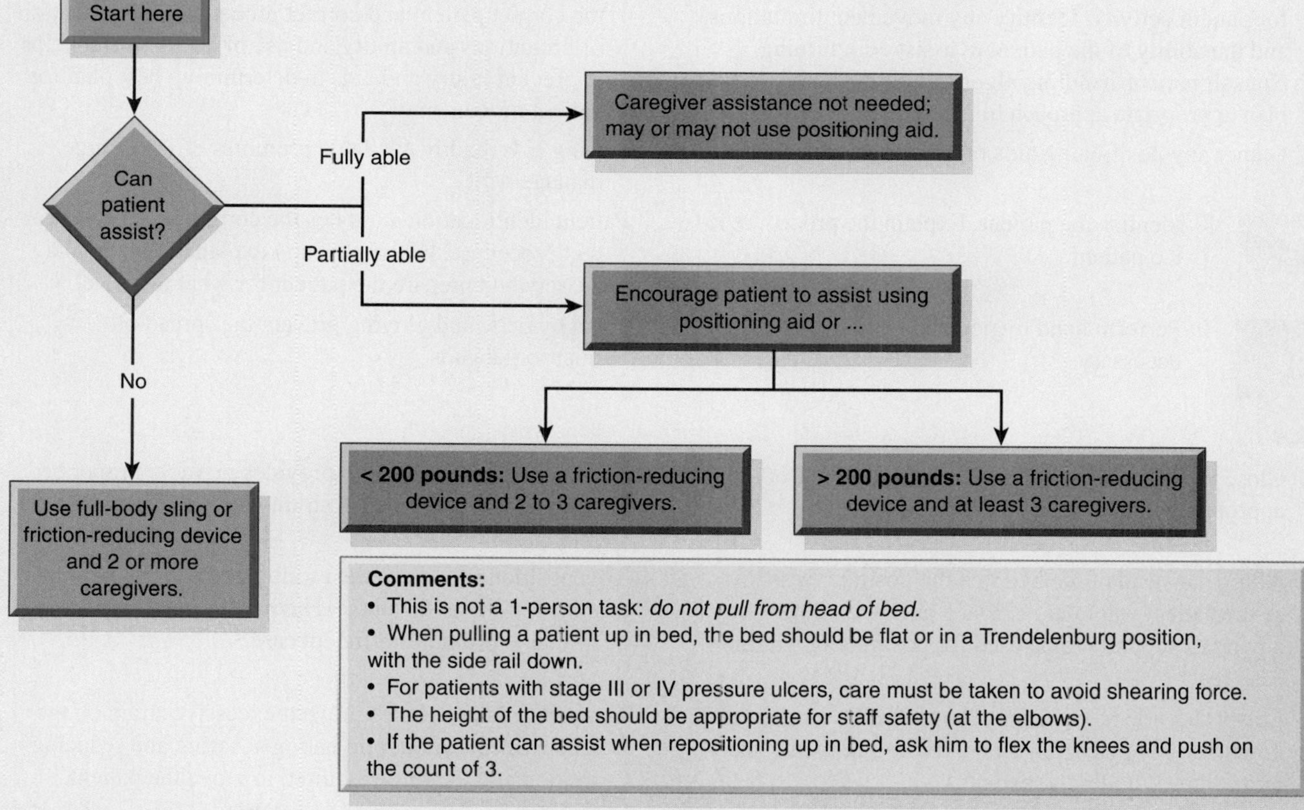

Figure 1. Step-by-step procedure or algorithm used to outline safe technique for repositioning a patient in bed. (From VISN8 Patient Safety Center of Inquiry. (2005). Safe patient handling and movement algorithms. Tampa, FL: Author. Available at www.VISN8.med.va.gov/patientsafetycenter/SPHMAlg050105.pdf.

(continued)

SKILL 9-1 Assisting a Patient With Turning in Bed *(continued)*

NURSING DIAGNOSIS

Determine the related factors for the nursing diagnoses based on the patient's current status. Appropriate nursing diagnoses may include:

- Activity Intolerance
- Risk for Activity Intolerance
- Fatigue
- Risk for Injury
- Impaired Bed Mobility
- Acute Pain
- Chronic Pain
- Risk for Impaired Skin Integrity
- Impaired Skin Integrity

OUTCOME IDENTIFICATION AND PLANNING

The expected outcome to achieve when assisting a patient with turning in bed is that the activity takes place without injury to patient or nurse. An additional outcome is that the patient is comfortable and in proper body alignment.

IMPLEMENTATION

ACTION	RATIONALE
1. Review the physician's orders and nursing plan of care for patient activity. Identify any movement limitations and the ability of the patient to assist with turning. Consult patient-handling algorithm, if available, to plan appropriate approach to moving the patient.	Checking the physician's order and plan of care validates the correct patient and correct procedure. Identification of limitations and ability and use of an algorithm helps to prevent injury and aids in determining best plan for patient movement.
2. Gather any positioning aids or supports, if necessary.	Having aids readily available promotes efficient time management.
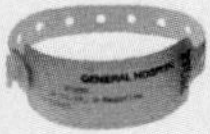 3. Identify the patient. Explain the procedure to the patient.	Patient identification validates the correct patient and correct procedure. Discussion and explanation help allay anxiety and prepare the patient for what to expect.
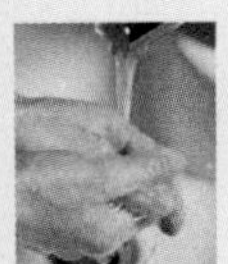 4. Perform hand hygiene and put on gloves, if necessary.	Hand hygiene and gloving prevent the spread of microorganisms.
5. Close the room door or curtains. Place the bed at an appropriate and comfortable working height.	Closing the door or curtain provides privacy. Proper bed height helps reduce back strain while performing the procedure.
6. Adjust the head of the bed to a flat position or as low as the patient can tolerate. Place pillows, wedges, or any other supports to be used for positioning within easy reach.	This position facilitates the turning maneuver and minimizes strain on the nurse. Having supports readily available promotes efficient care.
7. Lower the side rail nearest you if it has been raised. If not already in place, position a friction-reducing sheet or drawsheet under the patient.	Lowering side rail helps prevent excessive strain on the nurse. Sheets aid in preventing shearing and reducing friction and the force required to move the patient.
8. Using the friction-reducing sheet or drawsheet, move the patient to the edge of the bed, opposite the side to which he or she will be turned. Raise side rail and move to the opposite side of the bed.	With this placement, the patient will be on the center of the bed after turning is accomplished. Raising the opposite side rail prevents the patient from possible injury.

SKILL 9-1 Assisting a Patient With Turning in Bed *(continued)*

ACTION	RATIONALE
9. Stand on the side of the bed toward which the patient is turning. Lower the side rail nearest you.	This positions the nurse opposite the center of the body mass; lowering the near side rail prevents strain on the nurse.
10. **Place the patient's arms across his or her chest and cross his or her far leg over the leg nearest you (Figure 2).**	This facilitates the turning motion and protects the patient's arms during the turn.
11. Stand opposite the patient's center with your feet spread about shoulder width and with one foot ahead of the other (Figure 3). **Tighten your gluteal and abdominal muscles and flex your knees. Use your leg muscles to do the pulling.**	This helps avoid straining the nurse's lower back. The nurse is in a stable position with good body alignment and prepared to use large muscle masses to turn the patient.

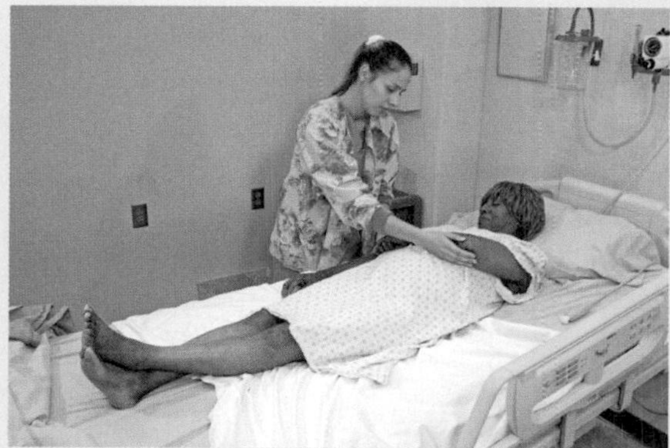

Figure 2. Placing patient's arms across chest and patient's far leg crossed over the leg nearest the nurse.

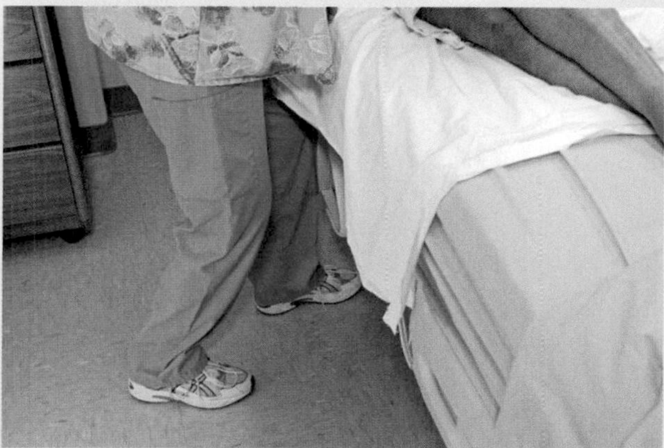

Figure 3. Standing opposite the patient's center with feet spread about shoulder width and with one foot ahead of the other.

ACTION	RATIONALE
12. If available, activate the bed mechanism to inflate the side of the bed opposite from where you are standing.	Activating the turn mechanism inflates the side of the bed for approx. 10 seconds, aiding in propelling the patient to turn, and reducing the work required by the nurse.
13. Position your hands on the patient's far shoulder and hip, and roll the patient toward you. Or, you may use the friction-reducing sheet or draw sheet to gently pull the patient over on his or her side (Figure 4).	This maneuver supports the patient's body and makes use of the nurse's weight to assist with turning.

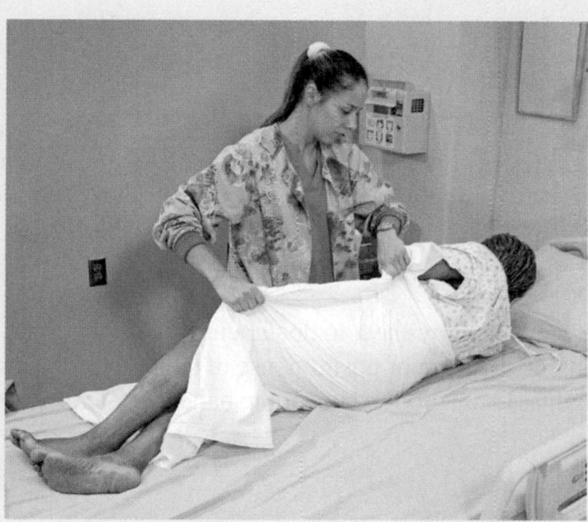

Figure 4. Using a drawsheet to pull patient over on her side.

(continued)

SKILL 9-1 Assisting a Patient With Turning in Bed *(continued)*

ACTION

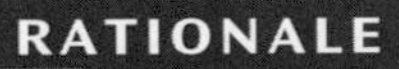

RATIONALE

14. Use a pillow or other support behind the patient's back. Pull the shoulder blade forward and out from under the patient.

    Pillow will provide support and help the patient maintain the desired position. Positioning the shoulder blade removes pressure from the bony prominence.

15. Make the patient comfortable and position in proper alignment, using pillows or other supports under the leg and arm as needed (Figure 5). Readjust the pillow under the patient's head. Elevate the head of the bed as needed for comfort.

    Positioning in proper alignment with supports ensures that the patient will be able to maintain the desired position and will be comfortable.

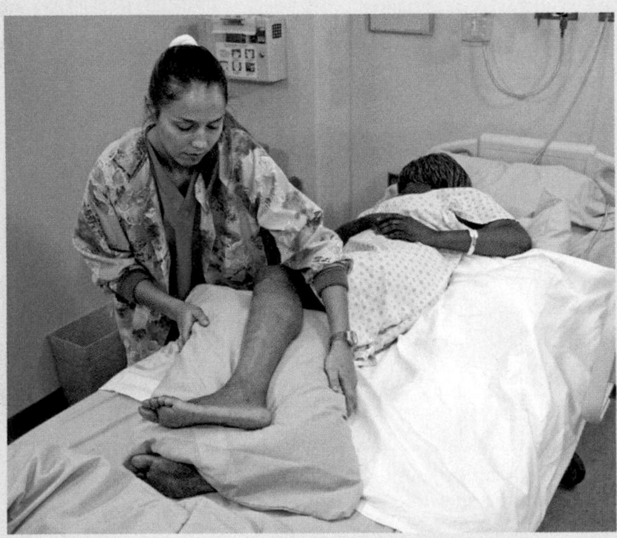

Figure 5. Making the patient comfortable.

16. Place the bed in the lowest position, with the side rails up. Make sure the call bell and other necessary items are within easy reach.

    Adjusting the bed height ensures patient safety.

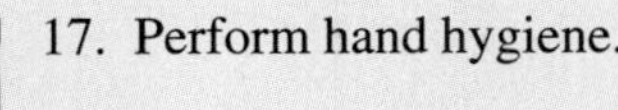

17. Perform hand hygiene.

    Hand hygiene prevents the spread of microorganisms.

EVALUATION

The expected outcome is met when the patient is turned and repositioned without injury to patient or nurse. The patient demonstrates proper body alignment and verbalizes comfort.

DOCUMENTATION

Guidelines

Many facilities provide areas on the bedside flow sheet to document repositioning. Be sure to document the time of the patient's change of position, use of supports, and any pertinent observations, including skin assessment. Document the patient's tolerance of the position change.

SKILL 9-1 Assisting a Patient With Turning in Bed *(continued)*

Sample Documentation

11/10/08 1130 Patient repositioned from right side to left side; alignment maintained with wedge support behind back and pillow between legs. Skin on pressure points on right side without signs of irritation, edema, or redness. Patient reports no pain with movement.—B. Clapp, RN

Unexpected Situations and Associated Interventions

- *You are turning a patient by yourself, but you realize that the patient cannot help as much as you thought and is heavier than you anticipated:* Use the call bell to summon assistance from a coworker. Alternatively, cover the patient, make sure all rails are up, lower the bed to the lowest position, and get someone to assist you. Consider using a friction-reducing sheet and two to three additional caregivers.

SKILL 9-2 Providing Range-of-Motion Exercises

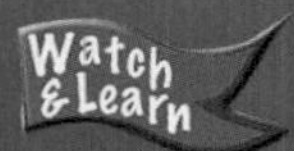

Range of motion (ROM) is the complete extent of movement of which a joint is normally capable. Taking part in routine activities of daily living helps to use muscle groups that keep many joints in an effective range of motion. When all or some of the normal activities are impossible, attention is given to the joints not being used or to those that have limited use. When the patient does the exercise for himself or herself, it is referred to as active range of motion. Exercises performed by the nurse without participation by the patient are referred to as passive range of motion. Exercises should be as active as the patient's physical condition permits. Allow the patient to do as much individual activity as his or her condition permits. Range-of-motion exercises should be initiated as soon as possible because body changes can occur after only 3 days of impaired mobility.

Equipment

No special equipment or supplies are necessary to perform range-of-motion exercises. If appropriate, nonsterile gloves may be worn.

ASSESSMENT

Review the medical record and nursing plan of care for any conditions or orders that will limit mobility. Perform a pain assessment before the time for the exercises. If the patient reports pain, administer the prescribed medication in sufficient time to allow for the full effect of the analgesic. Assess the patient's ability to perform range-of-motion exercises. Inspect and palpate joints for redness, tenderness, pain, swelling, or deformities.

NURSING DIAGNOSIS

Determine the related factors for the nursing diagnoses based on the patient's current status. Appropriate nursing diagnoses may include:

- Impaired Physical Mobility
- Impaired Bed Mobility
- Activity Intolerance
- Fatigue
- Risk for Injury
- Deficient Knowledge
- Acute Pain
- Chronic Pain
- Impaired Skin Integrity

(continued)

SKILL 9-2 Providing Range-of-Motion Exercises *(continued)*

OUTCOME IDENTIFICATION AND PLANNING

The expected outcome to achieve when performing range-of-motion exercises is that the patient maintains joint mobility. Other outcomes include improving or maintaining muscle strength, and preventing muscle atrophy and contractures.

IMPLEMENTATION

ACTION	RATIONALE
1. Review the physician's orders and nursing plan of care for patient activity. Identify any movement limitations.	Reviewing the order and plan of care validates the correct patient and correct procedure. Identification of limitations prevents injury.
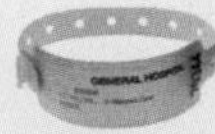 2. Identify the patient. Explain the procedure to the patient.	Patient identification validates the correct patient and correct procedure. Discussion and explanation help allay anxiety and prepare the patient for what to expect.
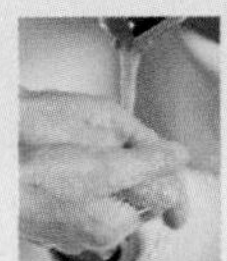 3. Perform hand hygiene and put on gloves, if necessary.	Hand hygiene and gloving prevent the spread of microorganisms.
4. Close the room door or curtains. Place the bed at an appropriate and comfortable working height. Adjust the head of the bed to a flat position or as low as the patient can tolerate.	Closing the door or curtains provides privacy. Proper bed height helps reduce back strain while performing the procedure.
5. Stand on the side of the bed where the joints are to be exercised. Lower side rail on that side, if in place. Uncover only the limb to be used during the exercise.	Standing on the side to be exercised and lowering the side rail prevents strain on the nurse's back. Proper draping provides for privacy and warmth.
6. Perform the exercises slowly and gently, providing support by holding the areas proximal and distal to the joint. Repeat each exercise two to five times, moving each joint in a smooth and rhythmic manner. **Stop movement if the patient complains of pain or if you meet resistance.**	Slow, gentle movements with support prevent discomfort and muscle spasms resulting from jerky movements. Repeated movement of muscles and joints improves flexibility and increases circulation to the body part. Pain may indicate the exercises are causing damage.
7. **While performing the exercises, begin at the head and move down one side of the body at a time.**	Proceeding from head to toe one side at a time promotes efficient time management and an organized approach to the task.
8. Move the chin down to rest on the chest (Figure 1). Return the head to a normal upright position (Figure 2). Tilt the head as far as possible toward each shoulder (Figure 3).	These movements provide for flexion, extension, and lateral flexion of the head and neck.
9. Move the head from side to side, bringing the chin toward each shoulder (Figure 4).	These movements provide for rotation of neck.
10. Start with the arm at the patient's side (Figure 5) and lift the arm forward to above the head (Figure 6). Return the arm to the starting position at the side of the body.	These movements provide for flexion and extension of the shoulder.

SKILL 9-2

Providing Range-of-Motion Exercises *(continued)*

ACTION

RATIONALE

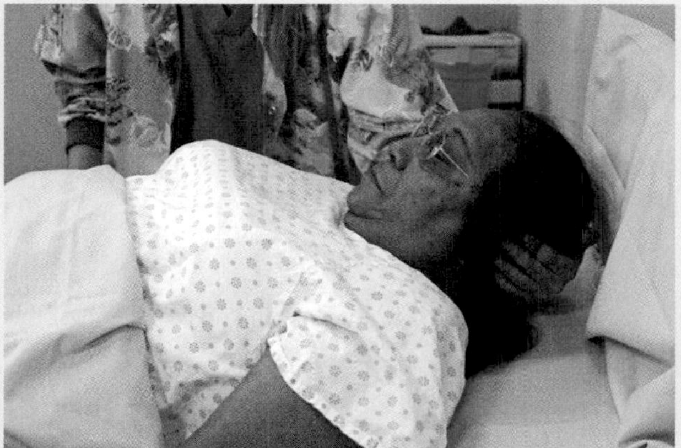

Figure 1. Moving patient's chin down to rest on chest.

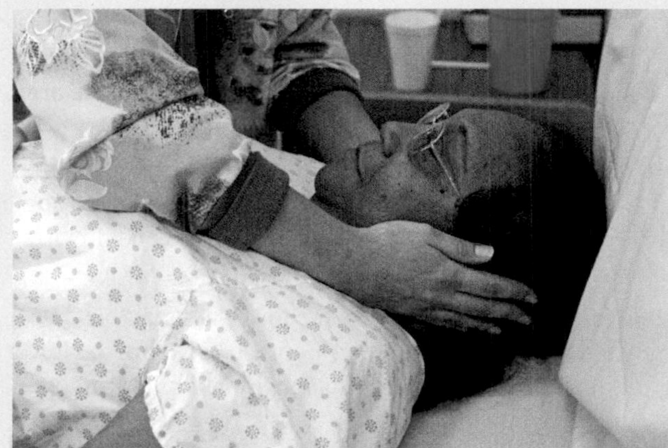

Figure 2. Holding patient's head upright and centered.

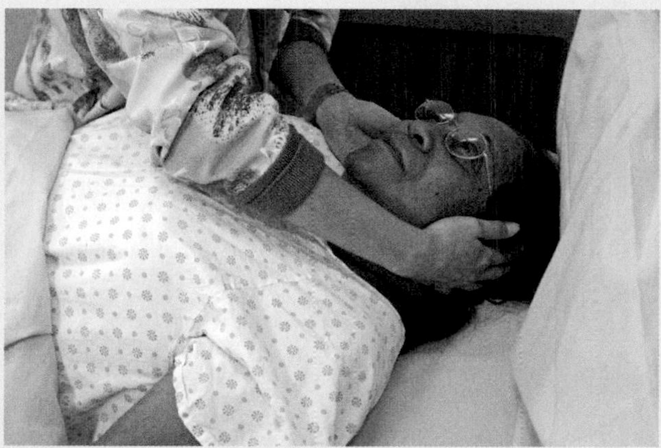

Figure 3. Moving patient's head to one shoulder.

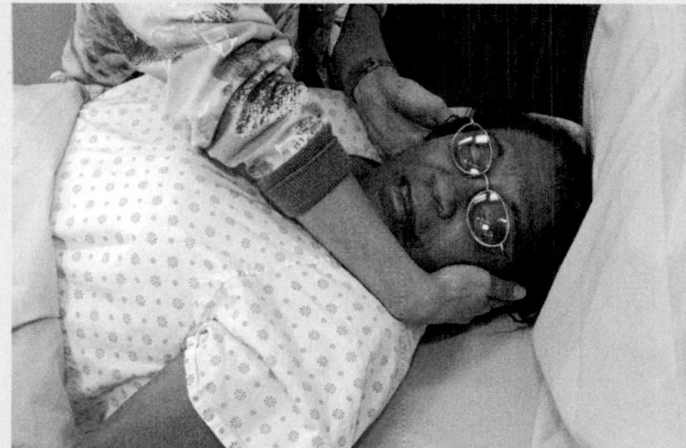

Figure 4. Moving patient's chin toward one shoulder.

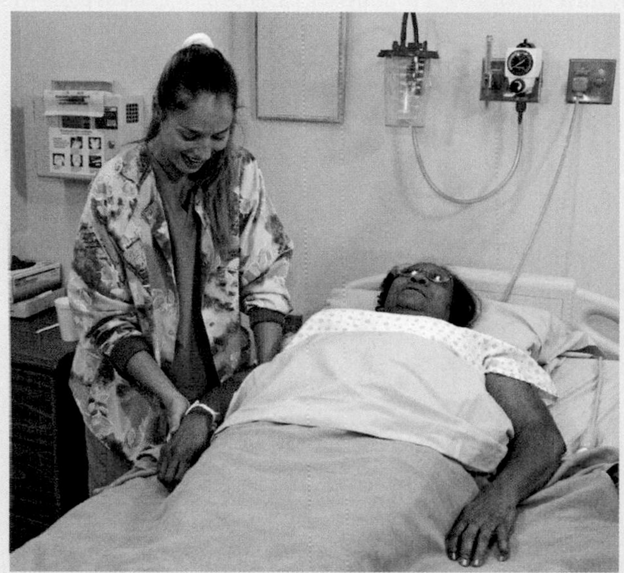

Figure 5. Holding patient's arm at side.

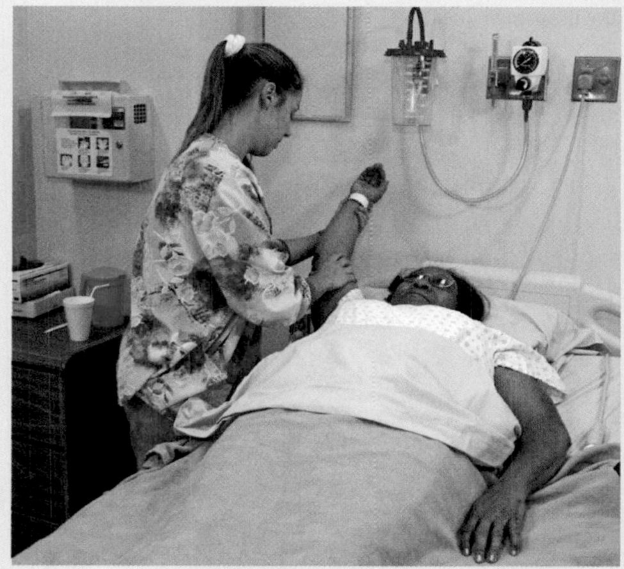

Figure 6. Lifting the arm forward to above the patient's head.

(continued)

SKILL 9-2 Providing Range-of-Motion Exercises *(continued)*

ACTION	RATIONALE
11. With the arm back at the patient's side, move the arm laterally to an upright position above the head (Figure 7), and then return to the original position. Move the arm across the body as far as possible (Figure 8).	These movements provide for abduction and adduction of the shoulder.
12. Raise the arm at the side until the upper arm is in line with the shoulder. Bend the elbow at a 90-degree angle (Figure 9) and move the forearm upward and downward, then return the arm to the side.	These movements provide for internal and external rotation of the shoulder.
13. Bend the elbow and move the lower arm and hand upward toward the shoulder (Figure 10). Return the lower arm and hand to the original position while straightening the elbow.	These movements provide for flexion and extension of the elbow.

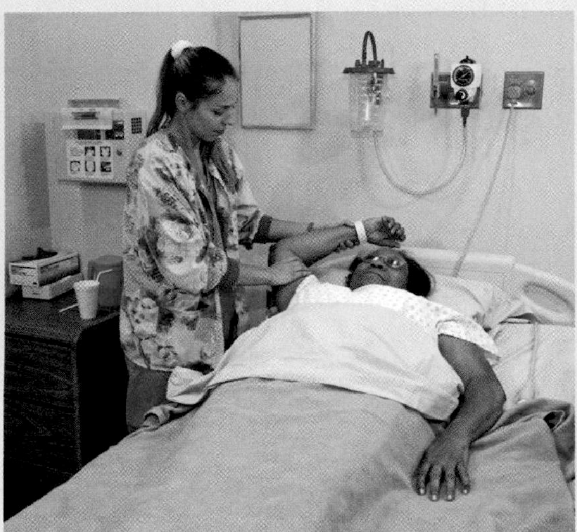

Figure 7. Moving the patient's arm laterally to an upright position above the patient's head.

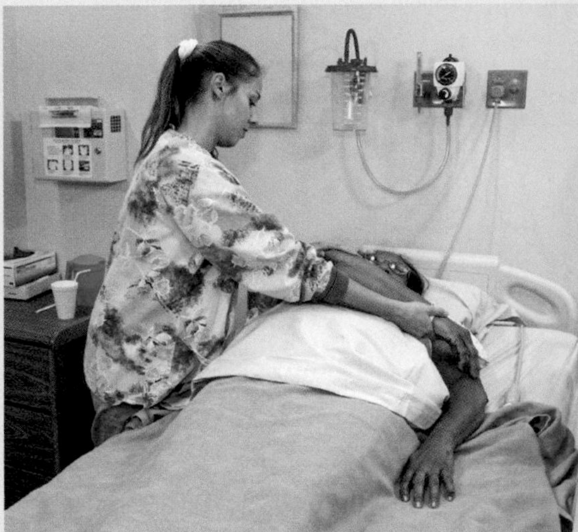

Figure 8. Moving the arm across the patient's body as far as possible.

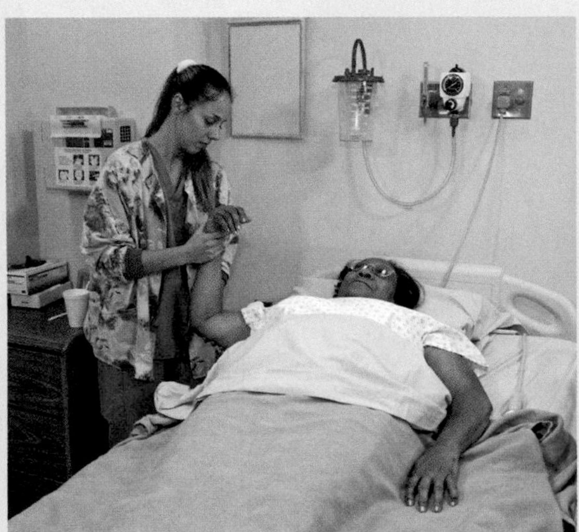

Figure 9. Raising the patient's arm until the upper arm is in line with the patient's shoulder, with elbow bent.

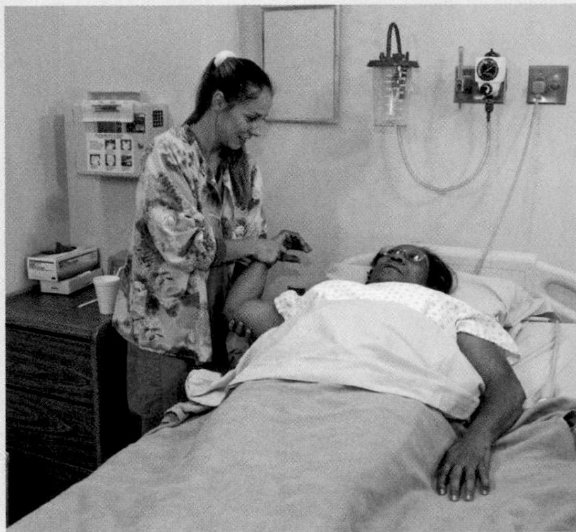

Figure 10. Bending the patient's elbow and move the lower arm and hand upward toward the shoulder.

SKILL 9-2 Providing Range-of-Motion Exercises *(continued)*

ACTION	RATIONALE
14. Rotate the lower arm and hand so the palm is up (Figure 11). Rotate the lower arm and hand so the palm of the hand is down.	These movements provide for supination and pronation of the forearm.

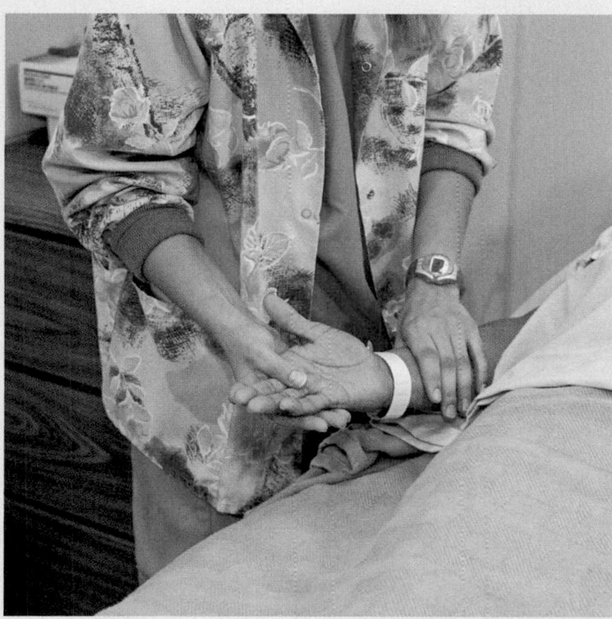

Figure 11. Rotating the patient's lower arm and hand so palm is up.

ACTION	RATIONALE
15. Move the hand downward toward the inner aspect of the forearm (Figure 12). Return the hand to a neutral position even with the forearm (Figure 13). Then move the dorsal portion of the hand backward as far as possible.	These movements provide for flexion, extension, and hyperextension of the wrist.

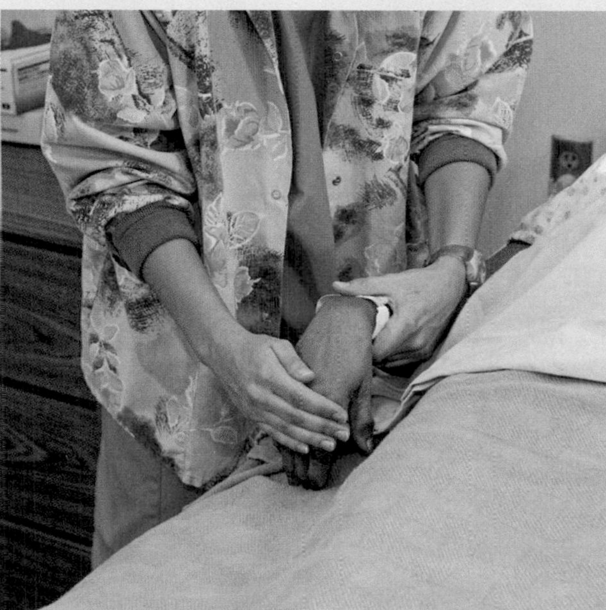

Figure 12. Moving the patient's hand downward toward the inner aspect of forearm.

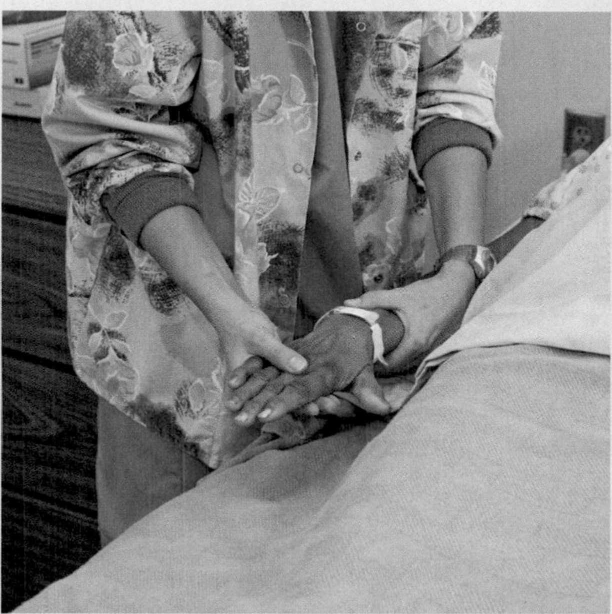

Figure 13. Returning hand to the neutral position.

(continued)

SKILL 9-2 Providing Range-of-Motion Exercises *(continued)*

ACTION	RATIONALE
16. Bend the fingers to make a fist (Figure 14), and then straighten them out (Figure 15). Spread the fingers apart (Figure 16) and return them back together. Touch the thumb to each finger on the hand (Figure 17).	These movements provide for flexion, extension, abduction, and adduction of the fingers.

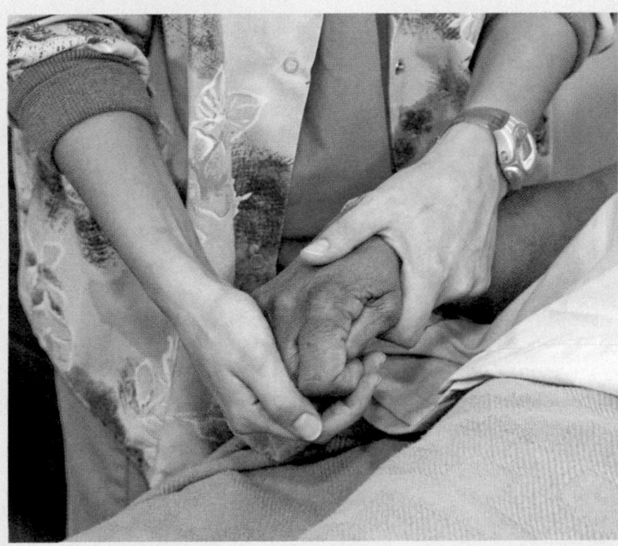

Figure 14. Bending patient's fingers to make a fist.

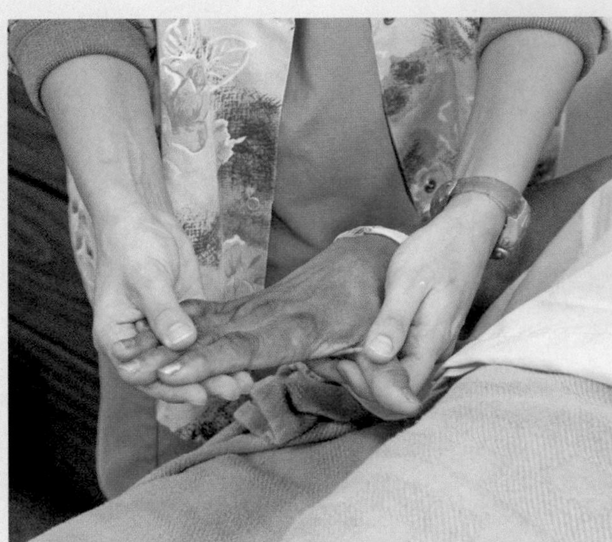

Figure 15. Straightening out patient's fingers.

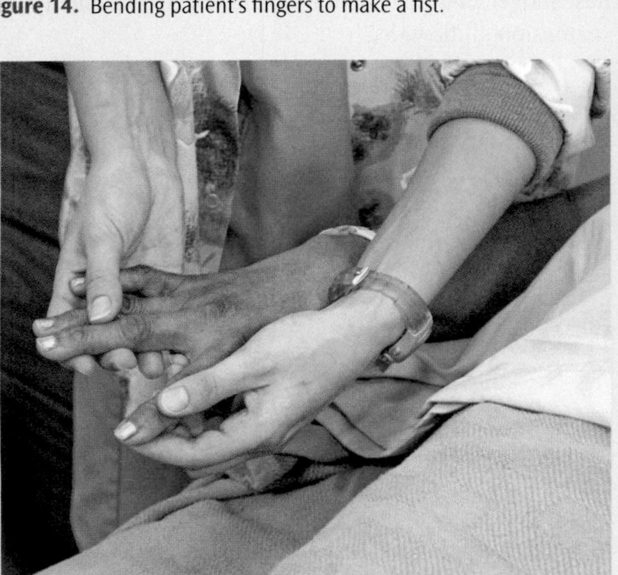

Figure 16. Spreading the patient's fingers apart.

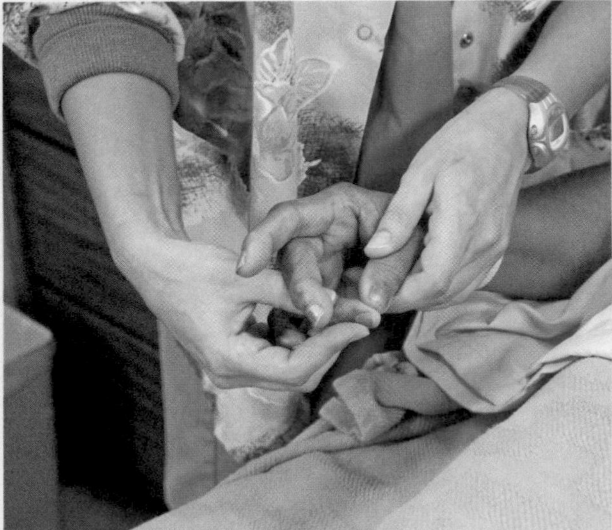

Figure 17. Assisting patient to touch thumb to each finger.

SKILL 9-2 Providing Range-of-Motion Exercises *(continued)*

ACTION	RATIONALE
17. Extend the leg and lift it upward (Figure 18). Return the leg to the original position beside the other leg.	These movements provide for flexion and extension of the hip.

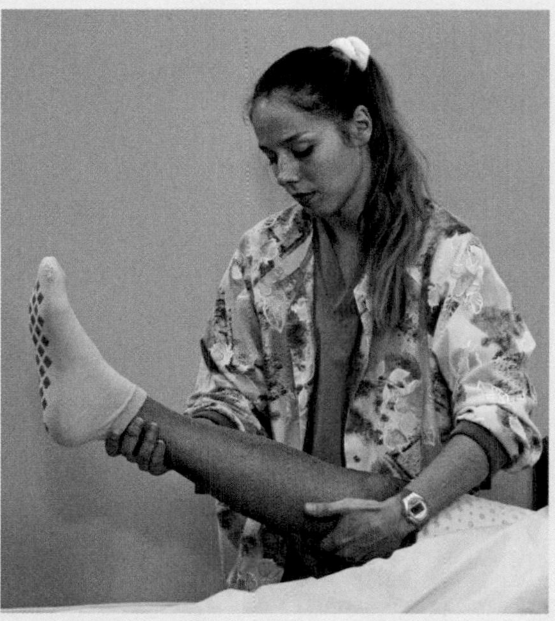

Figure 18. Extending and lifting the patient's leg.

ACTION	RATIONALE
18. Lift the leg laterally away from the patient's body (Figure 19). Return the leg back toward the other leg and try to extend it beyond the midline (Figure 20).	These movements provide for abduction and adduction of the hip.

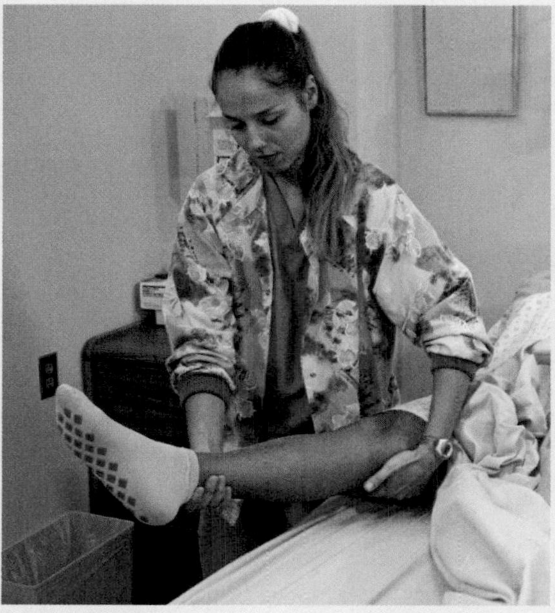

Figure 19. Lifting the patient's leg laterally away from the body (abduction).

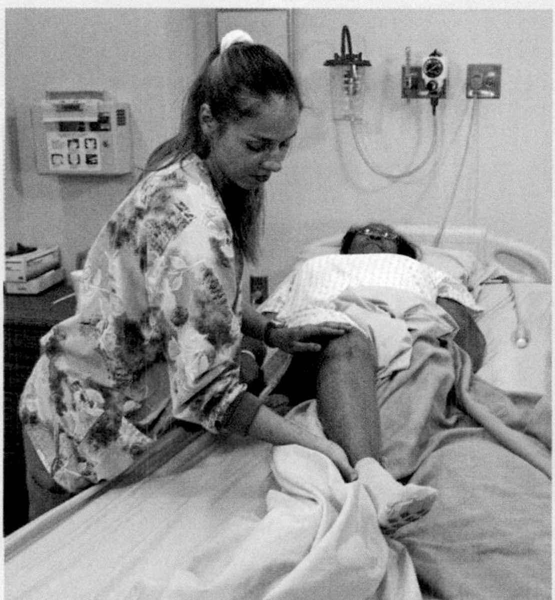

Figure 20. Returning the leg back toward the other leg and trying to extend it beyond the midline if possible.

(continued)

SKILL 9-2 Providing Range-of-Motion Exercises *(continued)*

ACTION	RATIONALE
19. Turn the foot and leg toward the other leg to rotate it internally (Figure 21). Turn the foot and leg outward away from the other leg to rotate it externally (Figure 22).	These movements provide for internal and external rotation of the hip.
20. Bend the leg and bring the heel toward the back of the leg (Figure 23). Return the leg to a straight position (Figure 24).	These movements provide for flexion and extension of the knee.

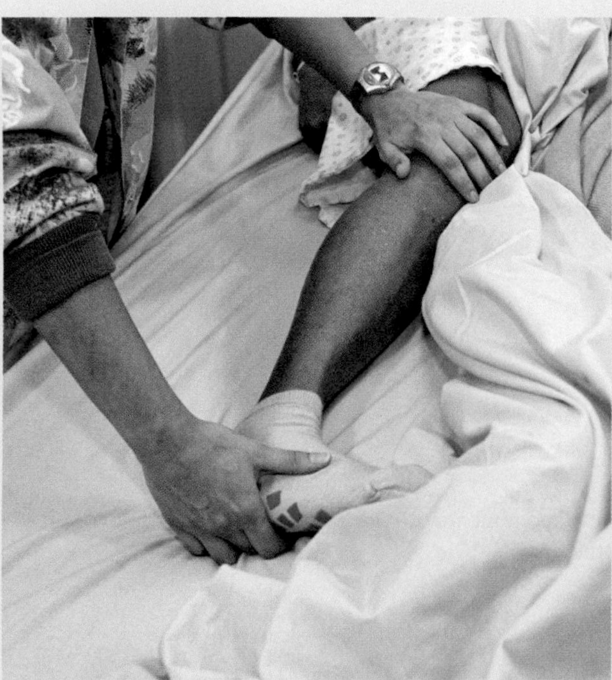

Figure 21. Turning the patient's foot and leg toward the opposite leg to rotate it internally.

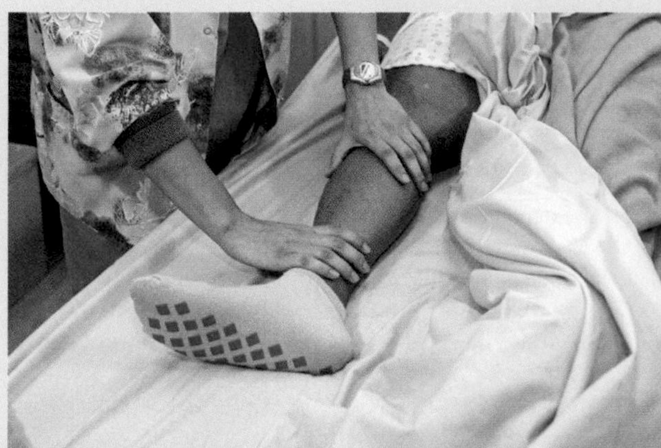

Figure 22. Moving the patient's foot and leg outward away from the opposite leg to rotate it externally.

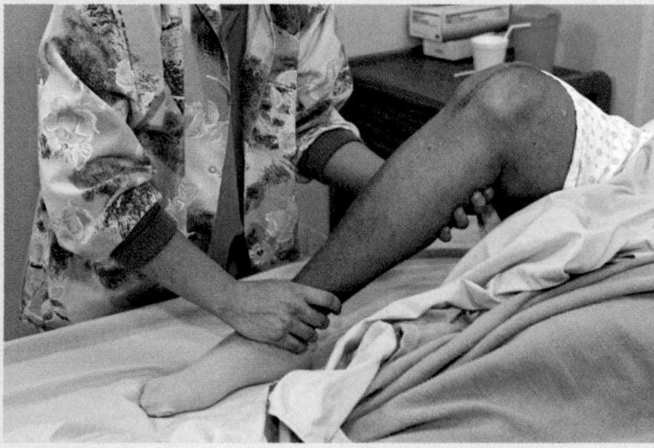

Figure 23. Bending the patient's leg and bringing the heel toward the back of the leg.

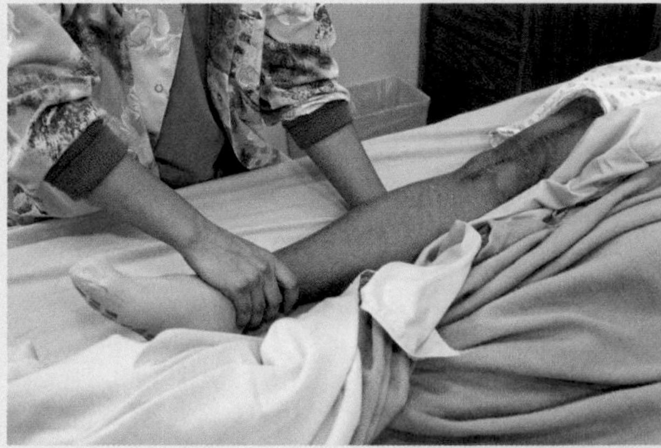

Figure 24. Returning the leg to a straight position.

SKILL 9-2 Providing Range-of-Motion Exercises *(continued)*

ACTION	RATIONALE
21. At the ankle, move the foot up and back until the toes are upright (Figure 25). Move the foot with the toes pointing downward (Figure 26).	These movements provide for dorsiflexion and plantar flexion of the ankle.
22. Turn the sole of the foot toward the midline (Figure 27). Turn the sole of the foot outward (Figure 28).	These movements provide for inversion and eversion of the ankle.

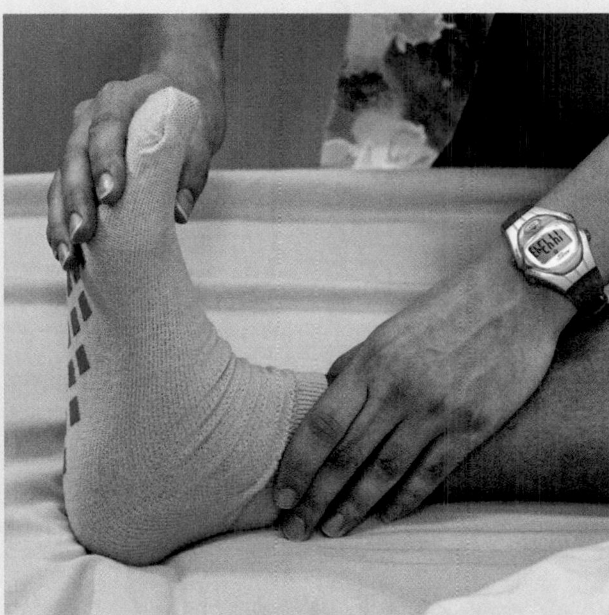

Figure 25. At the ankle, moving the patient's foot up and back until the toes are upright.

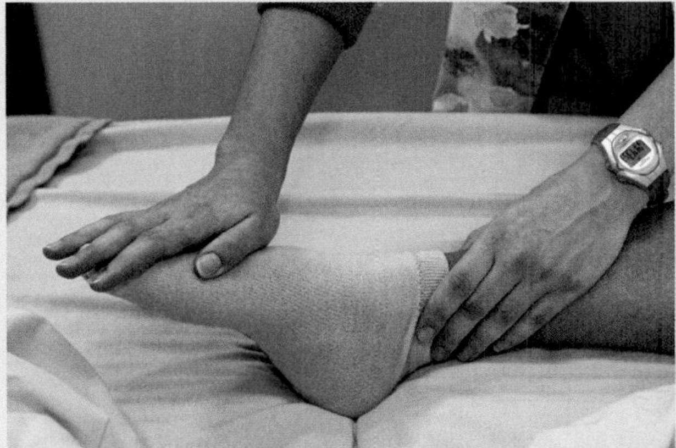

Figure 26. Moving the patient's foot with the toes pointing down.

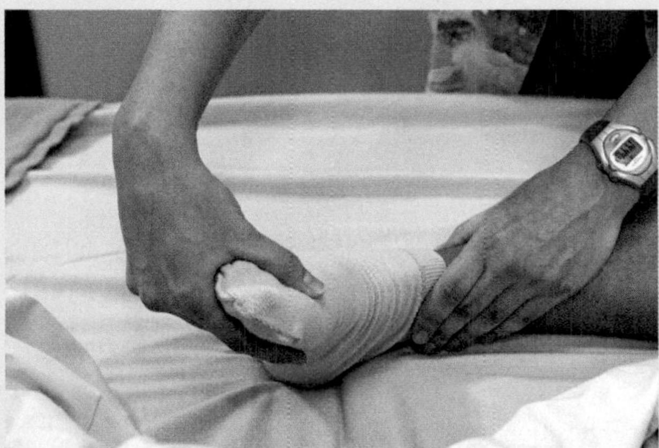

Figure 27. Turning the sole toward the midline.

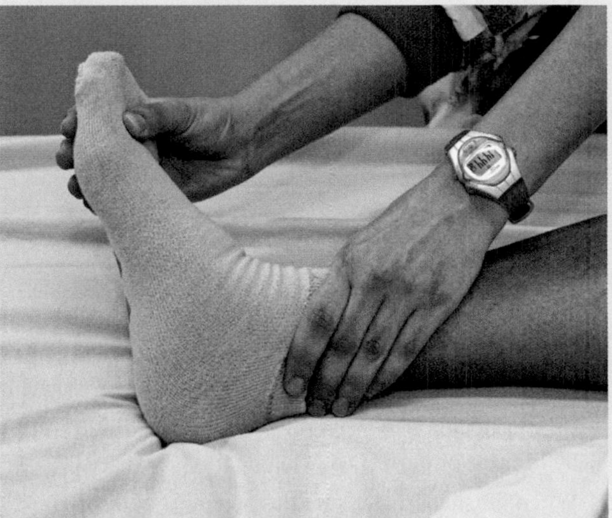

Figure 28. Turning the sole outward.

(continued)

SKILL 9-2

Providing Range-of-Motion Exercises *(continued)*

ACTION	RATIONALE
23. Curl the toes downward (Figure 29), and then straighten them out (Figure 30). Spread the toes apart (Figure 31) and bring them together (Figure 32).	These movements provide for flexion, extension, abduction, and adduction of the toes.

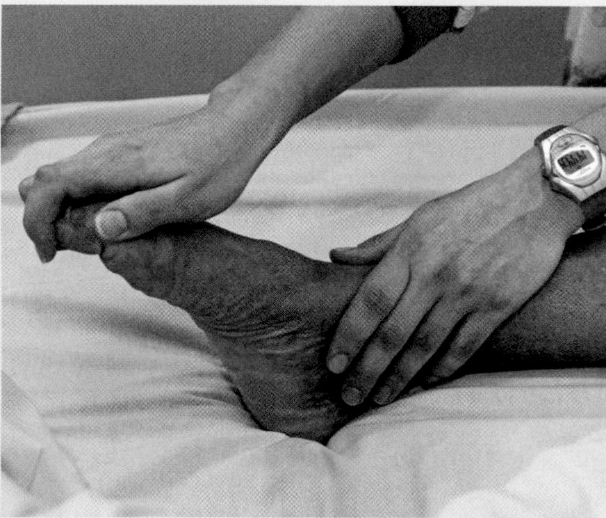

Figure 29. Curling the patient's toes down.

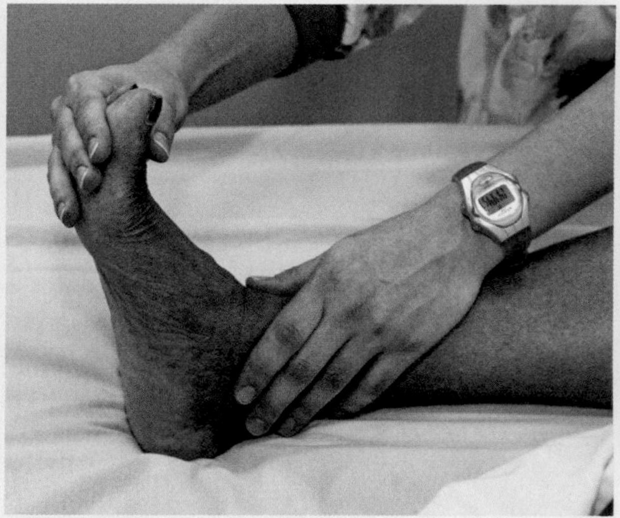

Figure 30. Straightening the patient's toes.

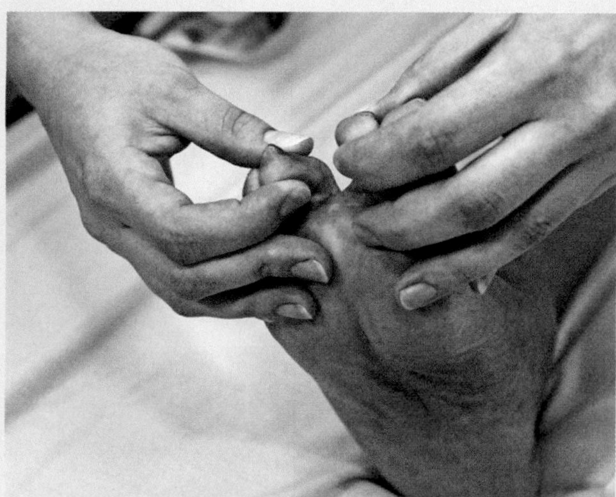

Figure 31. Spreading the patient's toes apart.

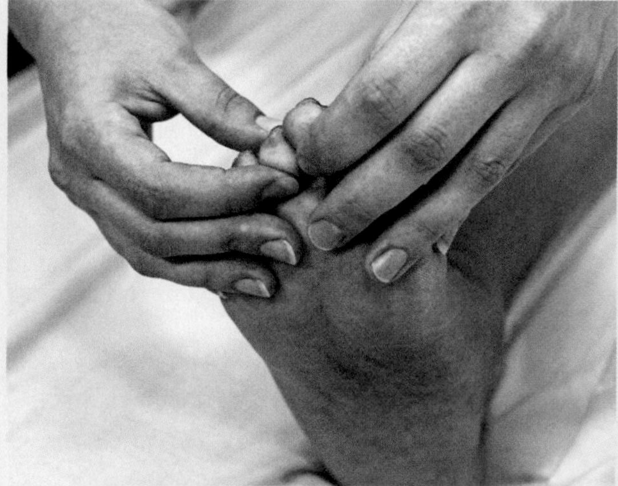

Figure 32. Bringing the patient's toes together.

ACTION	RATIONALE
24. Repeat these exercises on the other side of the body. Encourage the patient to do as many of these exercises by himself or herself as possible.	Repeating motions on the other side provides exercise for the entire body.
25. When finished, make sure the patient is comfortable, with the side rails up and the bed in the lowest position.	Proper positioning with raised side rails and proper bed height provides for patient comfort and safety.
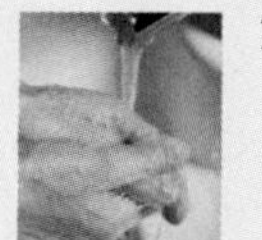 26. Remove gloves if used and perform hand hygiene.	Proper glove removal and hand hygiene prevent the spread of microorganisms.

SKILL 9-2 Providing Range-of-Motion Exercises *(continued)*

EVALUATION

The expected outcome is met when the patient maintains or improves joint mobility and muscle strength, and muscle atrophy and contractures are prevented.

DOCUMENTATION

Guidelines

Document the exercises performed, any significant observations, and the patient's reaction to the activities.

Sample Documentation

5/1/08 0945 Range-of-motion exercises performed to all joints. Patient able to perform active range of motion of head, neck, shoulders, and arms. Required moderate assistance with ROM to lower extremities. Denied any complaints of pain during exercises. Patient tolerated exercise session well. Sitting in semi-Fowler's position with side rails up, watching television.—J. Chrisp, RN

Unexpected Situations and Associated Interventions

- *While you are performing range-of-motion exercises, the patient complains of feeling tired:* Stop the activity for that time. Reevaluate the nursing plan of care. Space the exercises out at different times of the day. Schedule exercise times for the parts of the day the patient is typically feeling more rested.
- *While exercising your patient's leg, he complains of sudden, sharp pain:* Stop the exercises. Assess the patient for other symptoms. Notify the physician of the event and your findings. Joints should be moved until there is resistance but not pain. Uncomfortable reactions should be reported and exercises halted. The activity plan may have to be revised.

Special Considerations

General Considerations

- Many of these exercises can be incorporated into daily activities, such as during bathing.
- A physician's order and specific instructions should be obtained to perform range-of-motion exercises for patients with acute arthritis, fractures, torn ligaments, joint dislocation, acute myocardial infarction, and bone tumors or metastases.

Older Adult Considerations

- Avoid neck hyperextension and attempts to achieve full range of motion in all joints with older patients.

SKILL 9-3 Moving a Patient Up in Bed With the Assistance of Another Nurse

When a patient needs to be moved up in bed, it is important to avoid injuring yourself and the patient. The patient is at risk for injuries from shearing forces while being moved. Evaluate the patient's condition, any activity restrictions, the patient's ability to assist with positioning and ability to understand directions, the patient's body weight, and your strength to decide if additional assistance is needed. Safe Patient Handling Algorithm 4 (in Skill 9-1) can assist in making decisions about patient handling and movement. Using assistance, appropriate lifting and repositioning devices, good body mechanics, and correct technique are important to avoid injuries to yourself and the patient. Fundamentals Review 9-4 reviews examples of equipment and assistive devices that are available to aid in patient movement and handling.

(continued)

SKILL 9-3 Moving a Patient Up in Bed With the Assistance of Another Nurse *(continued)*

The procedure below describes moving a patient using a draw sheet; the Skill Variation at the end of the skill discusses using a full-body sling to reposition the patient.

Equipment

- Friction-reducing sheet or draw sheet
- Nonsterile gloves, if indicated
- Additional caregiver to assist
- Full-body sling lift and cover sheet, if necessary, based on assessment and availability

ASSESSMENT

Assess the situation to determine the need to move the patient up in the bed. Review the medical record and nursing plan of care for conditions that may influence the patient's ability to move or to be positioned. Assess for tubes, IV lines, incisions, or equipment that may alter the positioning procedure. Assess the patient's level of consciousness, ability to understand and follow directions, and ability to assist with moving. Assess the patient's weight and your strength to determine if a third individual is required to assist with the activity. Assess the patient's skin for signs of irritation, redness, edema, or blanching.

NURSING DIAGNOSIS

Determine the related factors for the nursing diagnoses based on the patient's current status. Appropriate nursing diagnosis may include:

- Activity Intolerance
- Risk for Injury
- Acute Pain
- Chronic Pain
- Impaired Tissue Integrity
- Impaired Skin Integrity
- Risk for Impaired Skin Integrity
- Impaired Bed Mobility

OUTCOME IDENTIFICATION AND PLANNING

The expected outcome to achieve when moving a patient up in bed with the assistance of another nurse is that the patient remains free from injury and maintains proper body alignment. Additional outcomes may include: the patient reports improved comfort; and the patient's skin is clean, dry, and intact, without any redness, irritation, or breakdown.

IMPLEMENTATION

ACTION	RATIONALE
1. Review the medical record and nursing plan of care for conditions that may influence the patient's ability to move or to be positioned. Assess for tubes, intravenous lines, incisions, or equipment that may alter the positioning procedure. Identify any movement limitations. Consult patient handling algorithm, if available, to plan appropriate approach to moving the patient.	Reviewing the order and plan of care validates the correct patient and correct procedure. Identification of limitations and ability and use of an algorithm helps to prevent injury and aids in determining best plan for patient movement.
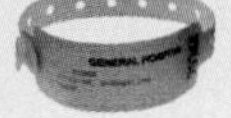 2. Identify the patient. Explain the procedure to the patient.	Patient identification validates the correct patient and correct procedure. Discussion and explanation help allay anxiety and prepare the patient for what to expect.
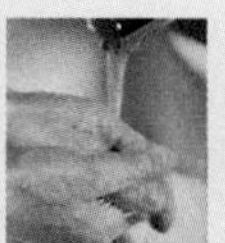 3. Perform hand hygiene and put on gloves, if necessary.	Hand hygiene and gloving prevent the spread of microorganisms.

SKILL 9-3

Moving a Patient Up in Bed With the Assistance of Another Nurse *(continued)*

ACTION	RATIONALE
4. Close the room door or curtains. Place the bed at an appropriate and comfortable working height. Adjust the head of the bed to a flat position or as low as the patient can tolerate. Placing the bed in slight Trendelenburg position aids movement, if the patient is able to tolerate it.	Closing the door or curtain provides for privacy. Proper bed height helps reduce back strain while you are performing the procedure. Flat positioning helps to decrease the gravitational pull of the upper body.
5. Remove all pillows from under the patient. Leave one at the head of the bed, leaning upright against the headboard.	Removing pillows from under the patient facilitates movement; placing a pillow at the head of the bed prevents accidental head injury against the top of the bed.
6. Position at least one nurse on either side of the bed, and lower both side rails.	Proper positioning and lowering the side rails facilitate moving the patient and minimize strain on the nurses.
7. If a friction-reducing sheet or drawsheet is not in place under the patient, place one under the patient's midsection (Figure 1).	A drawsheet supports the patient's weight and reduces friction during the lift.
8. Ask the patient (if able) to bend his or her legs and put his or her feet flat on the bed to assist with the movement.	Patient can use major muscle groups to push. Even if the patient is too weak to push on the bed, placing the legs in this fashion will assist with movement and prevent shearing of the skin on the heels.
9. **Have the patient fold the arms across the chest. Have the patient (if able) lift the head with chin on chest (Figure 2).**	Positioning in this manner provides assistance, reduces friction, and prevents hyperextension of the neck.

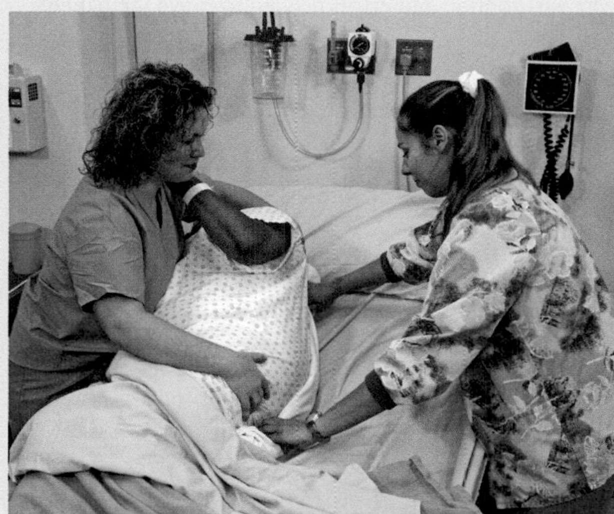

Figure 1. Placing drawsheet under the patient.

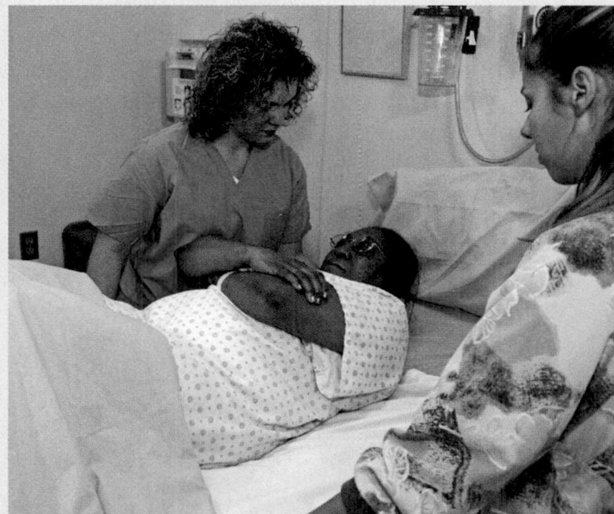

Figure 2. Assisting the patient to flex the neck with chin on chest.

(continued)

SKILL 9-3 Moving a Patient Up in Bed With the Assistance of Another Nurse *(continued)*

ACTION	RATIONALE
10. Position yourself at the patient's midsection with your feet spread shoulder width apart and one foot slightly in front of the other (Figure 3).	Doing so positions each nurse opposite the center of the body mass, lowers the center of gravity, and reduces the risk for injury.

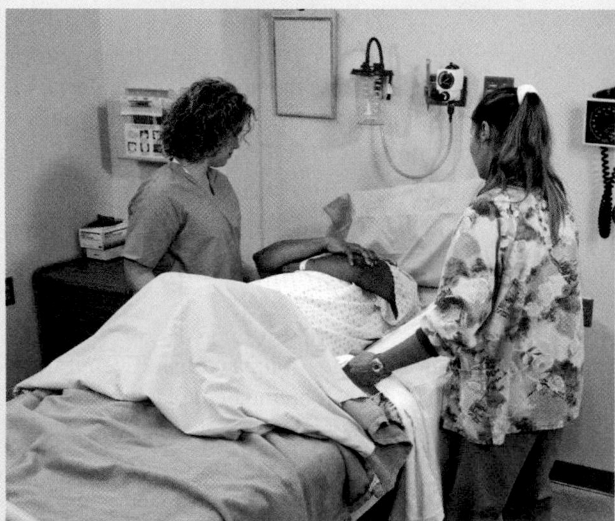

Figure 3. Nurses positioned at the patient's midsection.

ACTION	RATIONALE
11. If available on bed, engage mechanism to make the bed surface firmer for repositioning.	Decreases friction and effort needed to move the patient.
12. **Fold or bunch the drawsheet close to the patient before grasping it securely and preparing to move the patient (Figure 4).**	Having the drawsheet close to the body brings the patient's center of gravity closer to each nurse and provides for a secure hold.

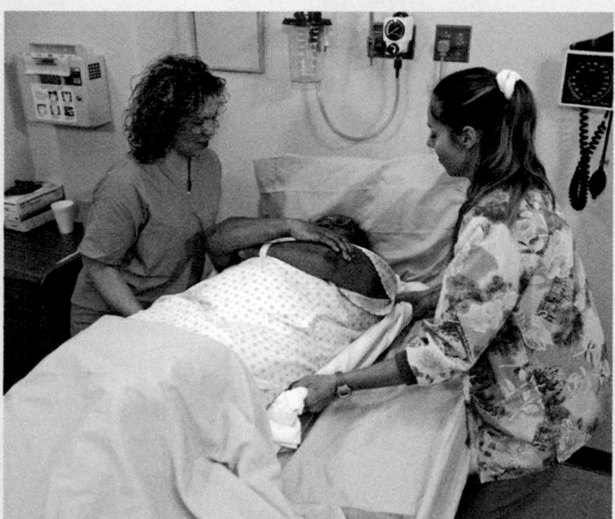

Figure 4. Folding drawsheet close to the patient.

SKILL 9-3 Moving a Patient Up in Bed With the Assistance of Another Nurse *(continued)*

ACTION	RATIONALE
13. Flex your knees and hips. Tighten your abdominal and gluteal muscles and keep your back straight.	Using the legs' large muscle groups and tightening muscles during transfer prevent back injury.
14. **Shift your weight back and forth from your back leg to your front leg and count to three. On the count of three, move the patient up in bed. If possible, the patient can assist with the move by pushing with the legs.** Repeat the process if necessary to get the patient to the right position (Figure 5).	The rocking motion uses the nurses' weight to counteract the patient's weight. Rocking develops momentum, which provides a smooth lift with minimal exertion by the nurses. If the patient assists, less effort is required by the nurses.

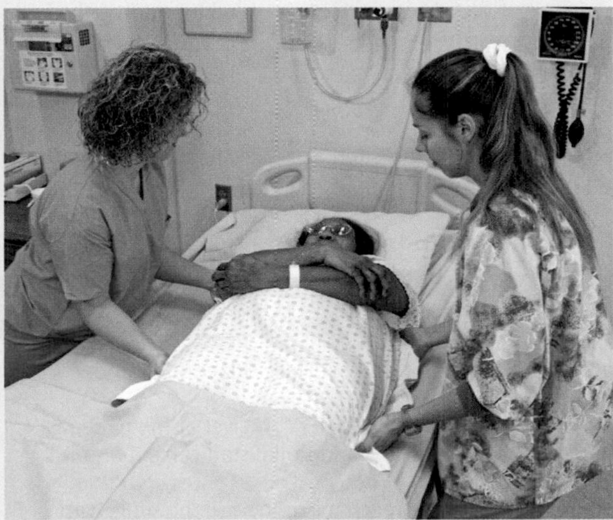

Figure 5. Moving the patient up in bed to a comfortable position.

ACTION	RATIONALE
15. Assist the patient to a comfortable position and readjust the pillows and supports as needed. Return bed surface to normal position, if necessary. Raise the side rails. Place the bed in the lowest position.	Readjusting the bed with supports and side rails ensures patient safety and comfort.
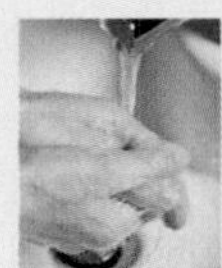 16. Remove gloves if used and perform hand hygiene.	Hand hygiene prevents the spread of microorganisms.

EVALUATION

The expected outcome is met when the patient is moved up in bed without injury and maintains proper body alignment, is comfortable, and demonstrates intact skin without evidence of any breakdown.

DOCUMENTATION

Guidelines

Many facilities provide areas on the bedside flow sheet to document repositioning. Document the time of the patient's change of position, use of supports, and any pertinent observations, including skin assessment. Document the patient's tolerance of the position change.

(continued)

SKILL 9-3 Moving a Patient Up in Bed With the Assistance of Another Nurse *(continued)*

Sample Documentation

11/10/08 1130 Patient repositioned from right side to left side; alignment maintained with wedge support behind back and pillow between legs. Skin on pressure points on right side without signs of irritation, edema, or redness. Patient reports no pain with movement.—B. Clapp, RN

Unexpected Situations and Associated Interventions

- *You are attempting to move a patient up in the bed with another nurse. Your first attempt is unsuccessful, and you realize the patient is too heavy for only two people to move:* Obtain the assistance of at least two other coworkers. Make use of available friction-reducing devices. Use full body lift if available. Position opposing pairs at the patient's shoulders and buttocks to distribute the weight. If necessary, have a fifth person lift the patient's legs or heels. The movement of very large patients is aided by putting the bed in a slight Trendelenburg position temporarily, provided the patient can tolerate it.

Special Considerations

General Considerations

- When moving a patient with a leg or foot problem, such as a cast, wound, or fracture, one assistant should be assigned to lift and move that extremity.

SKILL VARIATION Using Full Body Sling to Reposition Patient

- Review the medical record and nursing plan of care for conditions that may influence the patient's ability to move or to be positioned. Assess for tubes, intravenous lines, incisions, or equipment that may alter the positioning procedure. Identify any movement limitations.
- Check equipment for proper functioning.
- Identify the patient. Explain the procedure to the patient.
- Perform hand hygiene and put on gloves, if necessary.
- Close the room door or curtains. Place the bed at an appropriate and comfortable working height. Adjust the head of the bed to a flat position or as low as the patient can tolerate.
- Remove all pillows from under the patient. Leave one at the head of the bed, leaning upright against the headboard.
- Position at least one nurse on either side of the bed, and lower both side rails.
- Using the base-adjustment lever, widen the stance of the base of the device.
- Place cover sheet on sling surface. Place sling under patient.
- Position yourself and the other caregiver at the patient's midsection. If necessary, additional staff can support patient's legs.
- Crank or engage the mechanism to raise the sling, with the patient, up off the bed. Raise the patient just high enough to clear the bed surface.
- Guide the sling and relocate the patient to the appropriate place at the head of the bed.
- Release the sling slowly or activate the lowering device on the lift and slowly lower the patient to the bed surface.
- Remove the sling or leave in place for future use, based on facility policy.
- Assist the patient to a comfortable position and readjust the pillows and supports as needed. Raise the side rails. Place the bed in the lowest position.
- Remove gloves, if used, and perform hand hygiene.

SKILL 9-4 Transferring a Patient From the Bed to a Stretcher

While in the hospital, patients are often transported by stretcher to other areas for tests or procedures. Considerable care must be taken when moving someone from a bed to a stretcher or from a stretcher to a bed to prevent injury to the patient or staff. Refer to Figure 1, Safe Patient Handling Algorithm 2, to help in making decisions about safe patient handling and movement. Using assistance, appropriate lifting and repositioning devices, good body mechanics, and correct technique are important to avoid injuries to yourself and the patient. Be familiar with the proper way to use lateral-assist devices, based on the manufacturer's directions. Fundamentals Review 9-4 reviews examples of equipment and assistive devices that are available to aid in patient movement and handling.

Equipment

- Transport stretcher
- Friction-reducing sheet or draw sheet
- Lateral-assist device, such as a transfer board, roller board, or mechanical lateral-assist device, if available
- Bath blanket
- Regular blanket
- At least two assistants, depending on the patient's condition
- Nonsterile gloves, as needed

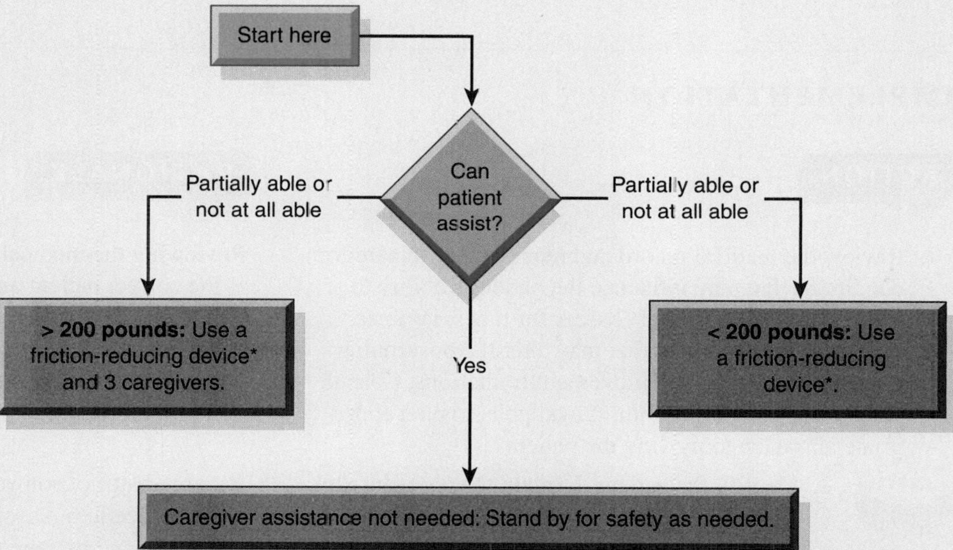
Algorithm 2: Lateral Transfer to and From: Bed to Stretcher, Trolley
Start here
Can patient assist?
Partially able or not at all able
Partially able or not at all able
> 200 pounds: Use a friction-reducing device* and 3 caregivers.
< 200 pounds: Use a friction-reducing device*.
Yes
Caregiver assistance not needed: Stand by for safety as needed.
Comments:
• Destination surface should be 1/2 inch lower for all lateral patient moves.
• For patients with stage III or IV pressure ulcers, care must be taken to avoid shearing force.
• During any patient transferring task, if any caregiver is required to lift more than 35 lbs. of a patient's weight, then the patient should be considered to be fully dependent and assistive devices should be used for the transfer.

Figure 1. Step-by-step procedure used to make safe decisions related to transferring a patient from bed to stretcher/trolley. (From VISN8 Patient Safety Center of Inquiry. [2005]. Safe patient handling and movement algorithms. Tampa, FL. Author. Available at www.VISN8.med.va.gov/patientsafetycenter/SPHMAlg050105.pdf.)

(continued)

SKILL 9-4 Transferring a Patient From the Bed to a Stretcher *(continued)*

ASSESSMENT

Review the medical record and nursing plan of care for conditions that may influence the patient's ability to move or to be transferred. Assess for tubes, IV lines, incisions, or equipment that may alter the transfer process. Assess the patient's level of consciousness, ability to understand and follow directions, and ability to assist with the transfer. Assess the patient's weight and your strength to determine if a fourth individual (or more) is required to assist with the activity. Assess the patient's comfort level; if needed, medicate as ordered with analgesics.

NURSING DIAGNOSIS

Determine the related factors for the nursing diagnoses based on the patient's current status. An appropriate nursing diagnosis is Risk for Injury. Other appropriate nursing diagnoses may include:

- Activity Intolerance
- Anxiety
- Risk for Falls
- Acute Pain
- Risk for Impaired Skin Integrity
- Impaired Transfer Ability

OUTCOME IDENTIFICATION AND PLANNING

The expected outcome to achieve when transferring a patient from the bed to a stretcher is that the patient is transferred without injury to patient or nurse.

IMPLEMENTATION

ACTION	RATIONALE
1. Review the medical record and nursing plan of care for conditions that may influence the patient's ability to move or to be positioned. Assess for tubes, IV lines, incisions, or equipment that may alter the positioning procedure. Identify any movement limitations. Consult patient-handling algorithm, if available, to plan appropriate approach to moving the patient.	Reviewing the medical record and plan of care validates the correct patient and correct procedure. Checking for interfering equipment helps reduce the risk for injury. Identification of limitations and ability and use of an algorithm helps to prevent injury and aids in determining best plan for patient movement.
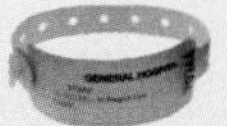 2. Identify the patient. Explain the procedure to the patient.	Patient identification validates the correct patient and correct procedure. Discussion and explanation help allay anxiety and prepare the patient for what to expect.
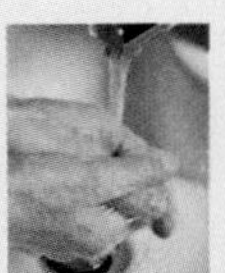 3. Perform hand hygiene and put on gloves, if necessary.	Hand hygiene and gloving prevent the spread of microorganisms.
4. Close the room door or curtains. Adjust the head of the bed to a flat position or as low as the patient can tolerate. Raise the bed to a height ½″ higher than the transport stretcher. Lower the side rails, if in place.	Closing the door or curtain provides privacy. Proper bed height and lowering side rails makes transfer easier and decreases the risk for injury.
5. Place the bath blanket over the patient and remove the top covers from underneath.	Bath blanket provides privacy and warmth.

SKILL 9-4 Transferring a Patient From the Bed to a Stretcher *(continued)*

ACTION	RATIONALE
6. If a friction-reducing sheet or drawsheet is not in place under the patient, place one under the patient's mid-section. Have patient fold arms against chest and move chin to chest. Use the drawsheet to move the patient to the side of the bed where the stretcher will be placed (Figure 2).	A drawsheet or other lateral-assist device supports the patient's weight, reduces friction during the lift, and provides for a secure hold. A transfer board or other lateral-assist device makes it easier to move the patient and minimizes the risk for injury to the patient and nurses.
7. Position the stretcher next to and parallel to the bed. **Lock the wheels on the stretcher and the bed.**	Positioning equipment makes the transfer easier and decreases the risk for injury. Locking the wheels keeps the bed and stretcher from moving.
8. Remove the pillow from the bed and place it on the stretcher. The two nurses should stand on the stretcher side of the bed. The third nurse should stand on the side of the bed without the stretcher.	Team coordination provides for patient safety during transfer.
9. Position the transfer board or other lateral-assist device under the patient. Use the drawsheet to roll the patient away from the stretcher. Slide the transfer board across the space between the stretcher and the bed, partially under the patient (Figure 3). Roll the patient onto his back, so he is partially on transfer board.	The transfer board or other lateral-assist device reduces friction, easing work load to move patient.
10. The nurse on the side of the bed without the stretcher should kneel on the bed, with his or her knee at the upper torso closer to the patient than the other knee. Fold or bunch the drawsheet close to the patient before grasping it securely in preparation for the transfer.	The nurse uses major muscle groups to assist in moving the patient.
11. Have one of the nurses on the stretcher side of the bed reach across the stretcher and grasp the drawsheet at the head and chest areas of the patient. If the transfer device used has long handles, each nurse should grasp two of the handles.	Doing so supports the patient's head and upper body.

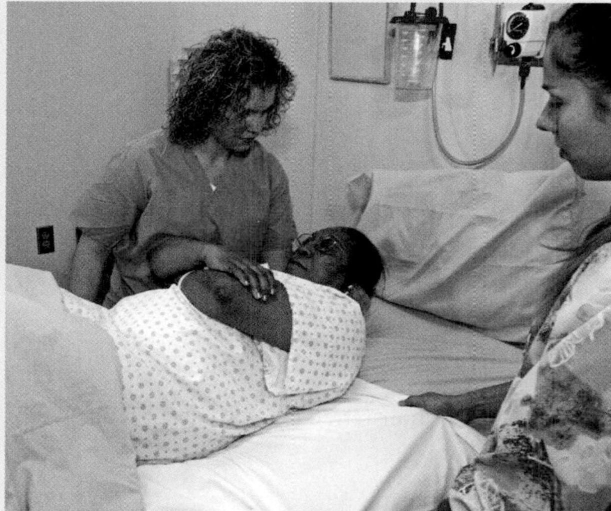

Figure 2. Using the drawsheet to move the patient to the side of the bed where the stretcher will be placed.

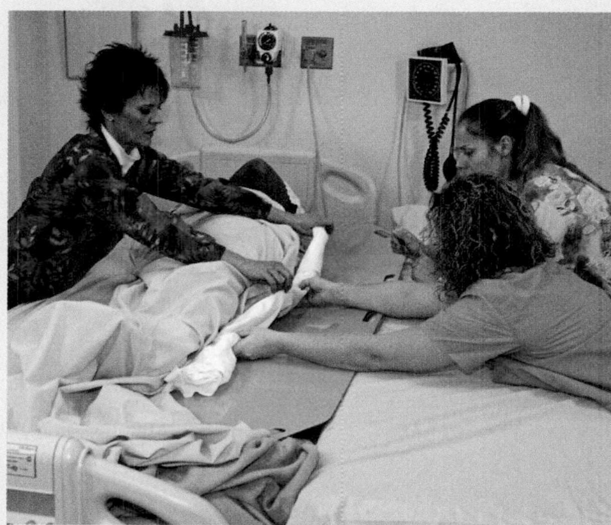

Figure 3. Ensuring that the transfer board is in position.

(continued)

SKILL 9-4 Transferring a Patient From the Bed to a Stretcher *(continued)*

ACTION	RATIONALE
12. Have the other nurse reach across the stretcher and grasp the drawsheet at the patient's waist and thigh area.	Doing so supports the lower part of the patient's body.
13. **At a signal given by one of the nurses, have the nurses standing on the stretcher side of the bed pull the sheet. At the same time, the nurse (or nurses) kneeling on the bed should lift the drawsheet, transferring the patient's weight toward the transfer board, and pushing the patient from the bed to the stretcher.**	Working in unison distributes the work of moving the patient and facilitates the transfer.
14. Once the patient is transferred to the stretcher, remove the transfer board, and secure the patient until the side rails are raised. Raise the side rails (Figure 4). Ensure the patient's comfort. Cover the patient with blanket and remove the bath blanket from underneath. Leave the friction-reducing sheet or drawsheet in place for the return transfer.	Side rails promote safety; blanket promotes comfort and warmth.

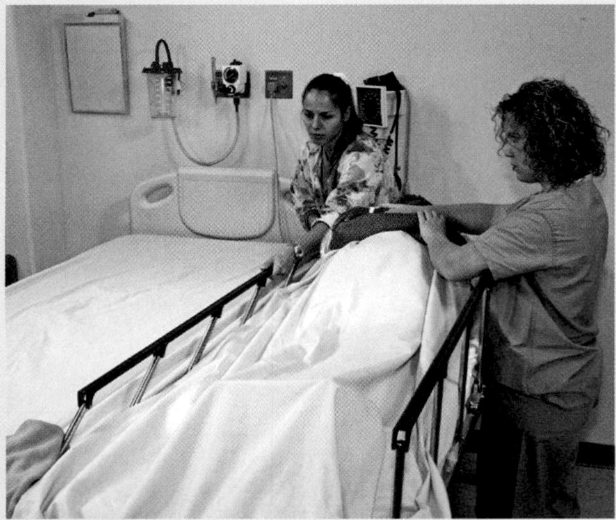

Figure 4. Securing the patient.

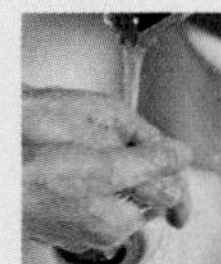

15. Remove gloves (if used) and perform hand hygiene.	Hand hygiene prevents the spread of microorganisms.

EVALUATION

The expected outcome is met when the patient is transferred to the stretcher without injury to patient or nurse.

DOCUMENTATION

Guidelines

Document the time and method of transport, and patient's destination, according to facility policy. Document the use of transfer aids and number of staff required for transfer.

SKILL 9-4 Transferring a Patient From the Bed to a Stretcher *(continued)*

Sample Documentation

5/12/08 1005 Patient transferred to stretcher via three-person assistance and lateral-assist transfer sheet. Transported to radiology for chest x-ray.—M. Joliet, RN

Unexpected Situations and Associated Interventions

- *Your patient needs to be transported to another department by stretcher. The patient is very heavy and somewhat confused, so you are concerned about his ability to cooperate with the transfer:* Obtain the assistance of three additional coworkers. Use a transfer board or mechanical lateral-assist device, if available, to move the patient. To place the transfer board, turn the patient on his side using the drawsheet, with his back toward the stretcher. Position the transfer board lengthwise and midway between the bed and the stretcher. Return the patient to his back with the drawsheet between the patient and the board. Using the drawsheet, move the patient across the transfer board and onto the stretcher. Reposition the patient on the stretcher, remove the board, and secure the patient on the stretcher.

Special Considerations

General Considerations

- Some mechanical lateral-transfer aids are motorized and others use a hand crank. If a mechanical lateral-assist device is used, follow the manufacturer's directions for safe movement of the patient. Be familiar with weight restrictions for individual pieces of equipment.
- Keep in mind that the transfer of patients is often delegated to unlicensed personnel. Before moving patients, all personnel need to complete instruction about this skill and must be able to provide return demonstrations of transfer skills. When a patient is being transferred, communicate clearly any mobility restrictions or special care needs.

SKILL 9-5 Transferring a Patient From the Bed to a Chair

Often, moving a patient from the bed to a chair helps him or her begin engaging in physical activity. Also, changing a patient's position will help prevent complications related to immobility. Safety and comfort are key concerns when assisting the patient out of bed. Assessing the patient's response to activity is a major nursing responsibility. Before performing the transfer, identify any restrictions related to the patient's condition and determine how activity levels may be affected. Figure 1, Safe Patient Handling Algorithm 1, can assist in making decisions about safe patient handling and movement. Using assistance, appropriate lifting and repositioning devices, good body mechanics, and correct technique are important to avoid injuries to yourself and the patient. Fundamentals Review 9-4 reviews examples of equipment and assistive devices that are available to aid in patient movement and handling.

Equipment

- Chair or wheelchair
- Gait belt
- Stand-assist aid, if available
- Additional staff person to assist
- Blanket to cover the patient in the chair
- Nonsterile gloves, if needed

(continued)

SKILL 9-5 Transferring a Patient From the Bed to a Chair *(continued)*

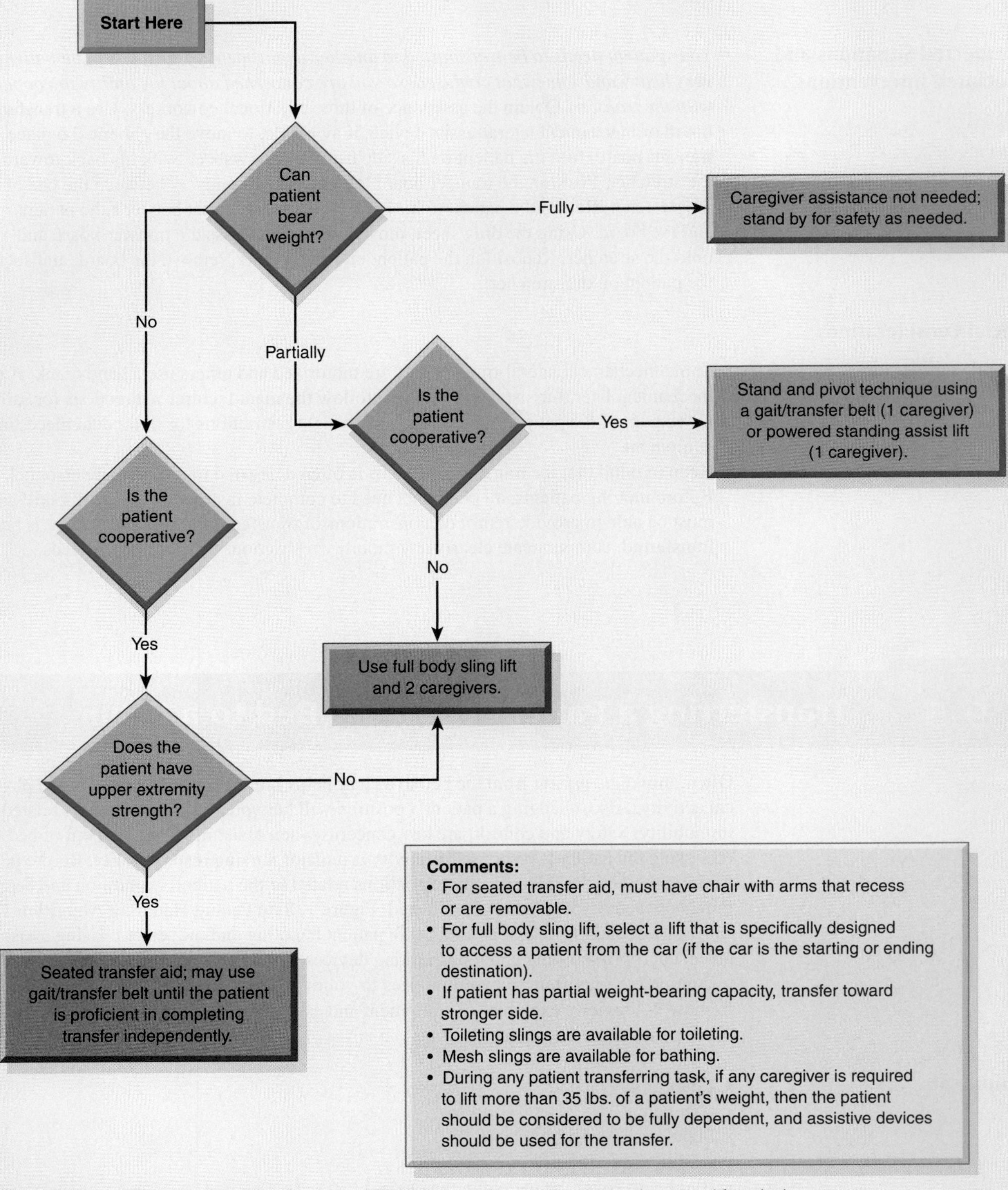

Figure 1. Step-by-step procedure used to make safe decisions related to transferring a patient to and from bed to chair, chair to toilet, chair to chair, or car to chair. (From VISN8 Patient Safety Center of Inquiry. [2005]. Safe patient handling and movement algorithms. Tampa, FL. Author. Available at www.VISN8.med. va.gov/patientsafetycenter/SPHMAlg050105.pdf.)

SKILL 9-5 Transferring a Patient From the Bed to a Chair *(continued)*

ASSESSMENT

Assess the situation to determine the need to get the patient out of bed. Review the medical record and nursing plan of care for conditions that may influence the patient's ability to move or to be transferred. Check for tubes, IV lines, incisions, or equipment that may require modifying the transfer procedure. Assess the patient's level of consciousness, ability to understand and follow directions, and ability to assist with the transfer. Assess the patient's weight and your strength to determine if additional assistance is needed. Assess the patient's comfort level; if needed, medicate as ordered with analgesics. If the patient is able to bear only partial weight, consider a second staff person to assist. If the patient is unable to bear even partial weight, or is uncooperative, use a full-body sling lift to move patient.

NURSING DIAGNOSIS

Determine the related factors for the nursing diagnoses based on the patient's current status. Appropriate nursing diagnoses may include:

- Activity Intolerance
- Risk for Activity Intolerance
- Anxiety
- Risk for Falls
- Impaired Transfer Ability
- Acute Pain
- Chronic Pain
- Impaired Physical Mobility
- Risk for Injury

OUTCOME IDENTIFICATION AND PLANNING

The expected outcome to achieve when transferring a patient from the bed to a chair is that the transfer is accomplished without injury to patient or nurse and the patient remains free of any complications of immobility.

IMPLEMENTATION

ACTION	RATIONALE
1. Review the medical record and nursing plan of care for conditions that may influence the patient's ability to move or to be positioned. Assess for tubes, IV lines, incisions, or equipment that may alter the positioning procedure. Identify any movement limitations. Consult patient-handling algorithm, if available, to plan appropriate approach to moving the patient.	Reviewing the medical record and plan of care validates the correct patient and correct procedure. Identification of limitations and ability and use of an algorithm helps to prevent injury and aids in determining best plan for patient movement.
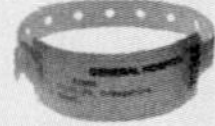 2. Identify the patient. Explain the procedure to the patient.	Patient identification validates the correct patient and correct procedure. Discussion and explanation help allay anxiety and prepare the patient for what to expect.
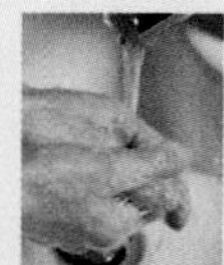 3. Perform hand hygiene and put on gloves, if necessary.	Hand hygiene and gloving prevent the spread of microorganisms.
4. If needed, move equipment to make room for the chair. Close the door or draw the curtains.	A clear pathway from the bed to the chair facilitates the transfer. Closing the door or curtain provides for privacy.

(continued)

SKILL 9-5 Transferring a Patient From the Bed to a Chair *(continued)*

ACTION	RATIONALE
5. Place the bed in the lowest position. Raise the head of the bed to a sitting position, or as high as the patient can tolerate.	Proper bed height and positioning facilitate the transfer. The amount of energy needed to move from a sitting position or elevated position to a sitting position is decreased.
6. **Make sure the bed brakes are locked. Put the chair next to the bed, facing the foot of the bed. If available, lock the brakes of the chair (Figure 2). If the chair does not have brakes, brace the chair against a secure object.**	Locking brakes or bracing the chair prevents movement during transfer and increases stability and patient safety.
7. Encourage the patient to make use of a stand-assist aid, either free-standing or attached to the side of the bed, if available, to move to the side of the bed and to a side-lying position, facing the side of the bed the patient will sit on.	Encourages independence, reduces strain for staff, and decreases risk for patient injury.
8. Lower the side rail if necessary and stand near the patient's hips. Stand with your legs shoulder width apart with one foot near the head of the bed, slightly in front of the other foot.	The nurse's center of gravity is placed near the patient's greatest weight to safely assist the patient to a sitting position.
9. Encourage the patient to make use of the stand-assist device. Assist the patient to sit up on the side of the bed; ask the patient to swing his or her legs over the side of the bed (Figure 3). At the same time, pivot on your back leg to lift the patient's trunk and shoulders. **Keep your back straight; avoid twisting.**	Gravity lowers the patient's legs over the bed. The nurse transfers weight in the direction of motion and protects his or her back from injury.
10. **Stand in front of the patient, and assess for any balance problems or complaints of dizziness. Allow legs to dangle a few minutes before continuing.**	Standing in front of the patient prevents falls or injuries from orthostatic hypotension. The sitting position facilitates transfer to the chair and allows the circulatory system to adjust to a change in position.

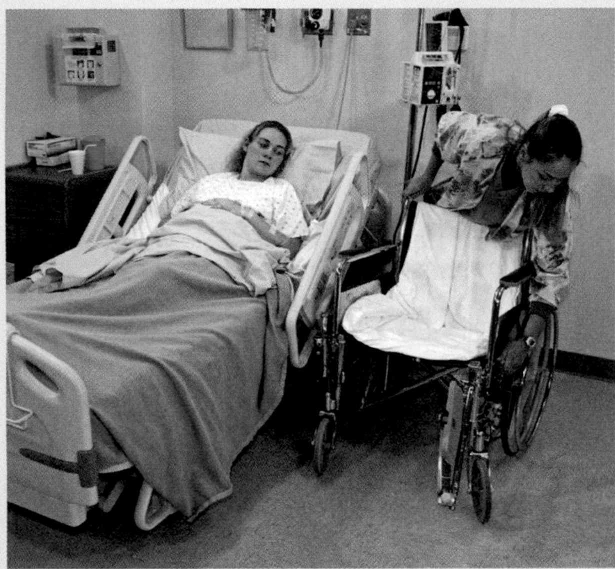

Figure 2. Putting the chair next to the bed, facing the foot of the bed, and locking the brakes.

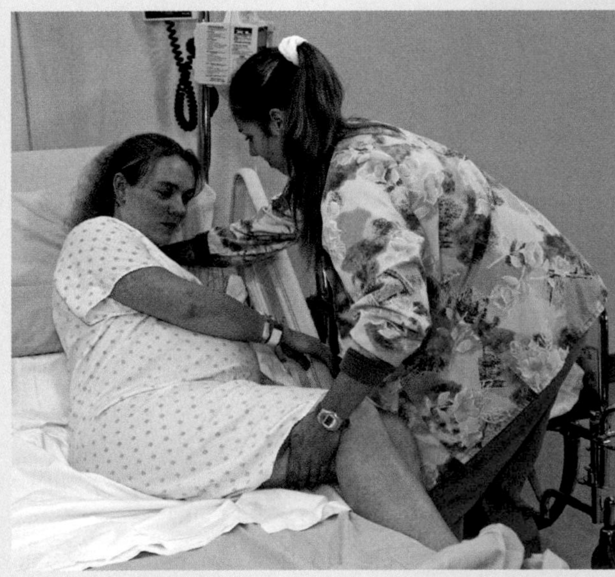

Figure 3. Assisting the patient to swing legs over side of bed.

SKILL 9-5 **Transferring a Patient From the Bed to a Chair** *(continued)*

ACTION	RATIONALE
11. Assist the patient to put on a robe and nonskid footwear.	Robe provides warmth and privacy. Nonskid soles reduce the risk for falling.
12. Wrap the gait belt around the patient's waist, based on assessed need and facility policy.	Gait belts improve the caregiver's grasp, reducing the risk of musculoskeletal injuries to staff and the patient. Provides firmer grasp for the caregiver if patient should lose his balance.
13. Stand facing the patient. Spread your feet about shoulder width apart and flex your hips and knees.	This position provides stability and allows for smooth movement using the legs' large muscle groups.
14. Ask the patient to slide his or her buttocks to the edge of the bed until the feet touch the floor. Position yourself as close as possible to the patient, with your foot positioned on the outside of the patient's foot. If a second staff person is assisting, have him/her assume a similar position.	Doing so provides balance and support.
15. Encourage the patient to make use of the stand-assist device. If necessary, have second staff person grasp gait belt on opposite side. Using the gait belt, assist the patient to stand. Rock back and forth while counting to three. **On the count of three, use your legs (not your back) to help raise the patient to a standing position (Figure 4). If indicated, brace your front knee against the patient's weak extremity as he or she stands.** Assess the patient's balance and leg strength. If the patient is weak or unsteady, return the patient to bed.	Holding at the gait belt prevents injury to the patient. Bracing your knee against a weak extremity prevents a weak knee from buckling and the patient from falling. Assessing balance and strength helps to identify need for additional assistance to prevent falling.

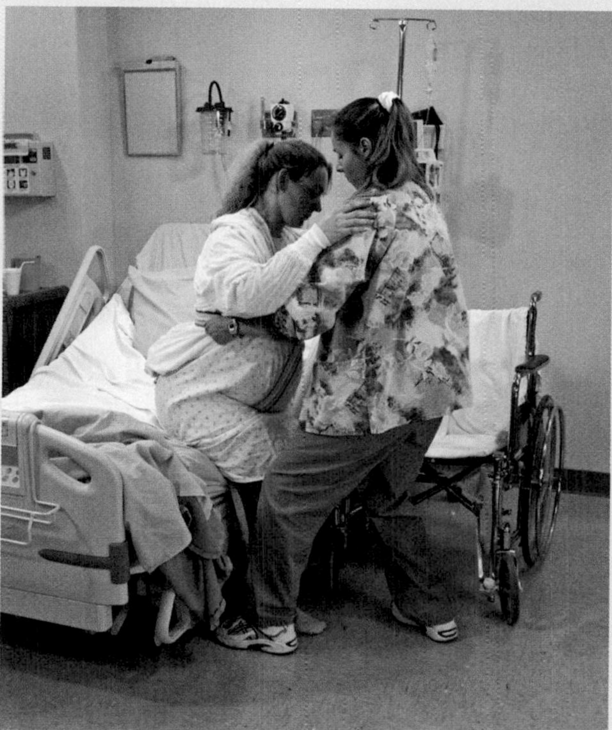

Figure 4. Nurse using her own legs to help raise the patient to a standing position.

(continued)

SKILL 9-5 Transferring a Patient From the Bed to a Chair *(continued)*

ACTION	RATIONALE
16. Pivot on your back foot and assist the patient to turn until the patient feels the chair against his or her legs.	This action ensures proper positioning before sitting.
17. Ask the patient to use an arm to steady himself or herself on the arm of the chair while slowly lowering to a sitting position. **Continue to brace the patient's knees with your knees and hold the gait belt. Flex your hips and knees when helping the patient sit in the chair (Figure 5).**	The patient uses his or her own arm for support and stability. Flexing hips and knees uses major muscle groups to aid in movement and reduce strain on the nurse's back.
18. Assess the patient's alignment in the chair (Figure 6). Remove gait belt, if desired. Depending on patient comfort, it could be left in place to use when returning to bed. Cover with a blanket if needed. Place the call bell close.	Assessment promotes comfort; blanket provides warmth and privacy; having the call bell readily available helps promote safety.

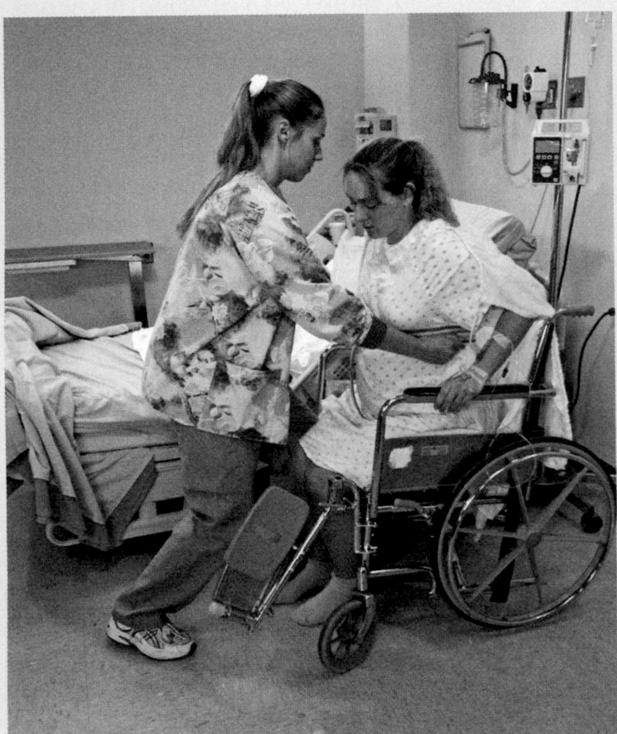

Figure 5. Assisting patient to sit.

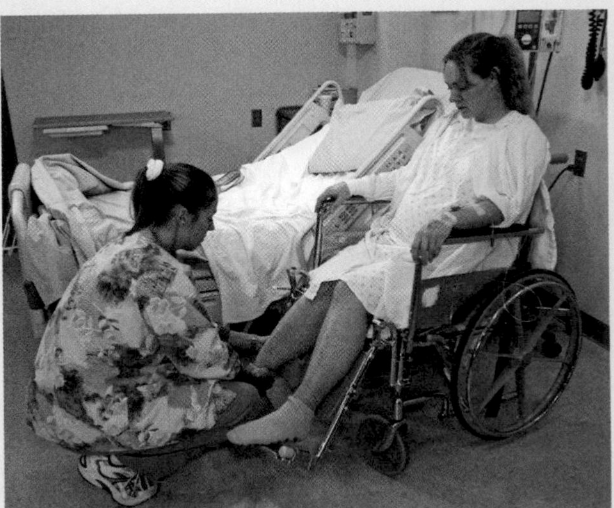

Figure 6. Assessing the patient's alignment in the chair.

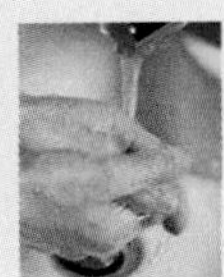

ACTION	RATIONALE
19. Remove gloves if used and perform hand hygiene.	Hand hygiene prevents the spread of microorganisms.

SKILL 9-5 **Transferring a Patient From the Bed to a Chair** *(continued)*

EVALUATION

The expected outcome is met when the patient transfers from the bed to the chair without injury and exhibits no signs and symptoms of problems or complications related to immobility. In addition, the nurse remains free of injury during the transfer.

DOCUMENTATION

Guidelines

Document the activity, including the length of time the patient sat in the chair, any observations, and the patient's tolerance of and reaction to the activity. Document the use of transfer aids and number of staff required for transfer.

Sample Documentation

5/13/08 1135 Patient dangled at side of bed for 5 minutes without complaints of dizziness or lightheadedness. Patient assisted out of bed to chair with minimal difficulty; gait belt in place. Tolerated sitting in chair for 30 minutes. Assisted back to bed, in semi-Fowler's position. Both side rails up.—J. Minkins, RN

Unexpected Situations and Associated Interventions

- *You are assisting a patient out of bed. The previous times the patient has gotten up, you have not had any difficulty helping him by yourself, so you are working alone this time. The patient is positioned on the side of the bed. You flex your hips and knees to help him stand. As you move to pivot to the chair, the patient becomes very lightheaded and weak and his knees buckle. The patient is too heavy for you to lift to the chair:* Do not continue the move to the chair. Lower the patient back to the side of the bed. Pivot him back into bed, cover him, and raise the side rails. Check vital signs and assess for any other symptoms. After his symptoms have subsided and you are ready to get him up again, arrange for the assistance of another staff member. Have the patient dangle his legs for a longer period of time before standing. Assess for lightheadedness or dizziness before helping him stand up. Notify the physician if there are any significant findings or if his symptoms persist.

Special Considerations

General Considerations

- Transfer of a patient to a chair or toilet can be accomplished using a powered stand-assist and repositioning lift, if available. These devices can be used with patients who have weight-bearing ability on at least one leg and who can follow directions and are cooperative. A simple sling is placed around the patient's back and under the arms. The patient rests his feet on the device's footrest and places his hands on the handle. The device mechanically assists the patient to stand, without any lifting by the nurse (see Fundamentals Review 9-4). Once the patient is standing, the device can be wheeled to a chair, the toilet, or bed. Some devices have removable foot rests and can be used as a walker. Some have scales incorporated into the device that can be used to weigh the patient.
- Patients who are unable to bear partial weight or full weight or who are uncooperative should be transferred using a full-body sling lift. Refer to Skill 9-6.
- The transfer of patients is often delegated to unlicensed personnel. Before moving patients, all personnel need to complete instruction and must be able to provide return demonstrations of transfer skills. Before the transfer, communicate clearly any mobility restrictions or special care needs.

SKILL 9-6 Transferring a Patient Using a Powered Full-Body Sling Lift

Powered full-body sling lift devices are used with patients who cannot bear any weight to move them out of bed, into and out of a chair, and to a commode or stretcher. A full-body sling is placed under the patient's body, including head and torso, and then the sling is attached to the lift. The device slowly lifts the patient. Some devices can be lowered to the floor to pick up a patient who has fallen. These devices are available on portable bases and ceiling-mounted tracks. Each manufacturer's device is slightly different, so review the instructions for your particular device. (See Fundamentals Review 9-4.)

Equipment

- Powered full-body sling lift
- Sheet or pad to cover the sling, if sling is not dedicated to only one patient
- Chair or wheelchair
- Additional staff person for assistance
- Nonsterile gloves, if necessary

ASSESSMENT

Assess the situation to determine the need to use the lift. Review the medical record and nursing plan of care for conditions that may influence the patient's ability to move or to be transferred. Assess for tubes, IV lines, incisions, or equipment that may alter the transfer procedure. Assess the patient's level of consciousness and ability to understand and follow directions. Assess the patient's comfort level; if needed, medicate as ordered with analgesics. Assess the condition of the equipment to ensure proper functioning before using with the patient.

NURSING DIAGNOSIS

Determine the related factors for the nursing diagnoses based on the patient's current status. Nursing diagnoses that may be appropriate include:

- Activity Intolerance
- Anxiety
- Fear
- Risk for Injury
- Acute Pain
- Chronic Pain
- Impaired Transfer Ability
- Risk for Falls

OUTCOME IDENTIFICATION AND PLANNING

The expected outcome to achieve when transferring a patient from the bed to a chair using a powered full-body sling lift is that the transfer is accomplished without injury to patient or nurse and the patient is free of any complications of immobility.

IMPLEMENTATION

ACTION	RATIONALE
1. Review the medical record and nursing plan of care for conditions that may influence the patient's ability to move or to be positioned. Assess for tubes, IV lines, incisions, or equipment that may alter the positioning procedure. Identify any movement limitations.	Reviewing the medical record and plan of care validates the correct patient and correct procedure. Checking for equipment and limitations reduces the risk for injury during the transfer.
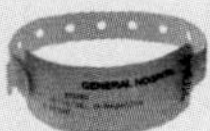 2. Identify the patient. Explain the procedure to the patient.	Patient identification validates the correct patient and correct procedure. Discussion and explanation allay anxiety and prepare the patient for what to expect.

SKILL 9-6

Transferring a Patient Using a Powered Full-Body Sling Lift *(continued)*

ACTION	RATIONALE
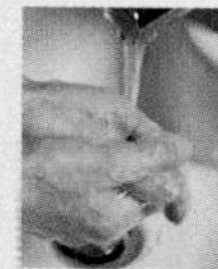 3. Perform hand hygiene and put on gloves, if necessary.	Hand hygiene and gloving prevent the spread of microorganisms.
4. If needed, move the equipment to make room for the chair. Close the door or draw the curtains.	Moving equipment out of the way provides a clear path and facilitates the transfer. Closing the door or curtain provides for privacy.
5. Adjust the bed to a comfortable working height. **Lock the bed brakes.**	Having the bed at the proper height prevents back and muscle strain. Locking the brakes prevents bed movement and ensures patient safety.
6. Lower the side rail, if in use, on the side of the bed you are working. If the sling is for use with more than one patient, place a cover or pad on the sling. Place the sling evenly under the patient. Roll the patient to one side and place half of the sling with the sheet or pad on it under the patient from shoulders to midthigh (Figure 1). Raise the rail and move to the other side. Lower the rail, if necessary. Roll the patient to the other side and pull the sling under the patient (Figure 2). Raise the side rail.	Lowering the side rail prevents strain on the nurse's back. Covering the sling prevents transmission of microorganisms. Some facilities, such as long-term care institutions, provide each patient with own transport sling. Rolling the patient positions the patient on the sling with minimal movement. Even distribution of the patient's weight in the sling provides for patient comfort and safety.

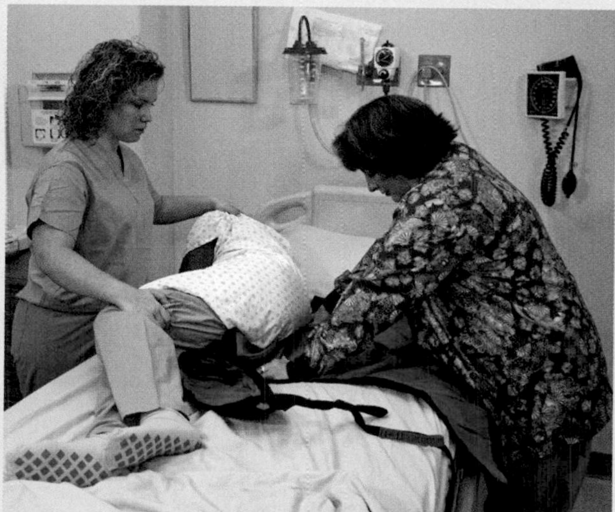

Figure 1. Rolling the patient to one side and placing the rolled sling underneath the patient.

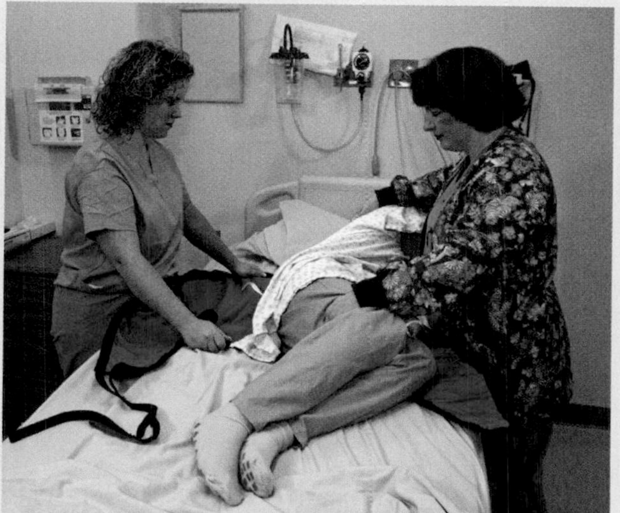

Figure 2. Rolling the patient to the opposite side and flattening out sling under the patient.

ACTION	RATIONALE
7. Bring the chair to the side of the bed. **Lock the wheels, if present.**	Bringing the chair close to the bed minimizes the distance needed for transfer. Locking the wheels prevents chair movement and ensures patient safety.
8. Lower the side rail on the chair side of the bed. **Roll the base of the lift under the side of the bed nearest to the chair. Center the frame over the patient. Lock the wheels of the lift.**	Lowering the rail allows for ease of transfer. Doing so reduces the distance necessary for transfer. Centering the frame helps maintain the balance of the lift. Locking the lift's wheels prevents the lift from rolling.

(continued)

SKILL 9-6 Transferring a Patient Using a Powered Full-Body Sling Lift *(continued)*

ACTION

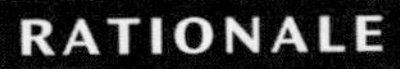

9. Using the base-adjustment lever, widen the stance of the base (Figure 3).

A wider stance provides greater stability and prevents tipping.

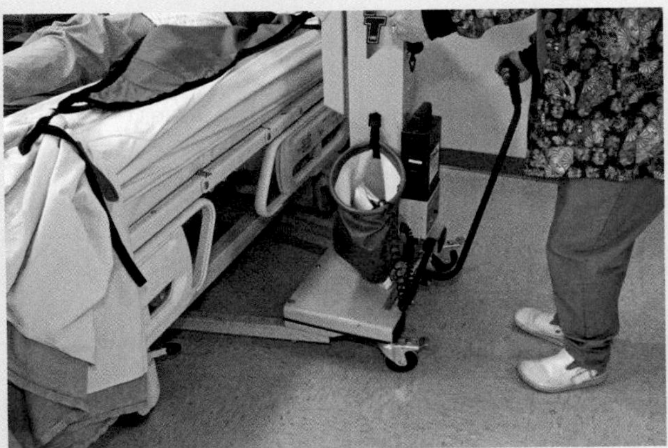

Figure 3. Widening the base of the lift.

10. Lower the arms close enough to attach the sling to the frame (Figure 4).

Lowering the arms is necessary to allow for the attachment of the sling's hooks.

11. Place the strap or chain hooks through the holes of the sling (Figure 5). Short straps attach behind the patient's back and long straps attach at the other end. Check the patient to make sure the hooks are not pressing into the skin. Some lifts have straps on the sling that attach to hooks on the frame. Check the manufacturer's instructions for each lift.

Connecting the straps or chains permits attachment of the sling to the lift. Checking the patient's skin for pressure from the hooks prevents injury.

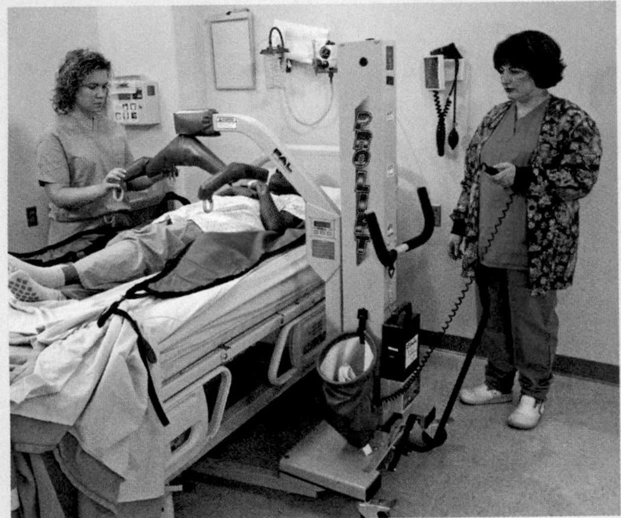

Figure 4. Lowering the arms of the lift.

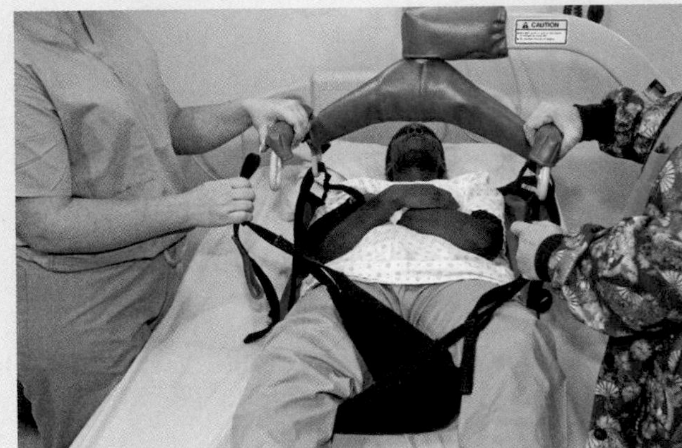

Figure 5. Connecting the straps to the lift.

12. Check all equipment, lines, and drains attached to the patient so that they are not interfering with the device. Have the patient fold his or her arms across the chest.

Ensuring that equipment and lines are free of the device prevents dislodgement and possible injury.

SKILL 9-6 Transferring a Patient Using a Powered Full-Body Sling Lift *(continued)*

ACTION	RATIONALE
13. With a person standing on each side of the lift, tell the patient that he or she will be lifted from the bed. Support injured limbs as necessary. Engage the pump to raise the patient about 6″ above the bed (Figure 6).	Having the necessary persons available provides for safety. Supporting injured limbs helps maintain stability. Informing the patient about what will occur reassures the patient and reduces fear.

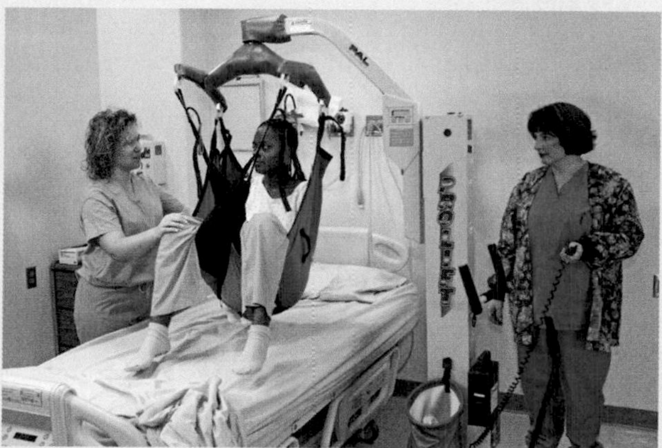

Figure 6. Raising the patient 6″ above the bed.

ACTION	RATIONALE
14. Unlock the wheels of the lift. **Carefully wheel the patient straight back and away from the bed.** Support the patient's limbs as needed.	Moving in this manner promotes stability and safety.
15. Position the patient over the chair with the base of the lift straddling the chair (Figure 7). Lock the wheels of the lift.	Proper positioning of the patient and device promotes stability and safety.
16. Gently lower the patient to the chair until the hooks or straps are slightly loosened from the sling or frame (Figure 8). Guide the patient into the chair with your hands as the sling lowers.	Gently lowering the patient in this manner places the patient fully in the chair and reduces the risk for injury.

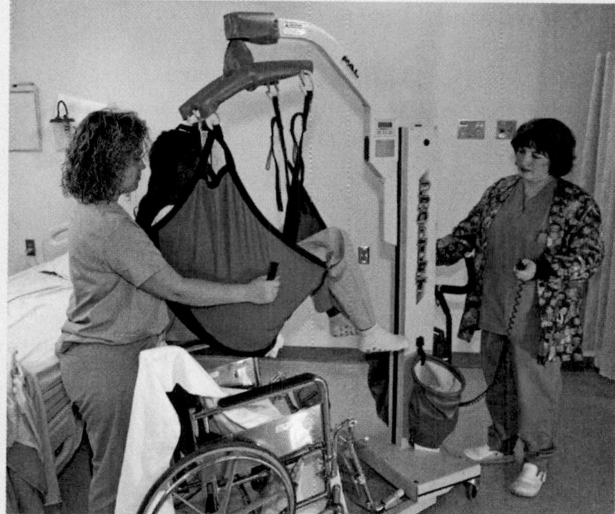

Figure 7. Positioning the patient in the sling over the chair.

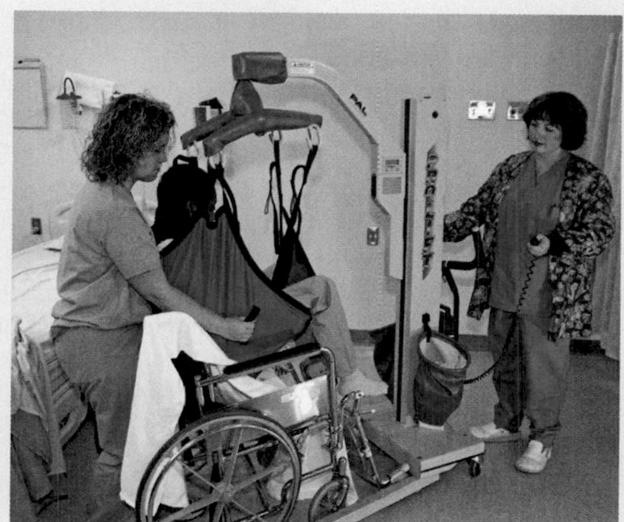

Figure 8. Lowering the patient in the sling into the chair.

(continued)

SKILL 9-6 Transferring a Patient Using a Powered Full-Body Sling Lift *(continued)*

ACTION	RATIONALE
17. Disconnect the hooks or strap from the frame. Keep the sling in place under the patient.	Disconnecting the hooks or straps allows the patient to be supported by the chair and promotes comfort. The sling will need to be reattached to the lift to move the patient back to bed.
18. Adjust the patient's position, using pillows if necessary. Check the patient's alignment in the chair. Cover the patient with a blanket if necessary. Place the call bell within reach. When it is time for the patient to return to bed, reattach the hooks or straps and reverse the steps.	Pillows and proper alignment provide for patient safety and comfort. Reattaching the hooks or straps allows the lift to support the patient for transfer back to bed.
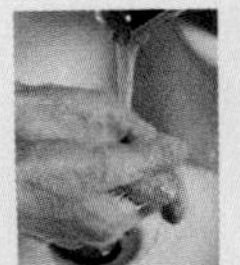 19. Remove gloves, if used, and perform hand hygiene.	Hand hygiene prevents the spread of microorganisms.

EVALUATION

The expected outcome is met when the transfer is accomplished without injury to patient or nurse, and the patient exhibits no evidence of complications of immobility.

DOCUMENTATION

Guidelines

Document the activity, transfer, any observations, the patient's tolerance of the procedure, and the length of time in the chair.

Sample Documentation

5/13/08 1430 Patient transferred out of bed to chair using powered full-body sling lift. Tolerated sitting in chair for 25 minutes without complaints of dizziness or pain. Assisted back to bed via lift. Left sitting in semi-Fowler's position with all four side rails up.—P. Jefferson, RN

Unexpected Situations and Associated Interventions

- *You are preparing to move a patient using a powered full-body sling lift. After you apply the sling and attach it to the frame, the patient becomes anxious and tells you she is afraid:* Acknowledge the patient's feelings and explain the procedure again. Reassure the patient about the safety of the device. Obtain an additional person to support the patient during the move by holding her hand or supporting her head. If possible, plan the transfer when a family member or friend is present to offer support.

Special Considerations

General Considerations

- The transfer of patients is often delegated to unlicensed personnel. Before moving patients, all personnel need to complete instruction and must be able to provide return demonstrations of transfer skills. Before the transfer, communicate clearly any mobility restrictions or special care needs.

SKILL 9-7 Assisting a Patient With Ambulation

Walking exercises most of the body's muscles and increases joint flexibility. It improves respiratory and gastrointestinal function. Ambulating also reduces the risk for complications of immobility. However, even a short period of immobility can decrease a person's tolerance for ambulating. If necessary, make use of appropriate equipment and assistive devices to aid in patient movement and handling. Refer to Fundamentals Review 9-4 for examples of assistive equipment and devices.

Equipment

- Gait belt, as necessary
- Nonskid shoes or slippers
- Stand-assist device as necessary, if available
- Additional staff for assistance as needed

ASSESSMENT

Assess the patient's ability to walk and the need for assistance. Review the patient's record for conditions that may affect ambulation. Perform a pain assessment before the time for the activity. If the patient reports pain, administer the prescribed medication in sufficient time to allow for the full effect of the analgesic. Take vital signs and assess the patient for dizziness or lightheadedness with position changes.

Nursing Diagnosis

Determine the related factors for the nursing diagnoses based on the patient's current status. Appropriate nursing diagnoses may include:

- Impaired Physical Mobility
- Risk for Injury
- Activity Intolerance
- Risk for Falls
- Fatigue
- Acute Pain
- Chronic Pain
- Impaired Walking

OUTCOME IDENTIFICATION AND PLANNING

The expected outcome to achieve when assisting a patient with ambulation is that the patient ambulates safely, without falls or injury. Additional appropriate outcomes include the patient demonstrates improved muscle strength and joint mobility; the patient's level of independence increases; and the patient remains free of complications of immobility.

IMPLEMENTATION

ACTION	RATIONALE
1. Review the medical record and nursing plan of care for conditions that may influence the patient's ability to move and ambulate. Assess for tubes, IV lines, incisions, or equipment that may alter the procedure for ambulation. Identify any movement limitations.	Reviewing the medical record and plan of care validates the correct patient and correct procedure. Checking for equipment and limitations reduces the risk for patient injury.
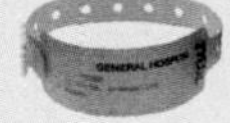 2. Identify the patient. Explain the procedure to the patient. Ask the patient to report any feelings of dizziness, weakness, or shortness of breath while walking. Decide how far to walk.	Patient identification validates the correct patient and correct procedure. Discussion and explanation help allay anxiety and prepare the patient for what to expect.

(continued)

SKILL 9-7 Assisting a Patient With Ambulation *(continued)*

ACTION	RATIONALE
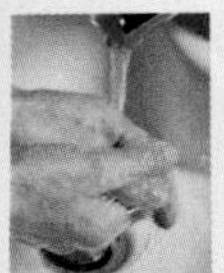 3. Perform hand hygiene.	Hand hygiene prevents the spread of microorganisms.
4. Place the bed in the lowest position.	Proper bed height ensures safety when getting the patient out of bed.
5. Encourage the patient to make use of a stand-assist aid, either free-standing or attached to the side of the bed, if available, to move to the side of the bed.	Encourages independence, reduces strain for staff, and decreases risk for patient injury.
6. Assist the patient to the side of the bed, if necessary. Have the patient sit on the side of the bed for several minutes and assess for dizziness or lightheadedness. Have the patient stay sitting until he or she feels secure.	Having the patient sit at the side of the bed minimizes the risk for blood pressure changes (orthostatic hypotension) that can occur with position change. Allowing the patient to sit until he or she feels secure reduces anxiety and helps prevent injury.
7. Assist the patient to put on footwear and a robe, if desired.	Doing so ensures safety and patient warmth.
8. Wrap the gait belt around the patient's waist, based on assessed need and facility policy.	Gait belts improve the caregiver's grasp, reducing the risk of musculoskeletal injuries to staff and the patient. The belt also provides a firmer grasp for the caregiver if patient should lose his balance.
9. Encourage the patient to make use of the stand-assist device. Assist the patient to stand, using the gait belt if necessary. Assess the patient's balance and leg strength. If the patient is weak or unsteady, return the patient to bed or assist to a chair.	Use of gait belt prevents injury to nurse and patient. Assessing balance and strength helps to identify need for additional assistance to prevent falling.
10. If you are the only nurse assisting, position yourself to the side and slightly behind the patient. Support the patient by the waist or transfer belt (Figure 1).	Positioning to the side and slightly behind the patient encourages the patient to stand and walk erect. It also places the nurse in a safe position if the patient should lose his or her balance or begin to fall.

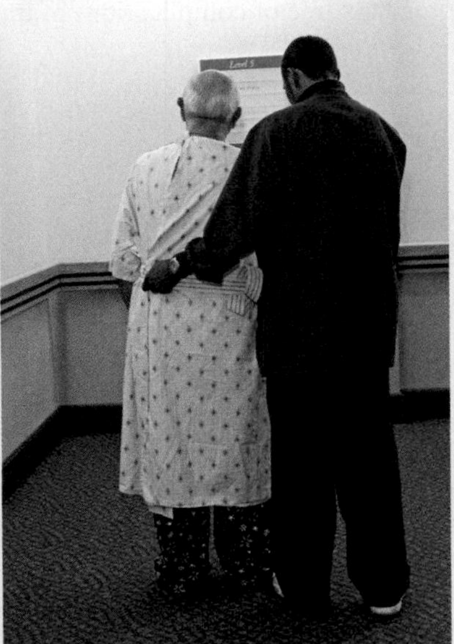

Figure 1. Nurse positioned to the side and slightly behind the patient while walking, supporting the patient by the waist or transfer belt.

SKILL 9-7 Assisting a Patient With Ambulation *(continued)*

ACTION	RATIONALE
When two nurses assist, position yourself to the side and slightly behind the patient, supporting the patient by the waist or gait belt. Have the other nurse carry or manage equipment or provide additional support from the other side.	Gait belts improve the caregiver's grasp, reducing the risk of musculoskeletal injuries to staff and the patient, and allow for a firmer grasp for the caregiver if patient should lose his balance.
Alternatively, when two nurses assist, stand at the patient's sides (one nurse on each side) with near hands grasping the gait belt and far hands holding the patient's lower arm or hand.	Gait belts improve the caregiver's grasp, reducing the risk of musculoskeletal injuries to staff and the patient, and allow for a firmer grasp for the caregiver if patient should lose his balance.
11. Take several steps forward with the patient. **Continue to assess the patient's strength and balance.** Remind patient to stand erect.	Taking several steps with the patient and standing erect promote good balance and stability. Continued assessment helps maintain patient safety.
12. Continue with ambulation for the planned distance and time. Return the patient to the bed or chair based on the patient's tolerance and condition.	Ambulation as prescribed promotes activity and prevents fatigue.
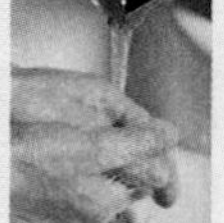 13. Remove gait belt. Perform hand hygiene.	Hand hygiene prevents the spread of microorganisms.

EVALUATION

The expected outcome is met when the patient ambulates safely for the prescribed distance and time and remains free from falls or injury. Additional outcomes are met when the patient exhibits increasing muscle strength, joint mobility, and independence and the patient remains free of any signs and symptoms of immobility.

DOCUMENTATION

Guidelines

Document the activity, any observations, the patient's tolerance of the procedure, and the distance walked.

Sample Documentation

5/14/08 1720 Patient ambulated with assistance in hallway for a distance of approximately 15 feet. Patient tolerated ambulation well; denied any complaints of dizziness, pain, or fatigue. Ambulated back to room and sitting in chair listening to music.—J. Minkins, RN

Unexpected Situations and Associated Interventions

- *You are walking with a postoperative patient in the hallway. She tells you she feels faint and begins to lean over as if she is going to fall:* Place your feet wide apart, with one foot in front. Rock your pelvis out on the side nearest the patient. This widens and stabilizes the base of support. Grasp the gait belt. This ensures a safe hold on the patient. Support the patient by pulling her weight backward against your body. Gently slide

(continued)

SKILL 9-7 Assisting a Patient With Ambulation *(continued)*

her down your body to the floor, protecting her head. This enables you to support the patient's weight with large muscle groups and protects you from back strain. Stay with the patient. Call for help. If another staff member was assisting you with ambulation, each of you should use one hand to grasp the gait belt and grasp the patient's hand or wrist with your other hands. Slowly lower her to the floor.

Special Considerations

General Considerations

- All equipment, such as indwelling urinary catheters, drains, or IV infusions, should be secured to a pole for ambulation. Do not carry equipment while helping the patient. Your hands should be free to provide support.

SKILL 9-8 Assisting a Patient With Ambulation Using a Walker

A walker is a lightweight metal frame with four legs. Nonskid caps cover the end of the legs to prevent slipping. Sometimes two or four of the leg caps are replaced with slides or wheels so the patient can push the walker instead of picking it up to move forward. Walkers provide stability and security for patients with insufficient strength and balance to use other ambulatory aids. There are several kinds of walkers; the choice of which to use is based on the patient's arm strength and balance. Regardless of the type used, the walker should extend from the floor to the patient's hip joint. The patient's elbows should be flexed about 30 degrees. Usually, the legs of the walker can be adjusted to the appropriate height.

Equipment

- Walker adjusted to the appropriate height
- Nonskid shoes or slippers
- Additional staff for assistance as needed
- Stand-assist device as necessary, if available
- Gait belt, if available

ASSESSMENT

Assess the patient's ability to walk and the need for assistance. Review the patient's record for conditions that may affect ambulation. Perform a pain assessment before the time for the activity. If the patient reports pain, administer the prescribed medication in sufficient time to allow for the full effect of the analgesic. Take vital signs and assess the patient for dizziness or lightheadedness with position changes. Assess the patient's knowledge regarding the use of a walker. Ensure that the walker is at the appropriate height for the patient.

NURSING DIAGNOSIS

Determine the related factors for the nursing diagnoses based on the patient's current status. Appropriate nursing diagnoses may include:

- Risk for Falls
- Impaired Walking
- Deficient Knowledge
- Risk for Injury
- Activity Intolerance
- Fatigue
- Acute Pain
- Chronic Pain

SKILL 9-8

Assisting a Patient With Ambulation Using a Walker *(continued)*

OUTCOME IDENTIFICATION AND PLANNING

The expected outcome to achieve when assisting a patient with ambulation using a walker is that the patient ambulates safely with the walker and is free from falls or injury. Additional appropriate outcomes include: the patient demonstrates proper use of the walker and states the need for the walker; the patient demonstrates increasing muscle strength, joint mobility, and independence; and the patient remains free of complications of immobility.

IMPLEMENTATION

ACTION	RATIONALE
1. Review the medical record and nursing plan of care for conditions that may influence the patient's ability to move and ambulate, and for specific instructions for ambulation such as distance. Assess for tubes, IV lines, incisions, or equipment that may alter the procedure for ambulation. Assess the patient's knowledge and previous experience regarding the use of a walker. Identify any movement limitations.	Reviewing the medical record and plan of care validates the correct patient and correct procedure. Checking for equipment and limitations helps minimize the risk for injury.
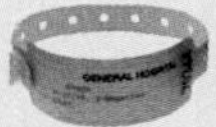 2. Identify the patient. Explain the procedure to the patient. Tell the patient to report any feelings of dizziness, weakness, or shortness of breath while walking. Decide how far to walk.	Patient identification validates the correct patient and correct procedure. Discussion and explanation help allay anxiety and prepare the patient for what to expect.
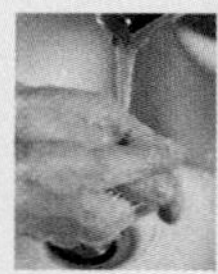 3. Perform hand hygiene.	Hand hygiene prevents the spread of microorganisms.
4. Place the bed in the lowest position.	Proper bed height ensures safety when getting the patient out of bed.
5. Encourage the patient to make use of a stand-assist aid, either free standing or attached to the side of the bed, if available, to move to the side of the bed.	Use of assistive devices encourages independence, reduces strain for staff, and decreases risk for patient injury.
6. Assist the patient to the side of the bed, if necessary. Have the patient sit on the side of the bed. Assess for dizziness or lightheadedness. Have the patient stay sitting until he or she feels secure.	Having the patient sit on the side of the bed minimizes the risk for blood pressure changes (orthostatic hypotension) that can occur with position change. Assessing patient complaints helps prevent injury.
7. Assist the patient to put on footwear and a robe, if desired.	Doing so ensures safety and warmth.
8. Wrap the gait belt around the patient's waist, based on assessed need and facility policy.	Gait belts improve the caregiver's grasp, reducing the risk of musculoskeletal injuries to staff and the patient and provide for a firmer grasp if patient should lose his balance.

(continued)

SKILL 9-8 Assisting a Patient With Ambulation Using a Walker *(continued)*

ACTION | **RATIONALE**

9. **Place the walker directly in front of the patient (Figure 1).** Ask the patient to push himself or herself off the bed or chair, make use of the stand-assist device, or assist the patient to stand (Figure 2). Once the patient is standing, have him or her hold the walker's hand grips firmly and equally. Stand slightly behind the patient, on one side.

   Proper positioning with the walker ensures balance. Standing within the walker and holding the hand grips firmly provide stability when moving the walker and helps ensure safety.

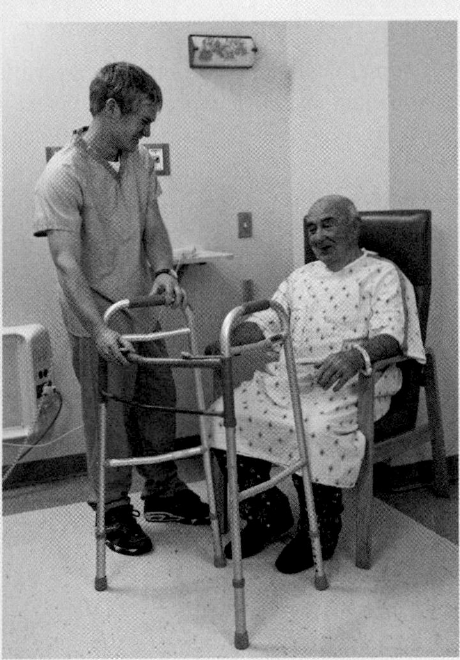

Figure 1. Setting the walker in front of a seated patient.

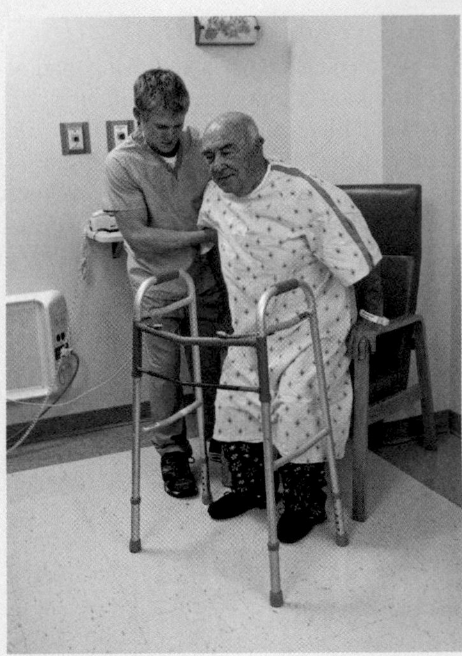

Figure 2. Assisting the patient to stand with the walker.

10. Have the patient move the walker forward 6″ to 8″ and set it down, making sure all four feet of the walker stay on the floor. Then, tell the patient to step forward with either foot into the walker, supporting himself or herself on his or her arms. Follow through with the other leg. **If one leg is weaker or impaired, have the patient step forward with the involved leg and follow with the uninvolved leg, again supporting himself or herself on his or her arms.**

    Having all four feet of the walker on the floor provides a broad base of support. Moving the walker and stepping forward moves the center of gravity toward the walker, ensuring balance and preventing tipping of the walker.

SKILL 9-8

Assisting a Patient With Ambulation Using a Walker *(continued)*

ACTION	RATIONALE
11. Move the walker forward again, and continue the same pattern. Continue with ambulation for the planned distance and time (Figure 3). Return the patient to the bed or chair based on the patient's tolerance and condition, ensuring that the patient is comfortable and call light is within reach.	Moving the walker promotes activity. Continuing for the planned distance and time prevents the patient from becoming fatigued.

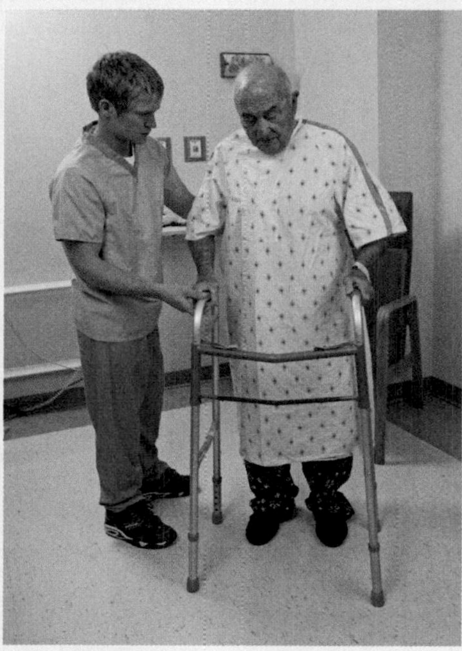

Figure 3. Assisting the patient to walk with the walker.

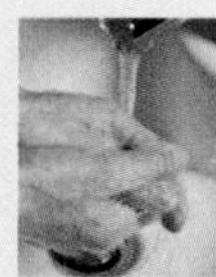

12. Remove gait belt. Perform hand hygiene.	Hand hygiene prevents the spread of microorganisms.

EVALUATION

The expected outcome is met when the patient uses the walker to ambulate safely and remains free of injury. Other outcomes are met when the patient exhibits increased muscle strength, joint mobility, and independence; demonstrates independent walker use; and exhibits no evidence of complications of immobility.

DOCUMENTATION

Guidelines

Document the activity, any observations, the patient's ability to use the walker, the patient's tolerance of the procedure, and the distance walked.

(continued)

SKILL 9-8 Assisting a Patient With Ambulation Using a Walker *(continued)*

Sample Documentation

5/15/08 0900 Patient ambulated with walker from bed to bathroom for morning care with minimal assistance; demonstrated proper steps in using walker. Able to ambulate back to bed using walker independently.—P. Collins, RN

Unexpected Situations and Associated Interventions

- *You are assisting a patient ambulating in the hallway using a walker. She becomes extremely tired and says she can't pick up the walker anymore ("it's too heavy"). However, she cannot walk without the walker:* Call for assistance. Have a coworker obtain a wheelchair to transport the patient back to her room. Assess the patient for other symptoms, if necessary. In the future, plan to ambulate for shorter distances to prevent her from becoming fatigued.

Special Considerations

General Considerations

- Never use a walker on the stairs.
- Wear nonskid shoes or slippers.
- If one leg is impaired, move that leg and the walker forward together for 6″ to 8″. Move the unaffected leg forward once body weight is securely supported by the walker and the impaired leg.
- Some walkers have wheels on the front legs. These walkers are best for patients with a gait that is too fast for a walker without wheels and for patients who have difficulty lifting a walker. Walkers also are available with wheels on all four legs. These can be used by patients who require a larger base of support and do not rely on the walker to bear weight. If full body weight is applied to this type of walker, it could roll away, resulting in a fall. Wheeled walkers are best for patients who need minimal weight bearing from the walker (Van Hook et al, 2003).
- Keep in mind, walkers often prove to be difficult to maneuver through doorways and congested areas. They should not be used on stairs (Van Hook et al, 2003).
- Advise the patient to check the walker before use for signs of damage, deformity of the frame, or loose or missing parts.
- Teach patients to use the arms of the chair or a stand-assist device for leverage when getting up from a chair. Patients should not pull on the walker to get up; the walker could tip or become unbalanced.

Older Adult Considerations

- Maintain close observation of older adults because they frequently develop dangerous walking patterns with a walker.

SKILL 9-9 Assisting a Patient With Ambulation Using Crutches

Crutches enable a patient to walk and remove weight from one or both legs. Crutches are often used when the patient has a sprain, fracture, or nonwalking cast. The patient uses the arms to support the body weight. Crutches can be used for the short or the long term. A short-term crutch, known as an underarm or axillary crutch, is a wooden or metal staff that extends from the floor to below the axilla. Long-term crutches, known as forearm support crutches, are metal and extend from the floor to the forearm, with metal bands encircling the forearms. Crutches used for the long term provide additional support for weak or paralyzed legs. This section will discuss short-term crutch use.

When ambulating with crutches, one of five specific crutch gaits or patterns are used. The four-point gait is used by patients who can bear weight on both legs. It is the safest

SKILL 9-9 Assisting a Patient With Ambulation Using Crutches *(continued)*

gait but requires good coordination. The two-point gait is used for patients with leg weakness but with good coordination and arm strength. The three-point gait is used with patients who are unable to bear weight or can only bear partial weight on one leg. The swing-to and swing-through gaits are used by patients with paralysis of the hips and legs.

Equipment

- Crutches with axillary pads, hand grips, and rubber suction tips
- Nonskid shoes or slippers
- Stand-assist device as necessary, if available

ASSESSMENT

Review the patient's record and nursing plan of care to determine the reason for using crutches and instructions for weight bearing. Check for specific instructions from physical therapy. Perform a pain assessment before the time for the activity. If the patient reports pain, administer the prescribed medication in sufficient time to allow for the full effect of the analgesic. Determine the patient's knowledge regarding the use of crutches and assess the patient's ability to balance on the crutches. Assess for muscle strength in the legs and arms. Determine the appropriate gait for the patient to use.

NURSING DIAGNOSIS

Determine the related factors for the nursing diagnoses based on the patient's current status. Appropriate nursing diagnoses may include:

- Risk for Injury
- Impaired Walking
- Deficient Knowledge
- Risk for Falls
- Activity Intolerance
- Acute Pain
- Chronic Pain

OUTCOME IDENTIFICATION AND PLANNING

The expected outcome to achieve when assisting a patient with ambulation using crutches is that the patient ambulates safely without experiencing falls or injury. Additional appropriate outcomes include: the patient demonstrates proper crutch-walking technique; the patient demonstrates increased muscle strength and joint mobility; and the patient exhibits no evidence of injury related to crutch use.

IMPLEMENTATION

ACTION	RATIONALE
1. Review the medical record and nursing plan of care for conditions that may influence the patient's ability to move and ambulate. Assess for tubes, IV lines, incisions, or equipment that may alter the procedure for ambulation. Assess the patient's knowledge and previous experience regarding the use of crutches. Determine that the appropriate size crutch has been obtained.	Reviewing the medical record and plan of care validates the correct patient and correct procedure. Assessment helps identify problem areas to minimize the risk for injury.
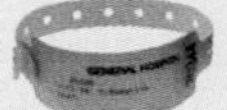 2. Identify the patient. Explain the procedure to the patient. Tell the patient to report any feelings of dizziness, weakness, or shortness of breath while walking. Decide how far to walk.	Patient identification validates the correct patient and correct procedure. Discussion and explanation help allay anxiety and prepare the patient for what to expect.

(continued)

SKILL 9-9

Assisting a Patient With Ambulation Using Crutches *(continued)*

ACTION / **RATIONALE**

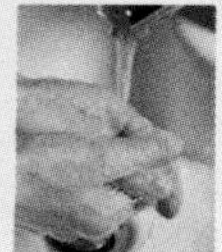

3. Perform hand hygiene.

Hand hygiene prevents the spread of microorganisms.

4. Encourage the patient to make use of the stand-assist device, if available. Assist the patient to stand erect, face forward in the tripod position (Figure 1). This means the patient holds the crutches 6″ in front of and 6″ to the side of each foot.

Stand-assist device reduces caregiver strain and decreases risk of patient injury. Positioning the crutches in this manner provides a wide base of support to increase stability and balance.

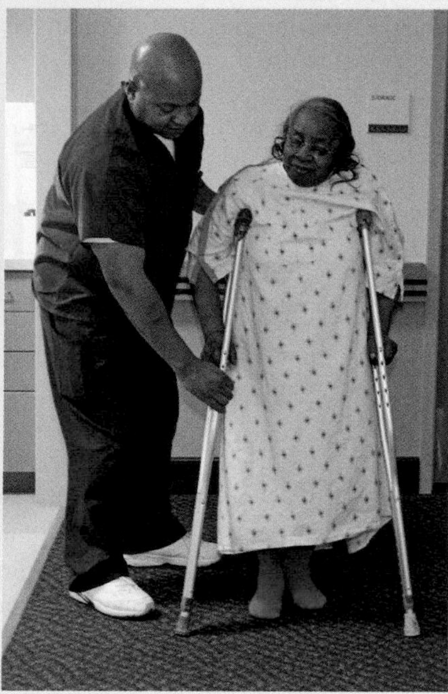

Figure 1. Assisting the patient to stand erect facing forward in the tripod position.

5. For the four-point gait:
   a. Have the patient move the right crutch forward 6″ and then move the left foot forward to the level of the right crutch.
   b. Then have the patient move the left crutch forward 6″ and then move the right foot forward to the level of the left crutch.

This movement ensures stability and safety.

6. For the three-point gait:
   a. Have the patient move the affected leg and both crutches forward about 6″.
   b. Have the patient move the stronger leg forward to the level of the crutches.

Patient bears weight on the stronger leg.

SKILL 9-9

Assisting a Patient With Ambulation Using Crutches *(continued)*

ACTION	RATIONALE
7. For the two-point gait: a. Have the patient move the left crutch and the right foot forward about 6″ at the same time. b. Have the patient move the right crutch and left leg forward to the level of the left crutch at the same time.	Patient bears partial weight on both feet.
8. For the swing-to gait: a. Have the patient move both crutches forward about 6″. b. Have the patient lift the legs and swing them to the crutches, supporting his or her body weight on the crutches.	Swing-to gait provides mobility for patients with weakness or paralysis of the hips or legs.
9. For the swing-through gait: a. Have the patient move both crutches forward about 6″. b. Have the patient lift the legs and swing through and ahead of the crutches, supporting his or her weight on the crutches.	The swing-through gait provides mobility for patients with weakness or paralysis of the hips or legs.
10. **Continue with ambulation for the planned distance and time. Return the patient to the bed or chair based on the patient's tolerance and condition, ensuring that the patient is comfortable and that the call light is within reach.**	Continued ambulation promotes activity. Adhering to the planned distance and time prevents the patient from becoming fatigued.
11. Perform hand hygiene.	Hand hygiene prevents the spread of microorganisms.

EVALUATION

The expected outcome is met when the patient demonstrates correct use of crutches to ambulate safely and without injury. Additional outcomes are met when the patient demonstrates increased muscle strength and joint mobility and exhibits no evidence of injury related to crutch use.

DOCUMENTATION

Guidelines

Document the activity, any observations, the patient's ability to use the crutches, the patient's tolerance of the procedure, and the distance walked.

Sample Documentation

5/10/08 1830 Patient instructed in crutch walking using four-point gait. Patient return-demonstrated gait, ambulating for approximately 15 feet in hallway, without difficulty.—H. Pointer, RN

(continued)

SKILL 9-9 Assisting a Patient With Ambulation Using Crutches *(continued)*

Unexpected Situations and Associated Interventions

- *You are assisting a patient ambulating in the hallway using crutches when the patient reports fatigue. You notice that the patient is bearing weight on the axillary area:* Call for assistance and have a coworker obtain a wheelchair to transport the patient back to the room. Once the patient is back in bed, reinforce instructions about avoiding pressure on the axillary area. In the future, plan for a shorter distance to prevent the patient from becoming fatigued. Talk with the multidisciplinary healthcare team about possible exercises for upper-extremity strengthening.

Special Considerations

General Considerations

- Crutches can be used when climbing stairs. The patient grasps both crutches as one on one side of the body and uses the stair railing. Have the patient stand in the tripod position facing the stairs. The patient transfers his or her weight to the crutches and holds the railing. The patient places the unaffected leg on the first stair tread. The patient then transfers his or her weight to the unaffected leg, moving up onto the stair tread. The patient moves the crutches and affected leg up to the stair tread and continues to the top of the stairs. Using this process, the crutches always support the affected leg.
- The crutch is appropriately sized when about 3 finger-widths remain between the axilla and the top of the crutch when the crutch is placed in a tripod position.
- Long-term use of the swing-to and swing-through gaits can lead to atrophy of the hips and legs. Appropriate exercises need to be included in the patient's plan of care to avoid this complication.
- Patients should not lean on the crutches. Prolonged pressure on the axillae can damage the brachial nerves, causing brachial nerve palsy, with resulting loss of sensation and inability to move the upper extremities.
- Patients using crutches should perform arm- and shoulder-strengthening exercises to aid with crutch walking.

SKILL 9-10 Assisting a Patient With Ambulation Using a Cane

Canes are useful for patients who can bear weight but need support for balance. They are also useful for patients who have decreased strength in one leg. Canes provide an additional point of support during ambulation. Canes are made of wood or metal and often have a rubberized cap on the tip to prevent slipping. Canes come in three variations: single-ended canes with half-circle handles (recommended for patients requiring minimal support and those who will be using stairs frequently); single-ended canes with straight handles (recommended for patients with hand weakness because the handgrip is easier to hold, but not recommended for patients with poor balance); canes with three (tripod) or four prongs (quad cane) or legs to provide a wide base of support (recommended for patients with poor balance).

The cane should rise from the floor to the height of the person's waist, and the elbow should be flexed about 30 degrees when holding the cane. The patient holds the cane in the hand opposite the weak or injured leg.

Equipment

- Cane of appropriate size with rubber tip
- Nonskid shoes or slippers
- Stand-assist aid, if necessary and available
- Gait belt, based on assessment and availability

SKILL 9-10 Assisting a Patient With Ambulation Using a Cane *(continued)*

ASSESSMENT

Assess the patient's upper body strength, ability to bear weight, ability to walk, and the need for assistance. Review the patient's record for conditions that may affect ambulation. Perform a pain assessment before the time for the activity. If the patient reports pain, administer the prescribed medication in sufficient time to allow for the full effect of the analgesic. Take vital signs and assess the patient for dizziness or lightheadedness with position changes. Assess the patient's knowledge regarding the use of a cane.

NURSING DIAGNOSIS

Determine the related factors for the nursing diagnoses based on the patient's current status. Appropriate nursing diagnoses may include:

- Risk for Falls
- Impaired Walking
- Deficient Knowledge
- Risk for Injury
- Activity Intolerance
- Acute Pain
- Chronic Pain

OUTCOME IDENTIFICATION AND PLANNING

The expected outcome to achieve when assisting a patient with ambulation using a cane is that the patient ambulates safely without falls or injury. Additional appropriate outcomes include: the patient demonstrates proper use of the cane; the patient demonstrates increased muscle strength, joint mobility, and independence; and the patient exhibits no evidence of injury from use of the cane.

IMPLEMENTATION

ACTION	RATIONALE
1. Review the medical record and nursing plan of care for conditions that may influence the patient's ability to move and ambulate. Assess for tubes, IV lines, incisions, or equipment that may alter the procedure for ambulation. Assess the patient's knowledge and previous experience regarding the use of a cane. Identify any movement limitations.	Review of the medical record and plan of care validates the correct patient and correct procedure. Identification of equipment and limitations helps reduce the risk for injury.
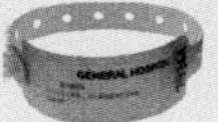 2. Identify the patient. Explain the procedure to the patient. Tell the patient to report any feelings of dizziness, weakness, or shortness of breath while walking. Decide how far to walk.	Patient identification validates the correct patient and correct procedure. Discussion and explanation help allay anxiety and prepare the patient for what to expect.
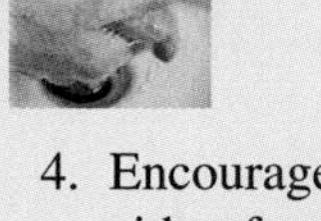 3. Perform hand hygiene.	Hand hygiene prevents the spread of microorganisms.
4. Encourage the patient to make use of a stand-assist aid, either free standing or attached to the side of the bed, if available, to move to and sit on the side of the bed.	Encourages independence, reduces strain for staff, and decreases risk for patient injury.

(continued)

SKILL 9-10 Assisting a Patient With Ambulation Using a Cane *(continued)*

ACTION	RATIONALE
5. Wrap the gait belt around the patient's waist, based on assessed need and facility policy.	Gait belts improve the caregiver's grasp, reducing the risk of musculoskeletal injuries to staff and the patient and provide firmer grasp for the caregiver if patient should lose his balance.
6. Encourage the patient to make use of the stand-assist device to stand with weight evenly distributed between the feet and the cane.	A stand-assist device reduces strain for caregiver and decreases risk for patient injury. Evenly distributed weight provides a broad base of support and balance.
7. Have the patient hold the cane on his or her stronger side, close to the body (Figure 1).	Holding the cane on the stronger side helps to distribute the patient's weight away from the involved side and prevents leaning.

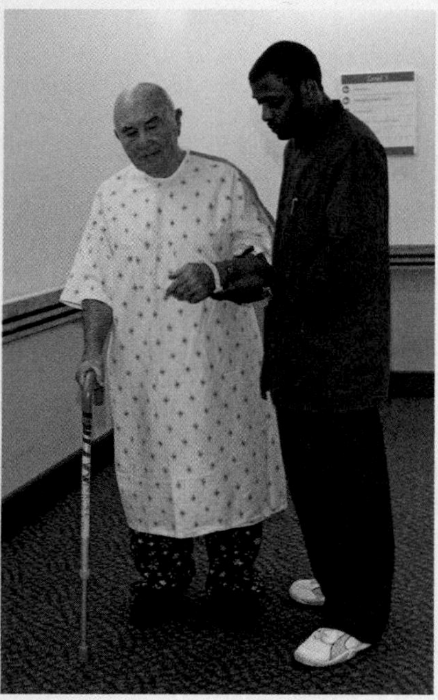

Figure 1. Standing with the patient with the cane held on the patient's stronger side, close to the body.

ACTION	RATIONALE
8. Tell the patient to advance the cane 4″ to 12″ (10–30 cm) and then, while supporting his or her weight on the stronger leg and the cane, advance the weaker foot forward, parallel with the cane.	Moving in this manner provides support and balance.
9. While supporting his or her weight on the weaker leg and the cane, have the patient advance the stronger leg forward ahead of the cane (heel slightly beyond the tip of the cane).	Moving in this manner provides support and balance.
10. Tell the patient to move the weaker leg forward until it is even with the stronger leg, and then advance the cane again.	This motion provides support and balance.

SKILL 9-10

Assisting a Patient With Ambulation Using a Cane *(continued)*

ACTION	RATIONALE
11. Continue with ambulation for the planned distance and time. Return the patient to the bed or chair based on the patient's tolerance and condition, ensuring the patient's comfort and that call light is within reach.	Continued ambulation promotes activity. Adhering to the planned distance and patient's tolerance prevents the patient from becoming fatigued.
12. Perform hand hygiene.	Hand hygiene prevents the spread of microorganisms.

EVALUATION

The expected outcome is met when the patient uses the cane to ambulate safely and is free from falls or injury. Additional outcomes are met when the patient demonstrates proper use of the cane; the patient exhibits increased muscle strength, joint mobility, and independence; and the patient experiences no injury related to cane use.

DOCUMENTATION

Guidelines

Document the activity, any observations, the patient's ability to use the cane, the patient's tolerance of the procedure, and the distance walked.

Sample Documentation

5/14/08 1330 Patient instructed in cane use. Patient return-demonstrated gait, ambulating approximately 10 feet in room. Patient needed continued reminders about leaning to one side. Requires continued instruction in cane use. Another teaching session planned for early evening.—J. Phelps, RN

Unexpected Situations and Associated Interventions

- *You are assisting a patient ambulating in the hallway using a cane when the patient says she can't walk any more:* Call for assistance. Have a coworker obtain a wheelchair to transport the patient back to her room. Assess the patient for possible causes, such as anxiety, fatigue, or a change in her condition. In the future, plan shorter distances to prevent her from becoming fatigued. Anticipate the need for referral to physical therapy for muscle strengthening.

Special Considerations

General Considerations

- Patients with bilateral weakness should not use a cane. Crutches or a walker would be more appropriate.
- To climb stairs, the patient should advance the stronger leg up the stair first, followed by the cane and with weaker leg. To descend, reverse the process.
- When less support is required from the cane, the patient can advance the cane and weaker leg forward simultaneously while the stronger leg supports the patient's weight.
- Patients should be taught to position their canes within easy reach when they sit down so that they can rise easily.

SKILL 9-11 Applying Pneumatic Compression Devices

Pneumatic compression devices (PCDs) consist of fabric sleeves containing air bladders that apply brief pressure to the legs. Intermittent compression pushes blood from the smaller blood vessels into the deeper vessels and into the femoral veins. This action enhances blood flow and venous return and promotes fibrinolysis, deterring venous thrombosis. The sleeves are attached by tubing to an air pump. The sleeve may cover the entire leg or may extend from the foot to the knee.

PCDs may be used in combination with antiembolism stockings and anticoagulant therapy to prevent thrombosis formation. They can be used preoperatively and postoperatively with patients at risk for blood clot formation. They are also prescribed for patients with other risk factors for clot formation, including inactivity or immobilization, chronic venous disease, and malignancies.

Equipment

- Compression sleeves of appropriate size based on the manufacturer's guidelines
- Inflation pump with connection tubing

ASSESSMENT

Assess the patient's history, medical record, and current condition and status to identify risk for development of deep-vein thrombosis. Assess the skin integrity of the lower extremities. Identify any leg conditions that would be exacerbated by the use of the compression device or would contraindicate its use. Review the patient's record and nursing plan of care to verify the physician's order for use.

NURSING DIAGNOSIS

Determine the related factors for the nursing diagnoses based on the patient's current status. Appropriate nursing diagnoses may include:

- Risk for Peripheral Neurovascular Dysfunction
- Impaired Physical Mobility
- Fatigue
- Delayed Surgical Recovery
- Risk for Injury

OUTCOME IDENTIFICATION AND PLANNING

The expected outcome to achieve when applying PCDs is that the patient maintains adequate circulation in extremities and is free from symptoms of neurovascular compromise.

IMPLEMENTATION

ACTION	RATIONALE
1. Review the medical record and nursing plan of care for conditions that may contraindicate the use of the PCD.	Reviewing the medical record and plan of care validates the correct patient and correct procedure and minimizes the risk for injury.
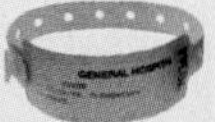 2. Identify the patient. Explain the procedure to the patient.	Patient identification validates the correct patient and correct procedure. Discussion and explanation help allay anxiety and prepare the patient for what to expect.
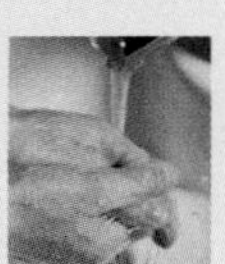 3. Perform hand hygiene.	Hand hygiene prevents the spread of microorganisms.

SKILL 9-11

Applying Pneumatic Compression Devices *(continued)*

ACTION	RATIONALE
4. Close the room door or curtains. Place the bed at an appropriate and comfortable working height.	Closing the door or curtains provides privacy. Proper bed height helps reduce back strain.
5. Hang the compression pump on the foot of the bed and plug it into an electrical outlet (Figure 1). Attach the connecting tubing to the pump.	Equipment preparation promotes efficient time management and provides an organized approach to the task.

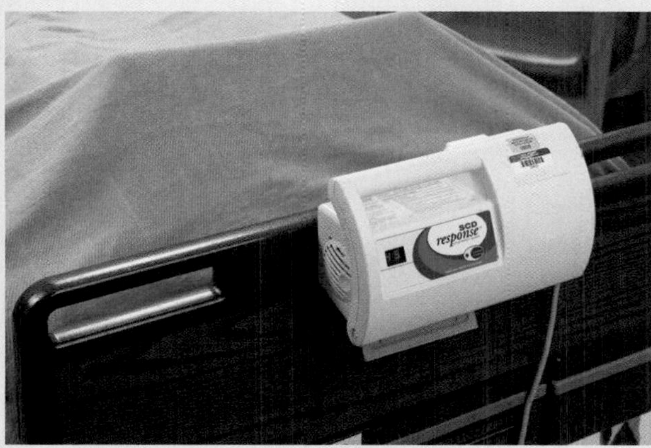

Figure 1. PCD machine at the foot of the bed.

ACTION	RATIONALE
6. Remove the compression sleeves from the package and unfold them. Lay the unfolded sleeves on the bed with the cotton lining facing up. Take note of the markings indicating the correct placement for the ankle and popliteal areas.	Proper placement of the sleeves prevents injury.
7. Apply antiembolism stockings if ordered. Place a sleeve under the patient's leg with the tubing toward the heel (Figure 2). Each one fits either leg. For total leg sleeves, place the behind-the-knee opening at the popliteal space to prevent pressure there. For knee-high sleeves, make sure the back of the ankle is over the ankle marking.	Proper placement prevents injury.

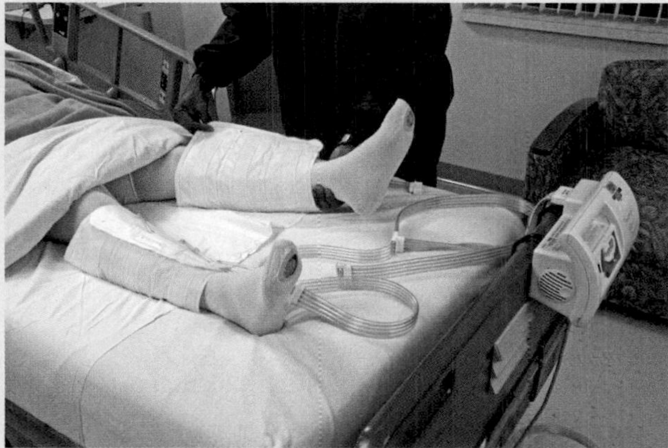

Figure 2. Placing PCD sleeves under the patient's legs with the tubing toward the heel.

(continued)

SKILL 9-11 Applying Pneumatic Compression Devices *(continued)*

ACTION | 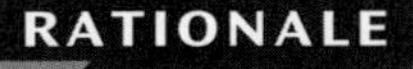 **RATIONALE**

8. Wrap the sleeve snugly around the patient's leg so that two fingers fit between the leg and the sleeve. Secure the sleeve with the Velcro fasteners. Repeat for the second leg, if bilateral therapy is ordered. Connect each sleeve to the tubing, following manufacturer's recommendations (Figure 3).

Correct placement ensures appropriate, but not excessive, compression of the extremity.

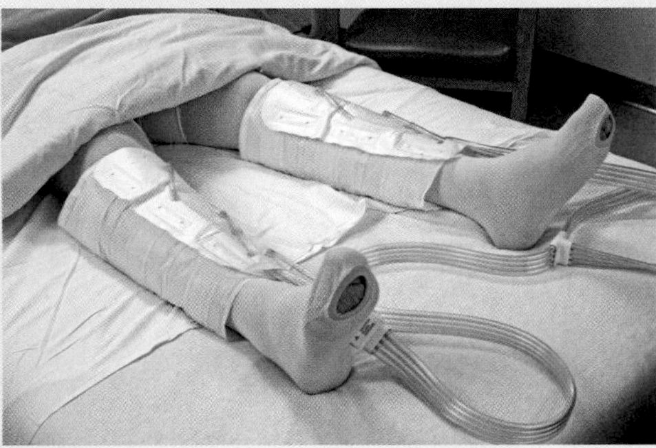

Figure 3. PCD sleeves snugly around the patient's legs.

9. Set the pump to the prescribed maximum pressure (usually 35–55 mm Hg). Make sure the tubing is free from kinks. Check that the patient can move about without interrupting the airflow. Turn on the pump. Initiate cooling setting, if available.

Proper pressure setting ensures patient safety and prevents injury. Some devices have a cooling setting available to increase patient comfort.

10. Observe the patient and the device during the first cycle. Check the audible alarms. Check the sleeves and pump at least once per shift or per facility policy.

Observation and frequent checking ensure proper fit and inflation and reduce the risk for injury from the device

11. Place the bed in the lowest position. Make sure the call bell and other necessary items are within easy reach.

Returning the bed to the lowest position and having the call bell and other items readily available promote patient safety.

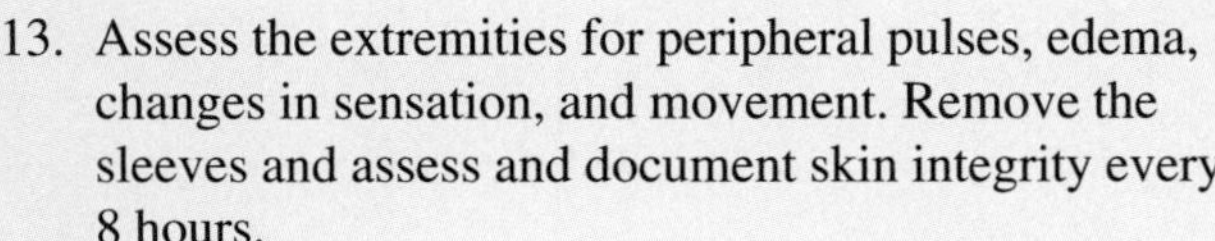

12. Perform hand hygiene.

Hand hygiene prevents the spread of microorganisms.

13. Assess the extremities for peripheral pulses, edema, changes in sensation, and movement. Remove the sleeves and assess and document skin integrity every 8 hours.

Assessment provides for early detection and prompt intervention for possible complications, including skin irritation.

EVALUATION

The expected outcome is met when the patient exhibits adequate circulation in extremities without symptoms of neurovascular compromise.

SKILL 9-11 Applying Pneumatic Compression Devices *(continued)*

DOCUMENTATION

Guidelines

Document the time and date of application of the PCD, the patient's response to the therapy, and the patient's understanding of the therapy. Document the status of the alarms and pressure settings. Note the use of the cooling setting, if appropriate.

Sample Documentation

4/27/08 1615 Patient instructed in reason for pneumatic compression device therapy; verbalizes understanding of therapy. Knee-high PCDs applied to both lower extremities; pressure set at 45 mm Hg as ordered. Patient denies any complaints of numbness or tingling. Feet and toes warm and pink; quick capillary refill; bilateral pedal pulses present and equal. Alarms and cooling settings as ordered.
—J. Trotter, RN

Unexpected Situations and Associated Interventions

- *Your postoperative patient is wearing PCDs on both legs. While you are performing a routine assessment, he tells you that he has started to have pain in his left leg, along with tingling and numbness:* Remove the PCDs and assess both lower extremities. Perform a skin and neurovascular assessment. Assess the extremities for peripheral pulses, edema, changes in sensation, and movement. Report the patient's symptoms and assessment to the physician.

Special Considerations

General Considerations

- PCDs are contraindicated in patients with suspected or existing deep-vein thrombosis. They should not be used for patients with arterial occlusive disease, severe edema, cellulitis, phlebitis, a skin graft, or an infection of the extremity.
- Use the cooling setting, if the unit has one. The skin under the sleeve can become wet with diaphoresis, which can increase the risk for impaired skin integrity.
- Generally, the PCDs should be worn continuously. They may be removed for bathing, walking, and physical therapy. Use is usually discontinued when the patient is ambulating consistently.
- The risk for deep-vein thrombosis formation and injury is greater if the sleeves are not applied correctly.

SKILL 9-12 Applying a Continuous Passive Motion Device

A continuous passive motion (CPM) device promotes range of motion, circulation, and healing of a joint. It is frequently used after total knee arthroplasty as well as after surgery on other joints, such as shoulders (Lynch et al., 2005). The amount of flexion and extension of the joint and the cycle rate (the number of revolutions per minute) are determined by the physician, but nurses place the patient in and out of the device and monitor the patient's response to the therapy.

Equipment

- CPM device
- Single-patient-use soft-goods kit
- Tape measure
- Goniometer
- Nonsterile gloves, if indicated

(continued)

SKILL 9-12 Applying a Continuous Passive Motion Device *(continued)*

ASSESSMENT

Review the medical record and nursing plan of care for orders for degrees of flexion and extension. Assess the neurovascular status of the involved extremity. Perform a pain assessment. Administer the prescribed medication in sufficient time to allow for the full effect of the analgesic before starting the device. Assess for proper alignment of the joint in the CPM device. Assess the patient's ability to tolerate the prescribed treatment.

NURSING DIAGNOSIS

Determine the related factors for the nursing diagnoses based on the patient's current status. Appropriate nursing diagnoses may include:

- Impaired Physical Mobility
- Activity Intolerance
- Anxiety
- Fatigue
- Risk for Injury
- Acute Pain
- Risk for Impaired Skin Integrity
- Delayed Surgical Recovery
- Risk for Peripheral Neurovascular Dysfunction

OUTCOME IDENTIFICATION AND PLANNING

The expected outcome to achieve when applying a CPM device is that the patient experiences increased joint mobility. Other outcomes include: the patient displays improved or maintained muscle strength; muscle atrophy and contractures are prevented; circulation is promoted in the affected extremity; effects of immobility are decreased; and healing is stimulated.

IMPLEMENTATION

ACTION	RATIONALE
1. Review the medical record and nursing plan of care for the appropriate degrees of flexion and extension, the cycle rate, and the length of time the CPM is to be used.	Reviewing the medical record and plan of care validates the correct patient and correct procedure and reduces the risk for injury.
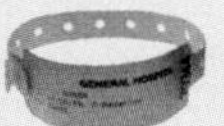 2. Identify the patient. Explain the procedure to the patient.	Patient identification validates the correct patient and correct procedure. Discussion and explanation help allay anxiety and prepare the patient for what to expect.
3. Obtain equipment. Apply the soft goods to the CPM device.	Equipment preparation promotes efficient time management and provides an organized approach to the task. The soft goods help to prevent friction to the extremity during motion.
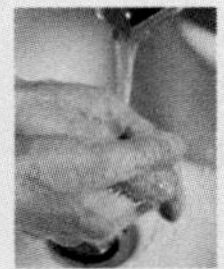 4. Perform hand hygiene, and put on gloves if indicated.	Hand hygiene prevents the spread of microorganisms. Gloves prevent contact with blood and body fluids.
5. Close the room door or curtains. Place the bed at an appropriate and comfortable working height.	Closing the door or curtains provides privacy. Proper bed height helps reduce back strain.
6. Using the tape measure, determine the distance between the gluteal crease and the popliteal space.	The thigh length on the CPM device is adjusted based on this measurement.

SKILL 9-12 Applying a Continuous Passive Motion Device *(continued)*

ACTION	RATIONALE
7. Measure the leg from the knee to ¼″ beyond the bottom of the foot.	The position of the footplate is adjusted based on this measurement.
8. Position the patient in the middle of the bed. The affected extremity should be in a slightly abducted position.	Proper positioning promotes correct body alignment and prevents pressure on the unaffected extremity.
9. Support the affected extremity and elevate it, placing it in the padded CPM device (Figure 1).	Support and elevation assist in movement of the affected extremity without injury.
10. Make sure the knee is at the hinged joint of the CPM device.	Proper positioning in the device prevents injury.
11. Adjust the footplate to maintain the patient's foot in a neutral position (Figure 2). Assess the patient's position to make sure the leg is not internally or externally rotated.	Adjustment helps ensure proper positioning and prevent injury.
12. Apply the restraining straps under the CPM device and around the leg. **Check that two fingers fit between the strap and the leg (Figure 3).**	Restraining straps maintain the leg in position. Leaving a space between the strap and leg prevents injury from excessive pressure from the strap.

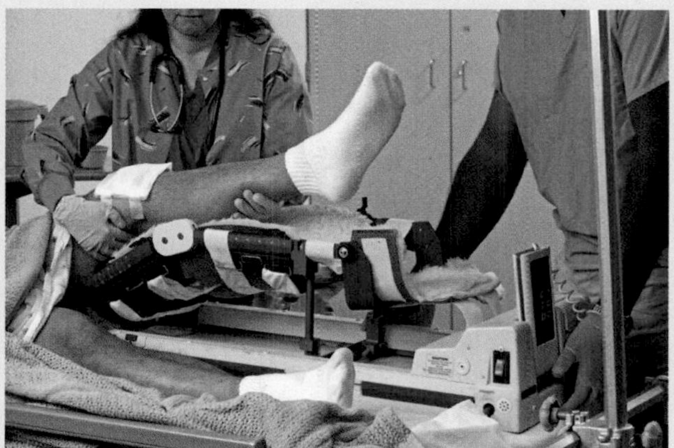

Figure 1. Placing the patient's leg into the CPM machine.

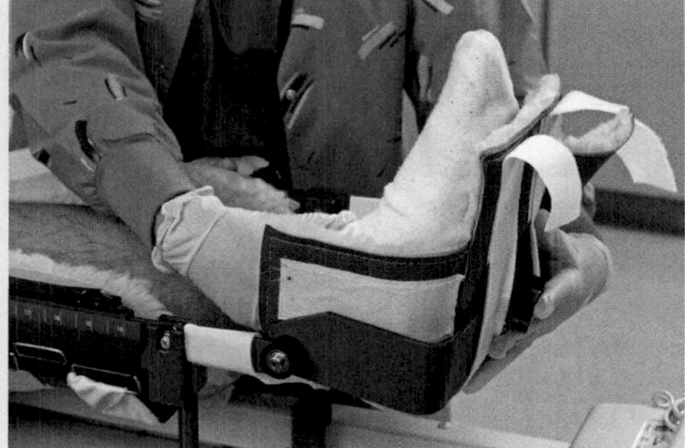

Figure 2. Adjusting the footplate to maintain the patient's foot in a neutral position.

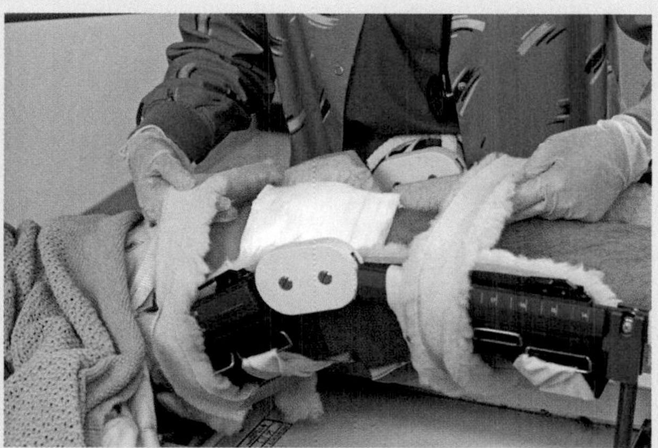

Figure 3. Using two fingers to check the fit between the straps and the leg.

(continued)

SKILL 9-12 Applying a Continuous Passive Motion Device *(continued)*

ACTION	RATIONALE
13. Explain the use of the STOP/GO button to the patient. Set the controls to the prescribed levels of flexion and extension and cycles per minute. Turn on the power to the CPM.	Explanation decreases anxiety by allowing the patient to participate in care.
14. Set the device to ON and start the therapy by pressing the GO button. Observe the patient and the device during the first cycle. Determine the angle of flexion when the device reaches its greatest height using the goniometer (Figure 4). Compare with prescribed degree.	Observation ensures that the device is working properly, thereby ensuring patient safety. Measuring with a goniometer ensures the device is set to the prescribed parameters.

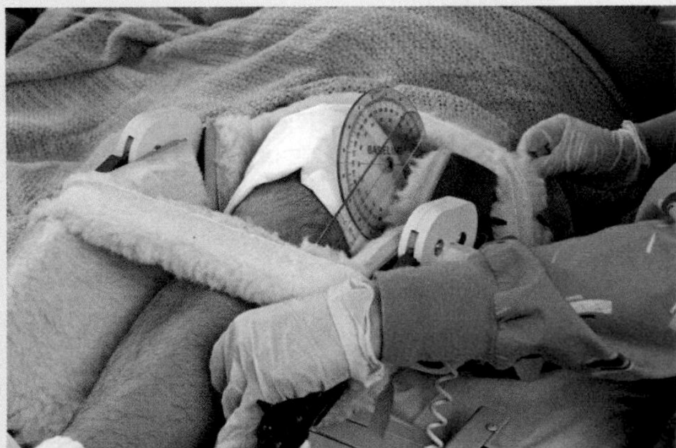

Figure 4. Using the goniometer, determining the angle of joint flexion when the device reaches its greatest height.

ACTION	RATIONALE
15. Check the patient's level of comfort and perform skin and neurovascular assessment at least every 8 hours or per facility policy.	Frequent assessments provide for early detection and prompt intervention should problems arise.
16. Place the bed in the lowest position, with the side rails up. Make sure the call bell and other necessary items are within easy reach.	Having the bed at the proper height and having the call bell and other items handy ensure patient safety.
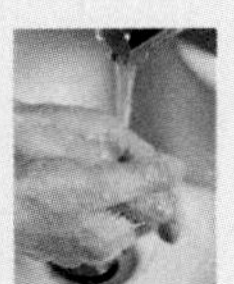 17. Remove gloves, if used, and perform hand hygiene.	Hand hygiene prevents the spread of microorganisms.

EVALUATION

The expected outcome is met when the patient demonstrates increased joint mobility. In addition, the patient exhibits improved muscle strength without evidence of atrophy or contractures.

DOCUMENTATION

Guidelines

Document the time and date of application of the CPM, the extension and flexion settings, the speed of the device, the patient's response to the therapy, and your assessment of the extremity.

SKILL 9-12 Applying a Continuous Passive Motion Device *(continued)*

Sample Documentation

5/03/08 1430 Right-knee incision clean and dry; dressing intact. Right toes pink and warm, with brisk capillary refill; equal to left. Pedal pulses present and equal bilaterally. CPM device applied with range of motion at 30 degrees of knee flexion, for 5 cycles per minute for 30 minutes. Patient complains of slight increase in pain from a rating of 4 out of 10 to 5 out of 10 but states, "I don't want anything for the pain right now." Plan to reassess in 15 minutes and offer analgesic as ordered.
—K. Dugas, RN

Unexpected Situations and Associated Interventions

- *A patient is prescribed therapy with a CPM device. After you initiate the prescribed flexion and extension of the joint, the patient complains of sudden pain in the joint:* Stop the CPM device. Check the settings to make sure the device is set correctly for the prescribed therapy. Assess the patient for other signs and symptoms and obtain vital signs. Perform a neurovascular assessment of the affected extremity. Notify the physician of the patient's pain and any other findings. When therapy is resumed, evaluate the need for premedication with analgesics. Continue pain intervention with analgesics as prescribed.

SKILL 9-13 Applying a Sling

A sling is a bandage that can provide support for an arm or immobilize an injured arm, wrist, or hand. Slings can be used to restrict movement of a fracture or dislocation and to support a muscle sprain. They may also be used to support a splint or secure dressings. Healthcare agencies usually use commercial slings. The sling should distribute the supported weight over a large area, not the back of the neck, to prevent pressure on the cervical spinal nerves.

Equipment

- Commercial arm sling
- ABD gauze pad

ASSESSMENT

Assess the situation to determine the need for a sling. Assess the affected limb for pain and edema. Perform a neurovascular assessment of the affected extremity. Assess body parts distal to the site for cyanosis, pallor, coolness, numbness, tingling, swelling, and absent or diminished pulses.

NURSING DIAGNOSIS

Determine the related factors for the nursing diagnoses based on the patient's current status. Appropriate nursing diagnoses may include:

- Impaired Physical Mobility
- Risk for Injury
- Acute Pain
- Risk for Peripheral Neurovascular Dysfunction
- Risk for Impaired Skin Integrity
- Dressing or Grooming Self-Care Deficit

(continued)

SKILL 9-13 Applying a Sling *(continued)*

OUTCOME IDENTIFICATION AND PLANNING

The expected outcome to achieve when applying a sling is that the arm is immobilized, and the patient maintains muscle strength and joint range of motion. In addition, the patient shows no evidence of contractures, venous stasis, thrombus formation, or skin breakdown.

IMPLEMENTATION

ACTION	RATIONALE
1. Review the medical record and nursing plan of care to determine the need for the use of a sling.	Reviewing the medical record and plan of care validates the correct patient and correct procedure and prevents injury.
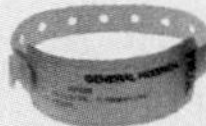 2. Identify the patient. Explain the procedure to the patient.	Patient identification validates the correct patient and correct procedure. Discussion and explanation help allay anxiety and prepare the patient for what to expect.
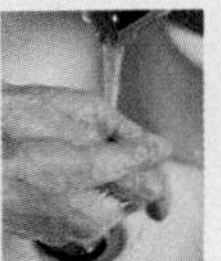 3. Perform hand hygiene.	Hand hygiene prevents the spread of microorganisms.
4. Close the room door or curtains. Place the bed at an appropriate and comfortable working height, if necessary.	Closing the door or curtain provides privacy. Proper bed height helps reduce back strain.
5. Assist the patient to a sitting position. Place the patient's forearm across the chest with the elbow flexed and the palm against the chest. Measure the sleeve length, if indicated.	Proper positioning facilitates sling application. Measurement ensures proper sizing of the sling and proper placement of the arm.
6. Enclose the arm in the sling, making sure the elbow fits into the corner of the fabric (Figure 1). Run the strap up the patient's back and across the shoulder opposite the injury, then down the chest to the fastener on the end of the sling (Figure 2).	This position ensures adequate support and keeps the arm out of a dependent position, preventing edema.

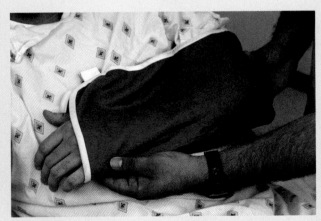

Figure 1. Placing the patient's arm into the canvas sling with the elbow flush in the corner of the sling.

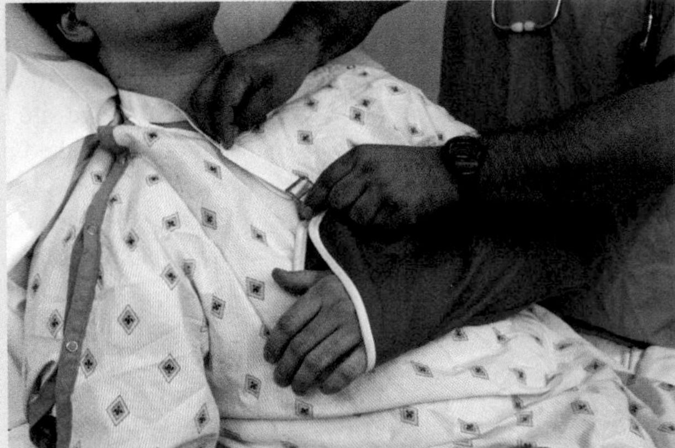

Figure 2. Placing the strap around the patient's neck.

SKILL 9-13 **Applying a Sling** *(continued)*

ACTION	RATIONALE
7. Place the ABD pad under the strap, between the strap and the patient's neck (Figure 3). Ensure that the sling and forearm are slightly elevated and at a right angle to the body (Figure 4).	Padding prevents skin irritation and reduces pressure on the neck. Proper positioning ensures alignment, provides support, and prevents edema.

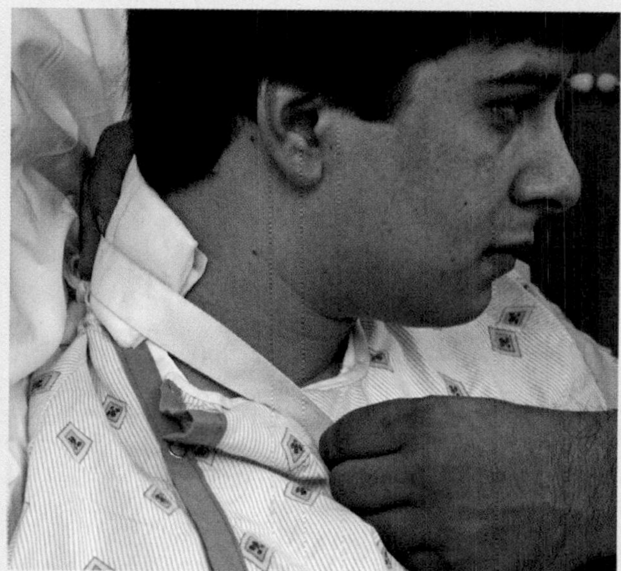

Figure 3. Placing padding between the strap and the patient's neck.

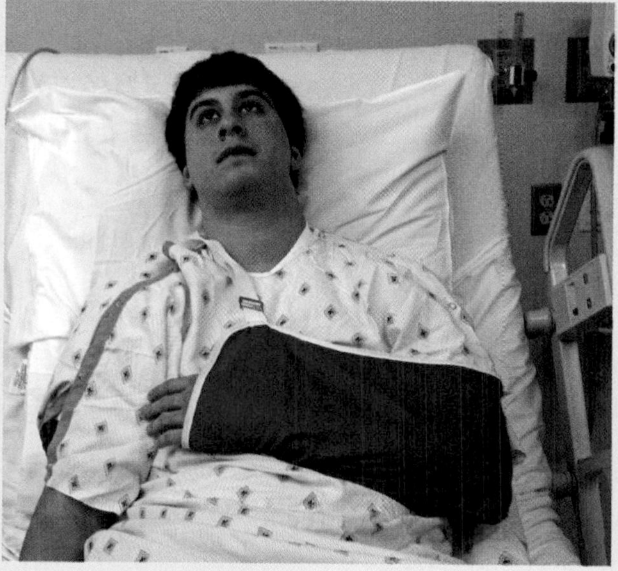

Figure 4. Patient with sling in place.

ACTION	RATIONALE
8. Place the bed in the lowest position, with the side rails up. Make sure the call bell and other necessary items are within easy reach.	Having the bed at proper height and leaving the call bell and other items within reach ensure patient safety.
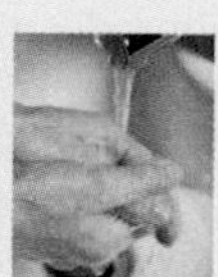 9. Perform hand hygiene.	Hand hygiene prevents the spread of microorganisms.
10. Check the patient's level of comfort, arm positioning, and neurovascular status of the affected limb every 4 hours or according to facility policy. Assess the axillary and cervical skin frequently for irritation or breakdown.	Frequent assessment ensures patient safety, prevents injury, and provides early intervention for skin irritation and other complications.

EVALUATION

The expected outcome is met when the patient demonstrates extremity in proper alignment with adequate muscle strength and joint range of motion. In addition, the patient demonstrates proper use of sling and remains free of complications, including contractures, venous stasis, thrombus formation, or skin breakdown.

DOCUMENTATION

Guidelines

Document the time and date the sling was applied. Document the patient's response to the sling and the neurovascular status of the extremity.

(continued)

SKILL 9-13 Applying a Sling *(continued)*

Sample Documentation

5/22/08 2015 Sling applied to left arm as ordered. Left hand and fingers warm to touch and pink. Brisk capillary refill. Left radial pulse present and equal to right. Patient denies any complaints of numbness, pain, or tingling of left upper extremity.—P. Peterson, RN

Unexpected Situations and Associated Interventions

- *Your patient needs a sling to support a wrist fracture, but you cannot obtain a commercially prepared sling:* Make a sling using a triangular bandage or cloth. Place the cloth or bandage on the chest with a corner of the cloth at the elbow. Place the affected arm across the chest with the elbow flexed and the palm on the chest. Wrap the end closest to the head around the neck, on the opposite side from the injured arm. Bring the end of the cloth that is farthest from the head up over the injured arm and tie it at the side of the neck. The sling and forearm should be slightly elevated and at a right angle to the body. Fold the material at the elbow and secure the sling with a safety pin above and behind the elbow.

Special Considerations

General Considerations

- Be sure that the patient's wrist is enclosed in the sling. Do not allow it to hang out and down over the edge. This prevents pressure on nerves and blood vessels and prevents muscle contractures, deformity, and discomfort.
- Assess circulation and comfort at regular intervals.

SKILL 9-14 Applying a Figure-Eight Bandage

Bandages are used to apply pressure over an area, immobilize a body part, prevent or reduce edema, and secure splints and dressings. Bandages can be elasticized or made of gauze, flannel, or muslin. In general, narrow bandages are used to wrap feet, the lower legs, hands, and arms, and wider bandages are used for the thighs and trunk. A roller bandage is a continuous strip of material wound on itself to form a roll. The free end is anchored and the roll is passed or rolled around the body part, maintaining equal tension with all turns. The bandage is unwound gradually and only as needed. The bandage should overlap itself evenly and by one-half to two-thirds the width the bandage. The figure-eight turn consists of oblique overlapping turns that ascend and descend alternately. It is used around the knee, elbow, ankle, and wrist.

Equipment

- Elastic or other bandage of the appropriate width
- Tape, pins, or self-closures
- Gauze pads
- Clean gloves, if indicated

ASSESSMENT

Review the medical record, physician's orders, and nursing plan of care and assess the situation to determine the need for a bandage. Assess the affected limb for pain and edema. Perform a neurovascular assessment of the affected extremity. Assess body parts distal to the site for evidence of cyanosis, pallor, coolness, numbness, tingling, and swelling and absent or diminished pulses. Assess the distal circulation of the extremity after the bandage is in place and at least every 4 hours.

SKILL 9-14

Applying a Figure-Eight Bandage *(continued)*

NURSING DIAGNOSIS

Determine the related factors for the nursing diagnoses based on the patient's current status. Appropriate nursing diagnoses may include:

- Impaired Physical Mobility
- Acute Pain
- Risk for Peripheral Neurovascular Dysfunction
- Risk for Impaired Skin Integrity
- Ineffective Tissue Perfusion
- Dressing or Grooming Self-Care Deficit

OUTCOME IDENTIFICATION AND PLANNING

The expected outcome to achieve when applying a figure-eight bandage is that the bandage is applied correctly without injury or complications. Other outcomes that may be appropriate include: patient maintains circulation to the affected part and remains free of neurovascular complications.

IMPLEMENTATION

ACTION	RATIONALE
1. Review the medical record and nursing plan of care to determine the need for a figure-eight bandage.	Reviewing the medical record and plan of care validates the correct patient and correct procedure and reduces risk for injury.
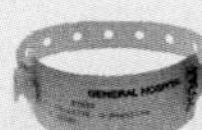 2. Identify the patient. Explain the procedure to the patient.	Patient identification validates the correct patient and correct procedure. Discussion and explanation help allay anxiety and prepare the patient for what to expect.
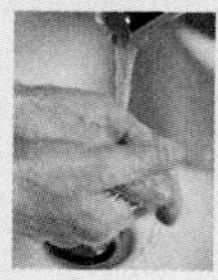 3. Perform hand hygiene and put on gloves if contact with drainage is possible.	Hand hygiene and gloving prevent the spread of microorganisms.
4. Close the room door or curtains. Place the bed at an appropriate and comfortable working height.	Closing the door or curtains provides privacy. Proper bed height helps reduce back strain.
5. Assist the patient to a comfortable position, with the affected body part in a normal functioning position.	Keeping the body part in a normal functioning position promotes circulation and prevents deformity and discomfort.
6. Hold the bandage roll with the roll facing upward in one hand while holding the free end of the roll in the other hand. Make sure to hold the bandage roll so it is close to the affected body part.	Proper handling of the bandage allows application of even tension and pressure.

(continued)

SKILL 9-14 Applying a Figure-Eight Bandage *(continued)*

ACTION / **RATIONALE**

7. Wrap the bandage around the limb twice, below the joint, to anchor it (Figure 1).

Anchoring the bandage ensures that it will stay in place.

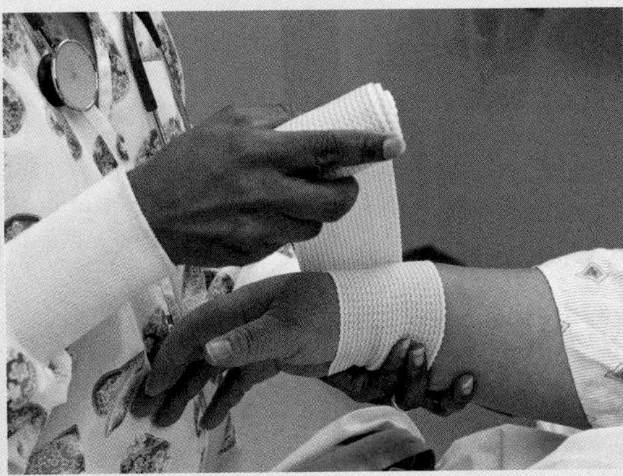

Figure 1. Wrapping the bandage around the patient's limb twice, below the joint, to anchor it.

8. Use alternating ascending and descending turns to form a figure eight (Figure 2). Overlap each turn of the bandage by one-half to two-thirds the width of the strip (Figure 3).

Making alternating ascending and descending turns helps to ensure the bandage will stay in place on a moving body part.

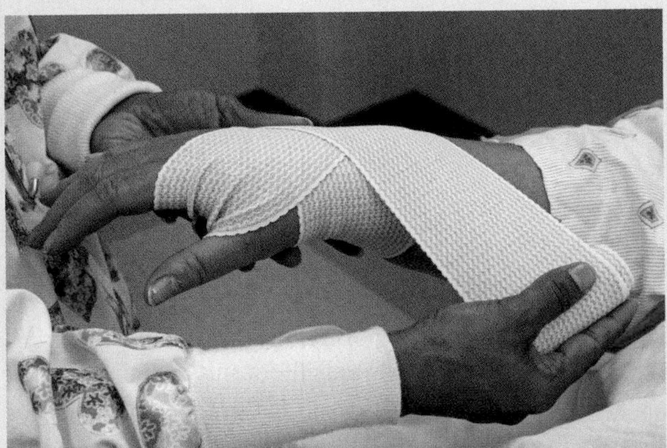

Figure 2. Using alternating ascending and descending turns to form a figure eight.

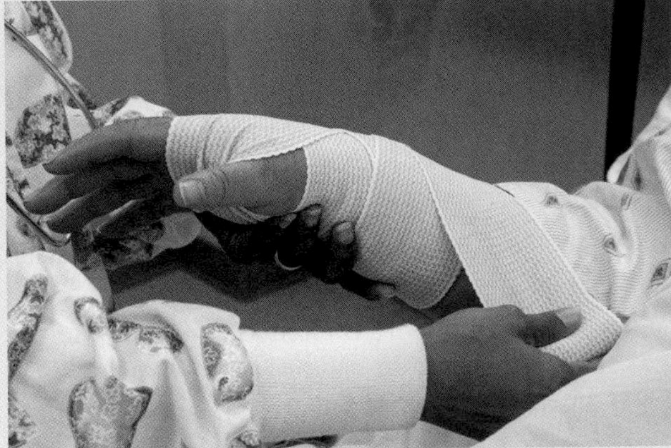

Figure 3. Overlapping each turn of the bandage by one-half to two-thirds the width of the strip.

9. **Unroll the bandage as you wrap, not before wrapping.**

Unrolling the bandage with wrapping prevents uneven pressure, which could interfere with blood circulation.

10. **Wrap firmly, but not tightly.** Assess the patient's comfort as you wrap. If the patient reports tingling, itching, numbness, or pain, loosen the bandage.

Firm wrapping is necessary to provide support and prevent injury, but wrapping too tightly interferes with circulation. Patient complaints are helpful indicators of possible circulatory compromise.

SKILL 9-14

Applying a Figure-Eight Bandage *(continued)*

ACTION	RATIONALE
11. After the area is covered, wrap the bandage around the limb twice, above the joint, to anchor it (Figure 4). Secure the end of the bandage with tape, pins, or self-closures. Avoid metal clips.	Anchoring at the end ensures the bandage will stay in place. Metal clips can cause injury.

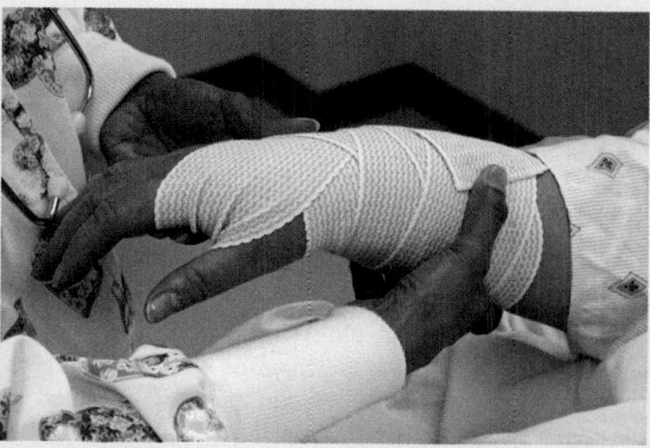

Figure 4. Wrapping the bandage around the patient's limb twice, above the joint, to anchor it, and secure the end of the bandage with tape, pins, or self-closures.

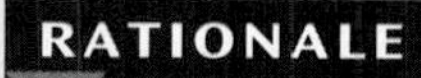

ACTION	RATIONALE
12. Remove your gloves, if worn, and discard them. Place the bed in the lowest position, with the side rails up. Make sure the call bell and other necessary items are within easy reach.	Repositioning the bed and having items nearby ensure patient safety.
13. Assess the distal circulation after the bandage is in place.	Elastic may tighten as it is wrapped. Frequent assessment of distal circulation ensures patient safety and prevents injury.
14. **Elevate the wrapped extremity for 15 to 30 minutes after application of the bandage.**	Elevation promotes venous return and reduces edema.
15. Lift the distal end of the bandage and assess the skin for color, temperature, and integrity. Assess for pain and perform a neurovascular assessment of the affected extremity after applying the bandage and at least every 4 hours, or per facility policy.	Assessment aids in prompt detection of compromised circulation and allows for early intervention for skin irritation and other complications.
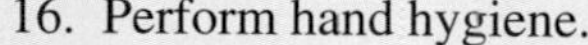 16. Perform hand hygiene.	Hand hygiene prevents the spread of microorganisms.

EVALUATION

The expected outcome is achieved when the patient exhibits a bandage that is applied correctly, without causing injury or neurovascular compromise. In addition, the patient demonstrates proper alignment of the bandaged body part; the patient remains free of evidence of complications; and the patient demonstrates understanding of signs and symptoms to report immediately.

(continued)

SKILL 9-14 Applying a Figure-Eight Bandage *(continued)*

DOCUMENTATION

Guidelines

Document the time, date, and site that the bandage was applied and the size bandage used. Include the skin assessment and care provided before application. Document the patient's response to the bandage and the neurovascular status of the extremity.

Sample Documentation

5/27/08 1615 3" bandage applied to right knee using figure-eight technique. Skin pink, warm, and dry, with quick capillary refill; pedal and dorsalis pedis pulses present and equal bilaterally. Patient denies any complaints of pain, numbness, or tingling. Patient instructed to report any complaints immediately. Right lower extremity resting on two pillows at present.—J. Wilkins, RN

Unexpected Situations and Associated Interventions

- *After you have applied a figure-eight bandage to a patient's elbow to hold dressings in place, the patient reports tingling, numbness, and pain in his hand during a routine assessment:* Remove the bandage, wait 30 minutes, and reapply the bandage with less tension. Continue to monitor the neurovascular status of the extremity. Symptoms should subside fairly quickly. If symptoms persist, notify the physician.
- *You remove the bandage on a patient's ankle and note the bandage is limp and less elastic than when it was applied:* Obtain a new bandage and apply it to the ankle. Launder the old bandage to restore its elasticity. Keep two bandages at the bedside: one can be applied while the other is laundered.

Special Considerations

General Considerations

- Keep in mind that a figure-eight bandage may be contraindicated if skin breakdown or lesions are present on the area to be wrapped.
- When wrapping an extremity, elevate it for 15 to 30 minutes before applying the bandage, if possible. This promotes venous return and prevents edema. Avoid applying the bandage to a dependent extremity.
- Place gauze pads or cotton between skin surfaces, such as toes and fingers, to prevent skin irritation. Skin surfaces should not touch after the bandage is applied.
- Include the heel when wrapping the foot, but do not wrap the toes or fingers unless necessary. Assess distal body parts to detect impaired circulation.
- Avoid leaving gaps in bandage layers or leaving skin exposed, as this may result in uneven pressure on the body part.
- Remove and change the bandage at least once a day, or per physician order or facility policy. Cleanse the skin and dry thoroughly before applying a new bandage. Assess the skin for irritation and breakdown.

SKILL 9-15 Assisting With Cast Application

A cast is a rigid external immobilizing device that encases a body part. Casts are used to immobilize a body part in a specific position and to apply uniform pressure on the encased soft tissue. They may be used to treat injuries, correct a deformity, stabilize weakened joints, or promote healing after surgery. Casts generally allow the patient mobility while restricting movement of the affected body part. Casts may be made of plaster or synthetic materials, such as fiberglass. Each material has advantages and disadvantages. Non-plaster casts set in 15 minutes and can sustain weight bearing or pressure in 15 to 30 minutes. Plaster casts

SKILL 9-15

Assisting With Cast Application *(continued)*

can take 24 to 72 hours to dry, with no weight bearing or pressure being applied during this period. Patient safety is of utmost importance during the application of a cast. Typically, a physician or other advanced practice professional applies the cast. Nursing responsibilities include preparing the patient and equipment and assisting during the application. The nurse provides skin care to the affected area before, during, and after the cast is applied. In some settings, nurses with special preparation may apply or change casts.

Equipment

- Casting materials, such as plaster rolls or fiberglass, depending on the type of cast being applied
- Padding material, such as stockinette, sheet wadding, or Webril®, depending on the type of cast being applied
- Plastic bucket or basin filled with warm water
- Disposable gloves and aprons
- Scissors
- Waterproof disposable pads

ASSESSMENT

Assess the skin condition in the affected area, noting redness, contusions, or open wounds. Assess the neurovascular status of the affected extremity, including distal pulses, color, temperature, presence of edema, capillary refill to fingers or toes, and sensation and motion. Perform a pain assessment. If the patient reports pain, administer the prescribed analgesic in sufficient time to allow for the full effect of the medication. Assess for muscle spasms and administer the prescribed muscle relaxant in sufficient time to allow for the full effect of the medication. Assess for the presence of disease processes that may contraindicate the use of a cast or interfere with wound healing, including skin diseases, peripheral vascular disease, diabetes mellitus, and open or draining wounds.

NURSING DIAGNOSIS

Determine the related factors for the nursing diagnoses based on the patient's current status. Appropriate nursing diagnoses may include:

- Risk for Peripheral Neurovascular Dysfunction
- Acute Pain
- Impaired Physical Mobility
- Risk for Injury
- Anxiety
- Disturbed Body Image
- Risk for Impaired Skin Integrity
- Ineffective Tissue Perfusion
- Deficient Knowledge

OUTCOME IDENTIFICATION AND PLANNING

The expected outcome to achieve when assisting with a cast application is that the cast is applied without interfering with neurovascular function and that healing occurs. Other outcomes that may be appropriate include that the patient is free from complications, the patient has knowledge of the treatment regimen, and the patient experiences increased comfort.

IMPLEMENTATION

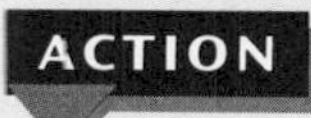

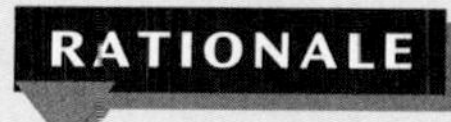

ACTION	RATIONALE
1. Review the medical record and medical orders to determine the need for the cast.	Reviewing the medical record and order validates the correct patient and correct procedure.

(continued)

SKILL 9-15 Assisting With Cast Application *(continued)*

ACTION	RATIONALE
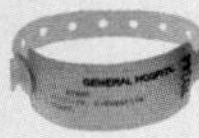 2. Identify the patient. Explain the procedure to the patient and verify area to be casted.	Patient identification validates the correct patient and correct procedure. Discussion and explanation help allay anxiety and prepare the patient for what to expect.
3. Perform a pain assessment and assess for muscle spasm. Administer prescribed medications in sufficient time to allow for the full effect of the analgesic and/or muscle relaxant.	Assessment of pain and analgesic administration ensure patient comfort and enhance cooperation.
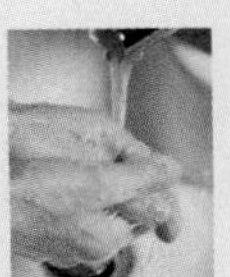 4. Perform hand hygiene and put on gloves, if necessary.	Hand hygiene and gloving prevent the spread of microorganisms; gloving also protects the nurse from residual casting materials collecting on hands.
5. Close the room door or curtains. Place the bed at an appropriate and comfortable working height, if necessary.	Closing the door or curtains provides privacy. Proper bed height helps reduce back strain while you are performing the procedure.
6. Position the patient as needed, depending on the type of cast being applied and the location of the injury. Support the extremity or body part to be casted.	Proper positioning minimizes movement, maintains alignment, and increases patient comfort.
7. Drape the patient with the waterproof pads.	Draping provides warmth and privacy and helps protect other body parts from contact with casting materials.
8. Cleanse and dry the affected body part.	Skin care before cast application helps prevent skin breakdown.
9. Position and maintain the affected body part in the position indicated by the physician as the stockinette, sheet wadding, and padding is applied (Figure 1). The stockinette should extend beyond the ends of the cast. As the wadding is applied, check for wrinkles.	Stockinette and other materials protect skin from casting materials and create a smooth, padded edge, protecting the skin from abrasion. Padding protects the skin, tissues, and nerves from the pressure of the cast.

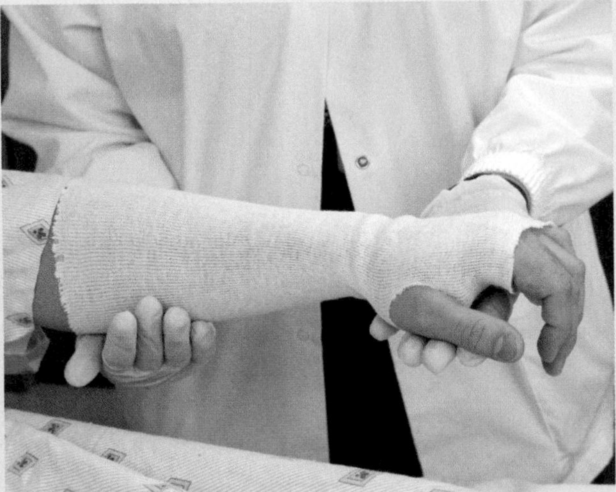

Figure 1. Stockinette in place.

SKILL 9-15 Assisting With Cast Application *(continued)*

ACTION	RATIONALE
10. Continue to position and maintain the affected body part in the position indicated by the physician or advanced practice professional as the casting material is applied (Figure 2). Assist with finishing by folding the stockinette or other padding down over the outer edge of the cast.	Smooth edges lessen the risk for skin irritation and abrasion.
11. **Support the cast during hardening.** Handle hardening plaster casts with the palms of hands, not fingers (Figure 3). Support the cast on a firm, smooth surface. Do not rest it on a hard surface or sharp edges. Avoid placing pressure on the cast.	Proper handling avoids denting of the cast and development of pressure areas.

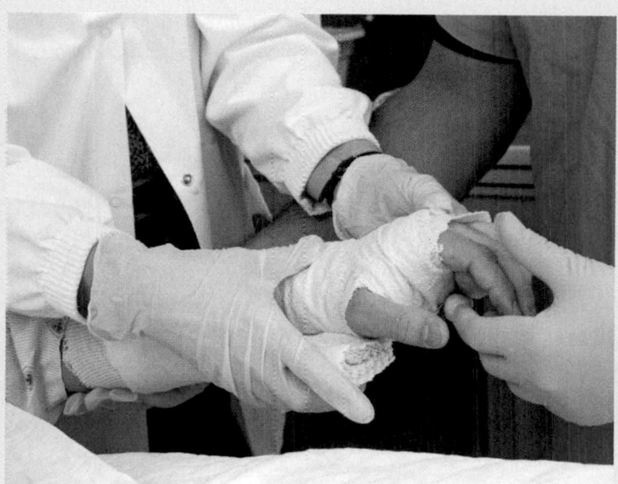
Figure 2. Casting material being applied.

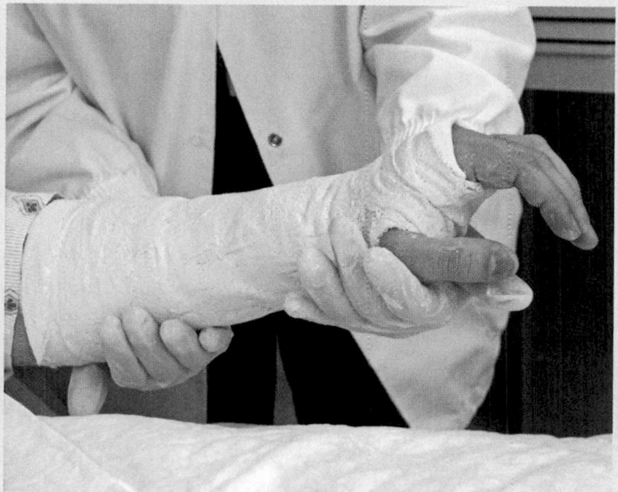
Figure 3. Using palms to move the casted limb.

ACTION	RATIONALE
12. **Elevate the injured limb above heart level with pillow or bath blankets as ordered, making sure pressure is evenly distributed under the cast.**	Elevation promotes venous return. Evenly distributed pressure prevents molding and denting of the cast and development of pressure areas.
13. Remove gloves and dispose of them properly; place the bed in the lowest position, if necessary.	Removing gloves properly reduces the risk for infection transmission and contamination of other items. Repositioning the bed promotes safety.
14. Obtain x-rays as ordered.	X-rays identify that the affected area is positioned properly.
15. **Instruct the patient to report pain, odor, drainage, changes in sensation, abnormal sensation, or the inability to move fingers or toes of the affected extremity.**	Pressure within a cast may increase with edema and lead to compartment syndrome. Patient complaints allow for early detection of and prompt intervention for complications such as skin irritation or impaired tissue perfusion.
16. Leave the cast uncovered and exposed to the air. Reposition the patient every 2 hours. Depending on facility policy, a fan may be used to dry the cast.	Keeping the cast uncovered promotes drying. Repositioning prevents development of pressure areas. Using a fan helps increase airflow and speeds drying.
17. Perform hand hygiene.	Hand hygiene prevents the spread of microorganisms.

(continued)

SKILL 9-15 Assisting With Cast Application *(continued)*

EVALUATION

The expected outcome is achieved when neurovascular function is maintained and healing occurs. In addition, the patient is free from complications, has knowledge of the treatment regimen, and experiences increased comfort.

DOCUMENTATION

Guidelines

Document the time, date, and site that the cast was applied. Include the skin assessment and care provided before application. Document the patient's response to the cast and the neurovascular status of the extremity.

Sample Documentation

6/1/08 1245 Fiberglass cast applied to right forearm from mid-upper arm to middle of hand. Cast clean and dry; edges padded. No signs of irritation noted. Patient able to move fingers freely. Fingers pale pink, warm, and dry. Capillary refill less than 2 seconds. Patient denies any numbness, tingling, or pain. Right forearm resting on two pillows. Patient instructed to report any complaints of pain, pressure, numbness, tingling, or decreased ability to move fingers.—P. Collins, RN

Unexpected Situations and Associated Interventions

- *Your patient, who has a cast on his hand and forearm, has been experiencing pain relief in the extremity with ice application and oral analgesics. He now reports pain unrelieved by the analgesic and a feeling of tightness in his arm. In addition, his fingers are cool, with sluggish capillary refill:* Compartment syndrome may be developing. Adjust the arm so that it is no higher than heart level. This enhances arterial perfusion and controls edema. Notify the physician of the situation immediately. Prepare for bivalving of the cast (cutting of the cast in half longitudinally) to relieve pressure.

Special Considerations

General Considerations

- Perform frequent, regular assessment of neurovascular status. Early recognition of diminished circulation and nerve function is essential to prevent loss of function. Be alert for the presence of compartment syndrome.
- Fiberglass casts dry quickly, usually within 5 to 15 minutes.
- If a fiberglass cast was applied, remove any fiberglass resin residue on the skin with alcohol or acetone.
- Synthetic casts are lightweight, easy to clean, and somewhat water resistant. If a Gore-Tex liner is used when the cast is applied, the cast may be immersed in water without affecting the cast integrity.

Infant and Child Considerations

- Synthetic casts come in different colors and with designs, such as cartoons and stripes. These features may make the experience more pleasant for a child.

SKILL 9-16 Caring for a Cast

A cast is a rigid external immobilizing device that encases a body part. Casts, made of plaster or synthetic materials such as fiberglass, are used to immobilize a body part in a specific position and to apply uniform pressure on the encased soft tissue. They may be used to treat injuries, correct a deformity, stabilize weakened joints, or promote healing after surgery. Casts generally allow the patient mobility while restricting movement of the affected body part. Nursing responsibilities after the cast is in place include maintaining the cast, preventing complications, and providing patient teaching related to cast care.

Equipment

- Washcloth
- Towel
- Skin cleanser
- Basin of warm water
- Waterproof pads
- Tape
- Pillows
- Nonsterile gloves, if indicated

ASSESSMENT

Review the patient's medical record and nursing plan of care to determine the need for cast care and care of the affected area. Perform a pain assessment and administer the prescribed medication in sufficient time to allow for the full effect of the analgesic before starting care. Assess the neurovascular status of the affected extremity, including distal pulses, color, temperature, presence of edema, capillary refill to fingers or toes, and sensation and motion. Assess the skin distal to the cast. Note any indications of infection, including any foul odor from the cast, pain, fever, edema, and extreme warmth over an area of the cast. Assess for complications of immobility, including alterations in skin integrity, reduced joint movement, decreased peristalsis, constipation, alterations in respiratory function, and signs of thrombophlebitis. Inspect the condition of the cast. Be alert for cracks, dents, or the presence of drainage from the cast. Assess the patient's knowledge of cast care.

NURSING DIAGNOSIS

Determine the related factors for the nursing diagnoses based on the patient's current status. Appropriate nursing diagnoses may include:

- Risk for Peripheral Neurovascular Dysfunction
- Disturbed Body Image
- Risk for Disuse Syndrome
- Risk for Falls
- Risk for Injury
- Deficient Knowledge
- Impaired Physical Mobility
- Acute Pain
- Self-Care Deficit (bathing/hygiene, feeding, dressing or grooming, or toileting)
- Risk for Impaired Skin Integrity
- Impaired Tissue Perfusion

OUTCOME IDENTIFICATION AND PLANNING

The expected outcome to achieve when caring for a patient with a cast is that the cast remains intact, and the patient does not experience neurovascular compromise. Other outcomes include that the patient is free from infection, the patient experiences only mild pain and slight edema or soreness, the patient experiences only slight limitations of range-of-joint motion, the skin around the cast edges remains intact, the patient participates in activities of daily living, and the patient demonstrates appropriate cast-care techniques.

(continued)

SKILL 9-16 Caring for a Cast *(continued)*

IMPLEMENTATION

ACTION	RATIONALE
1. Review the medical record and the nursing plan of care to determine the need for cast care and care for the affected body part.	Reviewing the medical record and plan of care validates the correct patient and correct procedure.
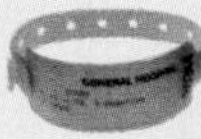 2. Identify the patient. Explain the procedure to the patient.	Patient identification validates the correct patient and correct procedure. Discussion and explanation help allay anxiety and prepare the patient for what to expect.
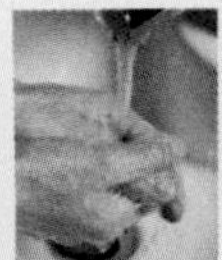 3. Perform hand hygiene and put on gloves, if necessary.	Hand hygiene and gloving prevent the spread of microorganisms. Gloves protect the nurse from residual casting materials collecting on hands.
4. Close the room door or curtains. Place the bed at an appropriate and comfortable working height, if necessary.	Closing the door or curtains provides privacy. Proper bed height helps reduce back strain while you are performing the procedure.
5. If a plaster cast was applied, handle the casted extremity or body area with the palms of your hands for the first 24 to 36 hours, until the cast is fully dry.	Proper handling of a plaster cast prevents dents in the cast, which may create pressure areas on the inside of the cast.
6. If the cast is on an extremity, elevate the affected area on pillows covered with waterproof pads (Figure 1). **Maintain the normal curvatures and angles of the cast.**	Elevation helps reduce edema and enhances venous return. Use of a waterproof pad prevents soiling of linen. Maintaining curvatures and angles maintains proper joint alignment, helps prevent flattened areas on the cast as it dries, and prevents pressure areas.

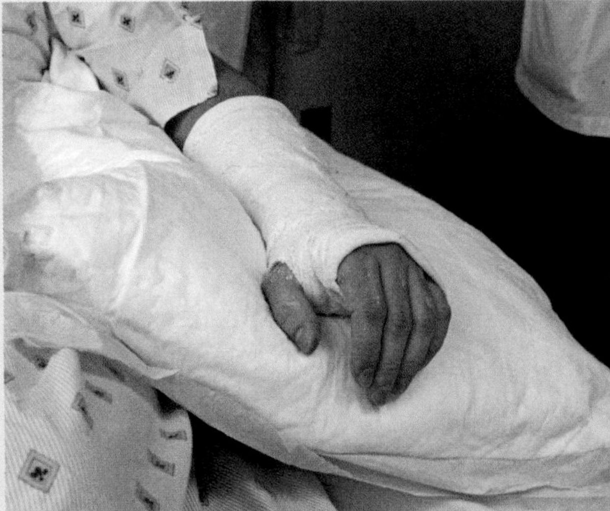

Figure 1. Elevating casted limb, maintaining the normal curvatures and angles of the cast.

ACTION	RATIONALE
7. Keep cast (plaster) uncovered until fully dry.	Keeping the cast uncovered allows heat and moisture to dissipate and air to circulate to speed drying.

SKILL 9-16 Caring for a Cast *(continued)*

ACTION | **RATIONALE**

8. Wash excess antiseptic or antimicrobial agents, such as povidone–iodine (Betadine), or residual casting material from the exposed skin. Dry thoroughly.

   Washing the area permits a clear area for inspection and reduces the risk for irritation and breakdown from the agent.

9. Assess the condition of the cast (Figure 2). Be alert for cracks, dents, or the presence of drainage from the cast. Perform skin and neurovascular assessment according to facility policy, as often as every 1 to 2 hours. **Check for pain, edema, inability to move body parts distal to the cast, pallor, pulses, and abnormal sensations. If the cast is on an extremity, compare it to the uncasted extremity (Figure 3).**

   Assessment helps detect abnormal neurovascular function or infection and allows for prompt intervention. Assessing the neurovascular status determines the circulation and oxygenation of tissues. Pressure within a cast may increase with edema and lead to compartment syndrome.

10. **If breakthrough bleeding or drainage is noted on the cast, mark the area on the cast (Figure 4). Indicate the date and time next to the area.** Follow physician orders or facility policy regarding the amount of drainage that needs to be reported to the physician.

    Marking the area provides a baseline for monitoring the amount of bleeding or drainage.

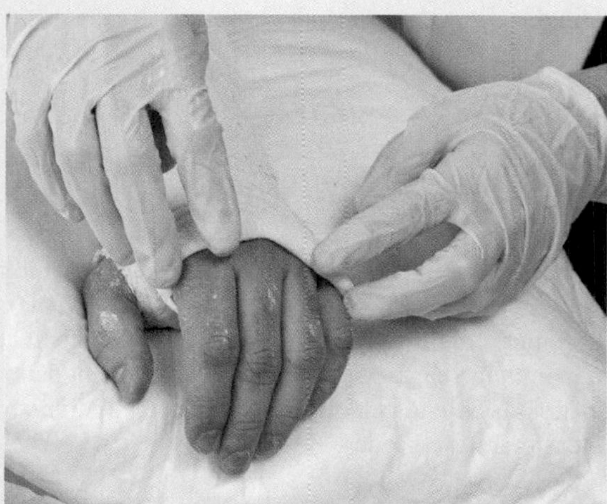

Figure 2. Assessing condition of cast.

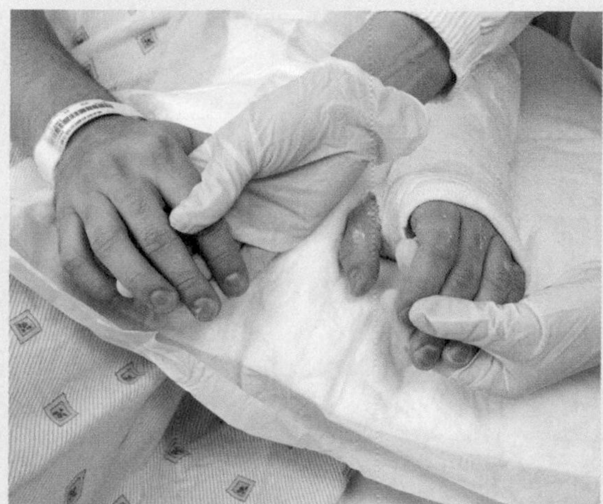

Figure 3. Assessing skin and neurovascular function; comparing with the uncasted extremity.

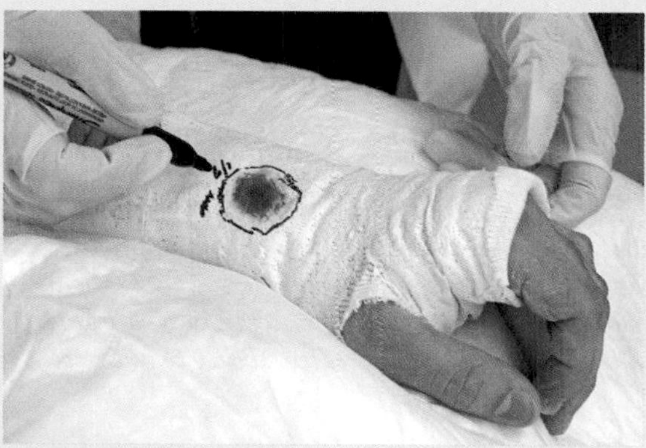

Figure 4. Marking any breakthrough bleeding on the cast, indicating the date and time.

(continued)

SKILL 9-16 Caring for a Cast *(continued)*

ACTION	RATIONALE
11. Assess for signs of infection. Monitor the patient's temperature. Assess for a foul odor from the cast, increased pain, or extreme warmth over an area of the cast.	Infection deters healing. Assessment allows for early detection and prompt intervention.
12. Reposition the patient every 2 hours. Provide back and skin care frequently. Encourage range of motion for unaffected joints. Encourage the patient to cough and deep breathe.	Repositioning promotes even drying of the cast and reduces the risk for the development of pressure areas under the cast. Frequent skin and back care prevents patient discomfort and skin breakdown. Range of motion maintains joint function of unaffected areas. Coughing and deep breathing reduce the risk for respiratory complications associated with immobility.
13. Instruct the patient to report pain, odor, drainage, changes in sensation, abnormal sensation, or the inability to move fingers or toes of the affected extremity.	Pressure within a cast may increase with edema and lead to compartment syndrome. Patient understanding of signs and symptoms allows for early detection and prompt intervention.
14. Remove gloves and dispose of them appropriately; place the bed in the lowest position, if necessary.	Proper glove removal and disposal reduce the risk for transmission of organisms; bed repositioning promotes safety.
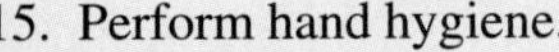 15. Perform hand hygiene.	Hand hygiene prevents the spread of microorganisms.

EVALUATION

The expected outcome is achieved when the patient exhibits a cast that is intact without evidence of neurovascular compromise to the affected body part. Other expected outcomes include: the patient remains free from infection; the patient verbalizes only mild pain and slight edema or soreness; the patient maintains range-of-joint motion; the patient demonstrates intact skin at cast edges; the patient is able to perform activities of daily living; and the patient demonstrates appropriate cast-care techniques.

DOCUMENTATION

Guidelines

Document all assessments and care provided. Document the patient's response to the cast, repositioning, and any teaching.

Sample Documentation

9/1/08 0845 Fiberglass cast in place on right lower extremity from just below knee to toes. Patient repositioned from right side to back. Cast clean and dry; edges padded. No signs of irritation noted. Patient able to move toes freely. Skin tone on right toes somewhat paler skin tone compared to left toes; toes warm and dry. Capillary refill less than 2 seconds. Patient denies any numbness, tingling, or pain. Right lower extremity elevated on two pillows. Patient instructed to report any complaints of pain, pressure, numbness, tingling, or decreased ability to move toes.
—P. Collins, RN

SKILL 9-16 Caring for a Cast *(continued)*

Unexpected Situations and Associated Interventions

- *Your patient, who has a cast on his hand and forearm, has been experiencing pain relief in the extremity with ice application and oral analgesics. He now reports pain unrelieved by the analgesic and a feeling of tightness in his arm. In addition, his fingers are cool, with sluggish capillary refill:* Compartment syndrome may be developing. Adjust the arm so that it is no higher than heart level. This enhances arterial perfusion and controls edema. Notify the physician of the situation immediately. Prepare for bivalving of the cast (cutting of the cast in half longitudinally) to relieve pressure.

Special Considerations

General Considerations

- Explain that itching under the cast is normal, but the patient should not stick objects down or in the cast to scratch.
- Begin patient teaching immediately after the cast is applied and continue until the patient or a significant other can provide care.
- If a cast is applied after surgery or trauma, monitor vital signs (the most accurate way to assess for bleeding).
- Synthetic casts are lightweight, easy to clean, and somewhat water resistant. If a Gore-Tex liner is used when the cast is applied, the cast may be immersed in water without affecting the cast integrity.

Infant and Child Considerations

- Do not allow the child to put anything inside the cast.
- Remove toys, hazardous floor rugs, pets, or other items that might cause the child to stumble.
- Keep in mind that synthetic casts come in different colors and with designs, such as cartoons and stripes. These features may make the experience more pleasant for a child.
- Cover a synthetic cast with a plastic bag for bathing.
- Instruct the parents/guardians of a child with a cast not to alter standard car seats to accommodate a cast. Specially designed car seats and restraints are available for travel in a car.

Older Adult Considerations

- Older adults may experience changes in circulation related to their age. They may have slow or poor capillary refill related to peripheral vascular disease. Obtain baseline information for comparison after the cast is applied. Use more than one neurovascular assessment to assess circulation. Compare extremities or sides of the body for symmetry.

SKILL 9-17 Applying Skin Traction and Caring for a Patient in Skin Traction

Traction is the application of a pulling force to a part of the body. It is used to reduce fractures, treat dislocations, correct or prevent deformities, improve or correct contractures, or decrease muscle spasms. It must be applied in the correct direction and magnitude to obtain the therapeutic effects desired.

With traction, the affected body part is immobilized by pulling with equal force on each end of the injured area, mixing traction and countertraction. Weights provide the pulling force or traction. The use of additional weights or positioning the patient's body weight against the traction pull provides the countertraction. Skin traction is applied directly to the skin, exerting indirect pull on the bone. The force may be applied using adhesive or nonadhesive traction tape or a boot, belt, or halter. Skin traction immobilizes a body part intermittently. See Box 9-1: Principles of Effective Traction.

(continued)

SKILL 9-17 Applying Skin Traction and Caring for a Patient in Skin Traction *(continued)*

BOX 9-1 Principles of Effective Traction

- Countertraction must be applied for effective traction.
- Traction must be continuous to be effective.
- Skeletal traction is never interrupted unless a life-threatening emergency occurs.
- Weights are not removed unless intermittent traction is prescribed.
- The patient must maintain good body alignment in the center of the bed.
- Ropes must be unobstructed.
- Weights must hang free.

Types of skin traction for adults include Buck's extension traction (lower leg), a cervical head halter, and the pelvic belt. Nursing care for skin traction includes setting the traction up, applying the traction, monitoring the application and patient response, and preventing complications from the therapy and immobility.

Equipment

- Bed with traction frame and trapeze
- Weights
- Velcro straps or other straps
- Rope and pulleys
- Boot with footplate
- Elastic hose
- Gloves
- Skin cleansing supplies

ASSESSMENT

Assess the patient's medical record, physician's orders, and the nursing plan of care to determine the type of traction, traction weight, and line of pull. Assess the traction equipment to ensure proper function, including inspecting the ropes for fraying and proper positioning. Assess the patient's body alignment. Perform a skin assessment and neurovascular assessment. Assess for complications of immobility, including alterations in respiratory function, skin integrity, urinary and bowel elimination, and muscle weakness, contractures, thrombophlebitis, pulmonary embolism, and fatigue.

NURSING DIAGNOSIS

Determine the related factors for the nursing diagnoses based on the patient's current status. Appropriate nursing diagnoses may include:

- Risk for Injury
- Ineffective Airway Clearance
- Anxiety
- Risk for Constipation
- Impaired Gas Exchange
- Deficient Knowledge
- Impaired Bed Mobility
- Acute Pain
- Impaired Physical Mobility
- Self-Care Deficit (bathing/hygiene, feeding, dressing or grooming, or toileting)
- Risk for Impaired Skin Integrity

SKILL 9-17

Applying Skin Traction and Caring for a Patient in Skin Traction *(continued)*

OUTCOME IDENTIFICATION AND PLANNING

The expected outcome to achieve when applying and caring for a patient in skin traction is that the traction is maintained with the appropriate counterbalance and the patient is free from complications of immobility. Other outcomes that may be appropriate include that the patient maintains proper body alignment, the patient reports an increased level of comfort, and the patient is free from injury.

IMPLEMENTATION

ACTION	RATIONALE
1. Review the medical record and the nursing plan of care to determine the type of traction being used and care for the affected body part.	Reviewing the medical record and plan of care validates the correct patient and correct procedure.
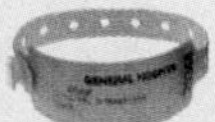 2. Identify the patient. Explain the procedure to the patient, emphasizing the importance of maintaining counterbalance, alignment, and position.	Patient identification validates the correct patient and correct procedure. Discussion and explanation help allay anxiety and prepare the patient for what to expect.
3. Perform a pain assessment and assess for muscle spasm. Administer prescribed medications in sufficient time to allow for the full effect of the analgesic and/or muscle relaxant.	Assessing pain and administering analgesics promote patient comfort.
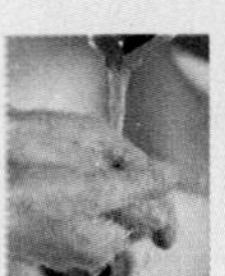 4. Perform hand hygiene.	Hand hygiene prevents the spread of microorganisms.
5. Close the room door or curtains. Place the bed at an appropriate and comfortable working height.	Closing the door or curtains provides for privacy. Proper bed height prevents back and muscle strain.
Applying Skin Traction	
6. Ensure the traction apparatus is attached securely to the bed. Assess the traction setup.	Assessment of traction setup and weights promotes safety.
7. Check that the ropes move freely through the pulleys. Check that all knots are tight and are positioned away from the pulleys. Pulleys should be free from the linens.	Checking ropes and pulleys ensures that weight is being applied correctly, promoting accurate counterbalance and function of the traction.
8. Place the patient in a supine position with the foot of the bed elevated slightly. The patient's head should be near the head of the bed and in alignment.	Proper patient positioning maintains proper counterbalance and promotes safety.
9. Cleanse the affected area. Place the elastic hose on the affected limb.	Skin care aids in preventing skin breakdown. Use of elastic hose prevents edema and neurovascular complications.

(continued)

SKILL 9-17 Applying Skin Traction and Caring for a Patient in Skin Traction *(continued)*

ACTION	RATIONALE
10. Place the traction boot over the patient's leg (Figure 1). Be sure the patient's heel is in the heel of the boot. Secure the boot with the straps.	The boot provides a means for attaching traction; proper application ensures proper pull.
11. Attach the traction cord to the footplate of the boot. Pass the rope over the pulley fastened at the end of the bed. Attach the weight to the hook on the rope, usually 5 to 10 pounds for an adult (Figure 2). Gently let go of the weight. **The weight should hang freely, not touching the bed or the floor.**	Attachment of weight applies the pull for the traction. Gently releasing the weight prevents a quick pull on the extremity and possible injury and pain. Properly hanging weights and correct patient positioning ensure accurate counterbalance and function of the traction.

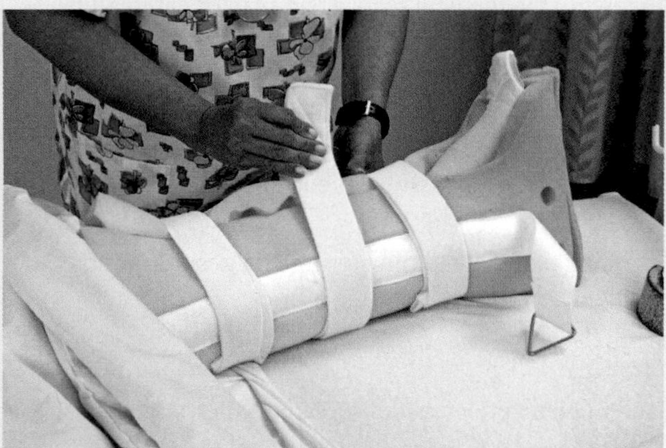

Figure 1. Applying the traction boot with an elastic stocking in place on the leg.

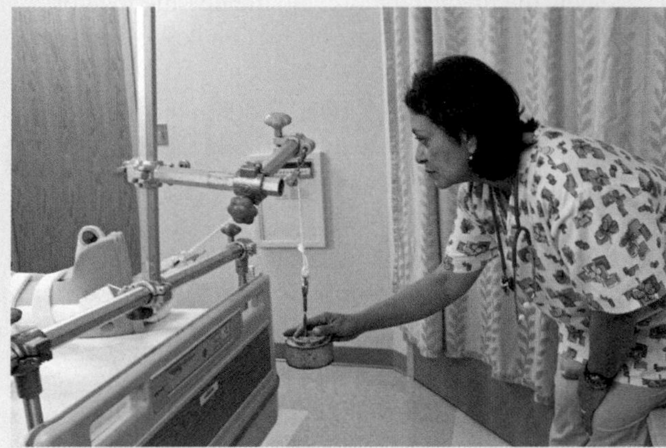

Figure 2. Applying the weight for the skin traction.

ACTION	RATIONALE
12. Check the patient's alignment with the traction.	Proper alignment is necessary for proper counterbalance and ensures patient safety.
13. Check the boot for placement and alignment. **Make sure the line of pull is parallel to the bed and not angled downward.**	Misalignment causes ineffective traction and may interfere with healing. A properly positioned boot prevents pressure on the heel.
14. Place the bed in the lowest position that still allows the weight to hang freely.	Proper bed positioning ensures effective application of traction without patient injury.
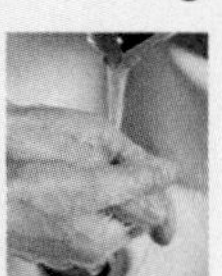 15. Perform hand hygiene.	Hand hygiene prevents the spread of microorganisms.

Caring for a Patient With Skin Traction

ACTION	RATIONALE
16. Perform a skin-traction assessment per facility policy. This assessment includes checking the traction equipment, examining the affected body part, maintaining proper body alignment, and performing a skin assessment and a neurovascular assessment.	Assessment provides information to determine proper application and alignment, thereby reducing the risk for injury. Misalignment causes ineffective traction and may interfere with healing.

SKILL 9-17

Applying Skin Traction and Caring for a Patient in Skin Traction *(continued)*

ACTION	RATIONALE
17. Remove the straps every 4 hours per the physician's order or facility policy. Check bony prominences for skin breakdown, abrasions, and pressure areas. Remove the boot per physician's order or facility policy every 8 hours. Put on gloves and wash, rinse, and thoroughly dry the skin.	Removing the straps provides assessment information for early detection and prompt intervention of potential complications should they arise. Washing the area enhances circulation to skin; thorough drying prevents skin breakdown. Using gloves prevents transfer of microorganisms.
18. Assess the extremity distal to the traction for edema, and assess peripheral pulses (Figure 3). Assess the temperature, color, and capillary refill (Figure 4), and compare with the unaffected limb. Check for pain, inability to move body parts distal to the traction, pallor, and abnormal sensations. Assess for indicators of deep-vein thrombosis, including calf tenderness, swelling, and a positive Homans' sign.	Doing so helps detect signs of abnormal neurovascular function and allows for prompt intervention. Assessing neurovascular status determines the circulation and oxygenation of tissues. Pressure within the traction boot may increase with edema.

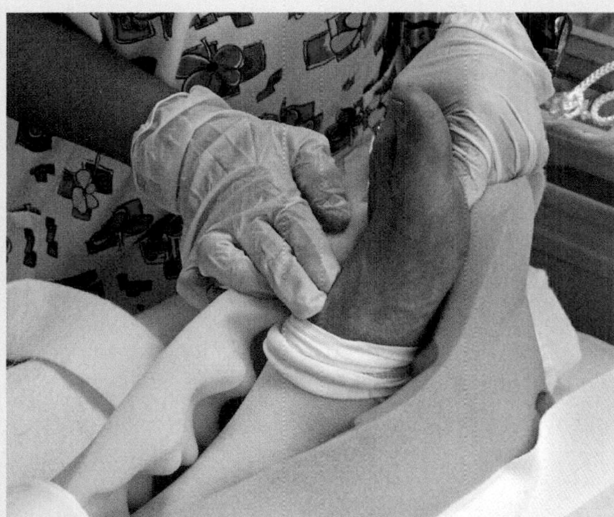
Figure 3. Assessing distal pulses.

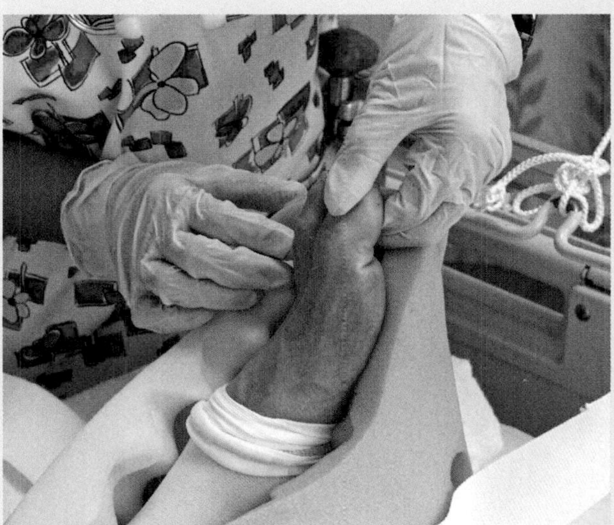
Figure 4. Assessing capillary refill.

ACTION	RATIONALE
19. Replace the traction and remove gloves and dispose of them appropriately.	Replacing traction is necessary to provide immobilization and facilitate healing. Proper disposal of gloves prevents the transmission of microorganisms.
20. Check the boot for placement and alignment. **Make sure the line of pull is parallel to the bed and not angled downward.**	Misalignment causes ineffective traction and may interfere with healing. A properly positioned boot prevents pressure on the heel.
21. **Ensure the patient is positioned in the center of the bed, with the affected leg aligned with the trunk of the patient's body.**	Misalignment interferes with the effectiveness of traction and may lead to complications.

(continued)

SKILL 9-17

Applying Skin Traction and Caring for a Patient in Skin Traction *(continued)*

ACTION	RATIONALE
22. Examine the weights and pulley system. **Weights should hang freely, off the floor and bed. Knots should be secure. Ropes should move freely through the pulleys. The pulleys should not be constrained by knots (Figure 5).**	Checking the weights and pulley system ensures proper application and reduces the risk for patient injury from traction application.

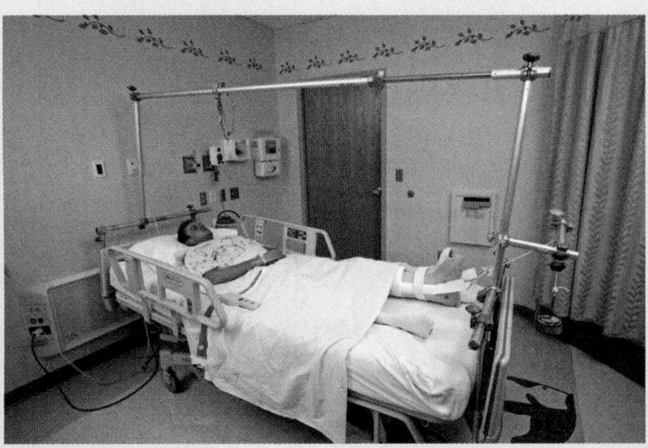

Figure 5. Skin traction in place.

ACTION	RATIONALE
23. Perform range-of-motion exercises on all unaffected joint areas, unless contraindicated. Encourage the patient to cough and deep breathe every 2 hours.	Range of motion maintains joint function. Coughing and deep breathing help to reduce the risk for respiratory complications related to immobility.
24. Raise the side rails. Place the bed in the lowest position that still allows the weight to hang freely.	Raising the side rails promotes patient safety. Proper bed positioning ensures effective application of traction without patient injury.
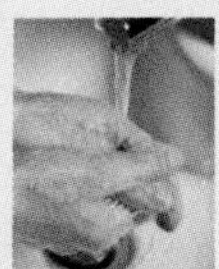 25. Perform hand hygiene.	Hand hygiene prevents the spread of microorganisms.

EVALUATION

The expected outcome is met when the patient demonstrates proper body alignment with traction applied and maintained with appropriate counterbalance. Other outcomes include: the patient verbalizes pain relief, with pain rated at lower numbers, and the patient remains free of injury.

Documentation

Guidelines

Document the time, date, type, amount of weight used, and the site where the traction was applied. Include the skin assessment and care provided before application. Document the patient's response to the traction and the neurovascular status of the extremity.

SKILL 9-17 Applying Skin Traction and Caring for a Patient in Skin Traction *(continued)*

Sample Documentation

6/3/08 1500 Patient complaining of pain in left hip due to fracture, rating it 7 out of 10. Administered oxycodone 2 tabs as ordered. Pain rated 3 out of 10, 30 minutes later. Buck's extension traction with 5 lb of weight applied to left extremity. Skin intact. Pedal pulses present and equal, feet pale pink, warm, and dry, with brisk capillary refill bilaterally. Patient able to wiggle toes freely. Denies numbness or tingling. Patient lying flat in bed with head of bed elevated approximately 15 degrees. Surgery planned for tomorrow.—L. James, RN

Unexpected Situations and Associated Interventions

- *Your patient is in Buck's traction and reports pain in the heel of the affected leg:* Remove traction and perform a skin and neurovascular assessment. Reapply the traction and reassess the neurovascular status in 15 to 20 minutes. Notify the physician.

Special Considerations

General Considerations

- Unless contraindicated, encourage the patient to do active flexion–extension ankle exercise and calf-pumping exercises at regular intervals to decrease venous stasis.
- Be alert for pressure on peripheral nerves with skin traction. Take care with Buck's traction to avoid pressure on the peroneal nerve at the point where it passes around the neck of the fibula just below the knee.
- Assess patients who are in traction for extended periods of time for development of helplessness, isolation, confinement, and loss of control. Diversional activities, therapeutic communication, and frequent visits by staff and significant others are an important part of care.

Older Adult Considerations

- Be extra vigilant with older adults in skin traction. Elderly patients are prone to alterations in skin integrity due to a decreased amount of subcutaneous fat and thinner, drier, more fragile skin.

SKILL 9-18 Caring for a Patient in Skeletal Traction

Skeletal traction provides pull to a body part by attaching weight directly to the bone, using pins, screws, wires, or tongs. It is used to immobilize a body part for prolonged periods. This method of traction is used to treat fractures of the femur, tibia, and cervical spine. Nursing responsibilities related to skeletal traction include maintaining the traction, maintaining body alignment, monitoring neurovascular status, promoting exercise, preventing complications from the therapy and immobility, and preventing infection by providing pin site care. Pin site care is performed frequently in the first 48 to 72 hours after application, when drainage may be heavy. Thereafter, pin site care may be done daily or weekly. Dressings are often applied for the first 48 to 72 hours, and then sites may be left open to air. There is little research evidence on which to base the management of skeletal pin sites (Baird Holmes & Brown, 2005). Skeletal pin site care varies based on physician and facility policy. Refer to specific patient medical orders and facility guidelines.

(continued)

SKILL 9-18 Caring for a Patient in Skeletal Traction *(continued)*

Equipment

- Sterile gloves
- Sterile applicators
- Cleansing agent for pin care, usually sterile normal saline or chlorhexidine, per physician order or facility policy
- Sterile container
- Antimicrobial ointment, if ordered
- Foam, nonstick, or gauze dressing, per medical order or facility policy

ASSESSMENT

Review the patient's medical record, physician's orders, and nursing plan of care to determine the type of traction, traction weight, and line of pull. Assess the traction equipment to ensure proper function, including inspecting the ropes for fraying and proper positioning. Assess the patient's body alignment. Perform a skin assessment and neurovascular assessment. Inspect the pin insertion sites for inflammation and infection, including swelling, cloudy or offensive drainage, pain, or redness. Assess for complications of immobility, including alterations in respiratory function, constipation, alterations in skin integrity, alterations in urinary elimination, and muscle weakness, contractures, thrombophlebitis, pulmonary embolism, and fatigue.

NURSING DIAGNOSIS

Determine the related factors for the nursing diagnoses based on the patient's current status. Appropriate nursing diagnoses may include:

- Impaired Skin Integrity
- Risk for Injury
- Ineffective Airway Clearance
- Anxiety
- Risk for Constipation
- Deficient Knowledge
- Impaired Bed Mobility
- Acute Pain
- Impaired Physical Mobility
- Self-Care Deficit (toileting, bathing or hygiene, or dressing or grooming)
- Risk for Infection
- Impaired Gas Exchange

OUTCOME IDENTIFICATION AND PLANNING

The expected outcome to achieve when caring for a patient in skeletal traction is that the traction is maintained appropriately and that the patient is free from complications of immobility and infection. Other outcomes that may be appropriate include: the patient maintains proper body alignment, the patient reports an increased level of comfort, and the patient is free from injury.

IMPLEMENTATION

ACTION	RATIONALE
1. Review the medical record and the nursing plan of care to determine the type of traction being used and the prescribed care.	Reviewing the medical record and plan of care validates the correct patient and correct procedure.

SKILL 9-18 Caring for a Patient in Skeletal Traction *(continued)*

ACTION	RATIONALE
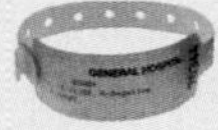 2. Identify the patient. Explain the procedure to the patient, emphasizing the importance of maintaining counterbalance, alignment, and position.	Patient identification validates the correct patient and correct procedure. Discussion and explanation help allay anxiety and prepare the patient for what to expect.
3. Perform a pain assessment and assess for muscle spasm. Administer prescribed medications in sufficient time to allow for the full effect of the analgesic and/or muscle relaxant.	Assessing for pain and administering analgesics promote patient comfort.
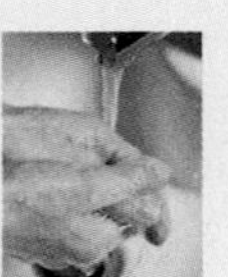 4. Perform hand hygiene.	Hand hygiene prevents the spread of microorganisms.
5. Close the room door or curtains. Place the bed at an appropriate and comfortable working height.	Closing the door or curtains provides for privacy. Proper bed height prevents back and muscle strain.
6. Ensure the traction apparatus is attached securely to the bed. Assess the traction setup, including application of the ordered amount of weight. **Be sure that the weights hang freely, not touching the bed or the floor.**	Proper traction application reduces the risk of injury by promoting accurate counterbalance and function of the traction.
7. Check that the ropes move freely through the pulleys. Check that all knots are tight and are positioned away from the pulleys. Pulleys should be free from the linens.	Free ropes and pulleys ensure accurate counterbalance and function of the traction.
8. Check the alignment of the patient's body as prescribed.	Proper alignment maintains an effective line of pull and prevents injury.
9. Perform a skin assessment. Pay attention to pressure points, including the ischial tuberosity, popliteal space, Achilles tendon, sacrum, and heel.	Skin assessment provides early intervention for skin irritation, impaired tissue perfusion, and other complications.
10. Perform a neurovascular assessment. Assess the extremity distal to the traction for edema and peripheral pulses. Assess the temperature and color and compare with the unaffected limb. Check for pain, inability to move body parts distal to the traction, pallor, and abnormal sensations. Assess for indicators of deep-vein thrombosis, including calf tenderness, swelling, and a positive Homans' sign.	Neurovascular assessment aids in early identification and allows for prompt intervention should compromised circulation and oxygenation of tissues develop.
11. Assess the site at and around the pins for redness, edema, and odor. Assess for skin tenting, prolonged or purulent drainage, elevated body temperature, elevated pin site temperature, and bowing or bending of the pins.	Pin sites provide a possible entry for microorganisms. Skin inspection allows for early detection and prompt intervention should complications develop.

(continued)

SKILL 9-18 Caring for a Patient in Skeletal Traction *(continued)*

ACTION	RATIONALE
12. Provide pin site care.	Performing pin site care prevents crusting at the site that could lead to fluid buildup, infection, and osteomyelitis.
a. Using sterile technique, open the applicator package and pour the cleansing agent into the sterile container.	Using sterile technique reduces the risk for transmission of microorganisms.
b. Put on the sterile gloves.	
c. Place the applicators into the solution.	
d. **Clean the pin site starting at the insertion area and working outward, away from the pin site (Figure 1).**	Cleaning from the center outward ensures movement from the least to most contaminated area.
e. **Use each applicator once. Use a new applicator for each pin site.**	Using an applicator once reduces the risk of transmission of microorganisms.

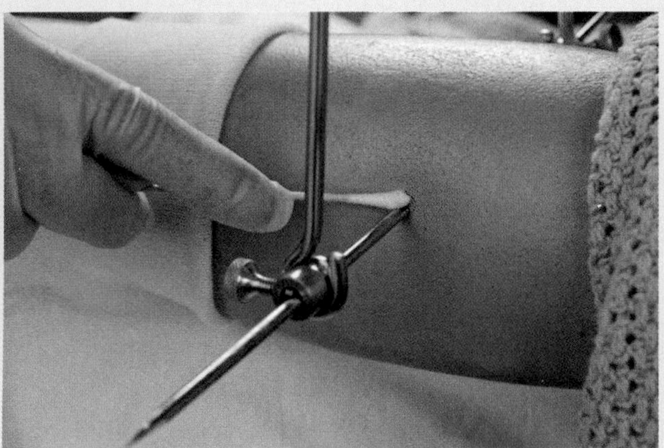

Figure 1. Cleaning around pin sites with normal saline on an applicator.

ACTION	RATIONALE
13. Depending on physician order and facility policy, apply the antimicrobial ointment to pin sites and apply a dressing.	Antimicrobial ointment helps reduce the risk of infection. A dressing aids in protecting the pin sites from contamination and contains any drainage.
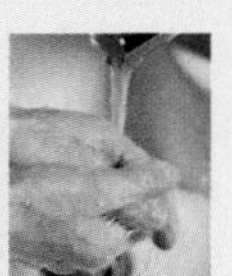 14. Remove gloves. Perform hand hygiene.	Gloves and hand hygiene deter the spread of microorganisms.
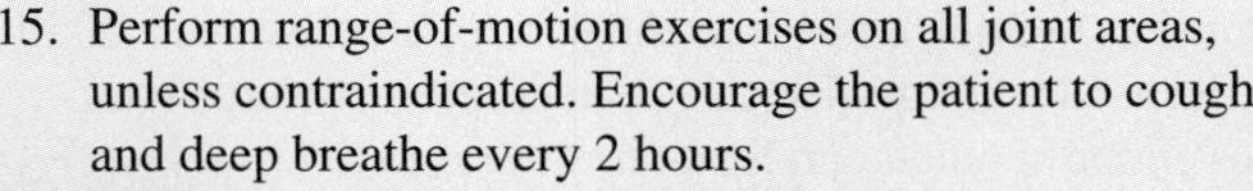 15. Perform range-of-motion exercises on all joint areas, unless contraindicated. Encourage the patient to cough and deep breathe every 2 hours.	Range-of-motion exercises promote joint mobility. Coughing and deep breathing reduce the risk of respiratory complications related to immobility.
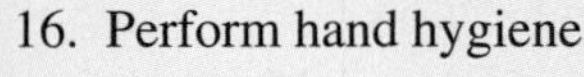 16. Perform hand hygiene.	Hand hygiene deters the spread of microorganisms.

SKILL 9-18 Caring for a Patient in Skeletal Traction *(continued)*

EVALUATION

The expected outcome is met when the patient demonstrates maintenance of skeletal traction with pin sites free of infection. In addition, the patient maintains proper body alignment and joint function, patient verbalizes pain relief, patient states signs and symptoms to report, and patient remains free of injury.

Documentation

Guidelines

Document the time, date, type of traction, and the amount of weight used. Include the skin assessment, pin site assessment, and pin site care. Document the patient's response to the traction and the neurovascular status of the extremity.

Sample Documentation

6/5/08 1020 Pin site care performed. Pin sites cleaned with normal saline and open to the air. Sites slightly red with serosanguineous crusting noted. Neurovascular status intact. Balanced suspension skeletal traction maintained as ordered.—M. Leroux, RN

Unexpected Situations and Associated Interventions

- *While performing a pin site assessment for your patient with skeletal traction, you note that several of the pins move and slide in the pin tract:* Assess the patient for other symptoms, including signs of infection at the pin sites, pain, and fever. Assess for neurovascular changes. Notify the physician of the findings.

Special Considerations

General Considerations

- If mechanical looseness or early signs of infection (swelling, cloudy or offensive drainage, pain or redness) are present, increase the frequency of pin site care (Baird Holmes & Brown, 2005).
- Assess the patient for chronic conditions, such as diabetes mellitus, peripheral vascular disease, and chronic obstructive pulmonary disease, which can significantly increase a patient's risk for complications when skeletal traction is in use.
- Never remove the weights from skeletal traction unless a life-threatening situation occurs. Removal of the weights interferes with therapy and can result in injury to the patient.
- Inspect the pin sites for inflammation and evidence of infection at least every 8 hours. Prevention of osteomyelitis is of utmost importance.

SKILL 9-19 Caring for a Patient With an External Fixation Device

External fixation devices are used to manage open fractures with soft-tissue damage. They consist of one of a variety of frames to hold pins that are drilled into or through bones. External fixators provide stable support for severe crushed or splintered fractures and access to and treatment for soft-tissue injuries. The use of these devices allows treatment of the fracture and damaged soft tissues while promoting patient comfort, early mobility, and active exercise of adjacent uninvolved joints. Complications related to disuse and immobility are minimized. Nursing responsibilities include reassuring the patient, maintaining the device, monitoring neurovascular status, promoting exercise, preventing complications from the therapy, preventing infection by providing pin site care, and providing teaching to ensure compliance and self-care. Pin site care is performed frequently in the

(continued)

SKILL 9-19

Caring for a Patient With an External Fixation Device *(continued)*

first 48 to 72 hours after application, when drainage may be heavy. Thereafter, pin site care may be done daily or weekly. Dressings are often applied for the first 48 to 72 hours, and then sites may be left open to air. There is little research evidence on which to base the management of pin sites (Baird Holmes & Brown, 2005). Pin site care varies based on physician and facility policy. Refer to specific patient medical orders and facility guidelines. Nurses play a major role in preparing the patient psychologically for the application of an external fixator. The devices appear clumsy and large. In addition, the nurse needs to clarify misconceptions regarding pain and discomfort associated with the device.

Equipment

Equipment varies with the type of fixator and the type and location of the fracture but may include:

- Sterile applicators
- Cleansing solution, usually sterile normal saline or chlorhexidine, per physician order or facility policy
- Ice bag
- Sterile gauze
- Foam, nonstick, or gauze dressing, per medical order or facility policy
- Analgesic, per physician order
- Antimicrobial ointment, per physician's order or facility policy

ASSESSMENT

Review the patient's medical record, physician's orders, and the nursing plan of care to determine the type of device being used and prescribed care. Assess the external fixator to ensure proper function and position. Perform a skin assessment and neurovascular assessment. Inspect the pin insertion sites for signs of inflammation and infection, including swelling, cloudy or offensive drainage, pain, or redness. Assess the patient's knowledge regarding the device and self-care activities and responsibilities.

NURSING DIAGNOSIS

Determine the related factors for the nursing diagnoses based on the patient's current status. Appropriate nursing diagnoses may include:

- Risk for Infection
- Impaired Skin Integrity
- Risk for Injury
- Anxiety
- Deficient Knowledge
- Acute Pain
- Self-Care Deficit (toileting, bathing or hygiene, or dressing or grooming)
- Impaired Physical Mobility

OUTCOME IDENTIFICATION AND PLANNING

The expected outcome to achieve when caring for a patient with an external fixator device is that the patient shows no evidence of complication such as infection, contractures, venous stasis, thrombus formation, or skin breakdown. Additional outcomes that may be appropriate include that the patient shows signs of healing, the patient experiences relief from pain, and the patient is free from injury.

SKILL 9-19 Caring for a Patient With an External Fixation Device *(continued)*

IMPLEMENTATION

ACTION	RATIONALE
1. Review the medical record and the nursing plan of care to determine the type of device being used and prescribed care.	Reviewing the medical record and plan of care validates the correct patient and correct procedure.
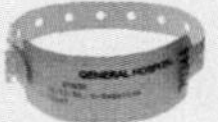 2. Identify the patient. Explain the procedure to the patient. Assure the patient that there will be little pain after the fixation device is in place. Reinforce that the patient will be able to adjust to the device and will be able to move about with the device, allowing him or her to resume normal activities more quickly.	Patient identification validates the correct patient and correct procedure. Discussion and explanation allay anxiety and prepare the patient psychologically for the application of the device.
3. After the fixation device is in place, **apply ice to the surgical site as ordered or per facility policy. Elevate the affected body part if appropriate (Figure 1).**	Ice and elevation help reduce swelling, relieve pain, and reduce bleeding.

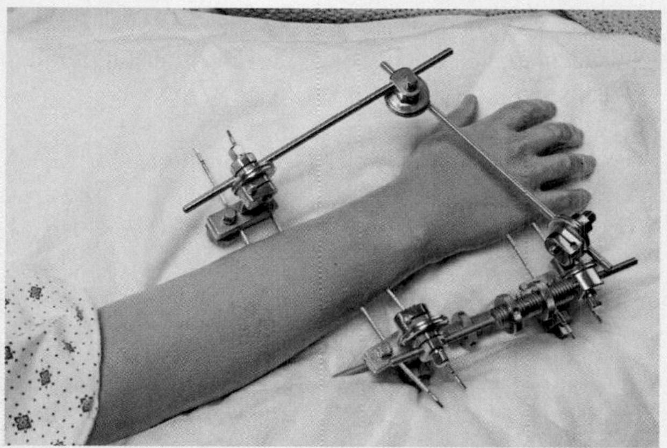

Figure 1. External fixation device in place.

ACTION	RATIONALE
4. Perform a pain assessment and assess for muscle spasm. Administer prescribed medications in sufficient time to allow for the full effect of the analgesic and/or muscle relaxant.	Pain assessment and analgesic administration help promote patient comfort.
5. Administer analgesics as ordered before exercising or mobilizing the affected body part.	Administration of analgesics promotes patient comfort and facilitates movement.
6. Perform neurovascular assessments per facility policy or physician's order, usually every 2 to 4 hours for 24 hours, then every 4 to 8 hours. Assess the affected body part for color, motion, sensation, edema, capillary refill, and pulses. If appropriate, compare with the unaffected side. Assess for pain not relieved by analgesics, burning, tingling, and numbness.	Assessment promotes early detection and prompt intervention of abnormal neurovascular function, nerve damage, or circulatory impairment. Assessment of neurovascular status determines the circulation and oxygenation of tissues.
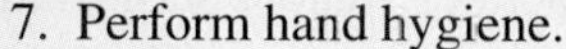 7. Perform hand hygiene.	Hand hygiene prevents the spread of microorganisms.

(continued)

SKILL 9-19 Caring for a Patient With an External Fixation Device *(continued)*

ACTION	RATIONALE
8. Close the room door or curtains. Place the bed at an appropriate and comfortable working height.	Closing the door or curtains provides for privacy. Proper bed height prevents back and muscle strain.
9. Assess the pin site for redness, tenting of the skin, prolonged or purulent drainage, swelling, and bowing, bending, or loosening of the pins. Monitor body temperature.	Assessing pin sites aids in early detection of infection and stress on the skin and allows for appropriate intervention.
10. Perform pin site care.	Performing pin site care prevents crusting at the site that could lead to fluid buildup, infection, and osteomyelitis.
a. Using sterile technique, open the applicator package and pour the cleansing agent into the sterile container.	Using sterile technique reduces the risk for transmission of microorganisms.
b. Put on the sterile gloves.	
c. Place the applicators into the solution.	
d. **Clean the pin site starting at the insertion area and working outward, away from the pin site (Figure 2).**	Cleaning from the center outward promotes movement from the least to most contaminated area.
e. **Use each applicator once. Use a new applicator for each pin site.**	Using each applicator only once prevents transfer of microorganisms.

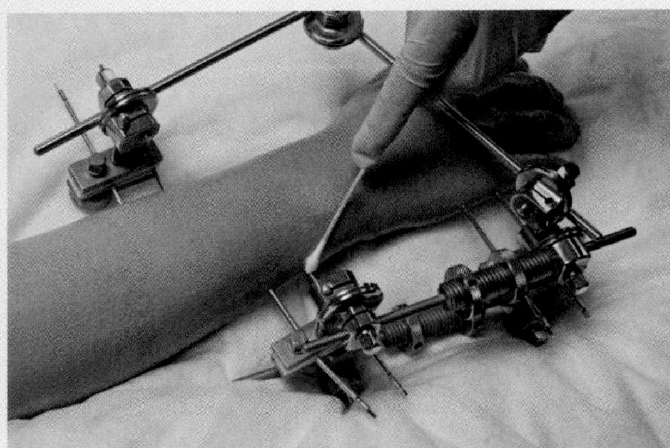

Figure 2. Cleaning around pin sites with normal saline on an applicator.

ACTION	RATIONALE
11. Depending on physician order and facility policy, apply the antimicrobial ointment to pin sites and apply a dressing.	Antimicrobial ointment prevents infection; applying a dressing helps contain drainage.
12. Remove gloves. Perform hand hygiene.	Hand hygiene prevents the spread of microorganisms.

EVALUATION

The expected outcome is met when the patient exhibits an external fixation device in place with pin sites that are clean, dry, and intact, without evidence of infection. The patient remains free of complications such as contractures, venous stasis, thrombus formation, or skin breakdown; the patient verbalizes pain relief; the patient remains free of injury, and the patient demonstrates knowledge of pin site care.

SKILL 9-19

Caring for a Patient With an External Fixation Device *(continued)*

DOCUMENTATION

Guidelines

Document the time, date, and type of device in place. Include the skin assessment, pin site assessment, and pin site care. Document the patient's response to the device and the neurovascular status of the affected area.

Sample Documentation

7/6/08 1020 External fixator in place on left forearm. Pin site care performed. Pin sites cleaned with normal saline and open to the air. Sites slightly red with serosanguineous crusting noted. Neurovascular status intact. Instruction given regarding range of motion to left fingers and elbow. Patient verbalizes understanding and able to demonstrate.—B. Clapp, RN

Special Considerations

General Considerations

- Teach the patient and significant others how to provide pin site care and how to recognize the signs of pin site infection. External fixator devices are in place for prolonged periods of time. Clean technique can be used at home.
- Patient and significant others should be able to identify early signs of infection, signs of a loose pin, and how to contact the orthopedic team, if necessary.
- Encourage the patient to refrain from smoking, if appropriate, to avoid delayed bone healing (Baird Holmes & Brown, 2005).
- Reinforce the importance of keeping the affected body part elevated when sitting or lying down to prevent edema.
- Do not adjust the clamps on the external fixator frame. It is the physician's or advanced practice professional's responsibility to adjust the clamps.
- Fractures often require additional treatment and stabilization with a cast or molded splint after the fixator device is removed.

The Taylor Suite offers these additional resources to enhance learning and facilitate understanding of this chapter:

- thePoint online resource, http://thepoint.lww.com/Lynn2E
- Student CD-ROM included with the book
- Skills Checklist to Accompany Taylor's Clinical Nursing Skills
- Taylor's Interactive Nursing: *Activity*
- Taylor's Video Guide to Clinical Nursing Skills: *Activity*

Developing Critical Thinking Skills

1. You are preparing to discharge Bobby Rowden from the emergency room. Discuss the teaching you should include for Bobby and his parents related to his injury and his plaster cast.
2. A pneumatic compression device has been ordered as part of the admission orders for Esther Levitz. You bring the pump and sleeves into the room, and she asks, "What is that? It looks like a torture machine!" How will you respond?
3. You are caring for Manuel Esposito the evening before his surgery. Your assessment of his affected extremity reveals skin that is warm to the touch, rapid capillary refill, and positive sensation and movement. What other assessments should you perform as part of your care for Mr. Esposito?

Bibliography

Altizer, L. (2004). Casting for immobilization. *Orthopaedic Nursing, 23*(2), 136–141.

ALS Association. Oregon and Southwest Washington Chapter. Range-of-Motion Exercises. Available at www.alsa-or.org/treatment/ROMExercises.htm. Accessed February 10, 2006.

American Nurses Association (ANA). (2003). Position statement on elimination of manual patient handling to prevent work-related musculoskeletal disorders. Silver Spring, MD: Author. Available at www.nursingworld.org/readroom/position/workplac/pathand.htm.

American Nurses Association (ANA). (2004). Handle with care. Silver Spring, MD: Author. Available at www.nursingworld.org/handlewithcare. Accessed January 27, 2006.

American Nurses Association (ANA). (2006). Handle with care. Fact sheet. Silver Spring, MD: Author. Available at www.nursingworld.org/handlewithcare/factsheet.htm. Accessed January 27, 2006.

Arthritis Foundation. (2004). Range-Of-Motion Exercises. Available at http://www.arthritis.org/conditions/onlinebrochures/ETR/ETR_ROM_brochure.pdf. Accessed February 10, 2006.

Baird Holmes, S., & Brown, S. (2005). National Association of Orthopaedic Nurses. Guidelines for orthopaedic nursing: Skeletal pin site care. *Orthopaedic Nursing, 24*(2), 99–107.

Beaupre, L. (2001). Exercise combined with continuous passive motion or slider board therapy compared with exercise only: A randomized controlled trial of patients following total knee arthroplasty. *Physical Therapy, 81*(4), 1029–1037.

Blocks, M. (2005). Practical solutions for safe patient handling. *Nursing, 35*(10), 44–45.

Brace, T. (2005). The dynamics of pushing and pulling in the workplace. Assessing and treating the problem. *AAOHN Journal, 53*(5), 224–229.

Converso, A., & Murphy, C. (2004). Winning the battle against back injuries. *RN, 67*(2), 52–57.

Craven, R., & Hirnle, C. (2003). *Fundamentals of nursing. Human health and function* (4th ed.). Philadelphia: Lippincott Williams & Wilkins.

Fletcher, K. (2005). Immobility: Geriatric self-learning module. *MEDSURG Nursing, 14*(1), 35–37.

Fort, C. W. (2002). Get pumped to prevent DVT. *Nursing, 32*(9), 50–52.

Geerts, W., Pineo, G., Heit, J., et al. (2004). Prevention of venous embolism: The Seventh ACCP Conference on Antithrombotic and Thrombolytic Therapy. *CHEST, 126*(3), Supplement, 338S–400S.

Geraghty, M. (2005). Nursing the unconscious patient. *Nursing Standard, 20*(1), 54–64.

Gillis, A., & MacDonald, B. (2005). Prevention: Deconditioning in the hospitalized elderly. *Canadian Nurse, 101*(6), 16–20.

Griffiths, H., & Gallimore, D. (2005). Positioning critically ill patients in hospital. *Nursing Standard, 19*(42), 56–64.

Gulanick, M., & Myers, J. (2003). *Nursing plans of care: Nursing diagnosis.* Philadelphia: Mosby.

Hockenberry, M. (2005). *Wong's essentials of pediatric nursing* (7th ed.). St. Louis, MO: Elsevier Mosby.

Hoenig, H. (2004). Assistive technology and mobility aids for the older patient with disability. *Annals of Long-Term Care, 12*(9), 12–19.

Lynch, D., Ferraro, M., Krol, J., et al. (2005). Continuous passive motion improves shoulder joint integrity following stroke. *Clinical Rehabilitation, 19*(6), 594–599.

McConnell, E. A. (1997). Clinical do's & don'ts: Assisting with cast application. *Nursing, 27*(12), 28.

McConnell, E. (2001). Clinical do's & don'ts: Teaching your patient to use a stationary walker. *Nursing, 31*(10), 17.

Mollabashy, A. (1997). Immobilization techniques for the cervical spine: Cervical orthoses, skeletal traction, and halo devices. *Topics in Emergency Medicine, 19*(3), 26–33.

Nelson, A., & Baptiste, A. (2004). Evidence-based practices for safe patient handling and movement. *Online Journal of Issues in Nursing, 9*(3), Manuscript 3. Available at www.nursingworld.org/ojin/topic25/tpc25_3.htm.

Nelson, A., Fragala, G., & Menzel, N. (2003). Myths and facts about back injuries in nursing. *American Journal of Nursing, 103*(2), 32–40.

Nelson, A., Owen, B., Lloyd, J., et al. (2003). Safe patient handling & movement: Preventing back injury among nurses requires careful selection of the safest equipment and techniques. *American Journal of Nursing, 103*(3), 32–43.

Pifer, G. (2000). Casting and splinting: Prevention of complications. *Topics in Emergency Medicine, 22*(3), 48–54.

Pullen, R. (2004). Logrolling a patient. *Nursing, 34*(2), 22.

Santulli, E. (2004). No strain? No pain! *Nursing, 34*(3), 32hn7–8.

Smeltzer, S., Bare, B., Hinkle, J. H., & Cheever, K. H. (2008). *Brunner & Suddarth's textbook of medical-surgical nursing* (11th ed.). Philadelphia: Lippincott Williams & Wilkins.

Tabone, S. (2005). Safe patient handling. *Texas Nursing, 79*(3), 10–11.

Taylor, C., Lillis, C., LeMone, P., et al. (2008). *Fundamentals of nursing. The art & science of nursing care* (6th ed.). Philadelphia: Lippincott Williams & Wilkins.

Trinkoff, A., Brady, B., & Nielsen, K. (2003). Workplace prevention and musculoskeletal injuries in nurses. *Journal of Nursing Administration, 33*(3), 153–158.

U.S. Department of Labor. Occupational Safety & Health Administration (OSHA). (2003). HealthCare Wide Hazards Module—Ergonomics. Washington, D.C.: Author. Available at www.osha.gov/SLTC/etools/hospital/hazards/ergo/ergo.html.

U.S. Preventive Services Task Force. (2003). Behavioral counseling in primary care to promote physical activity: Recommendation and rationale. *American Journal of Nursing, 103*(4), 101–107.

Van Hook, F., Demonbreun, D., & Weiss, B. (2003). Ambulatory devices for chronic gait disorders in the elderly. *American Family Physician, 67*(8), 1717–1724.

VISN 8 Patient Safety Center. (2005). Safe patient handling and movement algorithms. Tampa, FL: Author. Available at www.visn8.med.va.gov/patientsafetycenter/SPHMAlg050105.pdf.

Wright, K. (2005). Mobility and safe handling of people with dementia. *Nursing Times, 101*(17), 38–40.

CHAPTER 10

Comfort

Focusing on Patient Care

This chapter will help you develop the skills needed to meet the comfort needs of the following patients:

Mildred Simpson is a 75-year-old woman recovering from a total hip replacement.

Joseph Watkins comes to the emergency department because of acute pain in his lower back that started when he was moving furniture.

Jerome Batiste, age 60, has been diagnosed with bone cancer and is being discharged with an order for patient-controlled analgesia (PCA) at home.

Learning Objectives

After studying this chapter, you will be able to:

1. Promote patient comfort.
2. Give a back massage.
3. Apply a TENS unit.
4. Care for a patient receiving PCA.
5. Care for a patient receiving epidural analgesia.

Key Terms

acute pain: pain that is generally rapid in onset and varies in intensity from mild to severe

adjuvant: substances or treatments that enhance the effect of another treatment; especially substances that enhance the effect of drugs

allodynia: pain that occurs after a normally weak or nonpainful stimulus, such as a light touch or a cold drink; a characteristic feature of neuropathic pain

breakthrough pain: a temporary flare-up of moderate to severe pain that occurs even when the patient is taking around-the-clock medication for persistent pain

chronic pain: pain that may be limited, intermittent, or persistent but that lasts beyond the normal healing period

epidural route: administration of analgesia via an infusion catheter placed in the epidural space

gate control theory: theory that states that certain nerve fibers, those of small diameter, conduct excitatory pain stimuli toward the brain, while nerve fibers of a large diameter appear to inhibit the transmission of pain impulses from the spinal cord to the brain

intractable pain: pain that is resistant to therapy and persists despite a variety of interventions

neuropathic pain: pain that results from an injury to or abnormal functioning of peripheral nerves or the central nervous system

nonpharmacologic interventions: interventions without the use of medicine or drugs; interventions in addition to the use of medicines or drugs

pain threshold: the lowest intensity of a stimulus that causes the subject to recognize pain

pain tolerance: point beyond which a person is no longer willing to endure pain

perineural route: administration of local anesthetic for pain management via an infusion catheter placed along most or all of the length of a wound

Comfort is an important need, and ensuring a patient's comfort is a major nursing responsibility. Providing comfort can be as simple as straightening the patient's bed linens, offering to hold the patient's hand, or assisting with hygiene needs. Often, providing comfort means providing pain relief. A person in discomfort or pain often experiences it as an all-consuming reality and wants only one intervention—relief. No two people experience pain exactly the same way. Differences in individual pain perception and response to pain, as well as the multiple and diverse causes of pain, require the use of highly specialized abilities to promote comfort and relieve pain. The most important of these are the nurse's belief that the patient's pain is real, willingness to become involved in the patient's pain experience, and competence in developing effective pain management regimens.

Pain is an elusive and complex phenomenon, and despite its universality, its exact nature remains a mystery. It is one of the human body's defense mechanisms that indicates the person is experiencing a problem. The definition of pain that is probably of greatest benefit to nurses and patients is that offered by Margo McCaffery (1979, p. 11): "Pain is whatever the experiencing person says it is, existing whenever he (or she) says it does." This definition rests on the belief that the only one who can be a real authority on whether, and how, an individual is experiencing pain is that individual.

Pain is present whenever a person says it is, even when no specific cause of the pain can be found. Assessment of discomfort and pain includes identifying and evaluating potentially painful conditions and procedures, the patient's self-report, the report of family members or caregivers close to the patient, observing behaviors, and physiologic measures that may indicate pain, such as blood pressure or pulse rate (McCaffery & Pasero, 1999; Pasero & McCaffery, 2005b). Any indication of pain requires a thorough pain assessment. Fundamentals Review 10-1 outlines factors to include in a pain assessment. Fundamentals Review 10-2 is an example of a pain assessment tool.

A pain measurement scale should be part of the initial assessment and the continued assessment of pain and evaluation of pain control measures. Choosing an appropriate tool for patient assessment is necessary to obtain valid pain ratings. Because pain is subjective, self-report is generally considered the most reliable way to assess pain and should be used whenever possible (Spagrud et al, 2003). Fundamentals Review 10-3 provides examples of several tools for self reporting by adults and children. Infants, young children, and cognitively impaired adults, such as those with dementia, are at high risk for inadequate pain management as they are unable to describe their pain and may be poorly assessed (Merkel et al, 2002). Other tools are available to assess pain in people who cannot self-report discomfort and pain. Fundamentals Review 10-4 shows a tool that can be used to assess discomfort and pain in these patients.

This chapter will cover the skills to assist the nurse in providing for patient comfort, including pain relief. Fundamentals Review 10-5 and 10-6 provide a summary of additional information to assist in understanding the skills related to comfort and pain relief. Refer to a Fundamentals of Nursing textbook for further, in-depth discussions of the physiology, assessment, and treatment of pain.

Fundamentals Review 10-1

General Guidelines for Pain Assessment

Factors to Assess	Questions and Approaches
Characteristics of the pain Location	"Where is your pain? Is it external or internal?" (Asking the patient with acute pain to point to the painful area with one finger may help to localize the pain. Patients with chronic pain may have difficulty trying to localize their pain, however.)
Duration	"How long have you been experiencing pain? How long does a pain episode last? How often does a pain episode occur?"
Quantity	Ask the patient to indicate the degree (amount) of pain currently experienced on the scale below: 0 No pain — 1 — 2 Mild — 3 — 4 Moderate — 5 — 6 — 7 Severe — 8 — 9 — 10 Pain as bad as it can be It is also helpful to ask how much pain the patient has (on the same scale) when the pain is at its least and at its worst: Least__________ Worst__________
Quality	"What words would you use to describe your pain?"
Chronology	"How does the pain develop and progress?" (If pattern can be identified, interventions early in a pain sequence will often be far more effective than those used after the pain is well established.) "Has the pain changed since it first began? If so, how?"
Aggravating factors	"What makes the pain occur or increase in intensity?"
Alleviating factors	"What makes the pain go away or lessen? What methods of relief have you tried in the past? How long were they used? How effective were they?" (Methods of relief currently in effect for hospitalized patients should be apparent from the chart. It is important to verify the use of current orders and their effectiveness with the patient. Outpatients may need to be asked to record a medication profile, a thorough and accurate account of all medications they are taking.)
Associated phenomena	"Are there any other factors that seem to relate consistently to your pain? Any other symptoms that occur just before, during, or after your pain?"
Physiologic responses Vital signs (blood pressure, pulse, respirations) Skin color Perspiration Pupil size Nausea	Signs of sympathetic stimulation commonly occur with acute pain. Signs of parasympathetic stimulation (decreased blood pressure and pulse, rapid and irregular respirations, pupil constriction, nausea and vomiting, and warm, dry skin) may be present, especially in prolonged, severe pain, visceral, or deep pain.
Muscle tension	Observe. Ask the patient whether he or she is aware of any tight, tense muscles.
Anxiety	Are signs of anxiety evident? (May include decreased attention span or ability to follow directions, frequent asking of questions, shifting of topics of conversation, avoidance of discussion of feelings, acting out, somatizing.)

(continued)

Fundamentals Review 10-1

General Guidelines for Pain Assessment *(continued)*

Factors to Assess	Questions and Approaches
Behavioral responses	
Posture, gross motor activities	Does patient rub or support a particular area? Make frequent position changes? Walk, pace, kneel, or assume a rolled-up position? Does patient rest a particular body part? Protect an area from stimulation? Lie quietly? (In acute pain, postural and gross motor activities are often altered; in chronic pain, the only signs of change may be postures characteristic of withdrawal.)
Facial features	Does the patient have a pinched look? Are there facial grimaces? Knotted brow? Overall taut, anxious appearance? (A look of fatigue is more characteristic of chronic pain.)
Verbal expressions	Does the patient sigh, moan, scream, cry, repetitively use the same words?
Affective responses	
Anxiety	"Do you feel anxious? Are you afraid? If so, how bad are these feelings?"
Depression	"Do you feel depressed, down, or low? If so, how bad are these feelings? Are your feelings about yourself mostly good or bad? Do you have feelings of failure? Do you see yourself or your illness as a burden to those you care about?"
Interactions with others	How does the patient act when he or she is in pain in the presence of others? How does the patient respond to others when he or she is not in pain? How do significant others and caregivers respond to the patient when the patient is in pain? When the patient is not in pain?
Degree to which pain interferes with patient's life (use past performance as baseline)	"Does the pain interfere with sleep? If so, to what extent? Is fatigue a major factor in the pain experience? Is the conduct of intimate or peer relationships affected by the pain? Is work function affected? Participation in recreational–diversional activities?" (An activity diary is often helpful—sometimes crucial. One to several weeks of hourly activity recorded by the patient may be necessary. Levels of pain, intake of food, and sleep–rest periods are noted along with activities performed. Separate diaries for inpatient and outpatient episodes may be necessary because hospitalization markedly affects the nature and type of activities performed.)
Perception of pain and meaning to patient	"Are you worried about your illness? Do you see any connection between your pain and the nature or course of illness? If so, how do you see them as related? Do you find any meaning in your pain? If so, is this beneficial or detrimental to you? Are you struggling to find some meaning for your pain?"
Adaptive mechanisms used to cope with pain	"What do you usually do to relieve stress? How well do these things work? What techniques do you use at home to help cope with the pain? How well have they worked? Do you use these in the hospital? If not, why not?"
Outcomes	"What would you like to be doing right now, this week, this month, if the pain were better controlled? How much would the pain have to decrease (on the 0 to 10 scale) for you to begin to accomplish these goals?"

Fundamentals Review 10-2

Pain Assessment Tool

Date ____________

Patient's name ______________________ Age ________ Room ____________

Diagnosis ______________________ Physician ____________

Nurse ____________

1. LOCATION: Patient or nurse marks drawing.

Right Left Right Left Left Right Right Left R L L R Left Right Right Left Left Right

2. INTENSITY: Patient rates the pain. Scale used ____________
Present: ____________
Worst pain gets: ____________
Best pain gets: ____________
Acceptable level of pain: ____________
3. QUALITY: (Use patient's own words, e.g., prick, ache, burn, throb, pull, sharp)
____
4. ONSET, DURATION, VARIATION, RHYTHMS: ____________
5. MANNER OF EXPRESSING PAIN: ____________
6. WHAT RELIEVES THE PAIN? ____________
7. WHAT CAUSES OR INCREASES THE PAIN? ____________
8. EFFECTS OF PAIN: (Note decreased function, decreased quality of life.)
   - Accompanying symptoms (e.g., nausea) ____________
   - Sleep ____________
   - Appetite ____________
   - Physical activity ____________
   - Relationship with others (e.g., irritability) ____________
   - Emotions (e.g., anger, suicidal, crying) ____________
   - Concentration ____________
   - Other ____________
9. OTHER COMMENTS: ____________
10. PLAN: ____________

Self-reporting Pain Assessment Tools

Pain Distress Scales*

Simple Descriptive Pain Distress Scale

No Pain	Mild Pain	Moderate Pain	Severe Pain	Very Severe Pain	Worst Possible Pain

0–10 Numeric Pain Distress Scale

No Pain					Moderate Pain					Worst Possible Pain
0	1	2	3	4	5	6	7	8	9	10

Visual Analog Scale

No pain — Pain as bad as it could possibly be

Wong/Baker Faces Rating Scale for Use with Children†

1. Explain to the child that each face is for a person who feels happy because he or she has no pain (hurt, or whatever word the child uses) or feels sad because he or she has some or a lot of pain.
2. Point to the appropriate face and state, "This face . . .":
   0—"is very happy because he [or she] doesn't hurt at all."
   1—"hurts just a little bit."
   2—"hurts a little more."
   3—"hurts even more."
   4—"hurts a whole lot."
   5—"hurts as much as you can imagine, although you don't have to be crying to feel this bad."
3. Ask the child to choose the face that best describes how he or she feels. Be specific about which pain (eg, "shot" or incision) and what time (eg, Now? Earlier before lunch?)

**From ACHPR, Acute Pain Management Guide Panel, 1992.*

†From Wong, D. L., et al. (2001). Wong's essentials of pediatric nursing (6th ed.). St. Louis, MO: Mosby.

Fundamentals Review 10-4

FLACC Behavioral Scale

This display presents two ways of demonstrating the FLACC Behavioral Scale.

Categories	Scoring 0	1	2
Face	No particular expression or smile	Occasional grimace or frown, withdrawn, uninterested	Frequent to constant frown, clenched jaw, quivering chin
Legs	Normal position or relaxed	Uneasy, restless, tense	Kicking, or legs drawn up
Activity	Lying quietly, normal position, moves easily	Squirming, shifting back and forth, tense	Arched, rigid, or jerking
Cry	No cry (awake or asleep)	Moans or whimpers, occasional complaint	Crying steadily, screams or sobs, frequent complaints
Consolability	Content, relaxed	Reassured by occasional touching, hugging, or being talked to, distractable	Difficult to console or comfort

Each of the five categories (**F**) Face; (**L**) Legs; (**A**) Activity; (**C**) Cry; (**C**) Consolability is scored from 0–2, which results in a score between zero and 10.

Patients who are awake: Observe for at least 2 to 5 minutes. Observe legs and body uncovered. Reposition the patient or observe activity; assess body for tenseness and tone. Initiate consoling interventions if needed.
Patients who are asleep: Observe for at least 5 minutes. Observe body and legs uncovered. If possible, reposition the patient. Touch the body and assess for tenseness and tone.

Face

Score 0 points if patient has a relaxed face, eye contact, and interest in surroundings.
Score 1 point if patient has a worried look to face, with eyebrows lowered, eyes partially closed, cheeks raised, and/or mouth pursed.
Score 2 points if patient has deep furrows in forehead, with closed eyes, open mouth, and deep lines around the nose/lips.

Legs

Score 0 points if patient has usual tone and motion to limbs (legs and arms).
Score 1 point if patient has increased tone; rigidity; and/or tense, intermittent flexion/extension of limbs.
Score 2 points if patient has hypertonicity, legs pulled tight, and/or exaggerated flexion/extension of limbs.

Activity

Score 0 points if patient moves easily and freely, with normal activity/restrictions.
Score 1 point if patient shifts positions, is hesitant to move or is guarding, has tense torso with pressure on body part.
Score 2 points if patient is in fixed position, rocking, has side-to-side head movements, or is rubbing body part.

Cry

Score 0 points if patient has no cry/moan (awake or asleep).
Score 1 point if patient has occasional moans, cries, whimpers, or sighs.
Score 2 points if patient has frequent/continuous moans, cries, or grunts.

(continued)

Fundamentals Review 10-4

FLACC Behavioral Scale *(continued)*

Consolabilty

Score 0 points if patient is calm and does not require consoling.
Score 1 point if patient responds to comfort by touch or talk in 30 seconds to a minute.
Score 2 points if patient requires constant comforting or is unable to be consoled.

Whenever feasible, behavioral measurement of pain should be used in conjunction with self-report. When self-report is not possible, interpretation of pain behaviors and decision making regarding treatment of pain requires careful consideration of the context in which pain behaviors were observed.

Each category is scored on the 0–2 scale, which results in a total score of 0–10.

Assessment of Behavioral Scale

0 = Relaxed and comfortable
1–3 = Mild discomfort
4–6 = Moderate pain
7–10 = Severe discomfort/pain

Fundamentals Review 10-5

Additional Terms Used by Patients to Describe Pain

Quality

Sharp	Pain that is sticking in nature and that is intense.
Dull	Pain that is not as intense or acute as sharp pain, possibly more annoying than painful. It is usually more diffuse than sharp pain.
Diffuse	Pain that covers a large area. Usually, the patient is unable to point to a specific area without moving the hand over a large surface, such as the entire abdomen.
Shifting	Pain that moves from one area to another, such as from the lower abdomen to the area over the stomach.

Other terms used to describe the quality of pain include sore, stinging, pinching, cramping, gnawing, cutting, throbbing, shooting, viselike pressure.

Severity

Severe or excruciating Moderate Slight or mild	These terms depend on the patient's interpretation of pain. Behavioral and physiologic signs help assess the severity of pain. On a scale of 1 to 10, slight pain could be described as being between about 1 and 3; moderate pain, between about 4 and 7; and severe pain, between about 8 and 10.

Periodicity

Continuous	Pain that does not stop.
Intermittent	Pain that stops and starts again.
Brief or transient	Pain that passes quickly.

Common Responses to Pain

Behavioral (Voluntary) Responses

Moving away from painful stimuli
Grimacing, moaning, and crying
Restlessness
Protecting the painful area and refusing to move

Physiologic (Involuntary) Responses

Typical Sympathetic Responses When Pain Is Moderate and Superficial

Increased blood pressure
Increased pulse and respiratory rates
Pupil dilation
Muscle tension and rigidity
Pallor (peripheral vasoconstriction)
Increased adrenaline output
Increased blood glucose

Typical Parasympathetic Responses When Pain Is Severe and Deep

Nausea and vomiting
Fainting or unconsciousness
Decreased blood pressure
Decreased pulse rate
Prostration
Rapid and irregular breathing

Affective (Psychological) Responses

Exaggerated weeping and restlessness
Withdrawal
Stoicism
Anxiety
Depression
Fear
Anger
Anorexia
Fatigue
Hopelessness
Powerlessness

SKILL 10-1 Promoting Patient Comfort

Patient discomfort and pain can be relieved through various pain management therapies. Interventions may include the administration of analgesics, emotional support, comfort measures, and nonpharmacologic interventions. Nonpharmacologic methods of pain management can diminish the emotional components of pain, strengthen coping abilities, give patients a sense of control, contribute to pain relief, decrease fatigue, and promote sleep (McCaffery & Pasero, 1999). The following skill identifies potential interventions related to discomfort and pain. The interventions are listed sequentially for teaching purposes; the order is not sequential and should be adjusted based on patient assessment and nursing judgment. Not every intervention discussed will be appropriate for every patient.

Equipment

- Pain assessment tool and/or scale
- Oral hygiene supplies
- Nonsterile gloves, if necessary

ASSESSMENT

Review the patient's medical record and plan of care for information about the patient's status and contraindications to any of the potential interventions. Inquire about any allergies. Assess the patient's level of discomfort. Assess the patient's pain using an appropriate assessment tool. Assess the characteristics of any pain. Assess for other symptoms that often occur with the pain, such as headache or restlessness. Ask the patient what interventions have and have not been successful in the past to promote comfort and relieve pain. Assess the patient's vital signs. Check the patient's medication administration record for the time an analgesic was last administered. Assess cultural beliefs related to pain. Assess the patient's response to a particular intervention to evaluate effectiveness and presence of adverse effect.

NURSING DIAGNOSIS

Determine the related factors for the nursing diagnoses based on the patient's current status. Nursing diagnoses that may be appropriate include:

- Acute Pain
- Chronic Pain
- Disturbed Sleep Pattern
- Anxiety
- Fatigue
- Ineffective Coping
- Activity Intolerance
- Deficient Knowledge
- Self-Care Deficit

In addition, many other nursing diagnoses may require the use of this skill.

OUTCOME IDENTIFICATION AND PLANNING

The expected outcome to achieve is that the patient experiences relief from discomfort and/or pain without adverse effect. Other outcomes that may be appropriate include: the patient experiences decreased anxiety and improved relaxation; the patient is able to participate in activities of daily living; and the patient verbalizes an understanding of and satisfaction with the pain management plan.

SKILL 10-1 **Promoting Patient Comfort** *(continued)*

IMPLEMENTATION

ACTION	RATIONALE
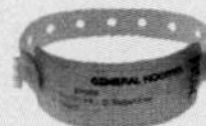 1. Identify the patient. Discuss pain with the patient, acknowledging that the patient's pain exists. Explain how pain medications and other pain management therapies work together to provide pain relief. Allow the patient to help choose interventions for pain relief.	Identifying the patient ensures the right patient receives the intervention and helps prevent errors. Pain discussion and patient involvement strengthen the nurse–patient relationship and promote pain relief (Taylor et al, 2008). Explanation encourages patient understanding and cooperation and reduces apprehension.
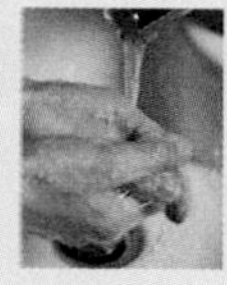 2. Perform hand hygiene. Put on nonsterile gloves, if necessary.	Hand hygiene deters the spread of microorganisms. Gloves are indicated if there is a potential for contact with blood or body fluids.
3. Assess the patient's pain, using an appropriate assessment tool and measurement scale (see Fundamentals Review 10-1 through 10-5).	Accurate assessment is necessary to guide treatment/relief interventions and evaluate the effectiveness of pain control measures.
4. Provide pharmacologic interventions, if indicated and ordered.	Analgesics and adjuvant drugs reduce perception of pain and alter responses to discomfort.
5. Adjust the patient's environment to promote comfort.	The environment can improve or detract from the patient's sense of well-being and can be a source of stimulation that aggravates pain and reduces comfort.
a. Adjust and maintain the room temperature per the patient's preference.	A too warm or too cool environment can be a source of stimulation that aggravates pain and reduces comfort.
b. Reduce harsh lighting, but provide adequate lighting per the patient's preference.	Harsh lighting can be a source of stimulation that aggravates pain and reduces comfort.
c. Reduce harsh and unnecessary noise. Avoid carrying out conversations immediately outside the patient's room.	Noise including talking can be a source of stimuli that aggravate pain and reduce comfort.
d. Close room door and/or curtain whenever possible.	Closing the door or curtain provides privacy and reduces noise and other extraneous stimuli that may aggravate pain and reduce comfort.
e. Provide good ventilation in the patient's room. Reduce unpleasant odors by promptly emptying bedpans, urinals, and emesis basins after use. Remove trash and laundry promptly.	Odors can be a source of stimuli that aggravate pain and reduce comfort.
6. Prevent unnecessary interruptions and coordinate patient activities to group activities together. Allow for and plan rest periods without disturbance.	Frequent interruptions and disturbances for assessment or treatment can be a source of stimuli that aggravate pain and reduce comfort. Fatigue reduces tolerance for pain and can increase the pain experience (Taylor et al, 2008).
7. Assist the patient to change position frequently. Assist the patient to a comfortable position, maintaining good alignment and supporting extremities as needed. Raise the head of the bed as appropriate. (See Chapter 9, Activity, for more information on positioning.)	Positioning in proper alignment with supports ensures that the patient will be able to maintain the desired position and reduces pressure.

(continued)

SKILL 10-1 Promoting Patient Comfort *(continued)*

ACTION	RATIONALE
8. Provide oral hygiene as often as necessary to keep the mouth and mucous membranes clean and moist, as often as every 1 or 2 hours if necessary. This is especially important for patients who cannot drink or are not permitted fluids by mouth. (See Chapter 7, Hygiene, for additional information about mouth care.)	Moisture helps maintain the integrity of mucous membranes. Dry mucous membranes can be a source of stimuli that aggravate pain and reduce comfort.
9. Ensure the availability of appropriate fluids for drinking, unless contraindicated. Make sure the patient's water pitcher is filled and within reach. Make other fluids of the patient's choice available.	Thirst and dry mucous membranes can be sources of stimuli that reduce comfort and aggravate pain.
10. Remove physical situations that may cause discomfort.	
a. Change soiled and/or wet dressings; replace soiled and/or wet bed linens.	Moisture can cause discomfort and irritation to skin.
b. Smooth wrinkles in bed linens.	Wrinkled bed linens apply pressure to skin and can cause discomfort and irritation to skin.
c. Ensure patient is not lying or sitting on tubes, tubing, wires or other equipment.	Tubing and equipment apply pressure to skin and can cause discomfort and irritation to skin.
11. Assist the patient as necessary with ambulation, active range of motion exercises, and/or passive range-of-motion exercises as appropriate (See Chapter 9, Activity, for more information about activity.).	Activity prevents stiffness and loss of mobility which can reduce comfort and aggravate pain.
12. Assess the patient's spirituality needs related to the pain experience. Ask the patient if he/she would like a spiritual counselor to visit.	Some individuals' spiritual beliefs facilitate positive coping with the effects of illness, including pain.
13. Consider the use of distraction. Distraction requires the patient to focus on something other than the pain.	Conscious attention often appears to be necessary to experience pain. Preoccupation with other things has been observed to distract the patient from pain. Distraction is thought to raise the threshold of pain and/or increase pain tolerance (Taylor et al, 2008).
a. Have the patient recall a pleasant experience or focus attention on an enjoyable experience.	
b. Offer age/developmentally appropriate games, toys, books, audiobooks, access to television and/or videos, or other items of interest to the patient.	
c. Encourage the patient to hold or stroke a loved person, pet, or toy.	
d. Offer access to music the patient prefers. Turn on the music when pain begins, or before anticipated painful stimuli. The patient can close his/her eyes and concentrate on listening. Raising or lowering the volume as pain increases or decreases can be helpful.	
14. Consider the use of guided imagery.	Guided imagery helps the patient to gradually become less aware of the discomfort or pain. Positive emotions evoked by the image help reduce the pain experience.
a. Help the patient to identify a scene or experience that the patient describes as happy, pleasant, or peaceful.	
b. Encourage the patient to begin with several minutes of focused breathing, relaxation, or meditation. (Refer to specific information in steps 15 and 16.)	
c. Help the patient concentrate on the peaceful, pleasant image.	

SKILL 10-1 **Promoting Patient Comfort** *(continued)*

ACTION	RATIONALE
d. If indicated, read a description of the identified scene or experience, using a soothing, soft voice.	
e. Encourage the patient to concentrate on the details of the image, such as its sight, sounds, smells, tastes, and touch.	
15. Consider the use of relaxation activities, such as deep breathing.	Relaxation techniques reduce skeletal muscle tension and lessen anxiety, which can reduce comfort and aggravate pain. Relaxation can also be a distraction, providing help in reducing the pain experience (LeMone & Burke, 2004; Schaffer & Yucha, 2004; Taylor et al, 2008).
a. Have the patient sit or recline comfortably and place hands on stomach. Close the eyes.	
b. Ask the patient to mentally count to maintain a comfortable rate and rhythm. Have the patient inhale slowly and deeply while letting the abdomen expand as much as possible. Have the patient hold his/her breath for a few seconds.	
c. Tell the patient to exhale slowly through mouth, blowing through puckered lips. Have the patient continue to count to maintain comfortable rate and rhythm, concentrating on the rise and fall of abdomen.	
d. When the patient's abdomen feels empty, have the patient begin again with a deep inhalation.	
e. Encourage patient to practice at least twice a day, for 10 minutes, and then use as needed to assist with pain management (Schaffer & Yucha, 2004).	
16. Consider the use of relaxation activities, such as progressive muscle relaxation.	Relaxation techniques reduce skeletal muscle tension and lessen anxiety, which can reduce comfort and aggravate pain. Relaxation can also be a distraction, providing help in reducing the pain experience (LeMone & Burke, 2004; Schaffer & Yucha, 2004; Taylor et al, 2008).
a. Assist the patient to a comfortable position.	
b. Direct the patient to focus on a particular muscle group. Start with the muscles of the jaw, then repeat with the neck muscles, shoulder muscles, upper and lower arm, hand, abdominal, buttocks, thigh, lower leg, and foot muscles.	
c. Ask the patient to tighten the muscle group and note the sensation that the tightened muscles produce. After 5 to 7 seconds, tell the patient to relax the muscles all at once and concentrate on the sensation of the relaxed state, noting the difference in feeling in the muscles when contracted and relaxed.	
d. Have the patient continue to tighten–hold–relax each muscle group until entire body has been covered.	
e. Encourage patient to practice at least twice a day, for 10 minutes, and then use as needed to assist with pain management (Schaffer & Yucha, 2004).	

(continued)

SKILL 10-1 Promoting Patient Comfort *(continued)*

ACTION	RATIONALE
17. Consider the use of cutaneous stimulation, such as the intermittent application of heat or cold, or both. (See Chapter 8, Skin Integrity and Wound Care, for additional information on heat and cold therapy.)	Heat helps relieve pain by stimulating specific nerve fibers, closing the gate that allows the transmission of pain stimuli to centers in the brain. Heat accelerates the inflammatory response to promote healing, and reduces muscle tension to promote relaxation and to help to relieve muscle spasms and joint stiffness. Cold reduces blood flow to tissues and decreases the local release of pain-producing substances such as histamine, serotonin, and bradykinin, and reduces the formation of edema and inflammation. Cold reduces muscle spasm, alters tissue sensitivity (producing numbness), and promotes comfort by slowing the transmission of pain stimuli (Taylor et al, 2008).
18. Consider the use of cutaneous stimulation, such as massage. (See Skill 10-2.)	Cutaneous stimulation techniques stimulate the skin's surface, closing the gating mechanism in the spinal cord, decreasing the number of pain impulses that reach the brain for perception.
19. Discuss the potential for use of cutaneous stimulation such as TENS with the patient and primary care provider. (See Skill 10-3.)	Cutaneous stimulation techniques stimulate the skin's surface, closing the gating mechanism in the spinal cord, decreasing the number of pain impulses that reach the brain for perception.
20. Remove gloves, if worn, and perform hand hygiene.	Hand hygiene prevents transmission of microorganisms.
21. Evaluate the patient's response to interventions. Reassess level of discomfort or pain using original assessment tools. Reassess and alter plan of care as appropriate.	Evaluation allows for individualization of plan of care and promotes optimal patient comfort.

EVALUATION

The expected outcome is met when the patient experiences relief from discomfort and or pain without adverse effect; the patient experiences decreased anxiety and improved relaxation; the patient is able to participate in activities of daily living; and the patient verbalizes an understanding of and satisfaction with the pain management plan.

DOCUMENTATION

Guidelines

Document pain assessment and other significant assessments. Document pain relief therapies used and patient responses. Record alternative treatments to consider, if appropriate.

Sample Documentation

5/12/08 2030 Patient reports increased pain in lower extremities, rating the pain at 5/10, and described as burning and constant, consistent with previous pain. Medicated with oxycodone 5mg po as ordered for breakthrough pain. Patient using relaxation and deep-breathing techniques, as well as listening to music. Reviewed instructions for use of relaxation and deep breathing; patient verbalized understanding.—R. Curry, RN

5/12/08 2145 Patient reports pain reduced to 2/10. OOB to solarium with family. —R. Curry, RN

SKILL 10-1 Promoting Patient Comfort *(continued)*

Unexpected Situations and Associated Interventions

- *Patient reports or assessment reveals ineffective/or lack of pain relief:* Reassess pain and evaluate response to implemented therapies. Implement additional or alternate interventions until desired level of comfort is achieved.
- *Intervention increases patient discomfort or pain:* Immediately stop intervention. Document intervention used and the effect. Communicate changes in the patient's condition to the primary care provider, as appropriate. Revise plan of care, noting adverse effect of intervention, so other caregivers avoid using same intervention.

Special Considerations

General Considerations

- The use of alternate and adjunct therapies is often a 'try and see process.' Many interventions may be tried to achieve the best combination for a particular patient. Individuals respond to pain differently; what works for one person may not help another.

Infant and Child Considerations

- Assessment, measurement, and treatment of discomfort and pain in infants and children frequently involve the use of more than one technique. Communication with parents, guardians, or other significant others is vital for accurate pediatric pain assessment and management.
- Nonpharmacologic therapies can be very beneficial in decreasing the pain experience for these patients, including acute and chronic pain, as well as pain related to procedures (Hockenberry, 2005; Tanabe et al, 2002; Taylor et al, 2008).

Older Adult Considerations

- Older patients may report that their pain level is tolerable and that it only hurts when they move. These patients are at risk for developing conditions related to immobility. Effective pain relief should be provided to allow movement and participation in activities of daily living. The nursing plan of care should also include interventions related to 'Risk for Impaired Skin Integrity' (Tabloski, 2006).
- Older adults often view pain as a natural component of the aging process. They may not complain of pain due to fear of potential treatment or because they have accepted the pain as a part of their life; again, a part of the aging process (Taylor et al, 2008). Nurses need to be vigilant in performing pain assessment and forming a plan of care for these patients. Effective pain management will allow the patient to maintain dignity, functional capacity, and quality of life (American Geriatrics Society, 2002).

SKILL 10-2 Giving a Back Massage

Massage has many benefits, including general relaxation and increased circulation. Massage can help alleviate pain and can help reduce the amount of medication required to relieve pain (Roberson, 2003). A back massage can be incorporated into the patient's bath, as part of care before bedtime, or any time to promote increased patient comfort. Some nurses do not always give back massages to patients because they don't think they have enough time. However, giving a back massage provides an opportunity for the nurse to observe the skin for signs of breakdown. It improves circulation; decreases pain, symptom distress, and anxiety; improves sleep quality; and also provides a means of communicating with the patient through the use of touch. A back massage also provides cutaneous stimulation as a method of pain relief.

(continued)

SKILL 10-2 Giving a Back Massage *(continued)*

Because some patients consider the back massage a luxury and may be reluctant to accept it, communicate its importance and value to the patient. An effective back massage should take 4 to 6 minutes to complete. A lotion is usually used; warm it before applying to the back. Be aware of the patient's medical diagnosis when considering giving a back massage. A back massage is contraindicated, for example, when the patient has had back surgery or has fractured ribs. Position the patient on the abdomen or, if this is contraindicated, on the side for a back massage.

Equipment

- Massage lubricant or lotion
- Powder, if not contraindicated
- Bath blanket
- Towel
- Nonsterile gloves, if contact with blood or body fluids is likely

ASSESSMENT

Review the patient's medical record and plan of care for information about the patient's status and contraindications to back massage. Question the patient about any conditions that might require modifications or that might contraindicate a massage. Inquire about any allergies, such as to lotions or scents. Ask if the patient has any preferences for lotion or has his or her own lotion. Assess the patient's level of pain. Check the patient's medication administration record for the time an analgesic was last administered. If appropriate, administer an analgesic early enough so that it has time to take effect.

NURSING DIAGNOSIS

Determine the related factors for the nursing diagnoses based on the patient's current status. Appropriate nursing diagnoses may include:

- Acute Pain
- Chronic Pain
- Disturbed Sleep Pattern
- Risk for Impaired Skin Integrity
- Anxiety
- Activity Intolerance
- Deficient Knowledge

In addition, many other nursing diagnoses may require the use of this skill.

OUTCOME IDENTIFICATION AND PLANNING

The expected outcomes to achieve are that the patient reports increased comfort and/or decreased pain. and that the patient is relaxed. Other outcomes that may be appropriate include: the patient displays decreased anxiety and improved relaxation; skin breakdown is absent; and the patient understands the reasons for back massage.

IMPLEMENTATION

ACTION	RATIONALE
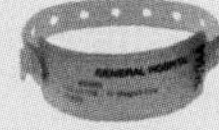 1. Identify the patient. Offer a back massage to the patient and explain the procedure.	Identifying the patient ensures the right patient receives the intervention and helps prevent errors. Explanation encourages patient understanding and cooperation and reduces apprehension.
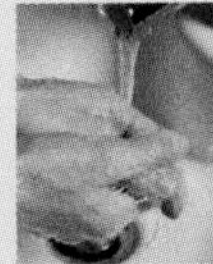 2. Perform hand hygiene and put on nonsterile gloves, if indicated.	Hand hygiene deters the spread of microorganisms. Gloves are not usually necessary. Gloves prevent contact with blood and body fluid.

SKILL 10-2 Giving a Back Massage *(continued)*

ACTION	RATIONALE
3. Close room door and/or curtain.	Closing the door or curtain provides privacy, promotes relaxation, and reduces noise and stimuli that may aggravate pain and reduce comfort.
4. Assess the patient's pain, using an appropriate assessment tool and measurement scale. (See Fundamentals Review 10-1 through 10-5.)	Accurate assessment is necessary to guide treatment/relief interventions and to evaluate the effectiveness of pain control measures.
5. Raise the bed to a comfortable working height and lower the side rail nearest you.	Proper bed height helps reduce back strain while performing the procedure.
6. Assist the patient to a comfortable position, preferably the prone or side-lying position. Remove the covers and move the patient's gown just enough to expose the patient's back from the shoulders to sacral area. Drape the patient as needed with the bath blanket.	This position exposes an adequate area for massage. Draping the patient provides privacy and warmth.
7. **Warm the lubricant or lotion in the palm of your hand, or place the container in small basin of warm water.**	Cold lotion causes chilling and discomfort.
8. Using light gliding strokes (*effleurage*), apply lotion to patient's shoulders, back, and sacral area (Figure 1).	Effleurage relaxes the patient and lessens tension.
9. Place your hands beside each other at the base of the patient's spine and stroke upward to the shoulders and back downward to the buttocks in slow, continuous strokes (Figure 2). Continue for several minutes.	Continuous contact is soothing and stimulates circulation and muscle relaxation.

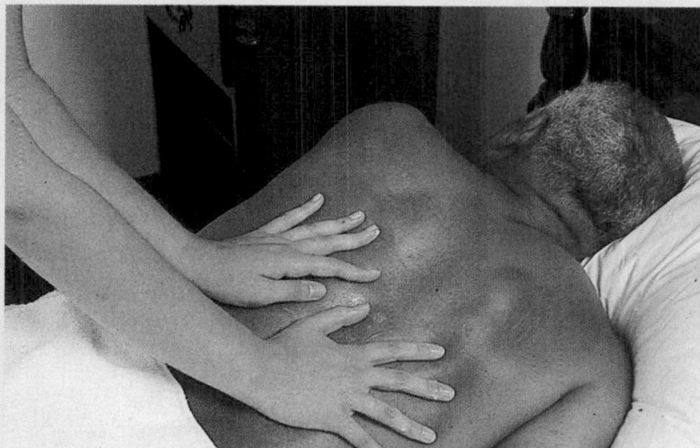

Figure 1. Using effleurage on a patient's back.

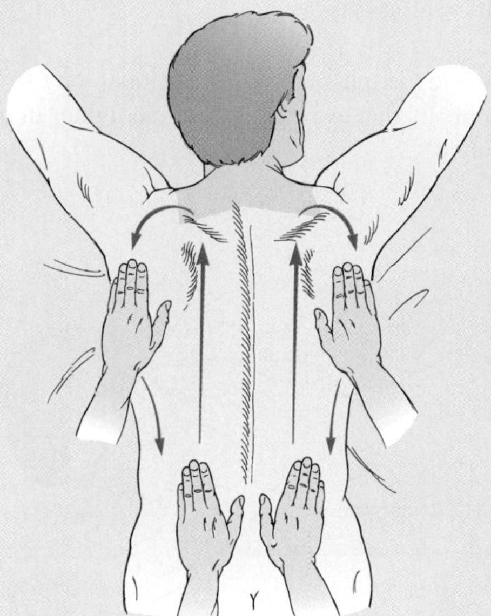

Figure 2. Stroking upward to the shoulders.

(continued)

SKILL 10-2 Giving a Back Massage *(continued)*

ACTION

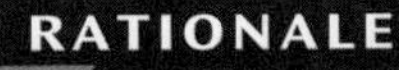

10. Massage the patient's shoulder, entire back, areas over iliac crests, and sacrum with circular stroking motions. **Keep your hands in contact with the patient's skin.** Continue for several minutes, applying additional lotion as necessary.

    A firm stroke with continuous contact promotes relaxation.

11. Knead the patient's skin by gently alternating grasping and compression motions (*pétrissage*) (Figure 3).

    Kneading increases blood circulation.

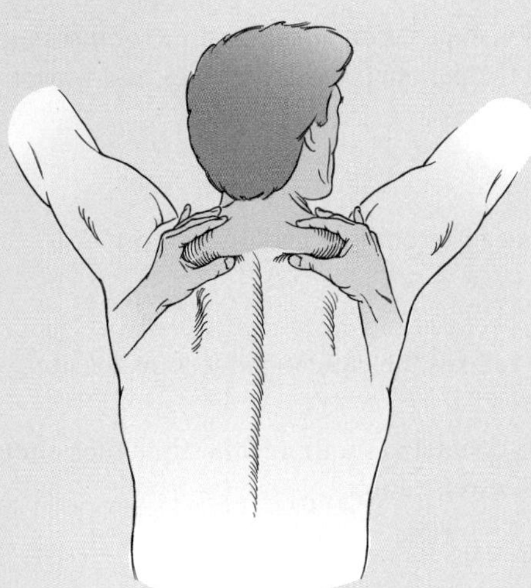

Figure 3. Using pétrissage.

12. Complete the massage with additional long stroking movements that eventually become lighter in pressure (Figure 4).

    Long stroking motions are soothing and promote relaxation; continued stroking with gradual lightening of pressure helps extend the feeling of relaxation.

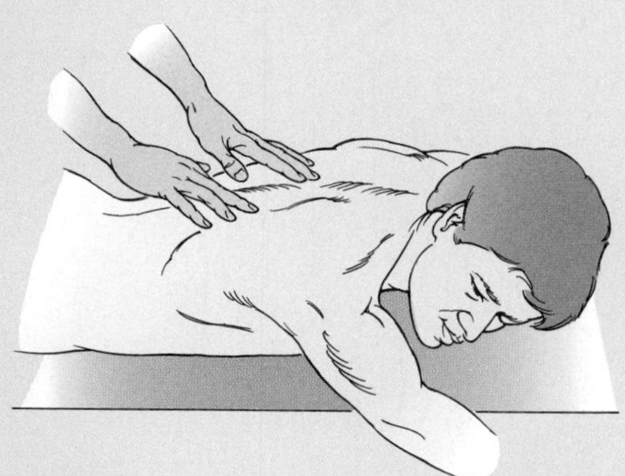

Figure 4. Using light strokes with lessening pressure.

13. During massage, observe the patient's skin for reddened or open areas. **Pay particular attention to the skin over bony prominences.**

    Pressure may interfere with circulation and lead to pressure ulcers.

SKILL 10-2 Giving a Back Massage *(continued)*

ACTION	RATIONALE
14. Use the towel to pat the patient dry and to remove excess lotion. Apply powder if the patient requests it.	Drying provides comfort and reduces the feeling of moisture on the back.
15. Reposition patient gown and covers. Raise side rail and lower bed. Assist patient to a position of comfort.	Repositioning bedclothes, linens, and the patient helps to promotes patient comfort and safety.
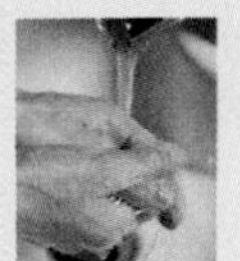 16. Remove gloves, if worn, and perform hand hygiene.	Hand hygiene deters the spread of microorganisms.
17. Evaluate the patient's response to interventions. Reassess level of discomfort or pain using original assessment tools. Reassess and alter plan of care as appropriate.	Reassessment allows for individualization of plan of care and promotes optimal patient comfort.

EVALUATION

The expected outcome is achieved when the patient reports increased comfort and/or decreased pain; the patient displays decreased anxiety and improved relaxation; skin breakdown is absent; and the patient verbalizes an understanding of the reasons for back massage.

DOCUMENTATION

Guidelines

Document pain assessment and other significant assessments. Document the use of and length of time of massage. and patient response. Record alternative treatments to consider, if appropriate.

Sample Documentation

12/6/08 2330 Patient reports inability to sleep and increased pain at surgical site, rated 3/10. Medicated with propoxyphene 100 mg and acetaminophen 650 mg as ordered. Back massage administered × 10 minutes. Patient reports increased comfort and relaxation; "I feel like I could sleep now."—B. Black, RN
12/6/08 2400 Patient reports pain level 0/10.—B. Black, RN

Unexpected Situations and Associated Interventions

- *Your patient cannot lie prone, so you are giving him a back massage while he is lying on his side. However, as you begin to massage the back, the patient cannot maintain the side-lying position:* If possible, have the patient hold on to the side rail on the side to which he is facing. If this is not possible or the patient cannot assist, use pillows and bath blankets to prevent the patient from rolling. If necessary, enlist the help of another person to maintain the patient's position. If possible, experiment with other positions based on the patient's condition and comfort, such as leaning forward against a pillow on the bedside table while sitting in a chair.
- *While massaging the patient's back, you notice a 2″ reddened area on the patient's sacrum:* Note this observation in the patient's medical record and report it to the physician. Do not massage the area. When the back massage is completed, position the patient off the sacral area, using pillows to maintain the patient's position, and institute a turning schedule.

(continued)

SKILL 10-2 Giving a Back Massage *(continued)*

Special Considerations

General Considerations

- Before giving a back massage, assess the patient's body structure and skin condition, and tailor the duration and intensity of the massage accordingly. If you are giving a back massage at bedtime, have the patient ready for bed beforehand so the massage can help him or her fall asleep.
- Use a separate bottle of lotion for each patient to prevent cross-contamination. If the patient has oily skin, substitute a talcum powder or lotion of the patient's choice. However, to avoid aspiration, do not use powder if the patient has an endotracheal or tracheal tube in place. Avoid using powder and lotion together because this may lead to skin maceration.
- When massaging the patient's back, stand with one foot slightly forward and your knees slightly bent to allow effective use of your arm and shoulder muscles.

Infant and Child Considerations

- Hold infants and small children in a comfortable, well-supported position, such as against the chest or across the lap.

Older Adult Considerations

- Be gentle with massage. The skin on the elderly is often fragile and dry.

SKILL 10-3 Applying a TENS Unit

Transcutaneous electrical nerve stimulation (TENS) is a noninvasive technique for providing pain relief that involves the electrical stimulation of large-diameter fibers to inhibit the transmission of painful impulses carried over small-diameter fibers. The TENS unit consists of a battery-powered portable unit, lead wires, and cutaneous electrode pads that are applied to the painful area (Figure 1). It is most beneficial when used to treat pain that is localized, and requires an order from the primary healthcare provider. The TENS unit may be applied intermittently throughout the day or worn for extended periods of time.

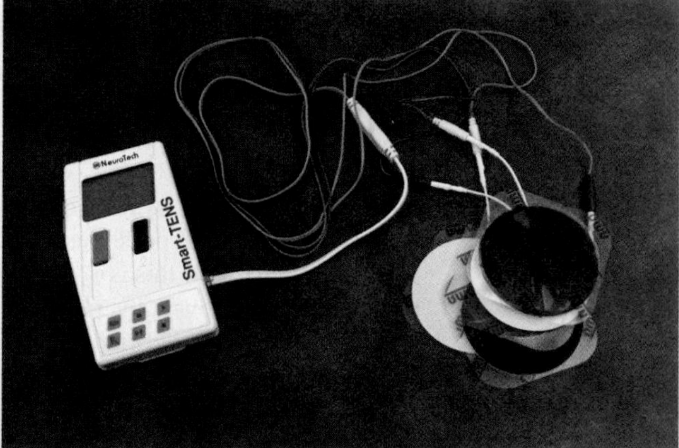

Figure 1. TENS unit.

Equipment

- TENS unit
- Electrodes
- Electrode gel (if electrodes are not pregelled)
- Tape (if electrodes are not self-adhesive)
- Skin cleanser and water
- Towel and washcloth

SKILL 10-3

Applying a TENS Unit *(continued)*

ASSESSMENT

Review the patient's medical record and plan of care for specific instructions related to TENS therapy, including the order and conditions indicating the need for therapy. Review the patient's history for conditions that might contraindicate therapy such as pacemaker insertion, cardiac monitoring, or electrocardiography. Determine the location of electrode placement in consultation with the ordering practitioner and on the patient's report of pain. Assess the patient's understanding of TENS therapy and the rationale for its use.

Inspect the skin of the area designated for electrode placement for irritation, redness, or breakdown. Assess the patient's pain and level of discomfort using an appropriate assessment tool. Assess the characteristics of any pain. Assess for other symptoms that often occur with the pain, such as headache or restlessness. Ask the patient what interventions have and have not been successful in the past to promote comfort and relieve pain. Assess the patient's vital signs. Check the patient's medication administration record for the time an analgesic was last administered. Assess the patient's response to a particular intervention to evaluate effectiveness and presence of adverse effect.

Check the unit to ensure proper functioning and review the manufacturer's instructions for use.

NURSING DIAGNOSIS

Determine the related factors for the nursing diagnoses based on the patient's current status. Appropriate nursing diagnoses may include:

- Acute Pain
- Chronic Pain
- Anxiety
- Ineffective Coping
- Deficient Knowledge
- Risk for Injury
- Risk for Impaired Skin Integrity

Many other nursing diagnoses may require the use of this skill.

OUTCOME IDENTIFICATION AND PLANNING

The expected outcome to achieve is that the patient verbalizes decreased discomfort and pain, without experiencing any injury or skin irritation or breakdown. Other appropriate outcomes may include: patient displays decreased anxiety, improved coping skills, and an understanding of the therapy and the reason for its use.

IMPLEMENTATION

ACTION	RATIONALE
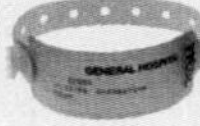 1. Identify the patient, show the patient the device, and explain the function of the device and the reason for its use.	Identifying the patient ensures the right patient receives the intervention and helps prevent errors. Explanation encourages patient understanding and cooperation and reduces apprehension.
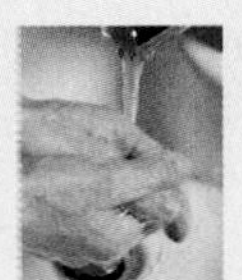 2. Perform hand hygiene.	Hand hygiene deters the spread of microorganisms.
3. Assess the patient's pain, using an appropriate assessment tool and measurement scale. (See Fundamentals Review 10-1 through 10-5.)	Accurate assessment is necessary to guide treatment/relief interventions and evaluate the effectiveness of pain control measures.

(continued)

SKILL 10-3 Applying a TENS Unit *(continued)*

ACTION	RATIONALE
4. Inspect the area where the electrodes are to be placed. Clean the patient's skin, using skin cleanser and water. Dry the area thoroughly.	Inspection ensures that the electrodes will be applied to intact skin. Cleaning and drying help ensure that electrodes will adhere.
5. Remove the adhesive backing from the electrodes and apply them to the specified location (Figure 2). **If the electrodes are not pregelled, apply a small amount of electrode gel to the bottom of each electrode.** If the electrodes are not self-adhering, tape them in place.	Application to the proper location enhances the success of the therapy. Gel is necessary to promote conduction of the electrical current.
6. **Check the placement of the electrodes; leave at least a 2″ (5 cm) space (about the width of one electrode) between them.**	Proper spacing is necessary to reduce the risk of burns due to the proximity of the electrodes.
7. **Check the controls on the TENS unit to make sure that they are off.** Connect the wires to the electrodes (if not already attached) and plug them into the unit.	This connection completes the electrical circuit necessary to stimulate the nerve fibers.
8. Turn on the unit and adjust the intensity setting to the lowest intensity and determine if the patient can feel a tingling, burning, or buzzing sensation (Figure 3). Then adjust the intensity to the prescribed amount or the setting most comfortable for the patient. Secure the unit to the patient.	Using the lowest setting at first introduces the patient to the sensations. Adjusting the intensity is necessary to provide the proper amount of stimulation.

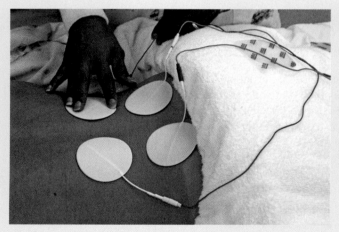

Figure 2. Applying the TENS electrodes.

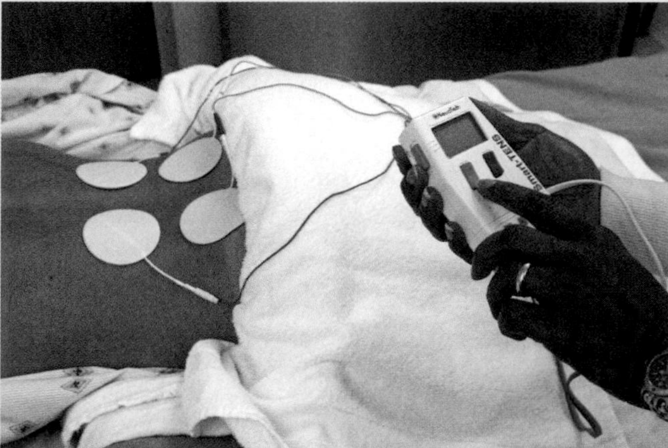

Figure 3. Turning on the unit.

ACTION	RATIONALE
9. Set the pulse width (duration of the each pulsation) as indicated or recommended.	The pulse width determines the depth and width of the stimulation.
10. Assess the patient's pain level during therapy.	Pain assessment helps evaluate the effectiveness of therapy.
a. If intermittent use is ordered, turn the unit off after the specified duration of treatment and remove the electrodes. Provide skin care to the area.	TENS therapy can be ordered for intermittent or continuous use. Skin care reduces the risk for irritation and breakdown.
b. If continuous therapy is ordered, periodically remove the electrodes from the skin (after turning the unit off) to inspect the area and clean the skin, according to facility policy. Reapply electrodes and continue therapy. Change electrodes according to manufacturer's directions.	Periodic removal of electrodes allows for skin assessment. Skin care reduces the risk for irritation and breakdown. Reapplication ensures continued therapy.

SKILL 10-3 **Applying a TENS Unit** *(continued)*

ACTION	RATIONALE
11. When therapy is discontinued, turn the unit off and remove the electrodes. Clean the patient's skin. Clean the unit and replace the batteries.	Turning the unit off and removing electrodes when therapy is discontinued reduces the risk of injury to the patient. Cleaning the unit and replacing the batteries ensures that the unit is ready for future use.
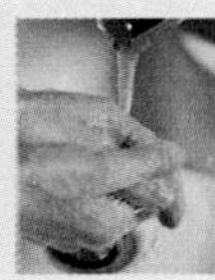 12. Perform hand hygiene.	Hand hygiene helps prevent the transmission of microorganisms.

EVALUATION

The expected outcome is achieved when the patient verbalizes pain relief. In addition, the patient remains free of signs and symptoms of skin irritation and breakdown and injury. The patient reports decreased anxiety and increased ability to cope with pain. The patient verbalizes information related to the functioning of the unit and reasons for its use.

DOCUMENTATION

Guidelines

Document the date and time of application; patient's initial pain assessment; electrode placement location; intensity and pulse width; duration of therapy; pain assessments during therapy and patient's response; and time of removal or discontinuation of therapy.

Sample Documentation

5/28/09 1105 Patient complaining of severe lower back pain, rating it as 9 out of 10 on pain rating scale. Identified lower sacral area as site of pain. TENS therapy ordered for 30 to 45 minutes. Electrodes applied to right and left sides of sacral area. Intensity initially set at 80 pulses per second with pulse width of 80 microseconds. Pain rating at 7 out of 10 after 15 minutes of therapy. Intensity increased to 100 pulses per second, with a pulse width increased to 100 microseconds. Pain rating at 5 out of 10 after 15 minutes at increased settings. Therapy continued for an additional 15 minutes and discontinued. Patient rated pain at 3 out of 10 at end of session. Skin on lower sacral area clean, dry, and intact without evidence of irritation or breakdown. Patient instructed to report increasing pain.—K. Lewin, RN

Unexpected Situations and Associated Interventions

- *While receiving TENS therapy, the patient reports pain and intolerable paresthesia:* Check the settings, connections, and placement of the electrodes. Adjust the settings and reposition the electrodes as necessary.
- *During a TENS therapy session, the patient reports muscle twitching:* Assess the patient and check the intensity setting. Readjust the intensity to a lower setting, because the patient is most likely experiencing overstimulation.
- *While assessing the skin where the electrodes are placed for a patient receiving continuous TENS therapy, you notice some irritation and redness:* Clean and dry the area thoroughly. Reposition the electrodes in the same area, but avoid the irritated and reddened area.

(continued)

SKILL 10-3 Applying a TENS Unit *(continued)*

Special Considerations

General Considerations

- Never place electrodes over the carotid sinus nerves or over laryngeal or pharyngeal muscles, over the eyes, or over the uterus of a pregnant woman.
- Do not use TENS when the etiology of the pain is unknown because it may mask a new pathology.
- Whenever electrodes are being repositioned or removed, turn the unit off first.
- For acute pain, use a recommended pulse width of 60 to 100 microseconds; for chronic or intense pain, a pulse width of 220 to 250 microseconds may be needed.
- Keep in mind that a conventional intensity setting ranges from 80 to 125 pulses per second.

SKILL 10-4 Caring for a Patient Receiving PCA Pump Therapy

Patient-controlled analgesia (PCA) allows patients to control the administration of their own medication within predetermined safety limits. This approach can be used with oral analgesic agents as well as with infusions of opioid analgesic agents by intravenous, subcutaneous, epidural, and perineural routes (Pasero, 2004; Smeltzer, Bare, et al., 2008). PCA provides effective individualized analgesia and comfort. This drug delivery system may be used to manage acute and chronic pain in a healthcare facility or the home.

The PCA pump permits the patient to self-administer continuous infusions of medication (basal rates) safely and to administer extra medication (bolus doses) with episodes of increased pain or painful activities. A PCA pump is electronically controlled by a timing device. The PCA system consists of a portable infusion pump containing a reservoir or chamber for a syringe that is prefilled with the prescribed medication, usually an opioid, or dilute anesthetic solutions in the case of epidural administration (Roman & Cabaj, 2005; Smeltzer, Bare, et al., 2008). When pain occurs, the patient pushes a button that activates the PCA device to deliver a small preset bolus dose of the analgesic. A lockout interval that is programmed into the PCA unit (usually 5–10 minutes) prevents reactivation of the pump and administration of another dose during that period of time. The pump mechanism can also be programmed to deliver only a specified amount of analgesic within a given time interval (basal rate; most commonly every hour or, occasionally, every 4 hours). These safeguards limit the risk for overmedication and allow the patient to evaluate the effect of the previous dose. PCA pumps also have a locked safety system that prohibits tampering with the device.

Nursing responsibilities for patients receiving medications via a PCA pump include patient/family teaching, initial setup of the device, monitoring the device to ensure proper functioning, and frequent assessment of the patient's response, including pain/discomfort control and presence of adverse effects. Additional information related to epidural infusions is discussed in Skill 10-5.

Equipment

- PCA system
- Syringe filled with medication
- PCA system tubing
- Antimicrobial swabs
- Appropriate label for syringe and tubing, based on facility policy and procedure
- Second nurse to verify medication and programmed pump information, if necessary, according to facility policy
- Nonsterile gloves, if appropriate

SKILL 10-4

Caring for a Patient Receiving PCA Pump Therapy *(continued)*

ASSESSMENT

Review the patient's medical record and plan of care for specific instructions related to PCA therapy, including the primary care provider's orders and conditions indicating the need for therapy. Check the medical order for the prescribed drug, initial loading dose, dose for self-administration, and lockout interval. Check to ensure proper functioning of the unit. Assess the patient's level of consciousness and understanding of PCA therapy and the rationale for its use.

Review the patient's history for conditions that might contraindicate therapy, such as respiratory limitations, history of substance abuse, or psychiatric disorder. Review the patient's medical record and assess for factors contributing to an increased risk for respiratory depression, such as the use of a basal infusion, the patient's age, obesity, upper abdominal surgery, sleep apnea, concurrent CNS depressants, and impaired organ functioning (Hagle et al, 2004). Determine the prescribed route for administration. Inspect the site to be used for the infusion for signs of infiltration or infection. If the route is via an intravenous infusion, ensure that the line is patent and the current solution is compatible with the drug ordered.

Assess the patient's pain and level of discomfort using an appropriate assessment tool. Assess the characteristics of any pain, and for other symptoms that often occur with the pain, such as headache or restlessness. Ask the patient what interventions have and have not been successful in the past to promote comfort and relieve pain. Assess the patient's vital signs. Assess the patient's respiratory status, including rate, depth, and rhythm, and oxygen saturation level using pulse oximetry. Also, assess the patient's sedation score (Table 10-1). Determine the patient's response to the intervention to evaluate effectiveness and for the presence of adverse effects.

TABLE 10-1 **Sedation Assessment Scale**

PATIENT ASSESSMENT CHARACTERISTICS	SEDATION SCORE
Sleeping, easy to arouse	S
Awake and alert	1
Slightly drowsy, easily aroused	2
Frequently drowsy, arousable, drifts off during conversation	3
Somnolent, minimal or no response to physical stimulation	4

(Used with permission. From Pasero, C., & McCaffery, M. [2005a]. Authorized and unauthorized use of PCA pumps. Clarifying the use of patient-controlled analgesia, in light of recent alerts. *American Journal of Nursing, 105*(7), 30–32. Copyright 1994, Chris Pasero.)

NURSING DIAGNOSIS

Determine the related factors for the nursing diagnoses based on the patient's current status. Appropriate nursing diagnoses may include:

- Acute Pain
- Chronic Pain
- Anxiety
- Fear
- Ineffective Coping
- Deficient Knowledge
- Risk for Injury

Many other nursing diagnoses may require the use of this skill.

OUTCOME IDENTIFICATION AND PLANNING

The expected outcome to achieve is that the patient reports increased comfort and/or decreased pain, without adverse effects, oversedation, and respiratory depression. Other appropriate outcomes may include: the patient displays decreased anxiety, improved coping skills, and an understanding of the therapy and the reason for its use.

(continued)

SKILL 10-4 Caring for a Patient Receiving PCA Pump Therapy *(continued)*

IMPLEMENTATION

ACTION	RATIONALE
1. Gather equipment. Check the medication order against the original physician's order according to agency policy. Clarify any inconsistencies. Check the patient's chart for allergies.	This comparison helps to identify errors that may have occurred when orders were transcribed. The physician's order is the legal record-of-medication orders for each agency.
2. Know the actions, special nursing considerations, safe dose ranges, purpose of administration, and adverse effects of the medications to be administered. Consider the appropriateness of the medication for this patient.	This knowledge aids the nurse in evaluating the therapeutic effect of the medication in relation to the patient's disorder and can also be used to educate the patient about the medication.
3. Prepare the medication syringe for administration. (See Chapter 5, Medications, for additional information.)	Proper preparation and administration procedure prevents errors.
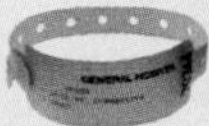 4. Identify the patient, show the patient the device, and explain the function of the device and reason for use. Explain the purpose and action of the medication to the patient.	Identifying the patient ensures the right patient receives the intervention and helps prevent errors. Explanation encourages patient understanding and cooperation and reduces apprehension.
5. Plug the PCA device into the electrical outlet, if necessary. Check status of battery power, if appropriate.	The PCA device requires a power source (electricity or battery) to run. Most units will alarm to acknowledge a low battery state.
6. Close the door to the room or pull the bedside curtain.	Provides patient privacy.
7. Complete necessary assessments before administering medication. Check allergy bracelet or ask patient about allergies. Assess the patient's pain, using an appropriate assessment tool and measurement scale. (See Fundamentals Review 10-1 through 10-5.)	Assessment is a prerequisite to administration of medications. Accurate assessment is necessary to guide treatment/relief interventions and evaluate the effectiveness of pain control measures.
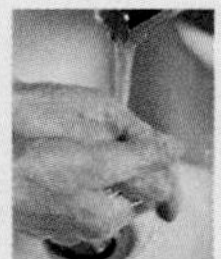 8. Perform hand hygiene and put on gloves, if indicated.	Hand hygiene deters the spread of microorganisms. Gloves are indicated if there is potential contact with blood or body fluids.
9. **Check the label on the prefilled drug syringe with the medication record and patient identification.** Obtain verification of information from second nurse, according to facility policy.	This action verifies that the correct drug and dosage will be administered to the correct patient. Confirmation of information by second nurse helps prevent errors.
10. If using a barcode administration system, scan the patient's barcode on the identification band, if required.	This provides additional check to ensure that the medication is given to the right patient.

SKILL 10-4

Caring for a Patient Receiving PCA Pump Therapy *(continued)*

ACTION	RATIONALE
11. Connect tubing to prefilled syringe (Figure 1) and place the syringe into the PCA device (Figure 2). **Prime the tubing (Figure 3).**	Doing so prepares the device to deliver the drug. Priming the tubing purges air from the tubing and reduces the risk for air embolism.

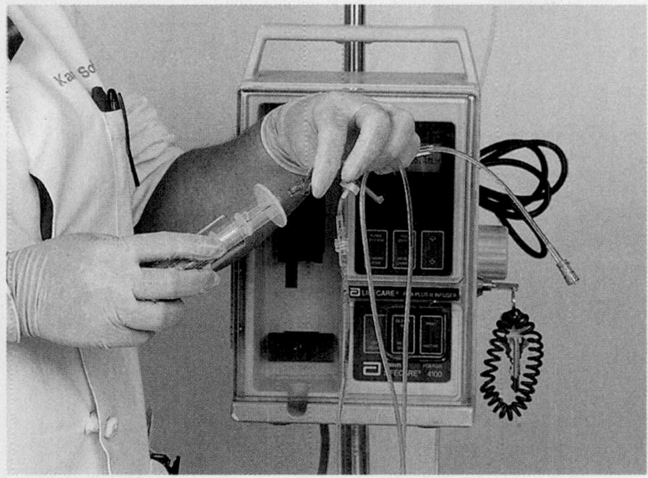

Figure 1. Connecting the tubing to the prefilled syringe. (Photo © B. Proud.)

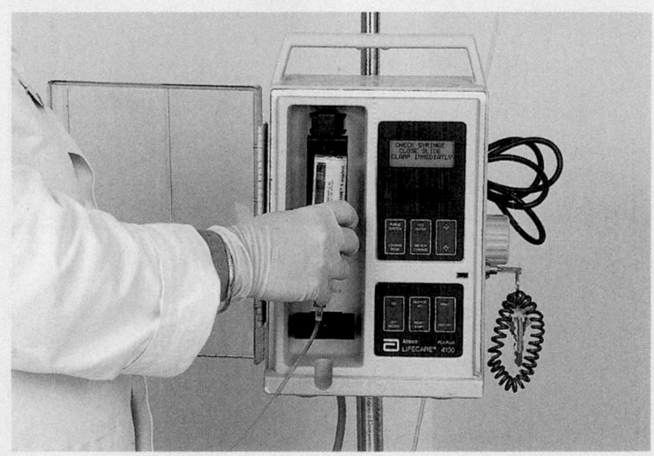

Figure 2. Loading the syringe into the PCA device. (Photo © B. Proud.)

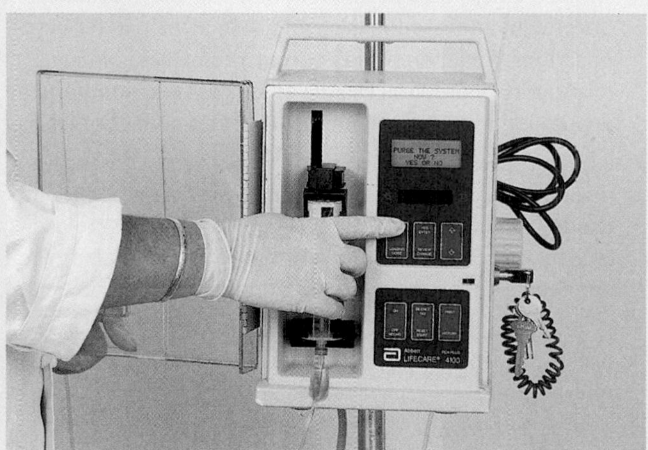

Figure 3. Priming the tubing. (Photo © B. Proud.)

ACTION	RATIONALE
12. Set the PCA device to administer the loading dose, if ordered, and then program the device based on the medical order for infusion dosage and lockout interval. Obtain verification of information from second nurse, according to facility policy.	These actions ensure that the appropriate drug dosage will be administered. Confirmation of information by second nurse helps prevent errors.
13. Using antimicrobial swab, clean connection port on intravenous infusion line or other site access, based on route of administration. Connect the PCA tubing to the patient's intravenous infusion line or appropriate access site, based on the specific site used. Secure the site per facility policy and procedure. Initiate the therapy by activating the appropriate button on the pump.	Cleaning the connection port reduces the risk of infection. Connection and initiation is necessary to allow drug delivery to the patient.

(continued)

SKILL 10-4 Caring for a Patient Receiving PCA Pump Therapy *(continued)*

ACTION | **RATIONALE**

14. Instruct the patient to press the button each time he or she needs relief from pain (Figure 4).

Instruction promotes correct use of the device.

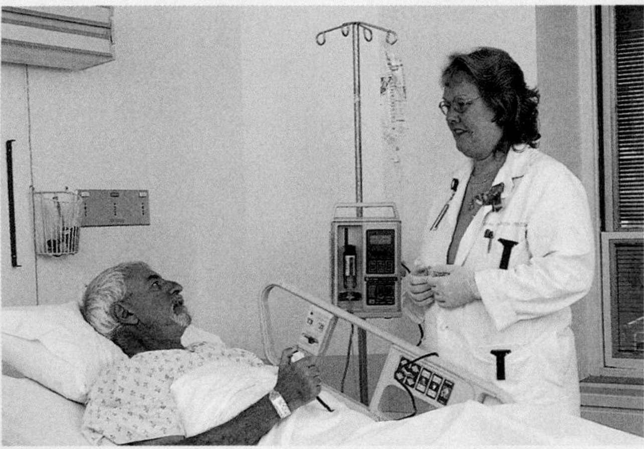

Figure 4. Instructing the patient to press the button each time he needs pain relief. (Photo © B. Proud.)

15. Assess the patient's pain at least every 1 to 2 hours. Monitor vital signs, especially respiratory status, including oxygen saturation. Assess the patient's sedation score (see Table 10-1).

Continued assessment at frequent intervals helps evaluate the effectiveness of the drug and reduce the risk for complications. Sedation occurs before clinically significant respiratory depression (Hagle et al, 2004). Respiratory depression may occur with the use of narcotic analgesics.

16. Assess the infusion site periodically, according to facility policy and nursing judgment. Assess the patient's use of the medication, noting number of attempts and number of doses delivered. Replace the drug syringe when it is empty.

Continued assessment of infusion site is necessary for early detection of problems. Continued assessment of patient's use of medication and effect is necessary to ensure adequate pain control without adverse effect. Replacing the syringe ensures continued drug delivery.

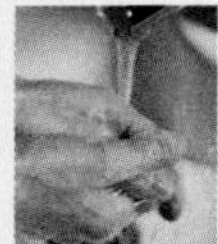

17. Make sure the patient control (dosing button) is within the patient's reach. Remove gloves, if worn, and perform hand hygiene.

Easy access to the control is essential for the patient's use of the device. Hand hygiene deters the spread of microorganisms.

EVALUATION

The expected outcome is achieved when the patient reports increased comfort and/or decreased pain, without adverse effects, oversedation, and respiratory depression; the patient displays decreased anxiety and improved coping skills; and the patient verbalizes an understanding of the therapy and the reason for its use.

DOCUMENTATION

Guidelines

Document the date and time PCA therapy was initiated, initial pain assessment, drug and loading dose administered, if appropriate, and individual dosing and time interval. Document continued pain, sedation level, vital sign assessments, and patient's response to therapy.

SKILL 10-4 Caring for a Patient Receiving PCA Pump Therapy *(continued)*

Sample Documentation

6/1/08 0645 Patient returned from surgery with PCA therapy with morphine sulfate 1 mg/mL in place via IV infusion. Device programmed to deliver 0.1 mg at 10-minute lockout intervals. Patient complaining of moderate to severe abdominal pain, rating pain as 6 to 8 out of 10 on a pain rating scale. Patient instructed to press PCA button for pain relief. Vital signs within acceptable parameters. Respiratory rate 16 breaths per minute. IV of 1000 cc D5LR infusing at 100 cc/minute; IV site clean and dry without evidence of infiltration or infection.—P. Joyner, RN

6/1/08 0700 Patient rates pain at 4. Respirations 16 breaths per minute. Encouraged patient to take deep breaths and cough. Lying on right side with the support of two pillows and head of bed elevated 30 degrees.—P. Joyner, RN

Unexpected Situations and Associated Interventions

- *While receiving PCA therapy, your patient's respiratory rate drops to 10 breaths per minute, with a sedation score of 3 via sedation scale (Pasero & McCaffery Sedation Scale):* Stop the PCA infusion if basal infusion is present. Notify the primary care provider. The basal infusion should be discontinued; if no basal infusion is being used, then the medication dosage should be reduced. Increase the frequency of sedation and respiratory rate monitoring to every 15 minutes. Arouse the patient every 15 minutes and encourage deep breathing (Hagle et al, 2004).
- *While receiving PCA therapy, your patient is somnolent, with a sedation score of 4 via sedation scale (Pasero & McCaffery Sedation Scale):* Stop the medication infusion immediately. Notify the primary care provider. Prepare to administer oxygen and a narcotic antagonist such as naloxone (Narcan). Because naloxone reverses all analgesia, as well as the respiratory depression, patients will experience extremely severe pain once the patient is awake and alert (Hagle et al, 2004).
- *The patient's intravenous infusion line becomes infiltrated:* Stop the PCA infusion and IV infusion. Remove the IV catheter and restart the IV line in another site. Once the site is established, resume the IV and PCA infusion.
- *The patient's subcutaneous infusion site becomes infiltrated:* Stop the PCA infusion. Remove the administration device and restart the infusion at another site. Once the site is established, resume the PCA infusion.

Special Considerations

General Considerations

- A wide variety of PCA devices are available on the market. Check the manufacturer's instructions before using the device.
- Adults and children who are cognitively and physically able to use the PCA equipment and are able to understand that pressing a button can result in pain relief are appropriate candidates for PCA therapy (Pasero & McCaffery, 2005a).
- PCA is considered safe because the analgesic administered most often is an opioid, which causes sedation before respiratory depression. A sedated patient can't self-administer a dose, reducing the risk of an overdose. (Hagle et al, 2004; Marders, 2004; Noah, 2003; Pasero & McCaffery, 2005a).
- Family members and nurses may need to remind the patient to push the button. If someone other than the patient delivers a dose, the risk for oversedation is increased (Hagle et al, 2004; Marders, 2004; Noah, 2003; Pasero & McCaffery, 2005a).
- Some facilities have developed clinical practice guidelines for nurse-controlled analgesia (NCA) and PCA by proxy. In these cases, one family member or primary nurse is designated as the primary pain manager and only that person can press the PCA button for the patient. In the case of family members, the primary pain manager must be chosen carefully and taught to asses for pain and the adverse effect of the medication.

(continued)

SKILL 10-4 Caring for a Patient Receiving PCA Pump Therapy *(continued)*

Additionally, nursing staff must be vigilant in assessing the patient's need for and response to the medication, following the same assessment guidelines previously discussed. It is very important to follow facility guidelines to ensure safe administration (Hagle, et al, 2004; Marders, 2004; Noah, 2003; Pasero & McCaffery, 2005a).

- If using a device that provides continuous and bolus doses, the cumulative doses per hour should not exceed the total hourly dose ordered by the physician.
- Vital-sign monitoring is crucial, especially when initiating therapy. Encourage the patient to practice coughing and deep breathing to promote ventilation and prevent pooling of secretions.
- A narcotic antagonist such as naloxone (Narcan) must be readily available in case the patient develops respiratory complications related to drug therapy.
- A fentanyl patient-controlled transdermal system (PCTS) is a new delivery technique for pain medication. The small device contains the medication in a reservoir in the patch and attaches to the patient's upper arm or chest with adhesive. When the patient pushes the button on the device, the medication is delivered by iontophoresis, an electrical current that introduces the medication into the tissues. The device is preprogrammed to deliver fixed 40-mcg doses of fentanyl. Each patch holds 80 doses, with a minimum time between doses of 10 minutes. The device will deliver the maximum 80 doses or will operate for 24 hours from the first dose, whichever occurs first. The patch then shuts off. If continued use is required, it is replaced with a new device, in another location. It is not for use with patients with implanted devices, such as pacemakers, that are sensitive to electricity (D'Arcy, 2005a; D'Arcy, 2005b; Koo, 2005).

Infant and Child Considerations

- PCA can be an effective method of pain control for a child. When determining the appropriateness of this therapy for a child, consider the child's chronologic age and developmental level, ability to understand (cognitive level), and motor skills.
- PCA has been shown to be very effective for adolescents because it gives them an increased feeling of control over the situation.

Home Care Considerations

- Be sure that the patient understands how to use the PCA device properly. Teach the patient how the device works, when to contact the physician, signs and symptoms of adverse reactions, and signs and symptoms of drug tolerance.
- Advise the patient to change positions gradually to prevent orthostatic hypotension, which may result from use of a narcotic analgesic.
- Ensure that there is a reliable adult who can provide backup assistance should the patient have difficulty.
- Consider a referral to a home healthcare agency to continue teaching and provide assessment of the therapy.

SKILL 10-5 Caring for a Patient Receiving Epidural Analgesia

Epidural analgesia is being used more commonly to provide pain relief during the immediate postoperative phase (particularly after thoracic, abdominal, orthopedic, and vascular surgery) and for chronic pain situations. Epidural pain management is also being used in children with terminal cancer and children undergoing hip, spinal, or lower extremity surgery. The anesthesiologist or radiologist usually inserts the catheter in the mid-lumbar region into the epidural space that exists between the walls of the vertebral canal and the dura mater or outermost connective tissue membrane surrounding the spinal cord. For temporary therapy, the catheter exits directly over the spine, and the tubing is positioned over the patient's shoulder with the end of the catheter taped to the chest. For long-term therapy, the catheter is usually tunneled subcutaneously and exits on the side of the body or on the abdomen (Figure 1).

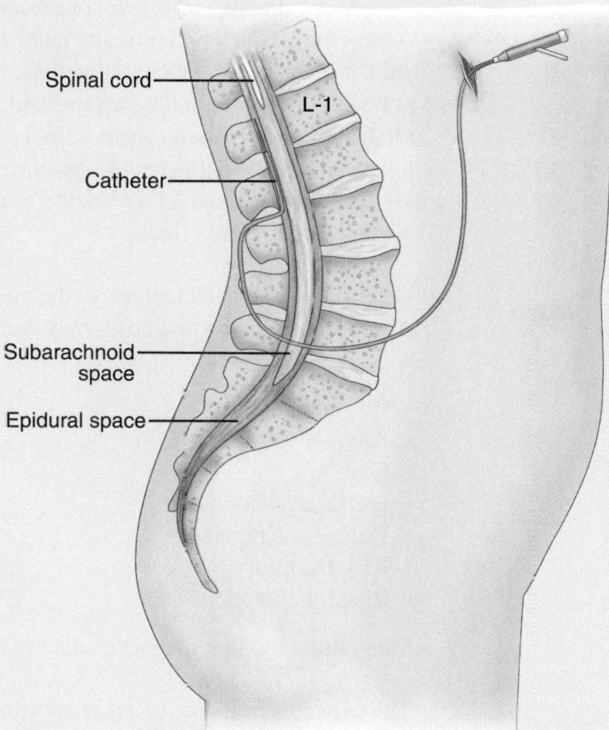

Figure 1. Placement of an epidural catheter for long-term use.

The epidural analgesia can be administered as a bolus dose (either one time or intermittent), via a continuous infusion pump, or by a patient-controlled epidural analgesia (PCEA) pump (D'Arcy, 2005; Pasero, 2003b; Roman & Cabaj, 2005). Additional information specific to PCA administration was discussed in Skill 10-4. Epidural catheters used for the management of acute pain are typically removed 36 to 72 hours after surgery, when oral medication can be substituted for relief of pain.

Equipment

- Volume infusion device
- Epidural infusion tubing
- Prescribed epidural analgesic solutions
- Transparent dressing or gauze pads
- Labels for epidural infusion line
- Tape

(continued)

SKILL 10-5 Caring for a Patient Receiving Epidural Analgesia *(continued)*

- Emergency drugs and equipment, such as naloxone, oxygen, endotracheal intubation set, handheld resuscitation bag, per facility policy
- Nonsterile gloves, if indicated

ASSESSMENT

Review the patient's medical record and plan of care for specific instructions related to epidural analgesia therapy, including the medical order for the drug and conditions indicating the need for therapy. Review the patient's history for conditions that might contraindicate therapy, such as local or systemic infections, neurologic disease, coagulopathy or use of anticoagulant therapy, spinal arthritis or spinal deformity, hypotension, marked hypertension, allergy to the prescribed medication, or psychiatric disorder. Check to ensure proper functioning of the unit. Assess the patient's level of consciousness and understanding of epidural analgesia therapy and the rationale for its use.

Assess the patient's level of discomfort and pain using an appropriate assessment tool. Assess the characteristics of any pain. Assess for other symptoms that often occur with the pain, such as headache or restlessness. Ask the patient what interventions have and have not been successful in the past to promote comfort and relieve pain. Assess the patient's vital signs and respiratory status, including rate, depth, and rhythm, and oxygen saturation level using pulse oximetry. Assess the patient's sedation score (see Table 10-1 in Skill 10-4). Assess the patient's response to the intervention to evaluate effectiveness and for the presence of adverse effects.

NURSING DIAGNOSIS

Determine the related factors for the nursing diagnoses based on the patient's current status. Appropriate nursing diagnoses may include:

- Acute Pain
- Chronic Pain
- Anxiety
- Fear
- Ineffective Coping
- Deficient Knowledge
- Risk for Injury
- Risk for Infection

Many other nursing diagnoses may require the use of this skill.

OUTCOME IDENTIFICATION AND PLANNING

The expected outcome to achieve is that the patient reports increased comfort and/or decreased pain, without adverse effects, oversedation, and respiratory depression. Other appropriate outcomes may include: the patient displays decreased anxiety; displays improved coping skills; remains free from infection; and verbalizes an understanding of the therapy and the reason for its use.

IMPLEMENTATION

ACTION	RATIONALE
1. Check the medication order against the original medical order according to agency policy. Clarify any inconsistencies. Check the patient's chart for allergies.	This comparison helps to identify errors that may have occurred when orders were transcribed. The physician's order is the legal record-of-medication orders for each agency.
2. Know the actions, special nursing considerations, safe dose ranges, purpose of administration, and adverse effects of the medications to be administered. Consider the appropriateness of the medication for this patient.	This knowledge aids the nurse in evaluating the therapeutic effect of the medication in relation to the patient's disorder and can also be used to educate the patient about the medication.

SKILL 10-5 Caring for a Patient Receiving Epidural Analgesia *(continued)*

ACTION	RATIONALE
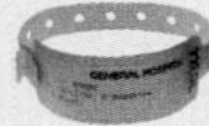 3. Identify the patient, show the patient the device, and explain the function of the device and reason for use. Explain the purpose and action of the medication to the patient.	Identifying the patient ensures the right patient receives the intervention and helps prevent errors. Explanation encourages patient understanding and cooperation and reduces apprehension.
4. Close the door to the room or pull the bedside curtain.	Closing the door or curtain provides patient privacy.
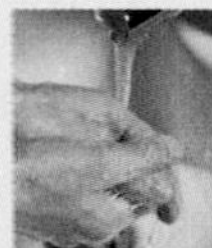 5. Perform hand hygiene. Put on nonsterile gloves, if indicated.	Hand hygiene deters the spread of microorganisms. Gloves are indicated for potential contact with blood or body fluids.
6. Complete necessary assessments before administering medication. Check allergy bracelet or ask patient about allergies. Assess the patient's pain, using an appropriate assessment tool and measurement scale (see Fundamentals Review 10-1 through 10-5).	Assessment is a prerequisite to administration of medications. Accurate assessment is necessary to guide treatment/relief interventions and evaluate the effectiveness of pain control measures.
7. **Have an ampule of 0.4-mg naloxone (Narcan) and a syringe at the bedside.**	Naloxone reverses the respiratory depressant effect of opioids.
8. After the catheter has been inserted and the infusion initiated by the anesthesiologist or radiologist, **check the label on the medication container and rate of infusion with the medication record and patient identification (Figure 2).** Obtain verification of information from second nurse, according to facility policy.	This action verifies that the correct drug and dosage will be administered to the correct patient. Confirmation of information by second nurse helps prevent errors.

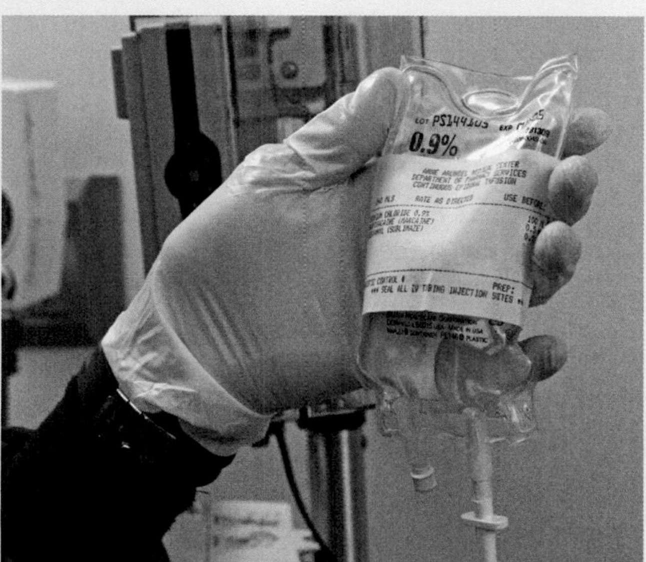

Figure 2. Checking the label on the medication container.

ACTION	RATIONALE
9. Tape all connection sites. Label the bag, tubing, and pump apparatus "For Epidural Infusion Only." **Do not administer any other narcotics or adjuvant drugs without the approval of the clinician responsible for the epidural injection.**	Taping prevents accidental dislodgement. Labeling prevents inadvertent administration of other intravenous medications through this setup. Additional medication may potentiate the action of the opioid, increasing the risk for respiratory depression.

(continued)

SKILL 10-5 Caring for a Patient Receiving Epidural Analgesia *(continued)*

ACTION	RATIONALE
10. Assess the exit site and apply a transparent dressing over the catheter insertion site, if not already in place (Figure 3). Monitor the infusion rate according to facility policy.	The transparent dressing protects the site while still allowing assessment. Monitoring the infusion rate prevents incorrect administration of the medication.

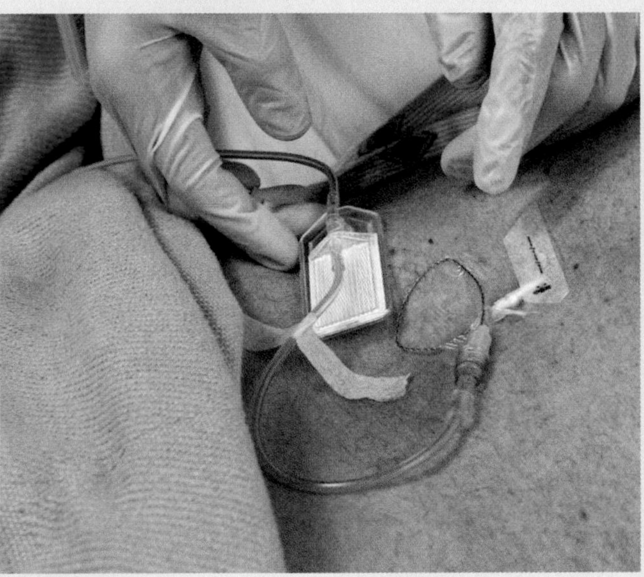

Figure 3. Assessing exit site.

ACTION	RATIONALE
11. Assess and record sedation level (see Table 10-1) and respiratory status every hour for the first 24 hours, then at 4-hour intervals (or according to agency policy). **Notify the physician if the sedation rating is 3 or 4, the respiratory depth decreases, or the respiratory rate falls below 8 breaths per minute.**	Opioids can depress the respiratory center in the medulla. A change in the level of consciousness is usually the first sign of altered respiratory function.
12. Keep the head of bed elevated 30 degrees unless contraindicated.	Elevation of the patient's head minimizes upward migration of the opioid in the spinal cord, thus decreasing the risk for respiratory depression.
13. Assess the patient's level of pain and the effectiveness of pain relief.	This information helps in determining the need for subsequent "breakthrough" pain medication.
14. Monitor urinary output and assess for bladder distention.	Opioids can cause urinary retention.
15. Assess motor strength every 4 hours.	The catheter may migrate into the intrathecal space and allow opioids to block the transmission of nerve impulses completely through the spinal cord to the brain.
16. Monitor for adverse effects (pruritus, nausea, and vomiting).	Opioids may spread into the trigeminal nerve, causing itching, or resulting in nausea and vomiting due to slowed gastrointestinal function or stimulation of a chemoreceptor trigger zone in the brain. Medications are available to treat these adverse effects.
17. Assess for signs of infection at the insertion site.	Inflammation or local infection may develop at the catheter insertion site.

SKILL 10-5 Caring for a Patient Receiving Epidural Analgesia *(continued)*

ACTION	RATIONALE
18. Change the dressing over the catheter exit site every 24 to 48 hours or as needed per agency policy using aseptic technique. Change the infusion tubing every 48 hours or as specified by agency policy.	Dressing and tubing changes using aseptic technique reduce the risk for infection.
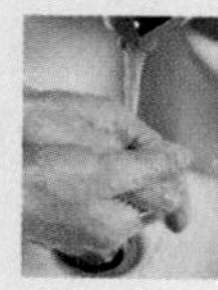 19. Remove gloves, if worn, and perform hand hygiene.	Proper disposal of gloves and hand hygiene deter the spread of microorganisms.

EVALUATION

The expected outcome is achieved when the patient verbalizes pain relief. In addition, the patient exhibits a dry, intact dressing, and the catheter exit site is free of signs and symptoms of complications, injury, or infection. The patient reports a decrease in anxiety and increased ability to cope with pain. The patient verbalizes information related to the functioning of the epidural catheter and the reasons for its use.

DOCUMENTATION

Guidelines

Document catheter patency, the condition of the insertion site and dressing, vital signs and assessment information, any change in infusion rate, solution, or tubing, analgesics administered, and the patient's response.

Sample Documentation

6/3/09 0935 Continuous morphine infusion via epidural catheter in place; see medication administration record. Exit site clean and slightly moist. Transparent dressing in place. Patient rates pain at 2 out of 10. Temperature 98.2° F; pulse, 76 beats per minute; respirations 16 breaths per minute and effortless; blood pressure, 110/70 mm Hg. Patient alert and quickly responds to verbal stimuli. Sedation score of 1. Bladder nonpalpable; urine output of 100 cc over the last 2 hours. Denies nausea, vomiting, or itching. Able to detect sensation of cold in lower extremities bilaterally. Able to wiggle toes and flex and dorsiflex feet bilaterally. Lower extremity muscle strength equal and moderately strong bilaterally.— T. James, RN

Unexpected Situations and Associated Interventions

- *While receiving epidural analgesia, the patient's sedation score drops below 2 and/or has a respiratory rate ≤8 breaths, or has shallow respirations:* Immediately notify the anesthesiologist. Stop the epidural infusion, if indicated, according to facility procedure. Encourage the patient to take deep slow breaths if possible. Prepare to administer oxygen and a narcotic antagonist such as naloxone (Narcan) via a peripheral IV site.
- *The patient demonstrates weakness and loss of sensation in the lower extremities while receiving epidural analgesia:* Reassess the patient's lower extremities for motor and sensory function. If positive for sensorimotor loss, notify the physician and expect to decrease the epidural infusion.
- *While receiving epidural analgesia, the patient suddenly develops a severe headache. Inspection of the catheter site reveals clear drainage on the dressing:* Stop the epidural infusion and notify the physician immediately. The catheter may have migrated and entered the dura.

(continued)

SKILL 10-5

Caring for a Patient Receiving Epidural Analgesia *(continued)*

Special Considerations

General Considerations

- Notify the anesthesiologist/pain management team immediately if the patient exhibits any of the following: respiratory rate below 10 breaths per minute, continued complaints of unmanaged pain, leakage at the insertion site, fever, inability to void, paresthesia, itching, or headache (Roman & Cabaj, 2005).
- Do not administer other sedatives or analgesics unless ordered by the anesthesiologist/pain management team to avoid oversedation (Roman & Cabaj, 2005).
- Always ensure that the patient receiving epidural analgesia has a peripheral IV line in place, either as a continuous IV infusion or as an intermittent infusion device, to allow immediate administration of emergency drugs if warranted.
- Keep in mind that drugs given via the epidural route diffuse slowly and may cause adverse reactions, including excessive sedation, for up to 12 hours after the infusion has been discontinued.
- Remember that typically an anesthesiologist orders analgesics and removes the catheter. However, facility policy may allow a specially trained nurse to remove the catheter.
- No resistance should be felt during the removal of an epidural catheter.

The Taylor Suite offers these additional resources to enhance learning and facilitate understanding of this chapter:

- thePoint online resource, http://thepoint.lww/Lynn2E
- Student CD-ROM included with the book
- Skills Checklist to Accompany Taylor's Clinical Nursing Skills

Developing Critical Thinking Skills

1. Since her surgery, Mildred Simpson has been spending most of her time in bed. A special pillow is placed between her legs to keep her hips in abduction. The nurse offers to give Mrs. Simpson a back massage. What areas would be most important for the nurse to address when performing this skill?
2. The physician decides to admit Joseph Watkins to the hospital for evaluation of his back pain. Intermittent TENS therapy is ordered and is to be started in the emergency department. How would the nurse initiate this therapy?
3. Jerome Batiste and his wife are concerned about using the PCA device at home. What information would the nurse provide to help alleviate their concerns?

Bibliography

Agency for Health Care Policy and Research (AHCPR). (1992). *Acute pain management guide panel.* Available at www.ahcpr.gov/clinic/cpgarchv.htm.

American Geriatrics Society (AGS). Panel on Chronic Pain in Older Persons. (2002). The management of persistent pain on older persons. *Journal of the American Geriatrics Society, 50,* Suppl 6, S205–S224.

Arnstein, P. (2002). Optimizing perioperative pain management. *AORN, 76*(5), 812–818.

Berger, J. (2003). Music for your practice. *Home Healthcare Nurse, 21*(1), 25–30.

Beyer, J., et al. (1992). The creation, validation, and continuing development of the Oucher: A measure of pain intensity in children. *Journal of Pediatric Nursing, 7*(5), 335.

Clinical Update: New standards for assessment and treatment of pain instituted by JCAHO. (2001). *American Journal for Nurse Practitioners, 5*(1), 43–44.

Criste, A. (2003). AANA Journal course update for nurse anesthetists. *AANA Journal Course, 70*(6), 475–480.

D'Arcy, Y. (2005a). Conquering pain: Have you tried these new techniques? *Nursing, 35*(3), 36–41.

D'Arcy, Y. (2005b). Controlling pain: Patching together transdermal pain control options. *Nursing, 35*(9), 17.

Ellis, J. (2003). Keeping pediatric patients comfortable. *Nursing, 33*(7), 22.

Griffie, J. (2003). Addressing inadequate pain relief: Effective communication among the health care team is essential. *American Journal of Nursing, 103*(8), 61–63.

Hagle, M., Lehr, V., Brubakken, K., et al. (2004). Respiratory depression in adult patients with intravenous patient-controlled analgesia. *Orthopaedic Nursing, 23*(1), 18–29.

Hockenberry, M. (2005). *Wong's essentials of pediatric nursing* (7th ed.). St. Louis, MO: Elsevier Mosby.

Hseish, R., & Lee, W. (2002). One-shot percutaneous electrical nerve stimulation vs. transcutaneous electrical nerve stimulation for low back pain: Comparison of therapeutic effects. *American Journal of Physical Medicine and Rehabilitation, 81*(11), 838–843.

Joint Commission on Accreditation of Healthcare Organizations (2000). *Joint Commission on Accreditation of Healthcare Organizations pain standards for 2001.* Available at www.jcaho.org.

Koo, P. (2005). Postoperative pain management with a patient-controlled transdermal delivery system for fentanyl. *American Journal of Health-System Pharmacy, 62*(11), 1171–1176.

Krieger, D. (1999). Therapeutic touch in hospice care. *American Journal of Nursing, 99*(4), 46.

Lane, P. (2004). Assessing pain in patients with advanced dementia. *Nursing, 34*(8), 17.

Lane, P., Kuntupis, M., MacDonald, S., et al. (2003). A pain assessment tool for people with advanced Alzheimer's and other progressive dementias. *Home Healthcare Nurse, 21*(1), 32–37.

LeMone, P., & Burke, K. (2004). *Medical-surgical nursing: Critical thinking in client care* (3rd ed.). Upper Saddle River, NJ: Pearson/Prentice Hall.

Marders, J. (2004). Device safety: PCA by proxy: Too much of a good thing. *Nursing, 34*(4), 24.

McCaffery, M. (1979). *Nursing management of the patient with pain* (2nd ed.). Philadelphia: J. B. Lippincott.

McCaffery, M. (2003). Switching from IV to PO: Maintaining pain relief in the transition. *American Journal of Nursing, 103*(5), 62–63.

McCaffery, M., & Beebe, A. (1989). *Pain: Clinical manual for nursing practice.* St. Louis, MO: C. V. Mosby.

McCaffery, M., & Ferrell, B. (1999). Opioids and pain management: What do nurses know? *Nursing, 29*(3), 48–52.

McCaffery, M., Ferrell, B., & Pasero, C. (1998). When the physician prescribes a placebo. *American Journal of Nursing, 98*(1), 52–53.

McCaffery, M., & Pasero, C. (1999). *Pain clinical manual* (2nd ed.). St. Louis, MO: C. V. Mosby.

McCaffery, M., & Pasero, C. (2003). Breakthrough pain. *American Journal of Nursing, 103*(4), 83–86.

Melzak, R., & Wall, P. (1968). Gate control theory of pain. In A. Soulairac, J. Cahn, & J. Carpentier (Eds). *Pain: Proceedings of the International Association on Pain.* Baltimore: Williams & Wilkins.

Merkel, S., Voepel-Lewis, T., & Malviya, S. (2002). Pain assessment in infants and young children: The FLACC Scale: A behavioral tool to measure pain in young children. *American Journal of Nursing, 102*(10), 55–58.

Mezinskis, P., Keller, A., & Schmidt Luggen, A. (2004). Assessment of pain in the cognitively impaired older adult in long-term care. *Geriatric Nursing, 25*(2), 107–112.

Neafsey, P. (2005). Medication news: Efficacy of continuous subcutaneous infusion in patients with cancer pain. *Home Healthcare Nurse,* 23(7), 421–423.

Newshan, G., & Schuller-Civitella, D. (2003). Large clinical study shows value of therapeutic touch program. *Holistic Nursing Practice, 17*(4), 189–192.

Nichols, R. (2003). Pain management in patients with addictive disease: A new position paper provides guidance. *American Journal of Nursing, 103*(3), 87–90.

Nisbet, A. (2003). Alternative approach. Some like it hot! Closing the gate on pain with superficial heat application. *Virginia Nurses Today, 11*(2), 10.

Noah, V. (2003). Controlling pain: PCA by proxy: Minimizing the risks. *Nursing, 33*(12), 17.

North American Nursing Diagnosis Association. (2005). *NANDA nursing diagnosis: Definitions & classification: 2005–2006.* Philadelphia: Author.

Pasero, C. (1998a). How aging affects pain management. *American Journal of Nursing, 98*(6), 12–13.

Pasero, C. (1998b). Is laughter the best medicine? *American Journal of Nursing, 98*(12), 12–14.

Pasero, C. (2003a). Pain in the emergency department: Withholding pain medication is not justified. *American Journal of Nursing, 103*(7), 73–74.

Pasero, C. (2003b). Epidural analgesia for postoperative pain: Excellent analgesia and improved patient outcomes after major surgery. *American Journal of Nursing, 103*(10), 62–64.

Pasero, C. (2004). Pain control. Perineural local anesthetic infusion. *American Journal of Nursing, 104*(7), 89–93.

Pasero, C., Gordon, D., & McCaffery, M. (1999). JCAHO on assessing and managing pain. *American Journal of Nursing, 99*(7), 22.

Pasero, C., & McCaffery, M. (1999). Providing epidural analgesia. *Nursing, 29*(8), 34–39.

Pasero, C., & McCaffery, M. (2005a). Authorized and unauthorized use of PCA pumps: Clarifying the use of patient-controlled analgesia, in light of recent alerts. *American Journal of Nursing, 105*(7), 30–32.

Pasero, C., & McCaffery, M. (2005b). No self-report means no pain-intensity rating: Assessing pain in patients who cannot provide a report. *American Journal of Nursing, 105*(10), 50–53.

Pullen, R. (2003), Managing IV patient-controlled analgesia. *Nursing, 33*(7), 24.

Roberson, L. (2003). The importance of touch for the patient with dementia. *Home Healthcare Nurse, 21*(1), 16–19.

Roman, M., & Cabaj, T. (2005). Epidural analgesia. *MEDSURG Nursing, 14*(4), 257–259.

Rush, S. L., & Harr, J. (2001). Evidence-based pediatric nursing: Does it have to hurt? *AACN Clinical Issues, 12*(4), 597–605.

Salmore, R. (2002). Development of a new pain scale: Colorado behavioral numerical pain scale for sedated adult patients undergoing gastrointestinal procedures. *Gastroenterology Nurse 25*(6), 257–262.

Schaffer, S., & Yucha, C. (2004). Relaxation & pain management: The relaxation response can play a role in managing chronic and acute pain. *American Journal of Nursing, 104*(8), 75–82.

Shea, R., Brooks, J., Dayhoff, N., & Keck, J. (2002). Pain intensity and postoperative pulmonary complications among the elderly after abdominal surgery. *Heart & Lung, 31*(6), 440–449.

Smeltzer, S., Bare, B., Hinkle, J. H., & Cheever, K. H. (2008). Brunner & Suddarth's textbook of medical-surgical nursing (11th ed.). Philadelphia: Lippincott Williams & Wilkins.

Spagrud, L, Piira, T., & von Baeyer, C. (2003). Children's self-report of pain intensity: The Faces Pain Scale–revised. *American Journal of Nursing, 103*(12), 62–64.

Steefel, L. (2001). Treat pain in any culture. *Nursing Spectrum (Philadelphia), 10*(25), 20–21.

Tabloski, P. (2006). *Gerontological nursing.* Upper Saddle River, NJ: Pearson/Prentice Hall.

Tanabe, P., Ferket, K., Thomas, R., et al. (2002). The effect of standard care, ibuprofen, and distraction on pain relief and patient satisfaction in children with musculoskeletal trauma. *Journal of Emergency Nursing,* 28(2), 118–125.

Taylor, C., Lillis, C., LeMone, P, et al. (2008). *Fundamentals of nursing* (6th ed.). Philadelphia: Lippincott Williams & Wilkins.

Wong, D. (2003). Topical local anesthetics. *American Journal of Nursing, 103*(6), 42–44.

CHAPTER 11

Nutrition

Focusing on Patient Care

This chapter will help you develop some of the skills related to nutrition needed to care for the following patients:

Paula Williams, age 78, who is recovering from a cerebrovascular accident (CVA), or stroke. The nurse needs to feed her breakfast.

Jack Mason, a 62-year-old man who has had bowel surgery and requires a nasogastric tube for decompression.

Cole Brenau, age 12, has cystic fibrosis and needs to increase his caloric intake through gastrostomy tube feedings at nighttime.

Learning Objectives

After studying this chapter, you will be able to:

1. Provide assistance to patients as needed in consuming their diets.
2. Insert a nasogastric tube.
3. Administer a tube feeding.
4. Remove a nasogastric tube.
5. Irrigate a nasogastric tube connected to suction.
6. Care for a gastrostomy tube.

Key Terms

anorexia: lack or loss of appetite for food

basal metabolism: amount of energy required to carry out involuntary activities of the body at rest

body mass index (BMI): ratio of height to weight that more accurately reflects total body fat stores in the general population (weight in kg/height[2] in meters)

calorie: measure of heat, or energy; kilocalorie, commonly referred to as a calorie, is defined as the amount of heat required to raise 1 kg of water by 1°C

carbohydrate: organic compounds (commonly known as sugars and starches) that are composed of carbon, hydrogen, and oxygen; the most abundant and least expensive source of calories in the diet worldwide

cholesterol: fatlike substance, found only in animal tissues, that is important for cell membrane structure, a precursor of steroid hormones, and a constituent of bile

enteral nutrition: alternate form of feeding that involves passing a tube into the gastrointestinal tract to allow instillation of the appropriate formula

ketosis: catabolism of fatty acids that occurs when an individual's carbohydrate intake is not adequate; without adequate glucose, the catabolism is incomplete and ketones are formed, resulting in increased ketones

lipid: group name for fatty substances, including fats, oils, waxes, and related compounds

minerals: inorganic elements found in nature

nasogastric (NG) tube: a tube inserted through the nose and into the stomach

nasointestinal (NI) tube: a tube inserted through the nose and into the upper portion of the small intestine

NPO (nothing by mouth): nothing can be consumed by mouth, including medications, unless ordered otherwise

nutrient: specific biochemical substance used by the body for growth, development, activity, reproduction, lactation, health maintenance, and recovery from illness or injury

nutrition: study of the nutrients and how they are handled by the body, as well as the impact of human behavior and environment on the process of nourishment

obesity: weight greater than 20% above ideal body weight

partial or peripheral parenteral nutrition (PPN): nutritional therapy used for patients who have an inadequate oral intake and require supplementation of nutrients through a peripheral vein

percutaneous endoscopic gastrostomy tube (PEG): a surgically or laparoscopically placed gastrostomy tube

percutaneous endoscopic jejunostomy tube (PEJ): a surgically or laparoscopically placed jejunostomy tube

protein: vital component of every living cell; composed of carbon, hydrogen, oxygen, and nitrogen

recommended dietary allowance (RDA): recommendations for average daily amounts of essential nutrients that healthy people should consume over time

residual: as applied to tube feeding, the amount of gastric contents in the stomach after the administration of a tube feeding

total parenteral nutrition (TPN): nutritional therapy that bypasses the gastrointestinal tract; used in patients who cannot take food orally; meets the patient's nutritional needs by way of nutrient-filled solutions administered through a central vein

trans fat: product that results when liquid oils are partially hydrogenated; these oils then become more stable and solid; trans fats raise serum cholesterol levels

triglycerides: predominant form of fat in food and the major storage form of fat in the body; composed of one glyceride molecule and three fatty acids

vitamins: organic substances needed by the body in small amounts to help regulate body processes; are susceptible to oxidation and destruction

Nutrition is a basic human need that changes throughout the life cycle and along the wellness–illness continuum. Food provides nutrition for both the body and the mind. Eating has evolved from being a simple necessity. It may be a source of pleasure, a pastime, a social event, a political statement, a religious symbol, a cultural emblem, or an integral component of medical treatment. As such, food, eating, and nutrition take on different meanings to different people, and changing a person's eating behaviors may be a difficult and slow process.

Because nutrition is vital for life and health, a person's diet should be varied in content to provide all the essential nutrients (see Fundamentals Review 11-1 for sources and functions of carbohydrates, protein, and fats). Important nutrients, found in food, are needed for the body to function. Poor nutrition can seriously decrease one's level of wellness.

Because of the significant influence that adequate nutrition plays in maintaining health and disease prevention, the nurse integrates nutritional assessment into the care of the patient (Fundamentals Review 11-2). Ongoing data collection through various methods such as history taking, the physical examination, and laboratory data analysis (Fundamentals Review 11-3) can provide pertinent information for directing the nursing plan of care. Factors that may affect nutritional status are discussed in Fundamentals Review 11-4.

This chapter discusses the skills necessary to care for patients with nutritional needs. At times, a patient will be unable to meet nutritional needs through oral intake of an adequate diet. When this circumstance is present, selection of a feeding tube may be appropriate. Factors that will be considered related to selection of a feeding tube will include aspiration risk, the anticipated duration of the feeding tube, the function of the gastrointestinal (GI) tract, and the patient's overall condition and prognosis. Also, the ethical implications surrounding initiation of tube feedings need to be considered, which entail knowledge of the patient's wishes concerning this intervention.

Fundamentals Review 11-1

Sources, Functions, and Significance of Carbohydrates, Protein, and Fat

Nutrient	Sources	Functions	Significance
Carbohydrates Simple sugars and starch	Fruits Vegetables Grains: rice, pasta, breads, cereals Dried peas and beans Milk (lactose) Sugars: white and brown sugar, honey, molasses, syrup	Provide energy Spare protein so it can be used for other functions Prevent ketosis from inefficient fat metabolism	Provide about 46% of the calories in the typical American diet; many believe carbohydrate intake should be increased to 50%–60% of total calories Low carbohydrate intake can cause ketosis; high simple sugar intake increases the risk for dental caries
Cellulose and other water-insoluble fibers	Whole wheat flour and wheat bran Vegetables: cabbage, peas, green beans, wax beans, broccoli, brussels sprouts, cucumber skins, peppers, carrots Apples	Absorb water to increase fecal bulk Decrease intestinal transit time	Is nondigestible; therefore, it is excreted Helps relieve constipation North Americans are urged to eat more of all types of fiber Excess intake can cause gas, distention, and diarrhea
Water-soluble fibers	Oat bran and oatmeal Dried peas and beans Vegetables Prunes, pears, apples, bananas, oranges	Slow gastric emptying Lower serum cholesterol level Delay glucose absorption	Help improve glucose tolerance in diabetics
Protein	Milk and milk products Meat, poultry, fish Eggs Dried peas and beans Nuts	Tissue growth and repair Component of body framework: bones, muscles, tendons, blood vessels, skin, hair, nails Component of body fluids: hormones, enzymes, plasma proteins, neurotransmitters, mucus Helps regulate fluid balance through oncotic pressure Helps regulate acid–base balance Detoxifies harmful substances Forms antibodies Transports fat and other substances through the blood Provides energy when carbohydrate intake is inadequate	Most North Americans consume twice the RDA (RNI) for protein Experts recommend that we eat less animal protein and more vegetable protein. Protein deficiency is characterized by edema, retarded growth and maturation, muscle wasting, changes in the hair and skin, permanent damage to physical and mental development (in children), diarrhea, malabsorption, numerous secondary nutrient deficiencies, fatty infiltration of the liver, increased risk for infections, and high mortality Except for elderly people, fad dieters, hospitalized patients, and people of low income, protein deficiency is rare in the United States and Canada

(continued)

Fundamentals Review 11-1

Sources, Functions, and Significance of Carbohydrates, Protein, and Fat *(continued)*

Nutrient	Sources	Functions	Significance
Fat	Butter, oils, margarine, lard, salt pork, salad dressings, mayonnaise, bacon Whole milk and whole milk products High-fat meats Nuts	Provides energy Provides structure Insulates the body Cushions internal organs Necessary for the absorption of fat-soluble vitamins	Fat supplies about 37% of total calories in the typical North American diet; experts suggest a reduction to 30% or less of total calories High-fat diets increase the risk for heart disease and obesity and are correlated with an increased risk for colon and breast cancers

(Dudek, S. G. [2006]. *Nutrition essentials for nursing practice* [5th ed.]. Philadelphia: Lippincott Williams & Wilkins.)

Fundamentals Review 11-2

Clinical Observations for Nutritional Assessment

Body Area	Signs of Good Nutritional Status	Signs of Poor Nutritional Status
General appearance	Alert, responsive	Listless, apathetic, and cachexic
General vitality	Endurance, energetic, sleeps well, vigorous	Easily fatigued, no energy, falls asleep easily, looks tired, apathetic
Weight	Normal for height, age, body build	Overweight or underweight
Hair	Shiny, lustrous, firm, not easily plucked, healthy scalp	Dull and dry, brittle, loss of color, easily plucked, thin and sparse
Face	Uniform skin color; healthy appearance, not swollen	Dark skin over cheeks and under eyes, flaky skin, facial edema (moon face), pale skin color
Eyes	Bright, clear, moist, no sores at corners of eyelids, membranes moist and healthy pink color, no prominent blood vessels	Pale eye membranes, dry eyes (xerophthalmia); Bitot's spots, increased vascularity, cornea soft (keratomalacia), small yellowish lumps around eyes (xanthelasma), dull or scarred cornea
Lips	Good pink color, smooth, moist, not chapped or swollen	Swollen and puffy (cheilosis), angular lesion at corners of mouth or fissures or scars (stomatitis)

Fundamentals Review 11-2

Clinical Observations for Nutritional Assessment *(continued)*

Body Area	Signs of Good Nutritional Status	Signs of Poor Nutritional Status
Tongue	Deep red, surface papillae present	Smooth appearance, beefy red or magenta colored, swollen, hypertrophy or atrophy
Teeth	Straight, no crowding, no cavities, no pain, bright, no discoloration, well-shaped jaw	Cavities, mottled appearance (Fluorosis), malpositioned, missing teeth
Gums	Firm, good pink color, no swelling or bleeding	Spongy, bleed easily, marginal redness, recessed, swollen and inflamed
Glands	No enlargement of the thyroid, face not swollen	Enlargement of the thyroid (goiter), enlargement of the parotid (swollen cheeks)
Skin	Smooth, good color, slightly moist, no signs of rashes, swelling, or color irregularities	Rough, dry, flaky, swollen, pale, pigmented, lack of fat under the skin, fat deposits around the joints (xanthomas), bruises, petechiae
Nails	Firm, pink	Spoon shaped (koilonychia), brittle, pale, ridged
Skeleton	Good posture, no malformations	Poor posture, beading of the ribs, bowed legs or knock-knees, prominent scapulas, chest deformity at diaphragm
Muscles	Well developed, firm, good tone, some fat under the skin	Flaccid, poor tone, wasted, underdeveloped, difficulty walking
Extremities	No tenderness	Weak and tender, presence of edema
Abdomen	Flat	Swollen
Nervous system	Normal reflexes, psychological stability	Decrease in or loss of ankle and knee reflexes, psychomotor changes, mental confusion, depression, sensory loss, motor weakness, loss of sense of position, loss of vibration, burning and tingling of the hands and feet (paresthesia)
Cardiovascular system	Normal heart rate and rhythm, no murmurs, normal blood pressure for age	Cardiac enlargement, tachycardia, elevated blood pressure
GI system	No palpable organs or masses (liver edge may be palpable in children)	Hepatosplenomegaly, enlarged liver or spleen

(Adapted from Dudek, S. G. [2006]. *Nutrition essentials for nursing practice* [5th ed.]. Philadelphia: Lippincott William & Wilkins.)

Biochemical Data With Nutritional Implications

- Hemoglobin (normal = 12–18 g/dL)
  decreased → anemia
- Hematocrit (normal = 40%–50%)
  decreased → anemia
  increased → dehydration
- Serum albumin (normal = 3.3–5 g/dL)
  decreased → malnutrition (prolonged protein depletion), malabsorption
- Transferrin (normal = 240–480 mg/dL)
  decreased → anemia, protein deficiency
- Total lymphocyte count (normal = greater than 1800) decreased → impaired nutritional intake, severe debilitating disease
- Blood urea nitrogen (normal = 17–18 mg/dL)
  increased → starvation, high protein intake, severe dehydration
  decreased → malnutrition, overhydration
- Creatinine (normal = 0.4–1.5 mg/dL)
  increased → dehydration
  decreased → reduction in total muscle mass, severe malnutrition

(Fischbach, F. [2004]. *A manual of laboratory and diagnostic tests* [7th ed.]. Philadelphia: Lippincott Williams & Wilkins.)

Factors That May Affect Nutritional Status

- Socioeconomic status
- Psychosocial factors (meaning of food)
- Medical conditions that involve malabsorption, such as Crohn's disease or cystic fibrosis
- Age
- Medical conditions that may affect desire to eat, such as chemotherapy treatment or pregnancy accompanied by morning sickness
- Culture
- Medications
- Alcohol abuse
- Religion
- Megadoses of nutrient substances

(Fischbach, F. [2004]. *A manual of laboratory and diagnostic tests* [7th ed.]. Philadelphia: Lippincott Williams & Wilkins.)

SKILL 11-1 Assisting With Patient Feeding

Depending on the patient's condition, the physician will order a diet. Many patients are able to independently meet their nutritional needs by feeding themselves. Other patients, especially the very young and some elderly patients, such as those individuals with arthritis of the hands, may have some difficulty opening juice containers, etc. On these occasions, it is necessary for the nurse to provide whatever assistance is needed. Patients with such conditions as paralysis of the hands and advanced dementia may be unable to feed themselves. This skill is frequently delegated to nursing assistants. However, the nurse is responsible for the initial and ongoing assessment of the patient for potential complications related to feeding. Before this skill can be delegated, it is paramount that the nursing assistant has been educated to observe for any swallowing difficulties and in aspiration-prevention precautions.

Equipment

- Patient tray
- Wet wipes for hand hygiene
- Mouth care materials
- Patient's dentures, eyeglasses, hearing aid if needed
- Special adaptive utensils as needed
- Napkins, protective covering or towel

ASSESSMENT

Before assisting the patient, the nurse will check the type of diet that has been ordered for the patient. Also, it is important to assess for any food allergies and religious or cultural preferences, as appropriate. The nurse should check to make sure the patient does not have any scheduled laboratory or diagnostic studies that may impact whether he/she is able to eat a meal. Before beginning the feeding, assessment for any swallowing difficulties should be conducted.

NURSING DIAGNOSIS

- Deficient Knowledge
- Anxiety
- Risk for Aspiration
- Risk for Impaired Social Interaction
- Risk for Alteration in Nutrition
- Feeding Self-Care Deficit
- Risk for Impaired Swallowing
- Risk for Adult Failure to Thrive

OUTCOME IDENTIFICATION AND PLANNING

The expected outcome to achieve when assisting a patient with feeding is that the patient consumes 50% to 60% of the contents of the meal tray. Also, another outcome is achieved when the patient does not aspirate during or after the meal. Additionally, a desired outcome is accomplished when the patient expresses contentment related to eating, as appropriate.

IMPLEMENTATION

ACTION	RATIONALE
1. Check the physician's order for the type of diet.	Ensures the correct diet for the patient.
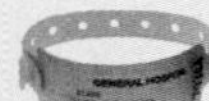 2. Identify the patient.	Identification of the patient ensures that the right patient receives the correct diet as ordered.
3. Explain procedure to patient.	Explanations provide reassurance and facilitate cooperation of the patient.

(continued)

SKILL 11-1 Assisting With Patient Feeding *(continued)*

ACTION	RATIONALE
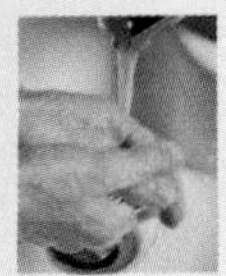 4. Perform hand hygiene.	Hand hygiene deters the spread of microorganisms.
5. Assess level of consciousness, for any physical limitations, decreased hearing or visual acuity. If patient uses a hearing aid or wears glasses or dentures, provide as needed. Ask if the patient has any cultural or religious preferences and food likes and dislikes, if possible.	Alertness is necessary for patient to swallow and consume food. Using a hearing aid, glasses, and dentures for chewing facilitates the intake of food. Patient preferences should be considered in food selection as much as possible to increase the intake of food and maximize the benefit of the meal.
6. Pull the patient's bedside curtain. Assess the abdomen. Ask the patient if he/she has any nausea. Ask the patient if he/she has any difficulty swallowing. Assess the patient for nausea or pain and administer an antiemetic or analgesic as needed.	Provide for privacy. A functioning GI tract is essential for digestion. The presence of pain or nausea will diminish appetite. If patient is medicated, wait for the appropriate time for absorption of the medication before beginning the feeding.
7. Offer to assist the patient with any elimination needs.	Promotes comfort and may avoid interruptions for toileting during meals.
8. Provide hand hygiene and mouth care as needed.	May improve appetite and promote comfort.
9. Remove any bedpans or undesirable equipment and odors if possible from the vicinity where meal will be eaten.	Unpleasant odors and equipment may decrease the appetite of the patient.
10. Open the patient's bedside curtain. Assist or position the patient in a high Fowler's or sitting position. Position the bed in the low position.	Proper positioning improves swallowing ability and reduces the risk of aspiration.
11. Place protective covering or towel over the patient if desired.	Prevents soiling of the patient's gown.
12. Check tray to make sure that it is the correct tray before serving. Place tray on the overbed table so patient can see food if able. Ensure that hot foods are hot and cold foods are cold. Use caution with hot beverages, allowing sufficient time for cooling if needed. Ask the patient for his/her preference related to what foods are desired first. Cut food into small pieces as needed. Observe swallowing ability throughout the meal.	Ensures that the correct tray is given to the patient. Encouraging the patient choice promotes patient dignity and respect.

SKILL 11-1

Assisting With Patient Feeding *(continued)*

ACTION	RATIONALE
13. If possible, sit facing the patient while feeding is taking place (Figure 1). It patient is able, encourage to hold finger foods and feed self as much as possible. Converse with patient during the meal as appropriate. Play relaxation music if patient desires.	In general, optimal meal time involves social interaction and conversation.

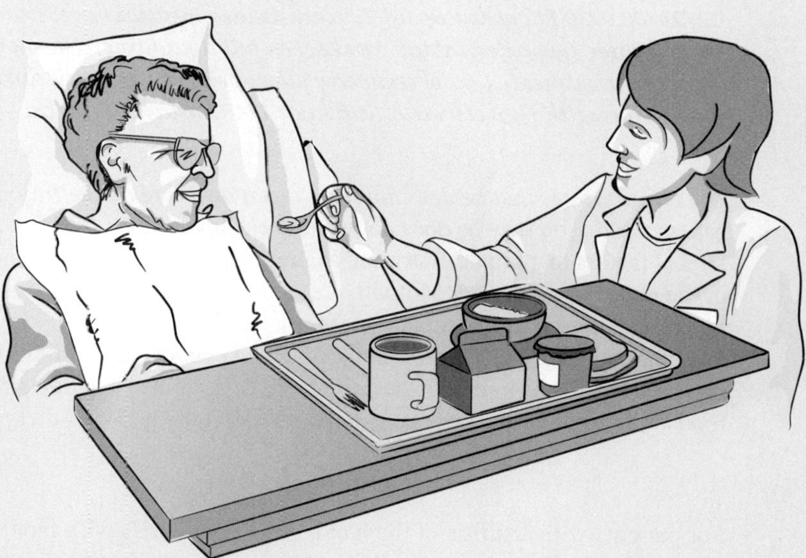

Figure 1. Assisting patient with eating.

ACTION	RATIONALE
14. Allow enough time for the patient to adequately chew and swallow the food. The patient may need to rest for short periods during eating.	Eating requires energy and disease can weaken patients. Rest can restore energy for eating.
15. **When the meal is completed or the patient is unable to eat any more, remove the tray from the room. Note the amount and types of food consumed.**	Nutrition plays an important role in healing and overall health. If the patient is not eating enough to meet nutritional requirements, alternative methods need to be considered.
16. Reposition the overbed table, remove the protective covering, offer hand hygiene as needed, and offer the bedpan. Assist the patient to a position of comfort and relaxation.	Promotes the comfort of the patient, meets possible elimination needs, and facilitates digestion.
17. Perform hand hygiene.	Hand hygiene reduces the transmission of microorganisms.

EVALUATION

The expected outcomes are met when the patient consumes an adequate amount of nutrients. In addition, the patient expresses an appetite for the food, relating likes and dislikes. Additionally, the patient experiences no nausea, vomiting, or aspiration episodes.

(continued)

SKILL 11-1 Assisting With Patient Feeding *(continued)*

DOCUMENTATION

Guidelines

Document the condition of the abdomen. Record that the HOB was elevated to at least 30 to 45 degrees. Note any swallowing difficulties and the patient's response to the meal. Document the percentage of the intake from the meal. If the patient had a poor intake, document the need for further consultation with the physician and dietitian as needed. Record any pertinent teaching that was conducted.

Sample Documentation

12/23/08 0730 Pt's abdomen SOFT, nondistended, positive bowel sounds. HOB elevated to 45 degrees. Gag reflex intact. Awake. Fed full liquid tray; consumed about 50%; ate most of the oatmeal, 4 oz. of cranberry juice. Some conversation during the meal. Pt remains with HOB elevated, watching TV. Call light in reach.—S. Essner, RN

Unexpected Situations and Associated Interventions

- *The patient states that he does not want to eat anything on the tray:* Explore with the patient the reason why he does not want to eat anything on the tray. Assess for psychological factors that impact nutrition. Malnutrition is sometimes found with depression in the elderly population. Mutually develop a plan to address the lack of nutritional intake and consult the dietitian as needed.
- *The patient states that she feels nauseated and cannot eat:* Remove the tray from the patient's room. Explore with the patient the desirability of eating small amounts of foods or liquids, such as crackers or ginger ale, if the patient's diet permits.

Special Considerations

General Considerations

- For patients with arthritis of the hands, special utensils with modified handles that facilitate an easier grip are available. Contact an occupational therapist for guidance on adaptive equipment.
- A visually impaired patient may be guided to feed him or herself through use of a "clock" pattern. For example, the chicken is placed at 6:00 o'clock; the vegetables at 3:00 o'clock.
- For the patient with dysphagia, suggest small bites of food such as puddings, ground meat, or cooked vegetables. Advise the patient not to talk while swallowing and to swallow twice after each bite.

SKILL 11-2 Inserting a Nasogastric Tube

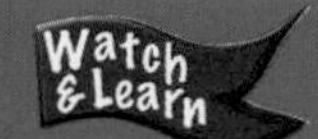

The nasogastric (NG) tube is passed through the nose and into the stomach. This type of tube permits the patient to receive nutrition through a tube feeding using the stomach as a natural reservoir for food. Another purpose of a NG tube may be to decompress or to drain unwanted fluid and air from the stomach. This application would be used, for example, to allow the intestinal tract to rest and promote healing after bowel surgery. The NG tube can also be used to monitor bleeding in the gastrointestinal (GI) tract, to remove undesirable substances (lavage) such as poisons, or to help treat an intestinal obstruction.

Equipment

- Nasogastric (polyurethane) tube of appropriate size (8–18 French)
- Stethoscope
- Small basin filled with ice or warm water (optional)

SKILL 11-2 Inserting a Nasogastric Tube *(continued)*

- Water-soluble lubricant
- Normal saline solution (for irrigation only)
- Tongue blade
- Asepto bulb syringe or Toomey syringe (20–50 mL)
- Flashlight
- Nonallergenic tape (1″ wide)
- Tissues
- Glass of water with straw
- Topical anesthetic (lidocaine spray or gel) (optional)
- Clamp
- Suction apparatus (if ordered)
- Bath towel or disposable pad
- Emesis basin
- Safety pin and rubber band
- Nonsterile disposable gloves
- Tincture of benzoin or skin adhesive
- pH paper

ASSESSMENT

Assess the patency of the patient's nares by asking the patient to occlude one nostril and breathe normally through the other. Select the nostril through which air passes more easily. Also, assess the patient's history for any recent facial trauma, polyps, blockages, or surgeries. Patients with facial fractures or facial surgeries present a higher risk for misplacement into the brain. Many institutions require a physician to place NG tubes in these patients. Inspect the abdomen for distention and firmness; auscultate for bowel sounds or peristalsis and palpate the abdomen for distention and tenderness. If the abdomen is distended, consider measuring the abdominal girth at the umbilicus to establish a baseline.

NURSING DIAGNOSIS

Determine the related factors for the nursing diagnoses based on the patient's current status. Nursing diagnoses may vary depending on the reason for the NG tube insertion. Possible nursing diagnoses may include:

- Imbalanced Nutrition, Less than Body Requirements
- Risk for Aspiration
- Impaired Swallowing
- Acute Pain
- Deficient Knowledge
- Risk for Disturbance in Body Image
- Nausea

OUTCOME IDENTIFICATION AND PLANNING

The expected outcome to achieve when inserting an NG tube is that the tube is passed into the patient's stomach without any complications. Other outcomes may include the following: the patient demonstrates weight gain, indicating improved nutrition; patient exhibits no signs and symptoms of aspiration; patient rates pain as decreased from prior to insertion; and patient verbalizes an understanding of the reason for NG tube insertion.

(continued)

SKILL 11-2 Inserting a Nasogastric Tube *(continued)*

IMPLEMENTATION

ACTION	RATIONALE
1. Check physician's order for insertion of NG tube and consider the risks associated with NG tube insertion.	This clarifies procedure and type of equipment required. Bronchial intubation is a possible complication.
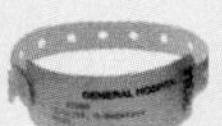 2. Identify the patient.	Identification of the patient ensures that the right patient receives the correct tube feeding as ordered.
3. Explain the procedure to the patient and provide the rationale as to why the tube is needed. Discuss the associated discomforts that may be experienced and possible interventions that may allay this discomfort. Answer any questions as needed.	Explanation facilitates patient cooperation. Some patient surveys report that of all routine procedures, the insertion of a NG tube is considered the most painful. Lidocaine gel or sprays are possible options to decrease discomfort during NG tube insertion.
4. Gather equipment including selection of the appropriate NG polyurethane tube.	This provides for organized approach to task. NG tubes should be radio-opaque, contain clearly visible markings for measurement, and have multiple ports for aspiration.
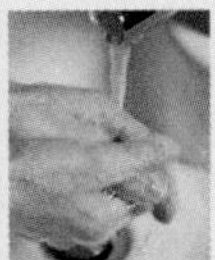 5. Perform hand hygiene. Put on nonsterile gloves.	Hand hygiene deters the spread of microorganisms.
6. Close the patient's bedside curtain or door. Raise the bed. Assist the patient to high Fowler's position or elevate the head of the bed 45 degrees if the patient is unable to maintain upright position (Figure 1). Drape chest with bath towel or disposable pad. Have emesis basin and tissues handy.	Closing curtains or door provides for patient privacy. Raising the bed promotes the comfort and proper body mechanics of the nurse. Upright position is more natural for swallowing and protects against bronchial intubation aspiration, if the patient should vomit. Passage of tube may stimulate gagging and tearing of eyes.

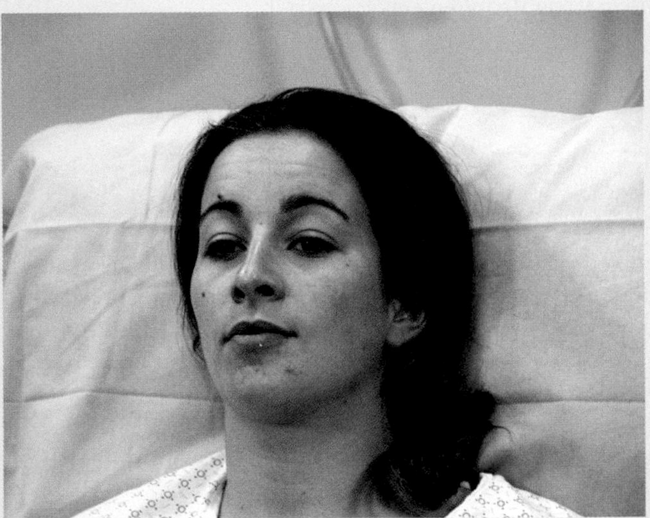

Figure 1. Placing patient in semi- to high Fowler's position in preparation for tube insertion.

SKILL 11-2 **Inserting a Nasogastric Tube** *(continued)*

ACTION	RATIONALE
7. **Measure the distance to insert tube by placing tip of tube at patient's nostril and extending to tip of ear lobe and then to tip of xiphoid process (Figures 2 and 3).** Mark tube with an indelible marker.	Measurement ensures that tube will be long enough to enter patient's stomach.

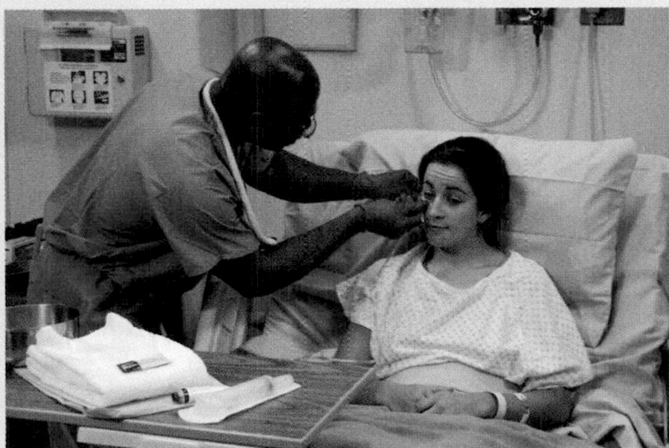

Figure 2. Measuring NG tube from nostril to tip of ear lobe.

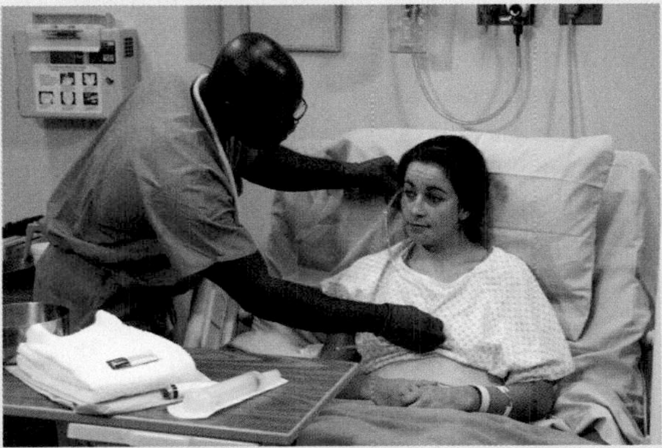

Figure 3. Measuring NG tube from tip of ear lobe to xiphoid process.

ACTION	RATIONALE
8. Lubricate tip of tube (at least 2″–4″) with water-soluble lubricant. Apply topical anesthetic to nostril and oropharynx, as appropriate.	Lubrication reduces friction and facilitates passage of the tube into stomach. Water-soluble lubricant will not cause pneumonia if tube accidentally enters the lungs. Topical anesthetics act as local anesthetics, reducing discomfort. Consult the physician for an order for a topical anesthetic such as lidocaine gel or spray if needed.
9. After selecting the appropriate nostril, ask patient to slightly flex head back against the pillow. Gently insert the tube into the nostril while directing the tube upward and backward along the floor of the nose (Figure 4). Patient may gag when tube reaches pharynx. Provide tissues for tearing or watering of eyes. Offer comfort and reassurance to the patient.	Following the normal contour of the nasal passage while inserting the tube reduces irritation and the likelihood of mucosal injury. The gag reflex is readily stimulated by the tube. Tears are a natural response as the tube passes into the nasopharynx. Many patients report that gagging and throat discomfort can be more painful then passing through the nostrils.

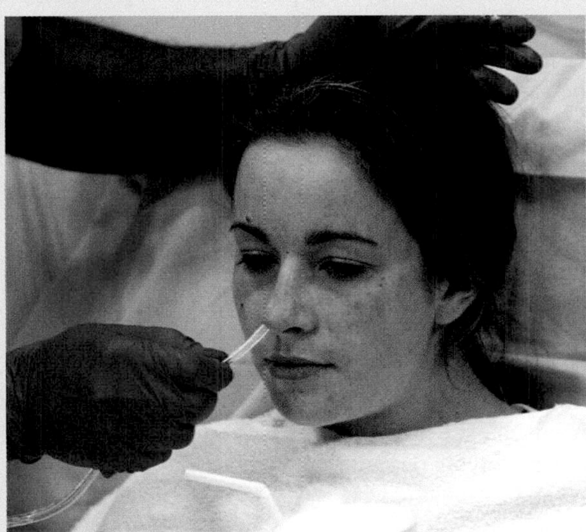

Figure 4. Beginning insertion with patient positioned with head up.

(continued)

SKILL 11-2 Inserting a Nasogastric Tube *(continued)*

ACTION	RATIONALE
10. **When pharynx is reached, instruct patient to touch chin to chest.** Encourage patient to sip water through a straw or swallow even if no fluids are permitted. Advance tube in downward and backward direction when patient swallows (Figure 5). Stop when patient breathes. **If gagging and coughing persist, stop advancing the tube and check placement of tube with tongue blade and flashlight.** If tube is curled, straighten the tube and attempt to advance again. Keep advancing tube until pen marking is reached. **Do not use force. Rotate tube if it meets resistance.**	Bringing the head forward helps close the trachea and open the esophagus. Swallowing helps advance the tube, causes the epiglottis to cover the opening of the trachea, and helps to eliminate gagging and coughing. Excessive coughing and gagging may occur if the tube has curled in the back of throat. Forcing the tube may injure mucous membranes.

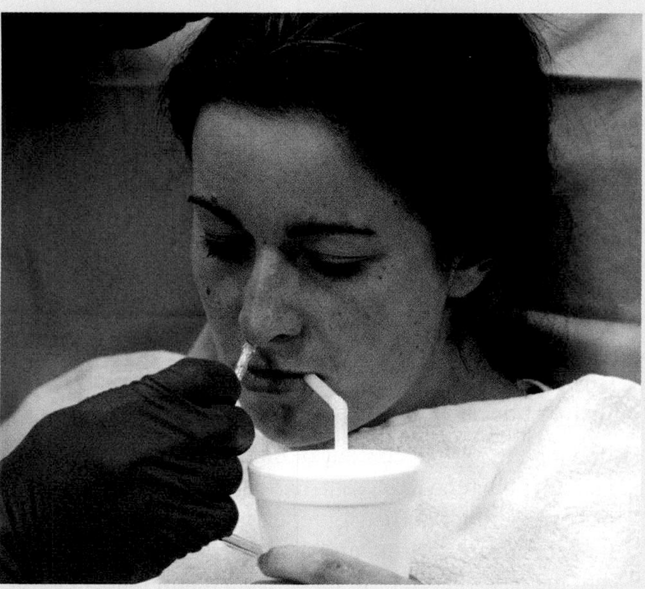

Figure 5. Advancing tube while patient drops chin to chest and swallows.

ACTION	RATIONALE
11. **Discontinue procedure and remove tube if there are signs of distress, such as gasping, coughing, cyanosis, and inability to speak or hum.**	The tube is in the airway if the patient shows signs of distress and cannot speak or hum. If after three attempts, nasogastric insertion is unsuccessful, another nurse may try or the patient should be referred to another healthcare professional.
12. **While keeping one hand on tube or temporarily securing with tape, determine that tube is in patient's stomach:**	Keeping one hand on the tube or temporarily securing with tape stabilizes the tube while position is being determined.
a. Attach syringe to end of tube and aspirate a small amount of stomach **contents.** (Figure 6).	The tube is in the stomach if its contents can be aspirated: pH of aspirate can then be tested to determine gastric placement. If unable to obtain specimen, reposition the patient and flush the tube with 30 mL of air. This action may be necessary several times. Current literature recommends that the nurse ensures proper placement of the NG tube by relying on multiple methods and not on one method alone.

SKILL 11-2 **Inserting a Nasogastric Tube** *(continued)*

ACTION	RATIONALE
b. Measure the pH of aspirated fluid using pH paper or a meter. Place a drop of gastric secretions onto pH paper or place small amount in plastic cup and dip the pH paper into it. Within 30 seconds, compare the color on the paper with the chart supplied by the manufacturer (Figure 7).	Current research demonstrates that the use of pH is predictive of correct placement. The pH of gastric contents is acidic (less than 5.5). If patient is taking an acid-inhibiting agent, the range may be 4.0 to 6.0. The pH of intestinal fluid is 7.0 or higher. The pH of respiratory fluid is 6.0 or higher. This method will not effectively differentiate between intestinal fluid and pleural fluid.
c. Visualize aspirated contents, checking for color and consistency.	Gastric fluid can be green with particles, off white, or brown if old blood is present. Intestinal aspirate tends to look clear or straw-colored to a deep golden-yellow color. Also, intestinal aspirate may be greenish-brown if stained with bile. Respiratory or tracheobronchial fluid is usually off-white to tan and may be tinged with mucus (Metheny & Titler, 2001). A small amount of blood-tinged fluid may be seen immediately after NG insertion.
d. Obtain radiograph (x-ray) of placement of tube (as ordered by physician).	The x-ray is considered the most reliable method for identifying the position of the NG tube.

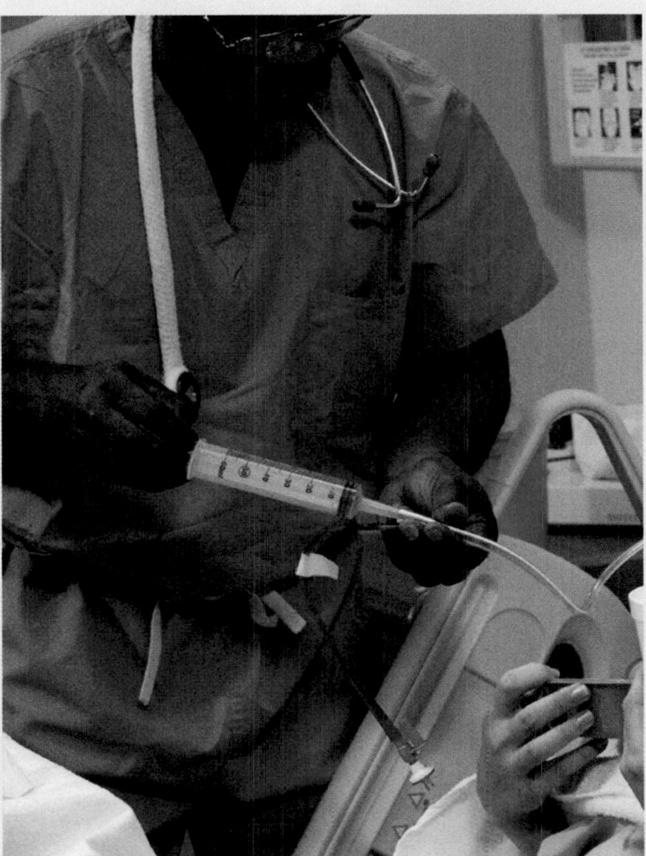
Figure 6. Aspirating to obtain gastric fluid.

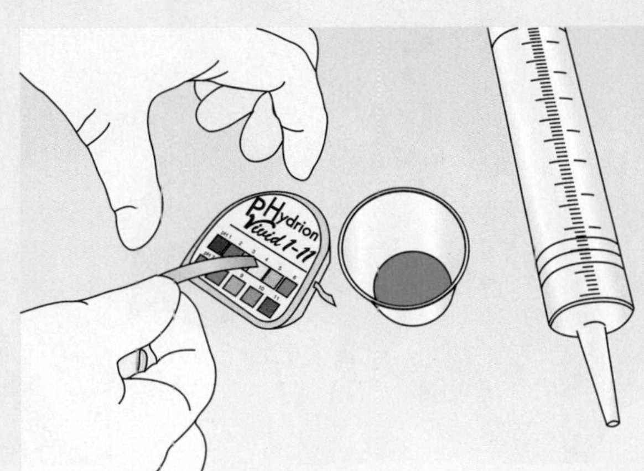

Figure 7. Checking pH of gastric fluid.

(continued)

SKILL 11-2 Inserting a Nasogastric Tube *(continued)*

ACTION | **RATIONALE**

13. Apply tincture of benzoin or other skin adhesive to tip of nose and allow to dry. Secure tube with tape to patient's nose:
    a. Cut a 4″ piece of tape and split bottom 2″ or use packaged nose tape for NG tubes (Figure 8).
    b. Place unsplit end over bridge of patient's nose (Figure 9).
    c. Wrap split ends under tubing and up and over onto nose (Figure 2). **Be careful not to pull tube too tightly against nose.**

Rationale: Tincture of benzoin or skin adhesive facilitates attachment of tape. Constant pressure of the tube against the skin and mucous membranes causes tissue injury.

14. Clamp tube and cap or attach tube to suction (Figure 11) according to the physician's orders.

Rationale: Suction provides for decompression of stomach and drainage of gastric contents.

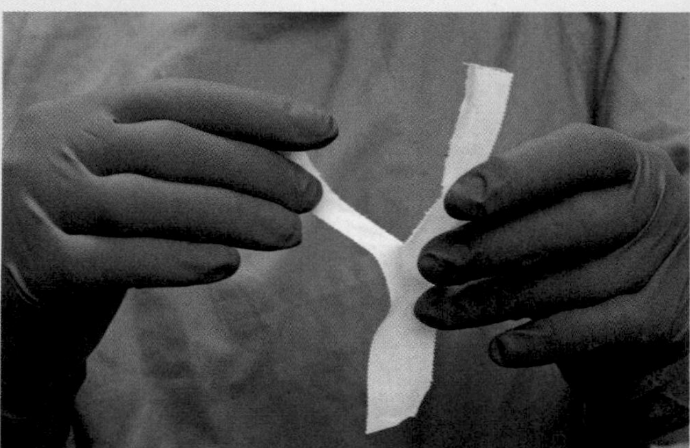

Figure 8. Making a 2″ cut into a 4″ strip of tape.

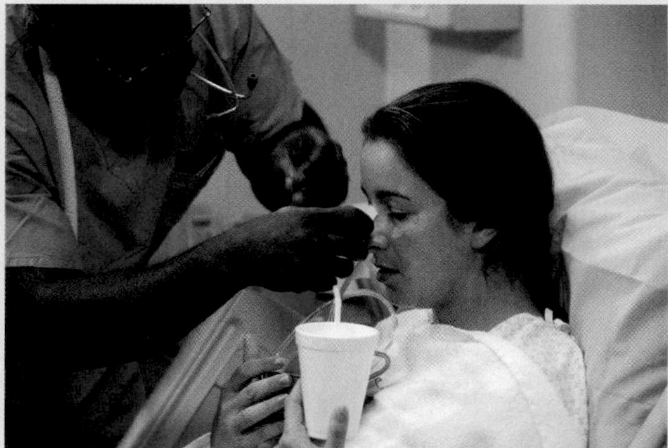

Figure 9. Applying tape to patient's nose.

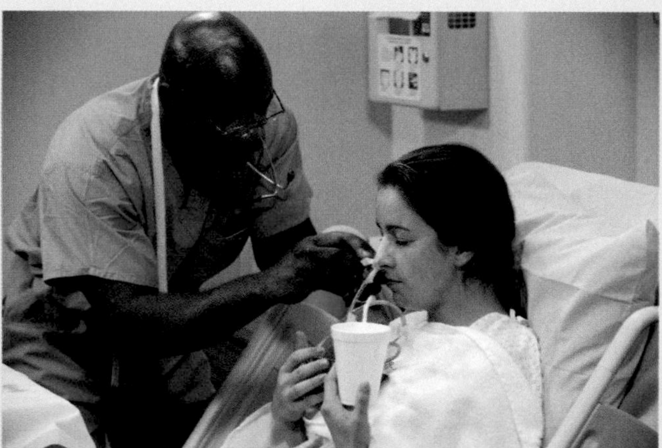

Figure 10. Wrapping split ends around NG tube.

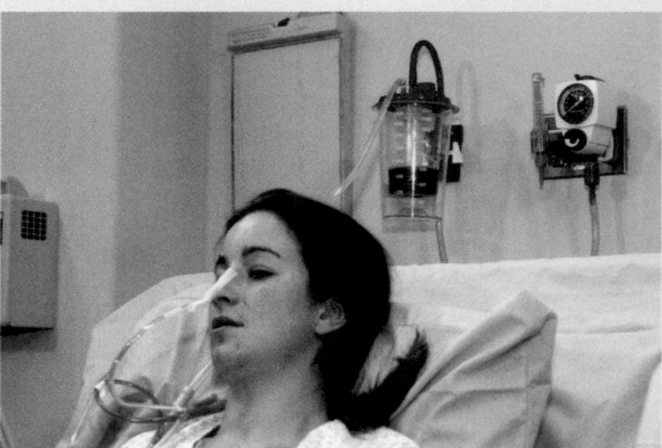

Figure 11. Attaching NG tube to wall suction.

SKILL 11-2 Inserting a Nasogastric Tube *(continued)*

ACTION	RATIONALE
15. Secure tube to patient's gown by using rubber band or tape and safety pin. For additional support, tube can be taped onto patient's cheek using a piece of tape. **If double-lumen tube (eg, Salem sump) is used, secure vent above stomach level.** Attach at shoulder level (Figure 12).	This prevents tension and tugging on the tube. Securing the double-lumen tube above stomach level prevents seepage of gastric contents and keeps the lumen clear for venting air.

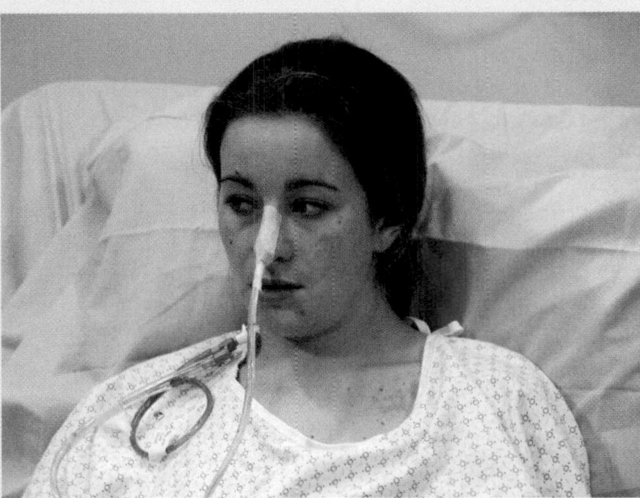

Figure 12. Patient with Salem sump tube (NG) secured. Note blue vent at patient's shoulder.

ACTION	RATIONALE
16. Assist with or provide oral hygiene at every 2- to 4-hour intervals. Lubricate the lips generously and clean nares and lubricate as needed. Offer analgesic throat lozenges or anesthetic spray for throat irritation if needed.	Oral hygiene keeps mouth clean and moist, promotes comfort, and reduces thirst.
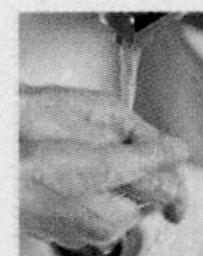 17. Remove all equipment, lower the bed, and make the patient comfortable. Remove non-sterile gloves and perform hand hygiene.	Hand hygiene deters the spread of microorganisms.

EVALUATION

The expected outcome is met when patient exhibits a nasogastric tube placed into the stomach without any complications. In addition, other outcomes are met when patient demonstrates weight gain, indicating improved nutrition; patient remains free of any signs and symptoms of aspiration; patient rates pain as decreased from prior to insertion; and patient verbalizes an understanding of the reason for NG tube insertion.

DOCUMENTATION

Guidelines

Document the size and type of NG tube that was inserted and the measurement from tip of the nose to the end of the tube. Also, document the results of an x-ray that was taken to confirm the position of the tube. Record a description of the gastric contents, including the pH of the contents. Document the naris where the tube is placed and the patient's response to the procedure. Include assessment data both subjective and objective related to the abdomen. Record the patient teaching that was discussed.

(continued)

SKILL 11-2 Inserting a Nasogastric Tube *(continued)*

Sample Documentation

10/4/08 0945 16 Fr. Salem sump tube inserted via R naris, 20 cm of tube from naris to end of tube; gastric contents aspirated, pH 4, contents light green; patient tolerated without incident; tube attached to low intermittent suction as ordered.—S. Essner, RN

Unexpected Situations and Associated Interventions

- *As tube is passing through pharynx, patient begins to retch and gag:* This is common during placement of an NG tube. Ask the patient if he/she wants the nurse to stop the procedure, allowing the patient to gain composure from the gagging episode. Continue to advance tube if the patient relates that he/she agrees. Have the emesis basin nearby in case patient begins to vomit.
- *The nurse is unable to pass the tube after trying a second time down the one nostril:* If the patient's condition permits, inspect the other nostril and attempt to pass the nasogastric tube down this nostril. If unable to pass down this nostril, consult another health professional.
- *As tube is passing through pharynx, patient begins to cough and shows signs of respiratory distress:* **Stop advancing the tube!** The tube is most likely entering the trachea. Pull tube back into nasal area. Support patient as he/she regains normal breathing ability and composure. If patient feels that he/she can tolerate another attempt, ask patient to keep chin on chest and swallow as tube is advanced to help prevent the tube from entering the trachea. Begin to advance tube, watching for any signs of respiratory distress.
- *No gastric contents can be aspirated:* If patient is comatose, check oral cavity. If tube is in gastric area, small air boluses may need to be given until gastric contents can be aspirated.

Special Considerations

Some patients require a nasointestinal tube. To insert a nasointestinal tube:

- Measure tube from tip of nose to ear lobe and from ear lobe to xiphoid process. Add 8″ to 10″ for intestinal placement. Mark tubing at desired point.
- Place patient on his or her right side. Nasointestinal tube is usually placed in the stomach and allowed to advance through peristalsis through the pyloric sphincter (may take up to 24 hours).
- Administer medications to enhance GI motility, such as metoclopramide (Reglan), if ordered.
- Test pH of aspirate when tube has advanced to marked point to confirm placement in intestine. Confirm position by radiograph. Secure with tape once placement is confirmed.

SKILL 11-3 Administering a Tube Feeding

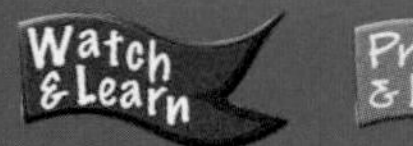

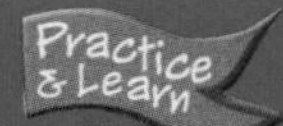

Depending on the patient's physical and psychosocial condition and nutritional requirements, a feeding through the NG tube or other GI tube might be ordered. The steps for administering feedings are similar regardless of the tube used.

Feeding can be provided on an intermittent or continuous basis. If the order calls for continuous feeding, an external feeding pump is needed to regulate the flow of formula. Intermittent feedings are delivered at regular intervals, using gravity for instillation or a feeding pump to administer the formula over a set period of time. Intermittent feedings might also be given as a bolus, using a syringe to instill the formula quickly in one large amount.

The below procedure describes using open systems and a feeding pump; the skill variation at the end of the skill describes using a closed system.

Equipment

- Tube feeding at room temperature
- Feeding bag or prefilled tube feeding set
- Stethoscope

SKILL 11-3 Administering a Tube Feeding *(continued)*

- Nonsterile gloves
- Alcohol preps
- Disposable pad or towel
- Asepto or Toomey syringe
- Enteral feeding pump (if ordered)
- Rubber band
- Clamp (Hoffman or butterfly)
- IV pole
- Water for irrigation and hydration as needed
- pH paper

ASSESSMENT

Assess abdomen by inspecting for presence of distention, auscultating for bowel sounds, and palpating the abdomen for firmness or tenderness. If the abdomen is distended, consider measuring the abdominal girth at the umbilicus. If the patient reports any tenderness or nausea, exhibits any rigidity or firmness of the abdomen, and if there is an absence of bowel sounds, confer with physician before administering the tube feeding. Assess for patient and/or family understanding if appropriate for the rationale for the tube feeding and address any questions or concerns expressed by the patient and family members. Consult physician if need for further explanation.

NURSING DIAGNOSIS

Determine the related factors for the nursing diagnoses based on the patient's current status. The most common nursing diagnosis would be Imbalanced Nutrition, Less than Body Requirements. Additional nursing diagnoses may include Risk for Aspiration, Deficient Knowledge, Risk for Impaired Social Interaction, Risk for Alteration in Nutrition, Risk for Body Image Disturbance.

OUTCOME IDENTIFICATION AND PLANNING

The expected outcome to achieve when administering a tube feeding is that the patient will receive the tube feeding without complaints of nausea or episodes of vomiting. Additional expected outcomes may include the following: the patient demonstrates an increase in weight; the patient exhibits no signs and symptoms of aspiration; and the patient verbalizes knowledge related to tube feeding.

IMPLEMENTATION

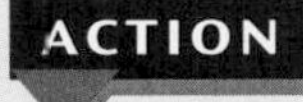

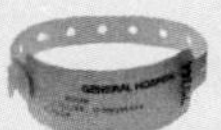

ACTION	RATIONALE
1. Identify the patient.	Identification of the patient ensures that the right patient receives the correct tube feeding as ordered.
2. Explain the procedure to the patient and why this intervention is needed. Raise the bed. Pull the patient's bedside curtain. Perform key abdominal assessments as described above.	Patient cooperation is facilitated when explanations are provided. Provide for privacy. Raising the bed promotes the comfort and proper body mechanics of the nurse. Due to changes in patient's condition, assessment is vital before initiating the intervention.
3. Assemble equipment. Check amount, concentration, type, and frequency of tube feeding on patient's chart. Check expiration date of formula.	This provides for organized approach to task. Checking ensures that correct feeding will be administered. Standard formulas consist of molecules of protein, carbohydrates, and fats; other formulas are available in simpler forms if patient's condition warrants. Outdated formula may be contaminated.

(continued)

SKILL 11-3 Administering a Tube Feeding *(continued)*

ACTION	RATIONALE
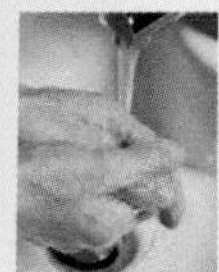 4. Perform hand hygiene. Put on nonsterile gloves.	Hand hygiene deters the spread of microorganisms. Gloves protect nurse from exposure to blood or body substances.
5. **Position patient with head of bed elevated at least 30 to 45 degrees or as near normal position for eating as possible.**	This position minimizes possibility of aspiration into trachea. Patients who are considered at high risk for aspiration should be assisted to a 45-degree position.
6. Unpin tube from patient's gown. **Check to see that the NG tube is properly located in the stomach, by first instilling air, then aspirate for gastric contents (Figure 1).** At times, due to the tendency of small-bore tubes to collapse upon aspiration, several attempts may be necessary to aspirate gastric contents. After repeated instillations of 30 mL of air, accompanied by repositioning the patient, if unable to aspirate gastric contents, the tube placement should be checked by radiograph verified by physician's order. Check the pH as described in Skill 11-2.	Even when initially positioned correctly, an NG tube left in place can become dislodged between feedings. The instillation of water or nourishment could lead to serious respiratory problems if a gastric tube is in the trachea or a bronchus rather than in the stomach. Research findings point out that aspiration is easier in small-bore tubes, such as a Dobhoff, when multiple ports rather than a single port are available. The testing for pH before the next feeding in intermittent feedings is conducted since the stomach has been emptied of the feeding formula. However, if the patient is receiving continuous feedings, the pH measurement is not useful since the formula raises the pH.

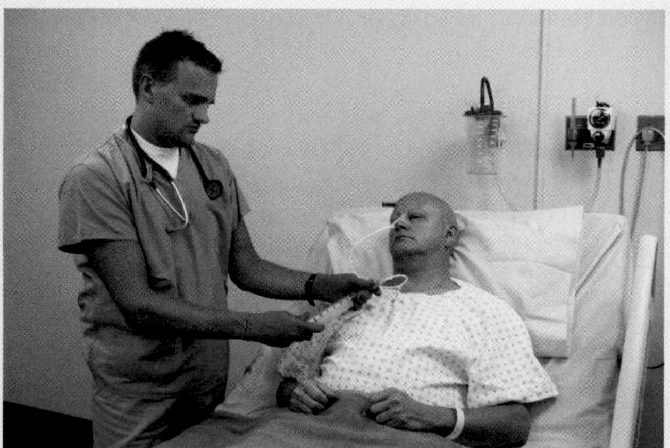

Figure 1. Aspirating gastric contents.

ACTION	RATIONALE
7. After multiple steps have been taken to ensure that the feeding tube is located in the stomach or small intestine, **aspirate all gastric contents with a syringe and measure to check for the residual amount of feeding in the stomach.** Flush tube with 30 mL of water for irrigation. Proceed with feeding if amount of residual does not exceed agency policy or physician's guideline. Disconnect syringe from tubing and cap end of tubing while preparing the formula feeding equipment. Remove gloves.	**Checking for residual before each feeding or every 4 to 6 hours during a continuous feeding according to institutional policy is implemented to identify delayed gastric emptying.** Capping the tube deters the entry of microorganisms and prevents leakage onto the bed linens.
8. Put on nonsterile gloves before preparing, assembling and handling any part of the feeding system.	
9. Administer feeding.	

SKILL 11-3

Administering a Tube Feeding *(continued)*

ACTION	RATIONALE
When Using a Feeding Bag (Open System)	
a. Hang bag on IV pole and adjust to about 12″ above the stomach. Clamp tubing.	Proper feeding bag height reduces risk of formula being introduced too quickly.
b. Check the expiration date of the formula. Cleanse top of feeding container with a disinfectant before opening it (Figure 2). **Pour formula into feeding bag and allow solution to run through tubing.** Close clamp.	Cleansing container top with alcohol minimizes risk for contaminants entering feeding bag. Formula displaces air in tubing.
c. Attach feeding setup to feeding tube, open clamp, and regulate drip according to physician's order, or allow feeding to run in over 30 minutes (Figure 3).	Introducing formula at a slow, regular rate allows the stomach to accommodate to the feeding and decreases GI distress.
d. **Add 30 to 60 mL (1–2 oz) of water for irrigation to feeding bag when feeding is almost completed and allow it to run through the tube (Figure 4).**	Water rinses the feeding from the tube and helps to keep it patent.
e. Clamp tubing immediately after water has been instilled. Disconnect from feeding tube. Clamp tube and cover end with cap (Figure 5).	Clamping the tube prevents air from entering the stomach. Capping tube deters entry of microorganisms and covering end of tube protects patient and linens from fluid leakage from tube.

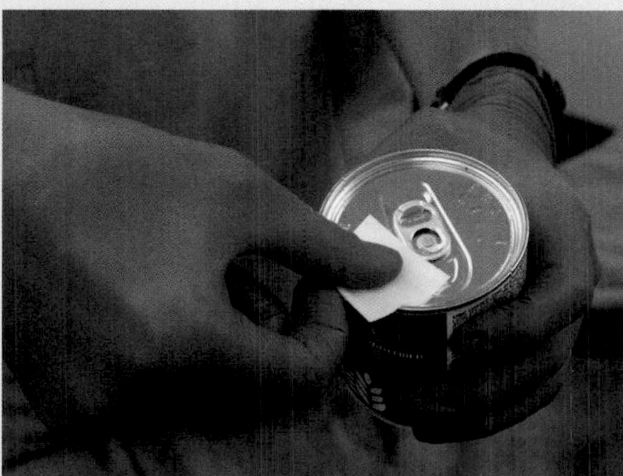

Figure 2. Cleaning top of feeding container with alcohol before opening it.

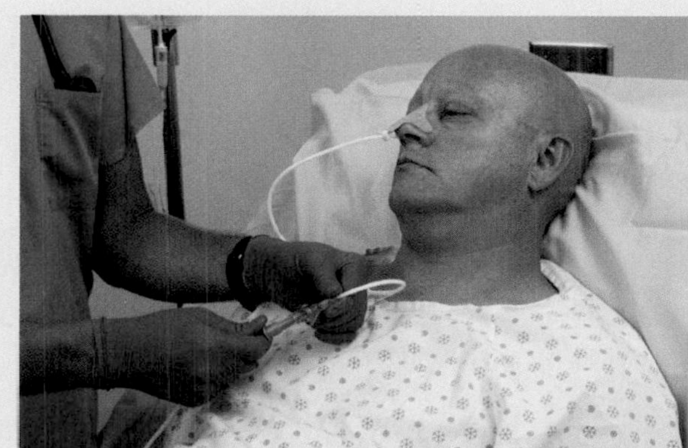

Figure 3. Attaching feeding bag tubing to NG tube.

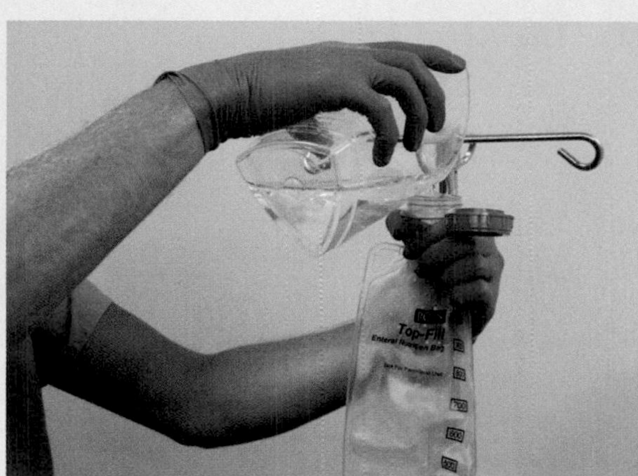

Figure 4. Pouring water into feeding bag.

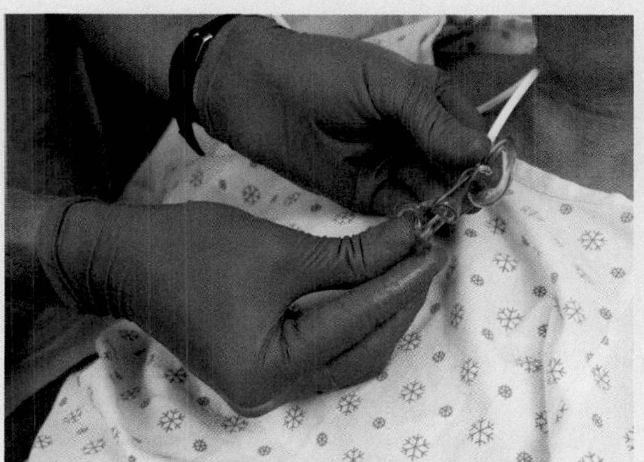

Figure 5. Capping NG tube after it is clamped.

(continued)

SKILL 11-3

Administering a Tube Feeding *(continued)*

ACTION	RATIONALE
When Using a Large Syringe (Open System)	
a. Remove plunger from 30- or 60-mL syringe (Figure 6).	
b. Attach syringe to feeding tube, pour premeasured amount of tube feeding into syringe (Figure 7), open clamp, and allow food to enter tube. **Regulate rate, fast or slow, by height of the syringe. Do not push formula with syringe plunger.**	Introducing the formula at a slow, regular rate allows the stomach to accommodate to the feeding and decreases GI distress. The higher the syringe is held, the faster the formula flows.
c. **Add 30 to 60 mL (1–2 oz) of water for irrigation to syringe (Figure 8) when feeding is almost completed, and allow it to run through the tube.**	Water rinses the feeding from the tube and helps to keep it patent.
d. When syringe has emptied, hold syringe high and disconnect from tube. Clamp tube and cover end with cap.	By holding syringe high, the formula will not backflow out of tube and onto patient. Clamping the tube prevents air from entering the stomach. Capping end of tube deters entry of microorganisms. Covering the end protects patient and linens from fluid leakage from tube.
	Continuous feedings permit gradual introduction of the formula into the GI tract, promoting maximal absorption. However, there is a risk of both reflux and aspiration with this method. Intermittent feedings are the preferred method introducing the formula over a set period of time via gravity or pump.

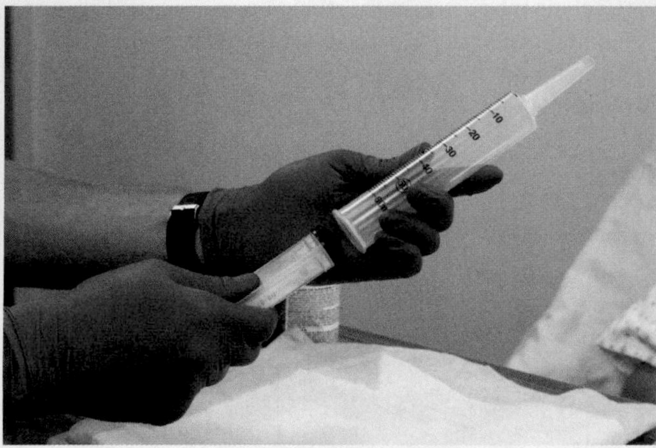

Figure 6. Removing plunger from a 60-cc syringe.

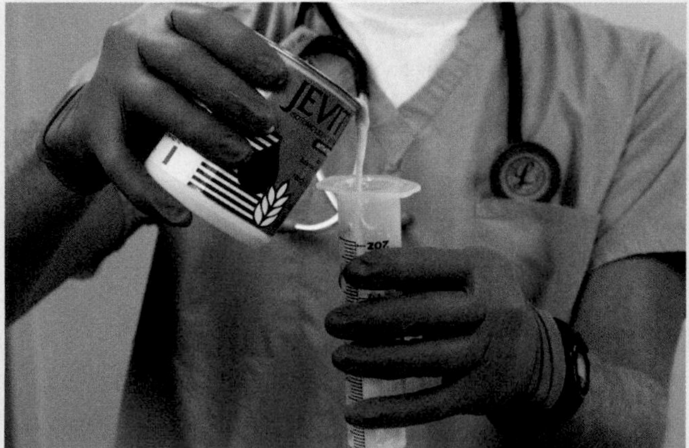

Figure 7. Pouring formula into syringe.

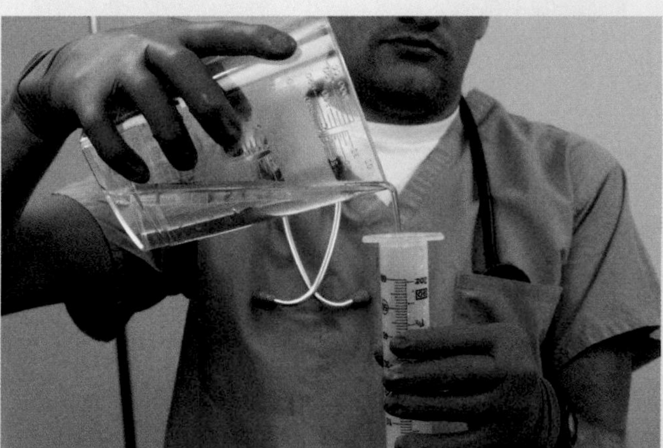

Figure 8. Pouring water into almost empty syringe.

SKILL 11-3 **Administering a Tube Feeding** *(continued)*

ACTION | **RATIONALE**

When Using an Enteral Feeding Pump

a. Close flow-regulator clamp on tubing and fill feeding bag with prescribed formula. Amount used depends on agency policy. Place label on container with patient's name, date, and time the feeding was hung.

Feeding intolerance is less likely to occur with smaller volumes. Hanging smaller amounts of feeding also reduces risk for bacteria growth and contamination of feeding at room temperature (when using open systems).

b. Hang feeding container on IV pole. **Allow solution to flow through tubing.**

This prevents air from being forced into the stomach or intestines.

c. Connect to feeding pump following manufacturer's directions. Set rate (Figure 9). Maintain the patient in the upright position throughout the feeding. If the patient needs to temporarily lie flat, the feeding should be paused. The feeding may be resumed after the patient's position has been changed back to 30 to 45 degrees.

Feeding pumps vary. Some of the newer pumps have built-in safeguards that protect the patient from complications. Safety features include cassettes that prevent free-flow of formula, automatic tube flush, safety tips that prevent accidental attachment to an IV setup, and various audible and visible alarms. Feedings are started at full strength rather than diluting the feeding, which was previously recommended. A smaller volume, 10 to 40 mL, of feeding infused per hour and gradually increased has been shown to be more easily tolerated by patients.

d. **Check residual every 4 to 8 hours.**

Checking verifies placement of the tube and proper absorption of the feeding and prevents distention, which could lead to aspiration. However, presence of large amounts of residual, such as more than 200 to 400 cc, should not be the sole criteria for stopping the enteral feeding as described in Step 7.

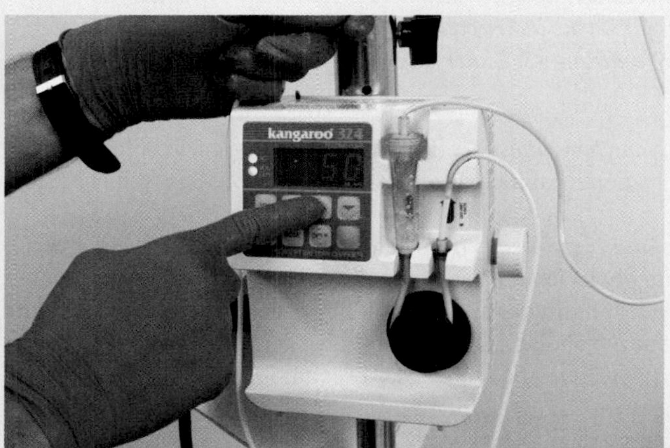

Figure 9. Setting up feeding pump with feeding bag and primed tubing.

10. Observe the patient's response during and after tube feeding and assess the abdomen at least once a shift.

Pain or nausea may indicate stomach distention, which may lead to vomiting. Physical signs such as abdominal distention and firmness or regurgitation of tube feeding may indicate intolerance.

11. **Have patient remain in upright position for at least 1 hour after feeding.**

This position minimizes risk for backflow and discourages aspiration, if any reflux or vomiting should occur.

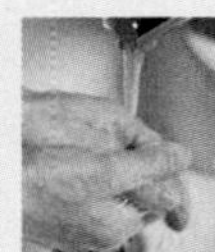

12. Wash and clean equipment or replace according to agency policy. Remove gloves and perform hand hygiene.

This prevents contamination and deters spread of microorganisms. Closed systems can be used up to 48 hours. Reusable systems are cleansed with soap and water every 24 hours and replaced every 24 hours. Refer to agency's policy and manufacturers' guidelines for specifics on equipment care.

(continued)

SKILL 11-3 Administering a Tube Feeding *(continued)*

EVALUATION

The expected outcome is achieved when the patient receives the ordered tube feeding without complaints of nausea or episodes of vomiting. The patient demonstrates an increase in weight; the patient remains free of any signs and symptoms of aspiration; and the patient voices knowledge related to tube feeding.

DOCUMENTATION

Guidelines

Document the type of nasogastric tube or gastrostomy/jejunostomy tube that is present. Record the criteria that were used to confirm proper placement before feeding was initiated, such as the tube length in inches or centimeters compared to the length on initial insertion. Document the aspiration of gastric contents and pH and bilirubin of the gastric contents when intermittent feeding is used. Note the components of the abdominal assessment, such as observation of the abdomen, presence of distention or firmness, and presence of bowel sounds. Include subjective data such as any reports from the patient such as abdominal pain or nausea or any other patient response. Record the amount of residual volume that was obtained. Document the position of the patient, the type of feeding, and the method and the amount of feeding. Include any relevant patient teaching.

Sample Documentation

10/29/08 1015 Position of NG tube was compared with initial measurement on insertion. Abdomen nondistended and soft; patient denies pain or nausea. HOB raised to 45 degrees. 150 mL of (Jevity 1.2 Cal.) administered via bolus feeding. 30 mL residual aspirated prior to feeding. Aspirate returned to stomach. Tube flushed with 60 mL water with ease. Patient instructed to call for nurse for pain or nausea or other concerns related to feeding.—S. Essner, RN

Unexpected Situations and Associated Interventions

- *Tube is found not to be in stomach or intestine:* Tube must be in stomach before feeding. If tube is in esophagus, patient is at increased risk for aspiration. See Skill 11-2 for steps to replace tube.
- *When checking for residue, nurse aspirates a large amount:* Before discarding or replacing residue, check with physician and agency policy. Replacing a large amount may increase patient's risk for vomiting and aspiration, while discarding a large amount may increase patient's risk for metabolic alkalosis. At times, the physician will order the nurse to replace half of the residue and recheck in a set amount of time.
- *Patient complains of nausea after tube feeding:* Ensure that head of bed remains elevated and that suction equipment is at bedside. Check medication record to see if any antiemetics have been ordered for patient. Consider notifying the physician for an order for an antiemetic.
- *When attempting to aspirate contents, nurse notes that tube is clogged:* Most obstructions are caused by coagulation of formula. Try using warm water and gentle pressure to remove clog. Carbonated sodas, such as Coca Cola, and meat tenderizers have not been shown effective in removing clogs in feeding tubes. Never use a stylet to unclog tubes. Tube may have to be replaced. To prevent clogs, ensure that adequate flushing is completed after feedings.

Special Considerations

General Considerations

- Step 7 above explains checking for the residual amount of feeding in the stomach. New research is suggesting to continue the feedings with residuals up to 400 mL. If greater than 400 mL, confer with physician or hold feedings according to agency policy. For patients who are experiencing gastric dysfunction or decreased level of consciousness, feedings may be held for smaller residual amounts (<400 mL) (Keithley & Swanson, 2004). Also, current research findings are inconclusive on the benefit of returning gastric

SKILL 11-3 Administering a Tube Feeding *(continued)*

volumes to the stomach or intestine to avoid fluid or electrolyte, which has been accepted practice. Consult agency policy concerning this practice. Some researchers point out that high residual volumes are not indicative of intolerance to the tube feeding. In contrast, low residual volumes do not guarantee that patients are tolerating enteral tube feedings and are not at risk for aspiration (McClave et al, 2005). Monitoring for trends in gradually increasing amounts of residual volumes and assessing for other signs of intolerance such as gastric pain or distention should be implemented.

- When the patient with dementia and family, as appropriate, is deciding on whether to agree to tube feeding nutrition, inform them that research is recommending that tube feedings not be used for this population of patients since they do not increase survival or prevent malnutrition or aspiration. It is suggested to use such methods to increase feeding assistance and change the food consistency as needed (Keithley & Swanson, 2004).

SKILL VARIATION Using a Prefilled Tube Feeding Set (Closed System)

Prefilled tube feeding solutions, which are considered closed systems, are frequently used to provide patient nourishment (Figure 1). Closed systems contain sterile feeding solutions in ready-to-hang containers. This method reduces the opportunity for bacterial contamination of the feeding formula. In general, these prefilled feedings are administered via an enteral pump.

- Verify the physician's order.
- Gather all equipment, checking the feeding solution and container for correct solution and expiration date. Label with patient's name, type of solution, and prescribed rate.
- Identify the patient and explain the procedure.
- Ensure the correct placement of the feeding tube through aspiration of stomach contents and checking for gastric or intestinal pH.
- Check for residual amount of feeding in the stomach and return residual as ordered.
- Flush tube with 30 mL of water.
- Put on nonsterile gloves and remove screw on cap, and attach administration setup with drip chamber and tubing.
- Hang feeding container on IV pole and connect to feeding pump, allowing solution to flow through tubing, following manufacturer's directions.
- Attach the feeding set-up to the patient's feeding tube.
- Open the clamp of the patient's feeding tube.
- Turn on the pump.
- Set the pump at the prescribed rate of flow and remove the nonsterile gloves.
- Observe the patient's response during the tube feeding.
- Continue to assess the patient for signs and symptoms of gastrointestinal distress, such as nausea, abdominal distention, or absence of bowel sounds.
- Have patient remain in the upright position throughout the feeding and for at least 1 hour after feeding. If patient's position needs to be changed to a supine position or turned in bed, pause the feeding pump during this time.
- After the prescribed amount of feeding has been administrated or according to agency policy, turn off the pump, put on nonsterile gloves, clamp the feeding tube, and disconnect the feeding tube from the feeding set tube, capping the end of the feeding set.
- Draw up 30 to 60 mL of water using a syringe.
- Attach the syringe to the feeding tube, unclamp the feeding tube, and instill the 30 to 60 mL of water into the feeding tube.
- Clamp the feeding tube.
- Remove equipment according to agency policy.
- Provide for any patient needs.
- Remove gloves and perform hand hygiene.

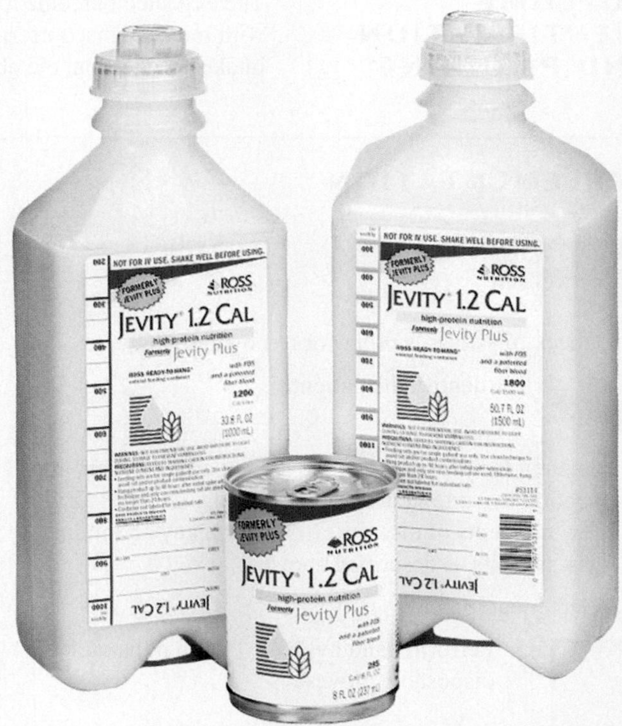

Prefilled tube feedings in plastic containers and ready-to-use feeding in a can. (Reprinted with permission from Abbott Laboratories, Ross Products Division.)

SKILL 11-4 Removing a Nasogastric Tube

When the NG tube is no longer necessary for treatment, the physician will order the tube to be removed. The NG tube is removed as carefully as it was inserted, to provide as much comfort as possible for the patient and to prevent complications. When the tube is removed, the patient must hold his or her breath to prevent aspiration of any secretions or fluid left in the tube as it is removed.

Equipment

- Tissues
- 50-mL syringe (optional)
- Nonsterile disposable gloves
- Stethoscope
- Disposable plastic bag
- Bath towel or disposable pad
- Normal saline solution for irrigation (optional)
- Emesis basin

ASSESSMENT

Perform an abdominal assessment by inspecting for presence of distention, auscultating for bowel sounds, and palpating the abdomen for firmness or tenderness. If the abdomen is distended, consider measuring the abdominal girth at the umbilicus. If the patient reports any tenderness or nausea, exhibits any rigidity or firmness with distention, and if there is an absence of bowel sounds, confer with physician before discontinuing the NG tube.

Also assess any output from the NG tube, noting amount, color, and consistency.

NURSING DIAGNOSIS

Determine the related factors for the nursing diagnoses based on the patient's current status. Possible nursing diagnoses may be Readiness for Enhanced Nutrition and Risk for Aspiration.

OUTCOME IDENTIFICATION AND PLANNING

The expected outcome to achieve when removing a NG tube is that the tube is removed with minimal discomfort to the patient, and the patient maintains an adequate nutritional intake. In addition, the abdomen remains free from distention and tenderness.

IMPLEMENTATION

ACTION	RATIONALE
1. Check physician's order for removal of NG tube.	This ensures correct implementation of physician's order.
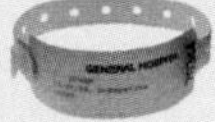 2. Identify the patient.	Identification of the patient ensures that the right patient receives the correct intervention as ordered.
3. Explain the procedure to the patient and why this intervention is warranted. Describe that it will entail a quick few moments of discomfort. Perform key abdominal assessments as described above.	Patient cooperation is facilitated when explanations are provided. Due to changes in patient's condition, assessment is vital before initiating intervention.
4. Gather equipment.	This provides for an organized approach to the task.
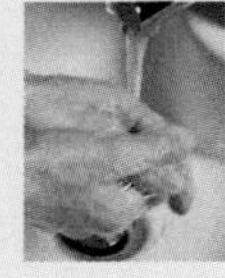 5. Perform hand hygiene. Put on nonsterile disposable gloves.	Hand hygiene deters the spread of microorganisms. Gloves protect nurse's hands from contact with abdominal secretions.

SKILL 11-4 Removing a Nasogastric Tube *(continued)*

ACTION	RATIONALE
6. Pull the patient's bedside curtain. Raise the bed to the appropriate height and place the patient in a 30- to 45-degree position. Place towel or disposable pad across patient's chest (Figure 1). Give tissues and emesis basin to patient.	Provide for privacy. Appropriate working height facilitates comfort and proper body mechanics for the nurse. This protects patient from contact with gastric secretions. Emesis basin is helpful if patient vomits or gags. Tissues are necessary if patient wants to blow his or her nose when tube is removed.
7. Discontinue suction and separate tube from suction. Unpin tube from patient's gown and carefully remove adhesive tape from patient's nose.	Disconnecting tube from suction and the patient allows for its unrestricted removal.
8. Check placement and **attach syringe and flush with 10 mL of water or normal saline solution (optional) or clear with 30 to 50 cc of air (Figure 2).**	Air or saline solution clears the tube of feeding or debris.

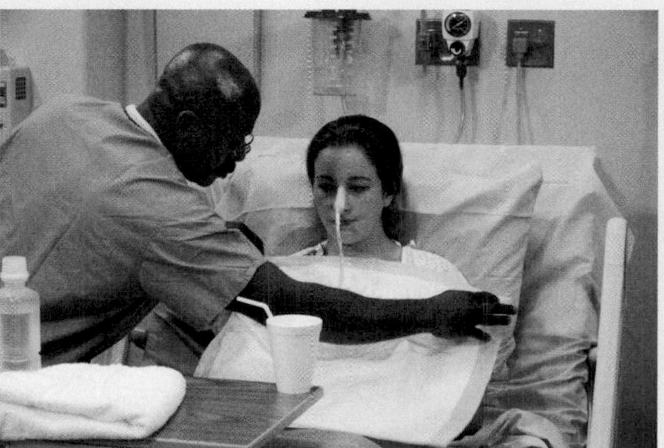

Figure 1. Placing towel or disposable pad across patient's chest.

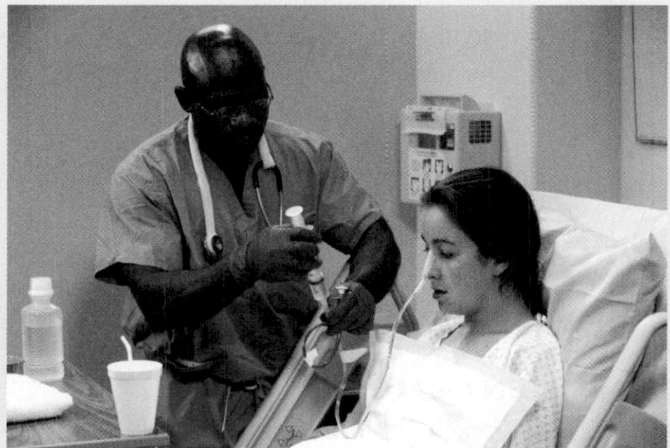

Figure 2. Flushing NG tube with 10 cc saline.

ACTION	RATIONALE
9. **Instruct patient to take a deep breath and hold it.**	This prevents accidental aspiration of gastric secretions in tube.
10. **Clamp tube with fingers by doubling tube on itself (Figure 3). Quickly and carefully remove tube while patient holds breath. Coil the tube in a disposable towel as you remove from the patient.**	Careful removal minimizes trauma and discomfort for patient. Clamping prevents drainage of gastric contents into the pharynx and esophagus. Containing the tube in a towel while removing prevents leakage onto the patient.
11. Dispose of tube per agency policy. Remove gloves and place in bag. Perform hand hygiene.	This prevents contamination with microorganisms. Follow the biohazard policy of the institution.
12. Offer mouth care to patient and facial tissue to blow nose. Lower the bed and assist the patient to a position of comfort as needed.	This provides for comfort.
13. Put on gloves and measure the amount of nasogastric drainage in the collection device and record on output flow record, subtracting irrigant fluids if necessary (Figure 4). Add solidifying agent to nasogastric drainage according to hospital policy.	Irrigation fluids are considered intake. To obtain the true nasogastric drainage, irrigant fluid amounts are subtracted from the total nasogastric drainage. Nasogastric drainage is recorded as part of the output of fluids from the patient. Solidifying agents added to liquid nasogastric drainage facilitate safe biohazard disposal.

(continued)

SKILL 11-4 Removing a Nasogastric Tube *(continued)*

ACTION | **RATIONALE**

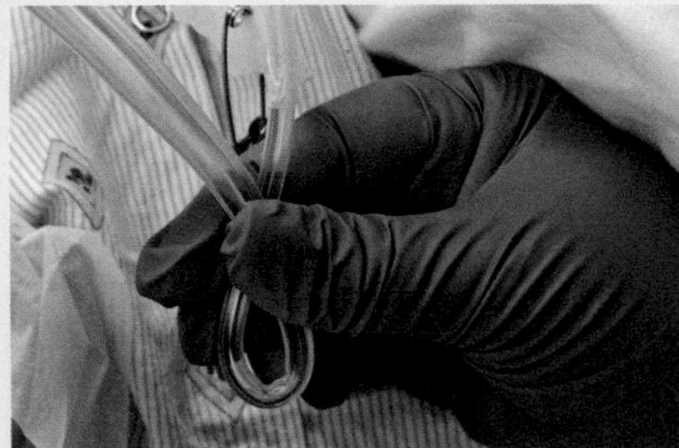

Figure 3. Doubling tube on itself.

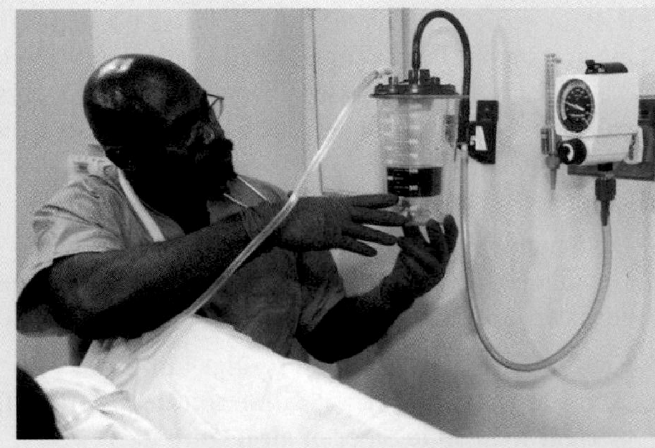

Figure 4. Measuring nasogastric drainage collection device.

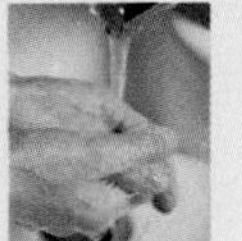

14. Remove gloves and perform hand hygiene.

Hand hygiene reduces transmission of microorganisms.

EVALUATION

The expected outcome is met when the patient experiences minimal discomfort and pain on NG tube removal. In addition, the patient's abdomen remains free from distention and tenderness, and the patient verbalizes measures to maintain an adequate nutritional intake.

DOCUMENTATION

Guidelines

Document assessment of the abdomen. If an abdominal girth reading was obtained, record this measurement. Document the removal of the nasogastric tube from the naris where it had been placed. Note if there is any irritation to the skin of the naris. Record the amount of NG drainage in the suction container on the patient's intake-and-output record as well as the color of the drainage. Record any pertinent teaching, such as instruction to patient to notify nurse if he/she experiences any nausea, abdominal pain, or bloating.

Sample Documentation

10/29/06 1320 NG tube removed from L naris without incident. 600 cc of dark brown liquid emptied from nasogastric tube. Patient's abdomen is 66 cm; abdomen is soft, nontender with hypoactive bowel sounds in all 4 quadrants.—S. Essner, RN

Unexpected Situations and Associated Interventions

- *Within 2 hours after NG tube removal, patient's abdomen is showing signs of distention:* Notify physician. Physician may order nurse to replace NG tube.
- *Epistaxis occurs with removal of NG tube:* Occlude both nares until bleeding has subsided. Ensure that patient is in upright position. Document epistaxis in patient's medical record.

SKILL 11-5 Irrigating a Nasogastric Tube Connected to Suction

NG tubes can be used to decompress the stomach and to monitor for GI bleeding. The tube is usually attached to suction when used for these reasons or the tube may be clamped. The tube must be kept free from obstruction or clogging and is usually irrigated every 4 to 8 hours.

Equipment

- NG tube connected to continuous or intermittent suction
- Normal saline solution for irrigation
- Nonsterile disposable gloves
- Irrigation set (Asepto or Toomey syringe and container or a 60-mL catheter-tip syringe and cup for irrigating solution)
- Clamp
- Disposable pad or bath towel
- Emesis basin
- pH paper and measurement scale

ASSESSMENT

Assess abdomen by inspecting for presence of distention, auscultating for bowel sounds, and palpating the abdomen for firmness or tenderness. If the abdomen is distended, consider measuring the abdominal girth at the umbilicus. If the patient reports any tenderness or nausea, confer with the physician. If the NG tube is attached to suction, assess suction to ensure that it is running at the prescribed pressure. Also, inspect drainage from NG tube, including color, consistency, and amount.

NURSING DIAGNOSIS

Determine the related factors for the nursing diagnoses based on the patient's current status. Possible nursing diagnoses may include Imbalanced Nutrition, Less than Body Requirements, and Risk for Injury, Nausea, Risk for Fluid Volume Deficit.

OUTCOME IDENTIFICATION AND PLANNING

The expected outcome to achieve when irrigating a patient's NG tube is that the tube will maintain patency with irrigation. In addition, the patient will not experience any trauma or injury.

IMPLEMENTATION

ACTION	RATIONALE
1. Check the physician's order.	This clarifies the schedule and irrigating solution.
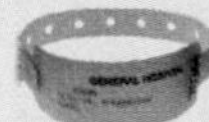 2. Identify the patient.	Identification of the patient ensures that the right patient receives the correct intervention as ordered.
3. Explain the procedure to the patient and why this intervention is warranted. Perform key abdominal assessments as described above.	Patient cooperation is facilitated when explanations are provided. Due to changes in patient's condition, assessment is vital before initiating intervention.
4. Gather necessary equipment. Check expiration dates on irrigating solution and irrigation set.	This provides for organized approach to task. Agency policy dictates safe interval for reuse of equipment.
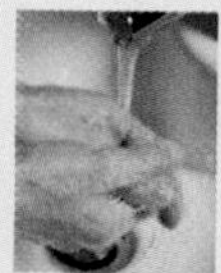 5. Perform hand hygiene. Put on gloves.	Hand hygiene and gloves deter the spread of microorganisms.
6. Pull the patient's bedside curtain. Raise the bed. Assist patient to 30- to 45-degree position, unless this is contraindicated.	Provide for privacy. Raising the bed promotes the comfort and proper body mechanics of the nurse. This position minimizes risk for aspiration.

(continued)

SKILL 11-5 Irrigating a Nasogastric Tube Connected to Suction *(continued)*

ACTION	RATIONALE
7. **Check placement of NG tube.** (Refer to Skill 11-2.)	
8. Pour irrigating solution into container. Draw up 30 mL of saline solution (or amount ordered by physician) into syringe (Figure 1).	This delivers measured amount of irrigant through tube. Saline solution (isotonic) compensates for electrolytes lost through nasogastric drainage.

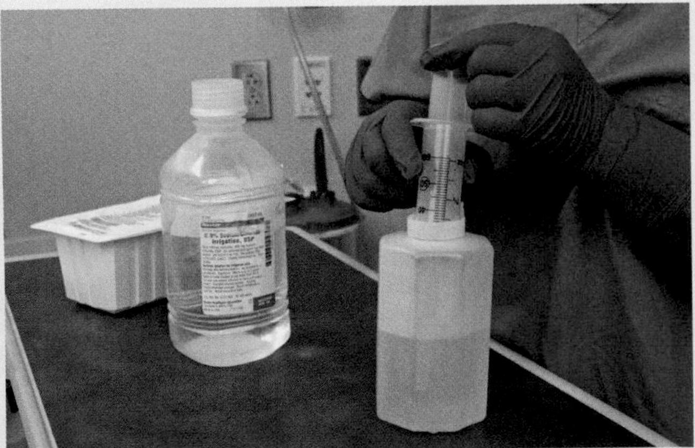

Figure 1. Preparing syringe with 30 mL saline for irrigation.

ACTION	RATIONALE
9. Clamp suction tubing near connection site (Figure 2). If needed, disconnect tube from suction apparatus and lay on disposable pad or towel, or hold both tubes upright in nondominant hand (Figure 3).	This protects patient from leakage of nasogastric drainage.

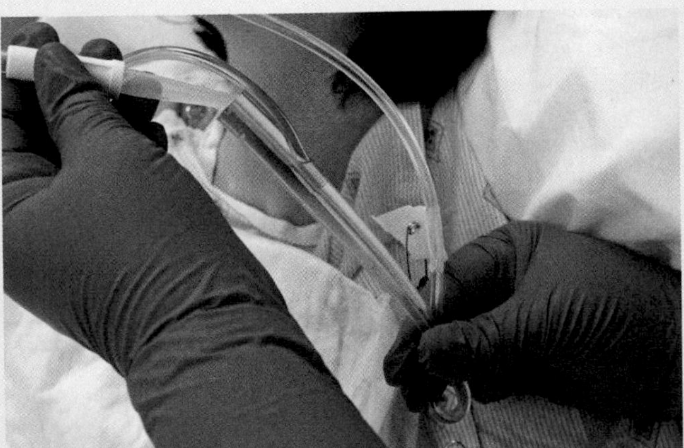

Figure 2. Clamping suction tube while disconnecting it from NG tube.

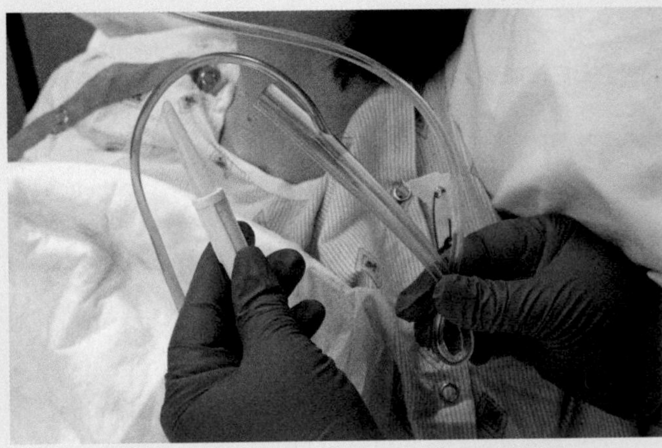

Figure 3. Holding both tubes upright to prevent backflow.

ACTION	RATIONALE
10. Place tip of syringe in tube. **If Salem sump or double-lumen tube is used, make sure that syringe tip is placed in drainage port and not in blue air vent.** Hold syringe upright and gently insert the irrigant (or allow solution to flow in by gravity if agency policy or physician indicates) (Figure 4). **Do not force solution into tube.**	Gentle insertion of saline solution (or gravity insertion) is less traumatic to gastric mucosa. The blue air vent acts to decrease pressure built up in the stomach when the Salem sump is attached to suction. It is not to be used for irrigation.

SKILL 11-5

Irrigating a Nasogastric Tube Connected to Suction *(continued)*

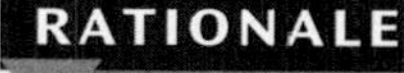

ACTION	RATIONALE

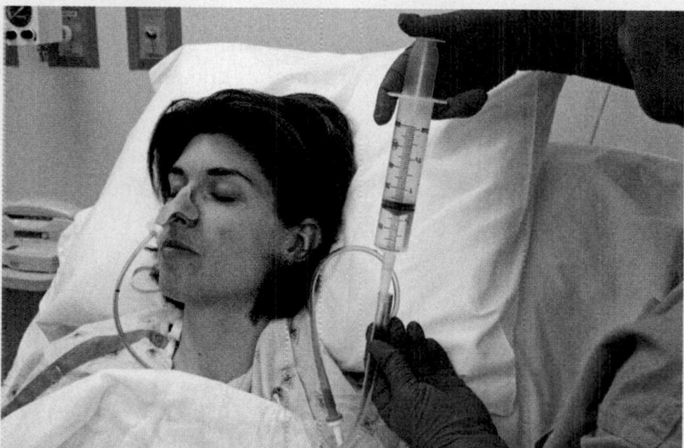

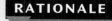

Figure 4. Gently instilling irrigation.

11. **If unable to irrigate tube, reposition patient and attempt irrigation again. Inject 10 to 20 cc of air and aspirate again (Figure 5). Check with physician or follow agency policy, if repeated attempts to irrigate tube fail.**

Tube may be positioned against gastric mucosa, making it difficult to irrigate. Injection of air may reposition end of tube.

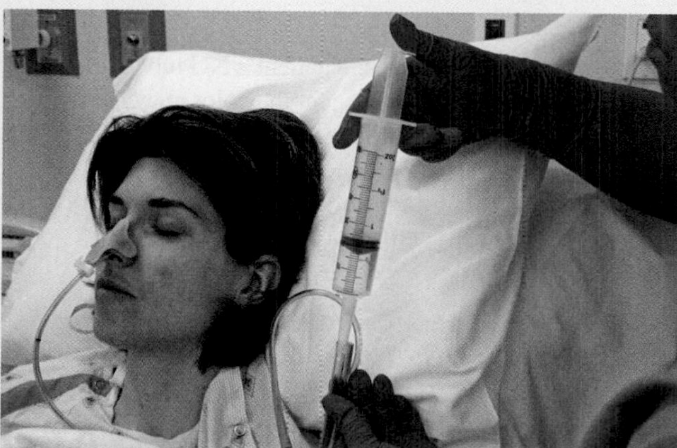

Figure 5. Injecting 10–20 cc of air into tube.

12. After irrigant has been instilled, observe for return flow of NG drainage into available container. Alternately, the nurse may reconnect the NG tube to suction and observe the return drainage as it drains into the suction container. **Inject air into blue air vent after irrigation is complete. Position the blue air vent above the patient's stomach.**

Return flow may be collected in an irrigating tray or other available container and measured. This amount will need to be subtracted from the irrigant to record the true NG drainage. A second method involves subtracting the total irrigant from the shift from the total NG drainage emptied over the entire shift, to find the true NG drainage. Check agency policy for guidelines.

Observation determines patency of tube and correct operation of suction apparatus.

Following irrigation, the blue air vent is injected with air to keep it clear. Positioning the blue air vent above the stomach prevents the stomach contents from leaking from the NG tube.

(continued)

SKILL 11-5 Irrigating a Nasogastric Tube Connected to Suction *(continued)*

ACTION	RATIONALE
13. Measure and record amount and description of irrigant and returned solution if measured at this time.	Irrigant placed in tube is considered intake; solution returned is recorded as output. Record on the intake and output record.
14. Rinse equipment if it will be reused. Label with the date, patient's name, room number, and purpose (for NG tube/irrigation). Remove gloves and perform hand hygiene.	This promotes cleanliness, infection control, and prepares equipment for next irrigation. Hand hygiene deters the spread of microorganisms.
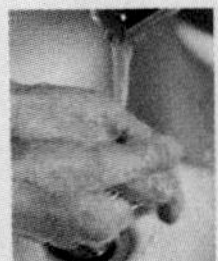 15. Lower the bed. Assist the patient to a position of comfort. Perform hand hygiene.	Lowering bed and assisting patient to a comfortable position promote safety and comfort. Hand hygiene deters the spread of microorganisms.

EVALUATION

The expected outcome is met when the patient demonstrates a patent and functioning NG tube. In addition, the patient reports no distress with irrigation. The patient remains free of any signs and symptoms of injury or trauma.

DOCUMENTATION

Guidelines

Document assessment of the patient's abdomen. Record if the patient's NG tube is clamped or connected to suction, including the type of suction. Document the color and consistency of the NG drainage. Record the solution used to irrigate the NG tube as well as ease of irrigation or if there was any difficulty related to the procedure. Record the patient's response to the procedure and any pertinent teaching points that were reviewed, such as to contact the nurse for any feelings of nausea, bloating, or abdominal pain.

Sample Documentation

10/15/08 1100 Abdomen slightly distended but soft, absent bowel sounds, denies nausea. NG tube placement confirmed; gastric contents Ph "4". NG irrigated with 30 mL of NS. NG reconnected to low intermittent suction. Clear drainage with brown flecks noted from tube. Patient tolerated irrigation without incident.—S. Essner, RN

Unexpected Situations and Associated Interventions

- *Flush solution is meeting a lot of force when plunger is pushed:* Inject 20 to 30 mL of free air into the abdomen in attempt to reposition the tube and enable the nurse to flush the tube.
- *Tube is connected to suction as ordered, but nothing is draining from tube:* First check the suction canister to ensure that the suction is working appropriately. Disconnect the NG tube from suction and place your gloved thumb over the end of the suction tubing. If there is suction present, the problem lies in the NG tube itself. Next, attempt to flush the tube to ensure patency of the tube.
- *After flushing the tube, the tube is not reconnected to suction as ordered:* Reconnect the tube to suction as soon as error is noticed. Assess the abdomen for distention and ask patient if he/she is experiencing any nausea or any abdominal discomfort. Complete any paperwork per institutional policy, such as an incident report.

SKILL 11-6 Caring for a Gastrostomy Tube

A gastrostomy tube may be inserted surgically via the abdomen into the stomach. Depending upon the patient's condition, this tube may be inserted into the jejunum. It is used for patients requiring long-term nutritional support. Special care is needed for the insertion site.

Equipment

- Nonsterile gloves
- Washcloth, towel, and soap
- Cotton-tipped applicators
- Sterile saline solution
- Gauze (if needed)

ASSESSMENT

Assess gastrostomy or jejunostomy tube site, noting any drainage, skin breakdown, or erythema. Check to ensure that the tube is securely stabilized and has not become dislodged. Also, assess the tension of the tube. If there is not enough tension, the tube may leak gastric or intestinal drainage around exit site. If the tension is too great, the internal anchoring device may erode through the skin.

NURSING DIAGNOSIS

Determine the related factors for the nursing diagnoses based on the patient's current status. Possible nursing diagnoses may include:

- Imbalanced Nutrition, Less than Body Requirements
- Impaired Skin Integrity
- Risk for Infection
- Deficient Knowledge
- Nausea
- Alteration in Comfort

OUTCOME IDENTIFICATION AND PLANNING

The expected outcome to achieve when caring for a gastrostomy tube is that the patient ingests an adequate diet and exhibits no signs and symptoms of irritation, excoriation, or infection at the tube insertion site. Also, that the patient verbalizes little discomfort related to tube placement. In addition, the patient will be able to verbalize the care needed for the gastrostomy tube.

IMPLEMENTATION

ACTION	RATIONALE
1. Check the physician's order.	Checking the physician's order verifies that the right patient receives the correct care.
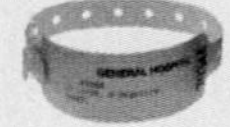 2. Identify the patient.	Identification of the patient ensures that the right patient receives the correct intervention as ordered.
3. Explain the procedure to the patient.	Explanations provide reassurance and facilitate cooperation of the patient.
4. Assess patient for presence of pain at the tube insertion site. If pain is present, offer patient analgesic medication per physician's order and wait for medication absorption before beginning insertion site care.	Feeding tubes can be uncomfortable, especially the first few days after insertion. Analgesic medication may permit the patient to tolerate the insertion site care more easily. After the first few days, it has been reported that the need for pain medication decreases.

(continued)

SKILL 11-6 Caring for a Gastrostomy Tube *(continued)*

ACTION	RATIONALE
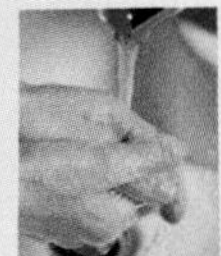 5. Perform hand hygiene. Put on nonsterile gloves.	Hand hygiene deters the spread of microorganisms. Gloves protect nurse from exposure to blood or bodily substances.
6. Raise the bed to the appropriate height. Pull the patient's bedside curtain.	Appropriate height promotes the comfort of the nurse and promotes proper body mechanics. Provides for privacy.
7. If gastrostomy tube is new and still has sutures holding it in place, dip cotton-tipped applicator into sterile saline solution and gently clean around the insertion site, removing any crust or drainage (Figure 1). Avoid adjusting or lifting the external disk for the first few days after placement except to clean the area. If the gastric tube insertion site has healed and the sutures are removed, wet a washcloth and apply a small amount of soap onto washcloth. Gently cleanse around the insertion, removing any crust or drainage (Figure 2). **Rinse site, removing all soap.**	Cleaning new site with sterile saline solution prevents the introduction of microorganisms into the wound. Crust and drainage can harbor bacteria and lead to skin breakdown. Removing soap helps to prevent skin irritation. If able, the patient may shower and cleanse the site with soap and water.

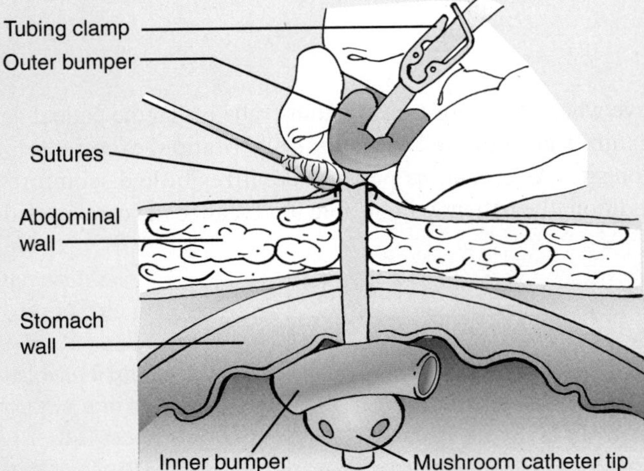

Figure 1. Wiping gastric tube site with cotton-tipped applicators.

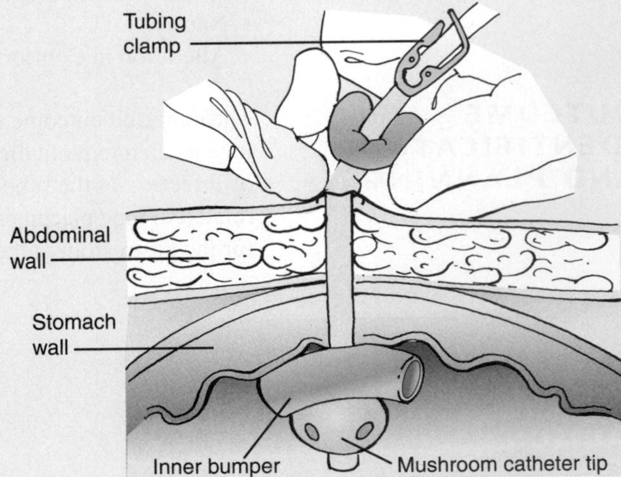

Figure 2. Cleaning site with soap, water, and washcloth.

ACTION	RATIONALE
8. Pat skin around insertion site dry.	Drying the skin thoroughly prevents skin breakdown.
9. If the sutures have been removed, gently **rotate the guard or external bumper 90 degrees at least once a day (Figure 3). Assess that the guard or external bumper is not digging into the surrounding skin. Avoid placing any tension on the feeding tube.**	Rotation of the guard or external bumper prevents skin breakdown and pressure ulcers. The risk of dislodgement is decreased when the tube has an external anchoring or bumper device.
10. Leave the stoma open to air unless there is drainage. If drainage is present, place one thickness of gauze pad under the external bumper and change as needed to keep the area dry. Use a skin protectant or substance such as zinc oxide to prevent skin breakdown.	The digestive enzymes from the gastric secretions may cause skin breakdown. Under normal conditions, expect only a minimal amount of drainage on a feeding tube dressing. Increased amounts of drainage should be explored for cause such as a possible gastric fluid leak.

SKILL 11-6 **Caring for a Gastrostomy Tube** *(continued)*

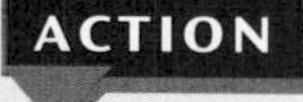

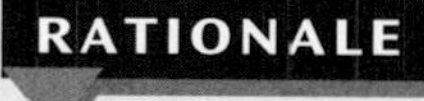

ACTION	RATIONALE

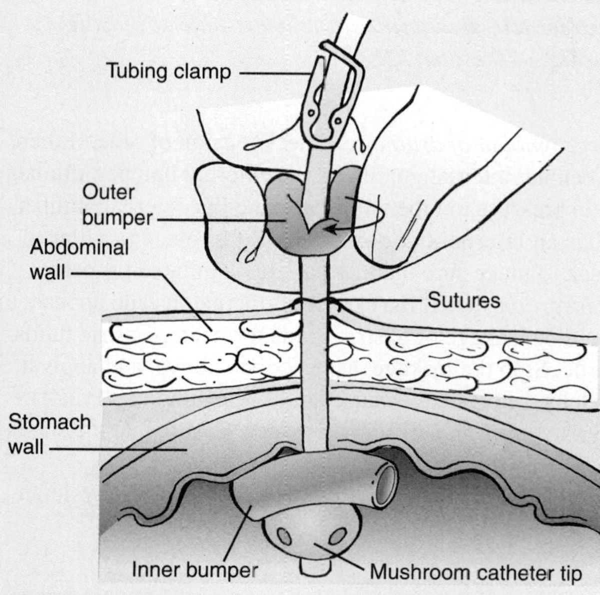

Figure 3. Turning or rotating guard 90 degrees.

ACTION	RATIONALE
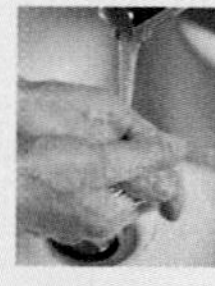 11. Remove gloves and perform hand hygiene.	Hand hygiene prevents the spread of microorganisms.
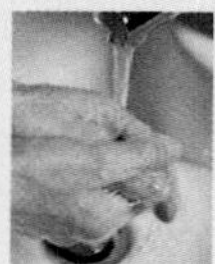 12. Lower the bed and assist the patient to a position of comfort as needed. Perform hand hygiene.	These actions ensure patient safety and comfort. Hand hygiene prevents the spread of microorganisms.

EVALUATION

The expected outcome is met when the patient exhibits a clean, dry, intact gastrostomy tube site without evidence of irritation, excoriation, or infection. Other expected outcomes may include the following: the patient verbalizes no pain when guard is rotated; skin remains pink without any sign of skin breakdown; and the patient participates in care measures.

DOCUMENTATION

Guidelines

Document the care that was given, including the substance used to cleanse the tube site. Record the condition of the site, including the surrounding skin. Note if any drainage was present, recording the amount and color. Note the rotation of the guard. Comment on the patient's response to the care, if the patient experienced any pain, and if an analgesic was given. Record any patient instruction that was given.

(continued)

SKILL 11-6 Caring for a Gastrostomy Tube *(continued)*

Sample Documentation

10/10/06 1145 Gastrostomy tube site cleansed with soap and water. Guard rotated. Skin surrounding site is pink without any signs of skin breakdown. Small amount of clear crust noted on tube. Patient tolerated without incident. Wife at bedside, actively participating in tube care.—S. Essner, RN

Unexpected Situations and Associated Interventions

- *Gastrostomy tube is leaking large amount of drainage:* Check tension of tube. If there is a large amount of slack between the internal guard and the external bumper, drainage can leak out of site. Apply gentle pressure to tube while pressing the external bumper closer to the skin. If the tube has an internal balloon holding it in place (similar to a urinary catheter balloon), check to make sure that the balloon is inflated properly.
- *Skin irritation is noted around insertion site:* If the skin is erythematous and appears to be broken down, the culprit could be leakage of gastric fluids from site. Gastric fluids have a low pH and are very acidic. Stop the leakage, as described above, and apply a skin barrier. If the skin has a patchy, red rash, the cause could be candidiasis (yeast). Notify the physician for an order to apply an antifungal powder. Ensure that the site is kept dry.
- *Site appears erythematous and patient complains of pain at site:* Notify physician; patient could be developing cellulitis at the site.

The Taylor Suite offers these additional sources to enhance learning and facilitate understanding of this chapter:

- thePoint online resource, http://thepoint.lww.com/Lynn2E
- Student CD-ROM included with the book
- Skills Checklist to Accompany Taylor's Clinical Nursing Skills
- Taylor's Interactive Nursing: *Nutrition*
- Taylor's Video Guide to Clinical Nursing Skills: *Nutrition*

Developing Critical Thinking Skills

1. Cole Brenau is concerned that his friends may see his gastrostomy tube. He confides to the nurse that he doesn't like the way the tube fits under his clothing. What can be done for him?
2. Jack Mason is concerned about how to clean the gastrostomy tube site and how he can prevent the tube site from getting wet while taking a shower.

Bibliography

Ackley, B., & Ladwig, G. (2006). *Nursing diagnosis handbook* (7th ed). Philadelphia: Mosby Elsevier.

Arbogast, D. (2002). Enteral feedings with comfort and safety. *Clinical Journal of Oncology Nursing,* 6,(5), 275–280.

Bauer, J. (2003). Enteral feeding pumps. *RN, 66*(8), 69–70.

Best, C. (2005). Caring for the patient with a nasogastric tube. *Nursing Standard, 20*(3), 59–65.

Bowers, S. (2000). All about tubes: Your guide to enteral feeding devices. *Nursing, 30*(12), 41–47.

DiMaria-Ghalili, R., & Amella, E. (2005). Nutrition in older adults. *American Journal of Nursing, 105*(3), 40–51.

Dochterman, J., & Bulechek, G. (Eds.). (2004). *Nursing interventions classification (NIC)* (4th ed.). St. Louis, MO: Mosby.

Ducharme, J., & Matheson, K. (2003). What is the best topical anesthetic for nasogastric insertion? *Journal of Emergency Medicine, 29*(5), 427–430.

Dudek, S. (2006). *Nutrition essentials for nursing practice* (5th ed.). Philadelphia: Lippincott Williams & Wilkins.

Earley, T. (2005). Using pH testing to confirm nasogastric tube position. *Nursing Times, 101*(38), 26–28.

Edwards, S., & Metheny, N. (2000). Measurement of gastric residual volume: State of the science. *MEDSURG Nursing, 9*(3), 125–128.

Ellet, M. (2004). What is known about methods of correctly placing gastric tubes in adults and children. *Gastroenterology Nursing, 27*(6), 253–261.

Ellis, J., & Bentz, P. (2007). *Modules for basic nursing skills* (7th ed.). Philadelphia: Lippincott Williams & Wilkins.

Fellows, L., Miller, E., Frederickson, M., Bly, B., & Felt, P. (2000). Evidence-based practice for enteral feedings: Aspiration prevention strategies, bedside detection, and practice change. *MEDSURG Nursing, 9*(1), 27–31.

Fischbach, F., & Dunning, M. (2004). *Common laboratory & diagnostic tests* (4th ed.). Philadelphia: Lippincott Williams & Wilkins.

Fluids & electrolytes. A 2-in-1 reference for nurses. (2006). Philadelphia: Lippincott Williams & Wilkins.

Holman, D., Roberts, S., & Nicol, M. (2005). Promoting adequate nutrition. *Nursing Older People, 17*(6), 31–32.

Keithley, J. K., & Swanson, B. (2004) Enteral nutrition: An update on practice recommendations. *Medsurg Nursing, 13*(2), 131.

Khair, J. (2005). Guidelines for testing the placing of nasogastric tubes. *Nursing Times, 101*(20), 26–27.

Kohn-Keeth, C. (2000). How to keep feeding tubes flowing freely. *Nursing, 30*(1), 58–59.

Maloney, J., Ryan, T., Brasel, K., Binion, D., Johnson, D., et al. (2002). Food dye use in enteral feedings: A review and a call for a moratorium. *Nutrition in Clinical Practice, 17*(3), 168–181.

Matlow, A., Wray, R., Goldman, C., Streitenberger, L., Freeman, R., & Kovach, D. (2003). Microbial contamination of enteral feed administration sets in a pediatric institution. *American Journal of Infection Control, 31*(1), 49–53.

McClave, S., Lukan, J., Stefater, J., Lowen, C., Looney, S., Matheson, P., Gleeson, K., & Spain, D. (2005). Poor validity of residual volumes as a marker for risk of aspiration in critically ill patients. *Critical Care Medicine, 33*(2), 324–330.

Metheny, N. (2002). Inadvertent intracranial nasogastric tube placement. *American Journal of Nursing, 102*(8), 25–27.

Metheny, N., & Stewart, B. (2002). Testing feeding tube placement during continuous tube feedings. *Applied Nursing Research, 15*(4), 254–258.

Metheny, N., & Titler, M. (2001). Assessing placement of feeding tubes. *American Journal of Nursing, 101*(5), 36–45.

Molle, E. (2005). Caring for older adults. Keep the upper GI tract from going downhill. *Nursing, 35*(10), 28–29.

Noble, K. (2003). Name that tube. *Nursing, 33*(3), 56–62.

North American Nursing Diagnosis Association. (2005). *Nursing diagnoses: Definitions and classification 2005–2006.* Philadelphia: Author.

Padula, C., Kenny, A., Olanchon, C., et al. (2004). Enteral feedings: What the evidence says: Avoid contamination of feedings and its sequelae with this research-based protocol. *American Journal of Nursing, 104*(7), 62–69.

Pullen, R. (2004). Clinical do's & don'ts. Measuring gastric residual volume. *Nursing, 34*(4), 18.

Roche, V. (2003). Percutaneous endoscopic gastrostomy: Clinical care of PEG tubes in older adults. *Geriatrics, 58*(11), 22–29.

Sanko, J. (2004). Aspiration assessment and prevention in critically ill enterally fed patients: Evidence-based recommendations for practice. *Gastroenterology Nursing, 27*(6), 279–285.

Smeltzer, S. C., Bare, B. G., Hinkle, J. H., & Cheever, K. H. (2008). *Brunner and Suddarth's textbook of medical surgical nursing* (11th ed.). Philadelphia: Lippincott Williams & Wilkins.

Sweeney, J. (2005). Clinical queries: How do I verify NG tube placement? *Nursing, 35*(8), 25.

CHAPTER 12

Urinary Elimination

Focusing on Patient Care

This chapter will help you develop some of the skills needed to care for the following patients:

Ralph Bellows is a 73-year-old man admitted with a stroke. Due to incontinence and skin breakdown, Ralph's nurse has decided to include the application of a condom catheter in his plan of care.

Grace Halligan, age 24, is pregnant and has been placed on bed rest. She needs to void but cannot get out of bed.

Mike Wimmer, age 36, receives peritoneal dialysis. Mike has noticed that the insertion site around his catheter is becoming tender and reddened.

Learning Objectives

After studying this chapter, you will be able to:

1. Assist with the use of a bedpan.
2. Assist with use of a urinal.
3. Assist with use of a bedside commode.
4. Assess bladder volume using an ultrasound bladder scanner.
5. Catheterize a female patient's urinary bladder.
6. Catheterize a male patient's urinary bladder.
7. Remove an indwelling urinary catheter.
8. Administer an intermittent closed-catheter irrigation.
9. Administer a closed continuous-bladder irrigation.
10. Apply an external condom catheter.
11. Change a stoma appliance on an ileal conduit.
12. Care for a suprapubic urinary catheter.
13. Care for a peritoneal dialysis catheter.
14. Care for hemodialysis access.

Key Terms

arteriovenous fistula: a surgically created passage connecting an artery and a vein, used in hemodialysis

arteriovenous graft: a surgically created connection between an artery and vein using synthetic material; used in hemodialysis

bruit: a sound caused by turbulent blood flow

external condom catheter: soft, pliable sheath made of silicone material, applied externally to the penis, connected to drainage tubing and a collection bag

fenestrated: having a window-like opening

hemodialysis: removal from the body, by means of blood filtration, of toxins and fluid that are normally removed by the kidneys

ileal conduit: a surgical diversion formed by bringing the ureters to the ileum; urine is excreted through a stoma

indwelling urethral catheter (retention or Foley catheters): a catheter (tube) through the urethra into the bladder for the purpose of continuous drainage of urine; a balloon is inflated to ensure that the catheter remains in the bladder once it is inserted

intermittent urethral catheter (straight catheter): a catheter through the urethra into the bladder to drain urine for a short period of time (5–10 minutes)

peritoneal dialysis: removal of toxins and fluid from the body by the principles of diffusion and osmosis; accomplished by introducing a solution (dialysate) into the peritoneal cavity

peritonitis: inflammation of the peritoneal membrane

sediment: precipitate found at the bottom of a container of urine

stoma: artificial opening on the body surface

suprapubic urinary catheter: a urinary catheter surgically inserted through a small incision above the pubic area into the bladder

symphysis pubis: the anterior midline junction of the pubic bones; the bony projection under the pubic hair

thrill: palpable feeling caused by turbulent blood flow

Elimination from the urinary tract helps to rid the body of waste products and materials that exceed bodily needs. See Fundamentals Review 12-1 for a review of the male and female genitourinary tract. A properly functioning urinary system is essential to physical and emotional well-being. Problems associated with urinary elimination, such as urinary incontinence, can be so embarrassing to patients that they may no longer leave their home. Nurses assisting patients with urinary elimination or intervening to resolve health problems related to urination need many specialized skills.

This chapter will cover skills that the nurse may use to promote urinary elimination. An assessment of the urinary system is required as part of the assessment related to many of the skills. Fundamentals Review 12-2 summarized factors that affect urinary elimination. The patient who has an indwelling catheter requires special care. Care of the patient with an indwelling catheter is summarized in Fundamentals Review 12-3.

Fundamentals Review 12-1

Anatomy of the Genitourinary Tract

- The main components of the urinary tract are the kidneys, ureters, bladder, and urethra.
- The average female urethra is 1.5″ to 2.5″ (3.7 to 6.2 cm) long, while the average male urethra is 7″ to 8″ (18 to 20 cm) long.
- The male urethra is divided into three segments: cavernous, membranous, and prostatic.
- The average age at which men begin to have prostatic enlargement is 50.

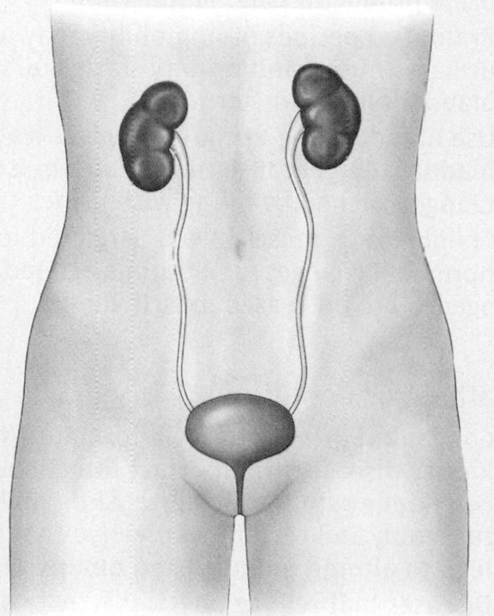

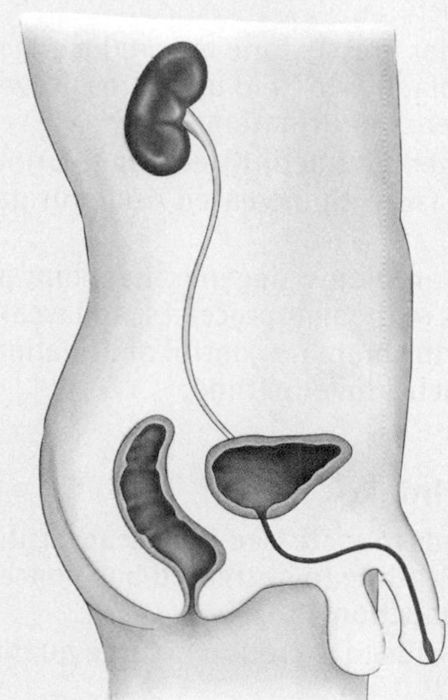

Urinary tract, showing kidneys, ureter, bladder, and urethra.

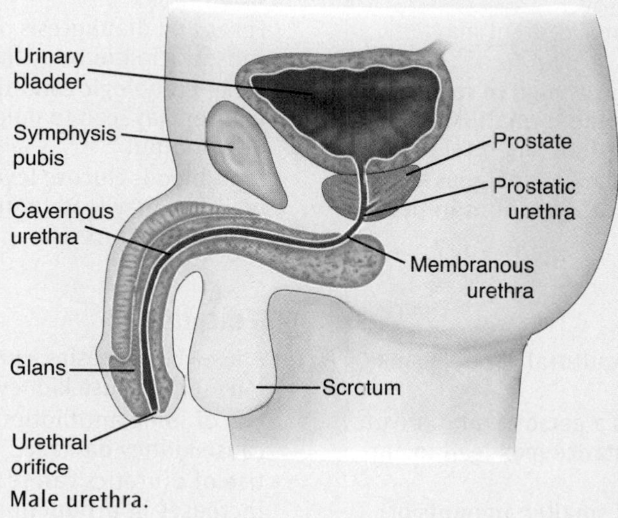

Male urethra.

Fundamentals Review 12-2

Factors Affecting Urinary Elimination

Numerous factors affect the amount and quality of urine produced by the body and the manner in which it is excreted.

Effects of Aging

- Diminished ability of kidneys to concentrate urine may result in nocturia.
- Decreased bladder muscle tone may reduce the capacity of the bladder to hold urine, resulting in increased frequency of urination.
- Decreased bladder contractility leading to urine retention and stasis with increased risk of urinary tract infection.
- Neuromuscular problems, degenerative joint problems, alterations in thought processes, and weakness may interfere with voluntary control of urination and the ability to reach a toilet in time.

Food and Fluid Intake

- Dehydration leads to increased fluid reabsorption by the kidneys, leading to decreased and concentrated urine production.
- Fluid overload leads to excretion of large quantity of dilute urine.
- Consumption of caffeine-containing beverages (cola, coffee, and tea) leads to increased urine production due to their diuretic effect.
- Consumption of alcoholic beverages leads to increased urine production due to their inhibition of antidiuretic hormone release.
- Ingestion of foods high in water content may increase urine production.
- Ingestion of foods and beverages high in sodium content leads to decreased urine formation due to sodium and water reabsorption and retention.
- Ingestion of certain foods, such as asparagus, onions, and beets, may lead to alterations in the odor or color of urine.

Psychological Variables

- Individual, family, and sociocultural variables may influence voiding habits.
- Patients may view voiding as a personal and private act. The need to ask for assistance may lead to embarrassment and/or anxiety.
- Stress may lead to voiding of smaller amounts of urine at more frequent intervals.
- Stress may lead to difficulty emptying the bladder due to its effects on relaxation of perineal muscles and the external urethral sphincter.

Activity and Muscle Tone

- Regular exercise increases metabolism and optimal urine production and elimination.
- Prolonged periods of immobility may lead to poor urinary control and urinary stasis due to decreased bladder and sphincter tone.
- Use of indwelling urinary catheters leads to loss of bladder tone because the bladder muscle is not being stretched by filling with urine.
- Childbearing, muscle atrophy related to menopausal hormonal changes, and trauma-related muscle damage lead to decreased muscle tone.

Pathologic Conditions

- Congenital urinary tract abnormalities, polycystic kidney disease, urinary tract infection, urinary calculi (kidney stones), hypertension, diabetes mellitus, gout, and certain connective tissue disorders lead to altered quantity and quality of urine.
- Diseases that reduce physical activity or lead to generalized weakness, such as arthritis, Parkinson's disease, and degenerative joint disease interfere with toileting.
- Cognitive deficits and psychiatric conditions may interfere with ability or desire to control urination voluntarily.
- Fever and diaphoresis (profuse perspiration) lead to conservation of body fluids.
- Other pathologic conditions, such as congestive heart failure, may lead to fluid retention and decreased urine output.
- High blood–glucose levels, such as with diabetes mellitus, may lead to increased urine output due to osmotic diuresis.

Medications

- Abuse of analgesics, such as aspirin or ibuprofen (Advil) can cause kidney damage (nephrotoxic).
- Use of some antibiotics, such as gentamicin, can cause kidney damage.
- Use of diuretics can lead to moderate to severe increases in production and excretion of dilute urine, related to their prevention of water

Fundamentals Review 12-2

Factors Affecting Urinary Elimination *(continued)*

and certain electrolyte reabsorption in the renal tubules.

- Use of cholinergic medications may lead to increased urination due to stimulation of detrusor muscle contraction.
- Use of some analgesics and tranquilizers interferes with urination due to the diminished effectiveness of the neural reflex for voiding because of suppression of the central nervous system.

Use of certain drugs causes changes to the color of urine. Anticoagulants may cause hematuria (blood in the urine) or a pink or red color. Diuretics can lighten the color of urine to pale yellow. Phenazopyridine (Pyridium) can cause orange or orange-red urine. Amitriptyline (Elavil) and B-complex vitamins can cause green or blue-green urine. Levodopa (L-dopa) and injectable iron compounds can cause brown or black urine.

Fundamentals Review 12-3

Guidelines for Care of the Patient With an Indwelling Catheter

- Use an indwelling catheter only when necessary.
- Employ strict hand hygiene principles.
- Use sterile technique when inserting a catheter.
- Secure the catheter properly to the patient's thigh or abdomen after insertion.
- Maintain a closed system whenever possible.
- If necessary, obtain urine samples using aseptic technique via a closed system.
- Keep the catheter free from obstruction to maintain free flow to the urine.
- Use the smallest appropriate-size catheter.
- Avoid irrigation unless needed to relieve or prevent obstruction.
- Ensure that patient maintains adequate fluid intake.
- Empty the drainage bad when half to two-thirds full or every 3 to 6 hours.
- Clean drainage bags daily using a commercial cleaning product or vinegar solution (1 part vinegar to 3 parts water).
- Provide daily routine personal hygiene as outlined in Chapter 7, Hygiene; there is no need to apply antibiotic ointment or betadine to the urethral meatus.

SKILL 12-1 Assisting With the Use of a Bedpan

Patients who cannot get out of bed because of physical limitations or physician's orders need to use a bedpan or urinal for voiding. Male patients confined to bed usually prefer to use the urinal for voiding and the bedpan for defecation; female patients usually prefer to use the bedpan for both. Many patients find it embarrassing and difficult to use the bedpan. When a patient uses a bedpan, promote comfort and normalcy as much as possible, while respecting the patient's privacy. Also be sure to provide skin care and perineal hygiene after bedpan use and maintain a professional manner.

Regular bedpans have a rounded, smooth upper end and a tapered, open lower end. The upper end fits under the patient's buttocks toward the sacrum, with the open end toward the foot of the bed (Figure 1). A special bedpan called a fracture bedpan is frequently used

(continued)

SKILL 12-1 Assisting With the Use of a Bedpan *(continued)*

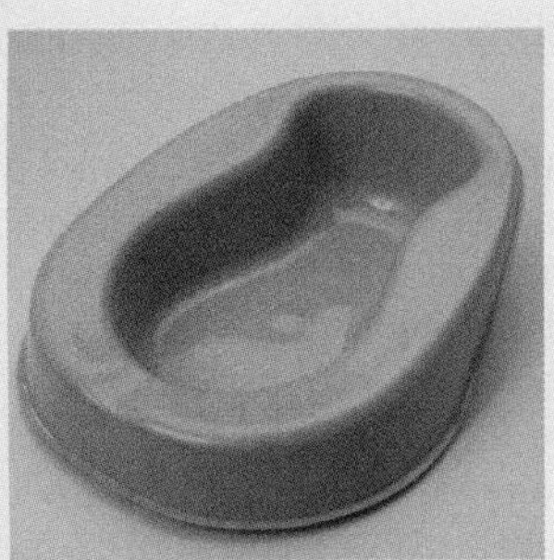

A. Regular bedpan

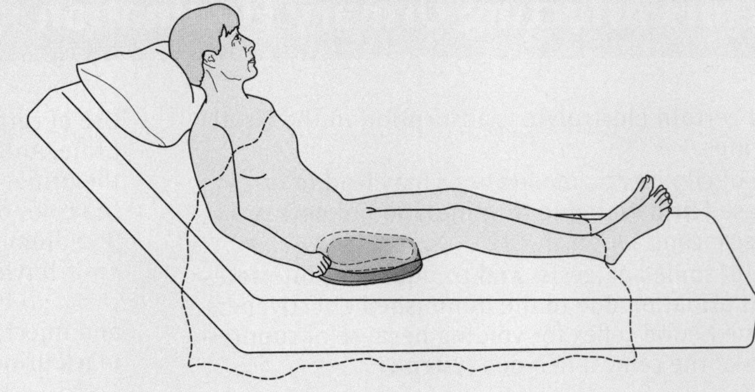

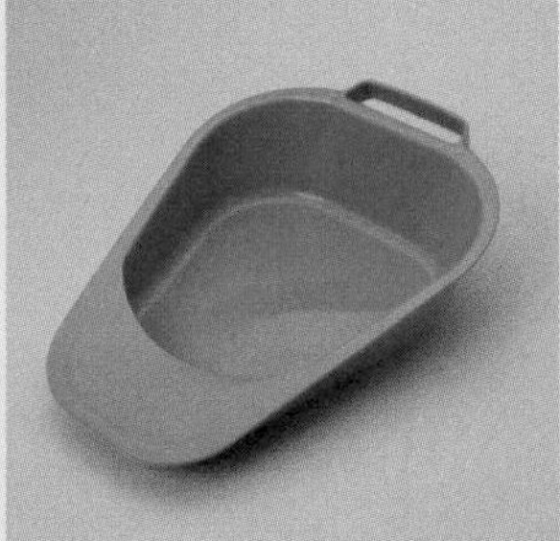

B. Fracture pan

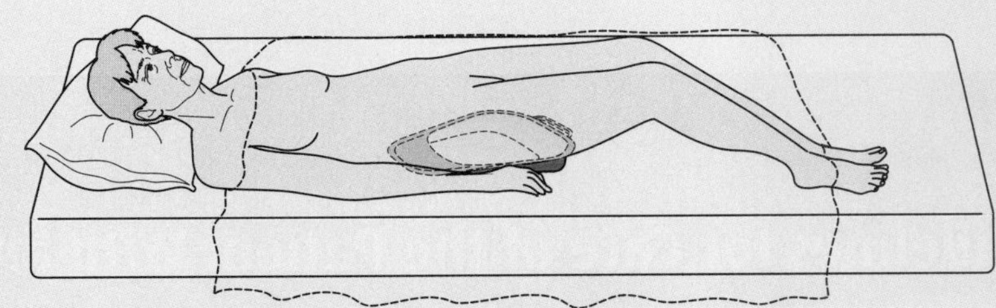

Figure 1. (**A**) Standard bedpan. Position a standard bedpan like a regular toilet seat—the buttocks are placed on the wide, rounded shelf, with the open end pointed toward the foot of the bed. (**B**) Fracture pan. Position a fracture pan with the thin edge toward the head of the bed.

by people with fractures of the femur or lower spine. Smaller and flatter than the ordinary bedpan, this type of bedpan is helpful for patients who cannot easily raise themselves onto the regular bedpan (see Fig. 1). Very thin or elderly patients often find it easier and more comfortable to use the fracture bedpan. The fracture pan has a shallow, narrow upper end with a flat wide rim, and a deeper, open lower end. The upper end fits under the patient's buttocks toward the sacrum, with the deeper, open lower end toward the foot of the bed.

Equipment

- Bedpan (regular or fracture)
- Toilet tissue
- Disposable clean gloves
- Cover for bedpan or urinal (disposable waterproof pad or cover)

ASSESSMENT

Assess the patient's normal elimination habits. Determine why the patient needs to use a bedpan, for example, a physician's order for strict bed rest or immobilization. Also assess the patient's degree of limitation and ability to help with activity. Assess for activity limitations, such as hip surgery or spinal injury, which would contraindicate certain actions by the patient. Check for the presence of drains, dressings, intravenous fluid infusion sites/equipment, traction, or any other devices that could interfere with the patient's ability to help with the procedure or that could become dislodged.

SKILL 12-1 Assisting With the Use of a Bedpan *(continued)*

NURSING DIAGNOSIS

Determine the related factors for the nursing diagnoses based on the patient's current status. The two most common nursing diagnoses are Impaired Urinary Elimination and Toileting Self-Care Deficit. Other appropriate nursing diagnoses may include:

- Impaired Physical Mobility
- Deficient Knowledge
- Functional Urinary Incontinence

OUTCOME IDENTIFICATION AND PLANNING

The expected outcome to achieve when offering a bedpan is that the patient is able to void with assistance. Other appropriate outcomes may include the following: the patient maintains continence, the patient demonstrates how to use the bedpan with assistance, and the patient maintains skin integrity.

IMPLEMENTATION

ACTION	RATIONALE
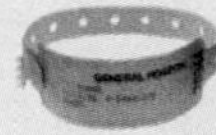 1. Identify the patient. Discuss procedure with patient and assess patient's ability to assist with the procedure, as well as personal hygiene preferences. Review chart for any limitations in physical activity. (See Skill Variation: When the Patient has Limited Movement.)	Identifying the patient ensures the right patient receives the intervention and helps prevent errors. This discussion promotes reassurance and provides knowledge about the procedure. Dialogue encourages patient participation and allows for individualized nursing care.
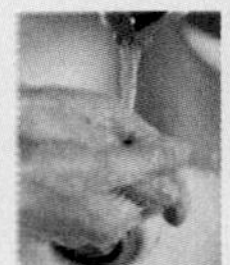 2. Bring bedpan and other necessary equipment to bedside. Perform hand hygiene. Put on disposable gloves.	Having equipment on hand saves time by avoiding unnecessary trips to storage area. Hand hygiene deters the spread of microorganisms. Gloves prevent exposure to blood and body fluids.
3. Warm bedpan, if it is made of metal, by rinsing it with warm water.	A cold bedpan feels uncomfortable and may make it difficult for the patient to void. Plastic bedpans do not require warming.
4. Unless contraindicated, apply powder to the rim of the bedpan.	Powder helps keep the bedpan from sticking to the patient's skin and makes it easier to remove. Powder is not applied if the patient has respiratory problems or is allergic to powder or if a urine specimen is needed (could contaminate the specimen).
5. Place bedpan and cover on chair next to bed. Close curtains around bed and close door to room if possible.	The bedpan on the chair allows for easy access. Closing the curtain or door provides for patient privacy.
6. If bed is adjustable, place it in high position. Place the patient in a supine position, with the head of the bed elevated about 30 degrees, unless contraindicated.	Having the bed in the high position reduces strain on the nurse's back while assisting the patient onto the bedpan. Supine position is necessary for correct placement on bedpan.

(continued)

SKILL 12-1 Assisting With the Use of a Bedpan *(continued)*

ACTION	RATIONALE
7. Fold top linen back just enough to allow placement of bedpan. If there is no waterproof pad on the bed and time allows, consider placing a waterproof pad under patient's buttocks before placing bedpan (Figure 2).	Folding back the linen in this manner minimizes unnecessary exposure while still allowing the nurse to place the bedpan. The waterproof pad will protect the bed should there be a spill.
8. Ask the patient to bend the knees. Have the patient lift his or her hips upward. Assist patient, if necessary, by placing your hand that is closest to the patient palm up, under the lower back and assist with lifting. Slip the bedpan into place with other hand (Figure 3).	The nurse uses less energy when the patient can assist by placing some of his or her weight on the heels.

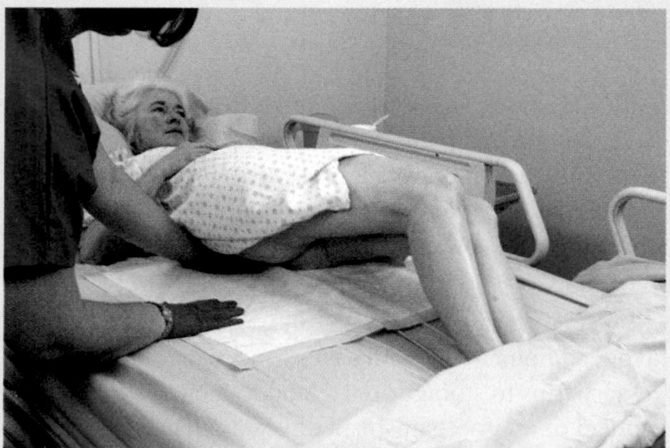

Figure 2. Placing waterproof pad under the patient's buttocks. *(Note: Covers should only be folded back just enough to work, not expose patient unnecessarily. Covers in this series of photos have been pulled back to show action.)*

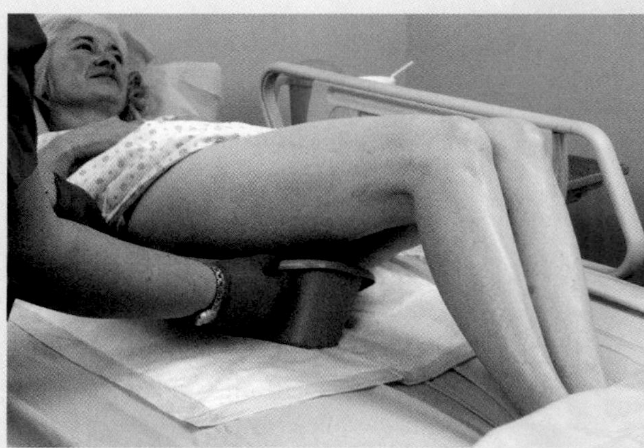

Figure 3. Assisting patient to raise self in bed to position the bedpan.

ACTION	RATIONALE
9. **Ensure that bedpan is in proper position and patient's buttocks are resting on the rounded shelf of the regular bedpan or the shallow rim of the fracture bedpan.**	Having the bedpan in the proper position prevents spills onto the bed, ensures patient comfort, and prevents injury to the skin from a misplaced bedpan.
10. Raise head of bed as near to sitting position as tolerated, unless contraindicated. Cover the patient with bed linens.	This position makes it easier for the patient to void or defecate, avoids strain on the patient's back, and allows gravity to aid in elimination. Covering promotes warmth and privacy.

SKILL 12-1 Assisting With the Use of a Bedpan *(continued)*

ACTION	RATIONALE
11. **Place call device and toilet tissue within easy reach. Place the bed in the lowest position.** Leave patient if it is safe to do so. Use side rails appropriately (Figure 4).	Falls can be prevented if the patient does not have to reach for items he or she needs. Placing the bed in the lowest position promotes patient safety. Leaving patient alone, if possible, promotes self-esteem and shows respect for privacy. Side rails assist the patient in repositioning.

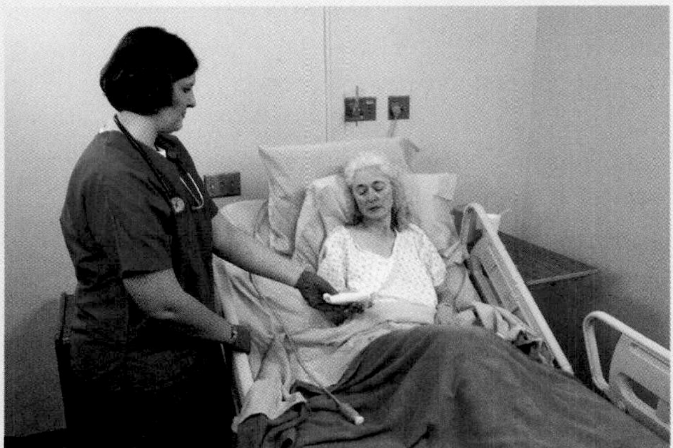

Figure 4. Placing call light within patient's reach and handing patient toilet tissue. Side rails are raised.

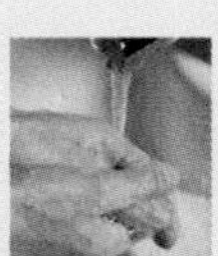

ACTION	RATIONALE
12. Remove gloves and perform hand hygiene.	Hand hygiene deters the spread of microorganisms.

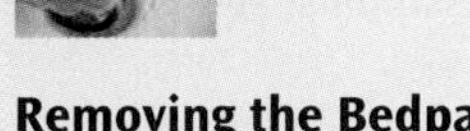

Removing the Bedpan

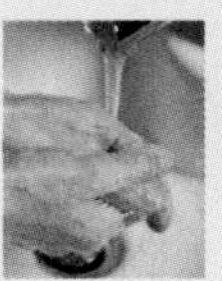

ACTION	RATIONALE
13. Perform hand hygiene and put on disposable gloves. Raise the bed to a comfortable working height. Have a receptacle, such as plastic trash bag, handy for discarding tissue.	Hand hygiene deters the spread of microorganisms. Gloves prevent exposure to blood and body fluids. Having the bed in the high position reduces strain on the nurse's back while assisting the patient off the bedpan.
14. Lower the head of the bed, if necessary, to about 30 degrees. Remove bedpan in the same manner in which it was offered, being careful to hold it steady. Ask the patient to bend the knees and lift the buttocks up from the bedpan. Assist patient, if necessary, by placing your hand that is closest to the patient palm up, under the lower back and assist with lifting. Place the bedpan on the bedside chair and cover it.	Holding the bedpan steady prevents spills. The nurse uses less energy when the patient can assist by placing some of his or her weight on the heels. Covering the bedpan helps to prevent the spread of microorganisms.
15. If patient needs assistance with hygiene, wrap tissue around the hand several times, and wipe patient clean, using one stroke from the pubic area toward the anal area. Discard tissue, and use more until patient is clean. Place patient on his or her side and spread buttocks to clean anal area.	Cleaning area from front to back minimizes fecal contamination of the vagina and urinary meatus. Cleaning the patient after he or she has used the bedpan prevents offensive odors and irritation to the skin.

(continued)

SKILL 12-1 Assisting With the Use of a Bedpan *(continued)*

ACTION	RATIONALE
16. Do not place toilet tissue in the bedpan if a specimen is required or if output is being recorded. Place toilet tissue in appropriate receptacle.	Mixing toilet tissue with a specimen makes laboratory examination more difficult and interferes with accurate output measurement.
17. Return the patient to a comfortable position. Make sure the linens under the patient are dry. Replace or remove pad under the patient as necessary. Remove your gloves and ensure that the patient is covered.	Positioning helps to promote patient comfort. Removing contaminated gloves prevents spread of microorganisms.
18. Raise side rail. Lower bed height and adjust head of bed to a comfortable position. Reattach call bell.	These actions promote patient safety.
19. Offer patient supplies to wash and dry his or her hands, assisting as necessary.	Washing hands after using the bedpan helps prevent the spread of microorganisms.
20. Put on clean gloves. Empty and clean the bedpan, measuring urine in graduated container, as necessary. Discard trash receptacle with used toilet paper per facility policy. Perform hand hygiene.	Gloves prevent exposure to blood and body fluids. Cleaning reusable equipment and hand hygiene help prevent the spread of microorganisms.

EVALUATION

The expected outcome is met when the patient voids using the bedpan. Other outcomes are met when the patient remains dry, the patient does not experience episodes of incontinence, the patient demonstrates measures to assist with using the bedpan, and the patient does not experience impaired skin integrity.

DOCUMENTATION

Guidelines

Document the patient's tolerance of the activity. Record the amount of urine voided on the intake and output record, if appropriate. Document any other assessments, such as unusual urine characteristics or alterations in the patient's skin.

Sample Documentation

12/06/08 0730 Patient placed on fracture bedpan with a 2-person assist. Voided 400 mL dark yellow urine, strong odor noted. Specimen sent for urinalysis as ordered.—S. Barnes, RN

Special Considerations

General Considerations

- A fracture bedpan is usually more comfortable for the patient, but it does not hold as large a volume as the regular bedpan.
- Bedpan should not be left in place for extended periods of time as this can result in excessive pressure and irritation to the patient's skin.

SKILL 12-1 Assisting With the Use of a Bedpan *(continued)*

SKILL VARIATION Assisting With Use of a Bedpan When the Patient Has Limited Movement

Patients who are unable to lift themselves onto the bedpan or who have activity limitations that prohibit the required actions can be assisted onto the bedpan in an alternate manner using these actions:

- Discuss procedure with patient and assess patient's ability to assist with the procedure, as well as personal hygiene preferences. Review chart for any limitations in physical activity.
- Bring bedpan and other necessary equipment to bedside. Perform hand hygiene. Put on disposable gloves.
- Warm bedpan, if it is made of metal, by rinsing it with warm water.
- Unless contraindicated, apply powder to the rim of the bedpan.
- Place bedpan and cover on chair next to bed. Close curtains around bed and close door to room if possible.
- If bed is adjustable, place it in high position. Place the patient in a supine position, with the head of the bed flat, unless contraindicated.
- Fold top linen just enough to turn the patient, while minimizing exposure. If there is no waterproof pad on the bed and time allows, consider placing a waterproof pad under patient's buttocks before placing bedpan.
- Assist the patient to roll to the opposite side or turn the patient into a side-lying position.
- Hold the bedpan firmly against the patient's buttocks, with the upper end of the bedpan under the patient's buttocks toward the sacrum, and down into the mattress (see Figure 1).
- Keep one hand against the bedpan. Apply gentle pressure to ensure the bedpan remains in place as you assist the patient to roll back onto the bedpan.
- Ensure that bedpan is in proper position and patient's buttocks are resting on rounded shelf of the regular bedpan or the shallow rim of the fracture bedpan.
- Raise head of bed as near to sitting position as tolerated, unless contraindicated. Cover the patient with bed linens.
- Place call device and toilet tissue within easy reach. Place the bed in the lowest position. Leave patient if it is safe to do so. Use side rails appropriately.
- Remove gloves and perform hand hygiene.
- To remove the bedpan, perform hand hygiene and put on disposable gloves. Raise the bed to a comfortable working height. Have a receptacle handy for discarding tissue.
- Lower the head of the bed. Grasp the closest side of the bedpan. Apply gentle pressure to hold the bedpan flat and steady. Assist the patient to roll to the opposite side or turn the patient into a side-lying position with the assistance of a second caregiver. Remove the bedpan and set on chair. Cover the bedpan.
- Wrap tissue around the hand several times, and wipe patient clean, using one stroke from the pubic area toward the anal area. Discard tissue in an appropriate receptacle, and use more until patient is clean. Do not place toilet tissue in the bedpan if a specimen is required or if output is being recorded. Spread buttocks to clean anal area.
- Return the patient to a comfortable position. Make sure the linens under the patient are dry and that the patient is covered.
- Remove your gloves. Offer patient supplies to wash and dry his or her hands, assisting as necessary.
- Raise side rail. Lower bed height and adjust head of bed to a comfortable position. Reattach call bell.
- Put on clean gloves. Empty and clean the bedpan, measuring urine in graduated container, as necessary. Perform hand hygiene.

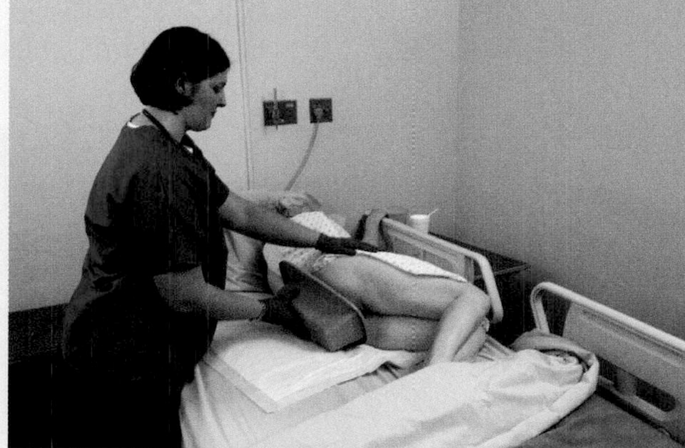

Figure 1. Rolling patient on side to place the bedpan *(Note: Covers should only be folded back just enough to work, not expose patient unnecessarily. Covers in photo pulled back to show action for photo.)*

SKILL 12-2 Assisting With the Use of a Urinal

Male patients confined to bed usually prefer to use the urinal for voiding. Often, male patients prefer to use the urinal at the bedside as a matter of convenience (Figure 1). The use of a urinal in the standing position facilitates emptying of the bladder. Patients who are unable to stand alone may benefit from assistance when voiding into a urinal. If the patient is unable to stand, the urinal may be used in bed. Patients may also use a urinal in the bathroom to facilitate measurement of urinary output. Many patients find it embarrassing to use the urinal. Promote comfort and normalcy as much as possible, while respecting the patient's privacy. Provide skin care and perineal hygiene after urinal use and maintain a professional manner.

Equipment

- Urinal with end cover (usually attached)
- Toilet tissue
- Disposable clean gloves

ASSESSMENT

Assess the patient's normal elimination habits. Determine why the patient needs to use a urinal, such as a physician's order for strict bed rest or immobilization. Also assess the patient's degree of limitation and ability to help with activity. Assess for activity limitations, such as hip surgery or spinal injury, which would contraindicate certain actions by the patient. Check for the presence of drains, dressings, intravenous fluid infusion sites/equipment, traction, or any other devices that could interfere with the patient's ability to help with the procedure or that could become dislodged.

NURSING DIAGNOSIS

Determine the related factors for the nursing diagnoses based on the patient's current status. The two most common nursing diagnoses are Impaired Urinary Elimination and Toileting Self-Care Deficit. Other appropriate nursing diagnoses may include:

- Impaired Physical Mobility
- Deficient Knowledge
- Functional Urinary Incontinence

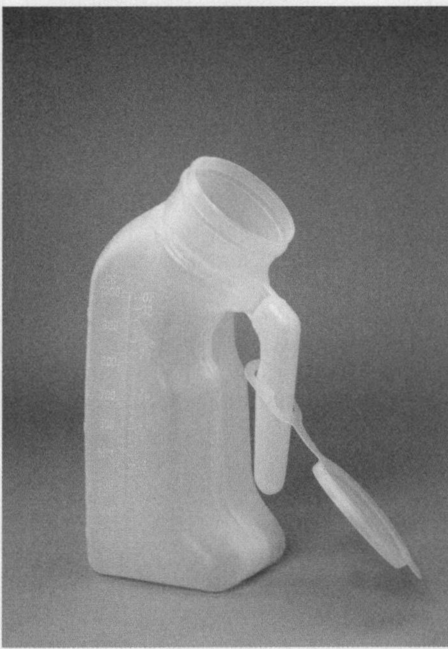

Figure 1. Urinal.

SKILL 12-2 Assisting With the Use of a Urinal *(continued)*

OUTCOME IDENTIFICATION AND PLANNING

The expected outcome to achieve when offering a urinal is that the patient is able to void with assistance. Other appropriate outcomes may include the following: the patient maintains continence, the patient demonstrates how to use the urinal, and the patient maintains skin integrity.

IMPLEMENTATION

ACTION	RATIONALE
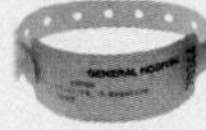 1. Identify the patient. Discuss procedure with patient and assess patient's ability to assist with the procedure, as well as personal hygiene preferences. Review chart for any limitations in physical activity.	Identifying the patient ensures the right patient receives the intervention and helps prevent errors. This discussion promotes reassurance and provides knowledge about the procedure. Dialogue encourages patient participation and allows for individualized nursing care.
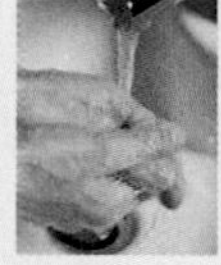 2. Bring urinal and other necessary equipment to bedside. Perform hand hygiene. Put on disposable gloves.	Having equipment on hand saves time by avoiding unnecessary trips to storage area. Hand hygiene deters the spread of microorganisms. Gloves prevent exposure to blood and body fluids.
3. Close curtains around bed and close door to room if possible.	Closing the curtain and door provides for patient privacy.
4. Assist the patient to an appropriate position as necessary: standing at the bedside, lying on one side or back, sitting in bed with the head elevated, or sitting on the side of the bed.	These positions facilitate voiding and emptying of the bladder.
5. If the patient remains in the bed, fold the linens just enough to allow for proper placement of the urinal.	Folding back the linen in this manner minimizes unnecessary exposure while still allowing the nurse to place the urinal.
6. If the patient is not standing, have him spread his legs slightly. **Hold the urinal close to the penis and position the penis completely within the urinal (Figure 2). Keep the bottom of the urinal lower than the penis. If necessary, assist the patient to hold the urinal in place.**	Slight spreading of the legs allows for proper positioning of the urinal. Placing penis completely within the urinal and keeping bottom low avoids urine spills.

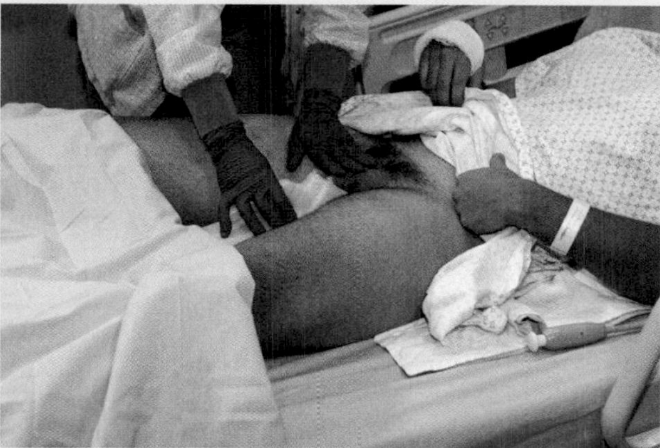

Figure 2. Positioning urinal in place for a male patient. (*Note: Covers should only be folded back just enough to work, not expose patient unnecessarily. Covers have been pulled back to show action.*)

(continued)

SKILL 12-2 Assisting With the Use of a Urinal *(continued)*

ACTION	RATIONALE
7. Cover the patient with the bed linens.	Covering promotes warmth and privacy.
8. Place call device and toilet tissue within easy reach. Have a receptacle, such as plastic trash bag, handy for discarding tissue. Place the bed in the lowest position. Leave patient if it is safe to do so. Use side rails appropriately.	Falls can be prevented if the patient does not have to reach for items he or she needs. Placing the bed in the lowest position promotes patient safety. Leaving patient alone, if possible, promotes self-esteem and shows respect for privacy. Side rails assist the patient in repositioning.
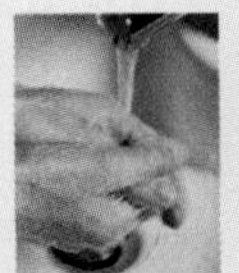 9. Remove gloves and perform hand hygiene.	Hand hygiene deters the spread of microorganisms.
Removing the Urinal	
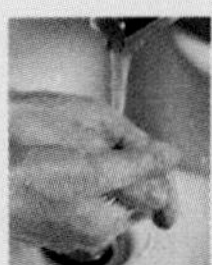 10. Perform hand hygiene and put on disposable gloves.	Hand hygiene deters the spread of microorganisms. Gloves prevent exposure to blood and body fluids.
11. Pull back the patient's bed linens just enough to remove the urinal. Cover the open end of the urinal. Place on the bedside chair. If patient needs assistance with hygiene, wrap tissue around the hand several times, and wipe patient clean. Place tissue in receptacle.	Covering the end helps to prevent the spread of microorganisms.
12. Return the patient to a comfortable position. Make sure the linens under the patient are dry. Remove your gloves and ensure that the patient is covered.	Proper positioning promotes patient comfort. Removing contaminated gloves prevents spread of microorganisms.
13. Ensure patient call bell is in reach.	Promotes patient safety.
14. Offer patient supplies to wash and dry his or her hands, assisting as necessary.	Washing hands after using the bedpan helps prevent the spread of microorganisms.
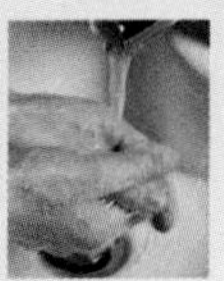 15. Put on clean gloves. Empty and clean the urinal, measuring urine in graduated container, as necessary. Discard trash receptacle with used toilet paper per facility policy. Remove gloves and perform hand hygiene.	Gloves prevent exposure to blood and body fluids. Hand hygiene helps prevent the spread of microorganisms.

EVALUATION

The expected outcome is met when the patient voids using the urinal. Other outcomes are met when the patient remains dry, the patient does not experience episodes of incontinence, the patient demonstrates measures to assist with using the urinal, and the patient does not experience impaired skin integrity.

DOCUMENTATION

Guidelines

Document the patient's tolerance of the activity. Record the amount of urine voided on the intake and output record, if appropriate. Document any other assessments, such as unusual urine characteristics or alterations in the patient's skin.

SKILL 12-2 Assisting With the Use of a Urinal *(continued)*

Sample Documentation

12/06/08 0730 Patient using urinal at bedside to void. Voided 600 mL yellow urine. Reinforced need for continued use of urinal for recording accurate output. Patient verbalized an understanding of instructions.—S. Barnes, RN

Special Considerations

General Considerations

- Urinal should not be left in place for extended periods of time, as pressure and irritation to the patient's skin can result. If patient is unable to use alone or with assistance, consider other interventions, such as commode or external condom catheter.
- It may be necessary to assist patients who have difficulty holding urinal in place, such as those with limited upper extremity movement or alteration in mentation, to prevent spillage of urine.
- The urinal may also be used standing or sitting at the bedside or in the patient's bathroom, if patient is able to do so.

SKILL 12-3 Assisting With the Use of a Bedside Commode

Patients who experience difficulty getting to the bathroom may benefit from the use of a bedside commode. Bedside commodes are portable toilet substitutes and can be used for voiding and defecation (Figure 1). A bedside commode can be placed close to the bed for easy use. Many have arm rests attached to the legs that may interfere with ease of transfer. The legs usually have some type of end cap on the bottom to reduce movement, but care must be taken to prevent the commode from moving during transfer, resulting in patient injury or falls.

Equipment

- Commode with cover (usually attached)
- Toilet tissue
- Disposable clean gloves

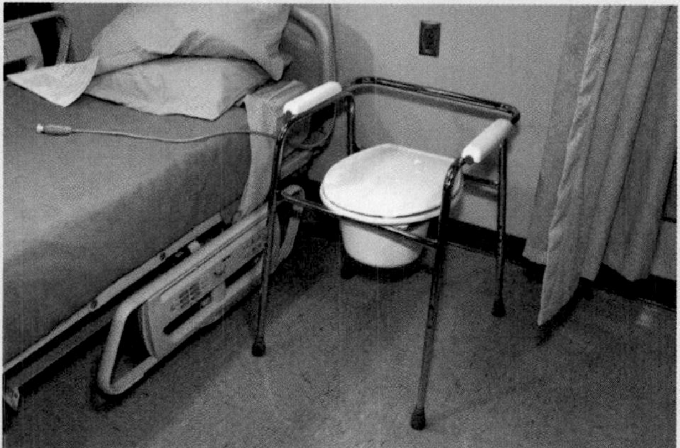

Figure 1. Bedside commode.

(continued)

SKILL 12-3 Assisting With the Use of a Bedside Commode *(continued)*

ASSESSMENT

Assess the patient's normal elimination habits. Determine why the patient needs to use a commode, such as weakness or unsteady gait. Assess the patient's degree of limitation and ability to help with activity. Check for the presence of drains, dressings, intravenous fluid infusion sites/equipment, or other devices that could interfere with the patient's ability to help with the procedure or that could become dislodged.

NURSING DIAGNOSIS

Determine the related factors for the nursing diagnoses based on the patient's current status. The two most common nursing diagnoses are Impaired Urinary Elimination and Toileting Self-Care Deficit. Other appropriate nursing diagnoses may include:

- Impaired Physical Mobility
- Deficient Knowledge
- Functional Urinary Incontinence
- Risk for Falls

OUTCOME IDENTIFICATION AND PLANNING

The expected outcome to achieve when assisting with the use of a commode is that the patient is able to void with assistance. Other appropriate outcomes may include the following: the patient maintains continence, the patient demonstrates how to use the commode, the patient maintains skin integrity, and the patient remains free from injury.

IMPLEMENTATION

ACTION	RATIONALE
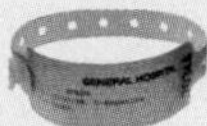 1. Identify the patient. Discuss procedure with patient and assess patient's ability to assist with the procedure, as well as personal hygiene preferences. Review chart for any limitations in physical activity.	Identifying the patient ensures the right patient receives the intervention and helps prevent errors. This discussion promotes reassurance and provides knowledge about the procedure. Dialogue encourages patient participation and allows for individualized nursing care. Physical limitations may require adaptations in performing the skill.
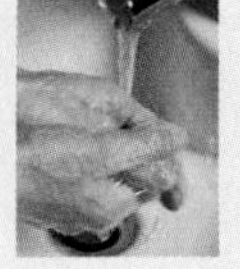 2. Bring the commode and other necessary equipment to bedside. Obtain assistance from another staff member, if necessary. Perform hand hygiene. Put on disposable gloves.	Having equipment on hand saves time by avoiding unnecessary trips to storage area. Assistance from additional staff member ensures patient safety and facilitates patient transfer. Hand hygiene deters the spread of microorganisms. Gloves prevent exposure to blood and body fluids.
3. Close curtains around bed and close door to room if possible.	Provides for patient privacy.
4. Place the commode close to and parallel with the bed. Raise or remove the seat cover. Refer to Figure 1.	Allows for easy access.
5. Assist the patient to a standing position and to pivot to the commode. **While bracing one commode leg with your foot, ask patient to place his or her hands one at a time on the arm rests. Assist the patient to slowly lower himself/herself onto the commode seat.**	Standing and then pivoting ensures safe patient transfer. Bracing the commode leg with a foot prevents the commode from shifting while the patient is sitting down.
6. Cover the patient with a blanket. Place call device and toilet tissue within easy reach. Leave patient if it is safe to do so.	Covering patient promotes warmth. Falls can be prevented if the patient does not have to reach for items he or she needs. Leaving patient alone, if possible, promotes self-esteem and shows respect for privacy.

SKILL 12-3

Assisting With the Use of a Bedside Commode *(continued)*

ACTION	RATIONALE
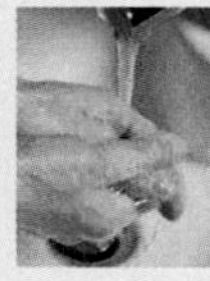 7. Remove gloves and perform hand hygiene.	Hand hygiene deters the spread of microorganisms.
Assisting Patient Off Commode	
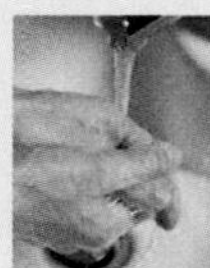 8. Perform hand hygiene and put on disposable gloves.	Hand hygiene deters the spread of microorganisms. Gloves prevent exposure to blood and body fluids.
9. Assist the patient to a standing position. If patient needs assistance with hygiene, wrap toilet tissue around your hand several times, and wipe patient clean, using one stroke from the pubic area toward the anal area. Discard tissue in an appropriate receptacle, according to facility policy, and continue with additional tissue until patient is clean.	Cleaning area from front to back minimizes fecal contamination of the vagina and urinary meatus. Cleaning the patient after he or she has used the commode prevents offensive odors and irritation to the skin.
10. Do not place toilet tissue in the commode if a specimen is required or if output is being recorded. Replace or lower the seat cover.	Mixing toilet tissue with a specimen makes laboratory examination more difficult and interferes with accurate output measurement. Covering the commode helps to prevent the spread of microorganisms.
11. Remove your gloves. Return the patient to the bed or chair. If the patient returns to the bed, raise side rails as appropriate. Ensure that the patient is covered and call device is readily within reach.	Removing contaminated gloves prevents spread of microorganisms. Returning the patient to the bed or chair promotes patient comfort. Side rails assist with patient movement in the bed. Having the call device readily available promotes patient safety.
12. Offer patient supplies to wash and dry his or her hands, assisting as necessary.	Washing hands after using the bedpan helps prevent the spread of microorganisms.
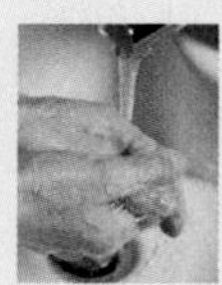 13. Put on clean gloves. Empty and clean the commode, measuring urine in graduated container, as necessary. Remove gloves and perform hand hygiene.	Gloves prevent exposure to blood and body fluids. Hand hygiene helps prevent the spread of microorganisms.

EVALUATION

The expected outcome is met when the patient successfully uses the bedside commode. Other outcomes are met when the patient remains dry, does not experience episodes of incontinence, demonstrates measures to assist with using the commode, and does not experience impaired skin integrity or falls.

DOCUMENTATION

Guidelines

Document the patient's tolerance of the activity, including his or her ability to use the commode. Record the amount of urine voided and/or stool passed on the intake and output record, if appropriate. Document any other assessments, such as unusual urine or stool characteristics or alterations in the patient's skin.

(continued)

SKILL 12-3 Assisting With the Use of a Bedside Commode *(continued)*

Sample Documentation

07/06/08 0730 Patient using commode at bedside to void with assistance of one for transfer. Voided 325 mL yellow urine. Reinforced need for continued use of commode related to patient's unsteady gait. Patient verbalized an understanding of instructions and states she will call for assistance when getting up to use commode.
—S. Barnes, RN

Special Considerations

General Considerations

- Commode can be left within patient's reach, to be used without assistance, if appropriate and safe to do so, based on patient's activity limitations and mobility. Adjust room door or curtain to provide privacy for the patient in the event the commode is used.

SKILL 12-4 Assessing Bladder Volume Using an Ultrasound Bladder Scanner

Portable bladder ultrasound devices are accurate, reliable, and noninvasive devices used to assess bladder volume. Bladder scanners do not pose a risk for the development of a urinary tract infection, unlike intermittent catheterization, which is also used to determine bladder volume. They are used when there is urinary frequency, absent or decreased urine output, bladder distention, or inability to void, and when establishing intermittent catheterization schedules. Protocols can be established to guide the decision to catheterize a patient. Some scanners offer the ability to print the scan results for documentation purposes.

Results are most accurate when the patient is in the supine position during the scanning. The device must be programmed for the gender of the patient by pushing the correct button on the device. If a female patient has had a hysterectomy, the male button is pushed (Corbett, 2004). A postvoid residual (PVR) volume less than 50 mL indicates adequate bladder emptying. A PVR of greater than 150 mL is often recommended as the guideline for catheterization, as residual urine volumes of greater than 150 mL have been associated with the development of urinary tract infections (Stevens, 2005).

Equipment

- Bladder scanner
- Ultrasound gel or bladder scan gel pad
- Alcohol wipe or other sanitizer recommended by the scanner manufacturer and/or facility policy
- Clean gloves
- Paper towel or washcloth

ASSESSMENT

Assess the patient for the need to check bladder volume, including evidence of signs of urinary retention, measurement of postvoid residual volume, verification that bladder is empty, identification of obstruction in an indwelling catheter, and evaluation of bladder distension to determine if catheterization is necessary. Verify physician order, if required by facility. Many facilities allow the use of a bladder scanner as a nursing judgment.

NURSING DIAGNOSIS

Determine the related factors for the nursing diagnoses based on the patient's current status. Appropriate nursing diagnoses may include:

- Impaired Urinary Elimination
- Urinary Retention

SKILL 12-4

Assessing Bladder Volume Using an Ultrasound Bladder Scanner *(continued)*

OUTCOME IDENTIFICATION AND PLANNING

The expected outcome to achieve when using a bladder scanner is that the volume of urine in the bladder will be accurately measured. Other appropriate outcomes may include the following: patient's urinary elimination will be maintained, with a urine output of at least 30 mL/hour; and the patient's bladder will not be distended.

IMPLEMENTATION

ACTION	RATIONALE
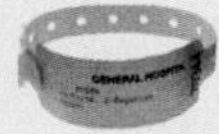 1. Identify the patient. Discuss procedure with patient. Review chart for any limitations in physical activity.	Identifying the patient ensures the right patient receives the intervention and helps prevent errors. This discussion promotes reassurance and provides knowledge about the procedure. Explanation encourages patient cooperation and reduces apprehension. Physical limitations will influence the positioning of the patient for the procedure.
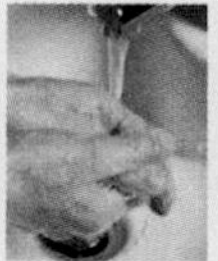 2. Bring the bladder scanner and other necessary equipment to bedside. Obtain assistance from another staff member, if necessary. Perform hand hygiene.	Having equipment on hand saves time by avoiding unnecessary trips to storage area. Assistance from additional staff member ensures patient safety and facilitates patient transfer. Hand hygiene deters the spread of microorganisms.
3. Close curtains around bed and close door to room if possible.	This action provides for patient privacy.
4. Raise the bed to a comfortable working height. Stand on the patient's right side if you are right handed, patient's left side if you are left handed.	Having the bed in the high position reduces strain on the nurse's back while performing the skill. Positioning allows for ease of use of dominant hand for the procedure.
5. Assist patient to a supine position. Drape patient.	Proper positioning allows accurate assessment of bladder volume. Keeping the patient covered as much as possible promotes patient comfort and privacy.
6. Put on clean gloves.	Gloves reduce the risk of exposure to blood and body fluids.
7. Press the 'On' button. Wait until the device warms up. Press the 'Scan' button to turn on the scanning screen.	Many devices require a few minutes to prepare the internal programs.
8. Press the appropriate gender button. The appropriate icon for male or female will appear on the screen (Figure 1).	The device must be programmed for the gender of the patient by pushing the correct button on the device. If a female patient has had a hysterectomy, the male button is pushed (Corbett, 2004).

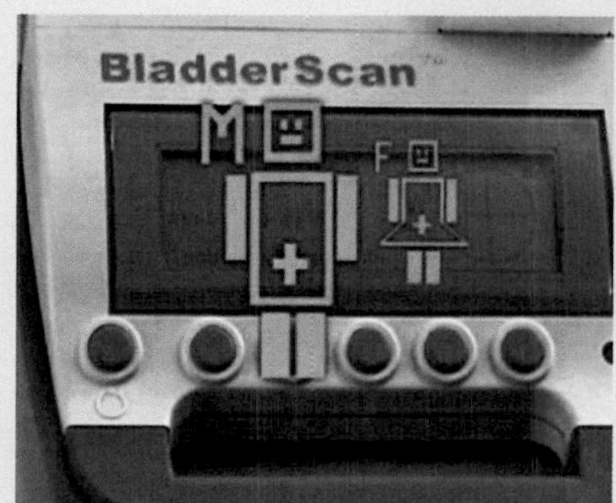

Figure 1. Identifying the icon for the patient's gender. From Patraca, K. (2005). Measure bladder volume without catheterization. *Nursing, 35*(4), 46.

(continued)

SKILL 12-4 Assessing Bladder Volume Using an Ultrasound Bladder Scanner *(continued)*

ACTION

9. Clean the scanner head with the appropriate cleaner (Figure 2).
10. **Gently palpate the patient's symphysis pubis (Figure 3). Place a generous amount of ultrasound gel or gel pad midline on the patient's abdomen, about 1″ to 1½″ above the symphysis pubis (anterior midline junction of pubic bones) (Figure 4).**

RATIONALE

Cleaning the scanner head deters transmission of microorganisms.

Palpation identifies the proper location and allows for correct placement of scanner head over the patient's bladder.

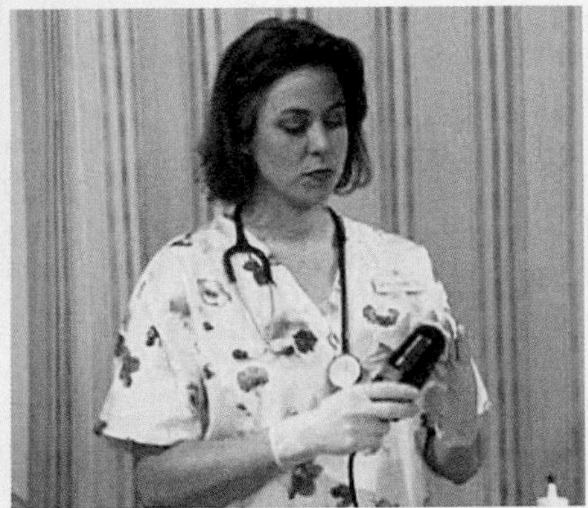

Figure 2. Cleaning scanner head. From Patraca, K. (2005). Measure bladder volume without catheterization. *Nursing, 35*(4), 46.

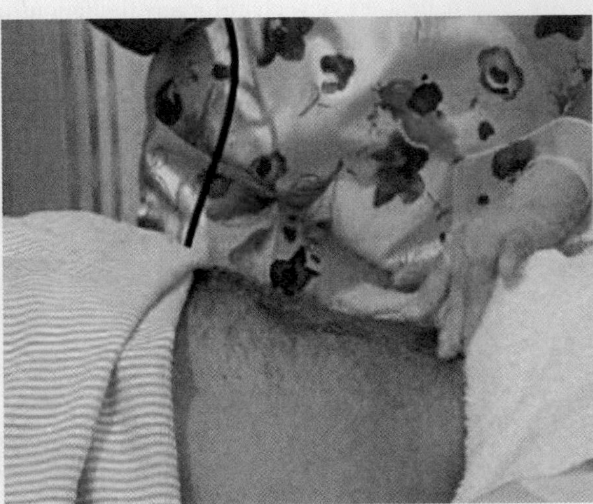

Figure 3. Palpating the patient's symphysis pubis. From Patraca, K. (2005). Measure bladder volume without catheterization. *Nursing, 35*(4), 46.

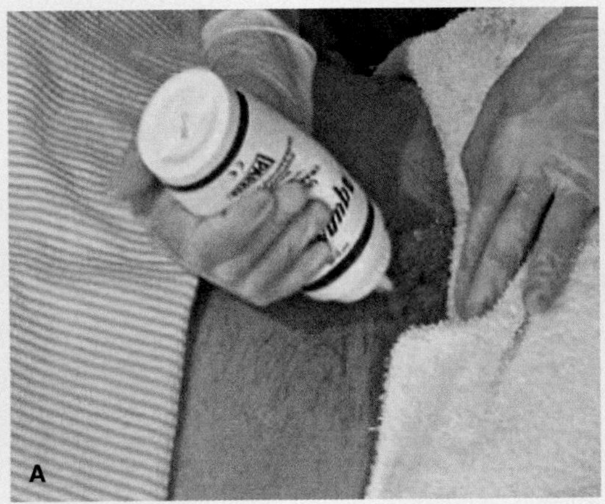

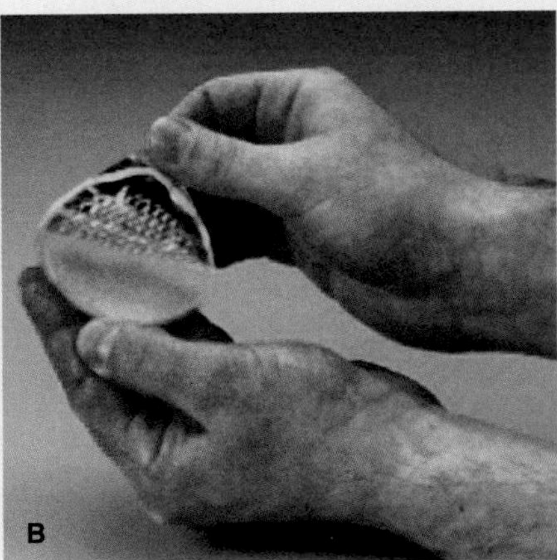

Figure 4. (**A**) Placing ultrasound gel about 1″ to 1½″ above symphysis pubis. (**B**) Gel pad. From Patraca, K. (2005). Measure bladder volume without catheterization. *Nursing, 35*(4), 47.

SKILL 12-4 Assessing Bladder Volume Using an Ultrasound Bladder Scanner *(continued)*

ACTION	RATIONALE
11. **Place the scanner head on the gel or gel pad, with the directional icon on the scanner head toward the patient's head. Aim the scanner head toward the bladder (point the scanner head slightly downward toward the coccyx) (Patraca, 2005). Press and release the 'Scan' button (Figure 5).**	Proper placement allows for accurate reading of urine in bladder.

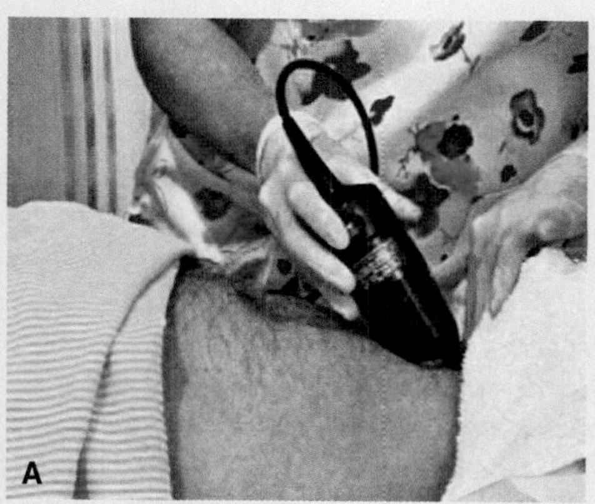

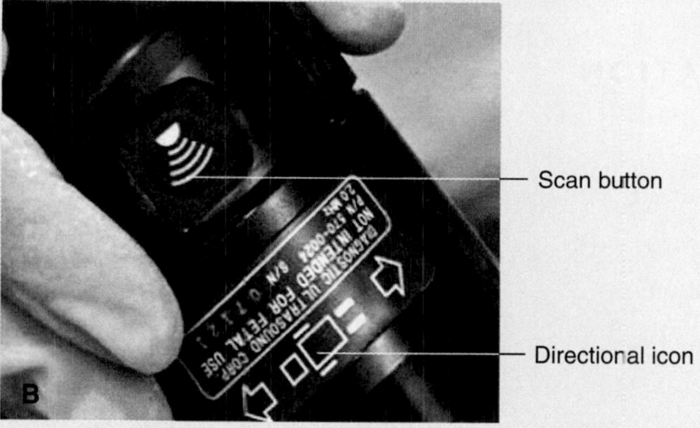

Figure 5. (**A**) Positioning the scanner head with directional icon toward the patient's head. (**B**) Pressing the scan button. From Patraca, K. (2005). Measure bladder volume without catheterization. *Nursing*, 35(4), 47.

ACTION	RATIONALE
12. Observe the image on the scanner screen. **Adjust the scanner head to center the bladder image on the crossbars (Figure 6).**	This action allows for accurate reading of urine in bladder.

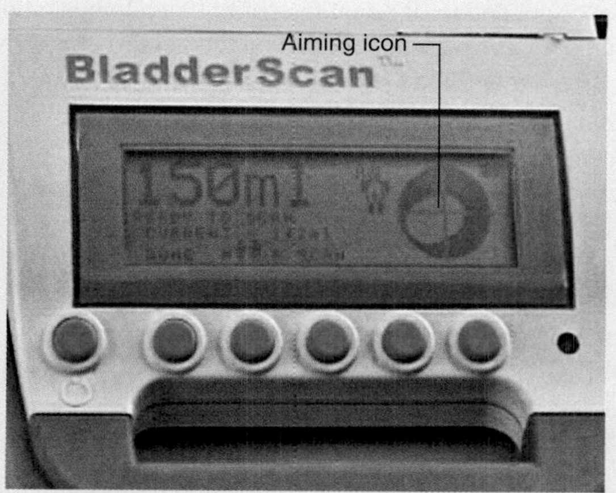

Figure 6. Centering the image on the crossbars. From Patraca, K. (2005). Measure bladder volume without catheterization. *Nursing, 35*(4), 47.

ACTION	RATIONALE
13. Press and hold the "Done" button until it beeps. Read the volume measurement on the screen. Print the results if required by pressing "Print."	This action provides for accurate documentation of reading.
14. Use a washcloth or paper towel to remove remaining gel from the patient's skin. Alternately, gently remove gel pad from patient's skin. Return the patient to a comfortable position. Remove your gloves and ensure that the patient is covered.	Removal of the gel promotes patient comfort. Removing contaminated gloves prevents spread of microorganisms.

(continued)

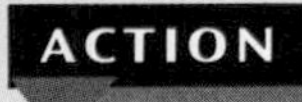

SKILL 12-4 Assessing Bladder Volume Using an Ultrasound Bladder Scanner *(continued)*

ACTION	RATIONALE
15. Lower bed height and adjust head of bed to a comfortable position. Reattach call bell if necessary.	These actions promote patient safety.

EVALUATION

The expected outcome is met when the volume of urine in the bladder is accurately measured, the patient's urinary elimination is maintained, with a urine output of at least 30 mL/hour; and the patient's bladder is not distended.

DOCUMENTATION

Guidelines

Document the assessment data that led to the use of the bladder scanner, the urine volume measured, and the patient's response.

Sample Documentation

7/06/08 1130 Patient has not voided 8 hours postcatheter removal. Patient denies feelings of discomfort, pressure, and pain. Bladder not palpable. Bladder scanned for 120 mL of urine. Patient encouraged to increase oral fluid intake to eight 6-oz. glasses today. Dr. Liu notified of assessment. Orders received to rescan in 4 hours if patient does not void.—B. Clapp, RN

Unexpected Situations and Associated Interventions

- *Nurse presses wrong icon for patient's gender when initiating scanner:* Turn scanner off and back on. Re-enter information using correct gender button.
- *Nurse has reason to believe bladder is full, based on assessment data, but scanner reveals little to no urine in bladder:* Ensure proper positioning of scanner head. Place a generous amount of ultrasound gel or gel pad midline on the patient's abdomen, about 1″ to 1½″ above the symphysis pubis. Place the scanner head on the gel or gel pad, with the directional icon on the scanner head toward the patient's head. Aim the scanner head toward the bladder (point the scanner head slightly downward toward the coccyx). Ensure that the bladder image is centered on the crossbars.

SKILL 12-5 Catheterizing the Female Urinary Bladder

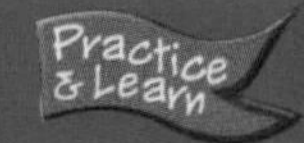

Urinary catheterization is the introduction of a catheter (tube) through the urethra into the bladder for the purpose of withdrawing urine. Catheterization is considered the most common cause of nosocomial infections (infections acquired in a hospital), so, whenever possible, catheterization should be avoided. When it is deemed necessary, it should be performed using careful, strict aseptic technique.

Intermittent urethral catheters, or straight catheters, are used to drain the bladder for shorter periods (5–10 minutes) (Figure 1B). If a catheter is to remain in place for continuous drainage, an **indwelling urethral catheter** is used. Indwelling catheters are also called retention or Foley catheters. The indwelling urethral catheter is designed so that it does not

SKILL 12-5 **Catheterizing the Female Urinary Bladder** *(continued)*

slip out of the bladder. A balloon is inflated to ensure that the catheter remains in the bladder once it is inserted. (Figure 1A). The following procedure reviews insertion of an indwelling catheter. The procedure for an intermittent catheter follows as a Skill Variation. Guidelines for caring for a patient with an indwelling catheter are summarized in Fundamentals Review 12-3.

Equipment

- Sterile catheter kit that contains:
  - Sterile gloves
  - Sterile drapes (one of which is fenestrated [having a window-like opening])
  - Sterile catheter
  - Antiseptic cleansing solution
  - Lubricant
  - Cotton balls or gauze squares
  - Forceps
  - Prefilled syringe with sterile water (sufficient to inflate indwelling catheter balloon)
  - Sterile basin (usually base of kit serves as this)
  - Sterile specimen container (if specimen is required)
- Flashlight or lamp
- Waterproof disposable pad
- Sterile disposable urine collection bag and drainage tubing (may be connected to catheter in catheter kit)
- Velcro leg strap or tape
- Disposable gloves
- Washcloth and warm water to perform perineal hygiene before and after catheterization

ASSESSMENT

Assess the patient's normal elimination habits. Assess the patient's degree of limitations and ability to help with activity. Assess for activity limitations, such as hip surgery or spinal injury, which would contraindicate certain actions by the patient. Assess for the presence of any other conditions that may interfere with passage of the catheter or contraindicate insertion of the catheter, such as urethral strictures or bladder cancer. Check for the presence of

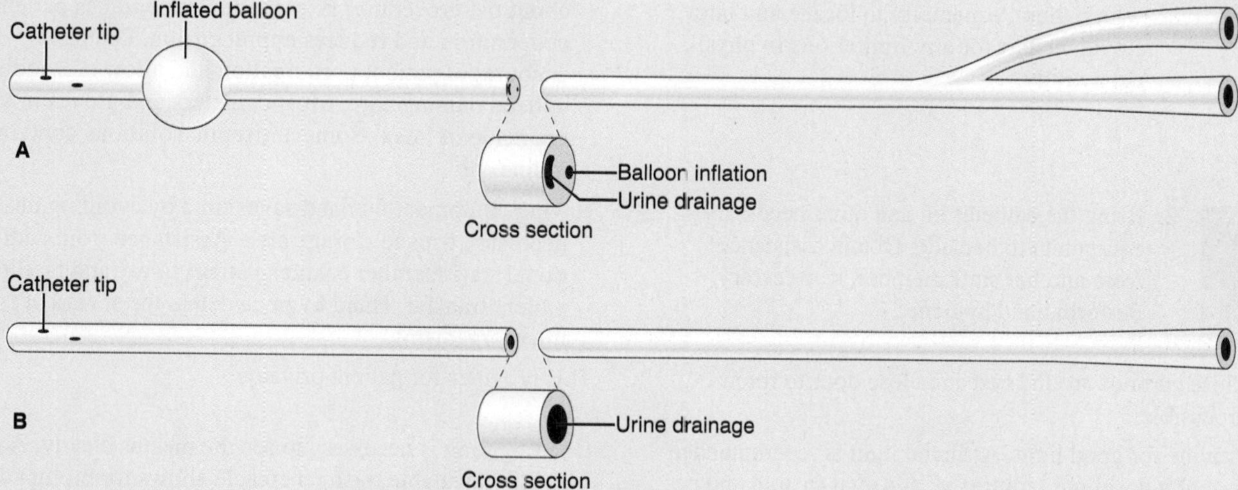

Figure 1. (**A**) Indwelling urethral catheter. (**B**) Intermittent urethral catheter.

(continued)

SKILL 12-5

Catheterizing the Female Urinary Bladder *(continued)*

drains, dressings, intravenous fluid infusion sites/equipment, traction, or any other devices that could interfere with the patient's ability to help with the procedure or that could become dislodged. Assess bladder fullness before performing procedure, either by palpation or with a handheld bladder ultrasound device. Question patient about any allergies, especially to latex and iodine. Ask patient if she has ever been catheterized. If she had an indwelling catheter previously, ask why and for how long it was used. The patient may have urethral strictures, which may make catheter insertion more difficult.

NURSING DIAGNOSIS

Determine the related factors for the nursing diagnoses based on the patient's current status. Appropriate nursing diagnoses may include:

- Impaired Urinary Elimination
- Urinary Retention
- Total Urinary Incontinence
- Risk for Infection
- Risk for Impaired Skin Integrity
- Risk for Injury

OUTCOME IDENTIFICATION AND PLANNING

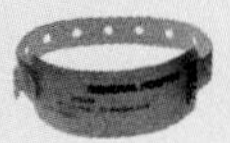

The expected outcome to achieve when inserting a female urinary catheter is that the patient's urinary elimination will be maintained, with a urine output of at least 30 mL/hour, and the patient's bladder will not be distended. Other appropriate outcomes may include the following: the patient's skin remains clean, dry, and intact, without evidence of irritation or breakdown; and the patient verbalizes an understanding of the purpose for and care of the catheter, as appropriate.

IMPLEMENTATION

ACTION	RATIONALE
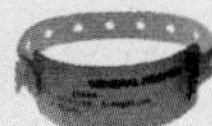 1. Identify the patient. Discuss procedure with patient and assess patient's ability to assist with the procedure. Discuss any allergies with patient, especially to iodine and latex. Review chart for any limitations in physical activity.	Identifying the patient ensures the right patient receives the intervention and helps prevent errors. This discussion promotes reassurance and provides knowledge about the procedure. Explanation encourages patient cooperation and reduces apprehension. Dialogue encourages patient participation and allows for individualized nursing care. Most catheters and gloves in kits are made of latex. Some antiseptic solutions contain iodine.
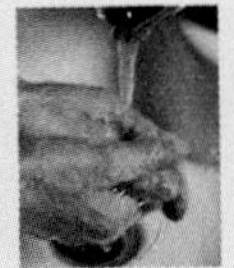 2. Bring the catheter kit and other necessary equipment to bedside. Obtain assistance from another staff member, if necessary. Perform hand hygiene.	Having equipment on hand saves time by avoiding unnecessary trips to storage area. Assistance from additional staff member ensures patient safety and facilitates patient transfer. Hand hygiene deters the spread of microorganisms.
3. Close curtains around bed and close door to room if possible.	This provides for patient privacy.
4. Provide for good light. Artificial light is recommended (use of a flashlight requires an assistant to hold and position it). Place a trash receptacle within easy reach.	Good lighting is necessary to see the meatus clearly. A readily available trash receptacle allows for prompt disposal of used supplies and reduces the risk of contaminating the sterile field.

SKILL 12-5 Catheterizing the Female Urinary Bladder *(continued)*

ACTION	RATIONALE
5. Raise the bed to a comfortable working height. Stand on the patient's right side if you are right handed, patient's left side if you are left handed.	Having the bed in the high position reduces strain on the nurse's back while performing the catheterization. Positioning allows for ease of use of dominant hand for catheter insertion.
6. Assist patient to dorsal recumbent position with knees flexed, feet about 2 feet apart, with her legs abducted. Drape patient (Figure 2). Alternately, the Sims', or lateral, position can be used. Place the patient's buttocks near the edge of the bed with her shoulders at the opposite edge and her knees drawn toward her chest (Figure 3). Allow the patient to lie on either side, depending on which position is easiest for the nurse and best for the patient's comfort. Slide waterproof pad under patient.	Proper positioning allows adequate visualization of the urinary meatus. Embarrassment, chilliness, and tension can interfere with catheter insertion; patient comfort will promote relaxation. The Sims' position may allow better visualization and be more comfortable for the patient, especially if hip and knee movements are difficult. The smaller area of exposure is also less stressful for the patient. The drape will protect bed linens from moisture.

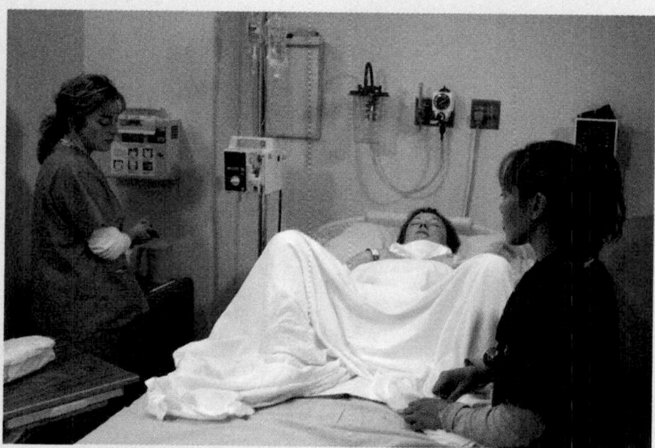

Figure 2. Patient in dorsal recumbent position and draped properly.

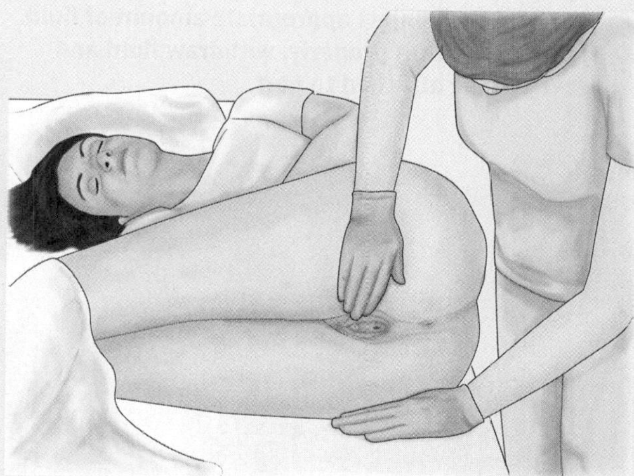

Figure 3. Demonstration of side-lying position.

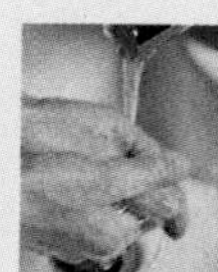

ACTION	RATIONALE
7. Put on clean gloves. Clean the perineal area with washcloth, skin cleanser, and warm water, using a different corner of the washcloth with each stroke. Wipe from above orifice downward toward sacrum (front to back). Rinse and dry. Remove gloves. Perform hand hygiene again.	Gloves reduce the risk of exposure to blood and body fluids. Cleaning reduces microorganisms near the urethral meatus and provides opportunity to visualize perineum and landmarks before procedure. Hand hygiene reduces the spread of microorganisms.
8. Prepare urine drainage setup if a separate urine collection system is to be used. Secure to bed frame according to manufacturer's directions.	This facilitates connection of the catheter to the drainage system and provides for easy access.
9. Open sterile catheterization tray on a clean overbed table using sterile technique.	Placement of equipment near worksite increases efficiency. Sterile technique protects patient and prevents spread of microorganisms.

(continued)

SKILL 12-5 Catheterizing the Female Urinary Bladder *(continued)*

ACTION	RATIONALE
10. Put on sterile gloves. Grasp upper corners of drape and unfold drape without touching unsterile areas. Fold back a corner on each side to make a cuff over gloved hands. Ask patient to lift her buttocks and slide sterile drape under her with gloves protected by cuff.	The drape provides a sterile field close to the meatus. Covering the gloved hands will help keep the gloves sterile while placing the drape.
11. Place a fenestrated sterile drape over the perineal area, exposing the labia (Figure 4).	The drape expands the sterile field and protects against contamination. Use of a fenestrated drape may limit visualization and is considered optional by some practitioners.
12. Place sterile tray on drape between patient's thighs.	This provides easy access to supplies.
13. Open all the supplies. **Test the catheter balloon by removing protective cap on tip of syringe and attaching syringe prefilled with sterile water to injection port (Figure 5). Inject appropriate amount of fluid. If balloon inflates properly, withdraw fluid and leave syringe attached to port.**	A balloon that does not inflate or that leaks needs to be replaced before insertion. Manufacturer provides appropriate amount of solution for the size of catheter in the kit; as a result, use entire syringe provided in the kit.

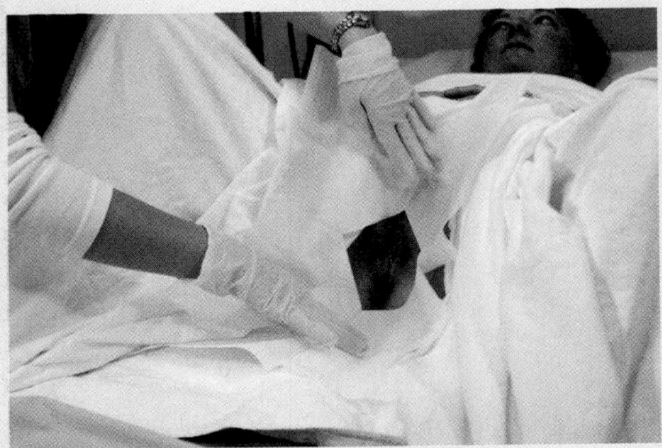

Figure 4. Patient with fenestrated drape in place over perineum.

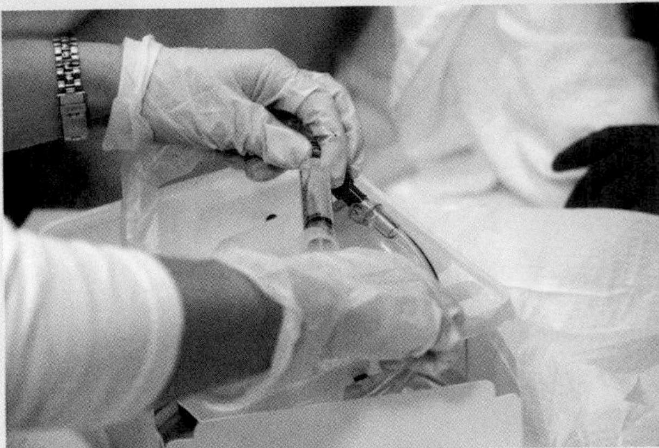

Figure 5. Testing balloon of indwelling catheter with syringe from catheter tray.

ACTION	RATIONALE
14. Fluff cotton balls in tray before pouring antiseptic solution over them. Alternately, open package of antiseptic swabs. Open specimen container if specimen is to be obtained.	It is necessary to open all supplies and prepare for the procedure while both hands are sterile.
15. Lubricate 1″ to 2″ of catheter tip.	Lubrication facilitates catheter insertion and reduces tissue trauma.

SKILL 12-5

Catheterizing the Female Urinary Bladder *(continued)*

ACTION

16. With thumb and one finger of nondominant hand, spread labia and identify meatus. **Be prepared to maintain separation of labia with one hand until catheter is inserted and urine is flowing well and continuously (Figure 6).** If the patient is in the side-lying position, lift the upper buttock and labia to expose the urinary meatus (Figure 7).

RATIONALE

Smoothing the area immediately surrounding the meatus helps to make it visible. Allowing the labia to drop back into position may contaminate the area around the meatus, as well as the catheter. Your nondominant hand is now contaminated.

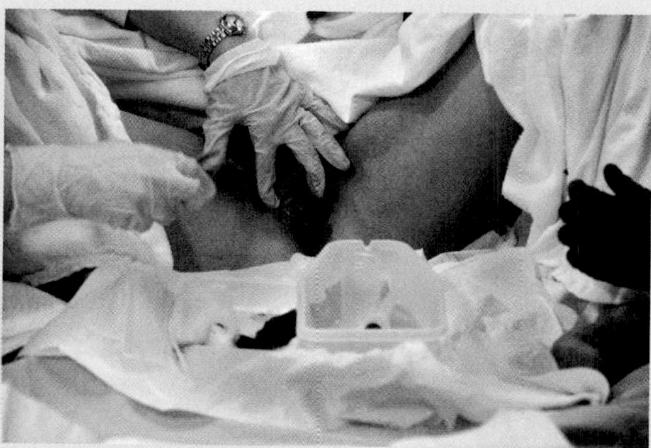

Figure 6. Using dominant hand to separate and hold labia open.

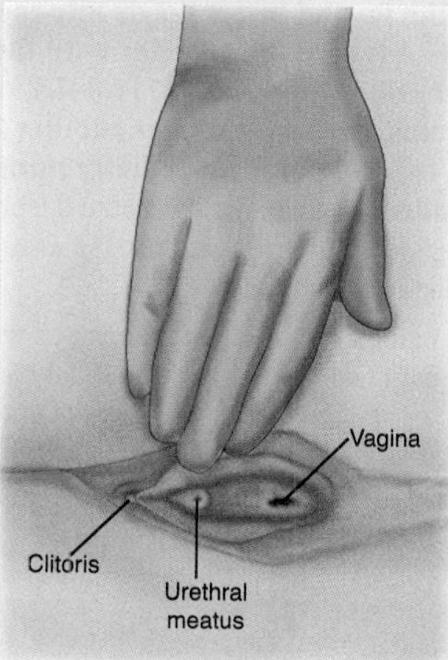

Figure 7. Exposing the urinary meatus with the patient in the side-lying position.

17. Use your dominant hand to pick up a cotton ball. **Clean one labial fold, top to bottom (from above the meatus down toward the rectum), then discard the cotton ball. Using a new cotton ball for each stroke, continue to clean the other labial fold, then directly over the meatus (Figure 8).**

Moving from an area where there is likely to be less contamination to an area where there is more contamination helps prevent the spread of microorganisms. Cleaning the meatus last helps reduce the possibility of introducing microorganisms into the bladder.

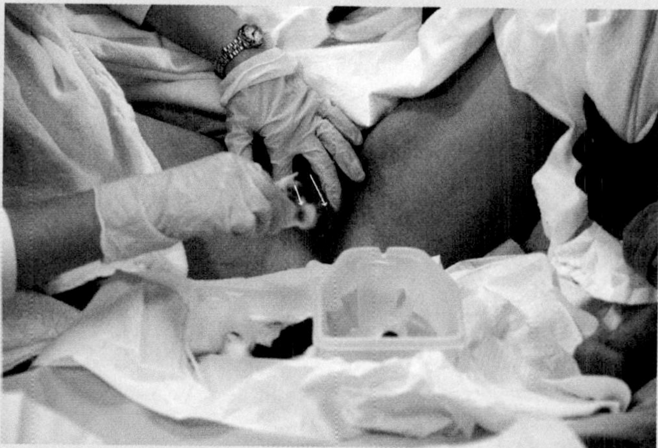

Figure 8. Wiping perineum with cotton ball held by forceps. Wipe in one direction from top to bottom.

(continued)

SKILL 12-5 Catheterizing the Female Urinary Bladder *(continued)*

ACTION	RATIONALE
18. With your uncontaminated, dominant hand, place drainage end of catheter in receptacle. If the catheter is preattached to sterile tubing and drainage container (closed drainage system), position catheter and setup within easy reach on sterile field. Ensure that clamp on drainage bag is closed.	This facilitates drainage of urine and minimizes risk of contaminating sterile equipment.
19. **Using your dominant hand, hold the catheter 2″ to 3″ from the tip and insert slowly into the urethra (Figure 9). Advance the catheter until there is a return of urine (approx. 2″–3″ [4.8–7.2 cm]). Once urine drains, advance catheter another 2″–3″ (4.8–7.2 cm). Do not force catheter through urethra into bladder.** Ask patient to breathe deeply, and rotate catheter gently if slight resistance is met as catheter reaches external sphincter.	The female urethra is about 1.5″–2.5″ (3.6–6.0 cm) long. Applying force on the catheter is likely to injure mucous membranes. The sphincter relaxes and the catheter can enter the bladder easily when the patient relaxes. Advancing an indwelling catheter an additional 2″–3″ (4.8–7.2 cm) ensures placement in the bladder and facilitates inflation of the balloon without damaging the urethra.
20. Hold the catheter securely at the meatus with your nondominant hand. Use your dominant hand to inflate the catheter balloon (Figure 10). Inject entire volume supplied in prefilled syringe.	Bladder or sphincter contraction could push the catheter out. The balloon anchors the catheter in place in the bladder. Sterile water is used to inflate the balloon as a precaution in case the balloon ruptures.

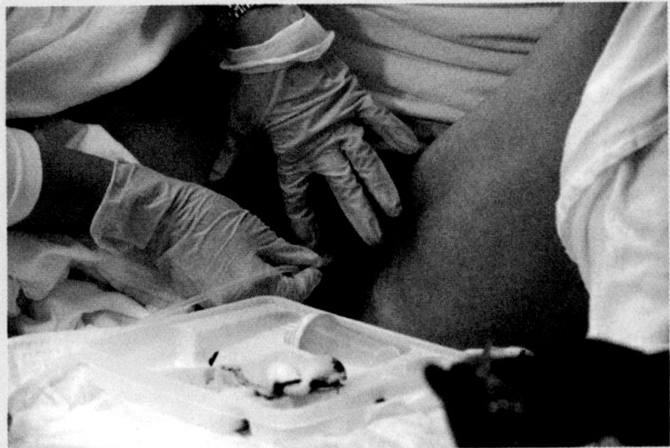

Figure 9. Inserting catheter with dominant hand while nondominant hand holds labia apart.

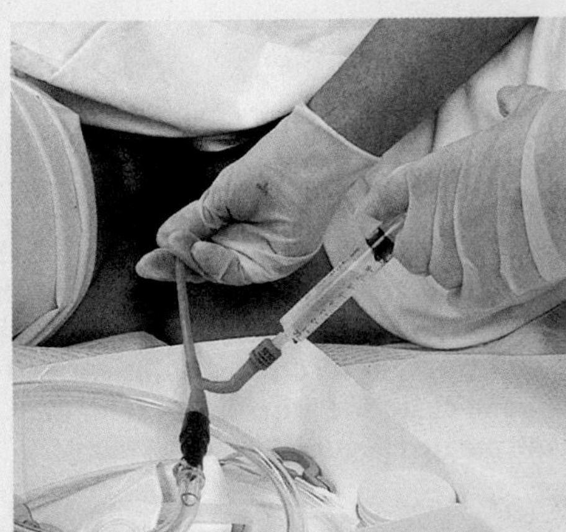

Figure 10. Inflating balloon of indwelling catheter.

ACTION	RATIONALE
21. Pull gently on catheter after balloon is inflated to feel resistance.	Improper inflation can cause patient discomfort and malpositioning of catheter.

SKILL 12-5

Catheterizing the Female Urinary Bladder *(continued)*

ACTION	RATIONALE
22. Attach catheter to drainage system if not already preattached. (Figure 11).	Closed drainage system minimizes the risk for microorganisms being introduced into the bladder.
23. Remove equipment and dispose of according to facility policy. Wash and dry the perineal area as needed.	Proper disposal prevents the spread of microorganisms. Cleaning promotes comfort and appropriate personal hygiene.
24. Remove gloves. **Secure catheter tubing to the patient's inner thigh with Velcro leg strap or tape (Figure 12).** Leave some slack in catheter for leg movement.	Proper attachment prevents trauma to the urethra and meatus from tension on the tubing. Whether to take the drainage tubing over or under the leg depends on gravity flow, patient's mobility, and comfort of the patient.

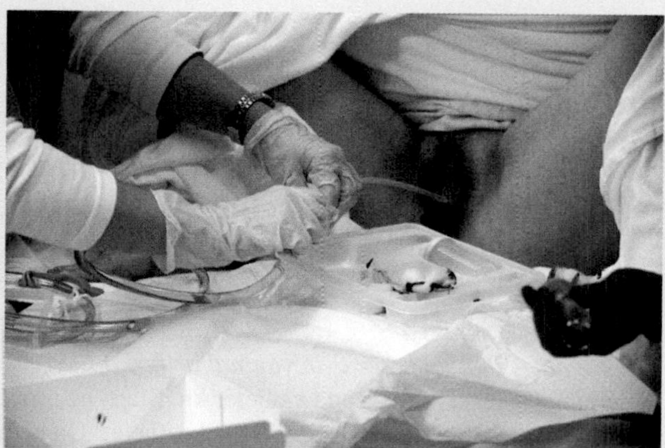

Figure 11. Attaching catheter to drainage bag.

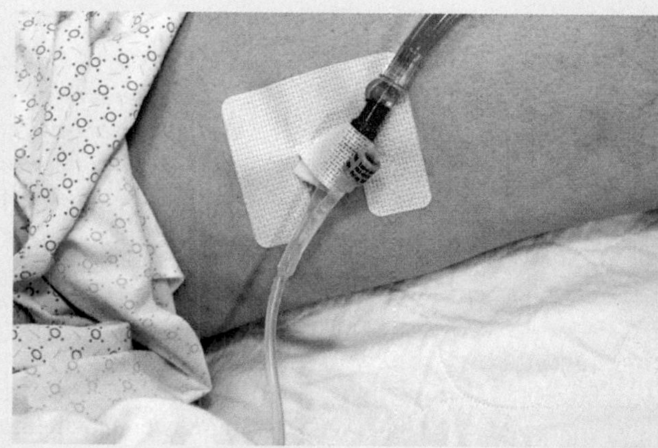

Figure 12. Catheter attached to leg.

ACTION	RATIONALE
25. Assist the patient to a comfortable position. Cover the patient with bed linens. Place the bed in the lowest position.	Positioning and covering provides warmth and promotes comfort.
26. Secure drainage bag below the level of the bladder. Check that drainage tubing is not kinked and that movement of side rails does not interfere with catheter or drainage bag.	This facilitates drainage of urine and prevents the backflow of urine.
27. Put on clean gloves. Obtain urine specimen immediately, if needed, from drainage bag. Label specimen. Send urine specimen to the laboratory promptly or refrigerate it.	Catheter system is sterile. Obtaining specimen immediately allows access to sterile system. Keeping urine at room temperature may cause microorganisms, if present, to grow and distort laboratory findings.
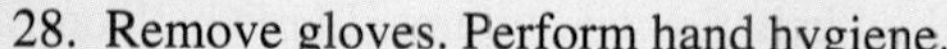 28. Remove gloves. Perform hand hygiene.	Hand hygiene deters the spread of microorganisms.

(continued)

SKILL 12-5 Catheterizing the Female Urinary Bladder *(continued)*

EVALUATION

The expected outcome is met when the catheter is inserted using sterile technique, results in the immediate flow of urine, and the bladder is not distended. Other outcomes are met when the patient does not experience trauma, reports little to no pain on insertion, and the perineal area remains clean and dry.

DOCUMENTATION

Guidelines

Document the type and size of catheter and balloon inserted, as well as the amount of fluid used to inflate the balloon. Document the patient's tolerance of the activity. Record the amount of urine obtained through the catheter and any specimen obtained. Document any other assessments, such as unusual urine characteristics or alterations in the patient's skin. Record urine amount on intake and output record, if appropriate.

Sample Documentation

7/14/08 0915 Physician notified of palpable bladder (3 cm below umbilicus) and patient's inability to void. 16 Fr. Foley catheter inserted without difficulty. 10 mL of sterile water injected into balloon port. 700 mL clear yellow urine returned. Patient states, "Oh, I feel much better now." Bladder is no longer palpable. Patient tolerated procedure without adverse event.—B. Clapp, RN

Unexpected Situations and Associated Interventions

- *No urine flow is obtained, and nurse notes that catheter is in vaginal orifice:* Leave catheter in place as a marker. Obtain new sterile gloves and catheter kit. Start the procedure over and attempt to place new catheter directly above misplaced catheter. Once the new catheter is correctly in place, remove the catheter in the vaginal orifice. Because of the risk of cross-infection, never remove a catheter from the vagina and insert it into the urethra (Robinson, 2004).
- *Patient moves legs during procedure:* If no supplies have been contaminated, ask patient to hold still and continue with procedure. If supplies have been contaminated, stop procedure and start over. If necessary, get an assistant to remind the patient to hold still.
- *Urine flow is initially well established and urine is clear, but after several hours flow dwindles:* Check tubing for kinking. If patient has changed position, the tubing and drainage bag may need to be moved to facilitate drainage of urine.
- *Patient complains of extreme pain when nurse is inflating balloon:* Stop inflation of balloon. Balloon is most likely still in urethra. Withdraw the solution from the balloon. Insert catheter an additional ½″ to 1″ (1.2–2.4 cm) and slowly attempt to inflate balloon again.
- *Urine leaks out of meatus around the catheter:* Do not increase the size of the indwelling catheter. Make sure the smallest sized catheter with a 10-mL balloon is used. Large catheters cause bladder and urethral irritation and trauma. Large balloon-fill volumes occupy more space inside the bladder and put added weight on the base of the bladder. Irritation of the bladder wall and detrusor muscle can cause leakage. If leakage

SKILL 12-5 **Catheterizing the Female Urinary Bladder** *(continued)*

persists, consider an evaluation for urinary tract infection. Ensure that the correct amount of solution was used to inflate the balloon. Underfilling the balloon can cause the catheter to dislodge into the urethra, causing urethral spasm, pain, and discomfort. If you suspect underfill, do not attempt to push the catheter further into the bladder. Remove the catheter and replace. Assess the patient for constipation. Bowel full of stool can cause pressure on the catheter lumen and prevent the drainage of urine. Implement interventions to prevent/treat constipation (Emr & Ryan, 2004; Robinson, 2004).

Special Considerations

General Considerations

- Be familiar with facility policy and/or primary practitioner guidelines for the maximum amount of urine to remove from bladder at the time of insertion.
- If patient is unable to lift buttocks or maintain required position for the procedure, the assistance of another staff member may be necessary to place the drape under the patient and to help the patient maintain the required position.
- Supplies can be opened and prepared on the overbed table, moving the tray onto the bed just before cleansing the patient.
- If there is not an immediate flow of urine after the catheter has been inserted, several measures may prove helpful:
  - Have the patient take a deep breath, which helps to relax the perineal and abdominal muscles.
  - Rotate the catheter slightly, because a drainage hole may be resting against the bladder wall.
  - Raise the head of the patient's bed to increase pressure in the bladder area.
  - Assess the patient' intake to ensure adequate fluid intake for urine production.
  - Assess the catheter and drainage tubing for kinks and occlusion.
- If the catheter cannot be advanced, have the patient take several deep breaths. Rotate the catheter half a turn and try to advance. If you are still unable to advance, remove the catheter. Notify the physician.
- Some catheter kits do not contain the catheter. This allows you to select a catheter and balloon size separately.

Infant and Child Considerations

- Size 5F to 8F is used for infants and young children. Size 8F to 12F catheters are commonly used for older children (Hockenberry, 2005).
- Distraction, such as blowing bubbles, deep breathing, or singing a song, can help the child relax.
- Lidocaine jelly is often used to anesthetize and lubricate the area before insertion of the catheter, decreasing the child's discomfort and anxiety.

Home Care Considerations

- Intermittent catheterization in the home is performed using clean technique. The bladder's natural resistance to the microorganisms normally found in the home makes sterile technique unnecessary. Catheters are washed, dried, and stored for repeated use.

(continued)

SKILL 12-5 Catheterizing the Female Urinary Bladder *(continued)*

SKILL VARIATION Intermittent Female Urethral Catheterization

- Identify the patient. Discuss procedure with patient and assess patient's ability to assist with the procedure. Discuss any allergies with patient, especially to iodine and latex. Review chart for any limitations in physical activity.
- Bring the catheter kit and other necessary equipment to bedside. Obtain assistance from another staff member, if necessary. Perform hand hygiene. Put on disposable gloves.
- Close curtains around bed and close door to room if possible.
- Provide for good light. Artificial light is recommended (use of a flashlight requires an assistant to hold and position it). Place a trash receptacle within easy reach.
- Raise the bed to a comfortable working height. Stand on the patient's right side if you are right handed, patient's left side if you are left handed.
- Assist patient to dorsal recumbent position with knees flexed, feet about 2 feet apart, with her legs abducted. Drape patient. Alternately, use the Sims', or lateral, position. Place the patient's buttocks near the edge of the bed with her shoulders at the opposite edge and her knees drawn toward her chest. Slide waterproof drape under patient.
- Put on clean gloves. Clean the perineal area with washcloth, skin cleanser, and warm water, using a different corner of the washcloth with each stroke. Wipe from above orifice downward toward sacrum (front to back). Rinse and dry. Remove gloves. Perform hand hygiene again.
- Open sterile catheterization tray on a clean overbed table using sterile technique.
- Put on sterile gloves. Grasp upper corners of drape and unfold drape without touching unsterile areas. Fold back a corner on each side to make a cuff over gloved hands. Ask patient to lift her buttocks and slide sterile drape under her with gloves protected by cuff.
- Place a fenestrated sterile drape over the perineal area, exposing the labia, if appropriate.
- Place sterile tray on drape between patient's thighs.
- Open all the supplies. Fluff cotton balls in tray before pouring antiseptic solution over them. Alternately, open package of antiseptic swabs. Open specimen container if specimen is to be obtained.
- Lubricate 1″ to 2″ of catheter tip.
- With thumb and one finger of nondominant hand, spread labia and identify meatus. If the patient is in the side-lying position, lift the upper buttock and labia to expose the urinary meatus. Be prepared to maintain separation of labia with one hand until catheter is inserted and urine is flowing well and continuously.
- Use your dominant hand to pick up a cotton ball. Clean one labial fold, top to bottom (from above the meatus down toward the rectum), then discard the cotton ball. Using a new cotton ball for each stroke, continue to clean the other labial fold, then directly over the meatus.
- With your uncontaminated, dominant hand, place drainage end of catheter in receptacle. If a specimen is required, place the end into the specimen container in the receptacle.
- Using your dominant hand, hold the catheter 2″ to 3″ from the tip and insert slowly into the urethra. Advance the catheter until there is a return of urine (approx. 2″ to 3″ [4.8–7.2 cm]). Do not force catheter through urethra into bladder. Ask patient to breathe deeply, and rotate catheter gently if slight resistance is met as catheter reaches external sphincter.
- Hold the catheter securely at the meatus with your nondominant hand while the bladder empties. If a specimen is being collected, remove the drainage end of the tubing from the specimen container after required amount is obtained and allow urine to flow into receptacle. Set specimen container aside and place lid on container.
- Allow the bladder to empty. Withdraw catheter slowly and smoothly after urine has stopped flowing. Remove equipment and dispose of according to facility policy. Wash and dry the perineal area as needed.
- Remove your gloves. Assist the patient to a comfortable position. Cover the patient with bed linens. Place the bed in the lowest position.
- Put on clean gloves. Secure the container lid and label specimen. Send urine specimen to the laboratory promptly or refrigerate it.
- Remove gloves. Perform hand hygiene.

SKILL 12-6 Catheterizing the Male Urinary Bladder

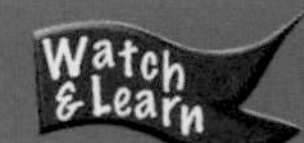

Urinary catheterization is the introduction of a catheter (tube) through the urethra into the bladder for the purpose of withdrawing urine. Catheterization is considered the most common cause of nosocomial infections (infections acquired in a hospital), so, whenever possible, catheterization should be avoided. When it is deemed necessary, it should be performed using careful, strict aseptic technique.

Intermittent urethral catheters, or straight catheters, are used to drain the bladder for shorter periods (5–10 minutes). If a catheter is to remain in place for continuous drainage,

SKILL 12-6 Catheterizing the Male Urinary Bladder *(continued)*

an indwelling urethral catheter is used. Indwelling catheters are also called retention or Foley catheters. The indwelling urethral catheter is designed so that it does not slip out of the bladder. A balloon is inflated to ensure that the catheter remains in the bladder once it is inserted (Figure 1, Skill 12-5).

The following procedure reviews insertion of an indwelling catheter. The procedure for an intermittent catheter follows as a Skill Variation. Guidelines for caring for a patient with an indwelling catheter are summarized in Fundamentals Review 12-3.

Equipment

- Sterile catheter kit that contains:
  - Sterile gloves
  - Sterile drapes (one of which is fenestrated)
  - Sterile catheter
  - Antiseptic cleansing solution
  - Lubricant, in a prefilled 10-mL syringe
  - Cotton balls or gauze squares
  - Forceps
  - Prefilled syringe with sterile water (sufficient to inflate indwelling catheter balloon)
  - Sterile basin (usually base of kit serves as this)
  - Sterile specimen container, if specimen is required
- Flashlight or lamp
- Waterproof disposable pad
- Sterile disposable urine collection bag and drainage tubing (may be connected to sterile indwelling catheter if a closed drainage system is used)
- Velcro leg strap or tape
- Disposable gloves
- Washcloth and warm water to perform perineal hygiene before and after catheterization

ASSESSMENT

Assess the patient's normal elimination habits. Assess the patient's degree of limitations and ability to help with activity. Assess for activity limitations, such as hip surgery or spinal injury, which would contraindicate certain actions by the patient. Assess for the presence of any other conditions that may interfere with passage of the catheter or contraindicate insertion of the catheter, such as urethral strictures or bladder cancer. Check for the presence of drains, dressings, intravenous fluid infusion sites/equipment, traction, or any other devices that could interfere with the patient's ability to help with the procedure or that could become dislodged. Assess bladder fullness before performing procedure, either by palpation or with a handheld bladder ultrasound device, and question patient about any allergies, especially to latex and iodine. Ask patient if he has ever been catheterized. If he had an indwelling catheter previously, ask why and for how long it was used. The patient may have urethral strictures, which may make catheter insertion more difficult. If the patient is 50 or older, ask if he has had any prostate problems. Prostate enlargement typically is noted around the age of 50 years.

NURSING DIAGNOSIS

Determine the related factors for the nursing diagnoses based on the patient's current status. Appropriate nursing diagnoses may include:

- Impaired Urinary Elimination
- Urinary Retention
- Total Urinary Incontinence

(continued)

SKILL 12-6 Catheterizing the Male Urinary Bladder *(continued)*

- Risk for Infection
- Risk for Impaired Skin Integrity
- Risk for Injury

OUTCOME IDENTIFICATION AND PLANNING

The expected outcome to achieve when inserting a male urinary catheter is that the patient's urinary elimination will be maintained, with a urine output of at least 30 mL/hour, and the patient's bladder will not be distended. Other appropriate outcomes may include the following: the patient's skin remains clean, dry, and intact, without evidence of irritation or breakdown; and the patient verbalizes an understanding of the purpose for and care of the catheter, as appropriate.

IMPLEMENTATION

ACTION	RATIONALE
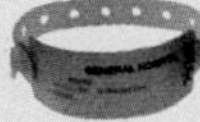 1. Identify the patient. Discuss procedure with patient and assess patient's ability to assist with the procedure. Discuss any allergies with patient, especially to iodine and latex. Review chart for any limitations in physical activity.	Identifying the patient ensures the right patient receives the intervention and helps prevent errors. This discussion promotes reassurance and provides knowledge about the procedure. Explanation encourages patient cooperation and reduces apprehension. Dialogue encourages patient participation and allows for individualized nursing care. Most catheters and gloves in kits are made of latex. Some antiseptic solutions contain iodine.
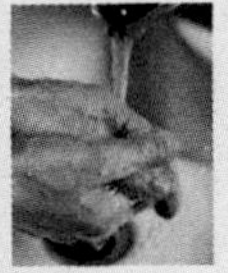 2. Bring the catheter kit and other necessary equipment to bedside. Obtain assistance from another staff member, if necessary. Perform hand hygiene. Put on disposable gloves.	Having equipment on hand saves time by avoiding unnecessary trips to storage area. Assistance from additional staff member ensures patient safety and facilitates patient transfer. Hand hygiene deters the spread of microorganisms. Gloves prevent exposure to blood and body fluids.
3. Close curtains around bed and close door to room if possible.	This action provides for patient privacy.
4. Provide for good light. Artificial light is recommended. Place a trash receptacle within easy reach.	Good lighting is necessary to perform the procedure properly. A readily available trash receptacle ensures appropriate disposal of used supplies and reduces the risk of contaminating the sterile field.
5. Raise the bed to a comfortable working height. Stand on the patient's right side if you are right handed, patient's left side if you are left handed.	Having the bed in the high position reduces strain on the nurse's back while performing the catheterization. Positioning allows for ease of use of dominant hand for catheter insertion.
6. Position patient on his back with thighs slightly apart. Drape patient so that only the area around the penis is exposed. Slide waterproof pad under patient.	This prevents unnecessary exposure and promotes warmth. The waterproof pad will protect bed linens from moisture.

SKILL 12-6 Catheterizing the Male Urinary Bladder *(continued)*

ACTION	RATIONALE
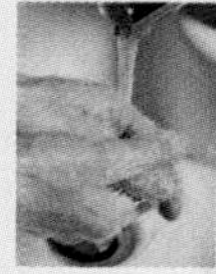 7. Put on clean gloves. Clean the genital area with washcloth, skin cleanser, and warm water. Clean the tip of the penis first, moving the washcloth in a circular motion from the meatus outward. Wash the shaft of the penis using downward strokes toward the pubic area. Rinse and dry. Remove gloves. Perform hand hygiene again.	Gloves reduce the risk of exposure to blood and body fluids. Cleaning the penis reduces microorganisms near the urethral meatus. Hand hygiene reduces the spread of microorganisms.
8. Prepare urine drainage setup if a separate urine collection system is to be used. Secure to bed frame according to manufacturer's directions.	This facilitates connection of the catheter to the drainage system and provides for easy access.
9. Open sterile catheterization tray on a clean overbed table, using sterile technique.	Placement of equipment near worksite increases efficiency. Sterile technique protects patient and prevents spread of microorganisms.
10. Put on sterile gloves. Open sterile drape and place on patient's thighs. Place fenestrated drape with opening over penis (Figure 1).	This maintains a sterile working area.

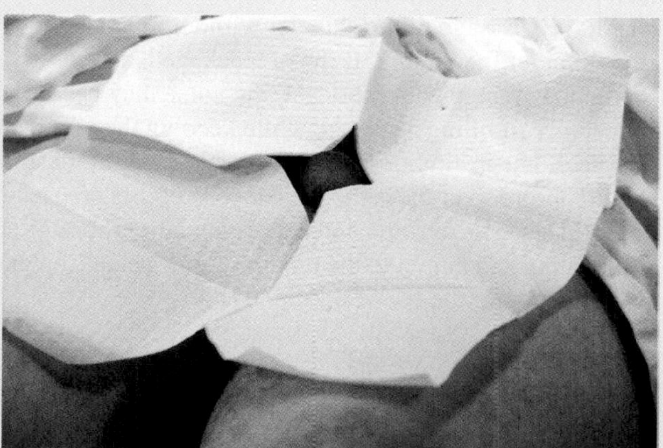

Figure 1. Patient lying supine with fenestrated drape over penis.

ACTION	RATIONALE
11. Place catheter set on or next to patient's legs on sterile drape.	Sterile setup should be arranged so that nurse's back is not turned to it, nor should it be out of the nurse's range of vision.
12. Open all the supplies. **Test the catheter balloon by removing protective cap on tip of syringe and attaching syringe prefilled with sterile water to injection port. Inject appropriate amount of fluid. If balloon inflates properly, withdraw fluid and leave syringe attached to port.**	A balloon that does not inflate or that leaks needs to be replaced before insertion. Manufacturer provides appropriate amount of solution for the size of catheter in the kit; as a result, use entire syringe provided in the kit.
13. Fluff cotton balls in tray before pouring antiseptic solution over them. Alternately, open package of antiseptic swabs. Open specimen container if specimen is to be obtained.	It is necessary to open all supplies and prepare for the procedure while both hands are sterile.

(continued)

SKILL 12-6 Catheterizing the Male Urinary Bladder *(continued)*

ACTION	RATIONALE
14. With your uncontaminated, dominant hand, place drainage end of catheter in receptacle. If the catheter is preattached to sterile tubing and drainage container (closed drainage system), position catheter and setup within easy reach on sterile field. Ensure that clamp on drainage bag is closed.	This facilitates drainage of urine and minimizes risk of contaminating sterile equipment.
15. Remove cap from syringe prefilled with lubricant.	
16. Lift penis with nondominant hand. Retract foreskin in uncircumcised patient. **Be prepared to keep this hand in this position until catheter is inserted and urine is flowing well and continuously. Using your dominant hand and the forceps, pick up a cotton ball. Using a circular motion, clean the penis, moving from the meatus down the glans of the penis (Figure 2). Repeat this cleansing motion two more times, using a new cotton ball each time. Discard each cotton ball after one use.**	The hand touching the penis becomes contaminated. Cleansing the area around the meatus and under the foreskin in the uncircumcised patient helps prevent infection. Moving from the meatus toward the base of the penis prevents bringing microorganisms to the meatus.
17. Hold penis with slight upward tension and perpendicular to patient's body. Use your dominant hand to pick up the lubricant syringe. **Gently insert tip of syringe with lubricant into urethra and instill the 10 mL of lubricant (Figure 3).**	The lubricant causes the urethra to distend slightly and facilitates passage of the catheter without traumatizing the lining of the urethra. If the prepackaged kit does not contain a syringe with lubricant, the nurse may need assistance in filling a syringe while keeping the lubricant sterile. Some institutions use lidocaine jelly for lubrication before insertion of the catheter. The jelly comes prepackaged in a sterile syringe and serves a dual purpose of lubricating and numbing the urethra. A physician's order is necessary for the use of lidocaine jelly.

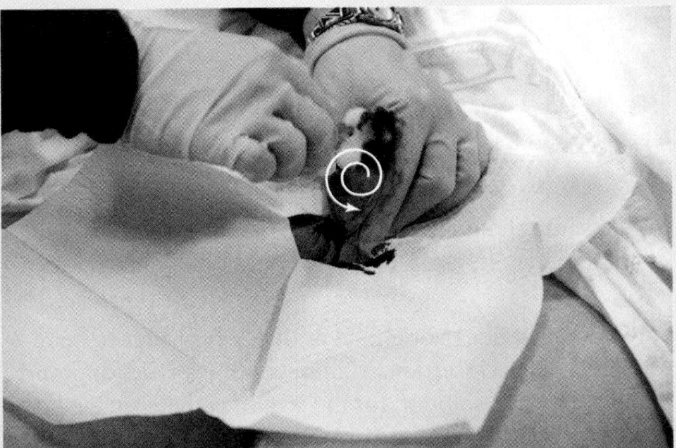

Figure 2. Lifting penis with gloved nondominant hand and cleaning meatus with cotton ball held with forceps in gloved dominant hand.

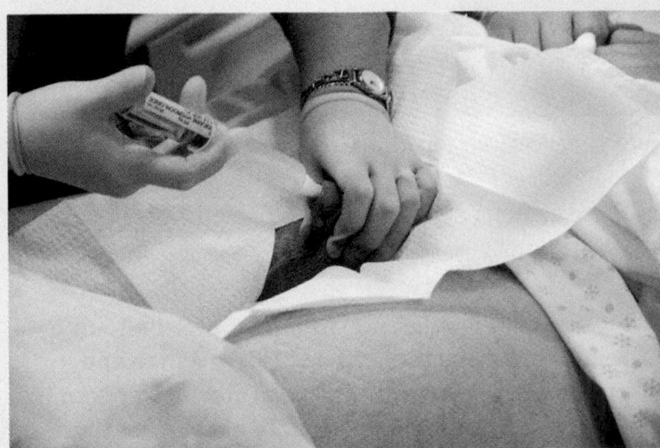

Figure 3. Inserting syringe with lubricant into urethra.

SKILL 12-6 Catheterizing the Male Urinary Bladder *(continued)*

ACTION	RATIONALE
18. Use your dominant hand to pick up the catheter and hold it an inch or two from the tip. Ask patient to bear down as if voiding. **Insert catheter tip into meatus (Figure 4). Ask the patient to take deep breaths as you advance the catheter to the bifurcation or "Y" level of the ports. Do not use force to introduce catheter.** If catheter resists entry, ask patient to breathe deeply and rotate catheter slightly.	Bearing down eases the passage of the catheter through the urethra. The male urethra is about 20 cm long. Having the patient take deep breaths or twisting the catheter slightly may ease the catheter past resistance at the sphincters. Advancing an indwelling catheter to the bifurcation ensures its placement in the bladder and facilitates inflation of the balloon without damaging the urethra.
19. Hold the catheter securely at the meatus with your nondominant hand. Use your dominant hand to inflate the catheter balloon. **Inject entire volume supplied in prefilled syringe. Once balloon is inflated, catheter may be gently pulled back into place. Replace foreskin over catheter.** Lower penis.	Bladder or sphincter contraction could push the catheter out. The balloon anchors the catheter in place in the bladder. Sterile water is used to inflate the balloon as a precaution in case the balloon ruptures.
20. Pull gently on catheter after balloon is inflated to feel resistance.	Improper inflation can cause patient discomfort and malpositioning of catheter.
21. Attach catheter to drainage system if necessary.	Closed drainage system minimizes the risk for microorganisms being introduced into the bladder.
22. Remove equipment and dispose of according to facility policy. Wash and dry the perineal area as needed.	Proper disposal prevents the spread of microorganisms. Promotes comfort and appropriate personal hygiene. Prevents tightening of the band behind the glans penis.
23. Remove gloves. Secure catheter tubing to the patient's inner thigh or lower abdomen (with the penis directed toward the patient's chest) with Velcro leg strap or tape (Figure 5). Leave some slack in catheter for leg movement.	Proper attachment prevents trauma to the urethra and meatus from tension on the tubing. Whether to take the drainage tubing over or under the leg depends on gravity flow, patient's mobility, and comfort of the patient.

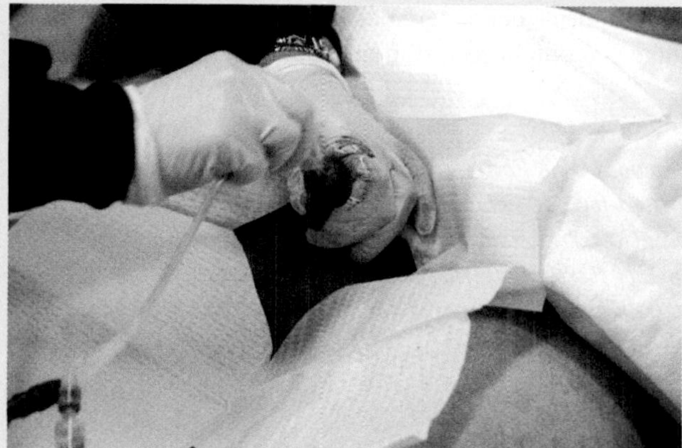
Figure 4. Inserting catheter with dominant hand.

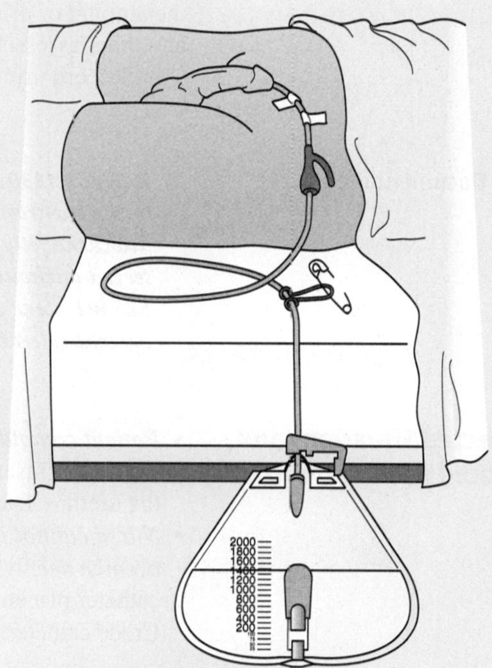
Figure 5. Securing tubing to patient's abdomen.

(continued)

SKILL 12-6 Catheterizing the Male Urinary Bladder *(continued)*

ACTION	RATIONALE
24. Assist the patient to a comfortable position. Cover the patient with bed linens. Place the bed in the lowest position.	Positioning and covering provides warmth and promotes comfort.
25. Secure drainage bag below the level of the bladder. Check that drainage tubing is not kinked and that movement of side rails does not interfere with catheter or drainage bag.	This facilitates drainage of urine and prevents the backflow of urine.
26. Put on clean gloves. Obtain urine specimen immediately, if needed, from drainage bag. Cover and label specimen. Send urine specimen to the laboratory promptly or refrigerate it.	Catheter system is sterile. Obtaining specimen immediately allows access to sterile system. Keeping urine at room temperature may cause microorganisms, if present, to grow and distort laboratory findings.
27. Remove gloves. Perform hand hygiene.	Hand hygiene deters the spread of microorganisms.

EVALUATION

The expected outcome is met when the catheter is inserted using sterile technique, results in the immediate flow of urine, and the bladder is not distended. Other outcomes are met when the patient does not experience trauma, reports little to no pain on insertion, and the perineal area remains clean and dry.

DOCUMENTATION

Guidelines

Document the type and size of catheter and balloon inserted, as well as the amount of fluid used to inflate the balloon. Document the patient's tolerance of the activity. Record the amount of urine obtained through the catheter and any specimen obtained. Document any other assessments, such as unusual urine characteristics or alterations in the patient's skin. Record urine amount on intake and output record, if appropriate.

Sample Documentation

7/14/08 1830 Patient unable to void × 8 hours and reports, "I feel like I have to go to the bathroom." Bladder scanned for 540 mL urine. Physician notified. 10 mL 2% lidocaine jelly instilled before catheterization per order. 14 Fr. Foley catheter inserted without difficulty. 10 mL of sterile water injected into 5-mL balloon port. 525 mL clear yellow urine returned. Patient reports decreased bladder pressure. Patient tolerated procedure without adverse event.—B. Clapp, RN

Unexpected Situations and Associated Interventions

- *Patient complains of intense pain when nurse begins to inflate balloon:* Stop inflation. Be sure to insert catheter all the way into the bifurcation. The balloon is probably still in the urethra. Damage to the urethra can result if balloon is inflated in urethra.
- *Nurse cannot insert catheter past 3" to 4"; rotating the catheter and having patient breathe deeply are of no help:* If still unable to place catheter, notify physician. Repeated catheter placement attempts can traumatize the urethra. Physician may order and insert a Credé catheter.

SKILL 12-6

Catheterizing the Male Urinary Bladder *(continued)*

- *Patient is obese or has retracted penis:* Have assistant available to place fingers on either side of the pubic area and press backward to bring the penis out of the pubic cavity. Hold patient's penis up and forward. The catheter still needs to be inserted to the bifurcation; the length of the urethra has not changed.
- *Urine flow initially contains a large amount of* ***sediment*** *(precipitate) and then suddenly stops; bladder remains palpable:* Catheter may be plugged with sediment. After obtaining a physician's order, gently irrigate the catheter to restore flow.
- *Urine leaks out of meatus around the catheter:* Do not increase the size of the indwelling catheter. Make sure the smallest sized catheter with a 10-mL balloon is used. Large catheters cause bladder and urethral irritation and trauma. Large balloon-fill volumes occupy more space inside the bladder and put added weight on the base of the bladder. Irritation of the bladder wall and detrusor muscle can cause leakage. If leakage persists, consider an evaluation for urinary tract infection. Ensure that the correct amount of solution was used to inflate the balloon. Underfilling the balloon can cause the catheter to dislodge into the urethra, causing urethral spasm, pain, and discomfort. If you suspect underfill, do not attempt to push the catheter further into the bladder. Remove the catheter and replace. Assess the patient for constipation. Bowel full of stool can cause pressure on the catheter lumen and prevent the drainage of urine. Implement interventions to prevent/treat constipation (Emr & Ryan, 2004; Robinson, 2004).
- *Urine flow is initially well established and urine is clear, but after several hours urine flow dwindles:* Check tubing for kinking. If patient has changed position, the tubing and drainage bag may need to be moved to facilitate drainage of urine.

Special Considerations

General Considerations

- Be familiar with facility policy and/or primary practitioner guidelines for the maximum amount of urine to remove from bladder at the time of insertion.
- Supplies can be opened and prepared on the overbed table, moving the tray onto the bed just before cleansing the patient.
- If there is not an immediate flow of urine after the catheter has been inserted, several measures may prove helpful:
  - Have the patient take a deep breath, which helps to relax the perineal and abdominal muscles.
  - Rotate the catheter slightly, because a drainage hole may be resting against the bladder wall.
  - Raise the head of the patient's bed to increase pressure in the bladder area.
  - Assess the patient's intake to ensure adequate fluid intake for urine production.
  - Assess the catheter and drainage tubing for kinks and occlusion.
- Urethral strictures, false passages, prostatic enlargement, and postsurgical bladder-neck contractures can make urethral catheterization difficult and may require the services of a urologist. If there is any question as to the location of the catheter, such as no return of urine, do not inflate the balloon. Remove the catheter and notify the physician (Society of Urologic Nurses and Associates, 2005c).
- If the catheter cannot be advanced, having the patient take several deep breaths may be helpful. Rotate the catheter half a turn, and try to advance. If you are still unable to advance, remove the catheter. Notify the physician.
- Some catheter kits do not contain the catheter. This allows you to select a catheter and balloon size separately.

Infant and Child Considerations

- Size 5F to 8F is used for infants and young children. Size 8F to 12F catheters are commonly used for older children (Hockenberry, 2005).
- Distraction, such as blowing bubbles, deep breathing, or singing a song, can be used to help the child relax.

(continued)

SKILL 12-6 Catheterizing the Male Urinary Bladder *(continued)*

- Lidocaine jelly is often used to anesthetize and lubricate the area before insertion of the catheter, decreasing the child's discomfort and anxiety.

Older Adult Considerations

- If resistance is met while inserting catheter and rotating does not help, the catheter is never forced. Enlargement of the prostate gland is commonly seen in men over age 50. A special crook-tipped catheter called a Credé catheter, inserted by the physician or advanced practice nurse, may be required to maneuver past the prostate gland.

Home Care Considerations

- Intermittent catheterization in the home is performed using clean technique. The bladder's natural resistance to the microorganisms normally found in the home makes sterile technique unnecessary. Catheters are washed, dried, and stored for repeated use.

SKILL VARIATION Intermittent Male Urethral Catheterization

- Identify the patient. Discuss procedure with patient and assess patient's ability to assist with the procedure. Discuss any allergies with patient, especially to iodine and latex. Review chart for any limitations in physical activity.
- Bring the catheter kit and other necessary equipment to bedside. Obtain assistance from another staff member, if necessary. Perform hand hygiene. Put on disposable gloves.
- Close curtains around bed and close door to room if possible.
- Provide for good light. Artificial light is recommended. Place a trash receptacle within easy reach.
- Raise the bed to a comfortable working height. Stand on the patient's right side if you are right handed, patient's left side if you are left handed.
- Position patient on his back with thighs slightly apart. Drape patient so that only the area around the penis is exposed. Slide waterproof pad under patient.
- Put on clean gloves. Clean the genital area with washcloth, skin cleanser, and warm water. Clean the tip of the penis first, moving the washcloth in a circular motion from the meatus outward. Wash the shaft of the penis using downward strokes toward the pubic area. Rinse and dry. Remove gloves. Perform hand hygiene again.
- Open sterile catheterization tray on a clean overbed table using sterile technique.
- Put on sterile gloves. Open sterile drape and place on patient's thighs. Place fenestrated drape with opening over penis.
- Place catheter set on or next to patient's legs on sterile drape.
- Open all the supplies. Fluff cotton balls in tray before pouring antiseptic solution over them. Alternately, open package of antiseptic swabs. Open specimen container if specimen is to be obtained.
- Remove cap from syringe prefilled with lubricant.
- Lift penis with nondominant hand. Retract foreskin in uncircumcised patient. Be prepared to keep this hand in this position until catheter is inserted and urine is flowing well and continuously.
- Using your dominant hand and the forceps, pick up a cotton ball. Using a circular motion, clean the penis, moving from the meatus down the glans of the penis. Repeat this cleansing motion two more times, using a new cotton ball each time. Discard each cotton ball after one use.
- Hold penis with slight upward tension and perpendicular to patient's body. Use your dominant hand to pick up the lubricant syringe. Gently insert tip of syringe with lubricant into urethra and instill the 10 mL of lubricant.
- With your uncontaminated, dominant hand, place drainage end of catheter in receptacle. If a specimen is required, place the end into the specimen container in the receptacle.
- Use your dominant hand to pick up the catheter and hold it an inch or two from the tip. Ask patient to bear down as if voiding. Insert catheter tip into meatus. Ask the patient to take deep breaths as you advance the catheter 6″ to 8″ (14.4–19.2 cm) or until urine flows.
- Hold the catheter securely at the meatus with your nondominant hand while the bladder empties. If a specimen is being collected, remove the drainage end of the tubing from the specimen container after required amount is obtained and allow urine to flow into receptacle. Set specimen container aside.
- Allow the bladder to empty. Withdraw catheter slowly and smoothly after urine has stopped flowing. Remove equipment and dispose of according to facility policy. Wash and dry the genital area as needed. Replace foreskin in forward position if necessary.
- Remove your gloves. Assist the patient to a comfortable position. Cover the patient with bed linens. Place the bed in the lowest position.
- Put on clean gloves. Cover and label specimen. Send urine specimen to the laboratory promptly or refrigerate it.
- Remove gloves. Perform hand hygiene.

SKILL 12-7 Removing an Indwelling Catheter

Removal of an indwelling catheter is performed using clean technique. Care must be taken to prevent trauma to the urethra during the procedure. The catheter balloon must be completely deflated before catheter removal to avoid irritation and damage to the urethra and meatus. The patient may experience burning or irritation the first few times he/she voids after removal, due to urethral irritation. If the catheter was in place for more than a few days, decreased bladder muscle tone and swelling of the urethra may cause the patient to experience difficulty voiding or an inability to void. Monitor the patient for urinary retention. It is important to encourage adequate oral intake to promote adequate urinary output. Check facility policy regarding the length of time the patient is allowed to accomplish successful voiding after catheter removal. Then notify the primary healthcare provider.

Equipment

- Syringe large enough to accommodate the volume of solution used to inflate the balloon (balloon size is printed on the balloon inflation valve on the catheter at the bifurcation)
- Waterproof disposable pad
- Disposable gloves
- Washcloth and warm water to perform perineal hygiene after catheter removal

ASSESSMENT

Check the medical record for an order to remove the catheter. Assess for discharge or encrustation around the urethral meatus. Assess urine output, including color and current amount in drainage bag.

NURSING DIAGNOSIS

Determine the related factors for the nursing diagnoses based on the patient's current status. Appropriate nursing diagnoses may include:

- Impaired Urinary Elimination
- Urinary Retention
- Risk for Injury

OUTCOME IDENTIFICATION AND PLANNING

The expected outcome to achieve when removing an indwelling catheter is that the catheter will be removed without difficulty and with minimal patient discomfort. Other appropriate outcomes include the following: the patient voids without discomfort postcatheter removal; the patient voids a minimum of 250 mL of urine within 6 to 8 hours of catheter removal; the patient's skin remains clean, dry, and intact, without evidence of irritation or breakdown; and the patient verbalizes an understanding of the need to maintain adequate fluid intake, as appropriate.

IMPLEMENTATION

ACTION	RATIONALE
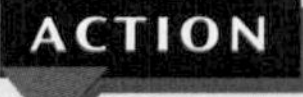 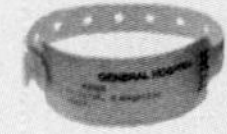 1. Identify the patient. Discuss procedure with patient.	Identifying the patient ensures the right patient receives the intervention and helps prevent errors. This discussion promotes reassurance and provides knowledge about the procedure. Explanation encourages patient cooperation and reduces apprehension.
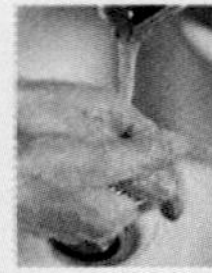 2. Perform hand hygiene.	Hand hygiene deters the spread of microorganisms.

(continued)

SKILL 12-7 Removing an Indwelling Catheter *(continued)*

ACTION	RATIONALE
3. Close curtains around bed and close door to room if possible.	This action provides for patient privacy.
4. Raise the bed to a comfortable working height. Stand on the patient's right side if you are right handed, patient's left side if you are left handed.	Having the bed in the high position reduces strain on the nurse's back while performing the procedure. Positioning allows for ease of use of dominant hand for catheter removal.
5. Position patient as for catheter insertion. Drape patient so that only the area around the catheter is exposed. Slide waterproof pad between the female patient's legs or over the male patient's thighs.	This prevents unnecessary exposure and promotes warmth. The drape will protect bed linens from moisture and serve as a receptacle for the used catheter after removal.
6. Remove the tape used to secure the catheter to the patient's thigh or abdomen.	This action permits removal of catheter and adhesive irritant from skin.
7. **Insert the syringe into the balloon inflation port. Aspirate the entire amount of fluid used to inflate the balloon (Figure 1).**	Aspiration of fluid deflates the balloon to allow for removal. All of the solution must be removed to prevent injury to the patient.

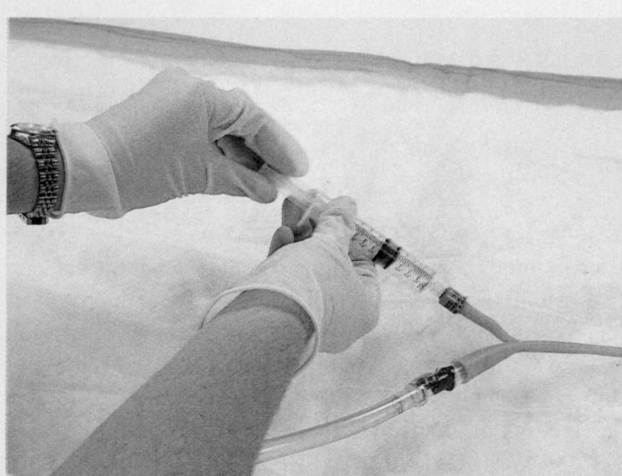

Figure 1. Aspirating fluid from balloon.

ACTION	RATIONALE
8. Ask the patient to take several slow deep breaths. **Slowly and gently remove the catheter.** Place it on the waterproof pad and wrap it in the pad.	Slow deep breathing helps to relax the sphincter muscles. Slow gentle removal prevents trauma to the urethra. Using a waterproof pad prevents contact with the catheter.
9. Wash and dry the perineal area as needed.	Cleaning promotes comfort and appropriate personal hygiene.
10. Remove gloves. Assist the patient to a comfortable position. Cover the patient with bed linens. Place the bed in the lowest position.	These actions provide warmth and promote comfort and safety.
11. Put on clean gloves. Remove equipment and dispose of according to facility policy. Note characteristics and amount of urine in drainage bag.	Proper disposal prevents the spread of microorganisms. Observing the characteristics ensures accurate documentation.
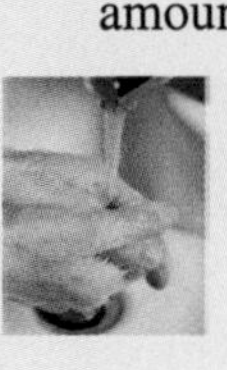 12. Remove gloves. Perform hand hygiene.	Hand hygiene deters the spread of microorganisms.

SKILL 12-7 Removing an Indwelling Catheter *(continued)*

EVALUATION

The expected outcomes are met when the catheter is removed without difficulty and with minimal patient discomfort; the patient voids without discomfort postcatheter removal; the patient voids a minimum of 250 mL of urine within 6 to 8 hours of catheter removal; the patient's skin remains clean, dry, and intact, without evidence of irritation or breakdown; and the patient verbalizes an understanding of the need to maintain adequate fluid intake, as appropriate.

DOCUMENTATION

Guidelines

Document the type and size of catheter removed and the amount of fluid removed from the balloon. Also document the patient's tolerance of the procedure. Record the amount of urine in the drainage bag. Note the time the patient is due to void. Document any other assessments, such as unusual urine characteristics or alterations in the patient's skin. Also record urine amount on intake and output record, if appropriate.

Sample Documentation

7/14/08 0800 15 mL fluid removed from catheter balloon. 14 F Foley removed without difficulty. 500 mL of clear yellow urine noted in drainage bag at time of removal. Patient due to void by 1600. Patient instructed to drink 6 to 8 6-oz. glasses of fluid in the course of the day, and that it may take some time for the passage of urine on his own; verbalized understanding of instructions. Urinal placed at bedside, with patient demonstrating appropriate use.—B. Clapp, RN

Unexpected Situations and Associated Interventions

- *Resistance is felt while attempting to pull catheter out:* Stop pulling the catheter. Reattach syringe to balloon inflation port and aspirate again to make sure all the fluid has been removed. Reattempt to continue removing catheter. If resistance is still present, stop removal and notify physician.

Special Considerations

General Considerations

- Have alternate toileting measures available, as necessary, based on patient assessment. A bedside commode, urinal, or bedpan may be necessary if the patient is unable to get to the bathroom.

SKILL 12-8 Performing Intermittent Closed Catheter Irrigation

Indwelling catheters at times require irrigation, or flushing, with solution to restore or maintain the patency of the drainage system. Sediment or debris as well as blood clots might block the catheter, preventing the flow of urine out of the catheter. Irrigations might also be used to instill medications that will act directly on the bladder wall. Irrigating a catheter through a closed system is preferred to opening the catheter because opening the catheter could lead to contamination and infection.

Equipment

- Sterile basin or container
- Sterile irrigating solution (at room temperature or warmed to body temperature)
- 30- to 60-mL syringe (with 18- or 19-gauge blunt-end needle, if catheter access port is not a needleless system)

(continued)

SKILL 12-8 Performing Intermittent Closed Catheter Irrigation *(continued)*

- Clamp for drainage tubing
- Bath blanket
- Disposable gloves
- Waterproof pad

ASSESSMENT

Check to ensure that a physician's order has been written, including the type and amount of solution to use for the irrigation. Before performing the procedure, assess catheter drainage and amount of urine in drainage bag. Also assess for bladder fullness either by palpation or with a handheld bladder ultrasound device. Assess for signs of adverse effects, which may include pain, bladder spasm, bladder distension/fullness, or lack of drainage from catheter.

NURSING DIAGNOSIS

Determine related factors for the nursing diagnoses based on the patient's current status. Appropriate nursing diagnoses may include:

- Impaired Urinary Elimination
- Risk for Infection

OUTCOME IDENTIFICATION AND PLANNING

The expected outcome to achieve when performing a closed catheter irrigation is that the patient exhibits the free flow of urine through the catheter. Other outcomes may include the following: the patient's bladder is not distended; the patient remains free from pain; and the patient remains free of any signs and symptoms of infection.

IMPLEMENTATION

ACTION	RATIONALE
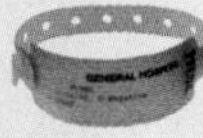 1. Identify the patient. Discuss procedure with patient.	Identifying the patient ensures the right patient receives the intervention and helps prevent errors. This discussion promotes reassurance and provides knowledge about the procedure. Explanation encourages patient cooperation and reduces apprehension.
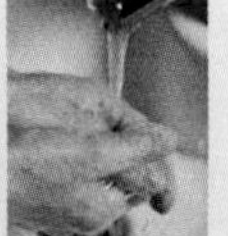 2. Perform hand hygiene.	Hand hygiene deters the spread of microorganisms.
3. Provide privacy by closing the curtains or door and draping patient with bath blanket.	The procedure may be embarrassing for the patient.
4. Raise the bed to a comfortable working height.	Having the bed in the high position reduces strain on the nurse's back while performing the procedure.
5. Empty the catheter drainage bag and measure the amount of urine, noting the amount and characteristics of the urine.	Emptying the drainage bag allows for accurate assessment of drainage after the irrigation solution is instilled. Assessment of urine provides baseline for future comparison.

SKILL 12-8 Performing Intermittent Closed Catheter Irrigation *(continued)*

ACTION	RATIONALE
6. Assist patient to comfortable position and expose access port on catheter setup (Figure 1). Place waterproof pad under catheter and aspiration port. Remove tape anchoring catheter to the patient.	This provides adequate visualization. Waterproof pad protects patient and bed from leakage. Removing the tape allows for manipulation of catheter.
7. Open supplies, using aseptic technique. Pour sterile solution into sterile basin. Aspirate the prescribed amount of irrigant (usually 30–60 mL) into sterile syringe (Figure 2) and attach capped, sterile, blunt-ended needle, if necessary. Put on gloves.	Use of aseptic technique ensures sterility of irrigating fluid and prevents spread of microorganisms. Gloves prevent contact with blood and body fluids.
8. **Cleanse the access port with antimicrobial swab (Figure 3).**	Cleaning the port reduces the risk of introducing organisms into the closed urinary system.
9. Clamp or fold catheter tubing below the access port (Figure 4).	This directs the irrigating solution into the bladder, preventing flow into the drainage bag.

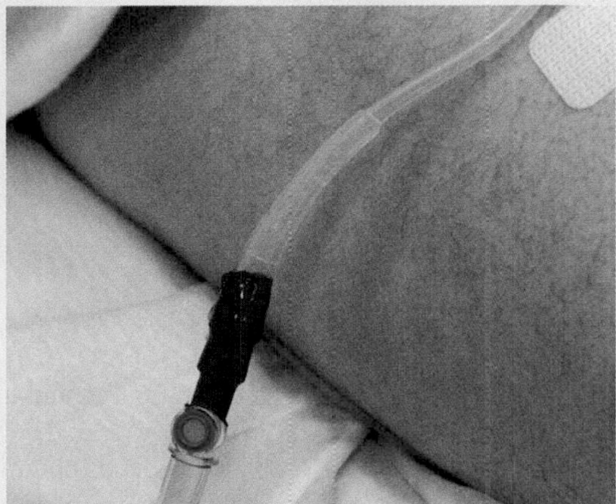

Figure 1. Aspiration port on catheter.

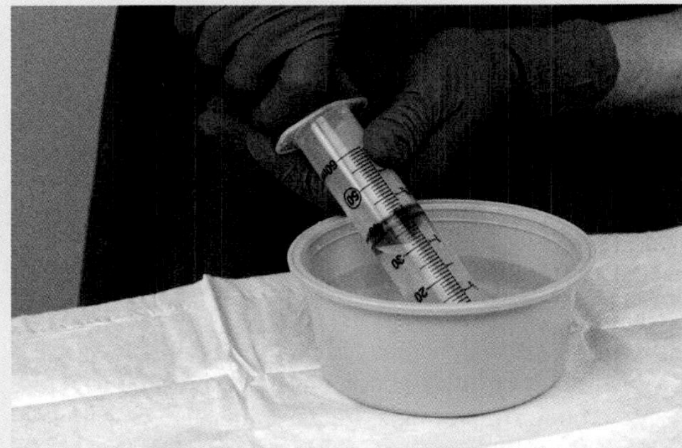

Figure 2. Drawing up irrigant from sterile basin into a 30-mL to 60-mL syringe.

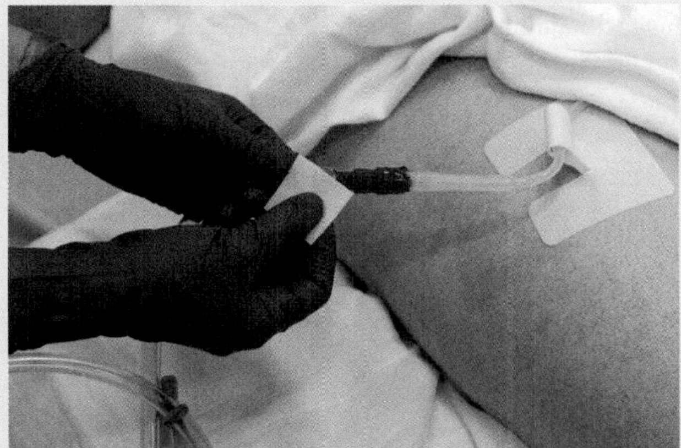

Figure 3. Wiping port on catheter.

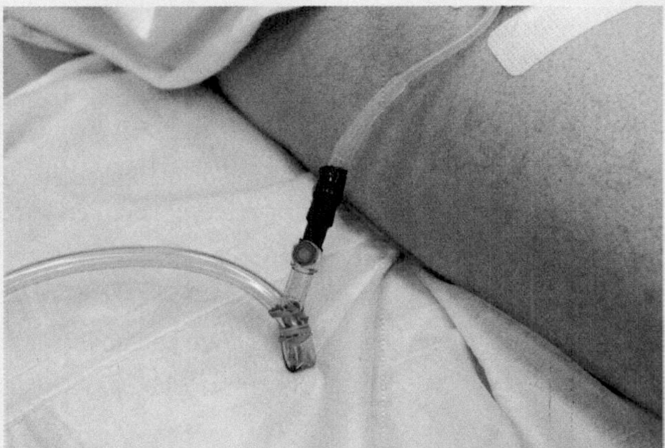

Figure 4. Urinary catheter with drainage tubing clamped or folded below port.

(continued)

SKILL 12-8 Performing Intermittent Closed Catheter Irrigation *(continued)*

ACTION	RATIONALE
10. Remove cap and insert needle into port (Figure 5). Alternately, attach the syringe to the port using a twisting motion, if needleless system is in place. **Gently instill solution into catheter.**	Gentle irrigation prevents damage to bladder lining. Instillation of fluid dislodges material blocking catheter.
11. Remove syringe/needle from port. Apply needle guard, if needle used. **Unclamp or unfold tubing and allow irrigant and urine to flow into the drainage bag (Figure 6).** Repeat procedure as necessary.	Gravity aids drainage of urine and irrigant from the bladder.

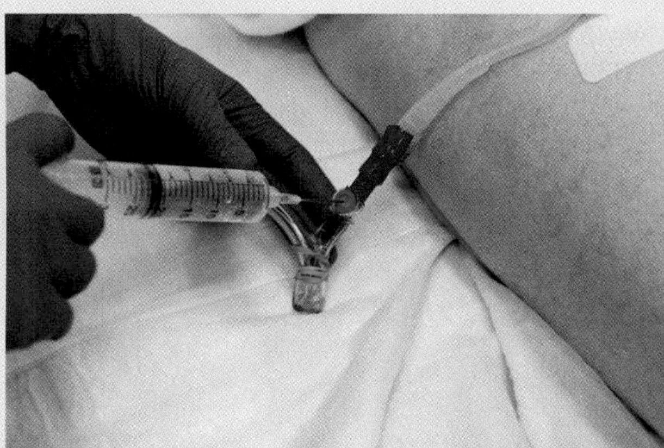

Figure 5. Inserting syringe into port.

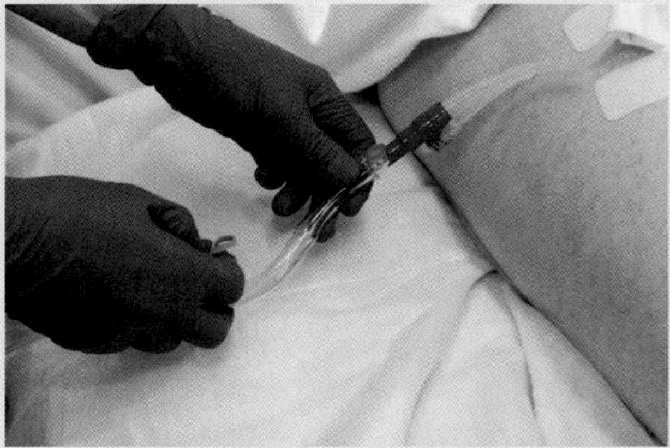

Figure 6. Fluid draining through tubing into drainage bag.

ACTION	RATIONALE
12. Remove gloves. Secure catheter tubing to the patient's inner thigh or lower abdomen (if a male patient) with Velcro leg strap or tape. Leave some slack in catheter for leg movement.	Proper attachment prevents trauma to the urethra and meatus from tension on the tubing. Whether to take the drainage tubing over or under the leg depends on gravity flow, patient's mobility, and comfort of the patient.
13. Assist the patient to a comfortable position. Cover the patient with bed linens. Place the bed in the lowest position.	Positioning and covering provide warmth and promote comfort.
14. Secure drainage bag below the level of the bladder. Check that drainage tubing is not kinked and that movement of side rails does not interfere with catheter or drainage bag.	This facilitates drainage of urine and prevents the backflow of urine.
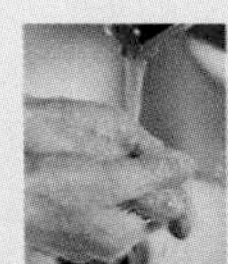 15. Remove equipment and discard needle and syringe in appropriate receptacle. Perform hand hygiene.	This provides accurate documentation of the procedure. Hand hygiene deters the spread of microorganisms.
16. Assess patient's response to procedure and quality and amount of drainage after the irrigation.	This provides accurate assessment of the patient's response to the procedure.

EVALUATION

The expected outcome is met when the patient exhibits the free flow of urine through the catheter; the irrigant and urine are returned into the drainage bag; the patient's bladder is not distended; the patient remains free from pain; and the patient remains free of any signs and symptoms of infection.

SKILL 12-8 Performing Intermittent Closed Catheter Irrigation *(continued)*

DOCUMENTATION

Guidelines

Document baseline assessment of patient. Document the amount and type of irrigation solution used and the amount and characteristics of drainage returned after the procedure. Document the ease of irrigation and the patient's tolerance of the procedure. Record urine amount emptied from the drainage bag before the procedure and the amount of irrigant used on intake and output record. Subtract irrigant amount from the urine output when totaling output to provide accurate recording of urine output.

Sample Documentation

7/22/08 1630 Urinary catheter irrigated with 60 mL of normal saline without difficulty. All of irrigation returned plus 200 mL of cloudy yellow urine. Patient tolerated procedure without adverse effect. Order received to notify physician if urine output <30 mL per hour.—B. Clapp, RN

Unexpected Situations and Associated Interventions

- *Irrigation solution will not enter the catheter:* Do not force the solution into the catheter. Notify physician. Prepare to change catheter.
- *Tubing was not clamped before introducing irrigation solution:* Repeat irrigation. If the tubing is not clamped, the irrigation solution will drain into the urinary drainage bag and not enter the catheter.

Special Considerations

General Considerations

- If irrigant is a medication intended for action in bladder, be aware of specific dwell time included in the order or determined by the action of the medication. Allow the appropriate amount of time to lapse before unclamping drainage tubing after instillation of irrigant.

SKILL 12-9 Administering a Continuous Closed Bladder Irrigation

Indwelling catheters sometimes require continuous irrigation, or flushing, with solution to restore or maintain the patency of the drainage system. Sediment or debris as well as blood clots might block the catheter, preventing the flow of urine out of the catheter. Irrigations might also be used to instill medications that will act directly on the bladder wall. Irrigating a catheter through a closed system is preferred to opening the catheter because opening the catheter could lead to contamination and infection. If the irrigation is to be continuous, a triple-lumen or three-way catheter is placed to maintain a closed system (Figure 1).

Equipment

- Sterile irrigating solution (at room temperature or warmed to body temperature)
- Sterile tubing with drip chamber and clamp for connection to irrigating solution
- IV pole
- IV pump (if bladder is being irrigated with a solution containing medication)
- Three-way indwelling catheter in place in patient's bladder
- Indwelling catheter drainage setup (tubing and collection bag)
- Alcohol swabs
- Bath blanket
- Disposable gloves

(continued)

SKILL 12-9

Administering a Continuous Closed Bladder Irrigation *(continued)*

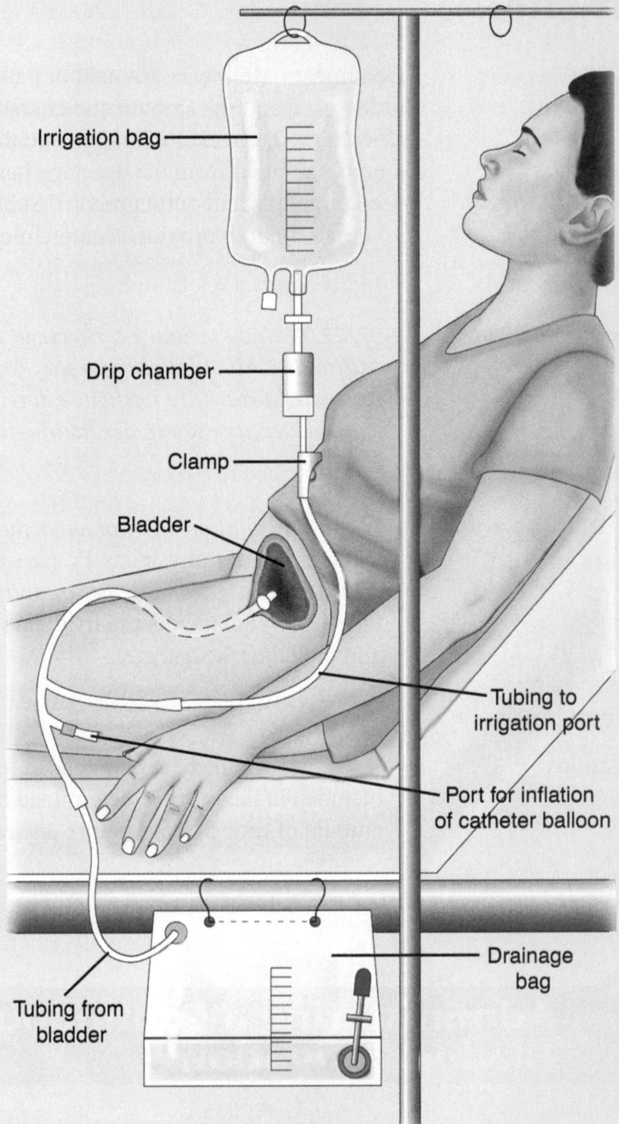

Figure 1. A continuous bladder irrigation (CBI) setup.

ASSESSMENT

Verify physician's order for continuous bladder irrigation, including type and amount of irrigant. Assess the catheter to ensure that it has an irrigation port (if the patient has an indwelling catheter already in place). Assess the characteristics of urine present in tubing and drainage bag. Review the patient's medical record for and ask the patient about any allergies to medications. Before performing the procedure, assess the bladder for fullness either by palpation or with a handheld bladder ultrasound device. Assess for signs of adverse effects, which may include pain, bladder spasm, bladder distension/fullness, or lack of drainage from catheter.

NURSING DIAGNOSIS

Determine related factors for the nursing diagnoses based on the patient's current status. Appropriate nursing diagnoses may include:

- Impaired Urinary Elimination
- Risk for Infection

SKILL 12-9 Administering a Continuous Closed Bladder Irrigation *(continued)*

OUTCOME IDENTIFICATION AND PLANNING

The expected outcome to achieve is that the patient exhibits free-flowing urine through the catheter. Initially, clots or debris may be noted. These should decrease over time, with the patient ultimately exhibiting urine that is free of clots or debris. Other outcomes may include the following: the continuous bladder irrigation continues without adverse effect; drainage is greater than the hourly amount of irrigation solution being placed in bladder; and the patient exhibits no signs and symptoms of infection.

IMPLEMENTATION

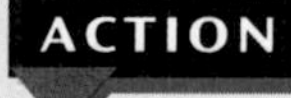

ACTION	RATIONALE
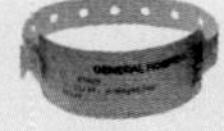 1. Assemble equipment and double-check physician's order. Identify the patient. Discuss procedure with patient.	Organization facilitates performance of tasks. Double-checking the order ensures that the correct procedure is to be performed. Identifying the patient ensures the right patient receives the intervention and helps prevent errors. This discussion promotes reassurance and provides knowledge about the procedure. Explanation encourages patient cooperation and reduces apprehension.
2. Calculate drip rate for prescribed infusion rate.	Solution must be administered at the appropriate rate as prescribed.
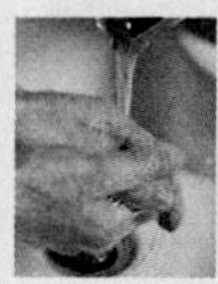 3. Perform hand hygiene.	Hand hygiene deters the spread of microorganisms.
4. Provide privacy by closing the curtains or door and draping patient with bath blanket.	The procedure may be embarrassing for the patient.
5. Raise the bed to a comfortable working height.	Having the bed in the high position reduces strain on the nurse's back while performing the procedure.
6. Empty the catheter drainage bag and measure the amount of urine, noting the amount and characteristics of the urine.	Emptying the drainage bag allows for accurate assessment of drainage after the irrigation solution is instilled. Assessment of urine provides baseline for future comparison.
7. Assist patient to comfortable position and expose the irrigation port on the catheter setup. Place waterproof pad under catheter and aspiration port. Remove tape anchoring catheter to patient.	This provides adequate visualization. Drape protects patient and bed from leakage. Removing the tape allows for manipulation of catheter.

(continued)

SKILL 12-9 Administering a Continuous Closed Bladder Irrigation *(continued)*

ACTION	RATIONALE
8. Prepare sterile irrigation bag for use as directed by manufacturer. Clearly label the solution as 'Bladder Irrigant.' Include the date and time on the label. Secure tubing clamp and attach sterile tubing with drip chamber to container using aseptic technique (Figure 2). Hang bag on IV pole 2 1/2′ to 3′ above level of patient's bladder. Release clamp and remove protective cover on end of tubing without contaminating it. Allow solution to flush tubing and remove air (Figure 3). Clamp tubing and replace end cover.	Proper labeling provided accurate information for caregivers. Sterile solution not used within 24 hours of opening should be discarded. Aseptic technique prevents contamination of solution irrigation system. Priming the tubing before attaching irrigation clears air from the tubing that might cause bladder distention.

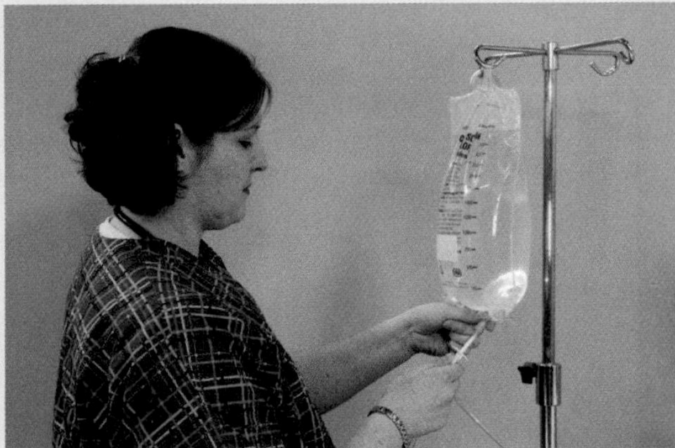

Figure 2. Spiking bag with tubing for irrigation.

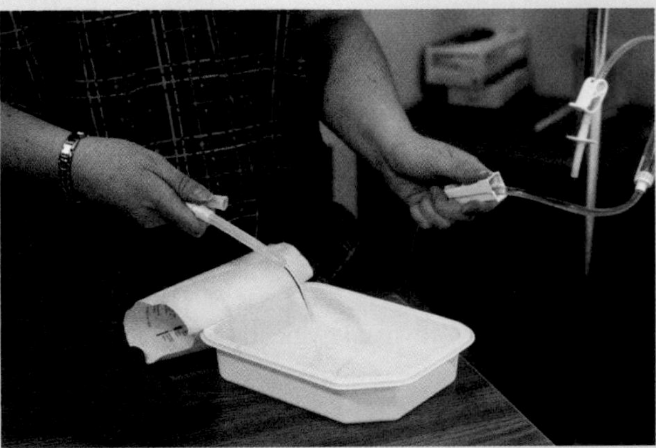

Figure 3. Regulating flow clamp to prime tubing.

ACTION	RATIONALE
9. Put on gloves. **Cleanse the irrigation port with an alcohol swab. Using aseptic technique, attach irrigation tubing to irrigation port of three-way indwelling catheter (Figure 4).**	Aseptic technique prevents the spread of microorganisms into the bladder.

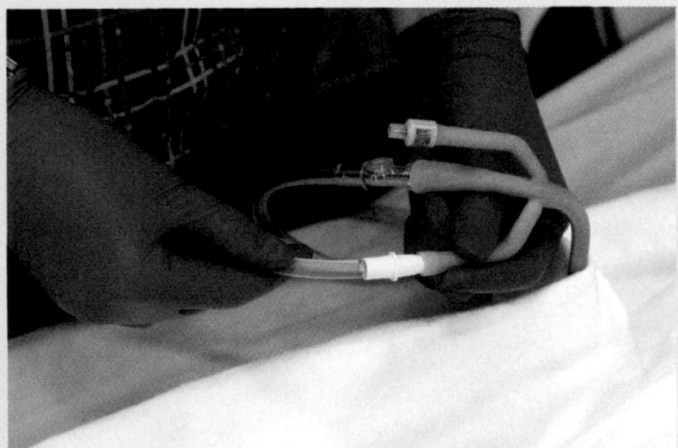

Figure 4. Attaching irrigation tubing to irrigation port on catheter.

SKILL 12-9 Administering a Continuous Closed Bladder Irrigation *(continued)*

ACTION	RATIONALE
10. Check the drainage tubing to make sure clamp, if present, is open.	An open clamp prevents accumulation of solution in the bladder.
11. **Release clamp on irrigation tubing and regulate flow at determined drip rate, according to physician's order (Figure 5).** At times, the physician may order the bladder irrigation to be done with a medicated solution. In these cases, use an IV pump to regulate the flow.	This allows for continual gentle irrigation without causing discomfort to the patient. An IV pump regulates the flow of the medication.

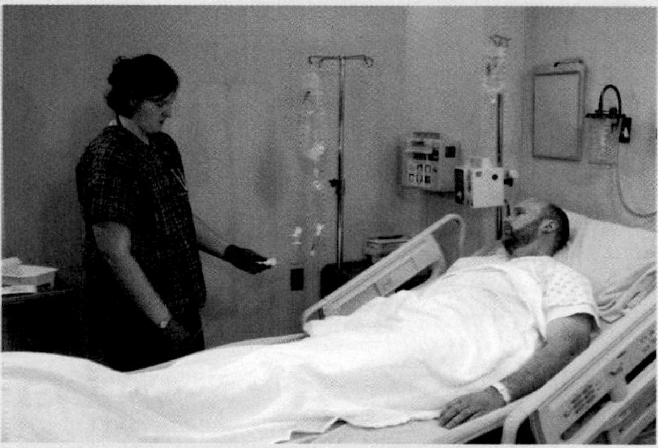

Figure 5. Regulating irrigation flow rate using flow clamp.

ACTION	RATIONALE
12. Remove gloves. Assist the patient to a comfortable position. Cover the patient with bed linens. Place the bed in the lowest position.	Positioning and covering provide warmth and promote comfort and safety.
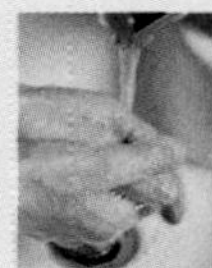 13. Perform hand hygiene.	Hand hygiene deters the spread of microorganisms.
14. Assess patient's response to procedure, and quality and amount of drainage.	Assessment is necessary to determine effectiveness of intervention and detection of adverse effects.
15. As irrigation fluid container nears empty, clamp the administration tubing. Do not allow drip chamber to empty. Disconnect empty bag and attach a new full irrigation solution bag. Continue as ordered by physician.	This eliminates the need to separate tubing from the catheter and clear air from the tubing. Opening the drainage system provides access for microorganisms. Gloves protect against exposure to blood, body fluids, and microorganisms.
16. Record amount of irrigant used on intake/output record. Put on gloves and empty drainage collection bag as each new container is hung and recorded.	This ensures accurate recording of urine output. Gloves protect against exposure to blood, body fluids, and microorganisms.

(continued)

SKILL 12-9 Administering a Continuous Closed Bladder Irrigation *(continued)*

EVALUATION

The expected outcome is met when urine flows freely through the catheter. Effectiveness of therapy is determined by the urine characteristics. Upon completion of the therapy with a continuous bladder irrigation, the patient should exhibit urine that is clear, without evidence of clots or debris. Other outcomes would include the following: the continuous bladder irrigation is administered without adverse effect; drainage is greater than the hourly amount of irrigation solution being instilled in bladder; and the patient exhibits no signs and symptoms of infection.

Documentation

Guidelines

Document baseline assessment of patient. Document the amount and type of irrigation solution used and the patient's tolerance of the procedure. Record urine amount emptied from the drainage bag before the procedure and the amount of irrigant used on intake and output record. Record the amount of urine and irrigant emptied from the drainage bag. Subtract the amount of irrigant instilled from the total volume of drainage to obtain the volume of urine output.

Sample Documentation

12/14/08 1330 Foley catheter replaced with 3-way Foley catheter. Bladder nonpalpable. Continuous bladder irrigation with normal saline initiated at 100 mL/hour. Patient tolerated procedure without adverse effect. Drainage from bladder slightly cloudy, light cherry colored. No evidence of clots.—B. Clapp, RN

Unexpected Situations and Associated Interventions

- *Continuous bladder irrigation begins and hourly drainage is less than amount of irrigation being given:* Palpate for bladder distention. If patient is lying supine, rolling the patient onto side may help increase the amount of drainage. Check to make sure that the tubing is not kinked. If return flow remains decreased, notify physician.
- *Bladder irrigation is not flowing at ordered rate, even with clamp wide open:* Check the tubing for kinks or pressure points. Raise the bag 3″ to 6″ and then check flow of irrigation solution. Frequently check flow rate of irrigation solution.

SKILL 12-10 Applying an External Condom Catheter

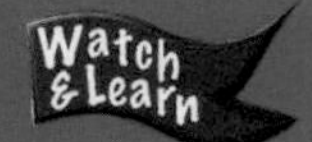

When voluntary control of urination is not possible for male patients, an alternative to an indwelling catheter is the **external condom catheter.** This soft, pliable sheath made of silicone material is applied externally to the penis. Most devices are self-adhesive. The condom catheter is connected to drainage tubing and a collection bag. The collection bag may be a leg bag. The risk for urinary tract infection with a condom catheter is lower that the risk associated with an indwelling urinary catheter. Nursing care of a patient with a condom catheter includes vigilant skin care to prevent excoriation. This includes removing the condom catheter daily, washing the penis with soap and water and drying carefully, and inspecting the skin for irritation. In hot and humid weather, more frequent changing is required (Newman, 2004). Always follow the manufacturer's instructions for applying the condom catheter because there are several variations. In all cases, care must be taken to fasten the condom securely enough to prevent leakage, yet not so tightly

SKILL 12-10 **Applying an External Condom Catheter** *(continued)*

as to constrict the blood vessels in the area. In addition, the tip of the tubing should be kept 1″ to 2″ (2.5–5 cm) beyond the tip of the penis to prevent irritation to the sensitive glans area.

Maintaining free urinary drainage is another nursing priority. Institute measures to prevent the tubing from becoming kinked and urine from backing up in the tubing. Urine can lead to excoriation of the glans, so position the tubing that collects the urine from the condom so that it draws urine away from the penis.

Always use a measuring or sizing guide supplied by the manufacturer to ensure the correct size of sheath is applied. Skin barriers, such as 3M® or Skin Prep® can be applied to the penis to protect penile skin from irritation and changes in integrity.

Equipment

- Condom sheath in appropriate size
- Skin protectant, such as 3M or Skin Prep
- Bath blanket
- Reusable leg bag with tubing or urinary drainage setup
- Basin of warm water and soap
- Disposable gloves
- Washcloth and towel
- Scissors

ASSESSMENT

Assess patient's knowledge of need for catheter. Ask patient about any allergies, especially to latex or tape. Assess the size of the patient's penis to ensure that the appropriate-sized condom catheter is used. Inspect the skin in the groin and scrotal area, noting any areas of redness, irritation, or breakdown. If any areas are observed, notify the physician.

NURSING DIAGNOSIS

Determine the related factors for the nursing diagnoses based on the patient's current status. Possible nursing diagnoses may include:

- Impaired Urinary Elimination
- Risk for Impaired Skin Integrity
- Total Urinary Incontinence
- Functional Urinary Incontinence

OUTCOME IDENTIFICATION AND PLANNING

The expected outcome to achieve when applying a condom catheter is that the patient's urinary elimination will be maintained, with a urine output of at least 30 mL/hour, and the bladder is not distended. Other outcomes may include the following: the patient's skin remains clean, dry, and intact, without evidence of irritation or breakdown.

IMPLEMENTATION

ACTION	RATIONALE
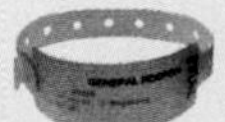 1. Identify the patient. Discuss procedure with patient and assess patient's ability to assist with the procedure. Discuss any allergies with patient, especially to latex.	This discussion promotes reassurance and provides knowledge about the procedure. Explanation encourages patient cooperation and reduces apprehension. Dialogue encourages patient participation and allows for individualized nursing care. Some condom catheters are made of latex.

(continued)

SKILL 12-10 Applying an External Condom Catheter *(continued)*

ACTION	RATIONALE
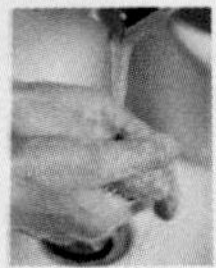 2. Bring the necessary equipment to bedside. Obtain assistance from another staff member, if necessary. Perform hand hygiene. Put on disposable gloves.	Having equipment on hand saves time by avoiding unnecessary trips to storage area. Assistance from additional staff member ensures patient safety and facilitates patient transfer. Hand hygiene deters the spread of microorganisms. Gloves prevent exposure to blood and body fluids.
3. Close curtains around bed and close door to room if possible.	This action provides for patient privacy.
4. Raise the bed to a comfortable working height. Stand on the patient's right side if you are right handed, patient's left side if you are left handed.	Having the bed in the high position reduces strain on the nurse's back while performing the catheterization. Positioning on one side allows for ease of use of dominant hand for catheter application.
5. Prepare urinary drainage setup or reusable leg bag for attachment to condom sheath (Figure 1).	This provides for an organized approach to the task.

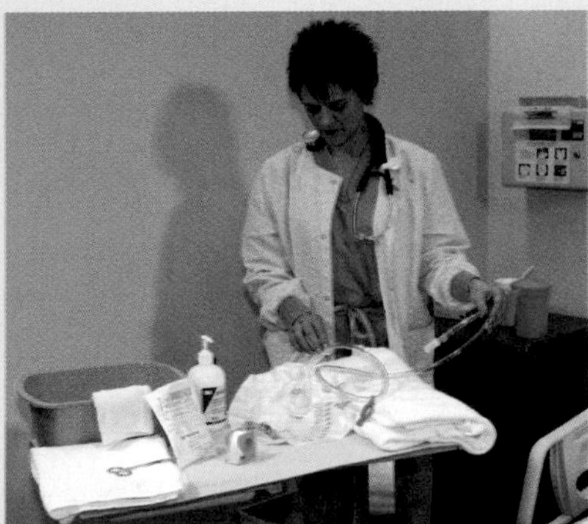

Figure 1. Preparing urinary drainage setup.

ACTION	RATIONALE
6. Position patient on his back with thighs slightly apart. Drape patient so that only the area around the penis is exposed. Slide waterproof pad under patient.	This prevents unnecessary exposure and promotes warmth. The waterproof pad will protect bed linens from moisture.
7. Put on disposable gloves. Trim any long pubic hair that is in contact with penis.	Trimming pubic hair prevents pulling of hair by adhesive without the risk of infection associated with shaving.
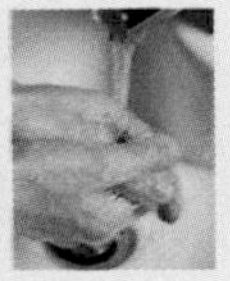 8. Clean the genital area with washcloth, skin cleanser, and warm water. If patient is uncircumcised, retract foreskin and clean glans of penis. Replace foreskin. Clean the tip of the penis first, moving the washcloth in a circular motion from the meatus outward. Wash the shaft of the penis using downward strokes toward the pubic area. Rinse and dry. Remove gloves. Perform hand hygiene again.	Gloves reduce the risk of exposure to blood and body fluids. Washing removes urine, secretions, and microorganisms. The penis must be clean and dry to minimize skin irritation. If the foreskin is left retracted, it may cause venous congestion in the glans of the penis, leading to edema. Hand hygiene reduces the spread of microorganisms.
9. Apply skin protectant to penis and allow to dry.	Skin protectant minimizes the risk of skin irritation from adhesive and moisture and increases adhesive's ability to adhere to skin.

SKILL 12-10 Applying an External Condom Catheter *(continued)*

ACTION	RATIONALE
10. Roll condom sheath outward onto itself. Grasp penis firmly with nondominant hand. **Apply condom sheath by rolling it onto penis with dominant hand (Figure 2). Leave 1″ to 2″ (2.5–5 cm) of space between tip of penis and end of condom sheath.**	Rolling the condom sheath outward allows for easier application. The space prevents irritation to tip of penis and allows free drainage of urine.
11. **Apply pressure to sheath at the base of penis for 10 to 15 seconds.**	Application of pressure ensures good adherence of adhesive with skin.
12. Connect condom sheath to drainage setup (Figure 3). Avoid kinking or twisting drainage tubing.	The collection device keeps the patient dry. Kinked tubing encourages backflow of urine.

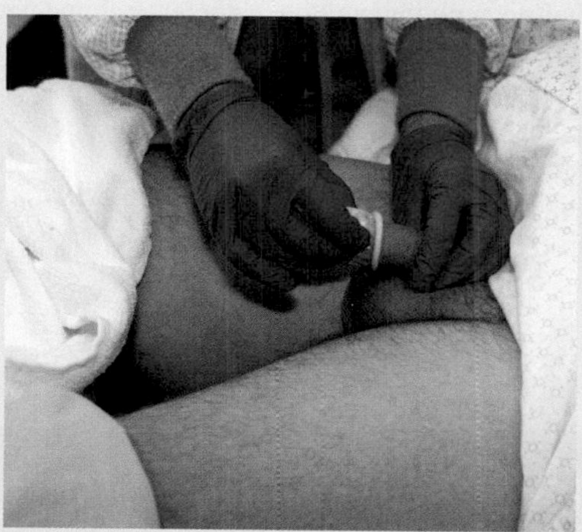

Figure 2. Grasping penis firmly and unrolling condom sheath onto penis.

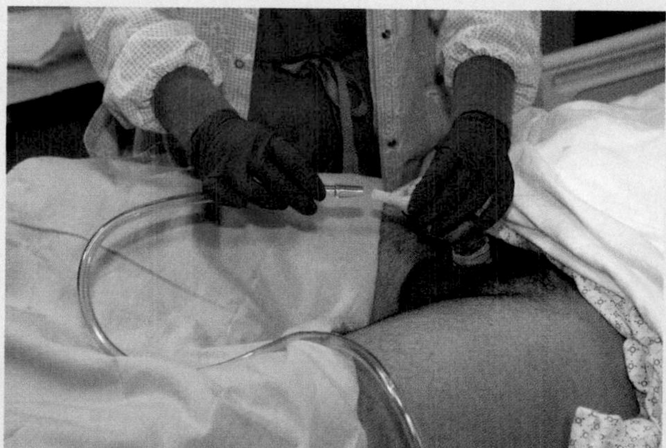

Figure 3. Attaching condom to drainage setup.

ACTION	RATIONALE
13. Remove gloves. Secure drainage tubing to the patient's inner thigh with Velcro leg strap or tape. Leave some slack in tubing for leg movement.	Proper attachment prevents tension on the sheath and potential inadvertent removal.
14. Assist the patient to a comfortable position. Cover the patient with bed linens. Place the bed in the lowest position.	Positioning and covering provide warmth and promote comfort.
15. Secure drainage bag below the level of the bladder. Check that drainage tubing is not kinked and that movement of side rails does not interfere with the drainage bag.	This facilitates drainage of urine and prevents the backflow of urine.

EVALUATION

The expected outcome is met when the condom catheter is applied without adverse effect; the patient's urinary elimination is maintained, with a urine output of at least 30 mL/hour; and the patient's skin remains clean, dry, and intact, without evidence of irritation or breakdown.

DOCUMENTATION

Guidelines

Document the application of the condom catheter and the condition of the patient's skin. Record urine output on the intake and output record.

(continued)

SKILL 12-10 Applying an External Condom Catheter *(continued)*

Sample Documentation

7/12/08 1910 Patient incontinent of urine; states "It just comes too fast. I can't get to the bathroom in time." Perineal skin slightly reddened. Discussed rationale for use of condom catheter. Patient and wife agreeable to trying condom catheter. Medium-sized condom catheter applied. 200 mL of clear urine returned. Leg bag in place for daytime use. Patient verbalized understanding of need to call for assistance to empty drainage bag.—B. Clapp, RN

Unexpected Situations and Associated Interventions

- *Condom catheter leaks with every voiding:* Check size of condom catheter. If it is too big or too small, it may leak. Check space between tip of penis and end of condom sheath. If this space is too small, the urine has no place to go and will leak out.
- *Condom catheter will not stay on patient:* Ensure that condom catheter is correct size and that penis is thoroughly dried before applying condom catheter. Remind patient that condom catheter is in place, so that patient does not tug at tubing. If the patient has a retracted penis, a condom catheter may not be the best choice; there are pouches made for patients with a retracted penis.
- *When assessing patient's penis, nurse finds a break in skin integrity:* Do not reapply condom catheter. Allow skin to be open to air as much as possible. If institution has a wound, ostomy, and continence nurse, a consult would be appropriate.

SKILL 12-11 Changing a Stoma Appliance on an Ileal Conduit

An ileal conduit is a cutaneous urinary diversion. An ileal conduit involves a surgical resection of the small intestine, with transplantation of the ureters to the isolated segment of small bowel. This separated section of the small intestine is then brought to the abdominal wall, where urine is excreted through a stoma, a surgically created opening on the body surface. Such diversions are usually permanent, and the patient wears an external appliance to collect the urine because elimination of the urine from the stoma cannot be voluntarily controlled. The frequency of changing the appliance depends on the type being used. The usual wear time is 5 days. The appliance usually is changed after a time of low fluid intake, such as in the early morning. Urine production is less at this time, making changing the appliance easier. Proper application minimizes the risk for skin breakdown around the stoma. Box 12-1 summarizes guidelines for care of the patient with a urinary diversion.

Equipment

- Basin with warm water,
- Skin cleanser, towel, washcloth
- Gauze squares
- Washcloth or cotton balls
- Skin protectant or barrier
- Ostomy appliance
- Stoma measuring guide
- Graduated container
- Ostomy belt (optional)
- Disposable gloves
- Small plastic trash bag

SKILL
12-11 Changing a Stoma Appliance on an Ileal Conduit *(continued)*

BOX 12-1 Guidelines for Care of the Patient With a Urinary Diversion

- Keep the patient as free of odors as possible. Empty the appliance frequently.
- Inspect the patient's stoma regularly. It should be dark pink to red and moist. A pale stoma may indicate anemia, and a dark or purple-blue stoma may reflect compromised circulation or ischemia. Bleeding around the stoma and its stem should be minimal. Notify the physician promptly if bleeding persists, is excessive, or if color changes occur in the stoma.
- Note the size of the stoma, which usually stabilizes within 6 to 8 weeks. Most stomas protrude 1/2″ to 1″ from the abdominal surface and may initially appear swollen and edematous. After 6 weeks, the edema usually subsides. If an abdominal dressing is in place at the incision site after surgery, check it frequently for drainage and bleeding.
- Keep the skin around the stoma site (peristomal area) clean and dry. If care is not taken to protect the skin around the stoma, irritation or infection may occur. A leaking appliance frequently causes skin erosion. Candida or yeast infections can also occur around the stoma if the area is not kept dry.
- Measure the patient's fluid intake and output. Careful monitoring of the patient's urinary output is necessary to monitor fluid balance.
- Monitor the return of intestinal function and peristalsis. Initially after surgery, peristalsis is inhibited. Remember, the patient had a bowel resection as part of the urinary diversion procedure.
- Watch for mucus in the urine from an ileal conduit, which is a normal finding. The isolated segment of small intestine continues to produce mucus as part of its normal functioning.
- Explain each aspect of care to the patient and explain what his or her role will be when he or she begins self-care. Patient teaching is one of the most important aspects of ostomy care and should include family members when appropriate. Teaching can begin before surgery so that the patient has adequate time to absorb information.
- Encourage the patient to participate in care and to look at the stoma. Patients normally experience emotional depression during the early postoperative period. Help the patient to cope by listening, explaining, and being available and supportive. A visit from a representative of the local ostomy support group may be helpful. Patients usually begin to accept their altered body image when they are willing to look at the stoma, make neutral or positive statements concerning the ostomy, and express interest in learning self-care.

ASSESSMENT

Assess current ileal conduit appliance, observing product style, condition of appliance, and stoma (if bag is clear). Note length of time the appliance has been in place. Determine the patient's knowledge of care of the ileal conduit, including level of self care and ability to manipulate equipment. After the appliance is removed, assess the skin surrounding the ileal conduit. Assess the condition of any abdominal scars or incisional areas, if surgery to create the urinary diversion was recent.

NURSING DIAGNOSIS

Determine the related factors for the nursing diagnoses based on the patient's current status. Possible nursing diagnoses may include:

- Impaired Urinary Elimination
- Risk for Impaired Skin Integrity
- Deficient Knowledge
- Disturbed Body Image

OUTCOME IDENTIFICATION AND PLANNING

The expected outcome to achieve when changing a patient's urinary stoma appliance is that the stoma appliance is applied correctly to the skin to allow urine to drain freely. Other outcomes may include the following: the patient exhibits a moist red stoma with intact skin surrounding the stoma; the patient demonstrates knowledge of how to apply the pouch; and the patient verbalizes positive self-image.

(continued)

SKILL 12-11 Changing a Stoma Appliance on an Ileal Conduit *(continued)*

IMPLEMENTATION

ACTION	RATIONALE
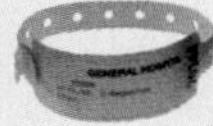 1. Identify the patient. Explain procedure and encourage patient to observe or participate if possible.	Identifying the patient ensures the right patient receives the intervention and helps prevent errors. This discussion promotes reassurance and provides knowledge about the procedure. Explanation encourages patient cooperation and reduces apprehension. Having the patient observe or assist encourages self-acceptance.
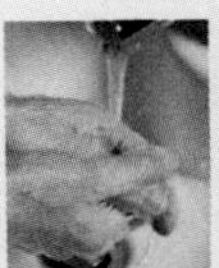 2. Perform hand hygiene.	Hand hygiene deters the spread of microorganisms.
3. Close curtains around bed and close door to room if possible.	This action provides for patient privacy.
4. Have patient sit or stand if able to assist with skill or assume supine position in bed. If in bed, raise the bed to a comfortable working height. Place waterproof pad under the patient at the stoma site.	These positions result in fewer abdominal folds and facilitate removal and application of the device. Having the bed in the high position reduces strain on the nurse's back while performing the procedure. A waterproof pad protects linens and patient from moisture.
5. Place a disposable waterproof pad on the overbed table. Set up the wash basin with warm water and the rest of the supplies. Place a trash bag within reach.	The pad protects the surface. Organization facilitates performance of procedure.
6. Put on nonsterile gloves. Empty pouch being worn into graduated container if it is not attached to straight drainage (Figure 1).	Gloves protect nurse from exposure to blood and body fluids. Emptying the pouch before handling it reduces the likelihood of spilling the excretions.

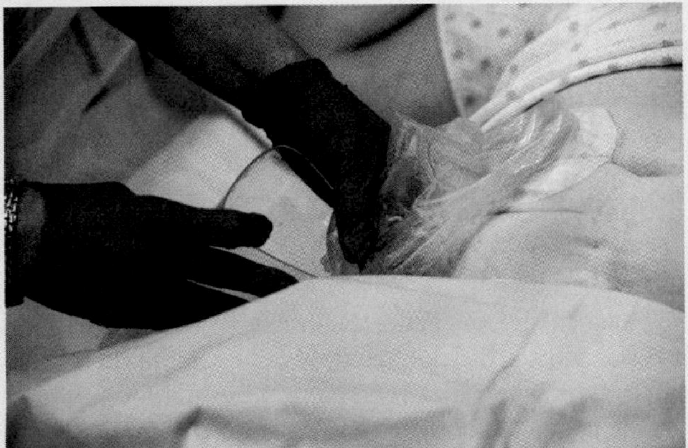

Figure 1. Emptying pouch into graduated container.

SKILL 12-11 Changing a Stoma Appliance on an Ileal Conduit *(continued)*

ACTION	RATIONALE
7. **Gently remove pouch faceplate from skin by pushing skin from appliance rather than pulling appliance from skin (Figures 2 and 3). Start at the top of the appliance, while keeping the abdominal skin taut. If resistance is felt, use warm water or adhesive remover to aid in removal.**	The seal between the surface of the faceplate and the skin must be broken before the faceplate can be removed. Harsh handling of the appliance can damage the skin and impair the development of a secure seal in the future. Pushing rather than pulling reduces irritation to the skin.
8. Place the used appliance in the trash bag, if disposable. If reusable, set aside to wash in lukewarm soap and water and allow to air dry after the new appliance is in place.	Thorough cleaning and airing of the appliance reduce odor and deterioration of appliance. For esthetic and infection-control purposes, used disposable appliances should be discarded appropriately.
9. Clean skin around stoma with mild soap and water or a cleansing agent and a washcloth (Figure 4). Remove all old adhesive from skin; use an adhesive remover if necessary.	Cleaning the skin removes excretions and old adhesive and skin protectant. Excretions or a buildup of other substances can irritate and damage the skin.
10. Gently pat area dry. **Make sure skin around stoma is thoroughly dry.** Assess stoma and condition of surrounding skin.	Careful drying prevents trauma to skin and stoma. An intact, properly applied urinary collection device protects skin integrity. Any change in color and size of the stoma may indicate circulatory problems.
11. Place one or two gauze squares over stoma opening (Figure 5).	Continuous drainage must be absorbed to keep skin dry during appliance change.

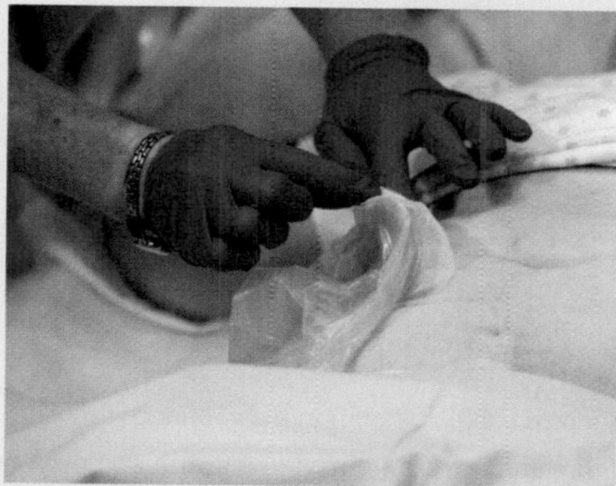

Figure 2. Removing pouch faceplate from skin.

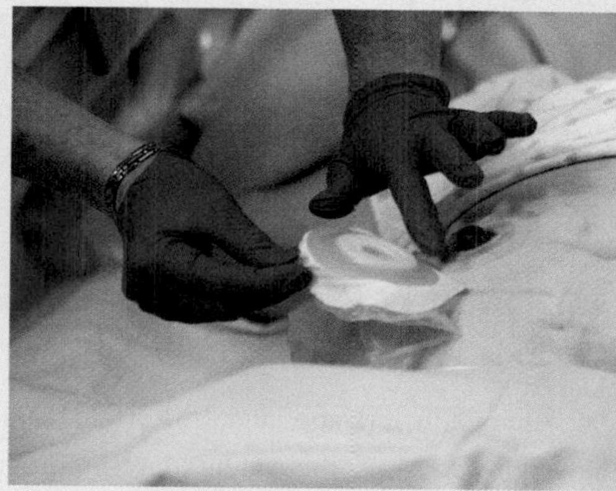

Figure 3. Pushing skin from appliance rather than pulling appliance from skin.

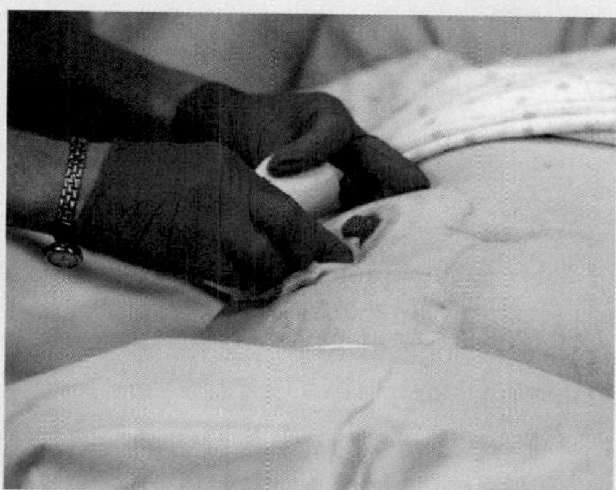

Figure 4. Cleaning stoma with cleansing agent and water and washcloth.

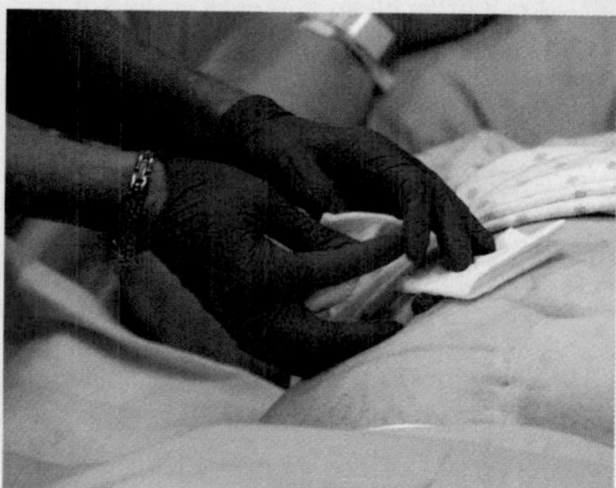

Figure 5. Placing one or two gauze squares over opening.

(continued)

SKILL 12-11 Changing a Stoma Appliance on an Ileal Conduit *(continued)*

ACTION	RATIONALE
12. Apply skin protectant to a 2″ (5-cm) radius around the stoma, and allow it to dry completely, which takes about 30 seconds.	The skin needs protection from the excoriating effect of the urine and appliance adhesive. The skin must be perfectly dry before the appliance is applied to ensure good adherence and prevent leaks.
13. Lift the gauze squares for a moment and measure the stoma opening, using the measurement guide. Replace the gauze. Trace the same size opening on the back center of the appliance. Cut the opening ⅛″ larger than the stoma size (Figure 6).	The appliance should fit snugly around the stoma, with only ⅛″ of skin visible around the opening. A faceplate opening that is too small can cause trauma to the stoma. If the opening is too large, exposed skin will be irritated by urine.
14. Remove the backing from the appliance. Quickly remove the gauze squares and discard appropriately; ease the appliance over the stoma. **Gently press onto the skin while smoothing over the surface (Figure 7). Apply gentle pressure to appliance for 5 minutes.**	The appliance is effective only if it is properly positioned and securely adhered.

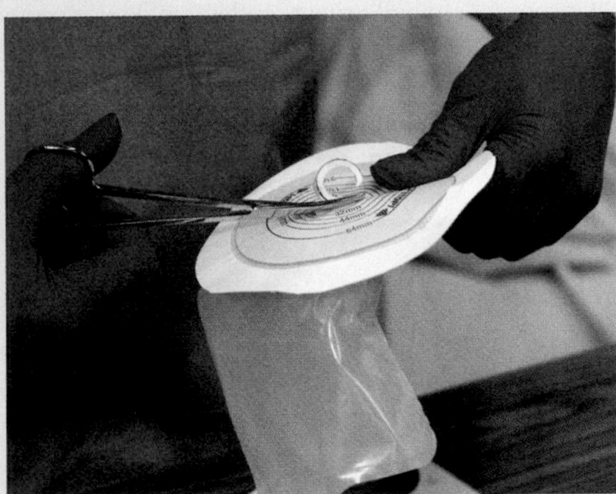

Figure 6. Cutting the faceplate opening ⅛″ larger than stoma size.

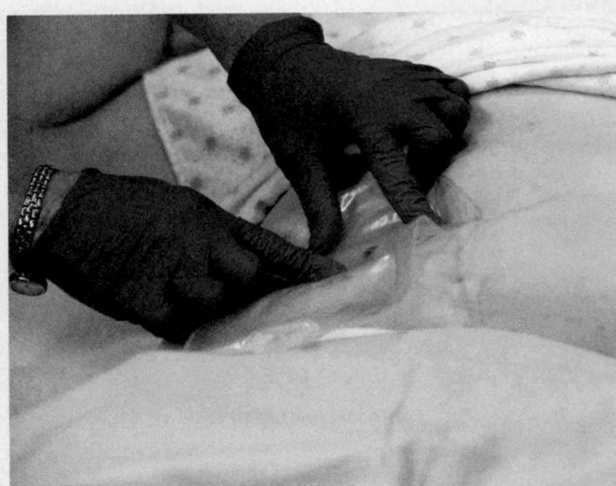

Figure 7. Applying faceplate over stoma.

ACTION	RATIONALE
15. Secure optional belt to appliance and around patient.	An elasticized belt helps support the appliance for some people.
16. Remove gloves. Assist the patient to a comfortable position. Cover the patient with bed linens. Place the bed in the lowest position.	Positioning and covering provide warmth and promote comfort and safety. Removing gloves reduces risk of infection transmission
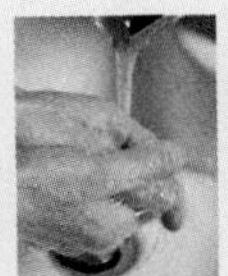 17. Put on clean gloves. Remove or discard any remaining equipment and assess patient's response to procedure. Remove gloves and perform hand hygiene.	The patient's response may indicate acceptance of the ostomy as well as the need for health teaching. Hand hygiene deters the spread of microorganisms.

EVALUATION

The expected outcome is met when the ileal conduit appliance is changed without trauma to stoma or peristomal skin, or leaking; urine is draining freely into the appliance; the skin surrounding the stoma is clean, dry, and intact; and the patient shows an interest in learning to perform the pouch change and verbalizes positive self-image.

SKILL 12-11 Changing a Stoma Appliance on an Ileal Conduit *(continued)*

DOCUMENTATION

Guidelines

Document the procedure, including the appearance of the stoma, condition of the peristomal skin, characteristics of the drainage, and the patient's response to the procedure.

Sample Documentation

7/23/08 1245 Ileal conduit appliance changed. Mr. Jones present. Mrs. Jones asking questions about care for ileal conduit, states, "I don't know if I'll ever be able to care for this thing at home." Tearful at times. Patient encouraged to express feelings. Patient agreed to talk with wound, ostomy, and continence nurse about concerns. Mr. Jones very supportive, also asking appropriate questions. Patient states would like to watch change one more time before she attempts to do it. Stoma is moist and red, peristomal skin intact, draining yellow urine with small amount of mucus. —B. Clapp, RN

Unexpected Situations and Associated Interventions

- *Nurse removes appliance and finds area of skin excoriated:* If institution has a wound, ostomy, and incontinence nurse, consider a consultation. Cleanse the skin thoroughly and pat dry. Apply products made for excoriated skin before placing appliance over stoma. Frequently check faceplate to ensure that a seal has formed and that there is no leakage. Document the excoriation in the patient's chart.
- *Faceplate is leaking after applying new appliance:* Remove appliance, clean the skin, and start over.
- *Nurse is ready to place faceplate and notices that opening is cut too large:* Discard appliance and begin over. A faceplate that is cut too big may lead to excoriation of the skin.

Special Considerations

General Considerations

- If using a two-piece appliance, after applying faceplate, snap the appliance pouch in place. Lay the pouch flange over the flange on the faceplate. Start at the bottom, and push as you run your fingers around the flange, snapping the pouch onto the flange.

SKILL 12-12 Caring for a Suprapubic Urinary Catheter

A suprapubic catheter is used for long-term continuous drainage. This type of catheter is surgically inserted through a small incision above the pubic area (Figure 1). Suprapubic bladder drainage diverts urine from the urethra when injury, stricture, prostatic obstruction, or gynecologic or abdominal surgery has compromised the flow of urine through the urethra. A suprapubic catheter is often preferred over indwelling urethral catheters for long-term urinary drainage. Suprapubic catheters are associated with decreased risk of contamination with organisms from fecal material, elimination of damage to the urethra, a higher rate of patient satisfaction, and lower risk of catheter-associated urinary tract infections (Newman, 2004). The drainage tube is secured with sutures or tape. Care of the patient with a suprapubic catheter includes skin care around the insertion site; care of the drainage tubing and drainage bag is the same as for an indwelling catheter.

(continued)

SKILL 12-12 Caring for a Suprapubic Urinary Catheter *(continued)*

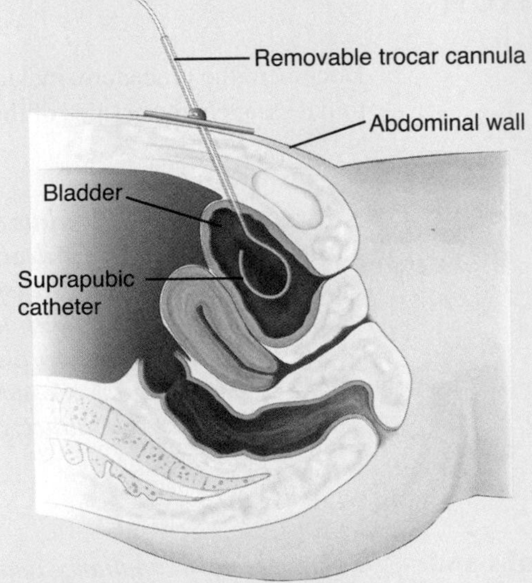

Figure 1. A suprapubic catheter positioned in the bladder.

Equipment

- Washcloth
- Gentle soap or skin cleanser
- Disposable gloves
- Velcro tube holder or tape to secure tube
- Drainage sponge (if necessary)
- Plastic trash bag
- Sterile cotton-tipped applicators and sterile saline solution (if the patient has a new suprapubic catheter)

ASSESSMENT

Assess the suprapubic catheter and bag, observing the condition of the catheter, the condition of the drainage bag connected to catheter, and the product style. If a dressing is in place at the insertion site, assess the dressing for drainage. Inspect the site around the suprapubic catheter, looking for drainage, erythema, or excoriation. Assess the method used to secure the catheter in place. If sutures are present, assess for intactness. Also, assess the characteristics of the urine in the drainage bag. Assess patient's knowledge of caring for a suprapubic catheter.

NURSING DIAGNOSIS

Determine the related factors for the nursing diagnoses based on the patient's current status. Possible nursing diagnoses may include:

- Impaired Urinary Elimination
- Risk for Impaired Skin Integrity
- Deficient Knowledge
- Risk for Infection

SKILL 12-12 Caring for a Suprapubic Urinary Catheter *(continued)*

OUTCOME IDENTIFICATION AND PLANNING

The expected outcomes to be achieved when caring for a suprapubic catheter are that the patient's skin remains clean, dry and intact, without evidence of irritation or breakdown; and the patient verbalizes an understanding of the purpose for and care of the catheter, as appropriate. Other appropriate outcomes include: the patient's urinary elimination is maintained, with a urine output of at least 30 mL/hour, and the patient's bladder is not distended.

IMPLEMENTATION

ACTION	RATIONALE
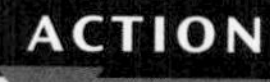 1. Identify the patient. Discuss procedure with patient. Encourage patient to observe or participate if possible.	Identifying the patient ensures the right patient receives the intervention and helps prevent errors. This discussion promotes reassurance and provides knowledge about the procedure. Explanation encourages patient cooperation and reduces apprehension. Observing or assisting with procedure encourages self-acceptance.
2. Assemble equipment.	Organization facilitates performance of task.
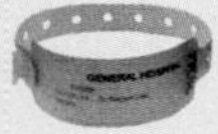 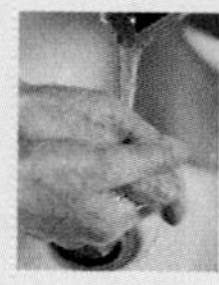 3. Perform hand hygiene.	Hand hygiene deters the spread of microorganisms.
4. Provide privacy by closing the curtains or door and draping patient with bath blanket.	The procedure may be embarrassing for the patient.
5. Raise the bed to a comfortable working height.	Having the bed in the high position reduces strain on the nurse's back while performing the procedure.
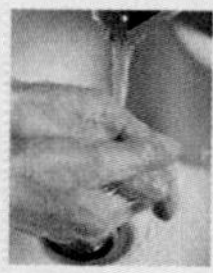 6. Put on clean gloves. Gently remove old dressing, if one is in place. Place dressing in trash bag. Remove gloves. Perform hand hygiene.	Gloves protect nurse from blood, body fluids, and microorganisms. Proper disposal of contaminated dressing and hand hygiene deter the spread of microorganisms.
7. Assess the insertion site and surrounding skin.	Any changes in assessment could indicate potential infection.
8. Wet washcloth with warm water and apply skin cleanser. **Gently cleanse around suprapubic exit site (Figure 2).** Remove any encrustations. If this is a new suprapubic catheter, sterile cotton-tipped applicators and sterile saline should be used to clean the site until incision has healed. **Moisten the applicators with the saline and clean in circular motion from the insertion site outward (Figure 3).**	Using a gentle soap or cleanser helps to protect the skin. The exit site is the most common area of skin irritation with a suprapubic catheter. If encrustations are left on the skin, they provide a medium for bacteria and an area of skin irritation.

(continued)

SKILL 12-12 Caring for a Suprapubic Urinary Catheter *(continued)*

ACTION | **RATIONALE**

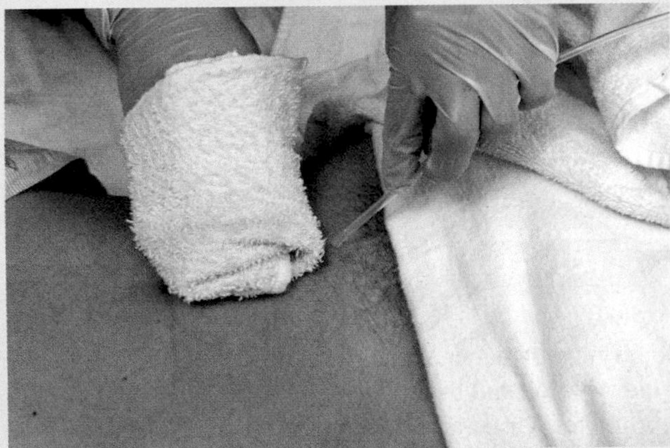

Figure 2. Cleaning area around catheter site with soap and water.

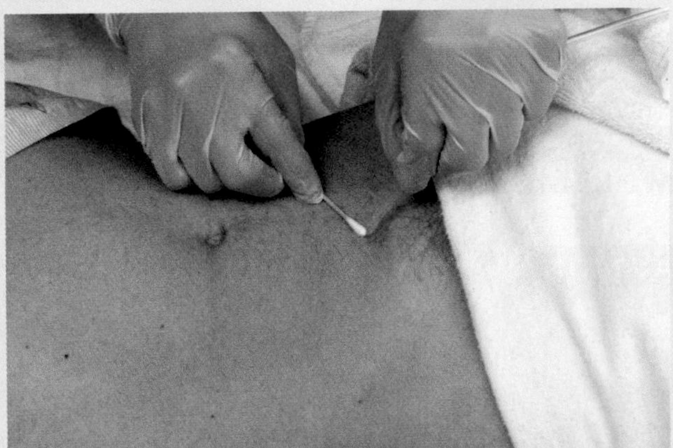

Figure 3. Using sterile cotton-tipped applicators for cleaning.

9. Rinse area of all cleanser. Pat dry.

If left on the skin, soap can cause irritation. The skin needs to be kept dry to prevent any irritation.

10. If exit site has been draining, place small drain sponge around catheter to absorb any drainage (Figure 4). Be prepared to change this sponge throughout the day, depending on the amount of drainage. Do not cut a 4 × 4 to make a drain sponge.

A small amount of drainage from the exit site is normal. The sponge needs to be changed when it becomes soiled to prevent skin irritation and breakdown. The fibers from the cut 4 × 4 may enter the exit site and cause irritation or infection.

11. Remove gloves. Form a loop in tubing and anchor the tubing on the patient's abdomen (Figure 5).

Anchoring the catheter and tubing absorbs any tugging, preventing tension on and irritation to the skin or bladder.

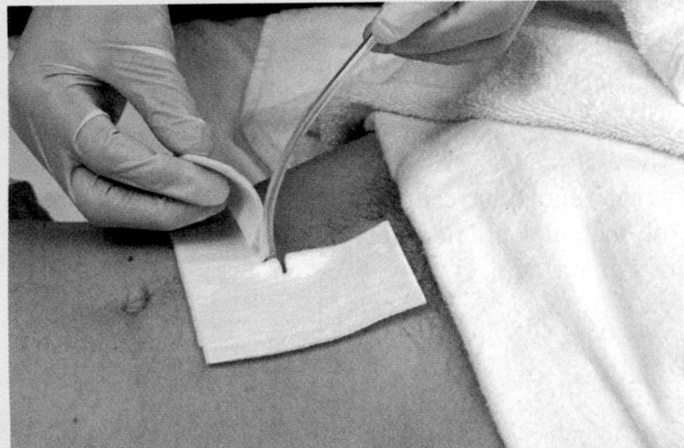

Figure 4. Applying small drain sponge around catheter.

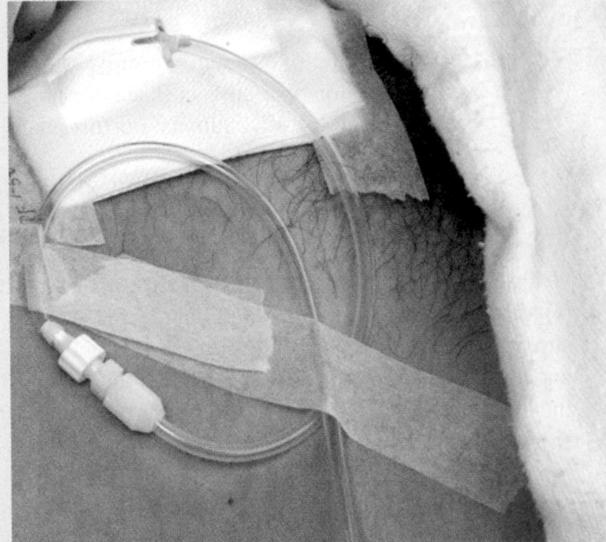

Figure 5. Forming a loop in tubing and taping to abdomen.

12. Assist the patient to a comfortable position. Cover the patient with bed linens. Place the bed in the lowest position.

Positioning and covering provide warmth and promote comfort.

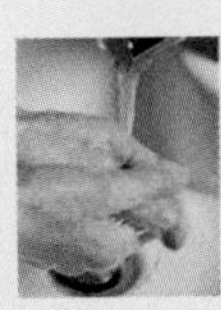

13. Put on clean gloves. Remove or discard equipment and assess patient's response to procedure. Remove gloves and perform hand hygiene.

The patient's response may indicate acceptance of the catheter or the need for health teaching. Hand hygiene deters the spread of microorganisms.

SKILL 12-12 Caring for a Suprapubic Urinary Catheter *(continued)*

EVALUATION

The expected outcomes are met when the patient's skin remains clean, dry and intact, without evidence of irritation or breakdown; the patient verbalizes an understanding of the purpose for and care of the catheter, as appropriate; the patient's urinary elimination is maintained, with a urine output of at least 30 mL/hour; and the patient's bladder is not distended.

Documentation

Guidelines

Document the appearance of catheter exit site and surrounding skin, urine amount and characteristics, as well as patient's reaction to procedure.

Sample Documentation

7/12/08 1845 Suprapubic catheter care performed. Patient assisted in care. Skin is slightly erythematous on R side where catheter was taped. Catheter taped to L side. Small amount of yellow, clear drainage noted on drain sponge. Patient would like to try to go without drain sponge at this time. Instructions given to call nurse if amount of drainage increases. Moderate amount of clear yellow urine continues to drain from catheter into collection bag.—B. Clapp, RN

Unexpected Situations and Associated Interventions

- *When cleaning site, catheter becomes dislodged and pulls out:* Notify physician. If this is a well-healed site, a new catheter can easily be replaced by the physician or advanced practice nurse. If this is a new suprapubic tube, the physician may want to assess for any trauma to the bladder wall.
- *Exit site is extremely excoriated:* Consult wound, ostomy, and incontinence nurse for evaluation. A skin protectant or barrier may need to be applied, as well as more frequent cleansing of the area and changing of the drain sponge (if applied).

Special Considerations

General Considerations

- Depending on the patient's situation, he/she may have both a suprapubic and indwelling urethral catheter. Urine will drain from both catheters; usually, drainage from the suprapubic catheter is the larger volume.
- If suprapubic is not draining into bag but, instead, has a valve at the end of the catheter, open the valve at least every 6 hours (or more frequently depending on physician order or institutional policy) to drain the urine from the bladder.

SKILL 12-13 Caring for a Peritoneal Dialysis Catheter

Peritoneal dialysis is a method of removing fluid and wastes from the body of a patient with kidney failure. A catheter inserted through the abdominal wall into the peritoneal cavity allows a special fluid (dialysate) to be infused and then drained from the body, removing waste products and excess fluid (Figure 1). The exit site is not disturbed initially after insertion, to allow for healing. Generally, this time frame is 7 to 10 days postinsertion (Redmond & Doherty, 2005). Once the exit site has healed, exit site care is an important part of patient care. The catheter insertion site is a site for potential infection, possibly leading to catheter tunnel infection and peritonitis (inflammation of the peritoneal membrane). Therefore, meticulous care is needed. The incidence of exit site infections can be reduced through a daily cleansing regimen by the patient or caregiver (Bernardini et al., 2005; Redmond & Doherty, 2005; Uttley et al., 2004). Often, in the acute care

(continued)

SKILL 12-13 Caring for a Peritoneal Dialysis Catheter *(continued)*

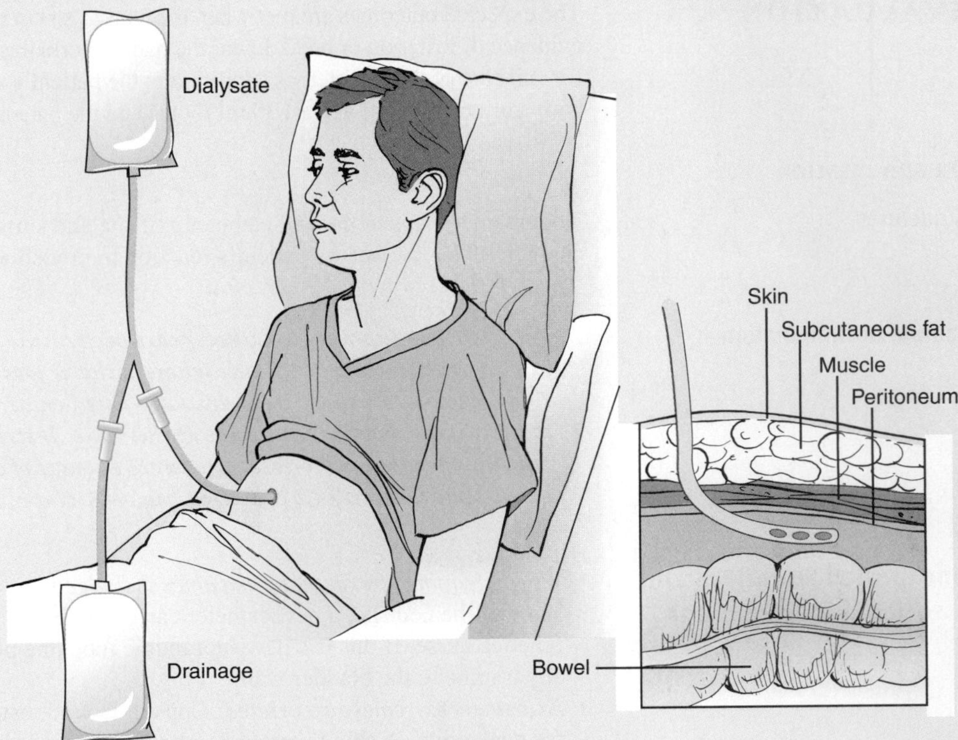

Figure 1. Position of catheter in peritoneal space. Patient is set up for peritoneal dialysis.

setting, catheter care is performed using aseptic technique, to reduce the risk for a hospital-acquired infection. At home, clean technique can be used by the patient and caregivers.

Equipment

- Face masks (2)
- Sterile gloves
- Nonsterile gloves
- Antimicrobial cleansing agent, per facility policy
- Sterile gauze squares (4)
- Sterile basin
- Sterile drain sponge
- Topical antibiotic, such as mupirocin or gentamicin, depending on order and policy
- Sterile applicator
- Plastic trash bag
- Bath blanket

ASSESSMENT

Inspect peritoneal dialysis catheter exit site for any erythema, drainage, bleeding, tenderness, swelling, skin irritation or breakdown, or leakage. These signs could indicate exit site or tunnel infection. Assess abdomen for tenderness, pain, and guarding. Assess the patient for nausea, vomiting, and fever, which could indicate peritonitis. Assess patient's knowledge about measures to care for exit site.

NURSING DIAGNOSIS

Determine the related factors for the nursing diagnoses based on the patient's current status. Possible nursing diagnoses include:

- Risk for Impaired Skin Integrity
- Risk for Infection

SKILL 12-13 Caring for a Peritoneal Dialysis Catheter *(continued)*

- Impaired Urinary Elimination
- Deficient Knowledge
- Excess Fluid Volume
- Deficient Fluid Volume

OUTCOME IDENTIFICATION AND PLANNING

The expected outcomes to achieve when performing care for a peritoneal dialysis catheter are as follows: the peritoneal dialysis catheter dressing change is completed using aseptic technique without trauma to the site or patient; the site is clean, dry, and intact, without evidence of inflammation or infection; and the patient exhibits fluid balance and participates in care as appropriate.

IMPLEMENTATION

ACTION	RATIONALE
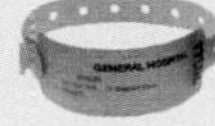 1. Identify the patient. Explain procedure and encourage patient to observe or participate if possible.	Identifying the patient ensures the right patient receives the intervention and helps prevent errors. This discussion promotes reassurance and provides knowledge about the procedure. Explanation encourages patient cooperation and reduces apprehension. Having the patient observe or assist encourages self-acceptance.
2. Bring the necessary equipment to the bedside. Close curtains around bed and close door to room if possible.	Provides for an organized approach to the procedure. Closing curtains and door provides for patient privacy.
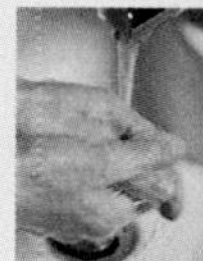 3. Perform hand hygiene and put on nonsterile gloves.	Hand hygiene deters the spread of microorganisms. Gloves protect nurse from contact with blood and bodily fluids.
4. Raise the bed to a comfortable working height.	Having the bed in the high position reduces strain on the nurse's back while performing the procedure.
5. Assist patient to supine position. Expose abdomen, draping the patient's chest with the bath blanket, exposing only the catheter site.	The supine position is usually the best way to gain access to the peritoneal dialysis catheter. Use of bath blanket provides patient warmth and avoids unnecessary exposure.
6. Put on one of the face masks; have patient put on the other mask.	The face masks deter the spread of microorganisms.
7. Gently remove old dressing, noting odor, amount and color of drainage, leakage, and condition of skin around catheter. Discard dressing in appropriate container.	Drainage, leakage, and skin condition can indicate problems with the catheter, such as infection.
8. Remove nonsterile gloves and discard. Set up sterile field. Open packages. Using aseptic technique, place two sterile 4 × 4s in basin with antimicrobial agent. Leave two sterile 4 × 4s opened on sterile field. Alternately (based on facility's policy), place sterile antimicrobial swabs on the sterile field. Place sterile applicator on field. Squeeze a small amount of the topical antibiotic on one of the gauze squares on the sterile field.	Until catheter site has healed, aseptic technique is necessary for site care to prevent infection.

(continued)

SKILL 12-13 Caring for a Peritoneal Dialysis Catheter *(continued)*

ACTION	RATIONALE
9. Put on sterile gloves.	Aseptic technique is necessary to prevent infection.
10. Pick up dialysis catheter with nondominant hand. **With the antimicrobial-soaked gauze or swab, cleanse the skin around the exit site using a circular motion, starting at the exit site and then slowly going outward 3″ to 4″. Gently remove crusted scabs if necessary.**	The antimicrobial cleanses the skin and removes any drainage or crust from the wound, reducing the risk for infection.
11. **Continue to hold catheter with nondominant hand. After skin has dried, clean the catheter with an antimicrobial-soaked gauze, beginning at exit site, going around catheter, and then moving up to end of catheter. Gently remove crusted secretions on the tube if necessary.**	Antimicrobial cleanses the catheter and removes any drainage or crust from the tube, reducing the risk for infection.
12. Using the sterile applicator, apply the topical antibiotic to the catheter exit site, if prescribed.	Application of mupirocin and gentamicin at catheter exit site prevents exit site infection and peritonitis (Bernardini et al., 2005; Uttley et al., 2004).
13. Place sterile drain sponge around exit site. Then place a 4 × 4 over exit site. Remove your gloves and secure edges of gauze pad with tape. Some institutions recommend placing a transparent dressing over the gauze pads instead of tape. Remove masks.	The drain sponge and 4 × 4 are used to absorb any drainage from the exit site. Occlusion of the site with a dressing deters contamination of site.
14. Coil the exposed length of tubing and secure to the dressing or patient's abdomen with tape.	Anchoring the catheter absorbs any tugging, preventing tension on and irritation to the skin or abdomen.
15. Assist the patient to a comfortable position. Cover the patient with bed linens. Place the bed in the lowest position.	Positioning and covering provide warmth and promote comfort. A bed in the low position promotes patient safety.
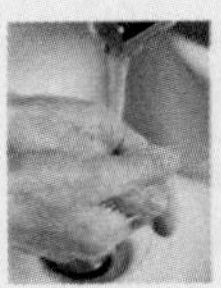 16. Put on clean gloves and dispose of equipment per facility policy. Remove gloves and perform hand hygiene.	These actions deter the spread of microorganisms.

EVALUATION

The expected outcome is met when the peritoneal dialysis catheter dressing change is completed using aseptic technique without trauma to the site or patient; the site is clean, dry, and intact, without evidence of redness, irritation, or excoriation; the patient's fluid balance is maintained; and the patient verbalizes appropriate measures to care for the site.

DOCUMENTATION

Guidelines

Document the dressing change, including condition of skin surrounding exit site, drainage, or odor, as well as patient's reaction to procedure, and any patient teaching provided.

SKILL 12-13 Caring for a Peritoneal Dialysis Catheter *(continued)*

Sample Documentation

8/22/08 1530 Peritoneal dialysis catheter dressing changed; skin surrounding catheter slightly erythematous but remains intact. Small amount of clear drainage approximately the size of a dime without odor noted on drain sponge. Pt asking appropriate questions regarding dressing change. Verbalized an understanding of explanations.—B. Clapp, RN

Unexpected Situations and Associated Interventions

- *Patient complains of pain when nurse palpates abdomen; purulent or cloudy drainage is present, or foul odor is noted when old dressing is removed:* Notify physician immediately. Any of these signs could indicate a site infection or peritonitis.
- *Nurse notes that old dressing is saturated with clear fluid:* Replace dressing to prevent skin breakdown. Notify physician. A frequent complication is leaking from exit site. Frequently check dressing, especially after patient has had solution placed in the abdominal cavity.

Special Considerations

General Considerations

- Patients with a peritoneal dialysis catheter should avoid baths and public pools.
- Patients performing own site care should be reminded of the importance of good hand washing before self-care.
- Once site is healed, some physicians do not require patients to wear a dressing unless the site is leaking. The patient may shower with an occlusive dressing over the exit site. The catheter exit site should be cleansed after showering.

Home Care Considerations

- Often, clean technique, instead of sterile technique, is used by the patient and caregivers in the home.

SKILL 12-14 Caring for a Hemodialysis Access (Arteriovenous Fistula or Graft)

Hemodialysis, a method of removing fluid and wastes from the body, requires access to the patient's vascular system. This is done via the insertion of a catheter into a vein or the creation of a fistula or graft. If a catheter is used, it is cared for in the same manner as a central venous access device (see Skill 15-7). An arteriovenous fistula is a surgically created passage that connects an artery and vein. An arteriovenous graft is a surgically created connection between an artery and vein using a synthetic material. The fistula or graft requires care by specialized personnel. Accessing a hemodialysis arteriovenous graft or fistula should be done only by specially trained healthcare team members. The following information should be taught to the patient to ensure that he or she cares for the site at home.

Equipment

- Stethoscope

ASSESSMENT

Ask the patient how much he or she knows about caring for the site. Ask the patient to describe important observations to be made. Note the location of the access site. Assess the site for signs of infection, including inflammation, edema, and drainage, and healing of the incision. Assess for patency by assessing for presence of bruit and thrill (refer to explanation in Step 4).

(continued)

SKILL 12-14 Caring for a Hemodialysis Access (Arteriovenous Fistula or Graft) *(continued)*

NURSING DIAGNOSIS

Determine the related factors for the nursing diagnoses based on the patient's current status. The primary nursing diagnosis is Deficient Knowledge. Another nursing diagnosis may be Risk for Injury.

OUTCOME IDENTIFICATION AND PLANNING

The expected outcomes to achieve when caring for a hemodialysis catheter are that the patient verbalizes appropriate care measures and observations to be made, the patient demonstrates care measures, and the graft or fistula remains patent.

IMPLEMENTATION

ACTION	RATIONALE
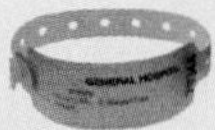 1. Identify the patient. Explain procedure and encourage patient to observe or participate if possible.	Identifying the patient ensures the right patient receives the intervention and helps prevent errors. This discussion promotes reassurance and provides knowledge about the procedure. Explanation encourages patient cooperation and reduces apprehension. Having the patient observe or assist encourages self-acceptance.
2. Close curtains around bed and close door to room if possible.	This action provides for patient privacy.
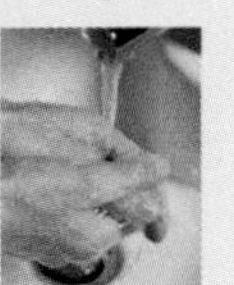 3. Perform hand hygiene.	Hand hygiene deters the spread of microorganisms.
4. **Inspect area over access site for any redness, warmth, tenderness, or blemishes. Palpate over access site, feeling for a thrill or vibration (Figure 1). Palpate pulses distal to the site. Auscultate over access site with bell of stethoscope, listening for a bruit or vibration.**	Inspection, palpation, and auscultation aid in determining the patency of the hemodialysis access. Assessment of distal pulse aids in determining the adequacy of circulation.

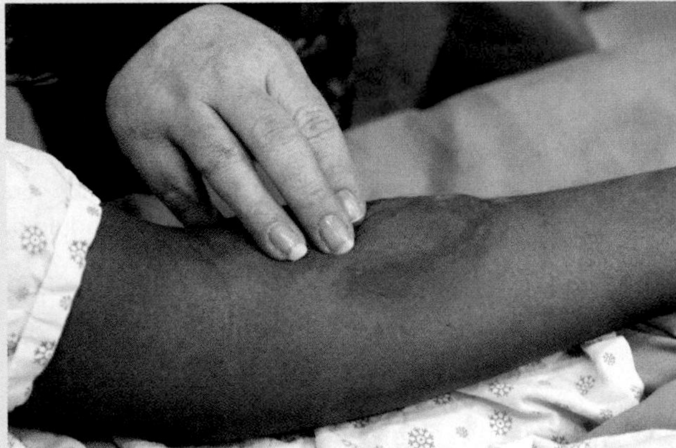

Figure 1. Palpating access site for thrill.

SKILL 12-14

Caring for a Hemodialysis Access (Arteriovenous Fistula or Graft) *(continued)*

ACTION	RATIONALE
5. Ensure that a sign is placed over head of bed informing the healthcare team which arm is affected. **Do not perform a venipuncture or start an IV on the access arm.**	The affected arm should not be used for any other procedures such as obtaining blood pressure, which could lead to clotting of the graft or fistula. Venipuncture or IV access could lead to an infection of the affected arm and could cause the loss of the graft or fistula.
6. Instruct patient not to sleep with the arm with the access site under head or body.	This could lead to clotting of the fistula or graft.
7. Instruct patient not to lift heavy objects with or put pressure on the arm with the access site. Advise the patient not to carry heavy bags (including purses) on the shoulder of that arm.	This could lead to clotting of the fistula or graft.
8. Remove gloves and perform hand hygiene.	Hand hygiene deters the spread of microorganisms.
9. Document assessment findings and any patient education performed.	A careful record is important for planning the patient's care.

EVALUATION

The expected outcome is met when the access site has an audible bruit and a palpable thrill; the site is without erythema, warmth, skin blemishes, or pain; and the patient verbalizes appropriate information about caring for the access site and observations to report.

DOCUMENTATION

Guidelines

Document assessment findings, including the presence or absence of a bruit and thrill. Document any patient education and patient response.

Sample Documentation

5/10/08 0830 Arteriovenous fistula patent in left upper arm. Area without redness, pain, and edema; skin at site similar to surrounding skin tone. Patient denies pain and tenderness. Positive bruit and thrill noted. Patient verbalized understanding of importance of avoiding venipuncture in left arm.—B. Clapp, RN

Unexpected Situations and Associated Interventions

- *Thrill is not palpable and/or bruit is not audible:* Notify the physician at once. The thrill and bruit are caused by arterial blood flowing into the vein. If these signs are not present, the access may be clotting off.
- *Site is warm to touch, erythematous, or painful or has a skin blemish:* Notify the physician. These signs can indicate a site infection.

The Taylor Suite offers these additional resources to enhance learning and facilitate understanding of this chapter:

- thePoint online resource, http://thepoint.lww.com/Lynn2E
- Student CD-ROM included with the book
- Skills Checklist to Accompany Taylor's Clinical Nursing Skills
- Taylor's Interactive Nursing: *Urinary Elimination*
- Taylor's Video Guide to Clinical Nursing Skills: *Urinary Elimination* and *Indwelling and Intermittent Catheters*

Developing Critical Thinking Skills

1. When checking Ralph Bellow's condom catheter, the nurse notices that although the catheter is still in place, Mr. Bellow's bed is soaked with urine and there is very little urine in the catheter tubing. What should the nurse do?

2. Grace Halligan is asking to go to the bathroom; she says, "I don't think I can go on a bedpan." The nurse rechecks the physician's orders and notices that Grace is on strict bed rest. How can the nurse help alleviate Grace's concerns about using a bedpan?

3. Mike Wimmer notices that his peritoneal dialysis catheter insertion site is reddened and tender. He phones the nurse to ask what should be done. What should the nurse tell Mike?

Bibliography

American Nephrology Nurses' Association, East Holly Avenue/Box 56, Pitman, NJ, 08071-0056; (856) 256-2320; available at http://www.annanurse.org.

Bernardini, J., Bender, F., Florio, T., et al. (2005). Randomized, double-blind trial of antibiotic exit site cream for prevention of exit site infection in peritoneal dialysis patients. *Journal of the American Society of Nephrology, 16*(2), 539–545.

Cohen, B., & Taylor, J. (2005). *Memmler's structure and function of the human body* (8th ed.). Philadelphia: Lippincott Williams & Wilkins.

Corbett, J. (2004). *Laboratory tests and diagnostic procedures* (6th ed.). Upper Saddle River, NJ: Pearson Prentice Hall.

Emr, K., & Ryan, R. (2004). Best practice for indwelling catheter in the home setting. *Home Healthcare Nurse, 22*(12), 820–828.

Hanchett, M. (2002). Techniques for stabilizing urinary catheters: Tape may be the oldest method, but it's not the only one. *American Journal of Nursing, 102*(3), 44–48.

Hockenberry, M. (2005). *Wong's essentials of pediatric nursing* (7th ed.). St. Louis, MO: Elsevier Mosby.

McConnell, E. (2002). Protecting a hemodialysis fistula. *Nursing, 32*(11), 18.

National Kidney and Urologic Diseases Information Clearinghouse, 3 Information Way, Bethesda, MD, 2092-3580; (301) 907-8906; available at http://kidney.niddk.nigh.gov.

Newman, D. (2004). Incontinence products and devices for the elderly. *Urologic Nursing, 24*(4), 316–334.

Newman, D., Fader, M., & Bliss, D. (2004.). Managing incontinence using technology, devices, and products: Directions for research. *Nursing Research, 53*(6S), Supplement. S42–S48.

Patraca, K. (2005). Measure bladder volume without catheterization. *Nursing, 35*(4), 46–47.

Phipps, W., Sands, J., & Marek, J. (2003). *Medical-surgical nursing: Concepts & clinical practice* (7th ed.). St. Louis, MO: C. V. Mosby.

Porth, C. (2005*). Pathophysiology: Concepts of altered health states* (7th ed.). Philadelphia: Lippincott Williams & Wilkins.

Redmond, A., & Doherty, E. (2005). Peritoneal dialysis. *Nursing Standard, 19*(40), 55–65.

Robinson, J. (2004). A practical approach to catheter-associated problems. *Nursing Standard, 14*(18), 38–42.

Smeltzer, S., Bare, B., Hinkle, J. H., & Cheever, K. H. (2008). *Brunner & Suddarth's textbook of medical–surgical nursing* (11th ed.). Philadelphia: Lippincott Williams & Wilkins.

Society of Urologic Nurses and Associates. (2005a). *Care of the patient with an indwelling catheter: Clinical practice guideline.* Available at suna.org/resources/indwellingCatheter.pdf. Accessed November 15, 2005.

Society of Urologic Nurses and Associates. (2005b). *Female urethral catheterization: Clinical practice guideline.* Available at suna.org/resources/femaleCatheterization.pdf. Accessed November 15, 2005.

Society of Urologic Nurses and Associates. (2005c). *Male urethral catheterization: Clinical practice guideline.* Available at suna.org/resources/maleCatheterization.pdf. Accessed November 15, 2005.

Sparks, A., Boyer, D., Gambrel, A., et al. (2004). The clinical benefits of the bladder scanner: A research synthesis. *Journal of Nursing Care Quality, 19*(3), 188–192.

Specht, J. (2005). 9 myths of incontinence in older adults. *American Journal of Nursing, 105*(6), 58–69.

Stevens, E. (2005). Bladder ultrasound: Avoiding unnecessary catheterizations. *MEDSURG Nursing, 14*(4), 249–253.

Toughill, E. (2005). Bladder matters. Indwelling urinary catheters: Common mechanical and pathogenic problems. *American Journal of Nursing, 105*(5), 35–37.

Trainor, B., Thompson, M., Boyd-Carson, W., et al. (2003). Changing an appliance . . . second in a series. *Nursing Standard, 18*(13), 41–42.

U.S. Department of Health and Human Services. Centers for Disease Control and Prevention. (2005). *Guidelines for prevention of catheter-associated urinary tract infections.* Available at http://www.cdc.gov/ncidod/dhqp/gl_catheter_assoc.html. Accessed December 14, 2005.

Uttley, L., Vardhan, A., Mahajan, S., et al. (2004). Decrease in infections with the introduction of mupirocin cream at the peritoneal dialysis catheter exit site. *Journal of Nephrology, 17*(2), 242–245.

Woods, A. (2005). Managing UTIs in older adults. *Nursing, 35*(3), 12.

CHAPTER 13

Bowel Elimination

Focusing on Patient Care

This chapter will help you develop some of the skills related to bowel elimination necessary to care for the following patients:

Hugh Levens is a 64-year-old man who has been placed on a bowel program after a fall left him paralyzed from the waist down.

Isaac Greenberg, age 9 years, has been having blood in his stools. He is scheduled for a colonoscopy as an outpatient. He and his mother need teaching about the preparation for the procedure, which includes a small-volume cleansing enema.

Maria Blakely, age 26, has recently received an ileostomy. She is having problems with her appliances and is concerned about excoriation.

Learning Objectives

After studying this chapter, you will be able to:

1. Insert a rectal tube.
2. Administer a large-volume cleansing enema.
3. Administer a small-volume cleansing enema.
4. Administer a retention enema.
5. Remove stool digitally.
6. Apply a fecal incontinence pouch.
7. Change and empty an ostomy appliance.
8. Irrigate a colostomy.

Key Terms

colostomy: artificial opening that permits feces from the colon to exit through the stoma

constipation: passage of dry, hard stools

defecation: emptying of the large intestine; also called a bowel movement

diarrhea: passage of excessively liquid, nonformed stool

enema: introduction of a solution into the large intestine

fecal impaction: prolonged retention or an accumulation of fecal material that forms a hardened mass in the rectum

flatus: intestinal gas

hemorrhoids: abnormally distended veins in the anal area

ileostomy: artificial opening created to allow liquid fecal content from the ileum to be eliminated through a stoma

ostomy: a surgically formed opening from the inside of an organ to the outside

stoma: the part of the ostomy that is attached to the skin; formed by suturing the mucosa to the skin

vagal stimulus or response: stimulation of the vagus nerve that causes an increase in parasympathetic stimulation, triggering a decrease in heart rate

Valsalva maneuver: voluntary contraction of the abdominal wall muscles, fixing of the diaphragm, and closing of the glottis that increases intra-abdominal pressure and aids in expelling feces

Elimination of the waste products of digestion is a natural process critical for human functioning. Patients differ widely in their expectations about bowel elimination, their usual pattern of defecation, and the ease with which they speak about bowel elimination or bowel problems. Although most people have experienced minor acute bouts of diarrhea or constipation, some patients experience severe or chronic bowel elimination problems affecting their fluid and electrolyte balance, hydration, nutritional status, skin integrity, comfort, and self-concept. Moreover, many illnesses, diagnostic tests, medications, and surgical treatments can affect bowel elimination. Nurses play an integral role in preventing and managing bowel elimination problems.

This chapter will cover skills to assist the nurse in promoting and assisting with bowel elimination. Understanding the anatomy of the gastrointestinal system is integral to performing the skills in this chapter (Fundamentals Review 13-1). An abdominal assessment is required as part of the assessment related to many of the skills (Fundamentals Review 13-2). Fundamentals Review 13-3 summarizes factors that affect elimination.

Fundamentals Review 13-1

Anatomy of the Gastrointestinal Tract

- The GI tract begins with the mouth and continues to the esophagus, the stomach, the small intestine, and the large intestine. It ends at the anus.
- From the mouth to the anus, the GI tract is approximately 9 m (30 feet) long.
- The small intestine consists of the duodenum, jejunum, and ileum.
- The large intestine consists of the cecum, colon (ascending, transverse, descending, and sigmoid), and rectum.
- Accessory organs of the GI tract include the teeth, salivary glands, gallbladder, liver, and pancreas.

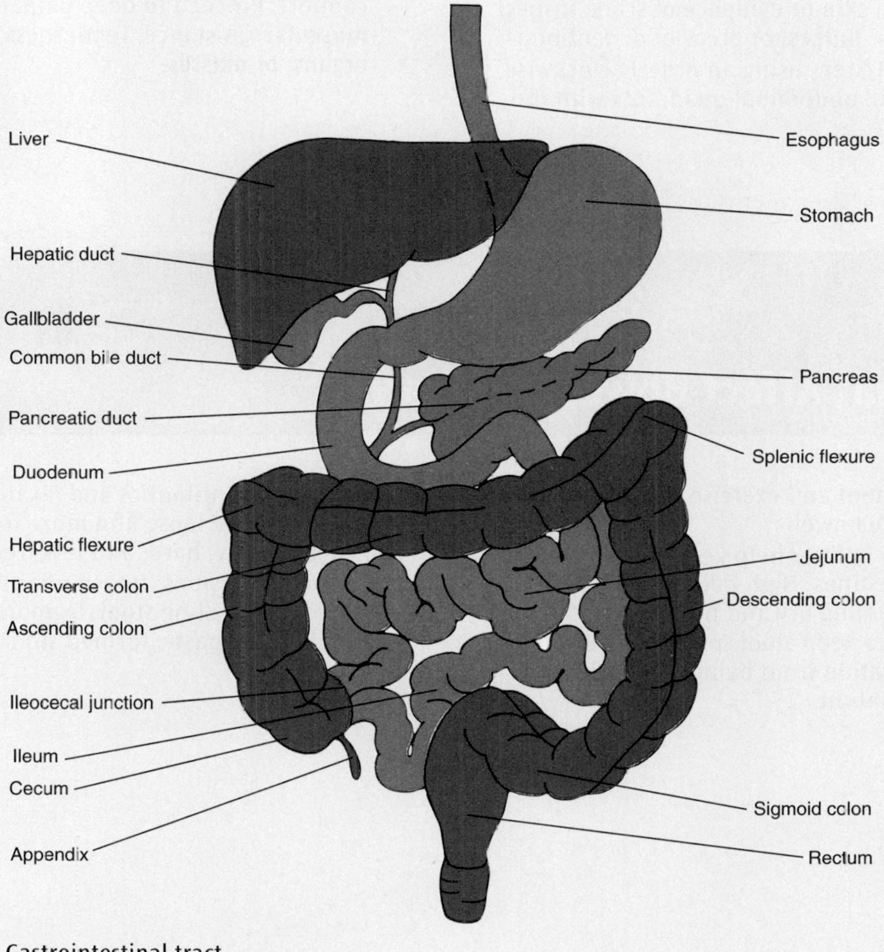

Gastrointestinal tract.

Assessment Techniques for the Abdomen

- Place patient in a supine position with knees slightly flexed.
- When assessing an infant or toddler, you may want to place the child on the parent's lap to prevent the child from becoming upset and crying.
- Perform the abdominal assessment in the following sequence: inspection, auscultation, percussion, palpation.
  - Inspection: Observe contour of abdomen; note any changes in skin or evidence of scars; inspect for any masses, bulges, or areas of distention.
  - Auscultation: Listen, using an orderly clockwise approach, in all abdominal quadrants with the diaphragm of the stethoscope; listen for bowel sounds (intermittent, soft click and gurgles); note the frequency of bowel sounds (should be 5 to 34 sounds per minute).
  - Percussion: Percuss, using an orderly clockwise approach in all abdominal quadrants; expect to hear tympany over most regions.
  - Palpation: Lightly palpate over abdominal quadrants, first checking for any areas of pain or discomfort. Proceed to deep palpation, noting any muscular resistance, tenderness, enlargement of organs, or masses.

Factors That Affect Bowel Elimination

- Mobility: Movement and exercise help to move stool through the bowel.
- Diet: Foods high in fiber help keep stool moving through the intestines. High fluid intake keeps stools from becoming dry and hard. Adequate fluid also helps fiber to keep stool soft and bulky and prevents dehydration from being a contributing factor to constipation.
- Medications: Antibiotics and laxatives may cause stool to become loose and more frequent. Diuretics may lead to dry, hard, and less frequent stools.
- Intestinal diversions: Ileostomies normally have liquid, foul-smelling stool. Sigmoid colostomies normally have pasty, formed stool.

SKILL 13-1 Inserting a Rectal Tube

Gases can build up in the stomach or intestine, causing flatulence. Moving about in bed or ambulating can help to promote peristalsis and the escape of gas. However, when these measures are ineffective, occasionally a rectal tube may be prescribed. This tube is inserted into the rectum to stimulate peristalsis and provide a passageway for gas to escape.

Equipment

- Disposable gloves
- Washcloth, soap, and towel
- Rectal tube (size 22–34 French for adults, 12–18 French for children)
- Water-soluble lubricant
- Disposable waterproof pad
- Tape
- Bedpan
- Paper towel
- Measuring tape

ASSESSMENT

Assess the rectal area for any fissures, hemorrhoids, sores, or rectal tears. If present, added care should be taken while inserting the tube. Assess the results of the patient's laboratory work, specifically the platelet count and white blood cell (WBC) count. A rectal catheter may irritate the gastrointestinal mucosa, causing bleeding, bowel perforation, or infection. Any unnecessary procedures that would place the patient at risk for bleeding or infection should not be performed. Measure the patient's abdominal girth with a tape measure at the umbilicus before inserting the tube. This measurement provides a baseline upon which to evaluate the effectiveness of the expulsion of gas. Measure again after the rectal tube has been removed, noting any decrease in abdominal girth. Percuss and palpate the abdomen. With excessive flatus, hyperresonance typically is noted. With increased flatulence or diarrhea, the abdomen may be firm, distended, or painful to deep and light palpation. Have the patient rate his or her level of pain before the rectal tube is inserted, and then compare this rating after the rectal tube is removed. Assess pulse rate before and during rectal tube insertion. Assess for dizziness, lightheadedness, diaphoresis, and clammy skin. The rectal tube may stimulate a vagal response, which increases parasympathetic stimulation, causing a decrease in heart rate.

NURSING DIAGNOSIS

Determine the related factors for the nursing diagnoses based on the patient's current status. Appropriate nursing diagnoses include:

- Acute Pain
- Risk for Injury

OUTCOME IDENTIFICATION AND PLANNING

The expected outcome to achieve when inserting a rectal tube is that the tube is inserted and removed without adverse effect, and the patient expels flatus. Other appropriate outcomes may include the following: the patient verbalizes decreased discomfort, and abdominal distention is absent.

IMPLEMENTATION

ACTION	RATIONALE
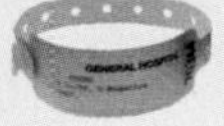 1. Identify the patient. Discuss the procedure with the patient and assess the patient's ability to assist with the procedure.	Identifying the patient ensures the right patient receives the intervention and helps prevent errors. This discussion promotes reassurance and provides knowledge about the procedure. Dialogue encourages patient participation and allows for individualized nursing care.

(continued)

SKILL 13-1 Inserting a Rectal Tube *(continued)*

ACTION	RATIONALE
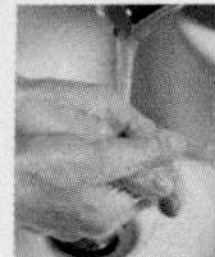 2. Bring rectal tube and other necessary equipment to bedside. Perform hand hygiene. Put on disposable clean gloves.	Having equipment on hand saves time by avoiding unnecessary trips to storage area. Hand hygiene deters the spread of microorganisms. Gloves prevent exposure to blood and body fluids.
3. Close curtains around bed and close door to room if possible.	This provides for patient privacy.
4. If bed is adjustable, place it in high position. Place the patient in a prone or knee–chest position, unless contraindicated. A right side-lying position is also acceptable.	Having the bed in the high position reduces strain on the nurse's back. Gas is lighter than fluids and solids and thus will rise.
5. Fold top linen back just enough to allow access to the patient's rectal area. Place a waterproof pad under the patient's hip.	Folding back the linen in this manner minimizes unnecessary exposure and promotes the patient's comfort and warmth. The waterproof pad will protect the bed.
6. Lubricate approximately 4″ (10 cm) of the rectal tube with water-soluble lubricant (Figure 1).	Lubrication reduces irritation to mucous membranes and facilitates insertion.

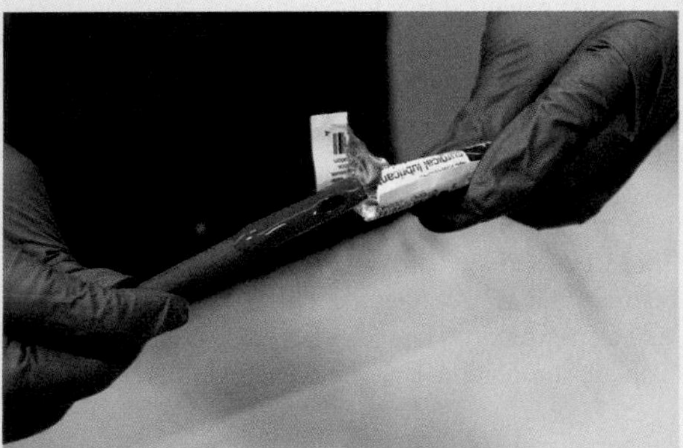

Figure 1. Lubricating rectal tube.

ACTION	RATIONALE
7. Separate buttocks so that anus is visible (Figure 2). Have patient take a slow, deep breath, inhaling through nose and exhaling through mouth. Gently insert the rectal tube beyond the anal canal into the rectum, angling toward the umbilicus (Figure 3), approximately 3″ to 4″ (10 cm) for an adult.	To remove flatus and to help stimulate peristalsis, the tube must be inserted into the rectum. The patient will concentrate on following directions, and this may help the patient to relax the anal sphincter.

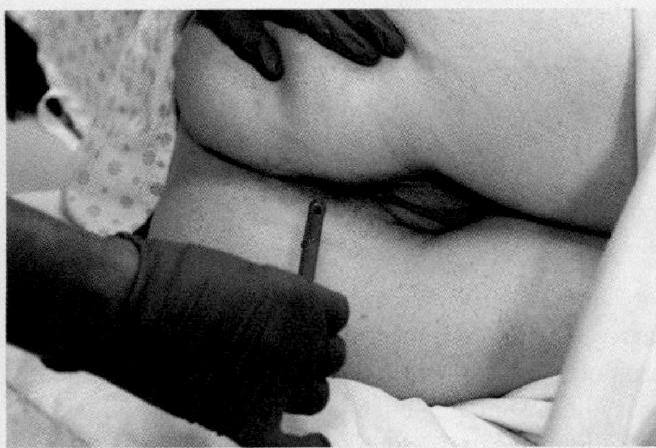

Figure 2. Separating the patient's buttocks, getting ready to insert rectal tube.

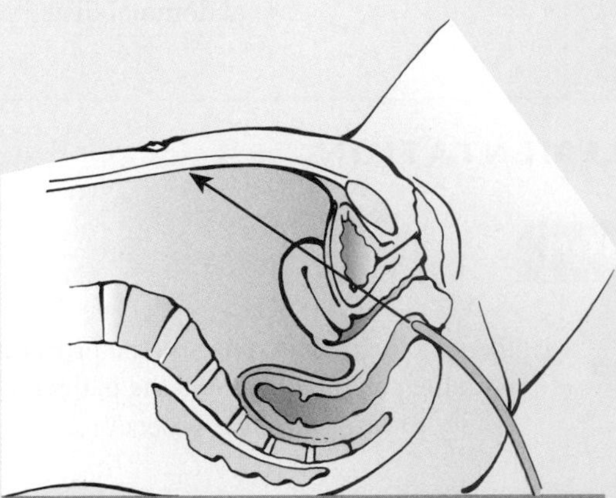

Figure 3. Gently inserting the tube into the rectum, angling toward the umbilicus.

SKILL 13-1

Inserting a Rectal Tube *(continued)*

ACTION	RATIONALE
8. Place end of rectal tube into the bedpan or waterproof pad (Figure 4). Instruct the patient to maintain his/her position while the tube is in place.	This will prevent any stool from leaking onto patient or bedding. Maintaining position prevents trauma to the rectum and mucosa.

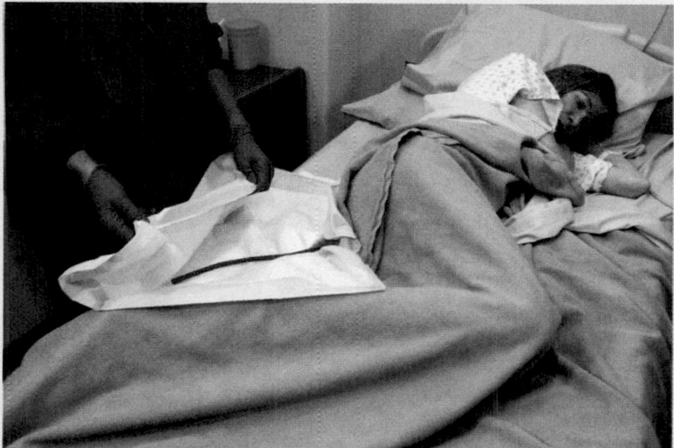

Figure 4. Securing waterproof pad to end of rectal tube already inserted.

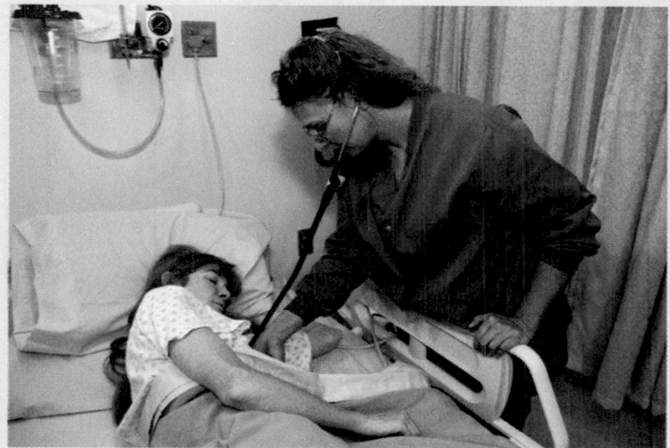

Figure 5. Monitoring the patient's heart rate.

ACTION	RATIONALE
9. Leave rectal tube in place for no longer than 20 minutes. Tube may be taped in place.	The tube will no longer act as a stimulant for peristalsis and may cause intestinal mucosal trauma if left in place longer.
10. Cover the patient with the bed linens.	Covering promotes warmth and privacy.
11. Stay with the patient while the tube is in place. While tube is in place, monitor patient for any change in heart rate or complaints of dizziness, lightheadedness, diaphoresis, and clammy skin (Figure 5).	The rectal tube may stimulate a vagal response, which increases parasympathetic stimulation, causing a decrease in heart rate. Tube should be removed.

Removing the Tube

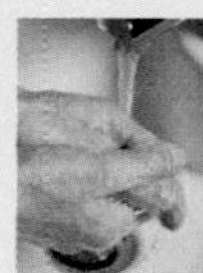

ACTION	RATIONALE
12. Perform hand hygiene and replace gloves if they have been removed.	Hand hygiene deters the spread of microorganisms. Gloves protect nurse from microorganisms in feces.
13. Have patient take a slow, deep breath, inhaling through nose and exhaling through mouth. Gently remove the tube at the same angle it was inserted.	The patient will concentrate on following directions, and this may help patient to relax anal sphincter. Prevents trauma to rectum and mucosa.
14. Wrap contaminated end of rectal tube in paper towel and discard (Figure 6).	Wrapping the end contains any feces that may be on the tip.
15. Clean perineal area.	Cleaning promotes comfort and helps to maintain skin integrity.
16. Return the patient to a comfortable position. Make sure the linens under the patient are dry. Remove your gloves and ensure that the patient is covered.	Promotes patient comfort. Removing contaminated gloves prevents spread of microorganisms.
17. Raise side rail. Lower bed height and adjust head of bed to a comfortable position.	These actions promote patient safety.

(continued)

SKILL 13-1 Inserting a Rectal Tube *(continued)*

ACTION	RATIONALE

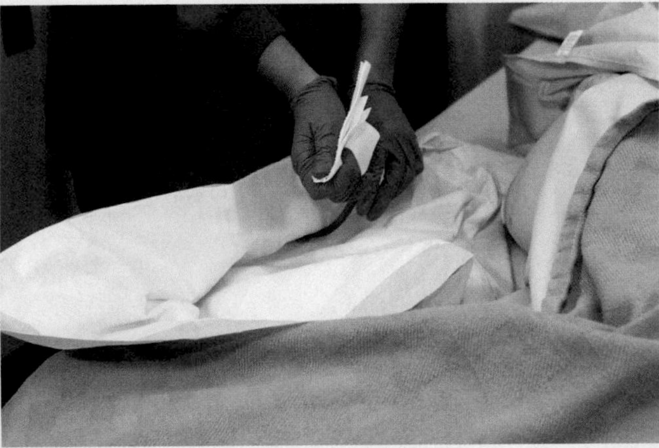

Figure 6. Wrapping contaminated rectal tube in paper towel to discard.

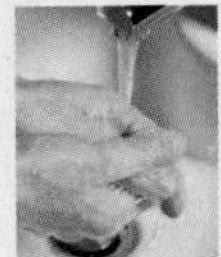

ACTION	RATIONALE
18. Remove any remaining equipment. Perform hand hygiene.	Hand hygiene deters the spread of microorganisms.

EVALUATION

The expected outcome is met when the tube is inserted and removed without adverse effect; the patient expels flatus; the patient verbalizes decreased discomfort; and abdominal distention is absent.

DOCUMENTATION

Guidelines

Document the size of rectal tube used; length of time tube was left in place; color, amount, and consistency of any stool removed; any changes noted in abdominal girth, abdominal assessment, or complaints of pain; patient's positions during procedure; and patient's reaction to procedure.

Sample Documentation

07/10/09 1145 Patient placed into side-lying Sims' position. Rectal tube 22 Fr. inserted and left in place for 15 minutes. Small amount of brown, soft stool removed. Patient's abdominal girth 42 cm prior to rectal tube; abdominal girth 40.5 cm after removal of tube. Abdomen remains slightly distended but is softer to palpation. Patient denies pain and discomfort.—K. Sanders, RN

Unexpected Situations and Associated Interventions

- *Abdominal girth has not changed and patient is still uncomfortable:* The rectal tube may be used intermittently every 2 to 3 hours, as ordered. Through repeated use, peristalsis may increase; however, irritation to gastrointestinal mucosa also increases with repeated use. Use caution to prevent irritation when using tube repeatedly.

SKILL 13-1 Inserting a Rectal Tube *(continued)*

Special Considerations

General Considerations

- If pain or resistance is encountered at any time during the procedure, stop, remove the tube, and contact the patient's physician.

Infant and Child Considerations

- Lubricate and insert the tube 2″ to 3″ for a child; 1″ to 1½″ for an infant.

SKILL 13-2 Administering a Large-Volume Cleansing Enema

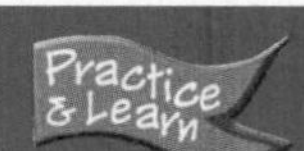

Cleansing enemas are given to remove feces from the colon. Some of the reasons for administering a cleansing enema include relieving constipation or fecal impaction, preventing involuntary escape of fecal material during surgical procedures, promoting visualization of the intestinal tract by radiographic or instrument examination, and helping to establish regular bowel function during a bowel training program. These enemas are classified as large-volume and small-volume cleansing enemas. Large-volume enemas are also known as hypotonic or isotonic, depending on the solution used. Hypotonic (tap water) and isotonic (normal saline solution) enemas are large-volume enemas that result in rapid colonic emptying. However, using such large volumes of solution (adults, 500 to 1000 mL; infants, 150 to 250 mL) may be dangerous for patients with weakened intestinal walls. These solutions often require special preparation and equipment.

This skill addresses administering a large-volume enema. See Table 13-1 for a list of commonly used enema solutions.

TABLE 13-1 Commonly Used Enema Solutions

SOLUTION	AMOUNT	ACTION	TIME TO TAKE EFFECT	ADVERSE EFFECTS
Tap water (hypotonic)	500–1000 mL	Distends intestine, increases peristalsis, softens stool	15 min	Fluid and electrolyte imbalance, water intoxication
Normal saline (isotonic)	500–1000 mL	Distends intestine, increases peristalsis, softens stool	15 min	Fluid and electrolyte imbalance, sodium retention
Soap	500–1000 mL (concentrate at 3–5 mL/1000 mL)	Distends intestine, irritates intestinal mucosa, softens stool	10–15 min	Rectal mucosa irritation or damage
Hypertonic	70–130 mL	Distends intestine, irritates intestinal mucosa	5–10 min	Sodium retention
Oil (mineral, olive, or cottonseed oil)	150–200 mL	Lubricates stool and intestinal mucosa	30 min	

Equipment

- Solution as ordered by the physician at a temperature of 105° to 110°F (40°–43°C) for adults in the prescribed amount. (Amount will vary depending on type of solution, patient's age, and patient's ability to retain the solution. Average cleansing enema for an adult may range from 750 to 1000 mL.)
- Disposable enema set, which includes a solution container and tubing

(continued)

SKILL 13-2 Administering a Large-Volume Cleansing Enema *(continued)*

- Water-soluble lubricant
- IV pole
- Necessary additives as ordered
- Waterproof pad
- Bath thermometer (if available)
- Bath blanket
- Bedpan and toilet tissue
- Disposable gloves
- Paper towel
- Washcloth, soap, and towel

ASSESSMENT

Ask the patient when he had his last bowel movement. Assess the patient's abdomen, including auscultating for bowel sounds, percussing, and palpating. Since the goal of a cleansing enema is to increase peristalsis, which should increase bowel sounds, assess the abdomen before and after the enema. Assess the rectal area for any fissures, hemorrhoids, sores, or rectal tears. If present, added care should be taken while inserting the tube. Assess the results of the patient's laboratory work, specifically the platelet count and white blood cell (WBC) count. An enema is contraindicated for patients with a low platelet count or low WBC count. An enema may irritate or traumatize the gastrointestinal mucosa, causing bleeding, bowel perforation, or infection. Any unnecessary procedures that would place the patient at risk for bleeding or infection should not be performed. Assess for dizziness, light-headedness, diaphoresis, and clammy skin. The enema may stimulate a vagal response, which increases parasympathetic stimulation, causing a decrease in heart rate. Enemas should not be administered to patients who have severe abdominal pain, bowel obstruction, bowel inflammation or bowel infection, or after rectal, prostate, and colon surgery.

NURSING DIAGNOSIS

Determine the related factors for the nursing diagnoses based on the patient's current status. Appropriate nursing diagnoses may include:

- Acute Pain
- Constipation
- Risk for Constipation
- Risk for Injury

OUTCOME IDENTIFICATION AND PLANNING

The expected outcome to be met when administering a cleansing enema is that the patient expels feces. Other appropriate outcomes may include the following: the patient verbalizes decreased discomfort; abdominal distention is absent; and the patient remains free of any evidence of trauma to the rectal mucosa or other adverse effects.

IMPLEMENTATION

ACTION	RATIONALE
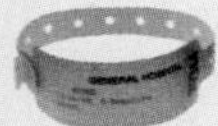 1. Verify the order for the enema. Identify the patient. Explain procedure to patient. Discuss where the patient will defecate. Have a bedpan, commode, or nearby bathroom ready for use.	Identifying the patient ensures the right patient receives the intervention and helps prevent errors. Verifying the physician's order is crucial to ensuring that the proper enema is administered to the right patient. Organization facilitates performance of tasks. Explanation helps to minimize anxiety. The patient is better able to relax and cooperate if he or she is familiar with the procedure and knows everything is in readiness when the urge to defecate is felt. Defecation usually occurs within 5 to 15 minutes.

SKILL 13-2 **Administering a Large-Volume Cleansing Enema** *(continued)*

IMPLEMENTATION

ACTION	RATIONALE
2. Warm solution in amount ordered, and check temperature with a bath thermometer if available. If bath thermometer is not available, warm to room temperature or slightly higher, and test on inner wrist. If tap water is used, adjust temperature as it flows from faucet (Figure 1).	Warming the solution prevents chilling the patient, adding to the discomfort of the procedure. Cold solution could cause cramping; too warm of solution could cause trauma to intestinal mucosa.

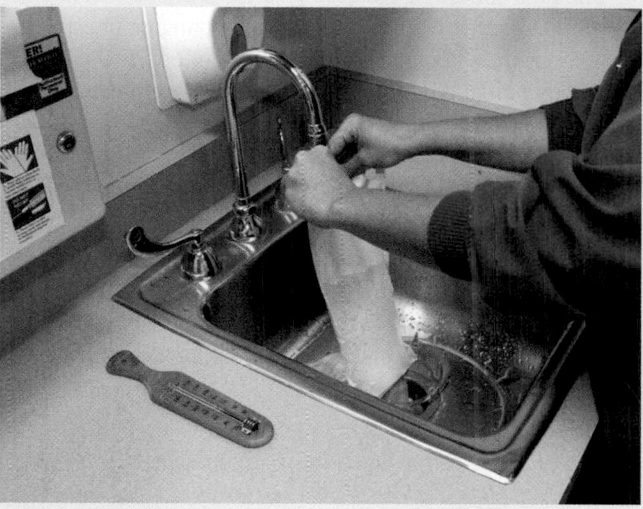

Figure 1. Preparing enema bag.

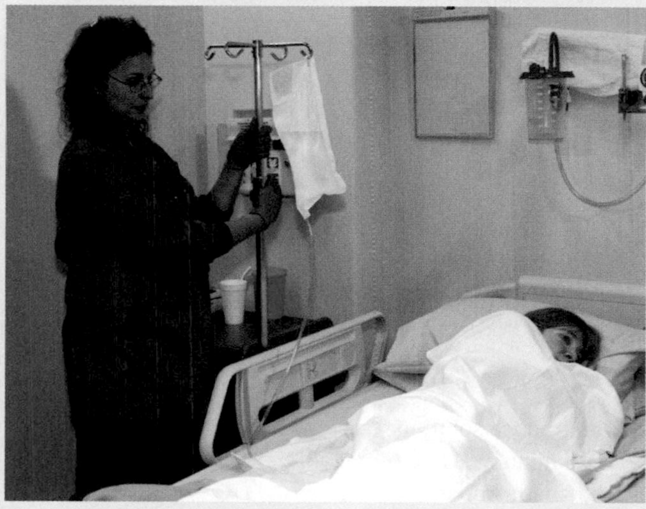

Figure 2. Adjusting the height of the solution container until it is 18″ above the patient.

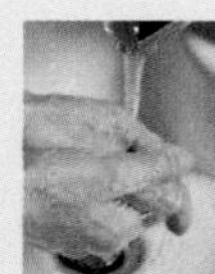

ACTION	RATIONALE
3. Perform hand hygiene.	Hand hygiene deters the spread of microorganisms.
4. Add enema solution to container. Release clamp and allow fluid to progress through tube before reclamping.	This causes any air to be expelled from the tubing. Although allowing air to enter the intestine is not harmful, it may further distend the intestine.
5. Pull the curtains around the bed and close the room door. If bed is adjustable, place it in high position.	Closing the curtains provides for privacy. Having the bed in the high position reduces strain on the nurse's back.
6. Position the patient on the left side (Sims' position), as dictated by patient comfort and condition. Fold top linen back just enough to allow access to the patient's rectal area. Place a waterproof pad under the patient's hip.	The exact position of the patient has not been found to alter the results of an enema significantly. Folding back the linen in this manner minimizes unnecessary exposure and promotes the patient's comfort and warmth. The waterproof pad will protect the bed.
7. Put on nonsterile gloves.	Gloves protect nurse from microorganisms in feces.
8. Elevate solution so that it is no higher than 18″ (45 cm) above level of anus (Figure 2). Plan to give the	Gravity forces the solution to enter the intestine. The amount of pressure determines the rate of flow and pres-

(continued)

SKILL 13-2 Administering a Large-Volume Cleansing Enema *(continued)*

ACTION	RATIONALE
solution slowly over a period of 5 to 10 minutes. The container may be hung on an IV pole or held in the nurse's hands at the proper height.	sure exerted on the intestinal wall. Giving the solution too quickly causes rapid distention and pressure, poor defecation, or damage to the mucous membrane.
9. Generously lubricate end of rectal tube 2″ to 3″ (5–7 cm). A disposable enema set may have a prelubricated rectal tube.	Lubrication facilitates passage of the rectal tube through the anal sphincter and prevents injury to the mucosa.
10. Lift buttock to expose anus. Slowly and gently insert the enema tube 3″ to 4″ (7–10 cm) for an adult. Direct it at an angle pointing toward the umbilicus, not bladder (Figure 3). Ask patient to take several deep breaths.	Good visualization of the anus helps prevent injury to tissues. The anal canal is about 1″ to 2″ (2.5–5 cm) long. The tube should be inserted past the external and internal sphincters, but further insertion may damage intestinal mucous membrane. The suggested angle follows the normal intestinal contour and thus will help to prevent perforation of the bowel. Slow insertion of the tube minimizes spasms of the intestinal wall and sphincters. Deep breathing helps relax the anal sphincters.
11. If resistance is met while inserting tube, permit a small amount of solution to enter, withdraw tube slightly, and then continue to insert it. Do not force entry of the tube. Ask patient to take several deep breaths.	Resistance may be due to spasms of the intestine or failure of the internal sphincter to open. The solution may help to reduce spasms and relax the sphincter, thus making continued insertion of the tube safe. Forcing a tube may injure the intestinal mucosa wall. Taking deep breaths helps relax the anal sphincter.
12. Introduce solution slowly over a period of 5 to 10 minutes. Hold tubing all the time that solution is being instilled.	Introducing the solution slowly helps prevent rapid distention of the intestine and a desire to defecate.
13. Clamp tubing or lower container if patient has desire to defecate or cramping occurs (Figure 4). Patient also may be instructed to take small, fast breaths or to pant.	These techniques help relax muscles and prevent premature expulsion of the solution.

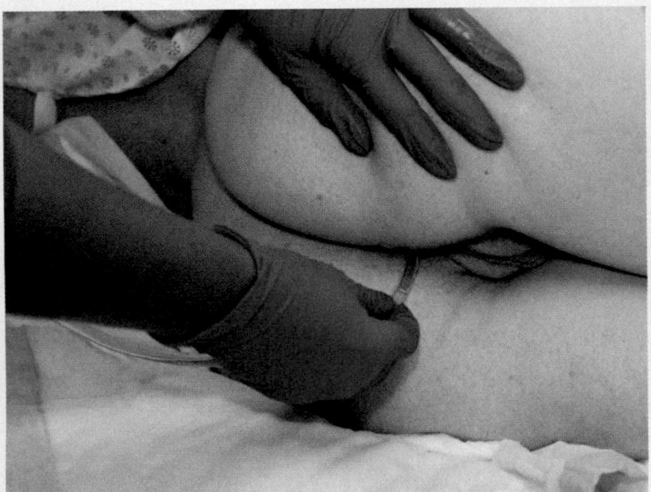

Figure 3. Inserting enema tip into anus, directing tip toward umbilicus.

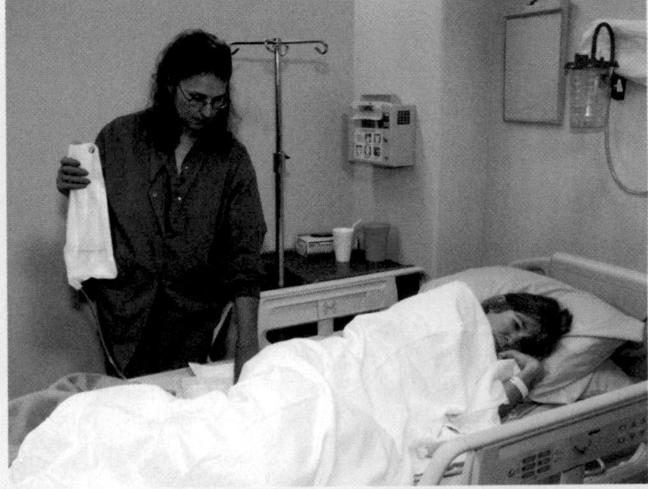

Figure 4. Holding bag lower to slow flow of enema solution.

ACTION	RATIONALE
14. After solution has been given, clamp tubing (Figure 5) and remove tube. Have paper towel ready to receive tube as it is withdrawn.	This amount of time usually allows muscle contractions to become sufficient to produce good results.

SKILL 13-2 Administering a Large-Volume Cleansing Enema *(continued)*

ACTION	RATIONALE
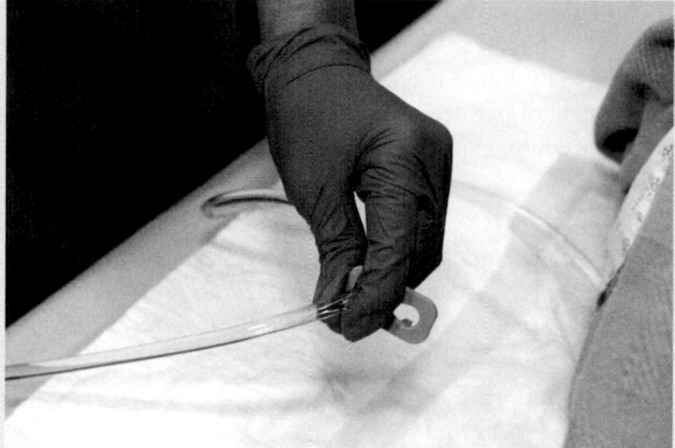 **Figure 5.** Clamping tubing before removing.	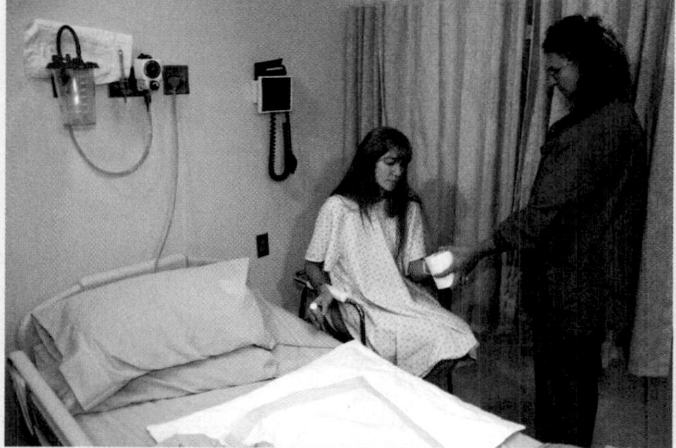 **Figure 6.** Offering toilet tissue to patient on bedside commode.
15. Return the patient to a comfortable position. Encourage the patient to hold the solution until the urge to defecate is strong, usually in about 5 to 15 minutes. Make sure the linens under the patient are dry. Remove your gloves and ensure that the patient is covered.	Promotes patient comfort. Removing contaminated gloves prevents spread of microorganisms.
16. Raise side rail. Lower bed height and adjust head of bed to a comfortable position.	Promotes patient safety.
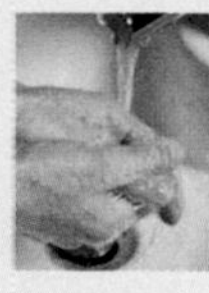 17. Remove any remaining equipment. Perform hand hygiene.	Hand hygiene deters the spread of microorganisms.
18. When patient has a strong urge to defecate, place him or her in a sitting position on a bedpan or assist to commode or bathroom (Figure 6). Stay with patient or have call light readily accessible.	The sitting position is most natural and facilitates defecation. Fall prevention is a high priority due to the urgency of reaching the commode.
19. Remind patient not to flush commode before nurse inspects results of enema.	The nurse needs to observe and record the results. Additional enemas may be necessary if physician has ordered enemas "until clear."
20. Put on gloves and assist patient if necessary with cleaning of anal area. Offer washcloths, soap, and water for handwashing. Remove gloves.	Cleaning the anal area and proper hygiene deter the spread of microorganisms.
21. Leave the patient clean and comfortable. Care for equipment properly.	Bacteria that grow in the intestine can be spread to others if equipment is not properly cleaned.
22. Perform hand hygiene.	Hand hygiene deters the spread of microorganisms.

(continued)

SKILL 13-2 Administering a Large-Volume Cleansing Enema *(continued)*

EVALUATION

The expected outcome is met when the patient expels feces; the patient verbalizes decreased discomfort; abdominal distention is absent; and the patient remains free of any evidence of trauma to the rectal mucosa or other adverse effect.

DOCUMENTATION

Guidelines

Document the amount and type of enema solution used; amount, consistency, and color of stool; pain assessment rating; assessment of perineal area for any irritation, tears, or bleeding; and patient's reaction to procedure.

Sample Documentation

7/22/09 1310 800 mL warm tap water enema given via rectum. Large amount of soft, brown stool returned. No irritation, tears, or bleeding noted in perineal area. Patient complained of "stomach cramping" relieved when enema was released. Rates pain as 0 after evacuation of enema.—K. Sanders, RN

Unexpected Situations and Associated Interventions

- *Solution does not flow into rectum:* Reposition rectal tube. If solution will still not flow, remove tube and check for any fecal contents.
- *Patient cannot retain enema solution for adequate amount of time:* Patient may need to be placed on bedpan in the supine position while receiving enema. The head of the bed may be elevated 30 degrees for the patient's comfort.
- *Patient cannot tolerate large amount of enema solution:* Amount and length of administration may have to be modified if patient begins to complain of pain.
- *Patient complains of severe cramping with introduction of enema solution:* Lower solution container and check temperature and flow rate. If the solution is too cold or flow rate too fast, severe cramping may occur.

Special Considerations

General Considerations

- If the patient experiences fullness or pain or if fluid escapes around the tube, stop administration. Wait 30 seconds to a minute and then restart the flow at a slower rate. If symptoms persist, stop administration and contact the patient's physician.
- If enema has been ordered to be given "until clear," check with the physician before administering more than three enemas. Severe fluid and electrolyte imbalances may occur if the patient receives more than three cleansing enemas. Results are considered clear whenever there are no more pieces of stool in enema return. The solution may be colored but still considered a clear return.

Infant and Child Considerations

- When administering an enema to a child, ensure that the volume of solution is appropriate and the solution is at a temperature of 100°F (37.7°C).
- Insert tubing into the rectum 2″ to 3″ for children, 1″ to 1½″ for infants.

Older Adult Considerations

- Older adult patients who cannot retain the enema solution should receive the enema while on the bedpan in the supine position. For comfort, the head of the bed can be elevated 30 degrees if necessary and pillows used appropriately.

SKILL 13-3 Administering a Small-Volume Cleansing Enema

Cleansing enemas are given to remove feces from the colon. Some of the reasons for administering a cleansing enema include relieving constipation or fecal impaction, preventing involuntary escape of fecal material during surgical procedures, promoting visualization of the intestinal tract by radiographic or instrument examination, and helping to establish regular bowel function during a bowel training program. These enemas are classified as large-volume and small-volume cleansing enemas. Small-volume enemas are also known as hypertonic enemas. Hypertonic solution preparations are available commercially and are administered in smaller volumes (adult, 70–130 mL). These solutions draw water into the colon, which stimulates the defecation reflex. They may be contraindicated in patients for whom sodium retention is a problem. They are also contraindicated for patients with renal impairment or reduced renal clearance, as these patients have compromised ability to excrete phosphate adequately, with resulting hyperphosphatemia (Davies, 2004). This skill addresses administering a small-volume enema.

Equipment

- Commercially prepared enema with rectal tip
- Water-soluble lubricant
- Waterproof pad
- Bath blanket
- Bedpan and toilet tissue
- Disposable gloves
- Paper towel
- Washcloth, soap, and towel

ASSESSMENT

Assess the patient's abdomen, including auscultating for bowel sounds, percussing, and palpating. Since the goal of a cleansing enema is to increase peristalsis, which should increase bowel sounds, the nurse will assess the abdomen before and after the enema. Inspect the rectal area for any fissures, hemorrhoids, sores, or rectal tears. If any of these are noted, added care should be taken while administering the enema. Check the results of the patient's laboratory work, specifically the platelet count and white blood cell (WBC) count. A normal platelet count ranges from 150,000 to 400,000/mm^3. A platelet count of less than 20,000 may seriously compromise the patient's ability to clot blood. Therefore, any unnecessary procedures that would place patient at risk for bleeding or infection should not be performed. A low WBC count places the patient at risk for infection. Enemas should not be administered to patients who have severe abdominal pain, bowel obstruction, bowel inflammation or bowel infection, or after rectal, prostate, and colon surgery.

NURSING DIAGNOSIS

Determine the related factors for the nursing diagnoses based on the patient's current status. Appropriate nursing diagnoses may include:

- Acute Pain
- Constipation
- Risk for Constipation
- Risk for Injury

OUTCOME IDENTIFICATION AND PLANNING

The expected outcome to be met when administering a cleansing enema is that the patient expels feces and reports a decrease in pain and discomfort. In addition, the patient remains free of any evidence of trauma to the rectal mucosa.

(continued)

SKILL 13-3 Administering a Small-Volume Cleansing Enema *(continued)*

IMPLEMENTATION

ACTION	RATIONALE
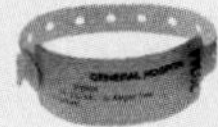 1. Verify the order for the enema. Identify the patient. Explain procedure to patient. Discuss where the patient will defecate. Have a bedpan, commode, or nearby bathroom ready for use.	Identifying the patient ensures the right patient receives the intervention and helps prevent errors. Verifying the physician's order is crucial to ensuring that the proper enema is administered to the right patient. Organization facilitates performance of tasks. Explanation helps to minimize anxiety. The patient is better able to relax and cooperate if he or she is familiar with the procedure and knows everything is in readiness when the urge to defecate is felt. Defecation usually occurs within 5 to 15 minutes.
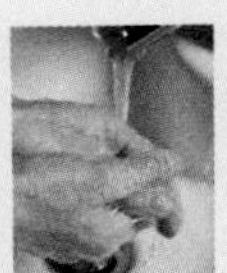 2. Perform hand hygiene.	Hand hygiene deters the spread of microorganisms.
3. Pull the curtains around the bed and close the room door. If bed is adjustable, place it in high position.	Provides for privacy. Having the bed in the high position reduces strain on the nurse's back.
4. Position the patient on the left side (Sims' position), as dictated by patient comfort and condition. Fold top linen back just enough to allow access to the patient's rectal area. Place a waterproof pad under the patient's hip.	The exact position of the patient has not been found to alter the results of an enema significantly. Folding back the linen in this manner minimizes unnecessary exposure and promotes the patient's comfort and warmth. The waterproof pad will protect the bed.
5. Put on nonsterile gloves.	Gloves protect nurse from microorganisms in feces.
6. Remove the cap and generously lubricate end of rectal tube 2″ to 3″ (5–7 cm) (Figure 1).	Lubrication facilitates passage of the rectal tube through the anal sphincter and prevents injury to the mucosa.

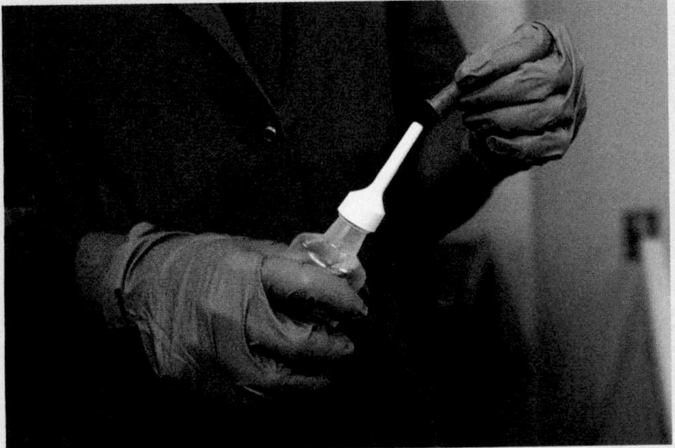

Figure 1. Removing cap from prepackaged enema solution container.

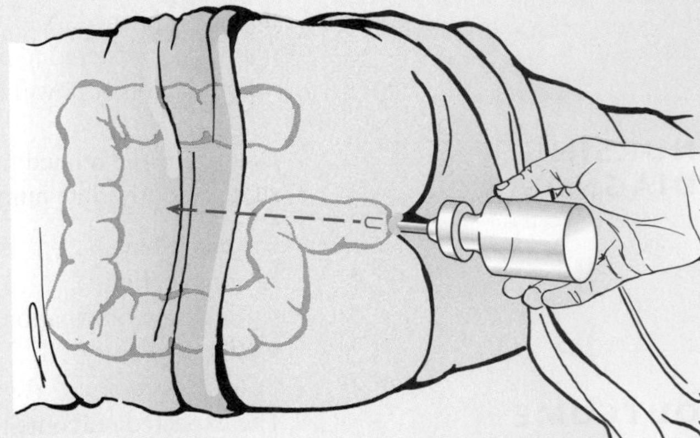

Figure 2. Inserting tube into rectum, directing toward umbilicus.

ACTION	RATIONALE
7. Lift buttock to expose anus. Slowly and gently insert the rectal tube 3″ to 4″ (7–10 cm) for an adult. Direct it at an angle pointing toward the umbilicus, not bladder (Figure 2). Ask patient to take several deep breaths.	Good visualization helps prevent injury to tissues. The anal canal is about 1″ to 2″ (2.5–5 cm) long. Insert the tube past the external and internal sphincters; further insertion may damage intestinal mucous membrane. The suggested angle follows the normal intestinal contour, helping prevent perforation of the bowel.

SKILL 13-3 **Administering a Small-Volume Cleansing Enema** *(continued)*

ACTION	RATIONALE
8. Do not force entry of the tube. Ask patient to take several deep breaths.	Forcing a tube may injure the intestinal mucosa wall. Taking deep breaths helps relax the anal sphincter.
9. Compress the container with your hands (Figure 3). Roll the end up on itself, toward the rectal tip. Administer all the solution in the container.	Rolling the container aids administration of all of the contents of the container.

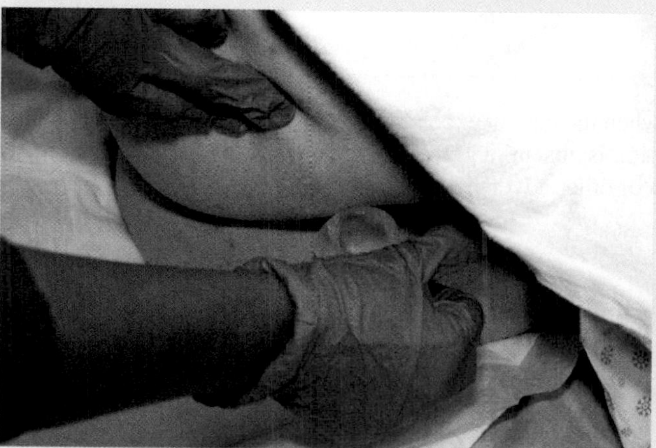

Figure 3. Compressing the container.

ACTION	RATIONALE
10. After solution has been given, remove tube, keeping the container compressed. Have paper towel ready to receive tube as it is withdrawn. Encourage the patient to hold the solution until the urge to defecate is strong, usually in about 5 to 15 minutes.	This amount of time usually allows muscle contractions to become sufficient to produce good results.
11. Remove gloves. Return the patient to a comfortable position. Make sure the linens under the patient are dry. Ensure that the patient is covered.	Promotes patient comfort. Removing contaminated gloves prevents spread of microorganisms.
12. Raise side rail. Lower bed height and adjust head of bed to a comfortable position.	Promotes patient safety.
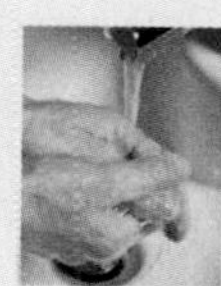 13. Remove any remaining equipment. Perform hand hygiene.	Hand hygiene deters the spread of microorganisms.
14. When patient has a strong urge to defecate, place him or her in a sitting position on a bedpan or assist to commode or bathroom. Stay with patient or have call light readily accessible.	The sitting position is most natural and facilitates defecation. Fall prevention is a high priority due to the urgency of reaching the commode.
15. Remind patient not to flush commode before nurse inspects results of enema.	The nurse needs to observe and record the results. Additional enemas may be necessary if physician has ordered enemas "until clear."
16. Put on gloves and assist patient if necessary with cleaning of anal area. Offer washcloths, soap, and water for handwashing. Remove gloves.	Cleaning the anal area and proper hygiene deter the spread of microorganisms.

(continued)

SKILL 13-3 Administering a Small-Volume Cleansing Enema *(continued)*

ACTION	RATIONALE
17. Leave the patient clean and comfortable. Care for equipment properly.	Bacteria that grow in the intestine can be spread to others if equipment is not properly cleaned.
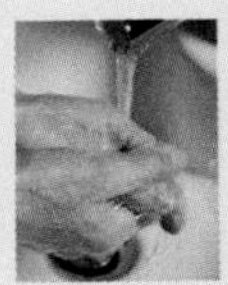 18. Perform hand hygiene.	Hand hygiene deters the spread of microorganisms.

EVALUATION

The expected outcome is met when the patient expels feces; the patient verbalizes decreased discomfort; abdominal distention is absent; and the patient remains free of any evidence of trauma to the rectal mucosa or other adverse effect.

DOCUMENTATION

Guidelines

Document the amount and type of enema solution used; amount, consistency, and color of stool; pain assessment rating; assessment of perineal area for any irritation, tears, or bleeding; and patient's reaction to procedure.

Sample Documentation

7/22/08 1310 210-mL Fleet enema given via rectum. Large amount of soft, brown stool returned. No irritation, tears, or bleeding noted in perineal area. Patient states "stomach fullness" relieved when enema was released. Rates pain as 0 after evacuation of enema.—K. Sanders, RN

Unexpected Situations and Associated Interventions

- *Patient cannot retain enema solution for adequate amount of time:* Patient may need to be placed on bedpan in the supine position while receiving enema. The head of the bed may be elevated 30 degrees for the patient's comfort.

Special Considerations

Infant and Child Considerations

- Insert tubing into the rectum 2″ to 3″ for children, 1″ to 1½″ for infants
- Enemas containing phosphates should be used with caution in children under 12 years of age (Davies, 2004).

Older Adult Considerations

- Enemas containing phosphates should be used with caution in frail older patients (Davies, 2004).

SKILL 13-4

Administering a Retention Enema

Retention enemas are ordered for various reasons. *Oil-retention* enemas help to lubricate the stool and intestinal mucosa, making defecation easier. *Carminative* enemas help to expel flatus from the rectum and relieve distention secondary to flatus. *Medicated* enemas are used to administer a medication rectally. *Anthelmintic* enemas are administered to destroy intestinal parasites. *Nutritive* enemas are administered to replenish fluids and nutrition rectally.

Equipment

- Enema solution (varies depending on reason for enema), often prepackaged, commercially prepared solutions
- Nonsterile gloves
- Waterproof pad
- Bath blanket
- Washcloth, soap, and towel
- Bedpan or commode
- Toilet tissue
- Water-soluble lubricant (if needed)

ASSESSMENT

Ask the patient when he had his last bowel movement. Assess the patient's abdomen, including auscultating for bowel sounds, percussing, and palpating. Since the goal of a cleansing enema is to increase peristalsis, which should increase bowel sounds, assess the abdomen before and after the enema. Assess the rectal area for any fissures, hemorrhoids, sores, or rectal tears. If present, added care should be taken while inserting the tube. Assess the results of the patient's laboratory work, specifically the platelet count and white blood cell (WBC) count. An enema is contraindicated for patients with a low platelet count or low WBC count. An enema may irritate or traumatize the gastrointestinal mucosa, causing bleeding, bowel perforation, or infection. Any unnecessary procedures that would place the patient at risk for bleeding or infection should not be performed. Assess for dizziness, lightheadedness, diaphoresis, and clammy skin. The enema may stimulate a vagal response, which increases parasympathetic stimulation, causing a decrease in heart rate. Enemas should not be administered to patients who have severe abdominal pain, bowel obstruction, bowel inflammation or bowel infection, or after rectal, prostate, and colon surgery.

NURSING DIAGNOSIS

Determine the related factors for the nursing diagnoses based on the patient's current status. Appropriate nursing diagnoses may include:

- Constipation
- Risk for Injury
- Acute Pain
- Risk for Infection
- Imbalanced Nutrition, Less than Body Requirements

OUTCOME IDENTIFICATION AND PLANNING

The expected outcome to be met when administering a retention enema is that the patient retains the solution for the prescribed, appropriate length of time and experiences the expected therapeutic effect of the solution. Other appropriate outcomes may include the following: the patient verbalizes decreased discomfort; abdominal distention is absent; patient demonstrates signs and symptoms indicative of a resolving infection; patient exhibits signs and symptoms of adequate nutrition; and the patient remains free of any evidence of trauma to the rectal mucosa or other adverse effect.

(continued)

SKILL 13-4 Administering a Retention Enema *(continued)*

IMPLEMENTATION

ACTION	RATIONALE
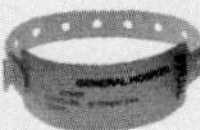 1. Verify physician's orders. Identify the patient. Explain to patient procedure and rationale for enema, including where he or she will defecate, and have a bedpan, commode, or nearby bathroom ready for use. Gather equipment. Allow solution to warm to room temperature.	Verifying the physician's order is crucial to ensuring that the proper enema is administered to the right patient. Identifying the patient ensures the right patient receives the intervention and helps prevent errors. Explanation decreases patient anxiety and facilitates cooperation. The patient will be better able to relax and cooperate if he or she is familiar with the procedure and knows everything is in readiness when the urge to defecate is felt. Organization facilitates performance of tasks. A cold solution can cause intestinal cramping.
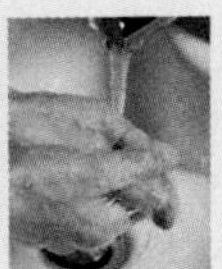 2. Perform hand hygiene.	Hand hygiene deters the spread of microorganisms.
3. Pull the curtains around the bed and close the room door. If bed is adjustable, place it in high position.	Provides for privacy. Having the bed in the high position reduces strain on the nurse's back.
4. Position the patient on the left side (Sims' position), as dictated by patient comfort and condition. Fold top linen back just enough to allow access to the patient's rectal area. Place a waterproof pad under the patient's hip.	The exact position of the patient has not been found to alter the results of an enema significantly. Folding back the linen in this manner minimizes unnecessary exposure and promotes the patient's comfort and warmth. The waterproof pad will protect the bed.
5. Put on nonsterile gloves.	Gloves prevent contact with blood and body fluids.
6. Remove cap of prepackaged enema solution and ensure that rectal tube is prelubricated. If not, apply a generous amount of lubricant to the tube.	Lubrication is necessary to minimize trauma on insertion.
7. Lift buttock to expose anus. Slowly and gently insert rectal tube 3″ to 4″ (7–10 cm) for an adult. Direct it at an angle pointing toward the umbilicus (Figure 1). Ask patient to take several deep breaths.	Good visualization of the anus helps prevent injury to tissues. The anal canal is about 1″ to 2″ (2.5–5 cm) long. The tube should be inserted past the external and internal sphincters, but further insertion may damage intestinal mucous membrane. The suggested angle follows the normal intestinal contour and thus will help to prevent perforation of the bowel. Slow insertion of the tube minimizes spasms of the intestinal wall and sphincters. Deep breathing helps relax the anal sphincters.

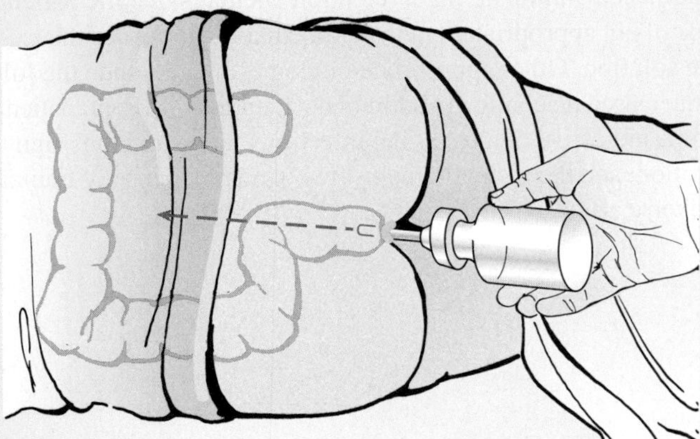

Figure 1. Inserting tube into rectum, directing toward umbilicus.

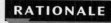

SKILL 13-4 Administering a Retention Enema *(continued)*

ACTION	RATIONALE
8. If resistance is met while inserting tube, permit a small amount of solution to enter, withdraw tube slightly, and then continue to insert it. **Do not force entry of tube.**	Resistance may be due to spasms of the intestine or failure of the internal sphincter to open. The solution may help to reduce spasms and relax the sphincter, thus making continued insertion of the tube safe. Forcing a tube may injure the intestinal mucosa wall.
9. Slowly squeeze enema container, emptying entire contents.	Compressing the container slowly allows the solution to enter the rectum and prevent rapid distention of the intestine and a desire to defecate.
10. **Remove container while keeping it compressed.** Have paper towel ready to receive tube as it is withdrawn.	If container is released, a vacuum will form, allowing some of the enema solution to re-enter the container.
11. **Instruct patient to retain enema solution for at least 30 minutes or as indicated.**	Solution needs to dwell for at least 30 minutes to provide quality results.
12. Return the patient to a comfortable position. Make sure the linens under the patient are dry. Remove your gloves and ensure that the patient is covered.	Promotes patient comfort. Removing contaminated gloves prevents spread of microorganisms.
13. Raise side rail. Lower bed height and adjust head of bed to a comfortable position.	Promotes patient safety.
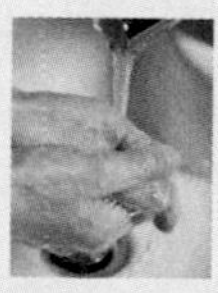 14. Remove any remaining equipment. Perform hand hygiene.	Hand hygiene deters the spread of microorganisms.
15. When patient has a strong urge to defecate, place him or her in a sitting position on bedpan or assist to commode or bathroom. Stay with patient or have call light readily accessible.	The sitting position is most natural and facilitates defecation. Fall prevention is a high priority due to the urgency of reaching the commode.
16. Remind patient not to flush commode before nurse inspects results of enema. Record character of stool and patient's reaction to enema.	The nurse needs to observe and record the results.
17. Assist patient if necessary with cleaning of anal area (putting on gloves if necessary). Offer washcloths, soap, and water for handwashing.	Proper cleansing deters spread of microorganisms and promotes hygiene.
18. Leave patient clean and comfortable. Care for equipment properly.	Bacteria that grow in the intestine can be spread to others if equipment is not properly cleaned.
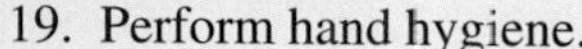 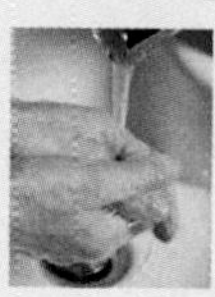 19. Perform hand hygiene.	Hand hygiene deters the spread of microorganisms.

EVALUATION

The expected outcome is met when the patient expels feces without evidence of trauma to the rectal mucosa. Depending on the reason for the retention enema, other outcomes met may include: patient verbalizes a decrease in pain after enema; patient demonstrates signs and symptoms indicative of a resolving infection; and patient exhibits signs and symptoms of adequate nutrition.

(continued)

SKILL 13-4 Administering a Retention Enema *(continued)*

DOCUMENTATION

Guidelines

Document the amount and type of enema solution used; length of time retained by the patient; amount, consistency, and color of stool; pain assessment rating; assessment of perineal area for any irritation, tears, or bleeding; and patient's reaction to procedure.

Sample Documentation

6/26/09 2030 100 mL of mineral oil administered as enema via rectum. Small amount of firm, black stool returned. Small (approx. 1 cm) tear noted at 2 o'clock position on anus. No erythema or bleeding noted. Physician notified of tear and stool color. Reports pain at 2 on a 0 to 10 rating scale after enema evacuated.—K. Sanders, RN

Unexpected Situations and Associated Interventions

- *Solution does not flow into rectum:* Reposition rectal tube; if solution still will not flow, remove and check for any fecal contents.
- *Patient cannot retain enema solution for adequate amount of time:* Patient may need to be placed on bedpan in supine position while receiving enema. The head of the bed may be elevated 30 degrees for the patient's comfort. If still unable to retain, notify physician.

Special Considerations

Infant and Child Considerations

- Insert tubing into the rectum 2″ to 3″ for children, 1″ to 1½″ for infants.

SKILL 13-5 Digital Removal of Stool

When a patient develops a fecal impaction (prolonged retention or an accumulation of fecal material that forms a hardened mass in the rectum), the stool must sometimes be broken up manually. Digital removal of feces is considered as a last resort after other methods of bowel evacuation have been unsuccessful (Kyle, Prynn, & Oliver, 2004). Patient discomfort and irritation of the rectal mucosa may occur.

Equipment

- Disposable gloves
- Water-soluble lubricant
- Waterproof pad
- Bedpan
- Toilet paper, washcloth, and towel
- Sitz bath (optional)

ASSESSMENT

Verify the time of the patient's last bowel movement by asking the patient and checking the patient's medical record. Assess the abdomen, including auscultating for bowel sounds, percussing, and palpating. Inspect the rectal area for any fissures, hemorrhoids, sores, or rectal tears. If any of these are noted, consult the prescriber for the appropriateness of the intervention. Assess the results of the patient's laboratory work, specifically the platelet count and white blood cell (WBC) count. Digital removal of stool is contraindicated for patients with a low platelet count or low WBC count. An enema may irritate or traumatize the gastrointestinal mucosa, causing bleeding, bowel perforation, or infection. Any unnecessary procedures that would place the patient at risk for bleeding or infection should not be performed. Assess for dizziness, lightheadedness, diaphoresis, and clammy skin. Assess pulse rate and blood

SKILL 13-5 Digital Removal of Stool *(continued)*

pressure before and after the procedure. The procedure may stimulate a vagal response, which increases parasympathetic stimulation, causing a decrease in heart rate and blood pressure. Digital removal of stool should not be performed on patients who have bowel inflammation or bowel infection, or after rectal, prostate, and colon surgery.

NURSING DIAGNOSIS

Determine the related factors for the nursing diagnoses based on the patient's current status. Appropriate nursing diagnosis may include:

- Constipation
- Acute Pain
- Risk for Injury

OUTCOME IDENTIFICATION AND PLANNING

The expected outcome to achieve when digitally removing stool is that the patient will expel feces with assistance. Other appropriate outcomes may include: the patient verbalizes decreased discomfort; abdominal distention is absent; and the patient remains free of any evidence of trauma to the rectal mucosa or other adverse effect.

IMPLEMENTATION

ACTION	RATIONALE
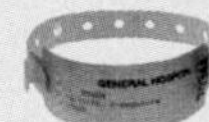 1. Verify physician's order. Identify the patient. Explain procedure to patient, discussing signs and symptoms of a slow heart rate. Instruct patient to alert you if any of these symptoms are felt during the procedure.	Digital removal of stool is considered an invasive procedure and requires a physician's order. Identifying the patient ensures the right patient receives the intervention and helps prevent errors. Explanation helps to minimize anxiety and foster cooperation. Rectal stimulation may cause a vagal response.
2. Gather necessary equipment.	Organization facilitates performance of task.
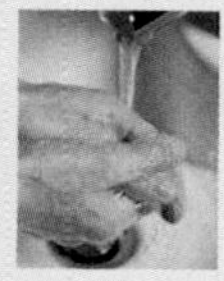 3. Perform hand hygiene.	Hand hygiene deters the spread of microorganisms.
4. Pull the curtains around the bed and close the room door. If bed is adjustable, place it in high position.	Provides for privacy. Having the bed in the high position reduces strain on the nurse's back.
5. Position the patient in a side-lying position, as dictated by patient comfort and condition. Fold top linen back just enough to allow access to the patient's rectal area. Place a waterproof pad under the patient's hip.	Folding back the linen in this manner minimizes unnecessary exposure and promotes the patient's comfort and warmth. The waterproof pad will protect the bed.
6. Put on nonsterile gloves.	This protects nurse from microorganisms in feces. The GI tract is not a sterile environment.
7. Generously lubricate index finger with water-soluble lubricant and insert finger (Figure 1) gently into anal canal, pointing toward the umbilicus.	Lubrication reduces irritation of the rectum. The presence of the finger added to the mass tends to cause discomfort for the patient if the work is not done slowly and gently.
8. Gently work the finger around and into the hardened mass to break it up (Figure 2) and then remove pieces of it. Instruct patient to bear down, if possible, while extracting feces to ease in removal. Place extracted stool in bedpan.	Fecal mass may be large and may need to be removed in smaller pieces.

(continued)

SKILL 13-5 Digital Removal of Stool *(continued)*

ACTION | **RATIONALE**

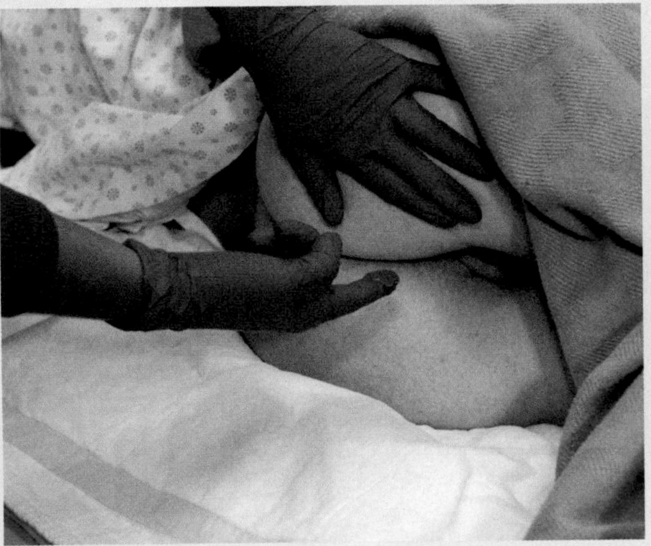

Figure 1. Inserting lubricated forefinger of dominant hand into anal canal.

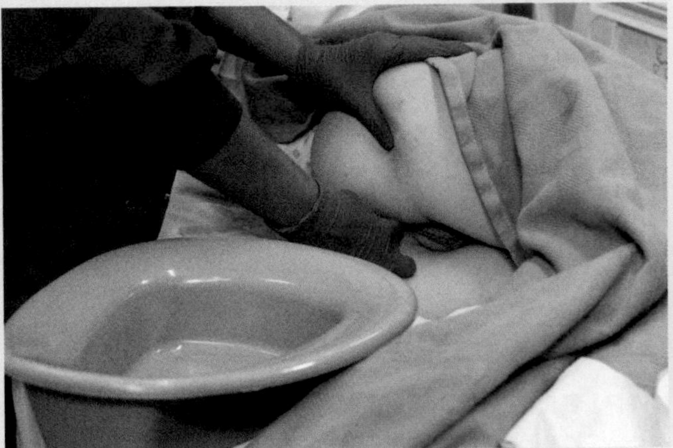

Figure 2. Gently working finger around to break up stool mass.

9. Remove impaction at intervals if it is severe. Instruct patient to alert you if he or she begins to feel lightheaded or nauseated. If patient reports either symptom, stop removal and assess patient.

This helps to prevent discomfort, irritation, and vagal nerve stimulation.

10. Put on clean gloves. Assist patient if necessary with cleaning of anal area (Figure 3). Offer washcloths, soap, and water for handwashing. If patient is able, offer sitz bath.

Cleaning deters the transmission of microorganisms and promotes hygiene. Sitz bath may relieve the irritated perianal area.

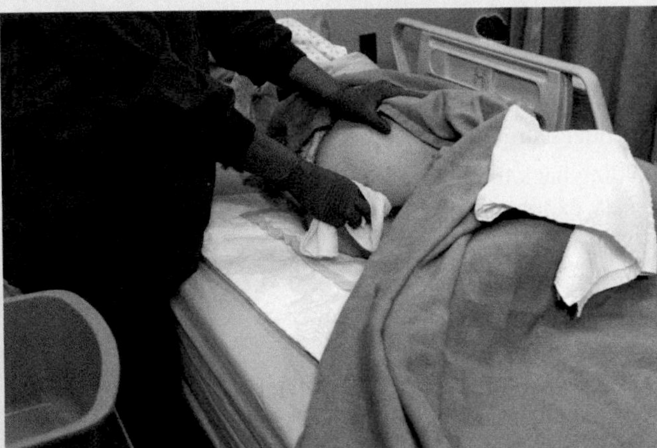

Figure 3. Helping to clean anal area with washcloth and soap.

11. Remove gloves. Return the patient to a comfortable position. Make sure the linens under the patient are dry. Ensure that the patient is covered.

Removing contaminated gloves prevents spread of microorganisms. The other actions promote patient comfort.

SKILL 13-5 Digital Removal of Stool *(continued)*

ACTION	RATIONALE
12. Raise side rail. Lower bed height and adjust head of bed to a comfortable position.	These promote patient safety.
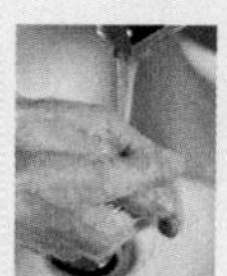 13. Perform hand hygiene.	Hand hygiene deters the spread of microorganisms.

EVALUATION

The expected outcome is met when the fecal impaction is removed and the patient expels feces with assistance; the patient verbalizes decreased discomfort; abdominal distention is absent; and the patient remains free of any evidence of trauma to the rectal mucosa or other adverse effect.

DOCUMENTATION

Guidelines

Document the following: color, consistency, and amount of stool removed; condition of perianal area after procedure; pain assessment rating; and patient's reaction to procedure.

Sample Documentation

6/29/09 1030 Large amount of hard, brown stool removed with digital exam. Perineal area remains free from tears, erythema, or bleeding. Patient denied any light-headedness or nausea during procedure. Rates pain at 1 on a scale of 0 to 10. —K. Sanders, RN

Unexpected Situations and Associated Interventions

- *Patient complains of being dizzy, lightheaded, or nauseated or begins to vomit:* Stop digital stimulation immediately. Vagal nerve might have been stimulated. Assess heart rate and blood pressure. Notify physician.
- *Patient experiences a large amount of pain during procedure:* Stop procedure and notify physician.

SKILL 13-6 Applying a Fecal Incontinence Pouch

A fecal incontinence pouch is used to protect the perianal skin from excoriation due to repeated exposure to liquid stool. Although best used before excoriation occurs, a skin barrier can be applied if excoriation already is present.

Equipment

- Fecal incontinence pouch
- Disposable gloves
- Washcloth and towel
- Urinary drainage (Foley) bag
- Scissors (optional)
- Skin protectant or barrier
- Bath blanket

(continued)

SKILL 13-6 Applying a Fecal Incontinence Pouch *(continued)*

ASSESSMENT

Assess the amount and consistency of stool being passed. Also assess the frequency. Inspect the perianal area for any excoriation, wounds, or hemorrhoids.

NURSING DIAGNOSIS

Determine the related factors for the nursing diagnoses based on the patient's current status. Appropriate nursing diagnosis may include:

- Bowel Incontinence
- Risk for Impaired Skin Integrity
- Impaired Skin Integrity
- Risk for Infection

OUTCOME IDENTIFICATION AND PLANNING

The expected outcome to achieve when applying a fecal incontinence pouch is that the patient expels feces into the pouch and maintains intact perianal skin. Other outcomes may include the following: patient demonstrates a decrease in the amount and severity of excoriation; patient verbalizes decreased discomfort; and patient remains free of any signs and symptoms of infection.

IMPLEMENTATION

ACTION	RATIONALE
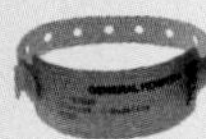 1. Gather necessary equipment. Identify the patient. Discuss reason for fecal incontinence bag with patient.	Organization facilitates performance of task. Identifying the patient ensures the right patient receives the intervention and helps prevent errors. Discussion promotes cooperation and helps to minimize anxiety.
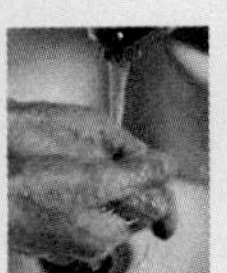 2. Perform hand hygiene.	Hand hygiene deters the spread of microorganisms.
3. Pull the curtains around the bed and close the room door. If bed is adjustable, place it in high position.	Provides for privacy. Having the bed in the high position reduces strain on the nurse's back.
4. Position the patient in a side-lying position, as dictated by patient comfort and condition. Fold top linen back just enough to allow access to the patient's rectal area. Place a waterproof pad under the patient's hip.	Folding back the linen in this manner minimizes unnecessary exposure and promotes the patient's comfort and warmth. The waterproof pad will protect the bed.
5. Put on nonsterile gloves. Cleanse perianal area. Pat dry thoroughly.	Gloves protect nurse from microorganisms in feces. The GI tract is not a sterile environment. Skin must be dry for pouch to adhere securely.
6. Trim perianal hair if needed.	It may be uncomfortable if the perianal hair is pulled by adhesive from the fecal pouch. Trimming with scissors minimizes the risk for infection compared with shaving.
7. Apply the skin protectant or barrier and allow to dry.	Skin protectant aids in adhesion of pouch and protects skin from irritation and injury from the adhesive. Skin must be dry for pouch to adhere securely.
8. Remove paper backing from adhesive of pouch (Figure 1).	Removing the paper backing is necessary so that the pouch can adhere to the skin.
9. With nondominant hand, separate buttocks. Apply fecal pouch to anal area with dominant hand, ensuring that opening of bag is over anus (Figure 2).	Opening should be over anus so that stool empties into bag and does not stay on patient's skin, which could lead to skin breakdown.

SKILL 13-6

Applying a Fecal Incontinence Pouch *(continued)*

ACTION	RATIONALE
10. Release buttocks. Attach connector of fecal incontinence pouch to urinary drainage bag (Figure 3). Hang drainage bag below patient (Figure 4).	Bag must be dependent for stool to drain into bag.

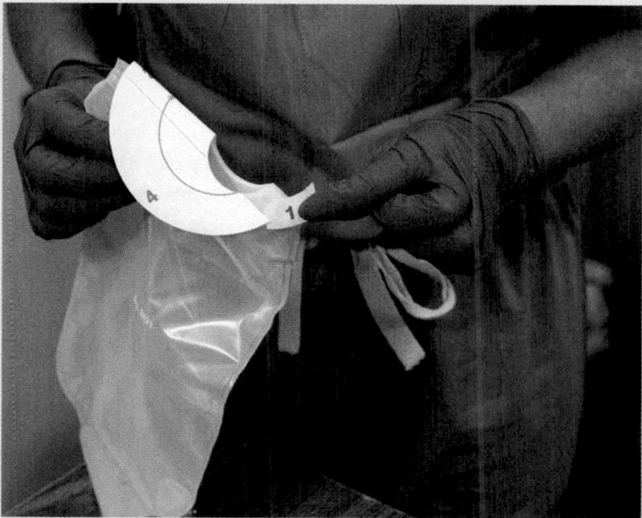

Figure 1. Removing paper backing from adhesive of rectal pouch.

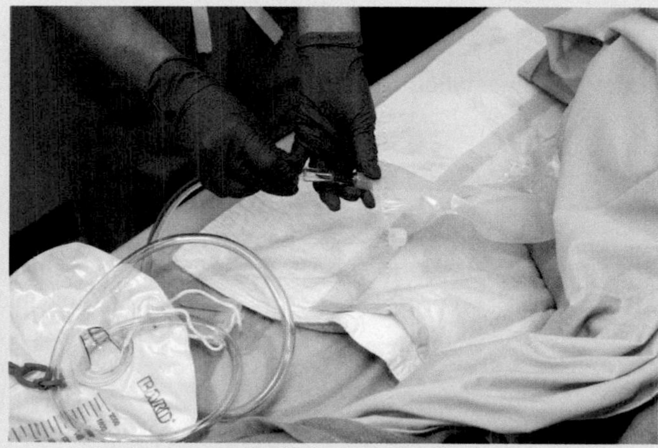

Figure 3. Attaching connector of fecal pouch to tubing of drainage bag.

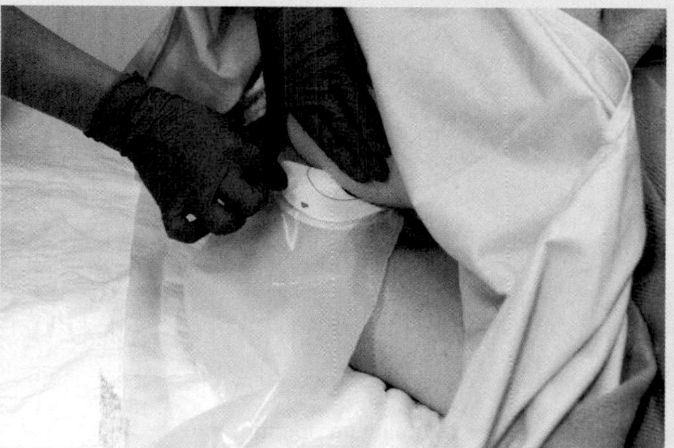

Figure 2. Applying pouch over anal opening.

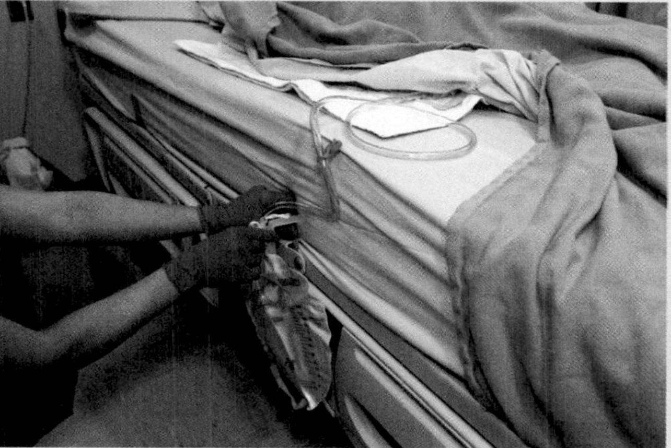

Figure 4. Checking that drainage bag is below the level of the patient.

ACTION	RATIONALE
11. Remove gloves. Return the patient to a comfortable position. Make sure the linens under the patient are dry. Ensure that the patient is covered.	Promotes patient comfort. Removing contaminated gloves prevents spread of microorganisms.
12. Raise side rail. Lower bed height and adjust head of bed to a comfortable position.	Promotes patient safety.
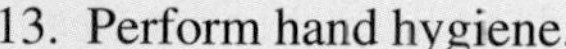 13. Perform hand hygiene.	Hand hygiene deters the spread of microorganisms.

(continued)

SKILL 13-6 Applying a Fecal Incontinence Pouch *(continued)*

EVALUATION

The expected outcome is met when the patient expels feces into the pouch and maintains intact perianal skin; patient demonstrates a decrease in the amount and severity of excoriation; patient verbalizes decreased discomfort; and patient remains free of any signs and symptoms of infection.

DOCUMENTATION

Guidelines

Document the date and time fecal pouch was applied; appearance of perianal area; color of stool; intake and output (amount of stool out); patient's reaction to procedure.

Sample Documentation

8/13/09 1210 Perianal area slightly erythematous. Fecal incontinence bag applied due to incontinence of large amounts of liquid stool and possible skin breakdown. Approximately 90 cc of liquid brown stool noted in drainage bag.—K. Sanders, RN

Unexpected Situations and Associated Interventions

- *Perianal area becomes excoriated:* Remove pouch. Thoroughly cleanse skin and apply skin barrier. Allow to dry completely. Reapply pouch. Monitor pouch adhesion and change pouch as soon as there is a break in adhesion.
- *Stool does not drain from pouch into urinary drainage bag:* Stool may be too thick. If stool no longer drains from pouch into drainage bag, remove pouch to prevent perianal skin breakdown.
- *Stool is leaking from around sides of fecal pouch:* Remove pouch. Thoroughly cleanse skin and apply skin barrier. Allow to dry completely. Reapply pouch. Monitor pouch adhesion and change pouch as soon as there is a break in adhesion.

Special Considerations

General Considerations

- Remove fecal pouch at least every 72 hours to check for signs of skin breakdown.

SKILL 13-7 Changing and Emptying an Ostomy Appliance

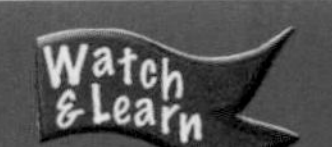

Sometimes patients undergo surgical procedures to create an opening into the abdominal wall for fecal elimination. The word *ostomy* is a term for a surgically formed opening from the inside of an organ to the outside. The intestinal mucosa is brought out to the abdominal wall, and a *stoma,* the part of the ostomy that is attached to the skin, is formed by suturing the mucosa to the skin. An *ileostomy* allows liquid fecal content from the ileum of the small intestine to be eliminated through the stoma. A *colostomy* permits formed feces in the colon to exit through the stoma. Colostomies are further classified by the part of the colon they originate from. Ostomy appliances or pouches are applied to the opening to collect stool. Ostomy appliances or pouches should be emptied promptly, usually when they are one-third to one-half full. If they are allowed to fill up, they may leak or become detached from the skin. Ostomy appliances are available in a one-piece or two-piece system and are usually changed every 3 to 7 days, although this could be done more often. Proper application minimizes the risk for skin breakdown around the stoma. Box 13-1 summarizes guidelines for care of the patient with a urinary diversion.

SKILL 13-7 Changing and Emptying an Ostomy Appliance *(continued)*

BOX 13-1 Guidelines for Ostomy Care

The ostomy requires specific physical care for which the nurse is initially responsible. The following guidelines help to promote the ostomy patient's physical and psychological comfort:

- Keep the patient as free of odors as possible. The application of a temporary appliance after surgery or during the time of the first dressing change postoperatively can eliminate much of the fecal odor from a bulky dressing. The ostomy appliance should be emptied frequently.
- Inspect the patient's stoma regularly. It should be dark pink to red and moist. A pale stoma may indicate anemia, and a dark or purple-blue stoma may reflect compromised circulation or ischemia. Bleeding around the stoma and its stem should be minimal. Notify the physician promptly if bleeding persists or is excessive, or if color changes occur in the stoma.
- Note the size of the stoma, which usually stabilizes within 6 to 8 weeks. Most stomas protrude ½″ to 1″ from the abdominal surface and may initially appear swollen and edematous. After 6 weeks, the edema has usually subsided. If an abdominal dressing is in place, check it frequently for drainage and bleeding.
- Keep the skin around the stoma site (peristomal area) clean and dry. If care is not taken to protect the skin around the stoma, irritation or infection may occur. A leaking appliance frequently causes skin erosion. Candida or yeast infections can also occur around the stoma if the area is not kept dry.
- Measure the patient's fluid intake and output. Check the ostomy appliance for the quality and quantity of discharge. Initially after surgery, peristalsis may be inhibited. As peristalsis returns, stool will be eliminated from the stoma. Record intake and output every 4 hours for the first 3 days after surgery. If the patient's output decreases while intake remains stable, report the condition promptly.
- Explain each aspect of care to the patient and explain what his or her role will be when he or she begins self-care. Patient teaching is one of the most important aspects of colostomy care and should include family members when appropriate. Teaching can begin before surgery so that the patient has adequate time to absorb information.
- Encourage the patient to participate in care and to look at the ostomy. Patients normally experience emotional depression during the early postoperative period. The nurse can help the patient to cope by listening, explaining, and being available and supportive. A visit from a representative of the local ostomy support group may be helpful. Patients usually begin to accept their altered body image when they are willing to look at the stoma, make neutral or positive statements concerning the ostomy, and express interest in learning self-care.

Equipment

- Basin with warm water
- Skin cleanser, towel, washcloth
- Gauze squares
- Washcloth or cotton balls
- Skin protectant or barrier
- Ostomy appliance
- Closure clamp, if required for appliance
- Stoma measuring guide
- Graduated container, toilet or bedpan
- Ostomy belt (optional)
- Disposable gloves
- Small plastic trash bag
- Waterproof disposable pad

ASSESSMENT

Assess current ileal conduit appliance, looking at product style, condition of appliance, and stoma (if bag is clear). Note length of time the appliance has been in place. Determine the patient's knowledge of care of the ileal conduit. After the appliance is removed, assess the skin surrounding the ileal conduit. Assess any abdominal scars, if surgery was recent. Assess the amount, color, consistency, and odor of stool from ostomy.

(continued)

SKILL 13-7 Changing and Emptying an Ostomy Appliance *(continued)*

NURSING DIAGNOSIS

Determine the related factors for the nursing diagnoses based on the patient's current status. Appropriate nursing diagnoses may include:

- Risk for Impaired Skin Integrity
- Deficient Knowledge
- Disturbed Body Image
- Ineffective Coping
- Constipation
- Diarrhea

OUTCOME IDENTIFICATION AND PLANNING

The expected outcome to be met when changing and emptying an ostomy appliance is that the stoma appliance is applied correctly to the skin to allow stool to drain freely. Other outcomes may include the following: the patient exhibits a moist red stoma with intact skin surrounding the stoma; the patient demonstrates knowledge of how to apply the appliance; patient demonstrates positive coping skills; patient expels stool that is appropriate in consistency and amount for the ostomy location, and the patient verbalizes positive self-image.

IMPLEMENTATION

ACTION	RATIONALE
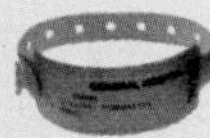 1. Gather necessary equipment. Identify the patient. Explain procedure and encourage patient to observe or participate if possible.	Organization facilitates performance of tasks. Identifying the patient ensures the right patient receives the intervention and helps prevent errors. This discussion promotes reassurance and provides knowledge about the procedure. Explanation encourages patient cooperation and reduces apprehension. Having the patient observe or assist encourages self-acceptance.
2. Close curtains around bed and close door to room if possible.	These provide for patient privacy.
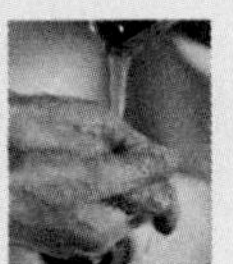 3. Perform hand hygiene.	Hand hygiene deters the spread of microorganisms.
4. Assist patient to a comfortable sitting or lying position in bed or a standing or sitting position in the bathroom.	Either position should allow the patient to view the procedure in preparation for learning to perform it independently. Lying flat or sitting upright facilitates smooth application of the appliance.
Emptying an appliance	
5. Put on disposable gloves. Remove clamp and fold end of pouch upward like a cuff (Figure 1).	Gloves prevent contact with blood, body fluids, and microorganisms. Creating a cuff before emptying prevents additional soilage and odor.
6. Empty contents into bedpan, toilet, or measuring device (Figure 2). Rinse appliance or pouch with tepid water in a squeeze bottle, per manufacturer's instructions.	Rinsing the inside provides a cleaner appearance and minimizes odor. Some appliances do not need rinsing because rinsing may reduce appliance's odor barrier.

SKILL 13-7

Changing and Emptying an Ostomy Appliance *(continued)*

ACTION	RATIONALE
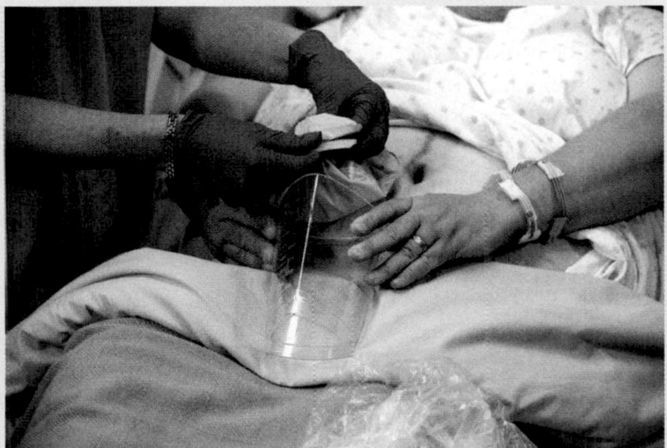 **Figure 1.** Removing clamp, getting ready to empty pouch.	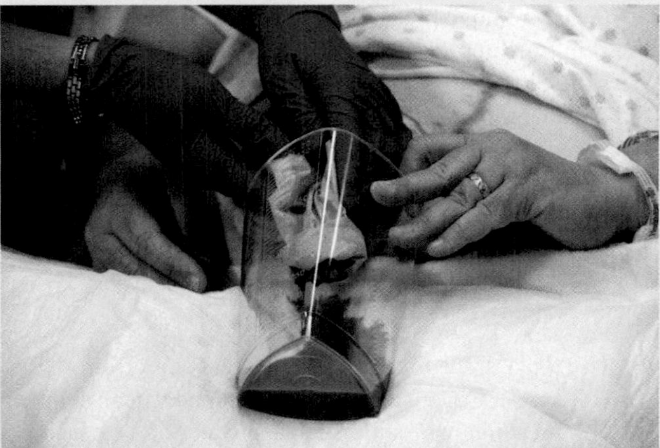 **Figure 2.** Emptying pouch into a measuring device.
7. Wipe the lower 2″ of the appliance or pouch with toilet tissue (Figure 3).	Drying the lower section removes any additional fecal material, thus decreasing odor problems.
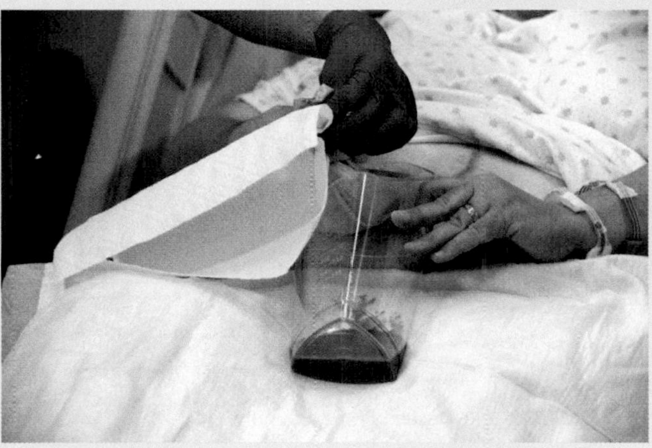 **Figure 3.** Wiping lower 2″ of pouch with toilet tissue.	
8. Uncuff edge of appliance or pouch and apply clip or clamp. Remove gloves. If appliance is not to be changed, perform hand hygiene. Assist patient to comfortable position.	The edge of the appliance or pouch should remain clean. The clamp secures closure. Hand hygiene deters spread of microorganisms. Ensures patient comfort.
Changing an Appliance	
9. Place a disposable pad on the work surface. Set up the wash basin with warm water and the rest of the supplies. Place a trash bag within reach.	Protects surface. Organization facilitates performance of procedure.
10. Put on clean gloves. Place waterproof pad under the patient at the stoma site. Empty the appliance as previously described.	Protects linens and patient from moisture. Emptying the contents before removal prevents accidental spillage of fecal material.

(continued)

SKILL 13-7 Changing and Emptying an Ostomy Appliance *(continued)*

ACTION	RATIONALE
11. Gently remove pouch faceplate from skin by pushing skin from appliance rather than pulling appliance from skin. Start at the top of the appliance, while keeping the abdominal skin taut. Push the skin from the appliance rather than pulling the appliance from the skin (Figure 4).	The seal between the surface of the faceplate and the skin must be broken before the faceplate can be removed. Harsh handling of the appliance can damage the skin and impair the development of a secure seal in the future. Reduces irritation to the skin. If resistance if felt, use warm water or adhesive remover to aid in removal.
12. Place the appliance in the trash bag, if disposable. If reusable, set aside to wash in lukewarm soap and water and allow to air dry after the new appliance is in place.	Thorough cleaning and airing of the appliance reduce odor and deterioration of appliance. For esthetic and infection-control purposes, used appliances should be discarded appropriately.
13. Use toilet tissue to remove any excess stool from stoma (Figure 5). Cover stoma with gauze pad. Clean skin around stoma with mild soap and water or a cleansing agent and a washcloth. Remove all old adhesive from skin; an adhesive remover may be used. Do not apply lotion to peristomal area.	Toilet tissue, used gently, will not damage the stoma. The gauze absorbs any drainage from the stoma while the skin is being prepared. Cleaning the skin removes excretions and old adhesive and skin protectant. Excretions or a buildup of other substances can irritate and damage the skin. Lotion will prevent a tight adhesive seal.

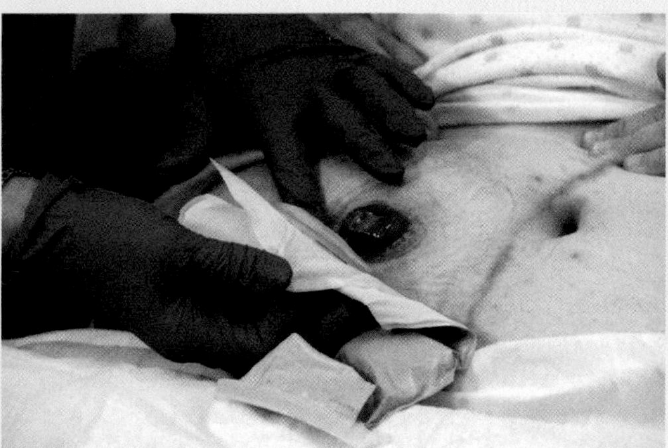

Figure 4. Removing appliance.

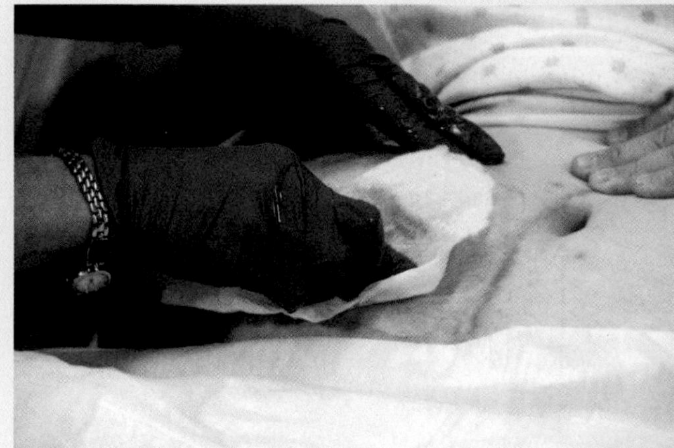

Figure 5. Using toilet tissue to wipe around stoma.

ACTION	RATIONALE
14. Gently pat area dry. Make sure skin around stoma is thoroughly dry. Assess stoma and condition of surrounding skin (Figure 6).	Careful drying prevents trauma to skin and stoma. An intact, properly applied urinary collection device protects skin integrity. Any change in color and size of the stoma may indicate circulatory problems.
15. Apply skin protectant to a 2″ (5-cm) radius around the stoma, and allow it to dry completely, which takes about 30 seconds.	The skin needs protection from the excoriating effect of the excretion and appliance adhesive. The skin must be perfectly dry before the appliance is placed to get good adherence and to prevent leaks.
16. Lift the gauze squares for a moment and measure the stoma opening, using the measurement guide (Figure 7). Replace the gauze. Trace the same-size opening on the back center of the appliance (Figure 8). Cut the opening ⅛″ larger than the stoma size (Figure 9).	The appliance should fit snugly around the stoma, with only ⅛″ of skin visible around the opening. A faceplate opening that is too small can cause trauma to the stoma. If the opening is too large, exposed skin will be irritated by urine.

SKILL 13-7

Changing and Emptying an Ostomy Appliance *(continued)*

ACTION | RATIONALE

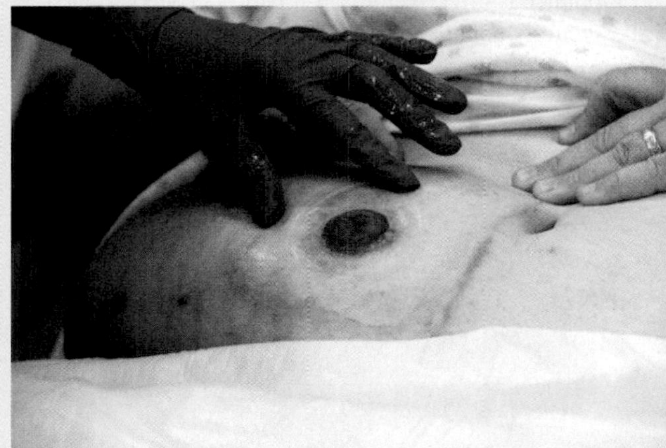

Figure 6. Assessing stoma and peristomal skin.

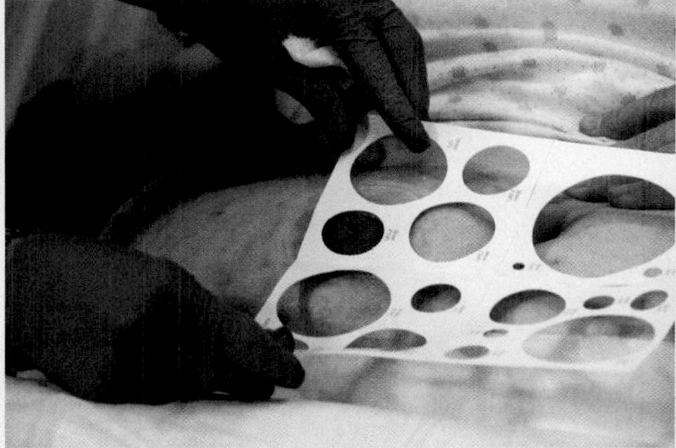

Figure 7. Using template to measure size of stoma.

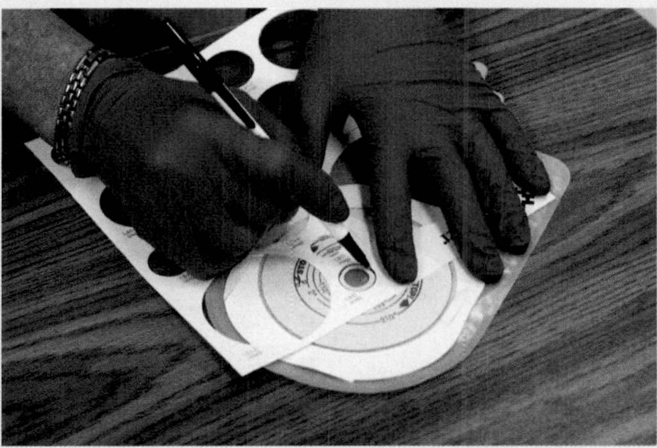

Figure 8. Tracing the same-sized circle on the back and center of skin barrier.

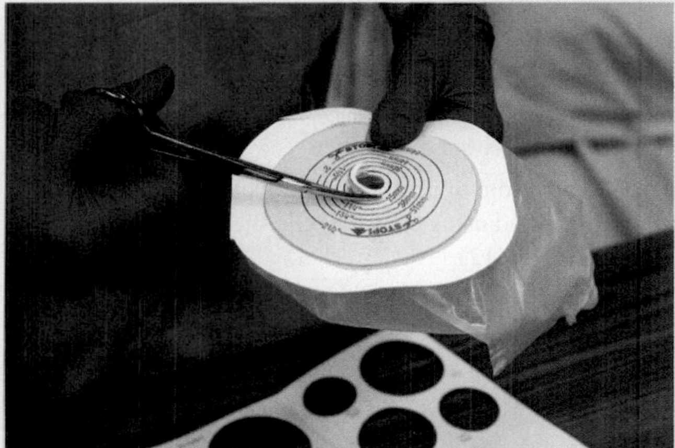

Figure 9. Cutting the opening 1/8″ larger than the stoma size.

(continued)

SKILL 13-7 Changing and Emptying an Ostomy Appliance *(continued)*

ACTION	RATIONALE
17. Remove the backing from the appliance (Figure 10). Quickly remove the gauze squares and ease the appliance over the stoma (Figure 11). Gently press onto the skin while smoothing over the surface. Apply gentle pressure to appliance for 5 minutes.	The appliance is effective only if it is properly positioned and securely adhered.

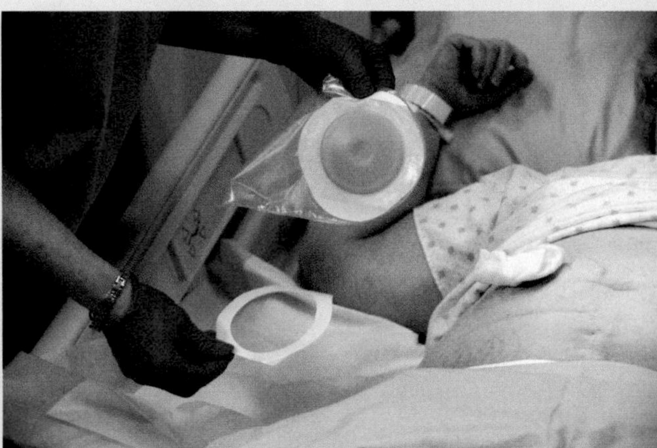

Figure 10. Removing paper backing on faceplate.

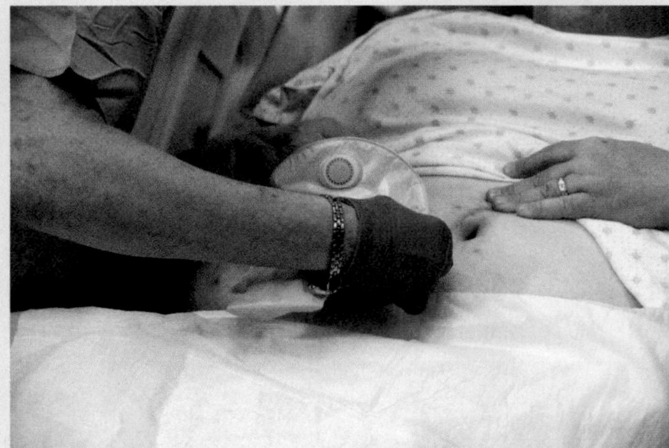

Figure 11. Easing appliance over the stoma.

ACTION	RATIONALE
18. Close bottom of appliance or pouch by folding the end upward and using clamp or clip that comes with product (Figure 12).	A tightly sealed appliance will not leak and cause embarrassment and discomfort for the patient.

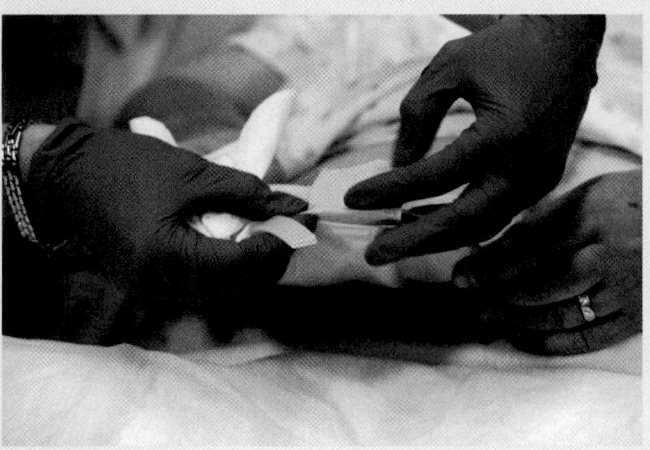

Figure 12. Closing bottom of pouch.

ACTION	RATIONALE
19. Remove gloves. Assist the patient to a comfortable position. Cover the patient with bed linens. Place the bed in the lowest position.	Provides warmth and promotes comfort and safety.
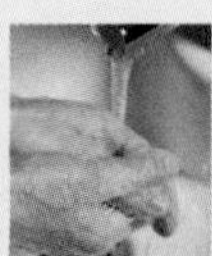 20. Put on clean gloves. Remove or discard equipment and assess patient's response to procedure. Remove gloves and perform hand hygiene.	The patient's response may indicate acceptance of the ostomy as well as the need for health teaching. Hand hygiene deters the spread of microorganisms.

SKILL 13-7 Changing and Emptying an Ostomy Appliance *(continued)*

EVALUATION

The expected outcomes are met when the patient tolerates the procedure without pain and the peristomal skin remains intact without excoriation. Odor is contained within the closed system. The patient participates in ostomy appliance care, demonstrates positive coping skills, and expels stool that is appropriate in consistency and amount for the location of the ostomy.

DOCUMENTATION

Guidelines

Document appearance of stoma, condition of peristomal skin, characteristics of drainage (amount, color, consistency, unusual odor), and patient's reaction to procedure.

Sample Documentation

7/22/08 1630 Colostomy bag changed due to leakage. Stoma is pink, moist, and flat against abdomen. No erythema or excoriation of surrounding skin. Moderate amount of pasty, brown stool noted in bag. Patient asking appropriate questions during bag application. States, "I'm ready to try the next one."—B. Clapp, RN

Unexpected Situations and Associated Interventions

- *Peristomal skin is excoriated or irritated:* Make sure that appliance is not cut too large. Skin that is exposed inside of the ostomy appliance will become excoriated. Assess for the presence of a fungal skin infection. If present, consult with prescriber to obtain appropriate treatment. Thoroughly cleanse skin and apply skin barrier. Allow to dry completely. Reapply pouch. Monitor pouch adhesion and change pouch as soon as there is a break in adhesion.
- *Patient continues to notice odor:* Check system for any leaks or poor adhesion. Clean outside of bag thoroughly when emptying.
- *Bag continues to come loose or fall off:* Thoroughly cleanse skin and apply skin barrier. Allow to dry completely. Reapply pouch. Monitor pouch adhesion and change pouch as soon as there is a break in adhesion.
- *Stoma is protruding into bag:* This is called a prolapse. Have patient rest for 30 minutes. If stoma is not back to normal size within that time, notify physician. If stoma stays prolapsed, it may twist, resulting in impaired circulation to the stoma.

SKILL 13-8 Irrigating a Colostomy

Irrigations may be used to help promote regular evacuation of feces from some colostomies. These colostomies typically are located in the right lower portion of the colon. When successful, irrigation can offer a regular, predictable elimination pattern for the patient, allowing for the use of a small covering over ostomy between irrigations instead of a regular appliance (Karadag, Mentes, & Ayaz, 2005).

Equipment

- Disposable irrigation system and irrigation sleeve
- Waterproof pad
- Bedpan or toilet
- Water-soluble lubricant
- IV pole
- Disposable gloves
- Lukewarm solution at a temperature of 105° to 110°F (40°–43°C) (as ordered by physician; normally tap water)
- Washcloth, soap, and towels
- Paper towel
- New appliance if needed

(continued)

SKILL 13-8 Irrigating a Colostomy *(continued)*

ASSESSMENT

Ask patient if he or she has been experiencing any abdominal discomfort. Ask patient about date of last irrigation and whether there have been any changes in stool pattern or consistency. If patient irrigates his or her ostomy at home, ask if he or she has any special routines during irrigation, such as reading the newspaper or listening to music. Also determine how much solution patient typically uses for irrigation. The normal amount of irrigation fluid varies but is usually around 750 to 1000 mL for an adult. If this is a first irrigation, the normal irrigation volume is around 250 to 500 mL.

Assess ostomy, ensuring that the diversion is a colostomy. Ileostomies are never irrigated because the fecal content is liquid and cannot be controlled. Note placement of ostomy on abdomen, color and size of ostomy, color and condition of stoma, and amount and consistency of stool.

NURSING DIAGNOSIS

Determine the related factors for the nursing diagnoses based on the patient's current status. Possible nursing diagnoses may include:

- Deficient Knowledge
- Anxiety
- Constipation
- Ineffective Coping
- Disturbed Body Image
- Risk for Injury

OUTCOME IDENTIFICATION AND PLANNING

The expected outcome to be met when irrigating a colostomy is that the patient expels soft formed stool. Other appropriate outcomes include: the patient remains free of any evidence of trauma to the stoma and intestinal mucosa; the patient demonstrates the ability to participate in care; the patient voices increased confidence with ostomy care; and the patient demonstrates positive coping mechanisms.

IMPLEMENTATION

ACTION	RATIONALE
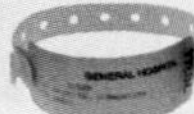 1. Assemble necessary equipment (Figure 1). Verify the order for the enema. Identify the patient. Explain procedure to patient. Plan where he or she will receive irrigation. Assist patient onto bedside commode or into nearby bathroom.	Organization facilitates task performance. Identifying the patient ensures the right patient receives the intervention and helps prevent errors. Verifying the physician's order is crucial to ensuring that the proper enema is administered to the right patient. Explanation helps to minimize anxiety and promote cooperation. The patient cannot hold the irrigation solution. A large immediate return of irrigation solution and stool usually occurs.

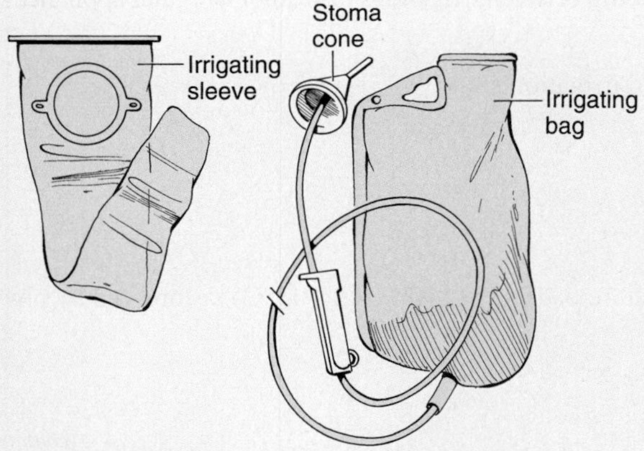

Figure 1. Irrigating sleeve and bag.

SKILL 13-8 Irrigating a Colostomy *(continued)*

ACTION	RATIONALE
2. Pull the curtains around the bed and close the room door. Drape the patient to keep him/her covered.	Provides for privacy. Minimizes unnecessary exposure and promotes the patient's comfort and warmth.
3. Warm solution in amount ordered, and check temperature with a bath thermometer if available. If bath thermometer is not available, warm to room temperature or slightly higher, and test on inner wrist. If tap water is used, adjust temperature as it flows from faucet.	If the solution is too cool, patient may experience cramps or nausea. Solution that is too warm or hot can cause irritation and trauma to intestinal mucosa.
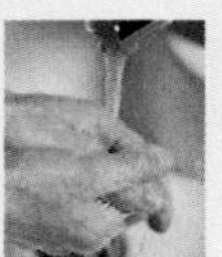 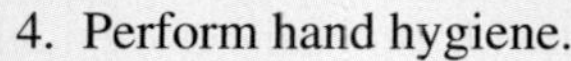 4. Perform hand hygiene.	Hand hygiene deters the spread of microorganisms.
5. Add irrigation solution to container. Release clamp and allow fluid to progress through tube before reclamping.	This causes any air to be expelled from the tubing. Although allowing air to enter the intestine is not harmful, it may further distend the intestine.
6. Hang container so that bottom of bag will be at patient's shoulder level when seated.	Gravity forces the solution to enter the intestine. The amount of pressure determines the rate of flow and pressure exerted on the intestinal wall.
7. Put on nonsterile gloves.	Gloves protect nurse from microorganisms in feces.
8. Remove ostomy appliance and attach irrigation sleeve (Figure 2). Place drainage end into toilet bowl or commode.	The irrigation sleeve directs all irrigation fluid and stool into the toilet or bedpan for easy disposal.
9. Lubricate end of cone with water-soluble lubricant.	This facilitates passage of the cone into the stoma opening.
10. Insert the cone into the stoma. Introduce solution slowly over a period of 5 to 6 minutes (Figure 3). Hold tubing (or if patient is able, allow patient to hold tubing) all the time that solution is being instilled. Control rate of flow by closing or opening the clamp.	If the irrigation solution is administered too quickly, the patient may experience nausea and cramps due to rapid distention and increased pressure in the intestine.

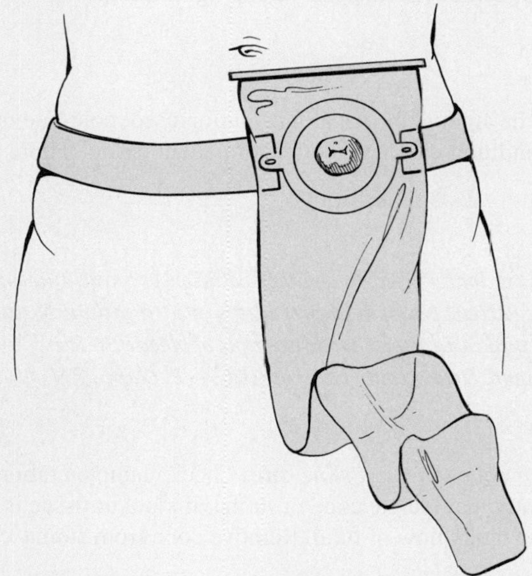

Figure 2. Positioning of irrigation sleeve on abdomen.

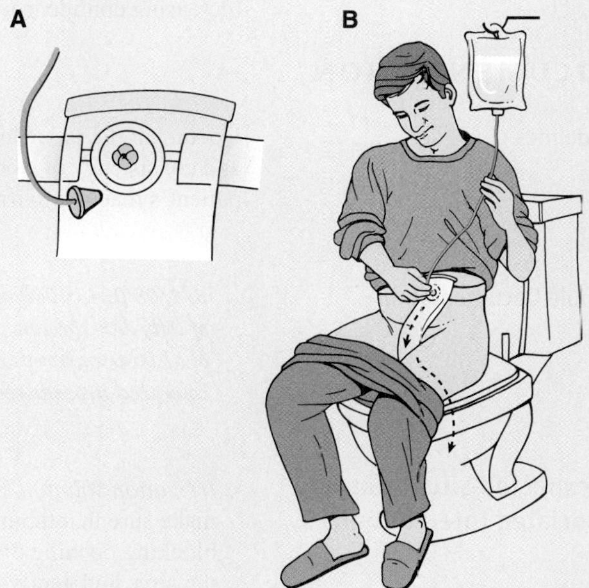

Figure 3. Colostomy irrigation. **(A)** Inserting irrigation cone. **(B)** Instilling irrigating fluid with sleeve in place.

(continued)

SKILL 13-8 Irrigating a Colostomy *(continued)*

ACTION	RATIONALE
11. **Hold cone in place for an additional 10 seconds after fluid is infused.**	This will allow a small amount of dwell time for the irrigation solution.
12. Remove cone. Patient should remain seated on toilet or bedside commode.	An immediate return of solution and stool will usually occur, followed by a return in spurts for up to 45 more minutes.
13. After majority of solution has returned, allow patient to clip (close) bottom of irrigating sleeve and continue with daily activities.	An immediate return of solution and stool will usually occur, followed by a return in spurts for up to 45 more minutes.
14. After solution has stopped flowing from stoma, put on clean gloves. Remove irrigating sleeve and cleanse skin around stoma opening with mild soap and water. Gently pat peristomal skin dry.	Gloves prevent contact with blood and body fluids. Peristomal skin must be clean and free of any liquid or stool before application of new appliance.
15. Attach new appliance to stoma or stoma cover (see Skill 13-7) as needed.	Some patients will not require an appliance, but may use a stoma cover. Protects stoma.
16. Remove gloves. Return the patient to a comfortable position. Make sure the linens under the patient are dry, if appropriate. Ensure that the patient is covered.	Promotes patient comfort. Removing contaminated gloves prevents spread of microorganisms.
17. Raise side rail. Lower bed height and adjust head of bed to a comfortable position.	Promotes patient safety.
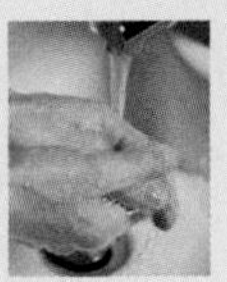 18. Perform hand hygiene.	Hand hygiene deters the spread of microorganisms.

EVALUATION

The expected outcome is achieved when the irrigation solution flows easily into the stoma opening and the patient expels soft formed stool; the patient remains free of any evidence of trauma to the stoma and intestinal mucosa; the patient participates in irrigation with increasing confidence; and the patient demonstrates positive coping mechanisms.

DOCUMENTATION

Guidelines

Document the procedure, including the amount of irrigating solution used; color, amount, and consistency of stool returned; condition of stoma; degree of patient participation; and patient's reaction to irrigation.

Sample Documentation

8/1/08 0945 1000 mL of warmed tap water used to irrigate colostomy. Large amount of soft, dark brown stool returned. Patient performed procedure with small amount of assistance from nurse. Stoma is pink and moist with no signs of bleeding. Patient tolerated procedure without incident. New ostomy bag applied.—B. Clapp, RN

Unexpected Situations and Associated Interventions

- *Irrigation solution is not flowing or is flowing at a slow rate:* Check clamp on tubing to make sure that tubing is open. Gently manipulate cone in stoma; if stool or tissue is blocking opening of cone, this may block flow of fluid. Remove cone from stoma, clean the area, and gently reinsert.
- Alternately, the patient may be assisted to side-lying or sitting position in bed. Place a waterproof pad under irrigation sleeve. Place drainage end of sleeve in bedpan.

The Taylor Suite offers these additional resources to enhance learning and facilitate understanding of this chapter:

- thePoint online resource, http://thepoint.lww.com/Lynn2E
- Student CD-ROM included with the book
- Skills Checklist to Accompany Taylor's Clinical Nursing Skills
- Taylor's Interactive Nursing: *Bowel Elimination*
- Taylor's Video Guide to Clinical Nursing Skills: *Bowel Elimination*

Developing Critical Thinking Skills

1. While you are digitally removing feces from Hugh Levens, he suddenly complains of feeling light-headed. You note that he is now diaphoretic. What should you do?
2. Isaac Greenberg is afraid that the enema is going to hurt. His mother worries about being able to prepare properly for his sigmoidoscopy. What information should you include when teaching the steps to administer a small-volume enema? What interventions should you include to promote Isaac's comfort and safety?
3. Maria Blakely has noted that an area of peristomal skin is becoming erythematous and excoriated. She asks you whether she should cut her ostomy bag bigger so that the adhesive does not irritate this skin. How should you reply?

Bibliography

Ahmed, D., Karch, A., & Karch, F. (2000). Hidden factors in occult blood testing. *American Journal of Nursing, 100*(12), 25.

Bryant, D., & Fleischer, I. (2000). Changing an ostomy appliance. *Nursing, 30*(11), 51–55.

Cohen, B., & Taylor, J. (2005). *Memmler's structure and function of the human body* (8th ed.). Philadelphia: Lippincott Williams & Wilkins.

Collett, K. (2002). Practical aspects of stoma management. *Nursing Standard, 17*(8), 45–52, 54–55.

Davies, C. (2004). The use of phosphate enemas in the treatment of constipation. *Nursing Times, 100*(18), 32–35.

Erwin-Toth, P. (2001). Caring for a stoma is more than skin deep. *Nursing, 31*(5), 36–40.

Hockenberry, M. (2005). *Wong's essentials of pediatric nursing* (7th ed.). St. Louis, MO: Elsevier Mosby.

Hyland, J. (2002). The basics of ostomies. *Gastroenterology Nursing, 25*(6), 241–244.

Ignatavicius, D., & Workman, M. (2002). *Medical-surgical nursing* (4th ed.). Philadelphia: W. B. Saunders Company.

Karadag, A., Mentes, B., & Ayaz, S. (2005). Colostomy irrigation: Results of 25 cases with particular reference to quality of life. *Journal of Clinical Nursing, 14*(4), 479–485.

Kyle, G., & Prynn, P. (2004). Guidelines for patients undergoing faecal occult blood testing. *Nursing Times, 100*(48), 62–64.

Kyle, G., Prynn, P., & Oliver, H. (2004). An evidence-based procedure for the digital removal of feces. *Nursing Times, 100*(48), 71.

McConnell, E. (2000). Myths & facts about rectal catheters. *Nursing, 30*(1), 73.

McConnell, E. (2002). Clinical do's & don'ts: Changing an ostomy appliance. *Nursing, 32*(3), 17.

Mitchell, S., Schaefer, D., & Dubagunta, S. (2004). A new view of occult and obscure gastrointestinal bleeding. *American Family Physician, 69*(4), 875–881.

Persson, E., Gustavsson, R. Hellstrom, A., et al. (2005). Ostomy patients' perceptions of quality care. *Journal of Advanced Nursing, 49*(1), 51–58.

Royal College of Nursing. (2004). *Digital rectal examination and manual removal of faeces. Guidance for nurses.* Publication code: 000943. London: Author. Available at www.rcn.org.uk/members/downloads/digitalrectalexamination000943.pdf. Accessed December 20, 2005.

Rushing, J. (2003). Administering an enema to an adult. *Nursing, 33*(11), 28.

Schmelzer, M., Schiller, L., Meyer, R., et al. (2004). Safety and effectiveness of large-volume enema solutions. *Applied Nursing Research, 17*(4), 265–274.

Secord, C., Jackman, M., & Wright, L. (2001). Adjusting to life with an ostomy. *Canadian Nurse, 97*(1), 29–32.

Smeltzer, S., Bare, B., Hinkle, J. H., & Cheever, K. H. (2008). *Brunner & Suddarth's textbook of medical-surgical nursing* (11th ed.). Philadelphia: Lippincott Williams & Wilkins.

Thompson, J. (2000). Part one: A practical ostomy guide. *RN, 63*(11), 61–68.

Trainor, B., Thompson, M., Boyd-Carson, W., et al. (2003). Changing an appliance . . . second in a series. *Nursing Standard, 18*(13), 41–42.

Van Orden, H. (2004). Constipation: An overview of treatment. *Journal of Pediatric HealthCare, 18*(6), 320–322.

Weber, J., & Kelley, J. (2007). *Health assessment in nursing* (3rd ed.). Philadelphia: Lippincott Williams & Wilkins.

CHAPTER 14

Oxygenation

Focusing on Patient Care

This chapter will help you develop some of the skills related to oxygenation necessary to care for the following patients:

Scott Mingus, age 12, who has a mediastinal chest tube after thoracic surgery

Saranam Srivastava, age 35, who has chest tube after a motor vehicle accident

Paula Cunningham, age 72, who is intubated and requires suctioning through her endotracheal tube

Learning Objectives

After studying this chapter, you will be able to:

1. Use a pulse oximeter.
2. Teach a patient to use an incentive spirometer.
3. Administer oxygen by nasal cannula.
4. Administer oxygen by mask.
5. Use an oxygen hood.
6. Use an oxygen tent.
7. Insert an oropharyngeal airway.
8. Insert a nasopharyngeal airway.
9. Suction the nasopharynx and oropharynx.
10. Suction an endotracheal tube using an open system.
11. Suction an endotracheal tube using a closed system
12. Secure an endotracheal tube.
13. Suction a tracheostomy.
14. Provide tracheostomy care.
15. Provide care of a chest drainage system.
16. Assist with chest tube removal.
17. Use a bag and mask (handheld resuscitation device) to deliver oxygen.

Key Terms

alveoli: small air sacs at the end of the terminal bronchioles that are the site of gas exchange

atelectasis: incomplete expansion or collapse of a part of the lungs

cilia: microscopic hairlike projections that propel mucus toward the upper airway so that it can be expectorated

dyspnea: difficult or labored breathing

endotracheal tube: polyvinylchloride airway that is inserted through the nose or mouth into the trachea, using a laryngoscope

expiration: act of breathing out

extubation: removal of a tube (in this case an endotracheal tube)

hemothorax: blood in the pleural space around the heart

hyperventilation: condition in which there is more than the normal amount of air entering and leaving the lungs as a result of increase in rate or depth of respiration or both

hypoventilation: decreased rate or depth of air movement into the lungs

hypoxia: inadequate amount of oxygen available to the cells

inspiration: act of breathing in

metered-dose inhaler (MDI)**:** device that delivers a controlled dose of medication with each compression of the canister

nasal cannula: disposable plastic device with two protruding prongs for insertion into the nostrils; used to administer oxygen

nasopharyngeal airway (nasal trumpet)**:** a curved, soft rubber or plastic tube inserted into the back of the pharynx through the mouth

nebulizer: method of delivering medication by dispersing fine particles of medication into the deeper passages of the respiratory tract

oropharyngeal airway: a semicircular tube of plastic or rubber inserted into the back of the pharynx through the mouth

perfusion: the process by which oxygenated capillary blood passes through the tissues of the body

pleurae: membranes that cover the lungs

pleural effusion: fluid in the pleural space

pneumothorax: air in the pleural space

pulse oximetry: noninvasive technique that measures the oxygen saturation (SpO_2) of arterial blood

respiration: gas exchange between the atmospheric air in the alveoli and the blood in the capillaries

spirometer: instrument used to measure lung capacity and volume; one type is used to encourage deep breathing (incentive spirometry)

subcutaneous emphysema: small pockets of air trapped in the subcutaneous tissue; usually found around chest tube insertion sites

tachypnea: rapid breathing

tracheostomy: curved tube inserted into an artificial opening made into the trachea; comes in varied angles and multiple sizes

ventilation (breathing)**:** the movement of air into and out of the lungs

Many people take respiratory function for granted, but a functioning respiratory system is necessary for life. The respiratory system (Figure 14-1) delivers oxygen to the cells and also removes carbon dioxide.

The respiratory system performs its functions through pulmonary ventilation, respiration, and perfusion. Normal functioning depends on three essential factors:

- The integrity of the airway system to transport air to and from the lungs
- A properly functioning alveolar system in the lungs to oxygenate venous blood and to remove carbon dioxide from the blood
- A properly functioning cardiovascular and hematologic system to carry nutrients and wastes to and from body cells

The air passages must remain patent (open) for oxygen to enter the system. Any condition that interferes with normal functioning must be minimized or eliminated to prevent pulmonary distress, which could lead to death. This chapter will cover the skills necessary for the nurse to promote oxygenation. While performing skills related to oxygenation, keep in mind factors that affect respiratory function (Fundamentals Review 14-1).

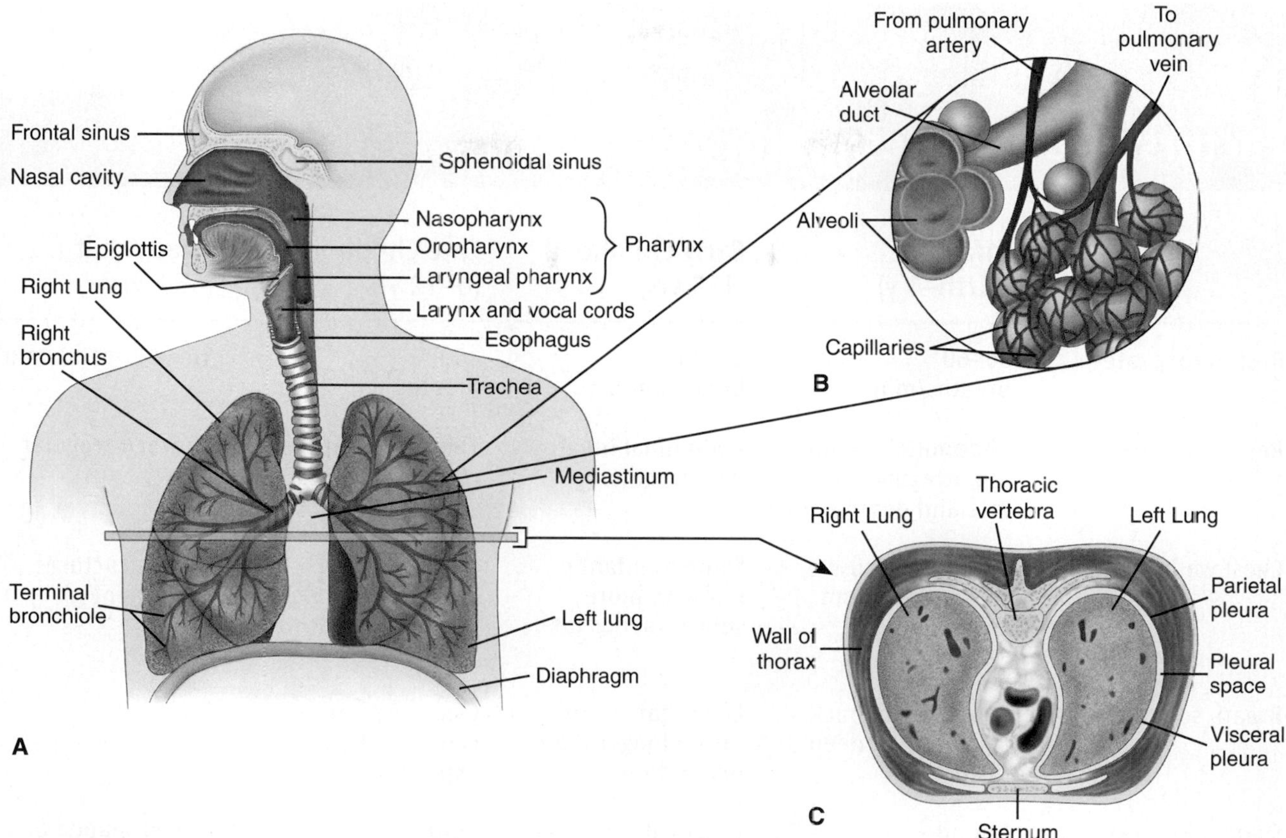

Figure 14-1. The organs of the respiratory tract. (**A**) Overview (**B**) Alveoli (air sacs) of the lungs and the blood capillaries (**C**) Transverse section through the lungs.

Factors Affecting Respiratory Function

A variety of factors can impact/affect respiratory functioning. This display reviews six common factors.

Level of Health

Acute and chronic illness can dramatically affect a person's respiratory function. Body systems, eg, the cardiovascular system and respiratory system or the musculoskeletal system and the respiratory system, work together, so alterations in one may affect the other. For example, alterations in muscle function contribute to inadequate pulmonary ventilation and respiration.

Developmental Level

Respiratory function varies across the life span. The table below summarizes variations.

(continued)

Factors Affecting Respiratory Function *(continued)*

	Infant (Birth–1 y)	Early Childhood (1–5 yrs)	Late Childhood (6–12 yrs)	Aged Adult (65+ yrs)
Respiratory rate	30–60 breaths/min	20–40 breaths/min	15–25 breaths/min	16–20 breaths/min
Respiratory pattern	Abdominal breathing, irregular in rate and depth	Abdominal breathing, irregular	Thoracic breathing, regular	Thoracic, regular
Chest wall	Thin, little muscle, ribs and sternum easily seen	Same as infant's but with more subcutaneous fat	Further subcutaneous fat deposited, structures less prominent	Thin, structures prominent
Breath sounds	Loud, harsh crackles at end of deep inspiration	Loud, harsh expiration longer than inspiration	Clear inspiration is longer than expiration	Clear
Shape of thorax	Round	Elliptical	Elliptical	Barrel shaped or elliptical

Medications

Many medications affect the function of the respiratory system. Many medications depress the respiratory system. The nurse should monitor patients taking certain medications, such as opioids, for rate and depth of respirations.

Life Style

Activity levels and habits can dramatically affect a person's respiratory status. For example, people who exercise can better respond to stressors to respiratory health. Cigarette smoking (active or passive) is a major contributor to lung disease and respiratory distress. Cigarette smoking is the most important risk factor for developing COPD (Boyle, 2004).

Environment

Research indicates that there is a high correlation between air pollution and occupational exposure to certain chemicals and lung disease. Additionally, people who have experienced an alteration in respiratory functioning often have difficulty continuing to perform self-care activities in a polluted environment.

Psychological Health

Many psychological factors can impact the respiratory system. Individuals responding to stress or anxiety may experience hyperventilation. In addition, patients with respiratory problems often develop some anxiety as a result of the hypoxia caused by the respiratory problem.

SKILL 14-1

Using a Pulse Oximeter

Pulse oximetry is a noninvasive technique that measures the arterial oxyhemoglobin saturation (SaO_2 or SpO_2) of arterial blood. A sensor, or probe, uses a beam of red and infrared light that travels through tissue and blood vessels. One part of the sensor emits the light and another part receives the light. The oximeter then calculates the amount of light that has been absorbed by arterial blood. Oxygen saturation is determined by the amount of each light absorbed; unoxygenated hemoglobin absorbs more red light and oxygenated hemoglobin absorbs more infrared light.

The nurse should know the patient's hemoglobin level before evaluating oxygen saturation because the test measures only the percentage of oxygen carried by the available hemoglobin. Thus, even a patient with a low hemoglobin could appear to have a normal SpO_2 because most of that hemoglobin is saturated. However, the patient may not have enough oxygen to meet body needs. A range of 95% to 100% is considered normal SpO_2; values less than 85% indicate that oxygenation to the tissues is inadequate.

Sensors are available for use on a finger, a toe, a foot (infants), an earlobe, and the bridge of the nose. Circulation to the sensor site must be adequate to ensure accurate readings. Pulse oximeters also display a measured pulse rate.

Pulse oximetry is useful for monitoring patients receiving oxygen therapy, titrating oxygen therapy, monitoring those at risk for hypoxia, and postoperative patients. Pulse oximetry does not replace arterial blood gas analysis. Desaturation indicates gas exchange abnormalities.

Equipment

- Pulse oximeter with an appropriate sensor or probe
- Alcohol wipe(s) or disposable cleansing cloth
- Nail polish remover (if necessary)

ASSESSMENT

Assess the patient's skin temperature and color, including the color of the nail beds. Temperature is a good indicator of blood flow. Warm skin indicates adequate circulation. In a well-oxygenated patient, the skin and nail beds are usually pink. Skin that is bluish or dusky indicates hypoxia (inadequate amount of oxygen available to the cells). Also check capillary refill: prolonged capillary refill indicates a reduction in blood flow. Assess the quality of the pulse proximal to the sensor application site. Auscultate the lungs (see Skill 2-3). Patients with clear lung sounds are expected to have a higher saturation than patients with coarse or wheezing lung sounds. Note the amount of oxygen and delivery method if the patient is receiving supplemental oxygen.

NURSING DIAGNOSIS

Determine the related factors for the nursing diagnosis based on the patient's current status. Appropriate nursing diagnoses may include:

- Ineffective Tissue Perfusion
- Impaired Gas Exchange
- Ineffective Airway Clearance
- Activity Intolerance

Other nursing diagnoses also may require the use of this skill, such as Decreased Cardiac Output, Excess Fluid Volume, Anxiety, and Risk for Aspiration.

OUTCOME IDENTIFICATION AND PLANNING

The expected outcome to achieve when caring for a patient with a pulse oximeter is that the patient will exhibit arterial blood oxygen saturation within acceptable parameters, or greater than 95%.

(continued)

SKILL 14-1 Using a Pulse Oximeter *(continued)*

IMPLEMENTATION

ACTION	RATIONALE
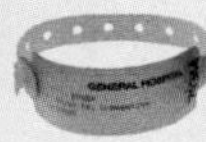 1. Identify the patient using at least two methods.	Positive identification of the patient is essential to ensure the intervention is administered to the correct patient.
2. Explain what you are going to do and why you are going to do it to the patient.	Explanation relieves anxiety and facilitates cooperation.
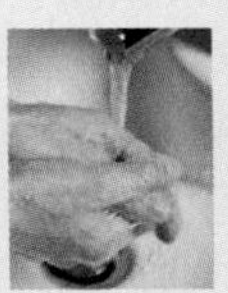 3. Perform hand hygiene.	Hand hygiene deters the spread of microorganisms.
4. Select an adequate site for application of the sensor.	Inadequate circulation can interfere with the oxygen saturation (SpO_2) reading.
a. Use the patient's index, middle, or ring finger (Figure 1).	Fingers are easily accessible.
b. Check the proximal pulse (Figure 2) and capillary refill (Figure 3) at the pulse closest to the site.	Brisk capillary refill and a strong pulse indicate that circulation to the site is adequate.
c. If circulation at site is inadequate, consider using the earlobe or bridge of nose.	These alternate sites are highly vascular alternatives.
d. Use a toe only if lower extremity circulation is not compromised.	Peripheral vascular disease is common in lower extremities.

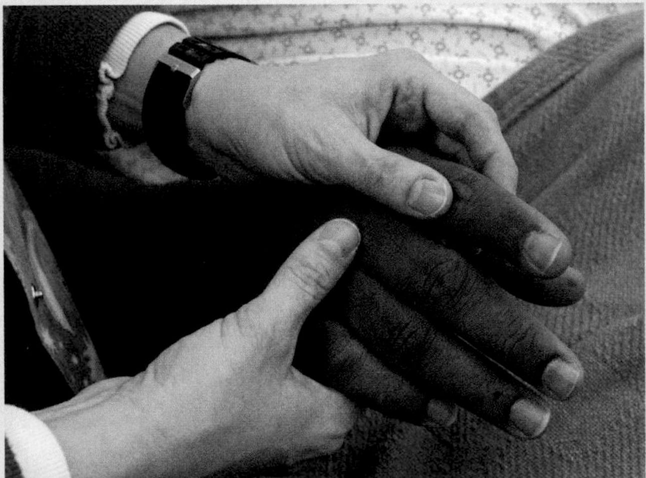

Figure 1. Selecting an appropriate finger.

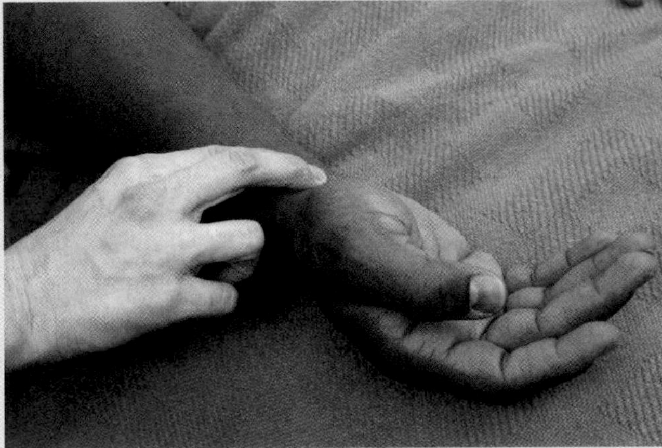

Figure 2. Assessing pulse.

ACTION	RATIONALE
5. Select proper equipment:	
a. If one finger is too large for the probe, use a smaller one. A pediatric probe may be used for a small adult.	Inaccurate readings can result if probe or sensor is not attached correctly.
b. Use probes appropriate for patient's age and size.	Probes come in adult, pediatric, and infant sizes.
c. Check if patient is allergic to adhesive. A nonadhesive finger clip or reflectance sensor is available.	A reaction may occur if patient is allergic to adhesive substance.

SKILL 14-1

Using a Pulse Oximeter *(continued)*

ACTION | **RATIONALE**

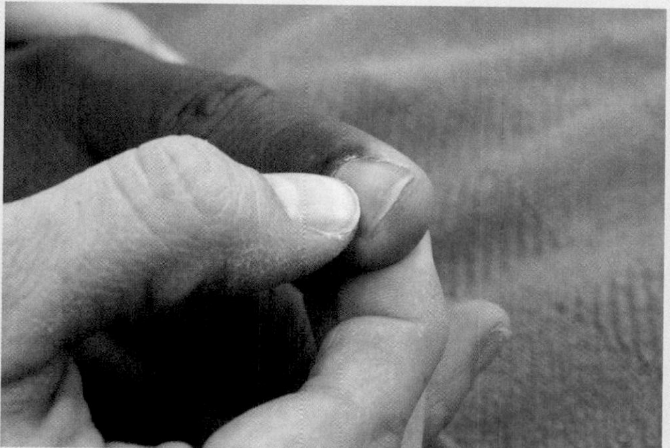

Figure 3. Assessing capillary refill.

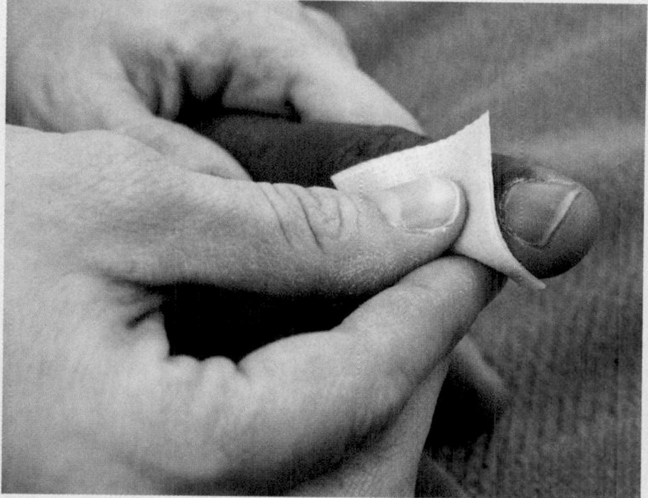

Figure 4. Cleaning the area.

6. Prepare the monitoring site. Cleanse the selected area with the alcohol wipe or disposable cleansing cloth (Figure 4). Allow the area to dry. If necessary, remove nail polish and artificial nails after checking manufacturer's instructions.

Skin oils, dirt, or grime on the site, polish, and artificial nails can interfere with the passage of light waves.

7. **Apply probe securely to skin (Figure 5). Make sure that the light-emitting sensor and the light-receiving sensor are aligned opposite each other (not necessary to check if placed on forehead or bridge of nose).**

Secure attachment and proper alignment promote satisfactory operation of the equipment and accurate recording of the SpO_2.

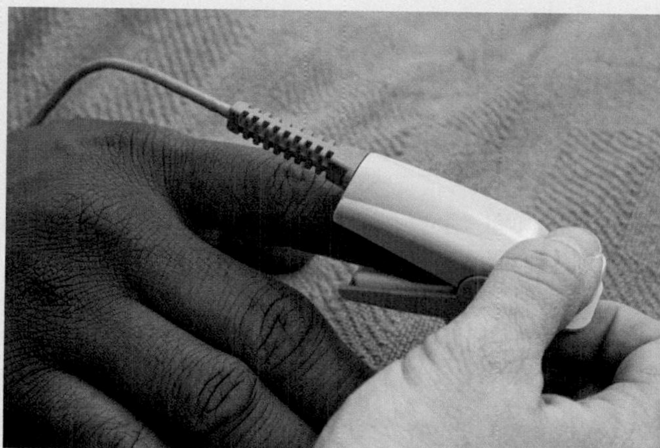

Figure 5. Attaching probe to patient's finger.

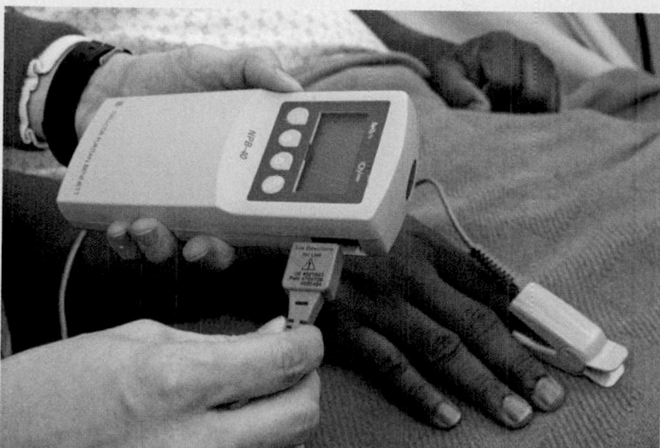

Figure 6. Connecting sensor probe to unit.

8. Connect the sensor probe to the pulse oximeter (Figure 6), turn the oximeter on, and check operation of the equipment (audible beep, fluctuation of bar of light or waveform on face of oximeter).

Audible beep represents the arterial pulse, and fluctuating waveform or light bar indicates the strength of the pulse. A weak signal will produce an inaccurate recording of the SpO_2. Tone of beep reflects SpO_2 reading. If SpO_2 drops, tone becomes lower in pitch.

(continued)

SKILL 14-1 Using a Pulse Oximeter *(continued)*

ACTION	RATIONALE
9. Set alarms on pulse oximeter. Check manufacturer's alarm limits for high and low pulse rate settings (Figure 7).	Alarm provides additional safeguard and signals when high or low limits have been surpassed.
10. **Check oxygen saturation at regular intervals (Figure 8), as ordered by physician and signaled by alarms. Monitor hemoglobin level.**	Monitoring SpO_2 provides ongoing assessment of patient's condition. A low hemoglobin level may be satisfactorily saturated yet inadequate to meet a patient's oxygen needs.

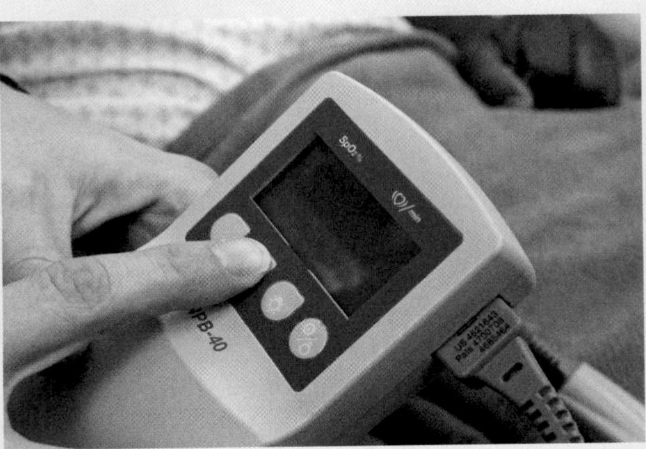

Figure 7. Checking alarms.

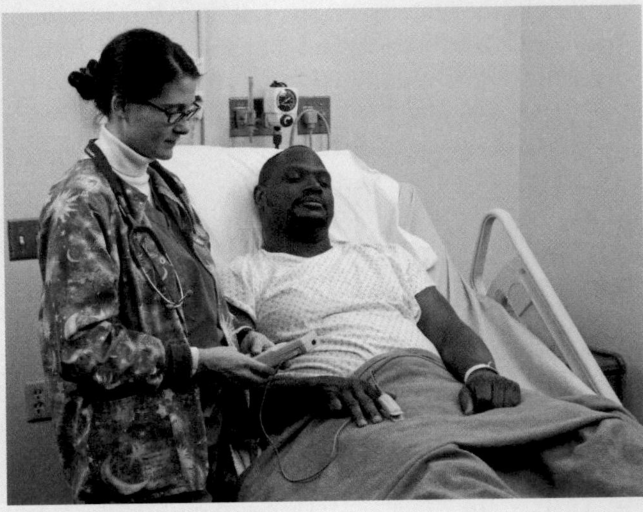

Figure 8. Reading pulse oximeter.

ACTION	RATIONALE
11. Remove sensor on a regular basis and check for skin irritation or signs of pressure (every 2 hours for spring tension sensor or every 4 hours for adhesive finger or toe sensor).	Prolonged pressure may lead to tissue necrosis. Adhesive sensor may cause skin irritation.
12. Clean nondisposable sensors according to the manufacturer's directions. Perform hand hygiene.	Each deters the spread of microorganisms and contaminants.

EVALUATION

The expected outcome is met when the patient exhibits an oxygen saturation level within acceptable parameters, or greater than 95%, and a heart rate that correlates with the pulse measurement.

DOCUMENTATION

Guidelines

Documentation should include the type of sensor and location used, the assessment of the proximal pulse and capillary refill, pulse oximeter reading, the amount of oxygen and delivery method if the patient is receiving supplemental oxygen, lung assessment, if relevant, and any other relevant interventions required as a result of the reading.

SKILL 14-1 Using a Pulse Oximeter *(continued)*

Sample Documentation

9/03/08 Pulse oximeter placed on patient's index finger on right hand. Radial pulse present with brisk capillary refill. Pulse oximeter reading 98% on oxygen at 2 L via nasal cannula. Heart rate measured by oximeter correlates with the radial pulse measurement—C. Bausler, RN

Unexpected Situations and Associated Interventions

- *Absent or weak signal:* Check vital signs and patient condition. If satisfactory, check connections and circulation to site. Hypotension makes an accurate recording difficult. Equipment (restraint, blood pressure cuff) may compromise circulation to site and cause venous blood to pulsate, giving an inaccurate reading. If extremity is cold, cover with a warm blanket.
- *Inaccurate reading:* Check prescribed medications and history of circulatory disorders. Try device on a healthy person to see if problem is equipment-related or patient-related. Drugs that cause vasoconstriction interfere with accurate recording of oxygen saturation.
- *A bright light (sunlight or fluorescent light) is suspected of causing equipment malfunction:* Cover probe with a dry washcloth. Bright light can interfere with operation of light sensors and cause unreliable report.

Special Considerations

General Considerations

- Accuracy of readings can be influenced by conditions that decrease arterial blood flow, such as peripheral edema, hypotension, and peripheral vascular disease. Excess motion of sensor probe site can also interfere with obtaining an accurate reading.

Infant and Child Considerations

- For infants, the oximeter probe may be placed on the toe or foot (Figure 9).

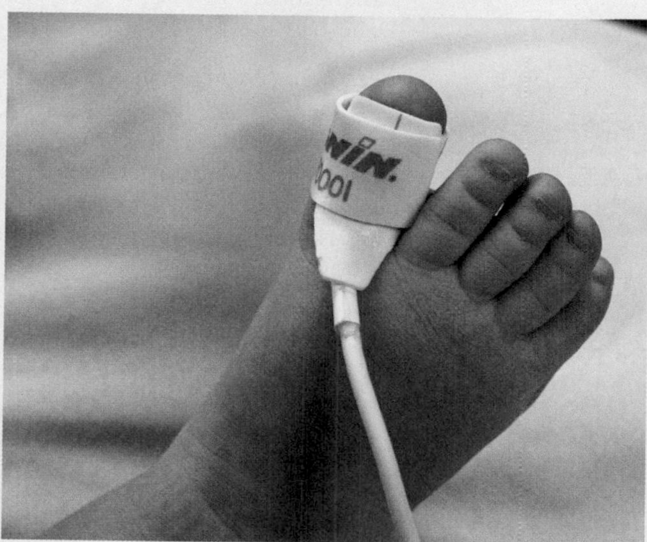

Figure 9. Oximetry probe on infant's toe.

Older Adult Considerations

- Careful attention to the patient's skin integrity and condition is necessary to prevent injury. Pressure or tension from the probe, as well as any adhesive used, can damage older, dry, thin skin.

Home Care Considerations

- Portable units are available for use in the home or an outpatient setting.

SKILL 14-2 Teaching Patient to Use an Incentive Spirometer

Incentive spirometry provides visual reinforcement for deep breathing by the patient. It assists the patient to breathe slowly and deeply, and to sustain maximal inspiration, while providing immediate positive reinforcement. Incentive spirometry encourages the patient to maximize lung inflation and prevent or reduce atelectasis. Optimal gas exchange is supported and secretions can be cleared and expectorated.

Equipment

- Incentive spirometer
- Stethoscope
- Folded blanket or pillow for splinting of chest or abdominal incision, if appropriate

ASSESSMENT

Assess the patient for pain and administer pain medication as prescribed if deep breathing may cause pain. Presence of pain may interfere with learning and performing required activities. Assess lung sounds pre- and postuse to establish a baseline and to determine the effectiveness of incentive spirometry. Incentive spirometry encourages patients to take deep breaths, and lung sounds may be diminished before using the incentive spirometer. Assess vital signs and oxygen saturation to provide baseline data to evaluate patient response. Oxygen saturation may increase due to reinflation of alveoli.

NURSING DIAGNOSIS

Determine the related factors for the nursing diagnosis based on the patient's current status. Appropriate nursing diagnoses may include:

- Ineffective Breathing Pattern
- Impaired Gas Exchange
- Acute Pain
- Activity Intolerance
- Risk for Injury
- Risk for Infection
- Deficient Knowledge

Other nursing diagnoses may require the use of this skill.

OUTCOME IDENTIFICATION AND PLANNING

The expected outcome is that the patient accurately demonstrates the procedure for using the spirometer. Other outcomes that may be appropriate include the following: patient demonstrates increased oxygen saturation level, patient reports adequate control of pain during use, and patient demonstrates increased lung expansion with clear breath sounds.

IMPLEMENTATION

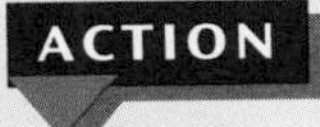

ACTION	RATIONALE
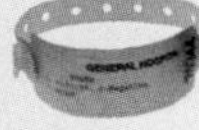 1. Identify the patient.	Positive identification of the patient is essential to ensure the intervention is administered to the correct patient.
2. Explain what you are going to do and the reason to the patient	Explanation relieves anxiety and facilitates cooperation.
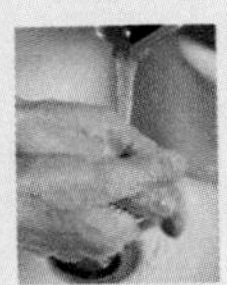 3. Perform hand hygiene.	Hand hygiene deters the spread of microorganisms.

SKILL 14-2 Teaching Patient to Use an Incentive Spirometer *(continued)*

ACTION	RATIONALE
4. Assist patient to an upright or semi-Fowler's position if possible. Remove dentures if they fit poorly. Administer pain medication as prescribed, if needed. Wait the appropriate amount of time for the medication to take effect. **If patient has recently undergone abdominal surgery, place a pillow or folded blanket over a chest or abdominal incision for splinting.**	Upright position facilitates lung expansion. Dentures may inhibit patient from taking deep breaths if patient is concerned that dentures may fall out. Pain may decrease patient's ability to take deep breaths. Deep breaths may cause patient to cough. Splinting the incision supports the area and helps reduce pain from the incision (Refer to Skill 6-1).
5. Demonstrate how to steady the device with one hand and hold mouthpiece with other hand (Figure 1). If patient cannot use hands, nurse may assist patient with the incentive spirometer.	This allows the patient to remain upright, visualize the volume of each breath, and stabilize the device.

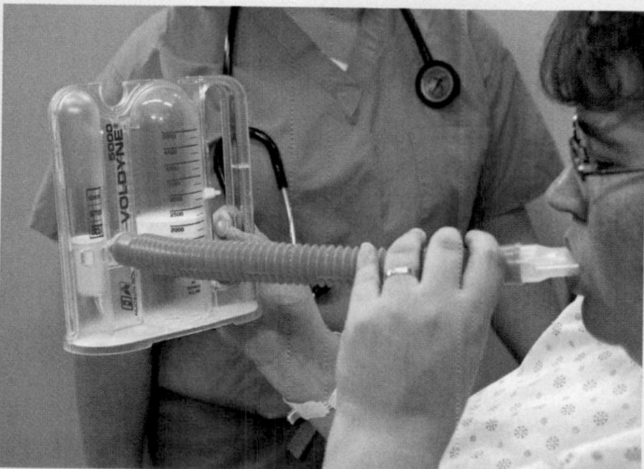

Figure 1. Patient using incentive spirometer.

ACTION	RATIONALE
6. Instruct patient to exhale normally and then place lips securely around the mouthpiece.	Patient should fully empty lungs so that maximum volume may be inhaled. A tight seal allows for maximum use of the device.
7. **Instruct patient to inhale slowly and as deeply as possible through the mouthpiece without using nose (if desired, a nose clip may be used).**	Inhaling through the nose would provide an inaccurate measurement of inhalation volume.
8. When the patient cannot inhale anymore, **the patient should hold his breath and count to three.** Check position of gauge to determine progress and level attained. If patient begins to cough, splint an abdominal or chest incision.	Holding breath for 3 seconds helps the alveoli to re-expand. Volume on incentive spirometry should increase with practice.
9. Instruct patient to remove lips from mouthpiece and exhale normally. **If patient becomes light-headed during the process, tell him or her to stop and take a few normal breaths before resuming incentive spirometry.**	Deep breaths may change the CO_2 level, leading to light-headedness.

(continued)

SKILL 14-2 Teaching Patient to Use an Incentive Spirometer *(continued)*

ACTION	RATIONALE
10. Encourage patient to perform incentive spirometry 5 to 10 times every 1 to 2 hours if possible.	This helps to reinflate the alveoli and prevent atelectasis due to hypoventilation.
11. Clean the mouthpiece with water and shake to dry. Perform hand hygiene.	These deter the spread of microorganisms and contaminants.

EVALUATION

The expected outcome is met when the patient demonstrates the steps for use of the incentive spirometer correctly and exhibits lung sounds that are clear and equal in all lobes. In addition, the patient demonstrates an increase in oxygen saturation levels, verbalizes adequate pain control and the importance of and need for incentive spirometry.

DOCUMENTATION

Guidelines

Documentation should include that the incentive spirometer was used by the patient, the number of repetitions, and the average volume reached. Document patient teaching and patient response, if appropriate. If the patient coughs, document whether the cough is productive or nonproductive. If productive cough is present, include the characteristics of the sputum, including consistency, amount, and color.

Sample Documentation

9/8/08 Incentive spirometry performed × 10, volume 1,500 mL obtained. Patient with nonproductive cough during incentive spirometry.—C. Bausler, RN

Unexpected Situations and Associated Interventions

- *Volume inhaled is decreasing:* Assess patient's pain and anxiety level. Patient may have pain and not be inhaling fully, or patient may have experienced pain previously during incentive spirometry and have an increased anxiety level. If ordered, medicate patient when pain is present. Discuss fears with patient and encourage him or her to inhale fully or to increase the volume by 100 each time incentive spirometry is performed.
- *Patient attempts to blow into incentive spirometer:* Compare the incentive spirometer to a straw. Remind patient to exhale before beginning each time.

Special Considerations

General Considerations

- Reinforce importance of continued use by postoperative patients upon discharge.

Older Adult Considerations

- Older adults have decreased muscle function and fatigue more easily. Encourage rest periods between repetitions.

SKILL 14-3 Suctioning the Nasopharyngeal and Oropharyngeal Airways

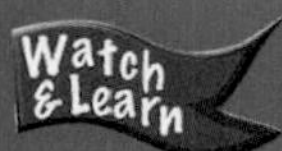

Suctioning of the pharynx is indicated to maintain a patent airway and remove saliva, pulmonary secretions, blood, vomitus, or foreign material from the pharynx. It helps a patient who can't successfully clear his airway by coughing and expectorating. When performing suctioning, position yourself on the appropriate side of the patient. If you are right handed, stand on the patient's right side; left handed, stand on the patient's left side. This allows for comfortable use of the dominant hand to manipulate the suction catheter.

Equipment

- Portable or wall suction unit with tubing
- A commercially prepared suction kit with an appropriate size catheter or
  - Sterile suction catheter with Y-port in the appropriate size (Adult: 10 Fr–16 Fr)
  - Sterile disposable container
  - Sterile gloves
- Sterile water or saline
- Towel or waterproof pad
- Goggles and mask or face shield
- Disposable, clean gloves
- Water-soluble lubricant

ASSESSMENT

Assess lung sounds. Patients who need to be suctioned may have wheezes, crackles, or gurgling present. Assess oxygenation saturation level. Oxygen saturation usually decreases when a patient needs to be suctioned. Assess respiratory status, including respiratory rate and depth. Patients may become tachypneic when they need to be suctioned. Assess patient for signs of respiratory distress, such as nasal flaring, retractions, or grunting. Assess effectiveness of coughing and expectoration. Patients with an ineffective cough and who are unable to expectorate secretions may need to be suctioned. Assess for history of deviated septum, nasal polyps, nasal obstruction, nasal injury, epistaxis (nasal bleeding), or nasal swelling.

NURSING DIAGNOSIS

Determine the related factors for the nursing diagnosis based on the patient's current status. Appropriate nursing diagnoses may include:

- Ineffective Airway Clearance
- Impaired Gas Exchange
- Ineffective Breathing Pattern
- Risk for Aspiration

OUTCOME IDENTIFICATION AND PLANNING

The expected outcome to achieve is that the patient will exhibit improved breath sounds and a clear, patent airway. Other outcomes that may be appropriate include the following: patient will exhibit an oxygen saturation level within acceptable parameters; patient will demonstrate a respiratory rate and depth within age-acceptable range; and patient will remain free of any signs of respiratory distress, including retractions, nasal flaring, or grunting.

IMPLEMENTATION

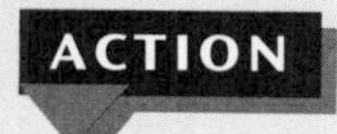

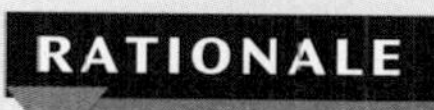

ACTION	RATIONALE
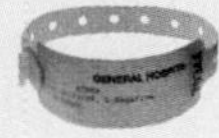 1. Identify the patient.	Positive identification of the patient is essential to ensure the intervention is administered to the correct patient.

(continued)

SKILL 14-3 Suctioning the Nasopharyngeal and Oropharyngeal Airways *(continued)*

ACTION	RATIONALE
2. Determine the need for suctioning. Verify the suction order in the patient's chart, if necessary. **For post-operative patient, administer pain medication before suctioning.**	To minimize trauma to airway mucosa, suctioning should be done only when secretions have accumulated or adventitious breath sounds are audible. Some facilities require an order for naso- and oropharyngeal suctioning. Suctioning stimulates coughing, which is painful for patients with surgical incisions.
3. Explain what you are going to do and the reason to the patient, even if the patient does not appear to be alert. Reassure patient you will interrupt procedure if he or she indicates respiratory difficulty.	Explanation alleviates fears. Even if patient appears unconscious, the nurse should explain what is happening. Any procedure that compromises respiration is frightening for the patient.
4. Perform hand hygiene.	Hand hygiene deters the spread of microorganisms.
5. Adjust bed to comfortable working position. Lower side rail closer to you. If patient is conscious, place him or her in a semi-Fowler's position. **If patient is unconscious, place him or her in the lateral position, facing you. Move the bed table close to your work area and raise to waist height.**	A sitting position helps the patient to cough and makes breathing easier. Gravity also facilitates catheter insertion. The lateral position prevents the airway from becoming obstructed and promotes drainage of secretions. Table provides work surface and helps maintain sterility of objects on work surface.
6. Place towel or waterproof pad across patient's chest.	This protects bed linens.
7. **Adjust suction to appropriate pressure (Figure 1).**	Higher pressures can cause excessive trauma, hypoxemia, and atelectasis.

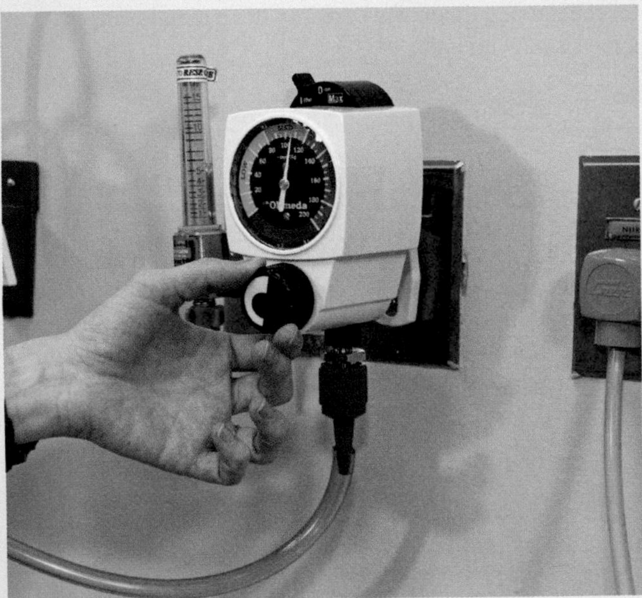

Figure 1. Adjusting wall suction.

SKILL 14-3

Suctioning the Nasopharyngeal and Oropharyngeal Airways *(continued)*

ACTION	RATIONALE
For a wall unit for an adult: 100–150 mm Hg; neonates: 60–80 mm Hg; infants: 80–100 mm Hg; children: 100–120 mm Hg For a portable unit for an adult: 10–15 cm Hg; neonates: 6–8 cm Hg; infants 8–10 cm Hg; children 10–12 cm Hg **Put on a disposable, clean glove and occlude the end of the connecting tubing to check suction pressure. Place the connecting tubing in a convenient location.**	
8. **Open sterile suction package using aseptic technique. The open wrapper or container becomes a sterile field to hold other supplies. Carefully remove the sterile container, touching only the outside surface. Set it up on the work surface and pour sterile saline into it.**	Sterile normal saline or water is used to lubricate the outside of the catheter, minimizing irritation of mucosa during introduction. It is also used to clear the catheter between suction attempts.
9. Place a small amount of water-soluble lubricant on the sterile field, taking care to avoid touching the sterile field with the lubricant package.	Lubricant facilitates passage of the catheter and reduces trauma to mucous membranes.
10. Increase the patient's supplemental oxygen level or apply supplemental oxygen per facility policy or physician order.	Suctioning removes air from the patient's airway and can cause hypoxemia. Hyperventilation can help prevent suction-induced hypoxemia.
11. Put on face shield or goggles and mask. Put on sterile gloves. **The dominant hand will manipulate the catheter and must remain sterile. The nondominant hand is considered clean rather than sterile and will control the suction valve (Y port) on the catheter.**	Handling the sterile catheter using a sterile glove helps prevent introducing organisms into the respiratory tract; the clean glove protects the nurse from microorganisms.
12. With dominant gloved hand, pick up sterile catheter. Pick up the connecting tubing with the nondominant hand and connect the tubing and suction catheter (Figure 2).	Sterility of the suction catheter is maintained.
13. Moisten the catheter by dipping it into the container of sterile saline (Figure 3). Occlude Y-tube to check suction.	Lubricating the inside of the catheter with saline helps move secretions in the catheter. Checking suction ensures equipment is working properly.

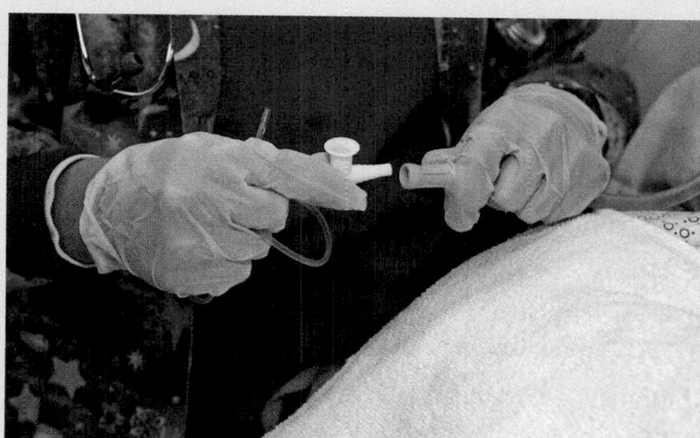

Figure 2. Connecting catheter to tubing.

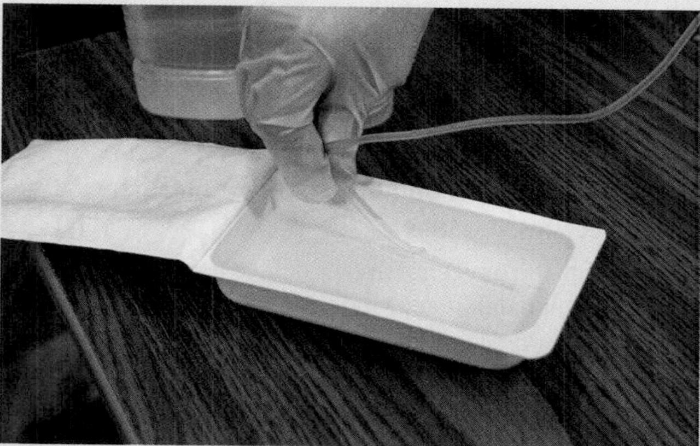

Figure 3. Dipping catheter into sterile saline.

(continued)

SKILL 14-3

Suctioning the Nasopharyngeal and Oropharyngeal Airways *(continued)*

ACTION / **RATIONALE**

14. Encourage the patient to take several deep breaths.

Suctioning removes air from the patient's airway and can cause hypoxemia. Hyperventilation can help prevent suction-induced hypoxemia.

15. Apply lubricant to the first 2″–3″ of the catheter, using the lubricant that was placed on the sterile field.

Lubricant facilitates passage of the catheter and reduces trauma to mucous membranes.

16. Remove the oxygen delivery device, if appropriate. Do not apply suction as the catheter is inserted. Hold the catheter between your thumb and forefinger.

Using suction while inserting the catheter can cause trauma to the mucosa and removes oxygen from the respiratory tract. Correct distance for insertion ensures proper placement of the catheter. The general guideline for determining insertion distance for nasopharyngeal suctioning for an individual patient is to estimate the distance from the patient's ear lobe to the nose.

For Nasopharyngeal Suctioning

Gently insert catheter through the naris and along the floor of the nostril toward trachea (Figure 4). Roll the catheter between your fingers to help advance it. Advance the catheter approximately 5″–6″ to reach the pharynx.

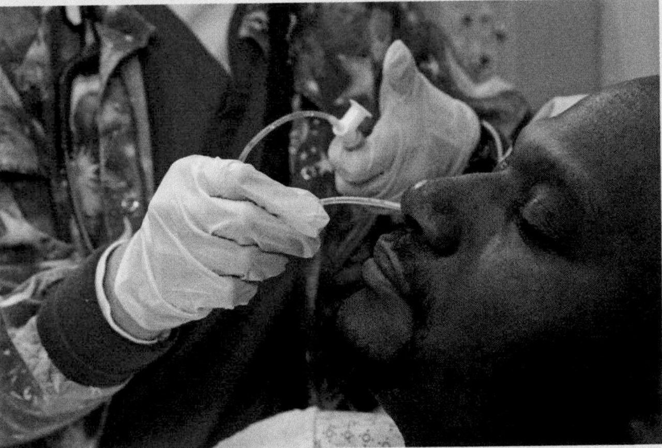

Figure 4. Inserting naris catheter into naris.

For Oropharyngeal Suctioning

Insert catheter through the mouth, along the side of the mouth toward trachea. Advance the catheter 3″–4″ to reach the pharynx. (For nasotracheal suctioning, see the accompanying Skill Variation display.)

17. Apply suction by intermittently occluding the Y port on the catheter with the thumb of your nondominant hand and gently rotate the catheter as it is being withdrawn (Figure 5). **Do not suction for more than 10 to 15 seconds at a time.**

Turning the catheter as it is withdrawn minimizes trauma to the mucosa. Suctioning for longer than 10 to 15 seconds robs the respiratory tract of oxygen, which may result in hypoxemia. Suctioning too quickly may be ineffective at clearing all secretions.

18. Replace the oxygen-delivery device using your nondominant hand, if appropriate, and have the patient take several deep breaths.

Suctioning removes air from the patient's airway and can cause hypoxemia. Hyperventilation can help prevent suction-induced hypoxemia.

19. Flush catheter with saline (Figure 6). Assess effectiveness of suctioning and repeat as needed and according to patient's tolerance.

Flushing clears catheter and lubricates it for next insertion. Reassessment determines need for additional suctioning.

SKILL 14-3

Suctioning the Nasopharyngeal and Oropharyngeal Airways *(continued)*

ACTION	RATIONALE
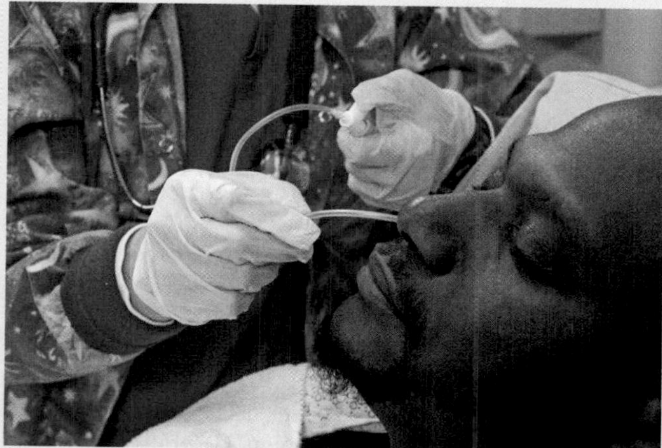 Figure 5. Suctioning nasopharynx.	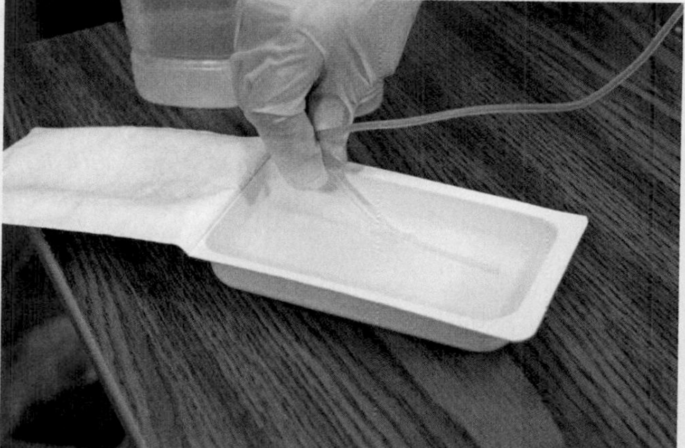 Figure 6. Rinsing catheter.
Wrap the suction catheter around your dominant hand between attempts.	Wrapping prevents inadvertent contamination of catheter.
20. **Allow at least a 30-seconds to 1-minute interval if additional suctioning is needed. No more than three suction passes should be made per suctioning episode. Alternate the nares, unless contraindicated, if repeated suctioning is required. Do not force catheter through the nares. Encourage patient to cough and deep breathe between suctioning.** Suction the oropharynx after suctioning the nasopharynx.	The interval allows for reventilation and reoxygenation of airways. Excessive suction passes contribute to complications. Alternating nares reduces trauma. Suctioning the oropharynx after the nasopharynx clears the mouth of secretions. More microorganisms are usually present in the mouth, so it is suctioned last to prevent transmission of contaminants.
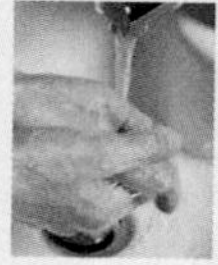 21. When suctioning is completed, remove gloves from dominant hand over the coiled catheter, pulling it off inside out. Remove glove from nondominant hand and dispose of gloves, catheter, and container with solution in the appropriate receptacle. Remove face shield or goggles and mask. Perform hand hygiene.	This technique reduces transmission of microorganisms. Hand hygiene prevents transmission of microorganisms.
22. Turn off suction. Remove supplemental oxygen placed for suctioning, if appropriate. Assist patient to a comfortable position. Raise bed rail.	Ensures patient comfort. Raising the bed rails helps maintain patient safety.
23. Offer oral hygiene after suctioning.	Respiratory secretions that are allowed to accumulate in the mouth are irritating to mucous membranes and unpleasant for the patient.
24. Reassess patient's respiratory status, including respiratory rate, effort, oxygen saturation, and lung sounds.	This assesses effectiveness of suctioning and the presence of complications.

EVALUATION

The expected outcome is met when the patient exhibits improved breath sounds and a clear and patent airway. In addition, the oxygen saturation level is within acceptable parameters, and the patient does not exhibit signs or symptoms of respiratory distress or complications.

(continued)

SKILL 14-3 Suctioning the Nasopharyngeal and Oropharyngeal Airways *(continued)*

DOCUMENTATION

Guidelines

Document the time of suctioning, your pre- and postintervention assessment, reason for suctioning, route used, and the characteristics and amount of secretions.

Sample Documentation

9/17/09 1440 Patient with gurgling on inspiration and weak cough; unable to clear secretions. Lungs with sonorous wheezes in upper airways. Nasopharyngeal suction completed with 12F catheter. Large amount of thick, yellow secretions obtained. After suctioning lung sounds clear in all lobes, respirations 18 breaths per min, no gurgling noted.—C. Bausler, RN

Unexpected Situations and Associated Interventions

- *The catheter or sterile glove touches an unsterile surface:* Stop the procedure. If the gloved hand is still sterile, ask call for assistance and have someone open another catheter, or remove the gloves and start the procedure over.
- *Patient vomits during suctioning:* If the patient gags or becomes nauseated, the catheter must be removed. It has probably inadvertently entered the esophagus. If the patient needs to be suctioned again, change catheters, as it is probably contaminated. Turn patient to the side and elevate the head of the bed to prevent aspiration.
- *Secretions appear to be stomach contents:* Ask the patient to extend the neck slightly. This helps to prevent the tube from passing into the esophagus.
- *Epistaxis is noted with continued suctioning:* Notify physician and anticipate the need for a nasal trumpet (see Skill 14-9). The nasal trumpet will protect the nasal mucosa from further trauma related to suctioning.

Special Considerations

Infant and Child Considerations

- For infants, use a 5 Fr to 6 Fr catheter
- For children, use a 6 Fr to 10 Fr catheter

SKILL VARIATION Nasotracheal Suctioning

Nasotracheal suctioning is indicated to maintain a patent airway and remove saliva, pulmonary secretions, blood, vomitus, or foreign material from the trachea. Tracheal suctioning can lead to hypoxemia, cardiac dysrhythmias, trauma, atelectasis, infection, bleeding, and pain. It is imperative to be diligent in maintaining aseptic technique and following facility guidelines and procedures to prevent potential hazards. To perform nasotracheal suctioning:

- Identify the patient.
- Determine the need for suctioning. For postoperative patient, administer pain medication before suctioning.
- Explain to the patient what you are going to do and the reason, even if the patient does not appear to be alert.
- Perform hand hygiene.
- Adjust bed to comfortable working position. Lower the side rail closer to you. **If patient is conscious, place him or her in a semi-Fowler's position. If patient is unconscious, place him or her in the lateral position, facing you.** Move overbed table close to your work area and raise to waist height.
- Place towel or waterproof pad across patient's chest.
- Turn suction to appropriate pressure. Put on a disposable, clean glove and occlude the end of the connecting tubing to check suction pressure. Place the connecting tubing in a convenient location.
- **Open sterile suction package using aseptic technique. The open wrapper becomes a sterile field to hold other supplies. Carefully remove the sterile container, touching only the outside surface. Set it up on the work surface and pour sterile saline into it.**
- Place a small amount of water-soluble lubricant on the sterile field, taking care to avoid touching the sterile field with the lubricant package.
- Increase the patient's supplemental oxygen level or apply supplemental oxygen per facility policy or physician order.
- Put on face shield or goggles and mask. Put on sterile gloves. **The dominant hand will manipulate the catheter and must remain sterile. The nondominant hand is considered clean rather than sterile and will control the suction valve.**
- With dominant gloved hand, pick up sterile catheter. Pick up the connecting tubing with the nondominant hand and connect the tubing and suction catheter.

SKILL 14-3 Suctioning the Nasopharyngeal and Oropharyngeal Airways *(continued)*

- Moisten the catheter by dipping it into the container of sterile saline. Occlude Y-tube to check suction.
- Encourage the patient to take several deep breaths.
- Apply lubricant to the first 2″–3″ of the catheter, using the lubricant that was placed on the sterile field.
- Remove the oxygen-delivery device, if appropriate. Do not apply suction as the catheter is inserted. Hold the catheter in your thumb and forefinger. Gently insert catheter through the naris and along the floor of the nostril toward trachea. Roll the catheter between your fingers to help advance it. Advance the catheter approximately 8″–9″ to reach the trachea. Resistance should not be met. If resistance is met, the carina or tracheal mucosa has been hit. Withdraw the catheter at least ½″ before applying suction.
- Apply suction by intermittently occluding the Y port on the catheter with the thumb of your nondominant hand, and gently rotate the catheter as it is being withdrawn. **Do not suction for more than 10 to 15 seconds at a time.**
- Replace the oxygen-delivery device using your nondominant hand and have the patient take several deep breaths.
- Flush catheter with saline. Assess effectiveness of suctioning and repeat as needed and according to patient's tolerance. Wrap the suction catheter around your dominant hand between attempts.
- **Allow at least a 30-seconds to 1-minute interval if additional suctioning is needed. No more than three suction passes should be made per suctioning episode. Alternate the nares, unless contraindicated, if repeated suctioning is required. Do not force catheter through the nares. Encourage patient to cough and deep breathe between suctioning. Suction the oropharynx after suctioning the trachea.**
- When suctioning is completed, remove glove from dominant hand over the coiled catheter, pulling it off inside out. Remove glove from nondominant hand and dispose of gloves, catheter, and container with solution in the appropriate receptacle. Remove face shield or goggles and mask. Perform hand hygiene.
- Turn off suction. Remove supplemental oxygen placed for suctioning, if appropriate. Assist patient to a comfortable position.
- Offer oral hygiene after suctioning.
- Reassess patient's respiratory status, including respiratory rate, effort, oxygen saturation, and lung sounds.
- Document the time of suctioning, your pre- and post-intervention assessment, the reason for suctioning, route used, and the characteristics and amount of secretions.

SKILL 14-4 Administering Oxygen by Nasal Cannula

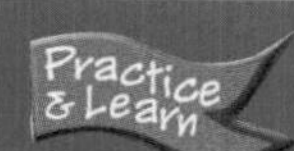

There are a variety of devices for delivering oxygen to the patient. Each has a specific function and oxygen concentration. Device selection is based on the patient's condition and oxygen needs. A nasal cannula, also called nasal prongs, is the most commonly used oxygen-delivery device. The cannula is a disposable plastic device with two protruding prongs for insertion into the nostrils. The cannula connects to an oxygen source with a flow meter and, many times, a humidifier. It is commonly used because the cannula does not impede eating or speaking and is easily used in the home. Disadvantages of this system are that it can easily be dislodged and can cause dryness of the nasal mucosa. A nasal cannula is used to deliver from 1 L per minute to 6 L per minute of oxygen. Table 14-1 compares amounts of delivered oxygen for these flow rates.

Equipment

- Flow meter connected to oxygen supply
- Humidifier with sterile distilled water (optional for low-flow system)
- Nasal cannula and tubing
- Gauze to pad tubing over ears (optional)

ASSESSMENT

Assess patient's oxygen saturation level before starting oxygen therapy to provide a baseline for evaluating the effectiveness of oxygen therapy. Assess patient's respiratory status, including respiratory rate, effort, and lung sounds. Note any signs of respiratory distress, such as tachypnea, nasal flaring, use of accessory muscles, or dyspnea.

(continued)

SKILL 14-4 Administering Oxygen by Nasal Cannula *(continued)*

TABLE 14-1 Oxygen Delivery Systems

METHOD	AMOUNT DELIVERED FiO_2 (FRACTION INSPIRED OXYGEN)	PRIORITY NURSING INTERVENTIONS
Nasal cannula	*Low Flow* 1 L/min = 24% 2 L/min = 28% 3 L/min = 32% 4 L/min = 36% 5 L/min = 40% 6 L/min = 44%	Check frequently that both prongs are in patient's nares. Never deliver more than 2–3 L/min to patient with chronic lung disease.
Simple mask	*Low Flow* 6–10 L/min = 35%–60% (5 L/min is minimum setting)	Monitor patient frequently to check placement of the mask. Support patient if claustrophobia is concern. Secure physician's order to replace mask with nasal cannula during meal time.
Partial rebreather mask	*Low Flow* 6–15 L/min = 70%–90%	Set flow rate so that mask remains two thirds full during inspiration. Keep reservoir bag free of twists or kinks.
Nonrebreather mask	*Low Flow* 6–15 L/min = 60%–100%	Maintain flow rate so reservoir bag collapses only slightly during inspiration. Check that valves and rubber flaps are functioning properly (open during expiration and closed during inhalation). Monitor SaO_2 with pulse oximeter.
Venturi mask	*High Flow* 4–10 L/min = 24%–55%	Requires careful monitoring to verify FiO_2 at flow rate ordered. Check that air intake valves are not blocked.

NURSING DIAGNOSIS

Determine the related factors for the nursing diagnosis based on the patient's current status. Appropriate nursing diagnoses may include:

- Impaired Gas Exchange
- Ineffective Breathing Pattern
- Ineffective Airway Clearance

Other nursing diagnoses that may be appropriate include:

- Risk for Activity Intolerance
- Decreased Cardiac Output
- Excess Fluid Volume

OUTCOME IDENTIFICATION AND PLANNING

The expected outcome is that the patient will exhibit an oxygen saturation level within acceptable parameters. Other outcomes that may be appropriate include the following: patient will not experience dyspnea; and patient will demonstrate effortless respirations in the normal range for age group, without evidence of nasal flaring or use of accessory muscles.

IMPLEMENTATION

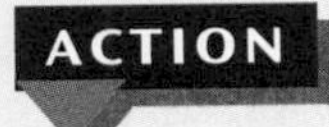

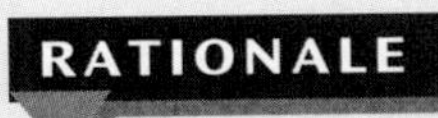

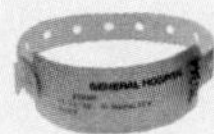

ACTION	RATIONALE
1. Identify the patient using at least two methods.	Positive identification of the patient is essential to ensure the intervention is administered to the correct patient.

SKILL 14-4 Administering Oxygen by Nasal Cannula *(continued)*

ACTION	RATIONALE
2. Explain what you are going to do and the reason to the patient. Review safety precautions necessary when oxygen is in use. Place "No Smoking" signs in appropriate areas.	Explanation relieves anxiety and facilitates cooperation. Oxygen supports combustion.
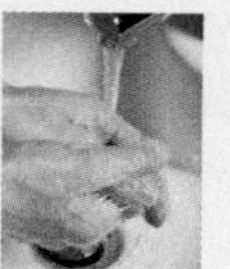 3. Perform hand hygiene.	Hand hygiene deters the spread of microorganisms.
4. **Connect nasal cannula to oxygen setup with humidification, if one is in use (Figure 1).** Adjust flow rate as ordered by physician (Figure 2). Check that oxygen is flowing out of prongs.	Oxygen forced through a water reservoir is humidified before it is delivered to the patient, thus preventing dehydration of the mucous membranes. Low-flow oxygen does not require humidification.

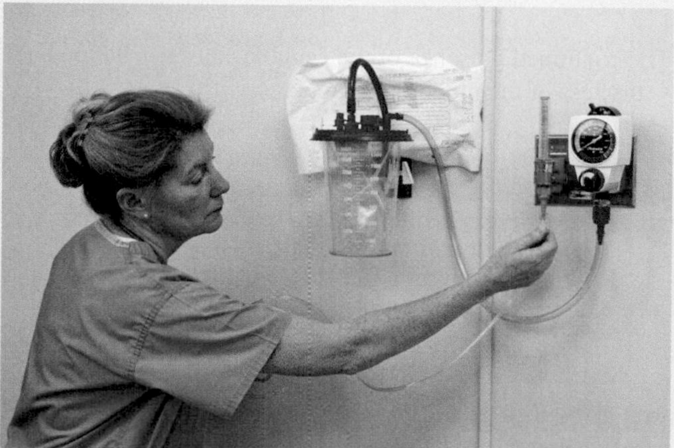
Figure 1. Connecting cannula to oxygen source.

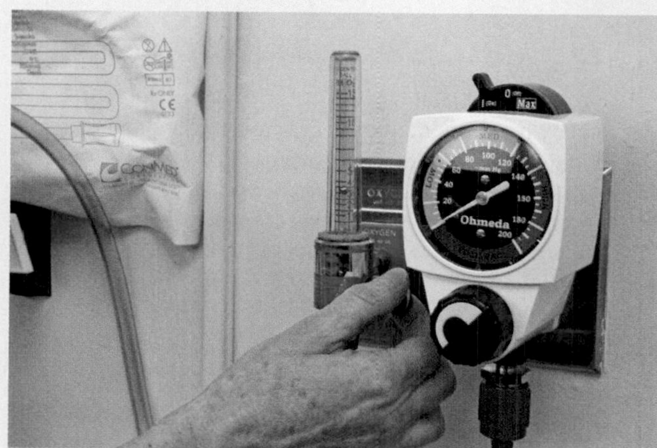

Figure 2. Adjusting flow rate.

ACTION	RATIONALE
5. Place prongs in patient's nostrils (Figure 3). Place tubing over and behind each ear with adjuster comfortably under chin or around the patient's head, with adjuster at the back of the head or neck. Place gauze pads at ear beneath the tubing as necessary (Figure 4).	Correct placement of the prongs and fastener facilitates oxygen administration and patient comfort. Pads reduce irritation and pressure and protect the skin.

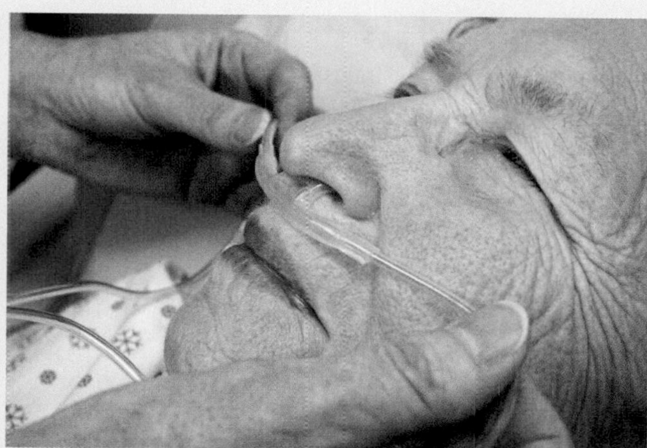
Figure 3. Applying cannula to nares.

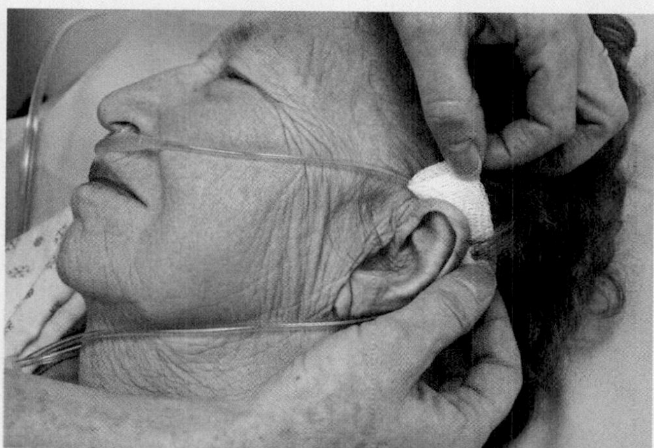
Figure 4. Placing gauze pad at ears.

(continued)

SKILL 14-4 Administering Oxygen by Nasal Cannula *(continued)*

ACTION	RATIONALE
6. Adjust the fit of the cannula as necessary (Figure 5). Tubing should be snug but not tight against the skin.	Proper adjustment maintains the prongs in the patient's nose. Excessive pressure from tubing could cause irritation and pressure to the skin.
7. **Encourage patient to breathe through the nose, with mouth closed.**	Nose breathing provides for optimal delivery of oxygen to patient. The percentage of oxygen delivered can be reduced in patients who breathe through the mouth.
8. Reassess patient's respiratory status, including respiratory rate, effort, and lung sounds. Note any signs of respiratory distress, such as tachypnea, nasal flaring, use of accessory muscles, or dyspnea.	These assess the effectiveness of oxygen therapy.
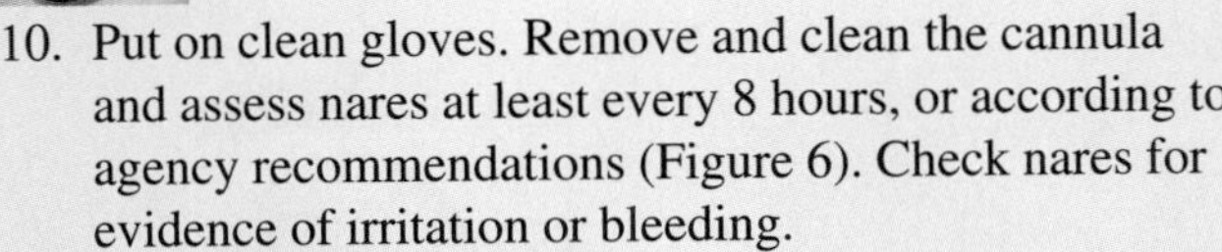 9. Perform hand hygiene.	Hand hygiene deters the spread of microorganisms.
10. Put on clean gloves. Remove and clean the cannula and assess nares at least every 8 hours, or according to agency recommendations (Figure 6). Check nares for evidence of irritation or bleeding.	The continued presence of the cannula causes irritation and dryness of the mucous membranes.

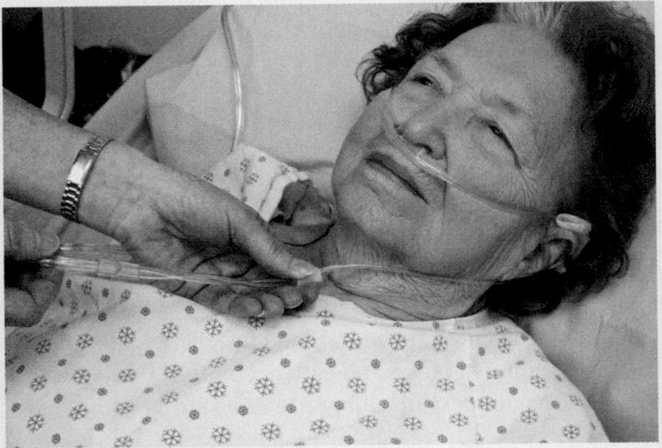

Figure 5. Adjusting cannula if needed.

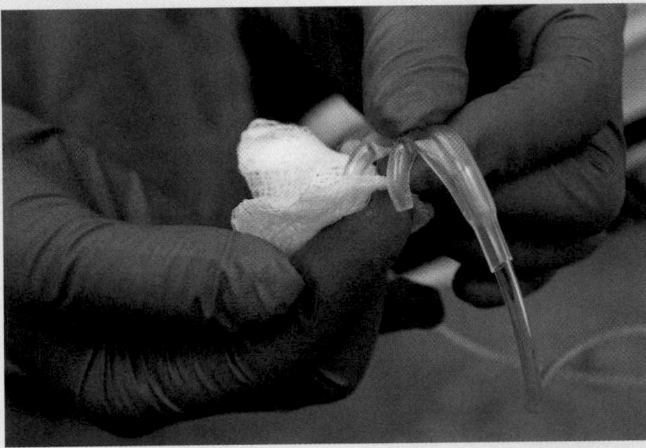

Figure 6. Cleaning cannula when indicated.

EVALUATION

The expected outcome is met when the patient demonstrates an oxygen saturation level within acceptable parameters. In addition, the patient remains free of dyspnea, nasal flaring, or accessory muscle use and demonstrates respiratory rate and depth within normal ranges.

DOCUMENTATION

Guidelines

Document your assessment pre- and postintervention. Document the amount of oxygen applied, the patient's respiratory rate, oxygen saturation, and lung sounds.

SKILL 14-4 Administering Oxygen by Nasal Cannula *(continued)*

Sample Documentation

9/17/08 1300 Oxygen via nasal cannula applied at 2 L/min. Humidification in place. Pulse oximeter before placing oxygen 92%; after oxygen at 2 L/min 98%. Respirations even and unlabored. Chest rises symmetrically. No nasal flaring or retractions noted. Lung sounds clear and equal all lobes.—C. Bausler, RN

Unexpected Situations and Associated Interventions

- *Patient was fine on oxygen delivered by nasal cannula but now is cyanotic, and the pulse oximeter reading is <93%:* Check to see that the oxygen tubing is still connected to the flow meter and the flow meter is still on the previous setting. Someone may have stepped on the tubing, pulling it from the flow meter, or the oxygen may have accidentally been turned off. Assess lung sounds to note any changes.
- *Areas over ear or back of head are reddened:* Ensure that areas are adequately padded and that tubing is not pulled too tight. If available, a skin care team may be able to offer some suggestions.
- *When dozing, patient begins to breathe through the mouth:* Temporarily place the nasal cannula near the mouth. If this does not raise the pulse oximeter reading, you may need to obtain an order to switch the patient to a mask while sleeping.

Special Considerations

Home Care Considerations

- Oxygen administration may need to be continued in the home setting. Portable oxygen concentrators are used most frequently. Caregivers require instruction concerning safety precautions with oxygen use and need to understand the rationale for the specific liter flow of oxygen.
- To prevent fires and injuries, take the following precautions:
  - Avoid open flames
  - Place "No Smoking" signs in conspicuous places in the patient's home. Instruct the patient and visitors about the hazard of smoking when oxygen is in use.
  - Check to see that electrical equipment used in the room is in good working order and emits no sparks.
  - Avoid using oils in the area. Oil can ignite spontaneously in the presence of oxygen.

SKILL 14-5 Administering Oxygen by Mask

When a patient requires a higher concentration of oxygen than a nasal cannula can deliver (6 L or 44% oxygen concentration), an oxygen mask is used (See Table 14-1 in Skill 14-4 for a comparison of different types of oxygen delivery systems). The mask is fitted carefully to the patient's face to avoid leakage of oxygen and should be comfortably snug but not tight against the face. Disposable and reusable face masks are available. The most commonly used types of masks are the simple face mask, the partial rebreather mask, the nonrebreather mask, and the Venturi mask. Figure 1 illustrates different types of oxygen masks.

(continued)

SKILL 14-5 Administering Oxygen by Mask *(continued)*

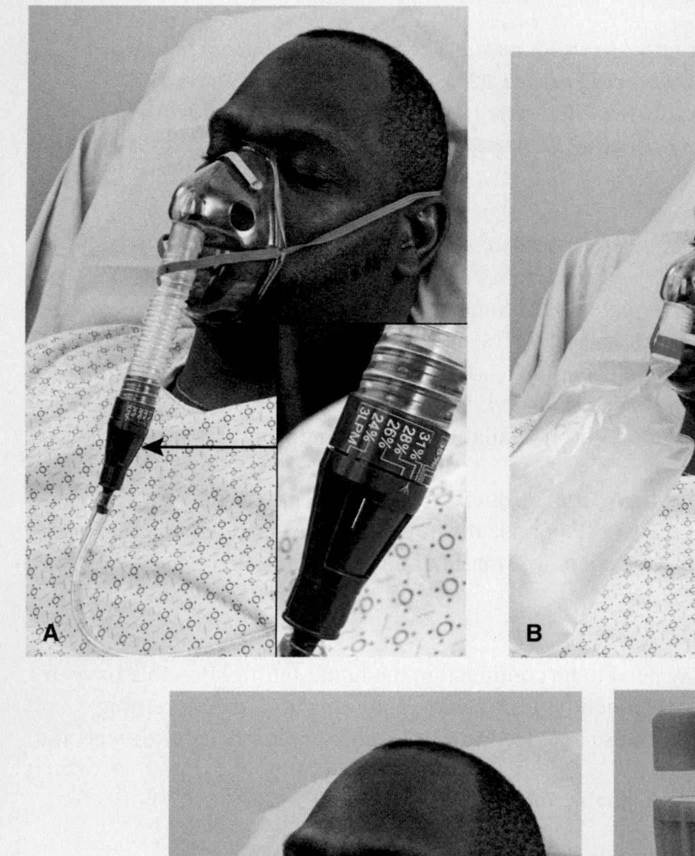

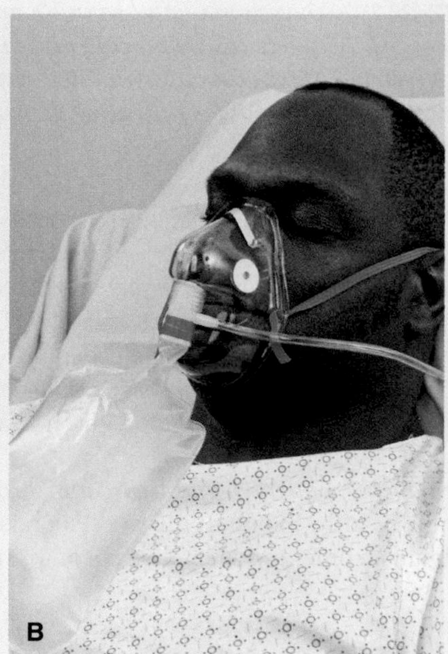

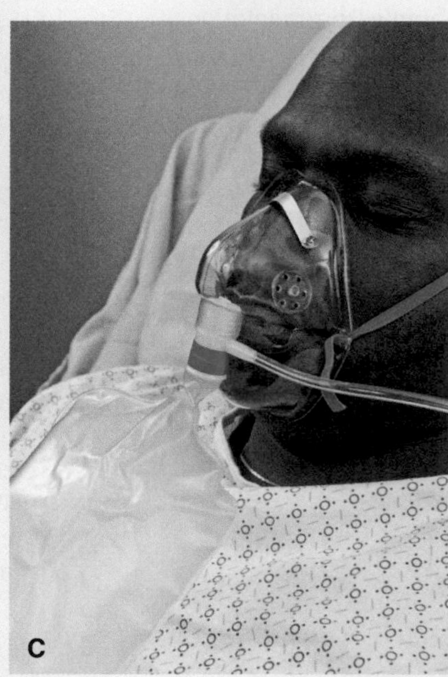

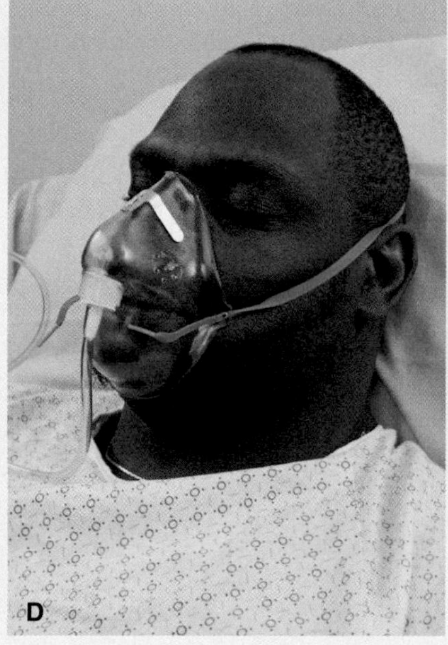

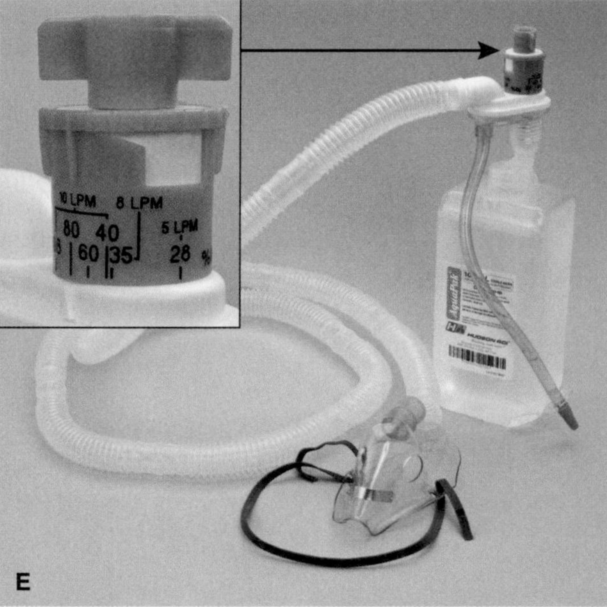

Figure 1. Types of oxygen masks. (**A**) Venturi mask. (**B**) Nonrebreather mask. (**C**) Partial rebreather mask. (**D**) Simple face mask. (**E**) High-flow oxygen face mask and bottle.

Equipment

- Flow meter connected to oxygen supply
- Humidifier with sterile distilled water, if necessary for the type of mask prescribed
- Face mask, specified by physician
- Gauze to pad elastic band (optional)

ASSESSMENT

Assess patient's oxygen saturation level before starting oxygen therapy to provide a baseline for determining the effectiveness of therapy. Assess patient's respiratory status, including respiratory rate and depth and lung sounds. Note any signs of respiratory distress, such as tachypnea, nasal flaring, use of accessory muscles, or dyspnea.

SKILL 14-5 Administering Oxygen by Mask *(continued)*

NURSING DIAGNOSIS

Determine the related factors for the nursing diagnosis based on the patient's current status. Appropriate nursing diagnoses may include:

- Impaired Gas Exchange
- Ineffective Breathing Pattern
- Ineffective Airway Clearance

Many other nursing diagnoses may be appropriate, possibly including:

- Risk for Activity Intolerance
- Decreased Cardiac Output
- Excess Fluid Volume

OUTCOME IDENTIFICATION AND PLANNING

The expected outcome is that patient exhibits an oxygen saturation level within acceptable parameters. Other outcomes that may be appropriate include the following: patient will remain free of signs and symptoms of respiratory distress; and respiratory status, including respiratory rate and depth, will be in the normal range for the patient's age.

IMPLEMENTATION

ACTION	RATIONALE
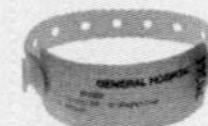 1. Identify the patient.	Positive identification of the patient is essential to ensure the intervention is administered to the correct patient.
2. Explain what you are going to do and the reason to the patient. Review safety precautions necessary when oxygen is in use. Place "No Smoking" signs in appropriate areas.	Explanation relieves anxiety and facilitates cooperation. Oxygen supports combustion.
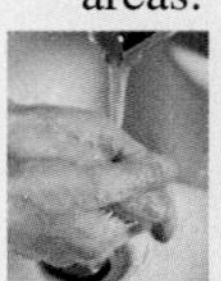 3. Perform hand hygiene.	Hand hygiene deters the spread of microorganisms.
4. Attach face mask to oxygen source (with humidification, if appropriate for the specific mask) (Figure 2). Start the flow of oxygen at the specified rate. For a mask with a reservoir, be sure to allow oxygen to fill the bag (Figure 3) before proceeding to the next step.	Oxygen forced through a water reservoir is humidified before it is delivered to the patient, thus preventing dehydration of the mucous membranes. A reservoir bag must be inflated with oxygen because the bag is the source of oxygen supply for the patient.
5. Position face mask over patient's nose and mouth (Figure 4). Adjust the elastic strap so that the mask fits snugly but comfortably on the face (Figure 5). Adjust the flow rate to the prescribed rate (Figure 6).	A loose or poorly fitting mask will result in oxygen loss and decreased therapeutic value. Masks may cause a feeling of suffocation, and the patient needs frequent attention and reassurance.
6. If the patient reports irritation or redness is noted, use gauze pads under the elastic strap at pressure points to reduce irritation to ears and scalp.	Pads reduce irritation and pressure and protect the skin.
7. Reassess patient's respiratory status, including respiratory rate, effort, and lung sounds. Note any signs of respiratory distress, such as tachypnea, nasal flaring, use of accessory muscles, or dyspnea.	This helps assess the effectiveness of oxygen therapy.

(continued)

SKILL 14-5 Administering Oxygen by Mask *(continued)*

ACTION | **RATIONALE**

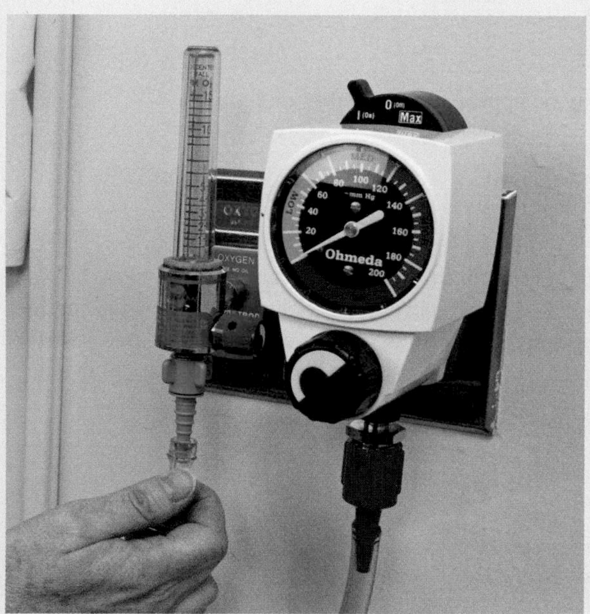

Figure 2. Connecting face mask to oxygen source.

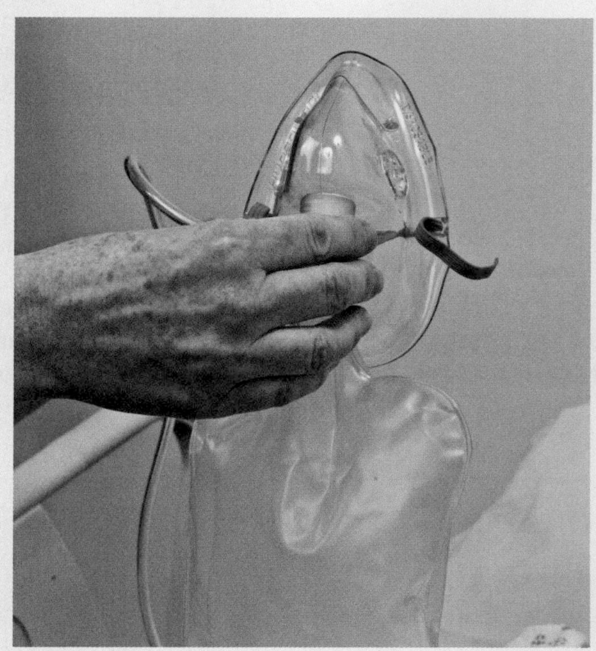

Figure 3. Allowing oxygen to fill the bag.

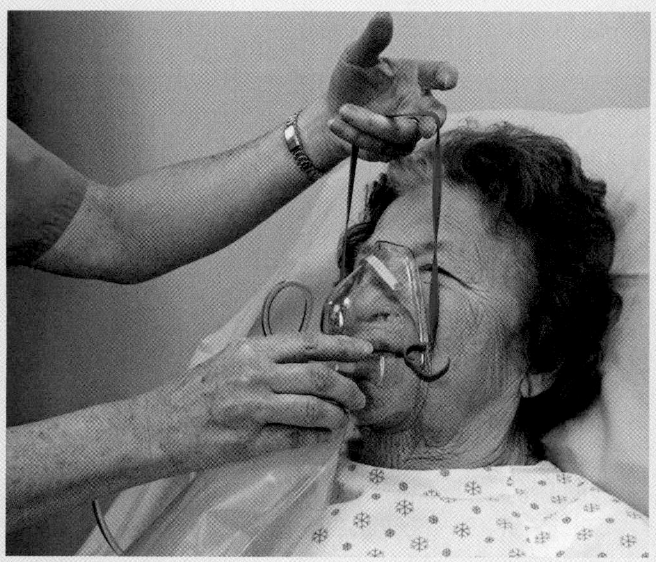

Figure 4. Applying face mask over nose and mouth.

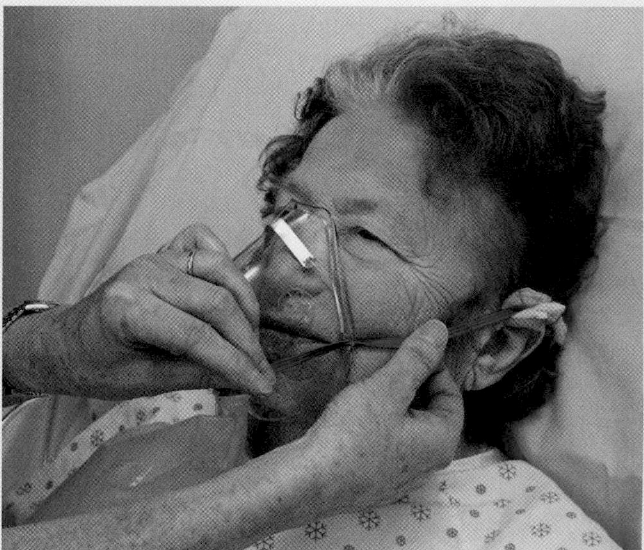

Figure 5. Adjusting elastic straps.

SKILL 14-5

Administering Oxygen by Mask *(continued)*

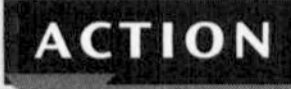
ACTION

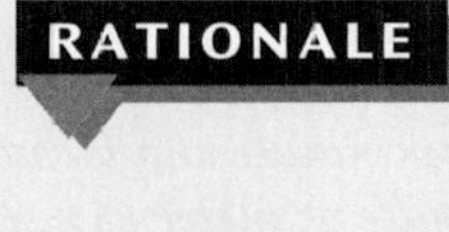
RATIONALE

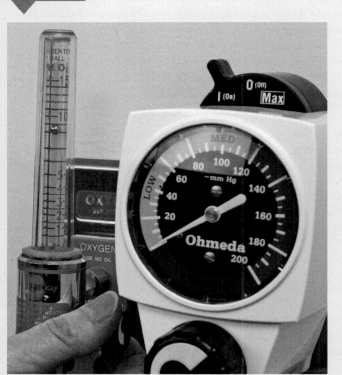

Figure 6. Adjusting flow rate.

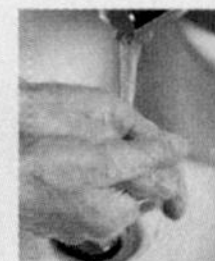

8. Perform hand hygiene. — Hand hygiene deters the spread of microorganisms.

9. **Remove the mask and dry the skin every 2 to 3 hours if the oxygen is running continuously. Do not use powder around the mask.** — The tight-fitting mask and moisture from condensation can irritate the skin on the face. There is a danger of inhaling powder if it is placed on the mask.

EVALUATION

The expected outcome is met when the patient exhibits an oxygen saturation level within acceptable parameters. In addition, the patient demonstrates an absence of respiratory distress and accessory muscle use and exhibits respiratory rate and depth within normal parameters.

DOCUMENTATION

Guidelines

Document type of mask used, amount of oxygen used, oxygen saturation level, lung sounds, and rate/pattern of respirations. Document your assessment pre- and postintervention.

(continued)

SKILL 14-5 Administering Oxygen by Mask *(continued)*

Sample Documentation

9/22/08 Patient reports feeling short of breath. Skin pale. Respirations 30 breaths per minute and labored. Lung sounds decreased throughout. Oxygen saturation via pulse oximeter 88%. Findings reported to Dr. Lu. Oxygen via nonrebreather face mask applied at 12 L/min as ordered. Patient's skin is pink after O_2 applied. Oxygen saturation increased to 98%. Respirations even and unlabored. Chest rises symmetrically. Respiratory rate 18 breaths per min. Lungs remain with decreased breath sounds throughout. Patient denies dyspnea.—C. Bausler, RN

Unexpected Situations and Associated Interventions

- *Patient was previously fine but now is cyanotic, and the pulse oximeter reading is <93%:* Check to see that the oxygen tubing is still connected to the flow meter and the flow meter is still on the previous setting. Someone may have stepped on the tubing, pulling it from the flow meter, or the oxygen may have accidentally been turned off. Assess lung sounds for any changes.
- *Areas over ear or back of head are reddened:* Ensure that areas are adequately padded and that tubing is not pulled too tight. If available, a skin-care team may be able to offer some suggestions.

Special Considerations

General Considerations

- Different types of face masks are available for use (Refer to Table 14-1 in Skill 14-3 for more information).
- It's important to ensure the mask fits snugly around the patient's face. If it's loose, it will not effectively deliver the right amount of oxygen.
- The mask must be removed for the patient to eat, drink, and take medications. Obtain an order for oxygen via nasal cannula for use during meal times and limit the amount of time the mask is removed to maintain adequate oxygenation.

SKILL 14-6 Using an Oxygen Hood

Oxygen hoods are generally used to deliver oxygen to infants. They supply an oxygen concentration that is almost 100%. The oxygen hood is placed over the infant's head and shoulders. The hoods are made of hard plastic or vinyl with a metal frame.

Equipment

- Oxygen source
- Oxygen hood
- Oxygen analyzer
- Humidification device

ASSESSMENT

Assess the patient's lung sounds. Many respiratory conditions may cause the patient's oxygen demand to increase. Assess the oxygen saturation level. The physician will usually order a baseline for the pulse oximeter (ie, deliver oxygen to keep pulse ox >95%). Assess skin color. A pale or cyanotic patient may not be receiving enough oxygen. Assess patient for any signs of respiratory distress such as nasal flaring, grunting, or retractions; oxygen-depleted patients often exhibit these signs.

NURSING DIAGNOSIS

Determine the related factors for the nursing diagnosis based on the patient's current status. Appropriate nursing diagnoses may include:

- Impaired Gas Exchange
- Ineffective Breathing Pattern
- Ineffective Airway Clearance

SKILL 14-6 Using an Oxygen Hood *(continued)*

Other nursing diagnoses may be appropriate, including:

- Risk for Activity Intolerance
- Decreased Cardiac Output
- Excess Fluid Volume
- Risk for Impaired Skin Integrity

OUTCOME IDENTIFICATION AND PLANNING

The expected outcome to achieve when administering oxygen via hood is that the patient exhibits an oxygen saturation level within acceptable parameters. Other outcomes that may be appropriate include the following: patient will remain free of signs and symptoms of respiratory distress; respiratory status, including respiratory rate and depth, will be in the normal range for the patient's age; and patient's skin will be pink, dry, and without evidence of breakdown.

IMPLEMENTATION

ACTION	RATIONALE
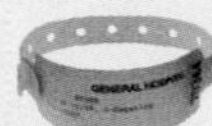 1. Identify the patient.	Positive identification of the patient is essential to ensure the intervention is administered to the correct patient.
2. Explain what you are going to do and the reason to the patient and parents/guardians. Review safety precautions necessary when oxygen is in use.	Explanation relieves anxiety and facilitates cooperation. Oxygen supports combustion.
3. Perform hand hygiene.	Hand hygiene deters the spread of microorganisms.
4. Calibrate the oxygen analyzer according to manufacturer's directions.	This ensures accurate readings and appropriate adjustments to therapy.
5. Place hood on crib. Connect humidifier to oxygen source in the wall. Connect the oxygen tubing to the hood. Adjust flow rate as ordered by physician. Check that oxygen is flowing into hood.	Oxygen forced through a water reservoir is humidified before it is delivered to the patient, thus preventing dehydration of the mucous membranes.
6. Turn analyzer on. **Place oxygen analyzer probe in hood.**	The analyzer will give an accurate reading of the concentration of oxygen in the hood or bed.
7. Adjust oxygen flow as necessary, based on sensor readings (Figure 1). Once oxygen levels reach the prescribed amount, place hood over patient's head (Figure 2). The hood should not rub against the infant's neck, chin, or shoulder.	Patient will receive oxygen once placed under the hood. Pressure and irritation could result in alterations in the infant's skin integrity.
8. If using the soft vinyl hood, roll small blankets or towels and place around edges where hood meets crib (if needed) to keep oxygen concentration at desired level. **Do not block hole in top of hood if present. If using a vinyl hood, the vent hole covering may need to be removed.**	The blankets help keep the edges of the hood sealed and prevent oxygen from escaping. This hole allows for the escape of carbon dioxide; blocking it may cause a buildup of carbon dioxide in the hood.
9. Instruct family members not to raise edges of the hood.	Every time the hood is raised, oxygen is released.
10. Reassess patient's respiratory status, including respiratory rate, effort, oxygen saturation, and lung sounds. Note any signs of respiratory distress, such as tachypnea, nasal flaring, grunting, retractions, or dyspnea.	This assesses the effectiveness of oxygen therapy.

(continued)

SKILL 14-6 Using an Oxygen Hood *(continued)*

ACTION | **RATIONALE**

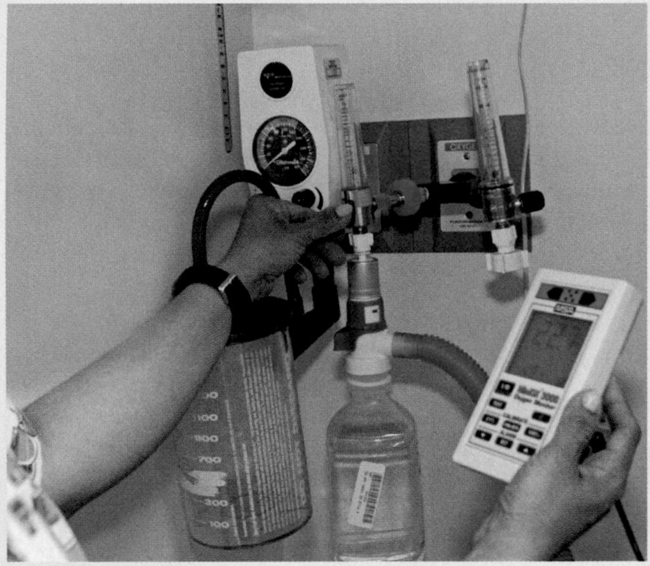

Figure 1. Adjusting oxygen based on sensor readings.

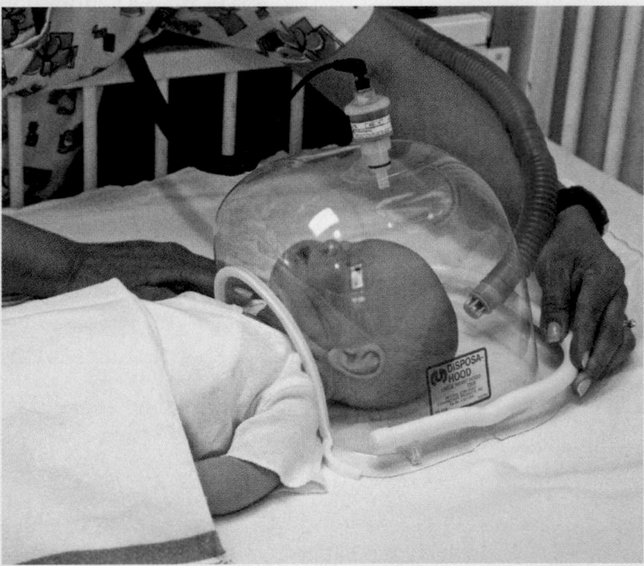

Figure 2. Placing oxygen hood over infant.

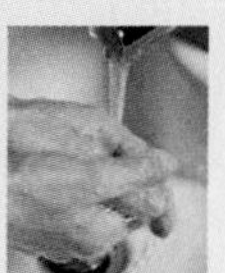

11. Perform hand hygiene.

Hand hygiene deters the spread of microorganisms.

12. Frequently check bedding and patient's head for moisture.

The humidification delivered in an oxygen hood makes cloth moist, which would be uncomfortable for the patient.

13. Monitor the patient's body temperature at regular intervals.

Hypothermia can result from administering cool oxygen.

EVALUATION

The expected outcome is met when the patient exhibits an oxygen saturation level within acceptable parameters. In addition, the patient remains free of dyspnea, nasal flaring, grunting, or use of accessory muscles when breathing, and respirations remain in normal range for age.

DOCUMENTATION

Guidelines

Document amount of oxygen applied, respiratory rate, oxygen saturation level, and your assessment pre- and postintervention.

Sample Documentation

9/17/09 Patient placed under oxygen hood at 35%. Pulse oximeter reading before placing under hood at 92%; increased to 99% after hood placement. Respirations even, unlabored, and symmetrical. No nasal flaring or retractions noted. Lung sounds clear and equal all lobes.—C. Bausler, RN

SKILL 14-6 Using an Oxygen Hood *(continued)*

Unexpected Situations and Associated Interventions

- *It is difficult to maintain oxygen at desired level:* Ensure that edges of hood are in contact with crib pad. If necessary, roll small blankets or towels and put around edges to prevent escape of oxygen. If you need to reach the baby's head for medication administration, feedings, and so forth, perform procedures together so that the hood remains in place for longer consecutive periods of time. Consider recalibrating the analyzer according to the manufacturer's directions.

SKILL 14-7 Using an Oxygen Tent

Oxygen tents are often used in children who will not leave a face mask or nasal cannula in place. The oxygen tent gives the patient freedom to move in the bed or crib while humidified oxygen is being delivered; however, it is difficult to keep the tent closed, since the child may want contact with his or her parents. It is also difficult to maintain a consistent level of oxygen and to deliver oxygen at a higher rate than 30% to 50%. Frequent assessment of the child's pajamas and bedding is necessary because the humidification quickly creates moisture, leading to damp clothing and linens, and possible hypothermia.

Equipment

- Oxygen source
- Oxygen tent
- Humidifier compatible with tent
- Oxygen analyzer
- Small blankets for blanket rolls

ASSESSMENT

Assess the patient's lung sounds. Secretions may cause the patient's oxygen demand to increase. Assess the oxygen saturation level. The physician will usually order a baseline for the pulse oximeter (ie, deliver oxygen to keep pulse ox >95%). Assess skin color. A pale or cyanotic patient may not be receiving enough oxygen. Assess patient for any signs of respiratory distress such as nasal flaring, grunting, or retractions; oxygen-depleted patients often exhibit these signs.

NURSING DIAGNOSIS

Determine the related factors for the nursing diagnosis based on the patient's current status. Appropriate nursing diagnoses may include:

- Impaired Gas Exchange
- Ineffective Breathing Pattern
- Ineffective Airway Clearance

Many other nursing diagnoses may be appropriate, possibly including:

- Risk for Activity Intolerance
- Decreased Cardiac Output
- Excess Fluid Volume
- Risk for Impaired Skin Integrity

OUTCOME IDENTIFICATION AND PLANNING

The expected outcome is that the patient exhibits an oxygen saturation level within acceptable parameters. Other outcomes that may be appropriate include the following: patient will remain free of signs and symptoms of respiratory distress; respiratory status, including respiratory rate and depth, will be in the normal range for the patient's age; and patient's skin will be pink, dry, and without evidence of breakdown.

(continued)

SKILL 14-7 Using an Oxygen Tent *(continued)*

IMPLEMENTATION

ACTION	RATIONALE
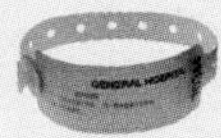 1. Identify the patient.	Positive identification of the patient is essential to ensure the intervention is administered to the correct patient.
2. Explain what you are going to do and the reason to the patient and parents/guardians. Review safety precautions necessary when oxygen is in use.	Explanation relieves anxiety and facilitates cooperation. Oxygen supports combustion.
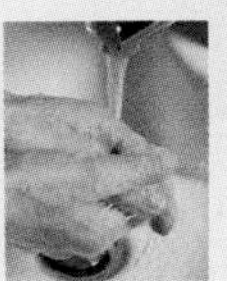 3. Perform hand hygiene.	Hand hygiene deters the spread of microorganisms.
4. Calibrate the oxygen analyzer according to manufacturer's directions.	Ensures accurate readings and appropriate adjustments to therapy.
5. Place tent over crib or bed. Connect the humidifier to the oxygen source in the wall and connect the tent tubing to the humidifier. Adjust flow rate as ordered by physician. Check that oxygen is flowing into tent.	Oxygen forced through a water reservoir is humidified before it is delivered to the patient, thus preventing dehydration of the mucous membranes.
6. Turn analyzer on. Place oxygen analyzer probe in tent, out of patient's reach.	The analyzer will give an accurate reading of the concentration of oxygen in the crib or bed.
7. Adjust oxygen as necessary, based on sensor readings (Figure 1). Once oxygen levels reach the prescribed amount, place patient in the tent (Figure 2).	Patient will receive oxygen once placed in the tent.

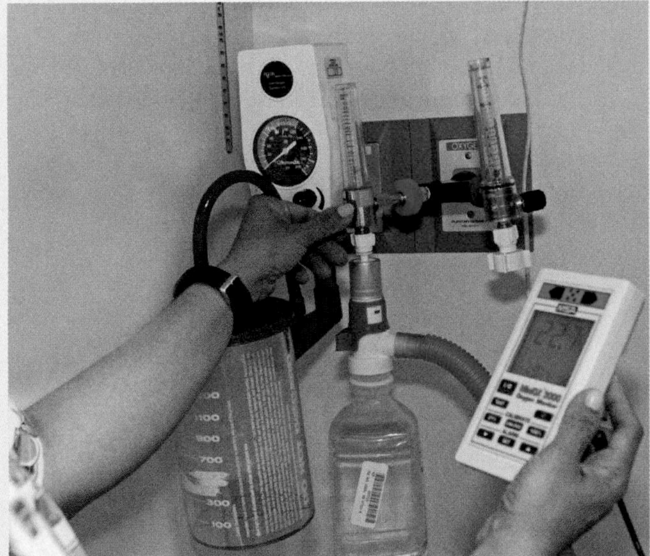

Figure 1. Adjusting oxygen flow.

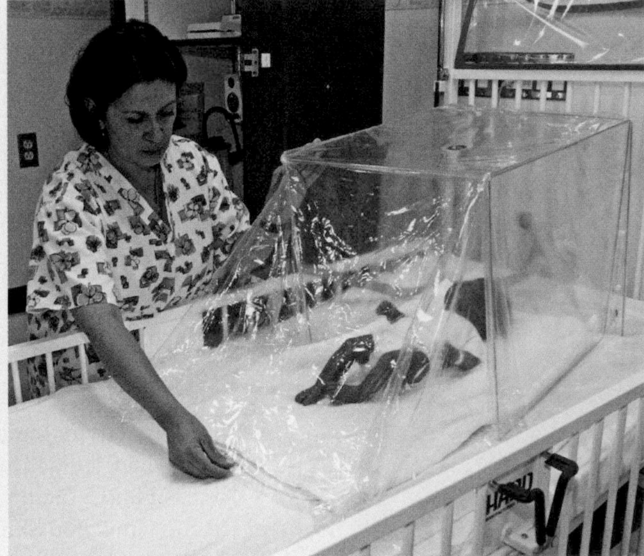

Figure 2. Placing patient in the tent.

ACTION	RATIONALE
8. Roll small blankets like a jelly roll and tuck tent edges under blanket rolls, as necessary. (Figure 3).	The blanket helps keep the edges of the tent flap from coming up and letting oxygen out.

SKILL 14-7 Using an Oxygen Tent *(continued)*

ACTION	RATIONALE
9. **Encourage patient and family members to keep tent flap closed.**	Every time the tent flap is opened, oxygen is released.

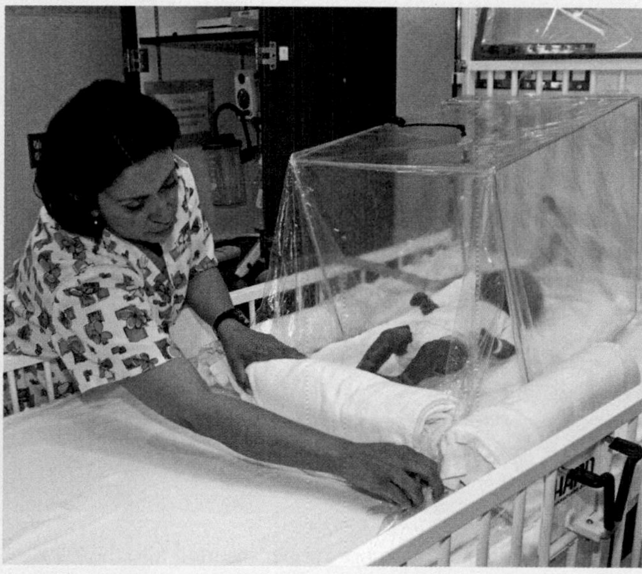

Figure 3. Tucking edges under blanket rolls.

ACTION	RATIONALE
10. Reassess patient's respiratory status, including respiratory rate, effort, and lung sounds. Note any signs of respiratory distress, such as tachypnea, nasal flaring, use of accessory muscles, grunting, retractions, or dyspnea.	This assesses the effectiveness of oxygen therapy.
11. Perform hand hygiene.	Hand hygiene deters the spread of microorganisms.
12. Frequently check bedding and patient's pajamas for moisture.	The large amount of humidification delivered in an oxygen tent quickly makes cloth moist, which would be uncomfortable for the patient.

EVALUATION

The expected outcome is met when the patient exhibits an oxygen saturation level within acceptable parameters. In addition, the patient remains free of dyspnea, nasal flaring, grunting, or use of accessory muscles when breathing; and respirations remain in normal range for age.

DOCUMENTATION

Guidelines

Document amount of oxygen applied, respiratory rate, oxygen saturation level, and your assessment pre- and postintervention.

(continued)

SKILL 14-7 Using an Oxygen Tent *(continued)*

Sample Documentation

9/17/08 Patient noted to have nasal flaring and grunting. Lung sounds clear and equal. Pulse oximeter reading 92%. Patient placed in oxygen tent at 45% per standing order. Pulse oximeter reading increased to 98% after placing in tent. Respirations even, unlabored, and symmetric. No nasal flaring or retractions noted. Lung sounds clear and equal all lobes.—C. Bausler, RN

Unexpected Situations and Associated Interventions

- *Child refuses to stay in tent:* Parent may play games in tent with child if this will help child to stay in tent. Alternative methods of oxygen delivery may need to be considered if child still refuses to stay in tent.
- *It is difficult to maintain an oxygen level above 40% in the tent:* Ensure that flap is closed and edges of tent are tucked under blanket. Check oxygen delivery unit to ensure that the rate has not been changed. Encourage patient to leave flaps closed. If still a problem, analyzer may need to be replaced or recalibrated.

SKILL 14-8 Inserting an Oropharyngeal Airway

An oropharyngeal airway is a semicircular tube of plastic or rubber inserted into the back of the pharynx through the mouth in a patient who is breathing spontaneously. The oropharyngeal airway can help protect the airway of an unconscious patient by preventing the tongue from falling back against the posterior pharynx and blocking it. Once the patient regains consciousness, the oropharyngeal airway is removed. Tape is not used to hold the airway in place because the patient should be able to expel the airway once he or she becomes alert. The nurse can insert this device at the bedside with little to no trauma to the unconscious patient. Oropharyngeal airways may also be used to aid in ventilation during a code situation and to facilitate suctioning an unconscious or semiconscious patient.

Equipment

- Oropharyngeal airway of appropriate size
- Disposable gloves
- Suction equipment
- Goggles or face shield (optional)
- Flashlight (optional)

ASSESSMENT

Assess patient's level of consciousness and ability to protect the airway. Assess amount and consistency of oral secretions. Auscultate lung sounds. If the tongue is occluding the airway, lung sounds may be diminished. Assess for loose teeth or recent oral surgery, which may contraindicate the use of an oropharyngeal airway.

NURSING DIAGNOSIS

Determine related factors for the nursing diagnosis based on the patient's current status. Appropriate nursing diagnoses may include:

- Risk for Aspiration
- Ineffective Airway Clearance
- Risk for Injury

Other nursing diagnoses may require the use of this skill.

SKILL 14-8 Inserting an Oropharyngeal Airway *(continued)*

OUTCOME IDENTIFICATION AND PLANNING

The expected outcome is that the patient will sustain a patent airway. Another outcome that may be appropriate includes the following: the patient remains free of aspiration and injury.

IMPLEMENTATION

ACTION	RATIONALE
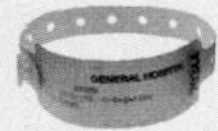 1. Identify the patient.	Positive identification of the patient is essential to ensure the intervention is administered to the correct patient.
2. Explain to the patient what you are going to do and the reason, even though the patient does not appear to be alert.	Explanation alleviates fears. Even though patient appears unconscious, the nurse should explain what is happening.
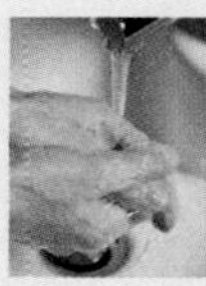 3. Perform hand hygiene.	Hand hygiene deters the spread of microorganisms.
4. Put on disposable gloves.	Gloves prevent contact with contaminants and body fluids.
5. Measure the oropharyngeal airway for correct size (Figure 1). The oropharyngeal airway is measured by holding the airway on the side of the patient's face. The airway should reach from the opening of the mouth to the back angle of the jaw.	Correct size ensures correct insertion and fit, allowing for conformation of the airway to the curvature of the palate.

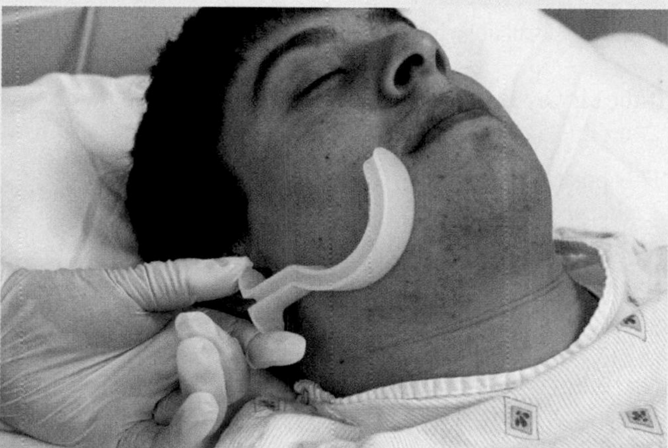

Figure 1. Measuring for oropharyngeal airway.

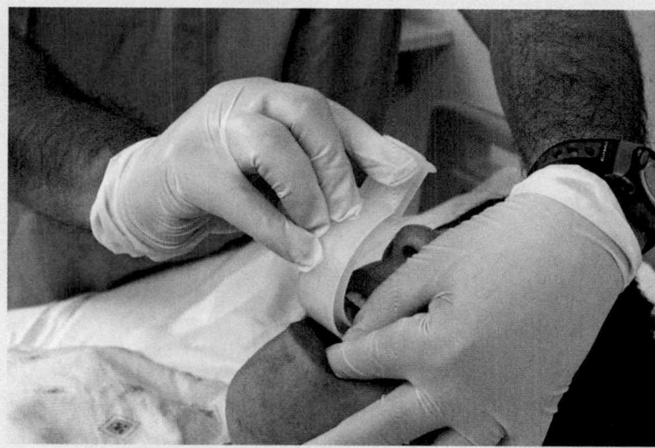

Figure 2. Sliding in the airway.

ACTION	RATIONALE
6. **Check mouth for any loose teeth, dentures, or other foreign material. Remove dentures or material if present.**	Prevents aspiration or swallowing of objects. During insertion, the airway may push any foreign objects in the mouth to the back of the throat.
7. Position patient in semi-Fowler's position.	This position facilitates airway insertion and helps prevent tongue from moving back against the posterior pharynx.
8. Suction patient if necessary.	This removes excess secretions and helps maintain patent airway.

(continued)

SKILL 14-8 Inserting an Oropharyngeal Airway *(continued)*

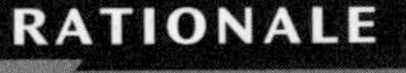

ACTION	RATIONALE
9. Open patient's mouth by using your thumb and index finger to gently pry teeth apart. **Insert the airway with the curved tip pointing up toward the roof of the mouth (Figure 2).**	This is done to advance the tip of the airway past the tongue, toward the back of the throat.
10. Slide the airway across the tongue to the back of the mouth. Rotate the airway 180 degrees as it passes the uvula (Figure 3). The tip should point down and the curvature should follow the contour of the roof of the mouth. A flashlight can be used to confirm the position of the airway with the curve fitting over the tongue.	This is done to shift the tongue anteriorly, thereby allowing the patient to breathe through and around the airway.

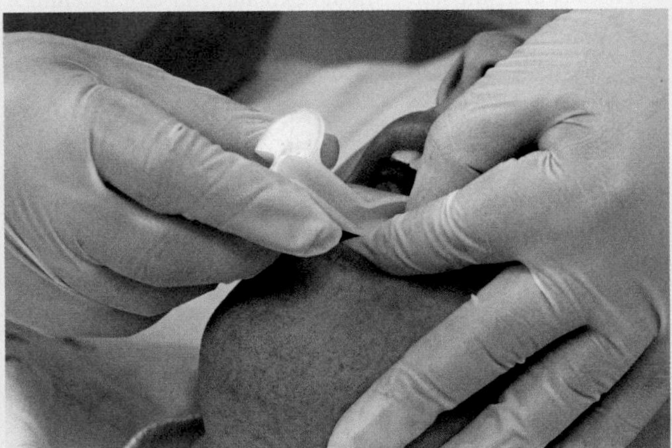

Figure 3. Rotating the airway.

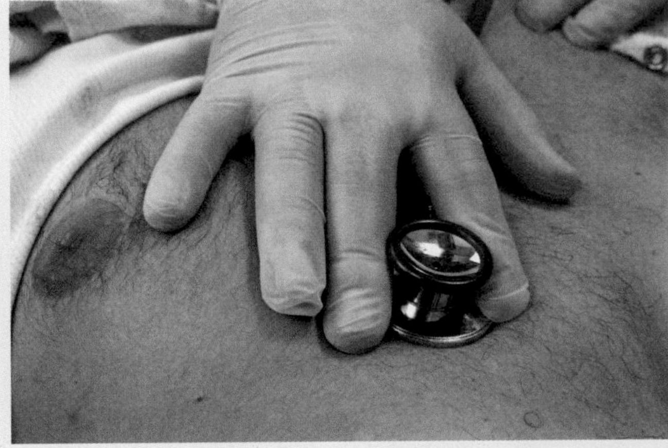

Figure 4. Auscultating breath sounds.

ACTION	RATIONALE
11. Ensure accurate placement and adequate ventilation by auscultating breath sounds (Figure 4).	If the airway is placed correctly, lung sounds should be audible and equal in all lobes.
12. Position patient on his or her side when airway is in place.	This position helps keep the tongue out of the posterior pharynx area, as well as helps to prevent aspiration if the unconscious patient should vomit.
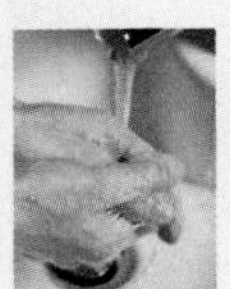 13. Remove gloves and perform hand hygiene.	Hand hygiene deters the spread of microorganisms.
14. Remove the airway for a brief period every 4 hours, or according to facility policy. Assess mouth, provide mouth care and clean the airway according to facility policy before reinserting it.	Tissue irritation and ulceration can result from prolonged use of an airway. Mouth care provides moisture to mucous membranes and helps maintain tissue integrity.

EVALUATION

The expected outcome is met when the patient exhibits a patent airway with oxygen saturation levels >95%. In addition, the patient remains free of injury and aspiration.

SKILL 14-8 Inserting an Oropharyngeal Airway *(continued)*

DOCUMENTATION

Guidelines

Document the placement of the airway, airway size, removal/cleaning, assessment pre- and postintervention, and oxygen saturation level.

Sample Documentation

9/22/08 1210 Patient noted to have 'gurgling' with respirations, tongue back in posterior pharynx. Difficult to suction oropharynx. Size 4 oropharyngeal airway inserted. Patient placed on left side. Lung sounds clear and equal all lobes. Pulse oximeter 98% on room air.—C. Bausler, RN

Unexpected Situations and Associated Interventions

- *The patient awakens:* Remove the oral airway once the patient is awake because it may be uncomfortable and cause vomiting. Conscious patients can usually protect their airway.
- *The tongue is sliding back into the posterior pharynx, causing respiratory difficulties:* Put on disposable gloves and remove the airway. Make sure the airway is the appropriate size for the patient.
- *Patient vomits as oropharyngeal airway is inserted:* Quickly position patient onto his or her side to prevent aspiration. Remove oral airway. Suction mouth if needed.

Special Considerations

General Considerations

- Wearing gloves, remove the airway briefly every 4 hours to provide mouth care. Assess the mouth and tongue for tissue irritation, tooth damage, bleeding, and ulceration. Ensure that the lips and tongue are not between the teeth and the airway to prevent injury.
- When reinserting the oropharyngeal airway, attempt to insert it on the other side of the mouth. This helps to prevent the tongue and mouth from irritation.
- Suction secretions, as needed, by manipulating around and through the oropharyngeal airway.

SKILL 14-9 Inserting a Nasopharyngeal Airway

Nasopharyngeal airways, frequently referred to as nasal trumpets, are curved soft rubber or plastic tubes inserted into the back of the pharynx through the mouth in patients who are breathing spontaneously. The nasal trumpet provides a route from the nares to the pharynx to help maintain a patent airway. These airways may be indicated if the teeth are clenched, the tongue is enlarged, or the patient needs frequent nasopharyngeal suctioning.

Equipment

- Nasal airway of appropriate size (size range for adolescent to adult is 24 Fr–36 Fr)
- Disposable gloves
- Water-soluble lubricant
- Suction equipment
- Mask (if necessary)
- Goggles (if necessary)

(continued)

SKILL 14-9 Inserting a Nasopharyngeal Airway *(continued)*

ASSESSMENT

Assess patient's lung sounds. If lung sounds are diminished, patient may need nasal airway to keep airway patent. If lung sounds are coarse or wheezing is noted, patient may need the nasal airway to help with suctioning. Assess patient's respiratory rate and effort. If patient is not getting enough air or if patient needs to be suctioned, the respiratory rate will generally increase and the patient may have retractions, nasal flaring, and grunting. Assess the oxygen saturation level. If the patient is not getting enough air or if the patient needs to be suctioned, the oxygen saturation level will generally decrease. Assess for the presence of nasal conditions, such as a deviated septum or recent nasal or oral surgery, and increased risk for bleeding, such as anticoagulant therapy, which would contraindicate the use of a nasopharyngeal airway.

NURSING DIAGNOSIS

Determine related factors for the nursing diagnosis based on the patient's current status. Appropriate nursing diagnoses may include:

- Risk for Aspiration
- Ineffective Airway Clearance
- Risk for Activity Intolerance
- Risk for Impaired Skin Integrity
- Risk for Infection
- Risk for Injury

OUTCOME IDENTIFICATION AND PLANNING

The expected outcome to achieve is that the patient will sustain and maintain a patent airway. Other outcomes that may be appropriate include the following: the patient demonstrates a respiratory rate and depth within normal limits and equal, clear lung sounds bilaterally.

IMPLEMENTATION

ACTION	RATIONALE
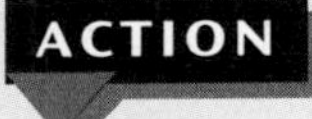 1. Identify the patient.	Positive identification of the patient is essential to ensure the intervention is administered to the correct patient.
2. Explain what you are going to do and the reason to the patient, even if the patient does not appear to be alert.	Explanation alleviates fears. Even if patient appears unconscious, the nurse should explain what is happening.
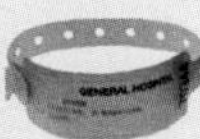 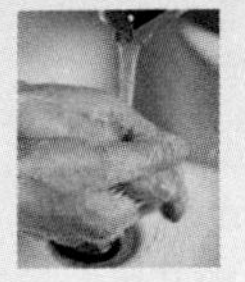 3. Perform hand hygiene.	Hand hygiene deters the spread of microorganisms.
4. Put on disposable gloves. If patient is coughing or has copious secretions, a mask and goggles should also be worn.	Gloves and personal protective equipment prevent contact with contaminants.
5. **Measure the nasopharyngeal airway for correct size (Figure 1).** The nasopharyngeal airway length is measured by holding the airway on the side of the patient's face. The airway should reach from the tragus of the ear to the nostril plus 1″. The diameter should be slightly smaller than the diameter of the nostril.	Correct size ensures correct insertion and fit, allowing for conformation of the airway to the curvature of the nasopharynx.

SKILL 14-9 Inserting a Nasopharyngeal Airway *(continued)*

ACTION	RATIONALE
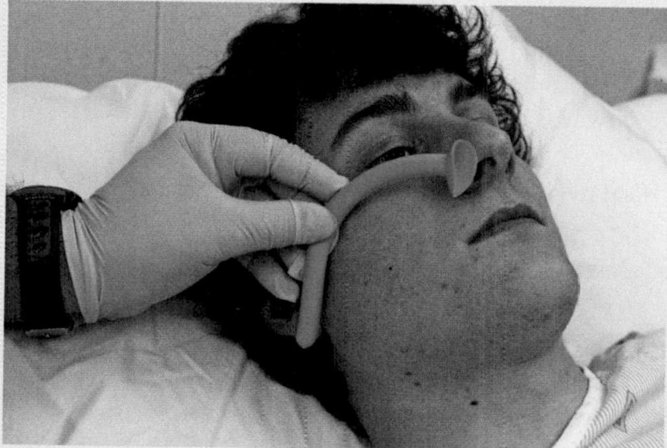 Figure 1. Measuring the nasopharyngeal airway.	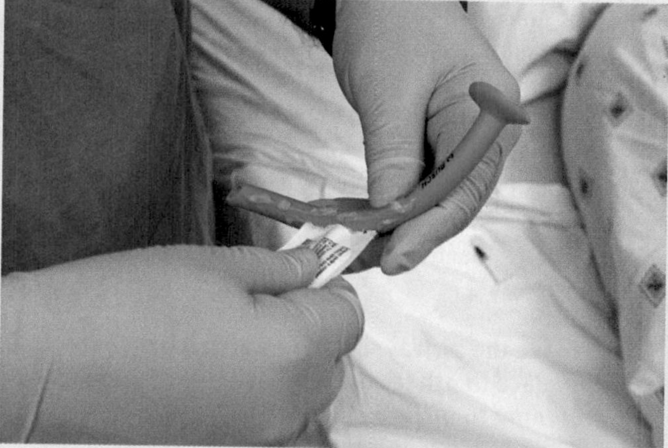 Figure 2. Lubricating nasopharyngeal airway.
6. Adjust bed to a comfortable working level. Lower side rail closer to you. If patient is awake and alert, position patient supine in semi-Fowler's position. If patient is not conscious or alert, position patient in a side-lying position.	By raising the head of the bed or placing patient in the side-lying position, the nurse is helping to protect the airway if the patient should vomit during the placement of the nasopharyngeal airway.
7. Suction patient if necessary.	Suctioning removes excess secretions and helps maintain patent airway.
8. Lubricate the nasopharyngeal airway generously with the water-soluble lubricant, covering the airway from the tip to the guard rim (Figure 2).	The water-soluble lubricant helps prevent injury to the mucosa as the airway is inserted.
9. Gently insert the airway into the naris (Figure 3), narrow end first, until the rim is touching the naris (Figure 4). If resistance is met, stop and try other naris.	To prevent injury, the airway should not be forced into the naris.
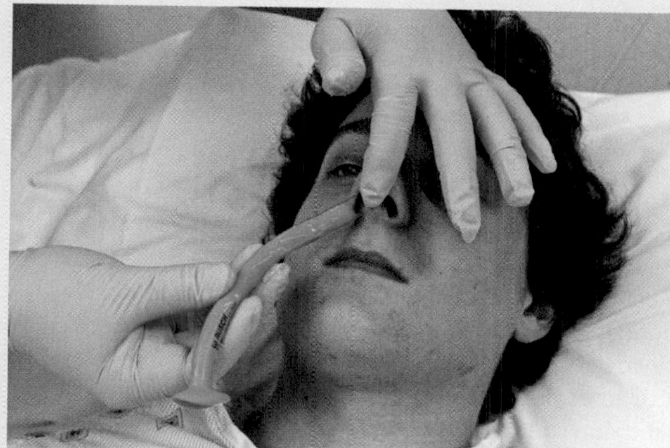 Figure 3. Inserting nasopharyngeal airway.	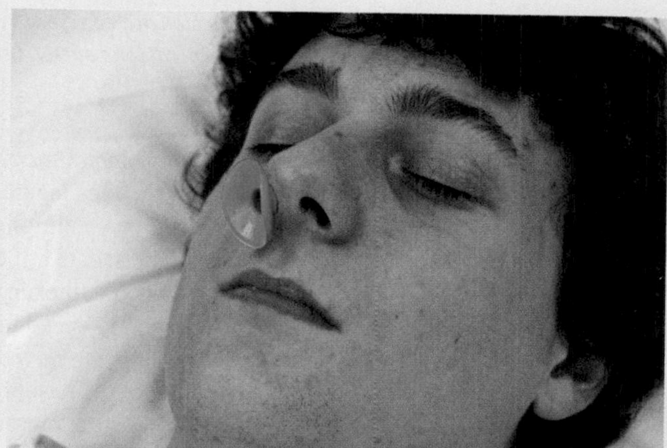 Figure 4. Nasopharyngeal airway inserted.

(continued)

SKILL 14-9

Inserting a Nasopharyngeal Airway *(continued)*

ACTION	RATIONALE
10. Check placement by closing the patient's mouth and place your fingers in front of the tube opening to check for air movement. Assess the pharynx to visualize the tip of the airway behind the uvula. Assess the nose for blanching or stretching of the skin.	This ensures correct placement and prevents injury. The skin should not be blanched or appear stretched due to the nasopharyngeal airway. If this occurs, a smaller size airway is needed.
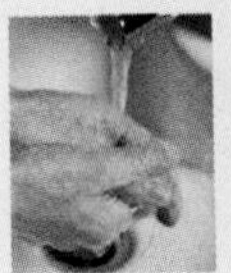 11. Remove gloves and other personal protective equipment. Raise bed rail. Perform hand hygiene.	Hand hygiene deters the spread of microorganisms.
12. **Remove the airway, clean in warm soapy water, and place in other naris at least every 8 hours, or according to facility policy.**	The nasopharyngeal airway may cause tissue trauma and skin breakdown if left in place for too long. Secretions can accumulate on surface and contribute to irritation and tissue trauma.

EVALUATION

The expected outcome is met when the patient maintains a clear, patent airway with minimal to no secretions. In addition, the patient exhibits an oxygen saturation level >95% and respiratory rate remains in the normal range. The patient experiences no trauma when suctioned.

DOCUMENTATION

Guidelines

Document the placement of the nasopharyngeal airway, including size of airway, nares used for placement, assessment pre- and postintervention, and removal/cleaning.

Sample Documentation

9/12/08 0430 24F nasal trumpet placed in right nares due to nasal mucosa trauma from frequent suctioning. Patient suctioned for copious amount of thin, white secretions after nasopharyngeal airway placement. Lung sounds before suctioning course throughout; after suctioning lung sounds clear all lobes. Respirations even/unlabored.—C. Bausler, RN

Unexpected Situations and Associated Interventions

- *Patient becomes tachypneic and anxious when nasal trumpet is placed:* Discuss with patient feelings regarding the nasal trumpet. Some patients feel fearful and uncomfortable, or even feelings of suffocation when the nasal trumpet is in place. Patient may need to be sedated, if ordered, or reassurance may be needed until patient becomes accustomed to the airway. If patient is unable to relax or tolerate the procedure, the physician may need to be notified and the airway discontinued.
- *When removing the nasopharyngeal airway, you note skin breakdown on the nares:* The size of the nasopharyngeal airway may need to be assessed. The airway may be too big, causing pressure on the skin surrounding the nares. Replace the airway in the opposite nares with a smaller-sized airway.

SKILL 14-9 Inserting a Nasopharyngeal Airway *(continued)*

Special Considerations

General Considerations

- If the patient coughs or gags on insertion, the nasal trumpet may be too long. Assess the pharynx. The tip of the airway should be visualized behind the uvula.

Older Adult Considerations

- The skin, mucous membranes, and tissues of older adults are more fragile and prone to injury and breakdown. Extra care on insertion to prevent injury and extra vigilance to provide oral hygiene and assessment of the area is necessary.

SKILL 14-10 Suctioning an Endotracheal Tube: Open System

The purpose of suctioning is to maintain a patent airway and remove pulmonary secretions, blood, vomitus, or foreign material from the airway. When suctioning via an endotracheal tube, the goal is to remove secretions that are not accessible to cilia bypassed by the tube itself. Remember that tracheal suctioning can lead to hypoxemia, cardiac dysrhythmias, trauma, atelectasis, infection, bleeding, and pain, so it is imperative to be diligent in maintaining aseptic technique and following facility guidelines and procedures to prevent potential hazards. Frequency of suctioning is based on clinical assessment.

Some consider open system suctioning to be the most efficient way to suction the endotracheal tube, arguing that there are no limitations to the movement of the suction catheter while suctioning. However, an open system may be unknowingly contaminated by the nurse during the procedure. In addition, with the open system, the patient must be removed from the ventilator during suctioning.

Suctioning removes secretions not accessible to bypassed cilia, so insertion of the catheter only as far as the end of the endotracheal tube is recommended. Catheter contact and suction cause tracheal mucosal damage, loss of cilia, edema, and fibrosis, as well as increasing the risk of infection and bleeding for the patient. Insertion of the suction catheter to a predetermined distance, no more than 1 cm past the length of the endotracheal tube, avoids contact with the trachea and carina, reducing the effects of tracheal mucosal damage (Pate, 2004; Pate & Zapata, 2002). Box 14-1 discusses several methods for determining appropriate suction catheter depth.

Equipment

- Portable or wall suction unit with tubing
- A commercially prepared suction kit with an appropriate size catheter (see General Considerations) or
  - Sterile suction catheter with Y-port in the appropriate size
  - Sterile disposable container
  - Sterile gloves
  - Towel or waterproof pad
  - Goggles and mask or face shield
  - Disposable, clean glove
  - Resuscitation bag connected to 100% oxygen
  - Assistant (optional)

(continued)

SKILL 14-10 Suctioning an Endotracheal Tube: Open System *(continued)*

BOX 14-1 Methods to Determine Suction Catheter Depth

Open Suction System

Method 1 (Endotracheal Tubes)

- Using a suction catheter with centimeter increments on it, insert the suction catheter into the endotracheal tube until the centimeter markings on both the endotracheal tube and catheter align.
- Insert the suction catheter no further than an additional 1 cm.

Method 2 (Endotracheal Tubes)

- Combine the length of the endotracheal tube and any adapter being used, and add an additional 1 cm.
- Document the determined length at the bedside or on the plan of care, according to facility policy.

Method 3 (Endotracheal and Tracheostomy Tubes)

- Using a spare endotracheal or tracheostomy tube of the same size as being used for the patient, insert the suction catheter to the end of the tube.
- Note the length of catheter used to reach the end of the tube.
- Document the determined length at the bedside or on the plan of care. Alternately, mark the distance on the suction catheter with permanent ink or tape and place the catheter at the bedside for reference. Refer to facility policy.

Closed Suction System (Endotracheal and Tracheostomy Tubes)

- Combine the length of the endotracheal or tracheostomy tube and any adapter being used, and add an additional 1 cm.
- Advance the catheter until the appropriate length can be seen through the catheter sheath or window.
- Document the depth of the catheter at the bedside or on the plan of care.

(Adapted from Pate, M. & Zapata, T. [2002]. Ask the experts: How deeply should I go when I suction an endotracheal tube or tracheostomy tube? *Critical Care Nurse, 22*[2], 130–131.)

ASSESSMENT

Assess lung sounds. Patients who need to be suctioned may have wheezes, crackles, or gurgling present. Assess oxygenation saturation level. Oxygen saturation usually decreases when a patient needs to be suctioned. Assess respiratory status, including respiratory rate and depth. Patients may become tachypneic when they need to be suctioned. Assess patient for signs of respiratory distress, such as nasal flaring, retractions, or grunting. Additional indications for suctioning via a tracheostomy tube include secretions in the tube, acute respiratory distress, and frequent or sustained coughing. Also assess for pain. If patient has had abdominal surgery or other procedures, pain medication should be administered before suctioning. Assess appropriate suction catheter depth.

NURSING DIAGNOSIS

Determine the related factors for the nursing diagnosis based on the patient's current status. Appropriate nursing diagnoses may include:

- Ineffective Airway Clearance
- Risk for Aspiration
- Risk for Infection
- Impaired Gas Exchange

OUTCOME IDENTIFICATION AND PLANNING

The expected outcome is that the patient will exhibit improved breath sounds and a clear, patent airway. Other outcomes that may be appropriate include the following: patient will exhibit an oxygen saturation level within acceptable parameters; patient will demonstrate a respiratory rate and depth within age-acceptable range; and patient will remain free of any signs of respiratory distress.

SKILL
14-10 Suctioning an Endotracheal Tube: Open System *(continued)*

IMPLEMENTATION

ACTION	RATIONALE
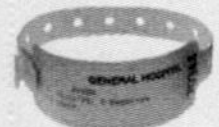 1. Identify the patient.	Positive identification of the patient is essential to ensure the intervention is administered to the correct patient.
2. Determine the need for suctioning. Verify the suction order in the patient's chart. **For postoperative patient, administer pain medication as prescribed before suctioning.**	To minimize trauma to airway mucosa, suctioning should be done only when secretions have accumulated or adventitious breath sounds are audible. Suctioning stimulates coughing, which is painful for patients with surgical incisions.
3. Explain what you are going to do and the reason to the patient, even if the patient does not appear to be alert. Reassure patient you will interrupt procedure if he or she indicates respiratory difficulty.	Explanation alleviates fears. Even if patient appears unconscious, the nurse should explain what is happening. Any procedure that compromises respiration is frightening for the patient.
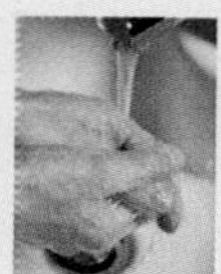 4. Perform hand hygiene.	Hand hygiene deters the spread of microorganisms.
5. Adjust bed to comfortable working position. Lower side rail closer to you. If patient is conscious, place him or her in a semi-Fowler's position. **If patient is unconscious, place him or her in the lateral position, facing you. Move the overbed table close to your work area and raise to waist height.**	A sitting position helps the patient to cough and makes breathing easier. Gravity also facilitates catheter insertion. The lateral position prevents the airway from becoming obstructed and promotes drainage of secretions. The overbed table provides work surface and maintains sterility of objects on work surface.
6. Place towel or waterproof pad across patient's chest.	This protects bed linens and the patient.
7. **Turn suction to appropriate pressure.** For a wall unit for an adult: 100–150 mm Hg; neonates: 60–80 mm Hg; infants: 80–100 mm Hg; children: 100–120 mm Hg For a portable unit for an adult: 10–15 cm Hg; neonates: 6–8 cm Hg; infants 8–10 cm Hg; children 1–12 cm Hg	Higher pressures can cause excessive trauma, hypoxemia, and atelectasis.
8. **Put on a disposable, clean glove and occlude the end of the connecting tubing to check suction pressure. Place the connecting tubing in a convenient location. Place the resuscitation bag connected to oxygen within convenient reach, if using.**	Glove prevents contact with blood and body fluids. Checking pressure ensures equipment is working properly. Allows for an organized approach to procedure.
9. **Open sterile suction package using aseptic technique. The open wrapper becomes a sterile field to hold other supplies. Carefully remove the sterile container, touching only the outside surface. Set it up on the work surface and pour sterile saline into it.**	Sterile normal saline or water is used to lubricate the outside of the catheter, minimizing irritation of mucosa during introduction. It is also used to clear the catheter between suction attempts.

(continued)

SKILL 14-10 Suctioning an Endotracheal Tube: Open System *(continued)*

ACTION	RATIONALE
10. Put on face shield or goggles and mask. Put on sterile gloves. **The dominant hand will manipulate the catheter and must remain sterile. The nondominant hand is considered clean rather than sterile and will control the suction valve (Y port) on the catheter.**	Handling the sterile catheter using a sterile glove helps prevent introducing organisms into the respiratory tract; the clean glove protects the nurse from microorganisms.
11. With dominant gloved hand, pick up sterile catheter. Pick up the connecting tubing with the nondominant hand and connect the tubing and suction catheter.	Sterility of the suction catheter is maintained.
12. Moisten the catheter by dipping it into the container of sterile saline, unless it is a silicone catheter. Occlude Y-tube to check suction.	Lubricating the inside of the catheter with saline helps move secretions in the catheter. Silicone catheters do not require lubrication. Checking suction ensures equipment is working properly.
13. Hyperventilate the patient using your nondominant hand and a manual resuscitation bag and delivering 3 to 6 breaths (Figure 1) or use the sigh mechanism on a mechanical ventilator.	Hyperoxygenation aids in preventing hypoxemia during suctioning.

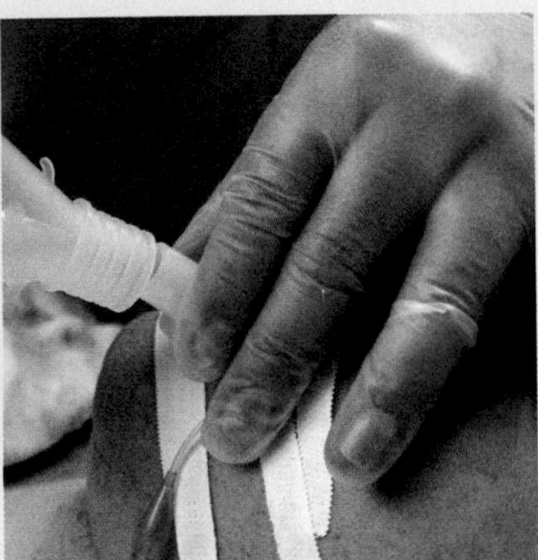

Figure 1. Removing ventilator tubing from endotracheal tube to hyperventilate the patient.

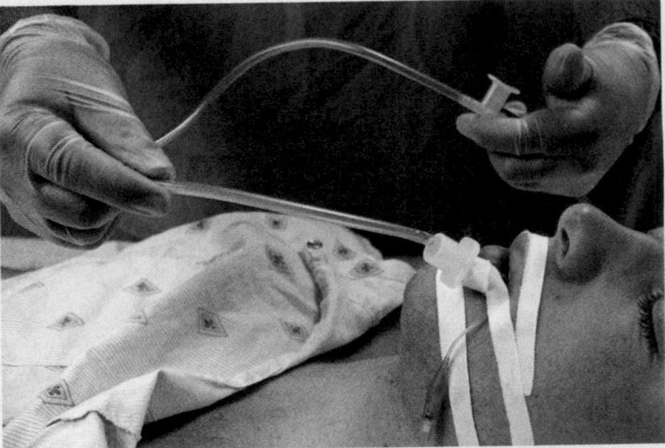

Figure 2. Inserting suction catheter into endotracheal tube.

ACTION	RATIONALE
14. Open the adapter on the mechanical ventilator tubing or remove the manual resuscitation bag with your nondominant hand.	This exposes tracheostomy tube without contaminating sterile gloved hand.
15. Using your dominant hand, gently and quickly insert catheter into trachea (Figure 2). **Advance the catheter to the predetermined length. Do not occlude Y-port when inserting catheter.**	Suctioning when inserting catheter increases the risk for trauma to airway mucosa and increases risk of hypoxemia. If resistance is met, the carina or tracheal mucosa has been hit. Withdraw the catheter at least ½″ before applying suction.
16. Apply suction by intermittently occluding the Y port on the catheter with the thumb of your nondominant hand, and gently rotate the catheter as it is being withdrawn (Figure 3). **Do not suction for more than 10 to 15 seconds at a time.**	Turning the catheter as it is withdrawn minimizes trauma to the mucosa. Suctioning for longer than 10 to 15 seconds robs the respiratory tract of oxygen, which may result in hypoxemia. Suctioning too quickly may be ineffective at clearing all secretions.

SKILL 14-10 **Suctioning an Endotracheal Tube: Open System** *(continued)*

ACTION	RATIONALE
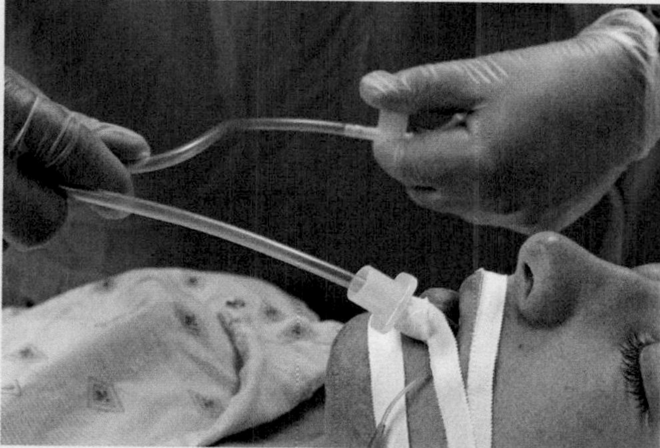 **Figure 3.** Withdrawing suction catheter and intermittently occluding Y port with thumb to apply suction.	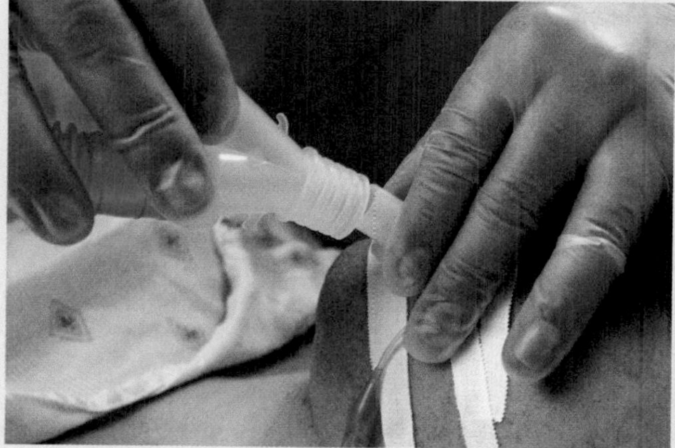 **Figure 4.** Reconnecting ventilator tubing to endotracheal tube.
17. Hyperventilate the patient using your nondominant hand and a manual resuscitation bag and delivering 3 to 6 breaths. Replace the oxygen delivery device, if applicable, using your nondominant hand and have the patient take several deep breaths. If the patient is mechanically ventilated, close the adapter on the mechanical ventilator tubing or replace ventilator tubing and use the sigh mechanism on a mechanical ventilator (Figure 4).	Suctioning removes air from the patient's airway and can cause hypoxemia. Hyperventilation can help prevent suction-induced hypoxemia.
18. Flush catheter with saline. Assess effectiveness of suctioning and repeat as needed and according to patient's tolerance.	Flushing clears catheter and lubricates it for next insertion. Reassessment determines need for additional suctioning.
Wrap the suction catheter around your dominant hand between attempts.	Wrapping the catheter prevents inadvertent contamination of catheter.
19. **Allow at least a 30-second to 1-minute interval if additional suctioning is needed. No more than three suction passes should be made per suctioning episode.** Suction the oropharynx after suctioning the trachea. Do not reinsert in the endotracheal tube after suctioning the mouth.	The interval allows for reventilation and reoxygenation of airways. Excessive suction passes contribute to complications. Suctioning the oropharynx clears the mouth of secretions. More microorganisms are usually present in the mouth, so it is suctioned last to prevent transmission of contaminants.
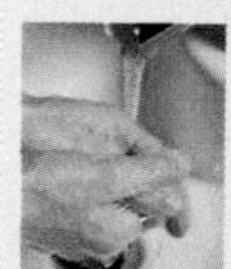 20. When suctioning is completed, remove glove from dominant hand over the coiled catheter, pulling it off inside out. Remove glove from nondominant hand and dispose of gloves, catheter, and container with solution in the appropriate receptacle. Remove face shield or goggles and mask. Perform hand hygiene.	All actions reduce transmission of microorganisms.
21. Turn off suction. Assist patient to a comfortable position. Raise bed rail. Offer oral hygiene after suctioning.	Respiratory secretions that are allowed to accumulate in the mouth are irritating to mucous membranes and unpleasant for the patient.

(continued)

SKILL 14-10 Suctioning an Endotracheal Tube: Open System *(continued)*

ACTION	RATIONALE
22. Reassess patient's respiratory status, including respiratory rate, effort, oxygen saturation, and lung sounds.	These assess effectiveness of suctioning and the presence of complications.

EVALUATION

The expected outcome is met when the patient exhibits improved breath sounds and a clear and patent airway. In addition, the oxygen saturation level is within acceptable parameters, and the patient does not exhibit signs or symptoms of respiratory distress or complications.

DOCUMENTATION

Guidelines

Document the time of suctioning, your pre- and postintervention assessment, reason for suctioning, oxygen saturation levels, and the characteristics and amount of secretions.

Sample Documentation

9/1/08 1850 Lung sounds coarse lower lobes, wheezes upper lobes bilaterally. Respirations 24 breaths per min. Intercostal retractions noted. Endotracheal tube suctioning completed with 12F catheter. Small amount of thin, white secretions obtained. Specimen for culture collected and sent. After suctioning lung sounds clear in all lobes, respirations 18 breaths per min, no intercostal retractions noted.—C. Bausler, RN

Unexpected Situations and Interventions

- *Catheter or sterile glove is contaminated:* Reconnect patient to ventilator. Discard gloves and suction catheter. Gather supplies and begin procedure again.
- *When suctioning, your eye becomes contaminated with respiratory secretions:* After attending to patient, perform hand hygiene and flush eye with large amount of sterile water. Contact employee health or house supervisor immediately for further treatment. Goggles or a face shield should be used when suctioning to prevent exposure to body fluids.

Special Considerations

General Considerations

- The size catheter used is determined by the size of the endotracheal tube. The external diameter of the suction catheter should not exceed half of the internal diameter of the endotracheal tube. Larger catheters can contribute to trauma and hypoxemia.
- Emergency equipment should be easily accessible at the bedside. Bag-valve mask, oxygen, and suction equipment should be kept at the bedside of a patient with an endotracheal tube at all times.

SKILL 14-11 Suctioning an Endotracheal Tube: Closed System

The purpose of suctioning is to maintain a patent airway and remove pulmonary secretions, blood, vomitus, or foreign material from the airway. When suctioning via an endotracheal tube, the goal is to remove secretions that are not accessible to cilia bypassed by the tube itself. Tracheal suctioning can lead to hypoxemia, cardiac dysrhythmias, trauma, atelectasis, infection, bleeding, and pain. It is imperative to be diligent in maintaining aseptic technique and following facility guidelines and procedures to prevent potential hazards. Suctioning frequency is based on clinical assessment to determine the need for suctioning. Closed system suction (Figure 1) may be used routinely or when a patient must be frequently and quickly suctioned due to an excess of secretions, depending on the policies of the institution. Closed system suctioning is thought to decrease the risk for contamination since the unit is self-contained. One drawback is thought to be the hindrance of the sheath when rotating the suction catheter upon removal.

Suctioning removes secretions not accessible to bypassed cilia, so insertion of the catheter only as far as the end of the endotracheal tube is recommended. Catheter contact and suction cause tracheal mucosal damage, loss of cilia, edema, and fibrosis, as well as increased risk of infection and bleeding for the patient. Insertion of the suction catheter to a predetermined distance, no more than 1 cm past the length of the endotracheal tube, avoids contact with the trachea and carina, reducing the effects of tracheal mucosal damage (Pate, 2004; Pate & Zapata, 2002). Box 14-1 (in Skill 14-10) shows several methods for nurses to use to determine appropriate suction catheter depth.

Equipment

- Portable or wall suction unit with tubing
- Closed suction device of appropriate size for patient
- 3-mL or 5-mL normal saline solution in dosette or syringe
- Sterile gloves

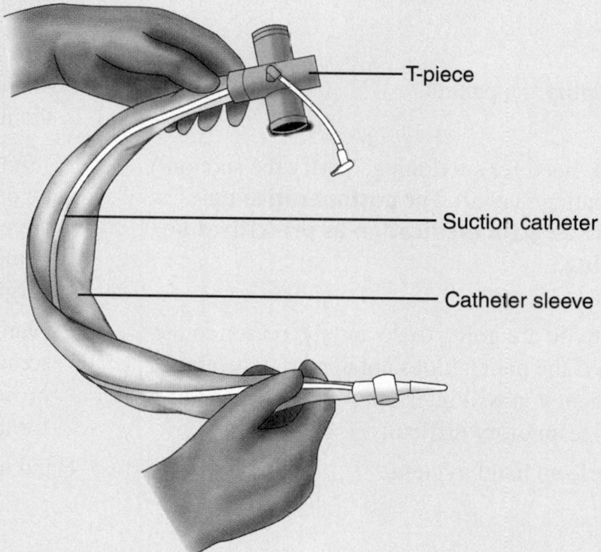

Figure 1. Closed suction device.

(continued)

SKILL 14-11 Suctioning an Endotracheal Tube: Closed System *(continued)*

ASSESSMENT

Assess lung sounds. Patients who need to be suctioned may have wheezes, crackles, or gurgling present. Assess oxygenation saturation level. Oxygen saturation usually decreases when a patient needs to be suctioned. Assess respiratory status, including respiratory rate and depth. Patients may become tachypneic when they need to be suctioned. Assess patient for signs of respiratory distress, such as nasal flaring, retractions, or grunting. Additional indications for suctioning via a tracheostomy tube include secretions in the tube, acute respiratory distress, and frequent or sustained coughing. Also assess for pain. If patient has had abdominal surgery or other procedures, pain medication should be administered before suctioning.

NURSING DIAGNOSIS

Determine the related factors for the nursing diagnosis based on the patient's current status. Appropriate nursing diagnoses may include:

- Ineffective Airway Clearance
- Risk for Aspiration
- Risk for Infection
- Impaired Gas Exchange

OUTCOME IDENTIFICATION AND PLANNING

The expected outcome is that the patient will exhibit improved breath sounds and a clear, patent airway. Other outcomes that may be appropriate include the following: patient will exhibit an oxygen saturation level within acceptable parameters; patient will demonstrate a respiratory rate and depth within age-acceptable range; and patient will remain free of any signs of respiratory distress.

IMPLEMENTATION

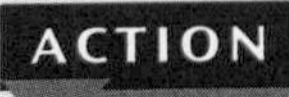

ACTION	RATIONALE
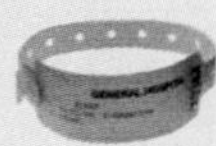 1. Identify the patient.	Positive identification of the patient is essential to ensure the intervention is administered to the correct patient.
2. Determine the need for suctioning. Verify the suction order in the patient's chart. **For postoperative patient, administer pain medication as prescribed before suctioning.**	To minimize trauma to airway mucosa, suctioning should be done only when secretions have accumulated or adventitious breath sounds are audible. Suctioning stimulates coughing, which is painful for patients with surgical incisions.
3. Explain what you are going to do and the reason to the patient, even if the patient does not appear to be alert. Reassure patient you will interrupt procedure if he or she indicates respiratory difficulty.	Explanation alleviates fears. Even if patient appears unconscious, the nurse should explain what is happening. Any procedure that compromises respiration is frightening for the patient.
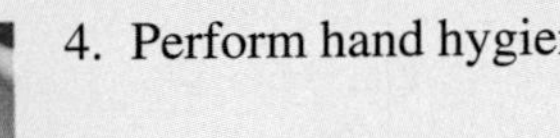 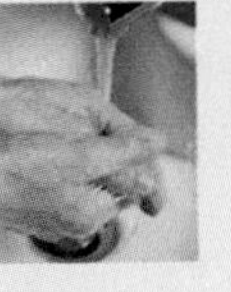 4. Perform hand hygiene.	Hand hygiene deters the spread of microorganisms.
5. Adjust bed to comfortable working position. Lower side rail closer to you. If patient is conscious, place him or her in a semi-Fowler's position. **If patient is unconscious, place him or her in the lateral position, facing you. Move the overbed table close to your work area and raise to waist height.**	A sitting position helps the patient to cough and makes breathing easier. Gravity also facilitates catheter insertion. The lateral position prevents the airway from becoming obstructed and promotes drainage of secretions. The overbed table provides work surface and maintains sterility of objects on work surface.

SKILL 14-11 Suctioning an Endotracheal Tube: Closed System *(continued)*

ACTION	RATIONALE
6. **Turn suction to appropriate pressure:** For a wall unit for an adult: 100–150 mm Hg; neonates: 60–80 mm Hg; infants: 80–100 mm Hg; children: 100–120 mm Hg. For a portable unit for an adult: 10–15 cm Hg; neonates: 6–8 cm Hg; infants 8–10 cm Hg; children 10–12 cm Hg. **Put on a disposable, clean glove and occlude the end of the connecting tubing to check suction pressure. Place the connecting tubing in a convenient location.**	Higher pressures can cause excessive trauma, hypoxemia and atelectasis.
7. Open the package of closed suction device using aseptic technique. **Make sure that the device remains sterile.**	The device must remain sterile to prevent a nosocomial infection.
8. Put on sterile gloves.	Gloves deter the spread of microorganisms.
9. Using nondominant hand, disconnect ventilator from endotracheal tube. **Place ventilator tubing in a convenient location so that the inside of the tubing remains sterile or continue to hold the tubing in your nondominant hand.**	This provides access to the endotracheal tube while keeping one hand sterile. The inside of the ventilator tubing should remain sterile to prevent a nosocomial infection.
10. **Using dominant hand and keeping device sterile, connect the closed suctioning device so that the suctioning catheter is in line with the endotracheal tube.**	Keeping the device sterile decreases the risk for a nosocomial infection.
11. **Keeping the inside of the ventilator tubing sterile, attach ventilator tubing to port perpendicular to the endotracheal tube.** Attach suction tubing to suction catheter.	The inside of the ventilator tubing must remain sterile to prevent a nosocomial infection. By connecting the ventilator tubing to the port, the patient does not need to be disconnected from the ventilator to be suctioned.
12. Pop top off sterile normal saline dosette. Open plug to port by suction catheter and insert saline dosette or syringe.	The saline will help to clean the catheter between suctioning.
13. **Hyperoxygenate or hyperventilate the patient by using the sigh button on the ventilator before suctioning.** Turn safety cap on suction button of catheter so that button is easily depressed.	Hyperoxygenating or hyperventilating before suctioning helps to decrease the effects of oxygen removal during suctioning. The safety button keeps the patient from accidentally depressing the button and decreasing the oxygen saturation.
14. Grasp suction catheter through protective sheath, about 6″ (15 cm) from the endotracheal tube. Gently insert the catheter into the endotracheal tube (Figure 2). Release the catheter while holding onto the protective sheath. Move hand further back on catheter. **Grasp catheter through sheath and repeat movement, advancing the catheter to the predetermined length. Do not occlude Y-port when inserting catheter.**	The sheath keeps the suction catheter sterile. Suctioning when inserting catheter increases the risk for trauma to airway mucosa and increases risk of hypoxemia. If resistance is met, the carina or tracheal mucosa has been hit. Withdraw the catheter at least ½″ before applying suction.

(continued)

SKILL 14-11 Suctioning an Endotracheal Tube: Closed System *(continued)*

ACTION

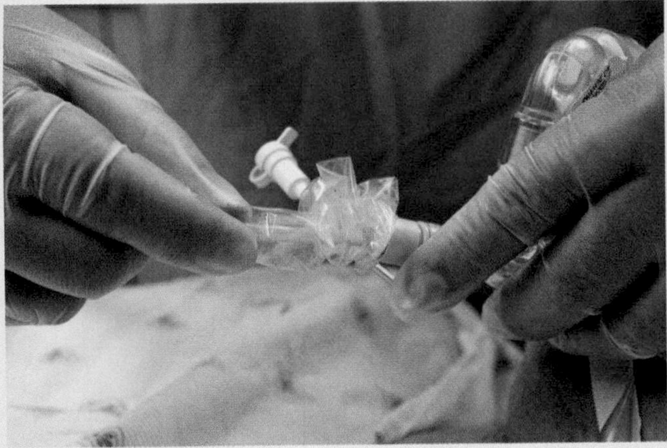

Figure 2. Inserting catheter through sheath and into endotracheal tube.

15. **Apply intermittent suction by depressing the suction button with thumb of nondominant hand (Figure 3). Gently rotate catheter with thumb and index finger of dominant hand as catheter is being withdrawn. Do not suction for more than 10 to 15 seconds at a time. Hyperoxygenate or hyperventilate with sigh button on ventilator as ordered.**
16. Once catheter is withdrawn back into sheath (Figure 4), depress the suction button while gently squeezing the normal saline dosette until catheter is clean. **Allow at least a 30-second to 1-minute interval if additional suctioning is needed. No more than three suction passes should be made per suctioning episode.**

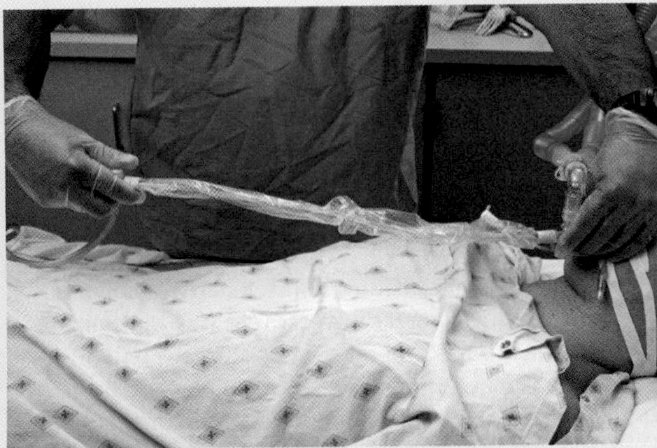

Figure 4. Removing suction catheter by pulling back into sheath.

17. **When procedure is completed, ensure that catheter is withdrawn into sheath, and turn safety button. Remove normal saline dosette and apply cap to port.**

RATIONALE

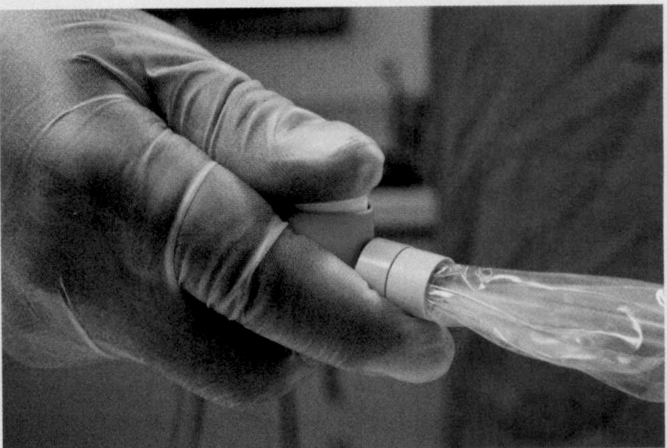

Figure 3. Pushing on suction button.

Turning the catheter while withdrawing it helps clean surfaces of respiratory tract and prevents injury to tracheal mucosa. Suctioning for longer than 10 to 15 seconds robs the respiratory tract of oxygen, which may result in hypoxemia. Suctioning too quickly may be ineffective at clearing all secretions. Hyperoxygenation and hyperventilation reoxygenates the lungs.

Flushing cleans and clears catheter and lubricates it for next insertion. Allowing time interval and replacing oxygen delivery setup help compensate for hypoxia induced by the suctioning. Excessive suction passes contribute to complications.

By turning safety button, the suction is blocked at the catheter so the suction cannot remove oxygen from the endotracheal tube.

SKILL 14-11 Suctioning an Endotracheal Tube: Closed System *(continued)*

ACTION	RATIONALE
18. Suction the oral cavity with a separate single-use, disposable catheter and perform oral hygiene.	Suctioning of the oral cavity removes secretions that may be stagnant in the mouth and pharynx, reducing the risk for infection. Oral hygiene offers comfort to the patient.
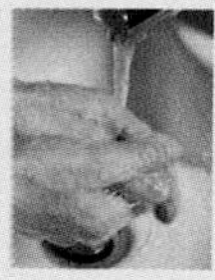 19. Remove gloves and perform hand hygiene.	This prevents transmission of microorganisms.
20. Adjust the patient's position and raise the side rail. Reassess patient's respiratory status, including respiratory rate, effort, oxygen saturation, and lung sounds.	These assess effectiveness of suctioning and the presence of complications.

EVALUATION

The expected outcome is met when the patient exhibits improved breath sounds and a clear and patent airway. In addition, the oxygen saturation level is within acceptable parameters, and the patient does not exhibit signs or symptoms of respiratory distress or complications.

DOCUMENTATION

Guidelines

Document the time of suctioning, your pre- and postintervention assessment, reason for suctioning, oxygen saturation levels, and the characteristics and amount of secretions.

Sample Documentation

9/1/08 1850 Lung sounds coarse lower lobes, wheezes upper lobes bilaterally. Respirations 24 breaths per min. Intercostal retractions noted. Endotracheal tube suctioning completed with 12F catheter. Small amount of thin, white secretions obtained. After suctioning, lung sounds clear in all lobes, respirations 18 breaths per min, no intercostal retractions noted.—C. Bausler, RN

Unexpected Situations and Associated Interventions

- *Patient is extubated during suctioning:* Remain with patient. Call for help to notify the physician. Assess patient's vital signs, ability to breathe without assistance, and oxygen saturation. Be ready to deliver assisted breaths with a bag-valve mask (Skill 14-17) or administer oxygen. Anticipate the need for reintubation.
- *Oxygen saturation level decreases after suctioning:* Hyperoxygenate patient. Auscultate lung sounds. If lung sounds are absent over one lobe, alert staff to notify physician. Remain with patient. Patient may have pneumothorax. Anticipate an order for a stat chest x-ray and chest tube placement.
- *When suctioning, you notice small yellow plugs in the secretions:* Assess patient's hydration status as well as the humidification on the ventilator. These mucous plugs may cause a ventilation-perfusion mismatch if not resolved. Patient may need more humidification.
- *Patient develops signs of intolerance to suctioning: oxygen saturation level decreases and remains low after hyperoxygenating, patient becomes cyanotic, or patient becomes bradycardic:* Stop suctioning. Auscultate lung sounds. Consider hyperventilating patient with manual resuscitation device. Remain with patient. Alert staff to notify physician.

SKILL 14-12 Securing an Endotracheal Tube

Endotracheal tubes provide an airway for patients who cannot maintain a sufficient airway on their own. A tube is passed through the mouth or nose into the trachea. Patients who have an endotracheal tube have a high risk for skin breakdown related to the securing of the endotracheal tube, compounded by the risk of increased secretions. The endotracheal tube should be retaped every 24 hours to prevent skin breakdown and to ensure that the tube is properly secured. Retaping an endotracheal tube requires two people. There are other ways of securing an endotracheal tube besides tape. To secure with another device, follow the manufacturer's recommendations. One example of taping an endotracheal tube is provided below, but this skill might be performed differently in your institution. Always refer to specific agency policy.

Equipment

- Assistant (nurse or respiratory therapist)
- Portable or wall suction unit with tubing
- Sterile suction catheter with Y-port
- 1″ tape (adhesive or waterproof tape)
- Disposable gloves
- Sterile suctioning kit
- Oral suction catheter
- Two 3-mL syringes or tongue blade
- Scissors
- Washcloth and cleaning agent
- Skin barrier (such as 3M® or Skin Prep®)
- Adhesive remover swab
- Towel
- Razor (optional)
- Shaving cream (optional)
- Sterile saline or water
- Hand-held pressure gauge

ASSESSMENT

Assess for the need for retaping: Loose or soiled tape, pressure on mucous membranes, or repositioning of tube. Assess endotracheal tube length. The tube has markings on the side to ensure it is not moved during the retaping. Assess lung sounds to obtain a baseline. Ensure that the lung sounds are still heard throughout the lobes. Assess oxygen saturation level. If the tube is dislodged, the oxygen saturation level may change. Assess the chest for symmetric rise and fall during respiration. If the tube is dislodged, the rise and fall of the chest will change. Assess patient's need for pain medication or sedation. The patient should be calm, free of pain, and relaxed during the retaping so that he or she does not move and cause an accidental extubation.

NURSING DIAGNOSIS

Determine the related factors for the nursing diagnosis based on the patient's current status. Appropriate nursing diagnoses may include:

- Risk for Impaired Skin Integrity
- Impaired Oral Mucous Membrane
- Risk for Infection
- Risk for Injury

OUTCOME IDENTIFICATION AND PLANNING

The expected outcome to achieve is that the tube remains in place, and the patient maintains bilaterally equal and clear lung sounds. Other outcomes may include: the patient demonstrates understanding about the reason for the endotracheal tube; skin remains intact; oxygen saturation remains >95%; chest rises symmetrically; and airway remains clear.

SKILL 14-12

Securing an Endotracheal Tube *(continued)*

IMPLEMENTATION

ACTION	RATIONALE
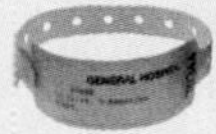 1. Identify the patient.	Positive identification of the patient is essential to ensure the intervention is administered to the correct patient.
2. Assess the need for endotracheal tube retaping. **Administer pain medication or sedation as prescribed before attempting to retape endotracheal tube.** Explain the procedure to the patient.	Explanation facilitates cooperation and provides reassurance for patient. Any procedure that compromises respiration is frightening for the patient. Retaping the endotracheal tube can stimulate coughing, which is painful for patients with surgical incisions.
3. Obtain the assistance of a second individual to hold the endotracheal tube in place while the old tape is removed and the new tape is placed.	This prevents accidental extubation.
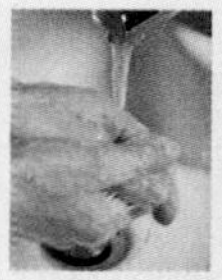 4. Perform hand hygiene.	Hand hygiene deters spread of microorganisms.
5. Adjust bed to comfortable working position. Lower side rail closer to you. If patient is conscious, place him or her in a semi-Fowler's position. **If patient is unconscious, place him or her in the lateral position, facing you. Move the overbed table close to your work area. Place a trash receptacle within easy reach of work area.**	A sitting position helps the patient to cough and makes breathing easier. The lateral position prevents the airway from becoming obstructed and promotes drainage of secretions. The overbed table provides work surface. Placing the trash receptacle within reach allows for organized approach to care.
6. Put on face shield or goggles and mask. Suction patient as described in Skill 14-10 or 14-11. Remove face shield or goggles and mask after suctioning.	Personal protective equipment prevents exposure to contaminants. Suctioning decreases the likelihood of patient coughing during the retaping of the endotracheal tube. If the patient coughs, the tube may become dislodged.
7. Measure a piece of tape for the length needed to reach around the patient's neck to the mouth plus 8″. Cut tape. Lay it adhesive side up on the table.	Extra length is needed so that tape can be wrapped around the endotracheal tube.
8. Cut another piece of tape long enough to reach from one jaw around the back of the neck to the other jaw. Lay this piece on the center of the longer piece on the table, matching the tapes' adhesive sides together.	This prevents the tape from sticking to the patient's hair and the back of the neck.
9. Take one 3-mL syringe or tongue blade and wrap the sticky tape around the syringe until the nonsticky area is reached. Do this for the other side as well.	This helps the nurse or respiratory therapist to manage the tape without it sticking to the sheets or the patient's hair.
10. Take one of the 3-mL syringes or tongue blades and pass it under the patient's neck so that there is a 3-mL syringe on either side of the patient's head.	This makes the tape easy to access when retaping the tube.
11. Put on disposable gloves. Have the assistant put on gloves as well.	Gloves protect hands from exposure to contaminants.
12. **Provide oral care, including suctioning the oral cavity.**	This helps to decrease secretions in the oral cavity and pharynx region.

(continued)

SKILL 14-12 Securing an Endotracheal Tube *(continued)*

ACTION / **RATIONALE**

13. Take note of the 'cm' position markings on the tube. Begin to unwrap old tape from around the endotracheal tube. After one side is unwrapped, have assistant hold the endotracheal tube as close to the lips or nares as possible to offer stabilization.

Assistant should hold tube to prevent accidental extubation. Holding tube as close to lips or nares as possible prevents accidental dislodgement of tube.

14. Carefully remove the remaining tape from the endotracheal tube (Figure 1). **After tape is removed, have assistant gently and slowly move endotracheal tube (if orally intubated) to the other side of the mouth (Figure 2). Assess mouth for any skin breakdown. Before applying new tape, make sure that markings on endotracheal tube are at same spot as when retaping began.**

The endotracheal tube may cause pressure ulcers if left in the same place over time. By moving the tube, the risk for pressure ulcers is reduced.

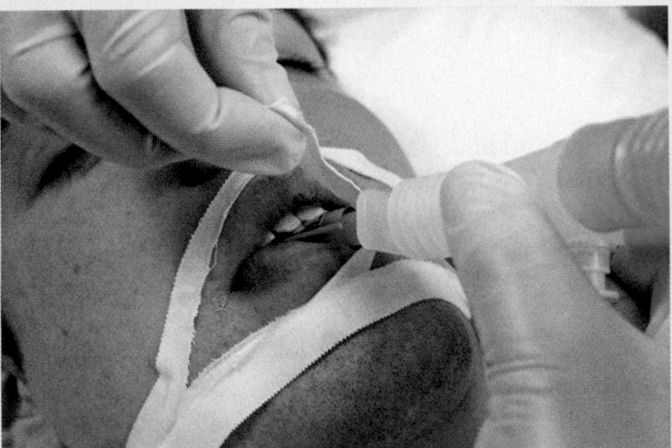

Figure 1. Ensuring endotracheal tube is stabilized and removing old tape.

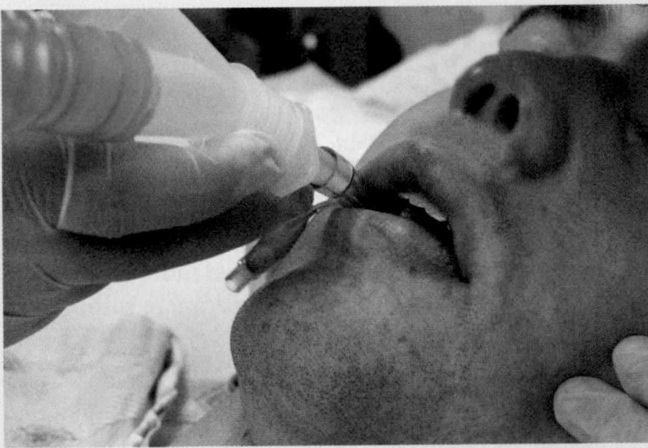

Figure 2. Moving endotracheal tube to other side of mouth.

15. Remove old tape from cheeks and side of face. Use adhesive remover to remove excess adhesive from tape (Figure 3). Clean the face and neck with washcloth and cleanser. If patient has facial hair, consider shaving cheeks. Pat cheeks dry with the towel.

To prevent skin breakdown, remove old adhesive. Shaving helps to decrease pain when tape is removed. Cheeks must be dry before new tape is applied to ensure that it sticks.

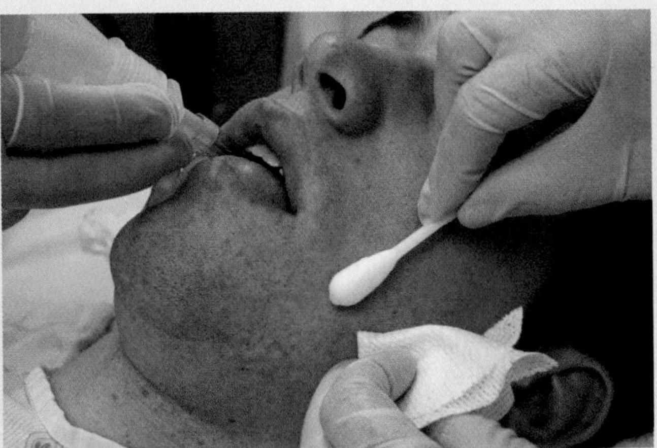

Figure 3. Cleaning cheeks at site of tape.

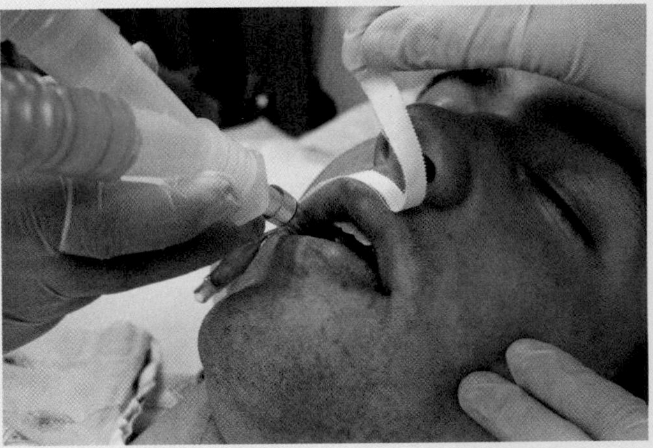

Figure 4. Putting new tape in place.

SKILL 14-12 Securing an Endotracheal Tube *(continued)*

ACTION	RATIONALE
16. Apply the skin barrier to the patient's face (under his nose, cheeks, under lower lip) where the tape will sit. Unroll one side of the tape. Ensure that nonsticky part of tape remains behind patient's neck while pulling firmly on the tape. **Place adhesive portion of tape snugly against patient's cheek.** Split the tape in half from the end to the corner of the mouth.	Skin barrier protects the skin from injury with subsequent tape removal and helps the tape adhere better to the skin. The tape should be snug to the side of the patient's face to prevent accidental extubation.
17. Place the top-half piece of tape under the patient's nose (Figure 4). Wrap the lower half around the tube in one direction, such as over and around the tube. Fold over tab on end of tape.	By placing one piece of tape on the lip and the other piece of tape on the tube, the tube remains secure. Tab makes tape removal easier.
18. Unwrap second side of tape. Split to corner of the mouth. Place the bottom-half piece of tape along the patient's lower lip. Wrap the top half around the tube in the opposite direction, such as below and around the tube. Fold over tab on end of tape (Figure 5).	Alternating the placement of the top and bottom pieces of tape provides more anchorage for the tube. Wrapping the tape in an alternating manner ensures that the tape will not accidentally be unwound.

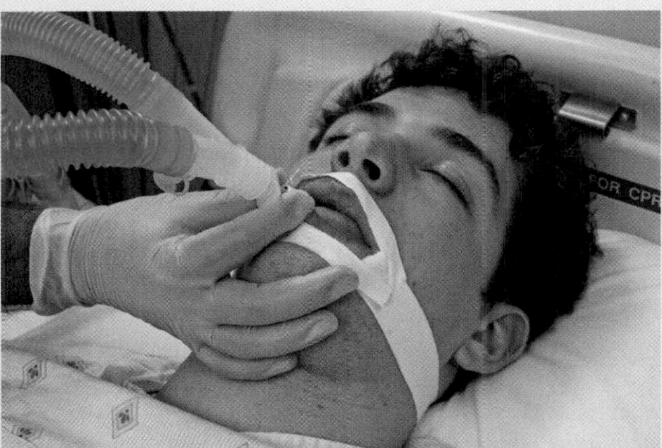

Figure 5. Ensuring tape is securely stabilizing the tube.

ACTION	RATIONALE
19. **Auscultate lung sounds. Assess for cyanosis, oxygen saturation, chest symmetry, and stability of endotracheal tube. Again check to ensure that the tube is at the correct depth.**	If tube has been moved from original place, the lung sounds may change, as well as oxygen saturation and chest symmetry. The tube should be stable and should not move with each respiration cycle.
20. **If endotracheal tube is cuffed, check pressure of balloon by attaching a hand-held pressure gauge to the pilot balloon of the endotracheal tube.**	Maximum cuff pressures should not exceed 24–30 cm H_20 to prevent tracheal ischemia and necrosis.
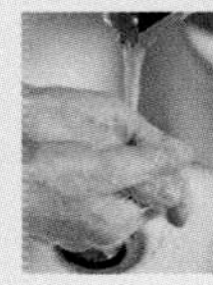 21. Remove face shield or goggles and mask. Remove gloves and perform hand hygiene. Assist patient to a comfortable position. Raise bed rail.	Hand hygiene deters the spread of microorganisms.

(continued)

SKILL 14-12 Securing an Endotracheal Tube *(continued)*

EVALUATION

The expected outcome is met when the endotracheal tube tape is changed without dislodgement or a depth change of the tube; lung sounds remain equal; no pressure ulcers are noted; airway remains clear; oxygen saturation remains >95%; chest rises symmetrically; skin remains acyanotic; and cuff pressure is maintained at 20 to 25 cm H_20.

DOCUMENTATION

Guidelines

Document the procedure, including the depth of the endotracheal tube from teeth or lips; the amount, consistency, and color of secretions suctioned; presence of any skin or mucous membrane changes or pressure ulcers; and pre- and postassessment, including lung sounds, oxygen saturation, skin color, cuff pressure, and chest symmetry.

Sample Documentation

9/27/08 1305 Endotracheal tube tape changed; tube remains 12 cm at lips; suctioned for tenacious, yellow secretions, copious in amount; 2-cm pressure ulcer noted on left side of tongue. Tube moved to right side of mouth; lung sounds clear and equal after retaping; pulse oximeter remains 98% on 35% FiO_2; skin pink; cuff pressure 22 cmH_2O; chest rises symmetrically.—C. Bausler, RN

Unexpected Situations and Associated Interventions

- *Patient is accidentally extubated during tape change:* Stay with patient. Instruct assistant to notify physician. Assess patient's vital signs, ability to breathe without assistance, and oxygen saturation. Be ready to deliver assisted breaths with a bag-valve mask (Skill 14-17) or administer oxygen. Anticipate the need for reintubation.
- *Tube depth changes during retaping:* Tube depth should be maintained at the same level unless otherwise ordered by the physician. Remove tape around tube, adjust tube to ordered depth, and reapply tape.
- *Air leak (air escaping around the balloon) is heard on inspiration cycle of ventilator:* Auscultate lung sounds and check depth of endotracheal tube to ensure that it has not dislodged. Obtain hand-held pressure gauge and check pressure. Air may need to be added to balloon to prevent air leak. If pressure is already 25 cm H_20, physician may need to be contacted before adding more air to balloon. Sometimes a change in the patient's position will resolve air leaks.
- *Patient is biting on endotracheal tube:* Obtain a bite block. With the help of an assistant, place the bite block around the endotracheal tube or in patient's mouth. If ordered, consider sedating the patient.
- *Depth of endotracheal tube changes with respiratory cycle:* Remove old tape. Repeat taping of the endotracheal tube, ensuring that tape is snug against patient's face.
- *Patient has trauma to face that prevents the use of tape when securing the endotracheal tube:* You may need to obtain a commercially prepared endotracheal tube holder. There are various types on the market; check with your institution for availability.
- *Lung sounds are greater on one side:* Check the depth of the endotracheal tube. If the tube has been advanced, the lung sounds will appear greater on the side on which the tube is further down. Remove tape and move tube so that it is properly placed. If the depth has not changed, assess patient's oxygen saturation, skin color, and respiratory rate. Notify physician. Anticipate the need for a chest x-ray.
- *Pressure ulcer is noted in the mouth or nares (if patient is intubated via nares):* If the ulcer is painful, you may obtain an order for a topical numbing medication such as lidocaine viscous jelly. Apply topically with cotton-tipped applicator. Keep area clean by performing more frequent oral or nasal care. Ensure that tubing is not pulling on endotracheal tube, thus applying pressure on the patient's skin.

SKILL 14-12 Securing an Endotracheal Tube *(continued)*

- *Pilot balloon is accidentally cut while caring for endotracheal tube:* Notify physician. Obtain a 22-gauge catheter and thread it into the pilot balloon tubing, being careful not to puncture the tubing with the needle, below the cut. Remove the needle from the catheter and apply a stopcock or needleless Luer-Lok to the catheter. If air is needed to reinflate the balloon, a syringe can be attached to the stopcock or Luer-Lok so that air may be added. Anticipate the need for a tube change.

Special Considerations

General Considerations

- Emergency equipment should be easily accessible at the bedside. Bag-valve mask, oxygen, and suction equipment should be kept at the bedside of a patient with an endotracheal tube at all times.

SKILL 14-13 Suctioning the Tracheostomy: Open System

Suctioning through a tracheostomy is indicated to maintain a patent airway. Tracheal suctioning can lead to hypoxemia, cardiac dysrhythmias, trauma, atelectasis, infection, bleeding, and pain. It is imperative to be diligent in maintaining aseptic technique and following facility guidelines and procedures to prevent potential hazards. Suctioning frequency is based on clinical assessment to determine the need for suctioning.

The purpose of suctioning is to remove secretions that are not accessible to bypassed cilia, so insertion of the catheter only as far as the end of the tracheostomy tube is recommended. Catheter contact and suction cause tracheal mucosal damage, loss of cilia, edema, and fibrosis, as well as increasing the risk of infection and bleeding for the patient. Insertion of the suction catheter to a predetermined distance, no more than 1 cm past the length of the tracheostomy tube, avoids contact with the trachea and carina, reducing the effects of tracheal mucosal damage (Pate, 2004; Pate & Zapata, 2002). Box 14-1 in Skill 14-10 shows several methods for nurses to use to determine appropriate suction catheter depth.

Note: In-line, closed systems are available to suction mechanically ventilated patients. The use of closed suction catheter systems may avoid some of the infection control issues and other complications associated with open suction techniques. This procedure is the same for patients with tracheostomy tubes and endotracheal tubes connected to mechanical ventilation. See Skill 14-11 for this procedure.

Equipment

- Portable or wall suction unit with tubing
- A commercially prepared suction kit with an appropriate size catheter (See General Considerations) or
  - Sterile suction catheter with Y-port in the appropriate size
  - Sterile disposable container
  - Sterile gloves
- Towel or waterproof pad
- Goggles and mask or face shield
- Disposable, clean gloves
- Resuscitation bag connected to 100% oxygen

(continued)

SKILL 14-13 Suctioning the Tracheostomy: Open System *(continued)*

ASSESSMENT

Assess lung sounds. Patients who need to be suctioned may have wheezes, crackles, or gurgling present. Assess oxygenation saturation level. Oxygen saturation usually decreases when a patient needs to be suctioned. Assess respiratory status, including respiratory rate and depth. Patients may become tachypneic when they need to be suctioned. Additional indications for suctioning via a tracheostomy tube include secretions in the tube, acute respiratory distress, and frequent or sustained coughing. Assess for pain. If patient has had abdominal surgery or other procedures, pain medication should be administered before suctioning.

NURSING DIAGNOSIS

Determine the related factors for the nursing diagnosis based on the patient's current status. Appropriate nursing diagnoses may include:

- Ineffective Airway Clearance
- Risk for Aspiration
- Impaired Gas Exchange
- Ineffective Breathing Pattern

OUTCOME IDENTIFICATION AND PLANNING

The expected outcome is that the patient will exhibit improved breath sounds and a clear, patent airway. Other outcomes that may be appropriate include the following: patient will exhibit an oxygen saturation level within acceptable parameters; patient will demonstrate a respiratory rate and depth within age-acceptable range; and patient will remain free of any signs of respiratory distress.

IMPLEMENTATION

ACTION	RATIONALE
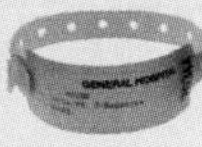 1. Identify the patient.	Positive identification of the patient is essential to ensure the intervention is administered to the correct patient.
2. Determine the need for suctioning. Verify the suction order in the patient's chart. **For postoperative patient, administer pain medication as prescribed before suctioning.**	To minimize trauma to airway mucosa, suctioning should be done only when secretions have accumulated or adventitious breath sounds are audible. Suctioning stimulates coughing, which is painful for patients with surgical incisions.
3. Explain to the patient what you are going to do and the reason, even if the patient does not appear to be alert. Reassure patient you will interrupt procedure if he or she indicates respiratory difficulty.	Explanation alleviates fears. Even if patient appears unconscious, the nurse should explain what is happening. Any procedure that compromises respiration is frightening for the patient.
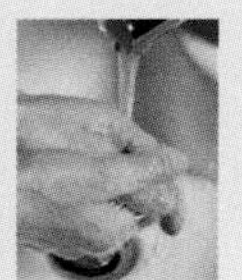 4. Perform hand hygiene.	Hand hygiene deters the spread of microorganisms.
5. Adjust bed to comfortable working position. Lower side rail closer to you. If patient is conscious, place him or her in a semi-Fowler's position (Figure 1). **If patient is unconscious, place him or her in the lateral position, facing you. Move the overbed table close to your work area and raise to waist height.**	A sitting position helps the patient to cough and makes breathing easier. Gravity also facilitates catheter insertion. The lateral position prevents the airway from becoming obstructed and promotes drainage of secretions. The overbed table provides a work surface and maintains sterility of objects on work surface.

SKILL 14-13 Suctioning the Tracheostomy: Open System *(continued)*

ACTION	RATIONALE
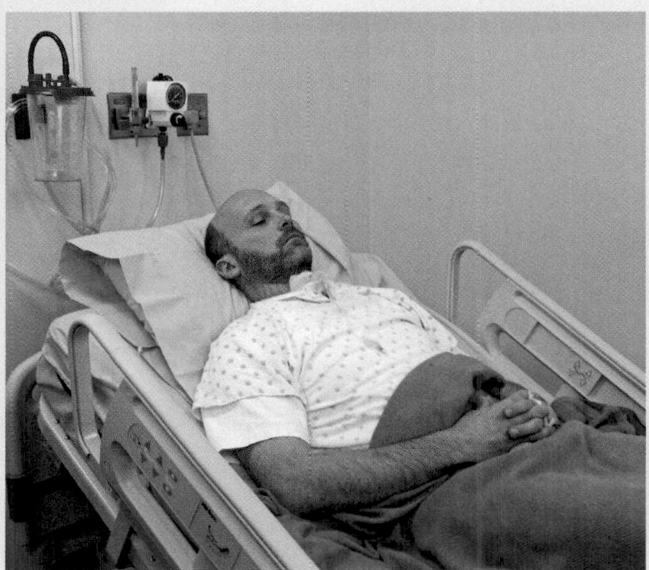 **Figure 1.** Patient in semi-Fowler's position.	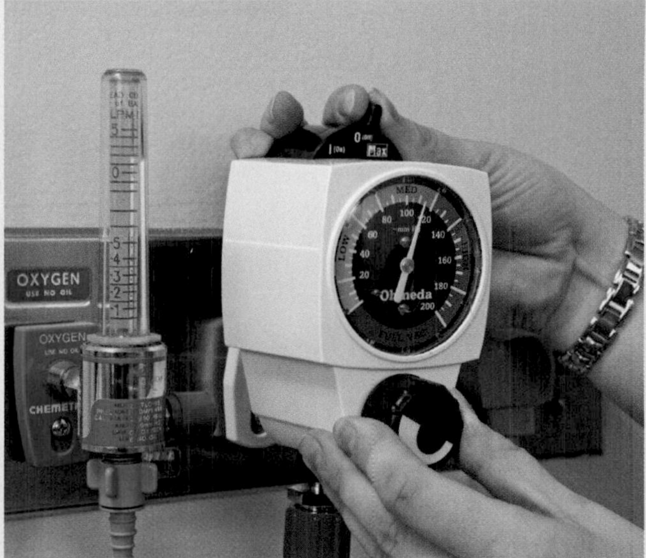 **Figure 2.** Turning suction device to the appropriate pressure.
6. Place towel or waterproof pad across patient's chest.	This protects bed linens and the patient.
7. **Turn suction to appropriate pressure (Figure 2):** For a wall unit for an adult: 100–150 mm Hg; neonates: 60–80 mm Hg; infants: 80–100 mm Hg; children: 100–120 mm Hg For a portable unit for an adult: 10–15 cm Hg; neonates: 6–8 cm Hg; infants 8–10 cm Hg; children 10–12 cm Hg **Put on a disposable, clean glove and occlude the end of the connecting tubing to check suction pressure. Place the connecting tubing in a convenient location. If using it, place resuscitation bag connected to oxygen within convenient reach.**	Higher pressures can cause excessive trauma, hypoxemia, and atelectasis.
8. **Open sterile suction package using aseptic technique. The open wrapper or container becomes a sterile field to hold other supplies. Carefully remove the sterile container, touching only the outside surface. Set it up on the work surface and pour sterile saline into it.**	Sterile normal saline or water is used to lubricate the outside of the catheter, minimizing irritation of mucosa during introduction. It is also used to clear the catheter between suction attempts.
9. Put on face shield or goggles and mask (Figure 3). Put on sterile gloves. **The dominant hand will manipulate the catheter and must remain sterile. The nondominant hand is considered clean rather than sterile and will control the suction valve (Y port) on the catheter.**	Handling the sterile catheter using a sterile glove helps prevent introducing organisms into the respiratory tract; the clean glove protects the nurse from microorganisms.

(continued)

SKILL 14-13 Suctioning the Tracheostomy: Open System *(continued)*

ACTION	RATIONALE

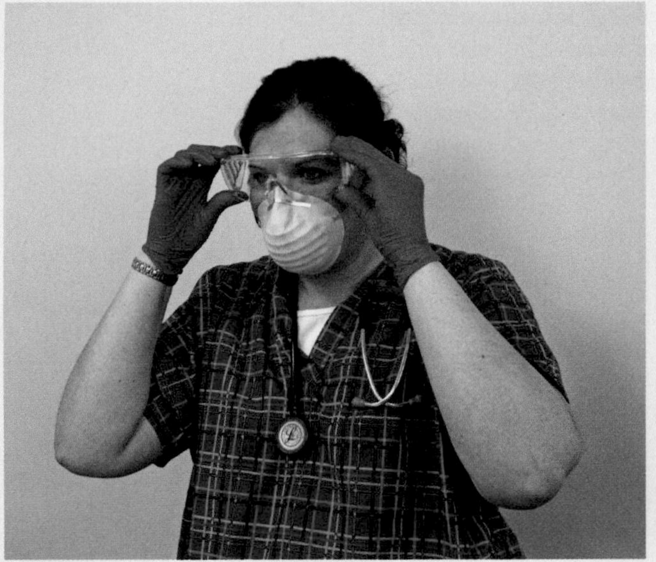

Figure 3. Putting on goggles and mask.

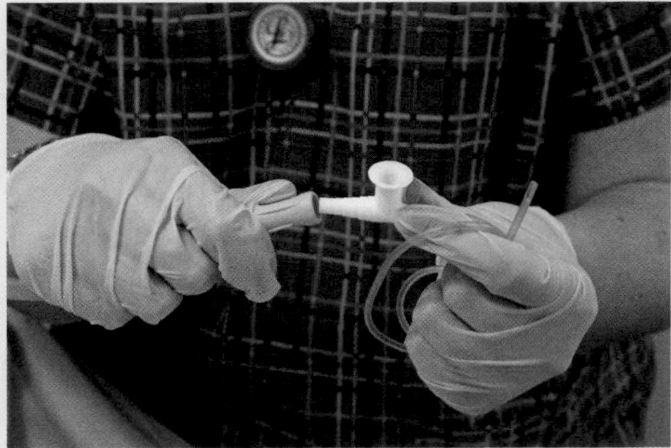

Figure 4. Connecting suction catheter to the suction tubing.

ACTION	RATIONALE
10. With dominant gloved hand, pick up sterile catheter. Pick up the connecting tubing with the nondominant hand and connect the tubing and suction catheter (Figure 4).	Sterility of the suction catheter is maintained.
11. Moisten the catheter by dipping it into the container of sterile saline, unless it is a silicone catheter (Figure 5). Occlude Y-tube to check suction (Figure 6).	Lubricating the inside of the catheter with saline helps move secretions in the catheter. Silicone catheters do not require lubrication. Checking ensures equipment is working properly.

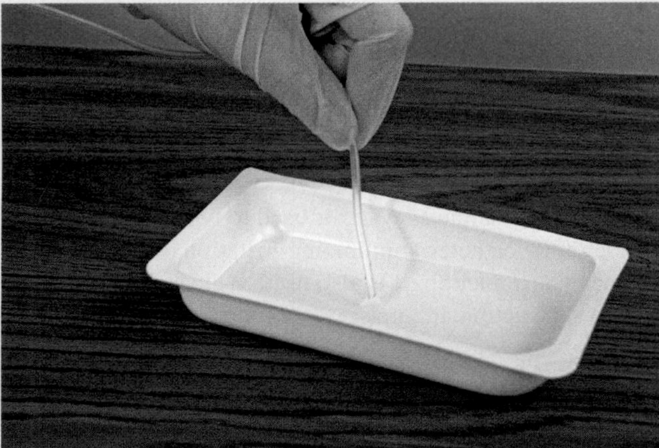

Figure 5. Moistening catheter in saline solution.

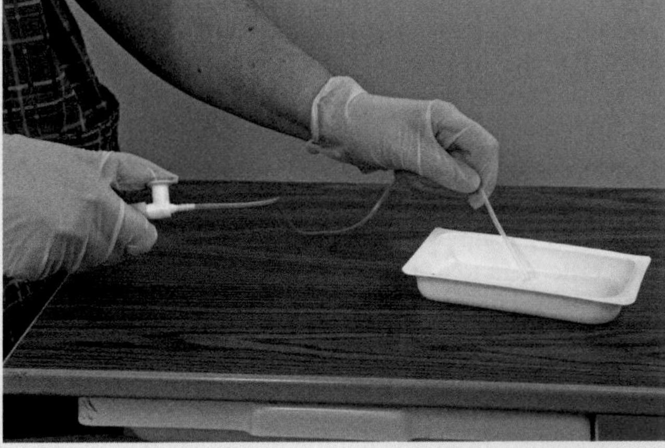

Figure 6. Occluding Y-port to check for proper suction.

ACTION	RATIONALE
12. Using your nondominant hand and a manual resuscitation bag, hyperventilate the patient delivering 3 to 6 breaths or use the sigh mechanism on a mechanical ventilator.	Hyperoxygenation aids in preventing hypoxemia during suctioning.

SKILL 14-13 Suctioning the Tracheostomy: Open System *(continued)*

ACTION	RATIONALE
13. Open the adapter on the mechanical ventilator tubing or remove oxygen delivery setup with your nondominant hand.	This exposes tracheostomy tube without contaminating sterile gloved hand.
14. Using your dominant hand, gently and quickly insert catheter into trachea. **Advance the catheter to the predetermined length. Do not occlude Y-port when inserting catheter.**	Suctioning when inserting catheter increases the risk for trauma to airway mucosa and increases risk of hypoxemia. If resistance is met, the carina or tracheal mucosa has been hit. Withdraw the catheter at least ½″ before applying suction.
15. Apply suction by intermittently occluding the Y port on the catheter with the thumb of your nondominant hand, and gently rotate the catheter as it is being withdrawn (Figure 7). **Do not suction for more than 10 to 15 seconds at a time.**	Turning the catheter as it is withdrawn minimizes trauma to the mucosa. Suctioning for longer than 10 to 15 seconds robs the respiratory tract of oxygen, which may result in hypoxemia. Suctioning too quickly may be ineffective at clearing all secretions.

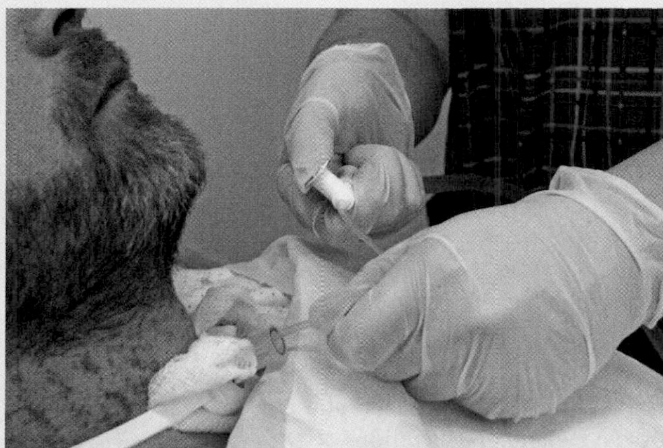
Figure 7. Applying intermittent suction while withdrawing catheter.

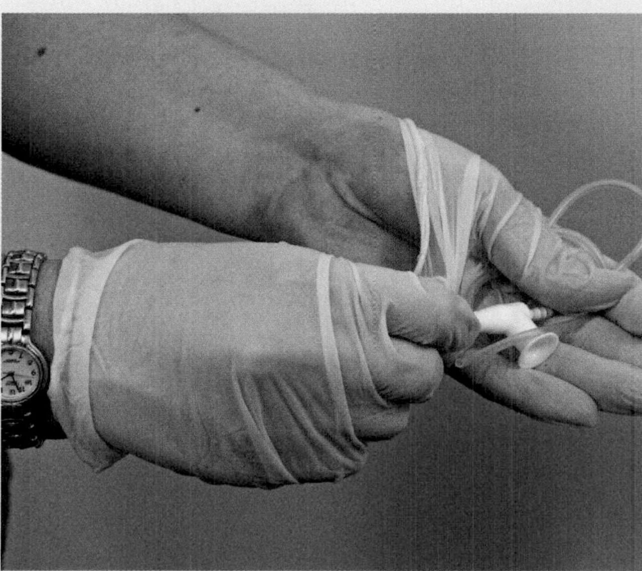
Figure 8. Removing gloves while keeping catheter inside.

ACTION	RATIONALE
16. Hyperventilate the patient using your nondominant hand and a manual resuscitation bag, delivering 3 to 6 breaths. Replace the oxygen delivery device, if applicable, using your nondominant hand and have the patient take several deep breaths. If the patient is mechanically ventilated, close the adapter on the mechanical ventilator tubing and use the sigh mechanism on a mechanical ventilator.	Suctioning removes air from the patient's airway and can cause hypoxemia. Hyperventilation can help prevent suction-induced hypoxemia.
17. Flush catheter with saline. Assess effectiveness of suctioning and repeat as needed and according to patient's tolerance. Wrap the suction catheter around your dominant hand between attempts.	Flushing clears catheter and lubricates it for next insertion. Reassessment determines need for additional suctioning. Prevents inadvertent contamination of catheter.

(continued)

SKILL 14-13 Suctioning the Tracheostomy: Open System *(continued)*

ACTION	RATIONALE
18. **Allow at least a 30-second to 1-minute interval if additional suctioning is needed. No more than three suction passes should be made per suctioning episode. Encourage patient to cough and deep breathe between suctionings.** Suction the oropharynx after suctioning the trachea. Do not reinsert in the tracheostomy after suctioning the mouth.	The interval allows for reventilation and reoxygenation of airways. Excessive suction passes contribute to complications. Alternating nares reduces trauma. Clears the mouth of secretions. More microorganisms are usually present in the mouth, so it is suctioned last to prevent transmission of contaminants.
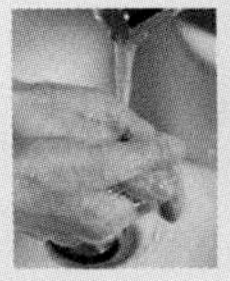 19. When suctioning is completed, remove glove from dominant hand over the coiled catheter, pulling it off inside out (Figure 8). Remove glove from nondominant hand and dispose of gloves, catheter, and container with solution in the appropriate receptacle. Remove face shield or goggles and mask. Perform hand hygiene.	All reduce transmission of microorganisms.
20. Turn off suction. Assist patient to a comfortable position. Raise bed rail. Offer oral hygiene after suctioning.	Respiratory secretions that are allowed to accumulate in the mouth are irritating to mucous membranes and unpleasant for the patient.
21. Reassess patient's respiratory status, including respiratory rate, effort, oxygen saturation, and lung sounds.	This assesses effectiveness of suctioning and the presence of complications.

EVALUATION

The expected outcome is met when the patient exhibits improved breath sounds and a clear and patent airway. In addition, the oxygen saturation level is within acceptable parameters, and the patient does not exhibit signs or symptoms of respiratory distress or complications.

DOCUMENTATION

Guidelines

Document the time of suctioning, your pre- and postintervention assessment, reason for suctioning, and the characteristics and amount of secretions.

Sample Documentation

9/1/08 1515 Lungs auscultated for wheezes in upper and lower lobes bilaterally. Respirations at 24 breaths per min. Weak, ineffective cough noted. Tracheal suction completed with 12F catheter. Large amount of thick, yellow secretions obtained. Specimen for culture collected and sent as ordered. After suctioning, lung sounds clear all lobes, oxygen saturation at 97%, respirations 18 breaths per min.—C. Bausler, RN

Unexpected Situations and Associated Interventions

- *Patient coughs hard enough to dislodge tracheostomy:* Spare tracheostomy and obturator should be kept at bedside. Insert obturator into tracheostomy tube and reinsert tracheostomy into stoma. Remove obturator. Secure ties and auscultate lung sounds. Palpate for any subcutaneous emphysema.
- *Lung sounds do not improve greatly and oxygen saturation remains low after three suctionings:* Allow patient time to recover from previous suctioning. If needed, hyperoxygenate again. Suction the patient again and assess whether the oxygen saturation increases, lung sounds improve, and secretion amount decreases.

SKILL 14-13 Suctioning the Tracheostomy: Open System *(continued)*

Special Considerations

General Considerations

- The size catheter used is determined by the size of the tracheostomy. The external diameter of the suction catheter should not exceed half of the internal diameter of the tracheostomy. Larger catheters can contribute to trauma and hypoxemia.
- Emergency equipment should be easily accessible at the bedside. Bag-valve mask, oxygen, and suction equipment should be kept at the bedside of a patient with a tracheostomy tube at all times.

SKILL 14-14 Providing Tracheostomy Care

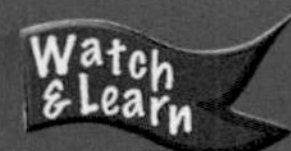

The nurse is responsible for either cleaning a nondisposable inner cannula or replacing a disposable one. The inner cannula requires cleaning or replacement to prevent accumulation of secretions that can interfere with respiration and occlude the airway. Because soiled tracheostomy dressings place the patient at risk for the development of skin breakdown and infection, regularly change dressings and ties. Use gauze dressings that are not filled with cotton to prevent aspiration of foreign bodies (eg, lint or cotton fibers) into the trachea. Clean the skin around a tracheostomy to prevent buildup of dried secretions and skin breakdown. Exercise care when changing the tracheostomy ties to prevent accidental decannulation or expulsion of the tube. Have an assistant hold the tube in place during the change or keep the soiled tie in place until a clean one is securely attached. Agency policy and patient condition determine specific procedures and schedules, but a newly inserted tracheostomy may require attention every 1 to 2 hours. Because the respiratory tract is sterile and the tracheostomy provides a direct opening, meticulous care using aseptic technique is necessary.

Equipment

- Disposable gloves
- Sterile gloves
- Goggles and mask or face shield
- Sterile tracheostomy cleaning kit (if available) or
  - Sterile basins (3)
  - Sterile brush/pipe cleaners
  - Sterile cotton-tipped applicators
  - Sterile gauze sponges
- Sterile cleaning solutions:
  - Hydrogen peroxide
  - Normal saline solution
- Sterile suction catheter and glove set
- Commercially prepared tracheostomy or drain dressing
- Tracheostomy ties (twill tape or Velcro™)
- Scissors
- Plastic disposal bag

(continued)

SKILL 14-14 Providing Tracheostomy Care

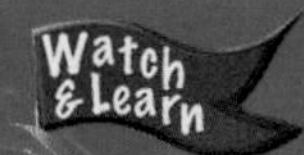

ASSESSMENT

Assess for signs and symptoms of the need to perform tracheostomy care, which include soiled dressings and ties, secretions in the tracheostomy tube, and diminished airflow through the tracheostomy, or in accordance with facility policy. Assess insertion site for any redness or purulent drainage; if present, these may signify an infection. Assess patient for pain. If tracheostomy is new, pain medication may be needed before performing tracheostomy care. Assess lung sounds and oxygen saturation levels. Lung sounds should be equal in all lobes, with an oxygen saturation level >93%. If tracheostomy is dislodged, lung sounds and oxygen saturation level will diminish. Inspect the area on the posterior portion of the neck for any skin breakdown that may result from irritation or pressure from tracheostomy ties.

NURSING DIAGNOSIS

Determine the related factors for the nursing diagnosis based on the patient's current status. Appropriate nursing diagnoses may include:

- Impaired Skin Integrity
- Risk for Infection
- Ineffective Airway Clearance
- Risk for Aspiration

OUTCOME IDENTIFICATION AND PLANNING

The expected outcome to achieve when performing tracheostomy care is that the patient will exhibit a tracheostomy tube and site free from drainage, secretions, and skin irritation or breakdown. Other outcomes that may be appropriate include the following: oxygen saturation levels will be within acceptable parameters, and patient will have no evidence of respiratory distress.

IMPLEMENTATION

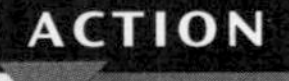

ACTION	RATIONALE
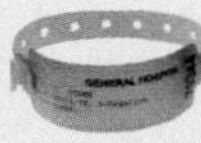 1. Identify the patient.	Positive identification of the patient is essential to ensure the intervention is administered to the correct patient.
2. Determine the need for tracheostomy care. **Assess patient's pain and administer pain medication, if indicated.**	If tracheostomy is new, pain medication may be needed before performing tracheostomy care.
3. Explain what you are going to do and the reason to the patient, even if the patient does not appear to be alert. Reassure patient you will interrupt procedure if he or she indicates respiratory difficulty.	Explanation alleviates fears. Even if patient appears unconscious, the nurse should explain what is happening. Any procedure that compromises respiration is frightening for the patient.
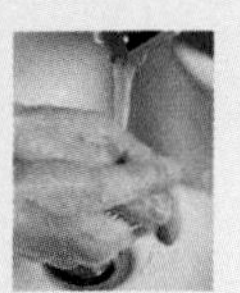 4. Perform hand hygiene. 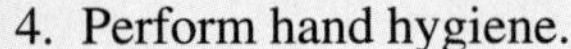	Hand hygiene deters the spread of microorganisms.
5. Adjust bed to comfortable working position. Lower side rail closer to you. If patient is conscious, place him or her in a semi-Fowler's position. **If patient is unconscious, place him or her in the lateral position, facing you. Move the overbed table close to your work area and raise to waist height. Place a trash receptacle within easy reach of work area.**	A sitting position helps the patient to cough and makes breathing easier. Gravity also facilitates catheter insertion. The lateral position prevents the airway from becoming obstructed and promotes drainage of secretions. The overbed table provides work surface and maintains sterility of objects on work surface. Trash receptacle within reach prevents reaching over sterile field or turning back to field to dispose of trash.

SKILL 14-14 Providing Tracheostomy Care *(continued)*

ACTION	RATIONALE
6. Put on face shield or goggles and mask. Suction tracheostomy if necessary. If tracheostomy has just been suctioned, remove soiled site dressing and discard before removal of gloves used to perform suctioning.	Personnel protective equipment prevents contact with contaminants. Suctioning removes secretions to prevent occluding outer cannula while the inner cannula is removed.
Cleaning the Tracheostomy: Nondisposable Inner Cannula.	
(See the accompanying Skill Variation for steps for replacing a disposable inner cannula.)	
7. Prepare supplies:	
a. Open tracheostomy care kit and separate basins, touching only the edges. If kit is not available, open three sterile basins.	Basins are sterile receptacles for cleaning solutions.
b. Fill one basin 0.5″ deep with hydrogen peroxide or half hydrogen peroxide and half saline, based on facility policy (Figure 1).	Hydrogen peroxide helps remove dry, encrusted secretions.
c. Fill other two basins 0.5″ deep with saline.	Saline rinses and removes hydrogen peroxide and lubricates the outer surface of the inner cannula for easier reinsertion.
d. Open sterile brush or pipe cleaners if they are not already available in a cleaning kit. Open additional sterile gauze pad.	Sterile brush or pipe cleaner provides friction to clean inner surface of cannula.

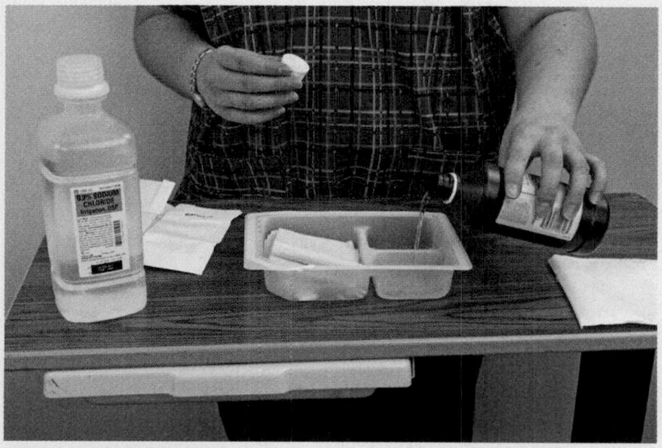

Figure 1. Preparing supplies.

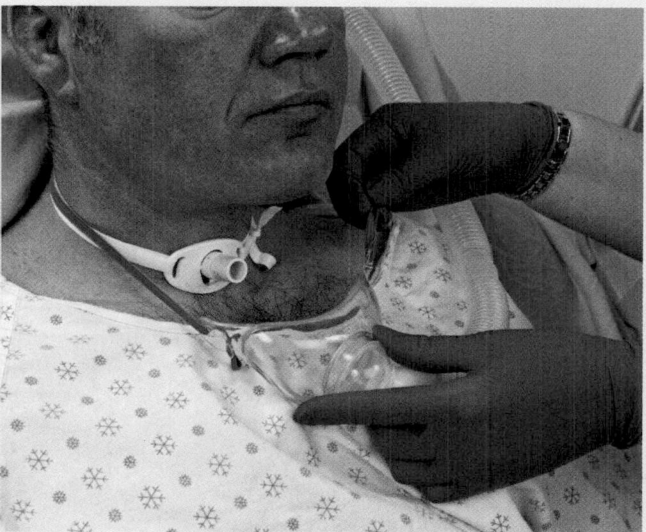

Figure 2. Removing oxygen source.

(continued)

SKILL 14-14

Providing Tracheostomy Care *(continued)*

ACTION | **RATIONALE**

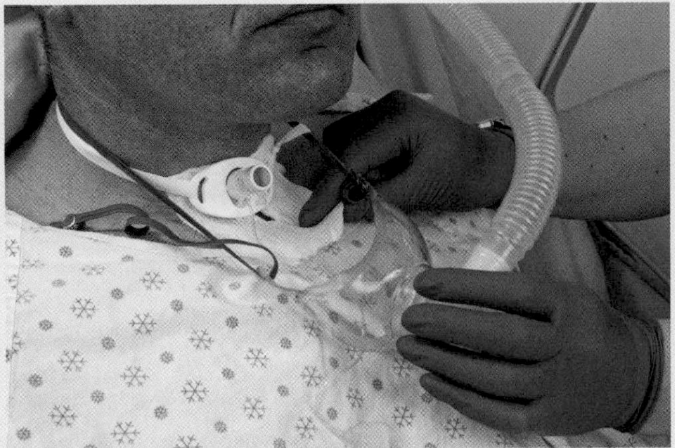

Figure 3. Removing soiled dressing.

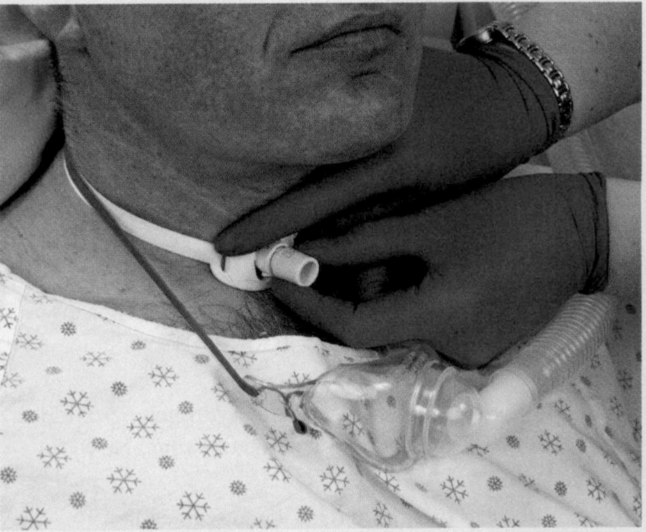

Figure 4. Rotating inner cannula while stabilizing outer cannula.

8. Put on disposable gloves.

Gloves protect against exposure to blood and body fluids.

9. Remove the oxygen source if one is present (Figure 2). If not already removed, remove site dressing and dispose of in the trash (Figure 3). Stabilize the outer cannula and faceplate of the tracheostomy with one hand. Rotate the lock on the inner cannula in a counterclockwise motion with your other hand to release it (Figure 4).

Stabilizing base plate prevents trauma to and pain from stoma. Releasing the lock permits removal of the inner cannula.

10. Continue to hold the faceplate. Gently remove the inner cannula (Figure 5) and carefully drop it in the basin with hydrogen peroxide. Replace the oxygen source over the outer cannula. Remove gloves and discard (Figure 6).

Soaking in hydrogen peroxide loosens dry, hardened secretions. Replacing the source maintains oxygen supply to the patient.

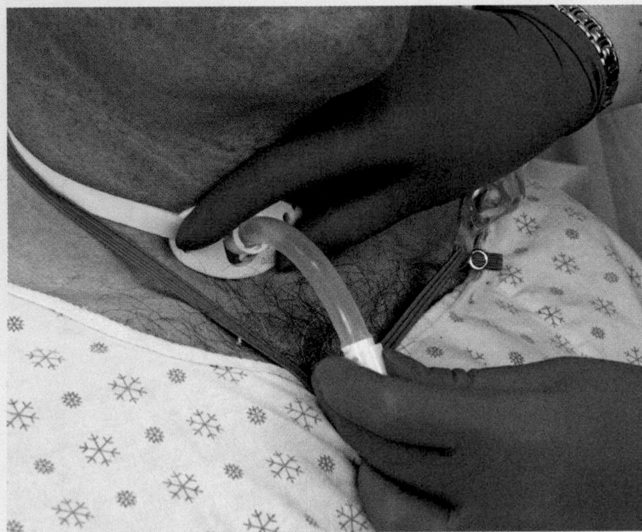

Figure 5. Removing inner cannula for cleaning.

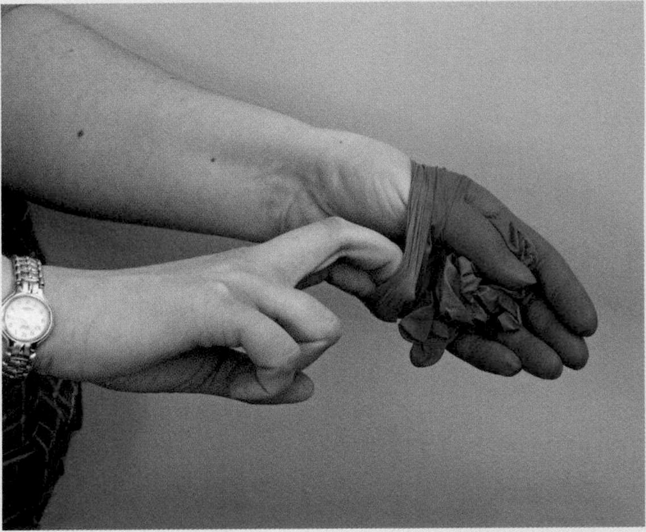

Figure 6. Removing gloves.

SKILL 14-14

Providing Tracheostomy Care *(continued)*

ACTION	RATIONALE
11. Clean the inner cannula as follows:	
a. Put on sterile gloves.	Sterile gloves maintain surgical asepsis.
b. Remove inner cannula from soaking solution. Moisten brush or pipe cleaners in saline and insert into tube, using back-and-forth motion (Figure 7).	Movement of brush creates friction and helps remove accumulated secretions.
c. Agitate cannula in saline solution (Figure 8). Remove and tap against inner surface of basin (Figure 9).	Saline rinses inner cannula. Tapping tube against basin removes excess saline in inner tube.
d. Place on sterile gauze pad.	Placing on sterile gauze maintains sterility and frees both hands for suctioning.

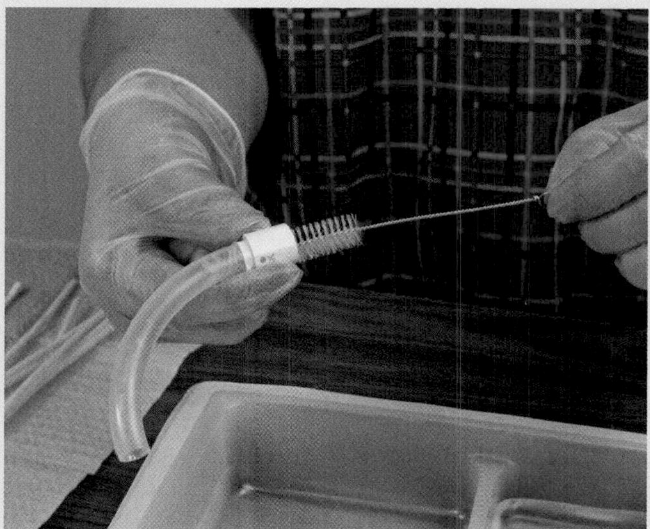
Figure 7. Using brush to clean inner cannula.

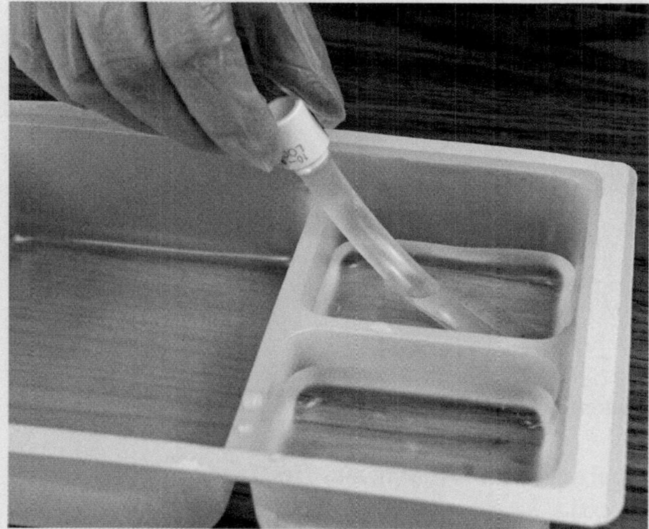
Figure 8. Rinsing cannula using an agitating motion.

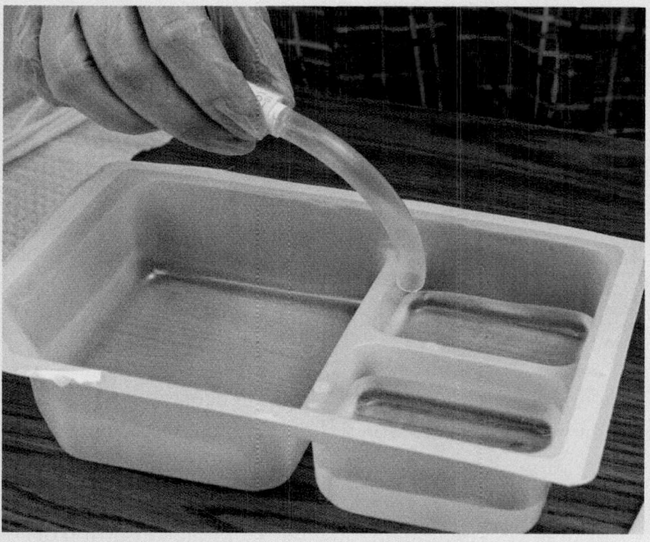
Figure 9. Tapping cannula to remove excessive moisture.

(continued)

SKILL 14-14

Providing Tracheostomy Care *(continued)*

ACTION	RATIONALE
12. **Suction outer cannula using sterile technique if necessary.**	Suctioning removes any remaining secretions.
13. Stabilize the outer cannula and faceplate with one hand. Replace inner cannula into outer cannula (Figure 10). Turn lock clockwise and check that inner cannula is secure. Reapply oxygen source if needed (Figure 11).	Clockwise motion secures inner cannula in place. Maintains oxygen supply to the patient.

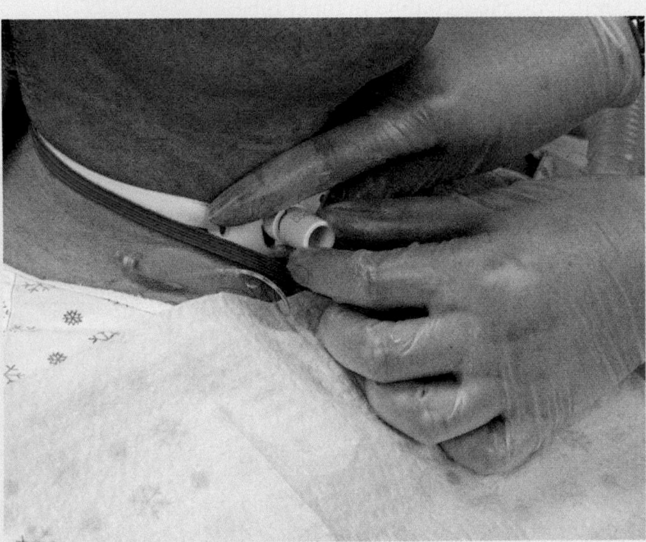

Figure 10. Replacing inner cannula.

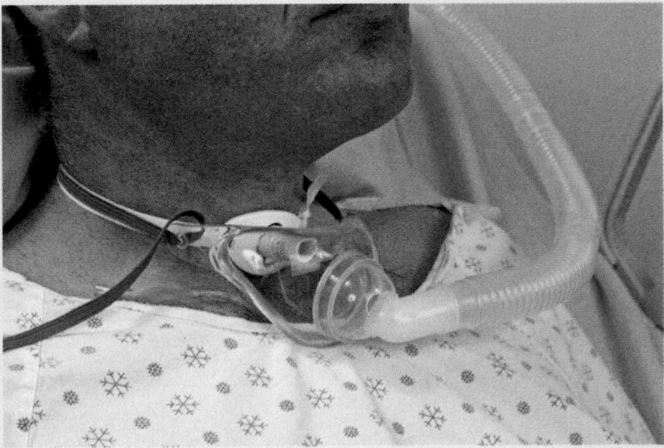

Figure 11. Reapplying oxygen source.

Applying Clean Dressing and Ties/Tape

(See accompanying Skill Variations for steps for an alternate site dressing if a commercially prepared sponge is not available and to secure a tracheostomy with a tracheostomy collar instead of ties/tape.)

ACTION	RATIONALE
14. Remove oxygen source. Dip cotton-tipped applicator or gauze sponge in second basin with sterile saline and clean stoma under faceplate. **Use each applicator or sponge only once, moving from stoma site outward (Figure 12).**	Saline is nonirritating to tissue. Cleansing from stoma outward and using each applicator only once promotes aseptic technique.
15. Pat skin gently with dry 4″ × 4″ gauze sponge (Figure 13).	Gauze removes excess moisture.
16. Slide commercially prepared tracheostomy dressing or prefolded non–cotton-filled 4″ × 4″ dressing under faceplate (Figure 14).	Lint or fiber from a cut cotton-filled gauze pad can be aspirated into the trachea, causing respiratory distress, or imbed in stoma and cause irritation or infection.
17. Change the tracheostomy tape:	
a. **Leave soiled tape in place until new one is applied.**	Leaving tape in place ensures that tracheostomy will not inadvertently be expelled if patient coughs or moves.
b. Cut piece of tape the length of twice the neck circumference plus 4″. Trim ends of tape on the diagonal (Figure 15).	This action provides for secure attachment with knot in front at neckplate. Diagonal cut facilitates insertion of tape into openings on faceplate.

SKILL 14-14 **Providing Tracheostomy Care** *(continued)*

ACTION	RATIONALE
c. Insert one end of tape through faceplate opening alongside old tape. Pull through until both ends are even length (Figure 16).	Doing so provides attachment for one side of faceplate.
d. Slide both ends of the tape under patient's neck and insert one end through remaining opening on other side of faceplate. Pull snugly and tie ends in double square knot (Figure 17). You should be able to fit one finger between the neck and the ties. Check to make sure that the patient can flex neck comfortably.	A secure tape prevents accidental expulsion of the tracheostomy tube. Allowing one finger-breadth under tape permits neck flexion that is comfortable and ensures that tape will not compromise circulation to the area.
e. Carefully remove old tape (Figure 18). Reapply oxygen source if necessary.	Removing old tape after application of new prevents accidental expulsion of the tracheostomy tube. Maintains oxygen supply to the patient.

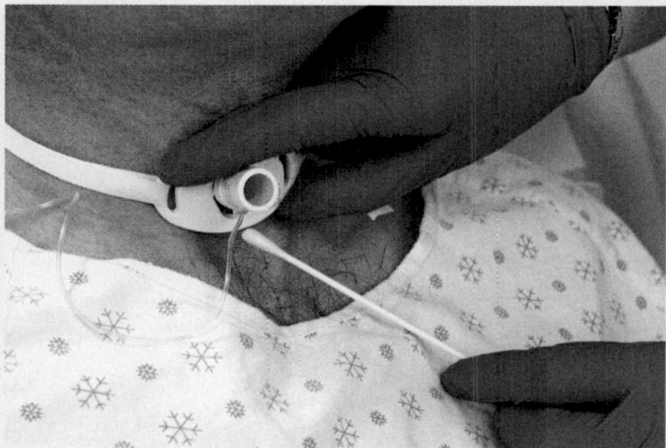
Figure 12. Cleaning with cotton-tipped applicators under faceplate.

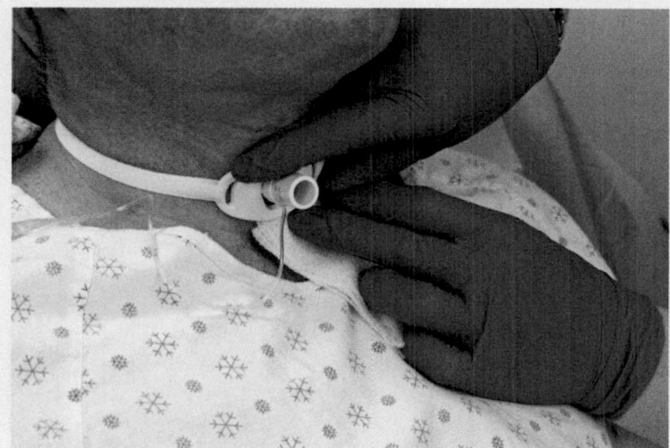
Figure 13. Patting skin around stoma gently.

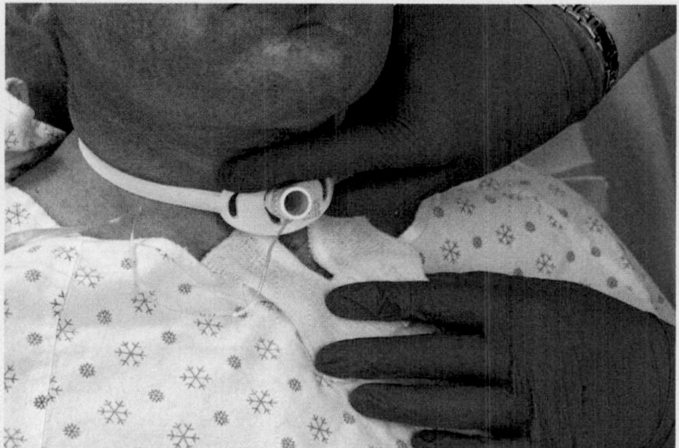
Figure 14. Sliding new tracheostomy dressing under faceplate.

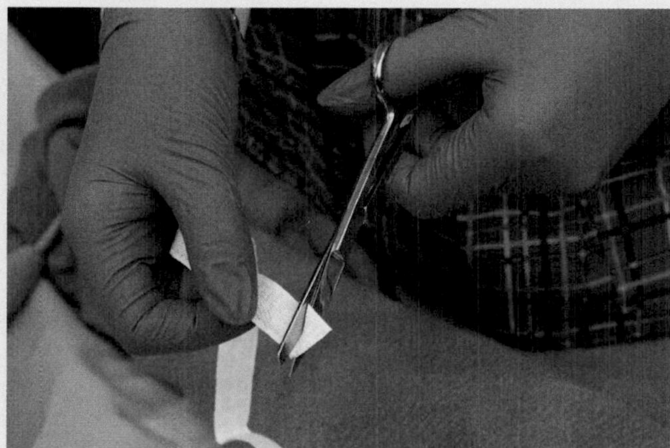
Figure 15. Cutting twill tape.

(continued)

SKILL 14-14 Providing Tracheostomy Care *(continued)*

ACTION | **RATIONALE**

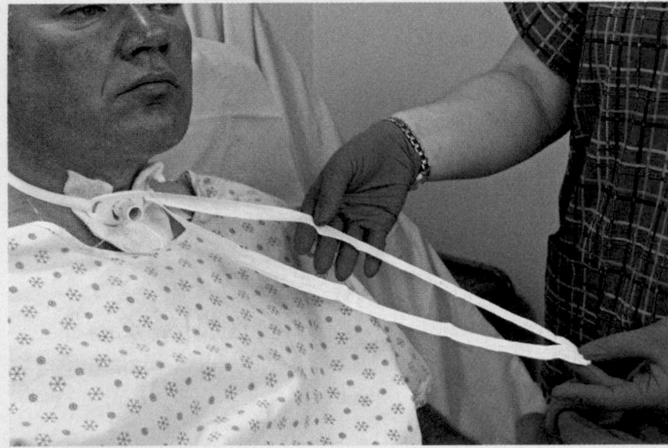

Figure 16. Pulling tape through alongside old tape.

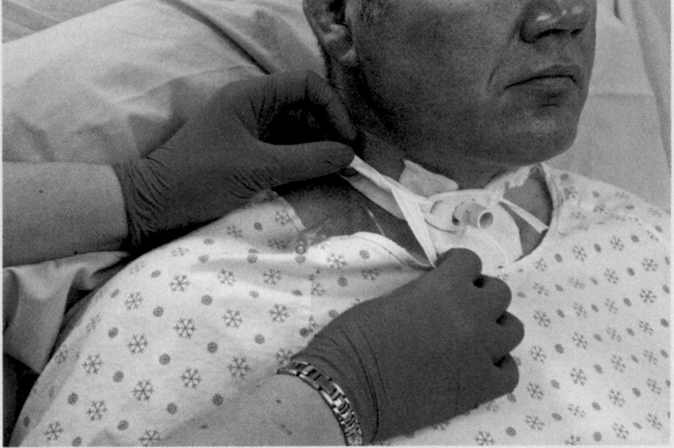

Figure 17. Tying ends with a double square knot.

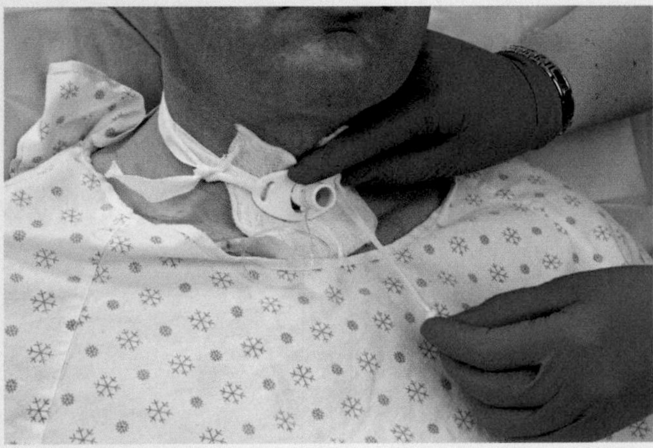

Figure 18. Removing old ties.

18. Remove face shield or mask and goggles. Remove gloves and discard. Perform hand hygiene. Reassess patient's respiratory status, including respiratory rate, effort, oxygen saturation, and lung sounds.

Hand hygiene prevents spread of microorganisms. Assessments determine the effectiveness of interventions and for the presence of complications.

EVALUATION

The expected outcome is met when the patient exhibits a tracheostomy tube and site free from drainage, secretions, and skin irritation or breakdown, oxygen saturation level within acceptable parameters, and is without evidence of respiratory distress. In addition, the patient verbalizes that site is free of pain and exhibits no evidence of skin breakdown on the posterior portion of the neck.

SKILL 14-14 Providing Tracheostomy Care *(continued)*

DOCUMENTATION

Guidelines

Document your pre- and postassessments, including site assessment, presence of pain, lung sounds, and oxygen saturation levels. Document presence of skin breakdown that may result from irritation or pressure from tracheostomy ties. Document care given.

Sample Documentation

9/26/08 1300 Tracheostomy care completed; lung sounds clear in all lobes; respirations even/unlabored; site without erythema or edema; small amount of thick yellow secretions noted at site.—C. Bausler, RN

Unexpected Situations and Associated Interventions

- *Patient coughs hard enough to dislodge tracheostomy:* A spare tracheostomy and obturator should be kept at bedside. Insert obturator into the new tracheostomy and insert tracheostomy into stoma. Remove obturator. Secure ties and auscultate lung sounds. Palpate for any subcutaneous emphysema.
- *On palpating around insertion site, you note a moderate amount of subcutaneous emphysema in tissue:* Assess for dislodgement of the tracheostomy tube. If the tube becomes displaced, a buildup of air in the subcutaneous portion of the skin is likely. Notify physician if the subcutaneous emphysema is a change in the status of the tracheostomy.

Special Considerations

General Considerations

- One nurse working alone should always place new tracheostomy ties in place before removing old ties to prevent accidental extubation of tracheostomy. If it is necessary to remove old ties first, obtain the assistance of a second person to hold the tracheostomy tube in place while the old tie is removed and the new tie is replaced.
- Emergency equipment should be easily accessible at the bedside. Bag-valve mask, oxygen, the obturator from the current tracheostomy, spare tracheostomy of the same size, spare tracheostomy one size smaller, and suction equipment should be kept at the bedside of a patient with an endotracheal tube at all times.
- If the patient is currently using a tracheostomy without a cuff, a spare tracheostomy of the same size with a cuff should be kept at the bedside for emergency use.

Home Care Considerations

- The patient and home caregiver should be instructed on how to perform tracheostomy care. The nurse should observe a return demonstration and provide feedback.
- Clean rather than sterile technique can be used in the home setting.
- Sterile saline can be made by mixing 1 teaspoon of table salt in 1 quart of water and boiling for 15 minutes. The solution is cooled and stored in a clean, dry container. Saline is discarded at the end of each day to prevent growth of bacteria.
- The patient who is performing self-care should use a mirror to view the steps in the procedure.

(continued)

SKILL 14-14 Providing Tracheostomy Care *(continued)*

SKILL VARIATION Replacing a Disposable Inner Cannula

Some tracheostomies use disposable inner cannulas, eliminating the need to clean the inner cannula. Disposable inner cannulas are simply removed and replaced, using aseptic technique.

- Identify the patient
- Determine the need for tracheostomy care. Assess patient's pain and administer pain medication, if indicated. Explain what you are going to do and the reason to the patient, even if the patient does not appear to be alert. Reassure patient you will interrupt procedure if he or she indicates respiratory difficulty.
- Perform hand hygiene.
- Adjust bed to comfortable working position. Lower side rail closer to you. If patient is conscious, place him or her in a semi-Fowler's position. If patient is unconscious, place him or her in the lateral position, facing you. Move the overbed table close to your work area and raise to waist height. Place a trash receptacle within easy reach of work area.
- Carefully open the package with the new disposable inner cannula, taking care not to contaminate the cannula the inside of the package.
- Suction tracheostomy if necessary. If tracheostomy has just been suctioned, remove soiled site dressing and discard before removing gloves used to perform suctioning.
- Put on disposable gloves.
- Remove the oxygen source if one is present. If not already removed, remove site dressing and dispose of in the trash. Stabilize the outer cannula and faceplate of the tracheostomy with your nondominant hand.
- Grasp the locking mechanism of the inner cannula with your dominant hand. Press the tabs and release lock (Figure A). Gently remove inner cannula and place in disposal bag.
- Discard gloves and put on sterile gloves. Pick up the new inner cannula with your dominant hand, stabilize the faceplate with your nondominant hand, and gently insert the new inner cannula into the outer cannula. Press the tabs to allow the lock to grab the outer cannula (Figure B).
- Continue with site care as detailed above.

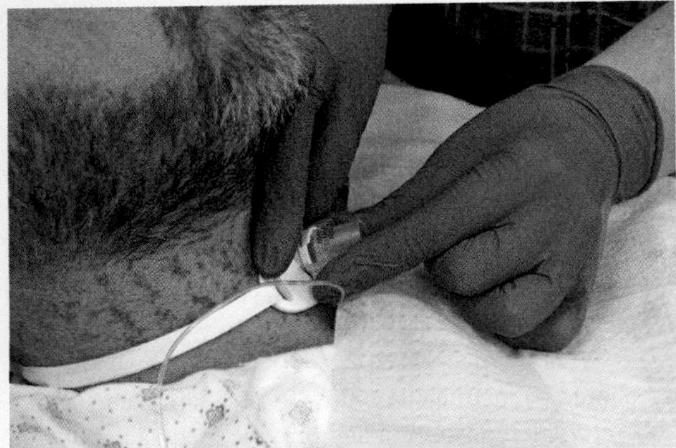

Figure A. Releasing lock on inner cannula.

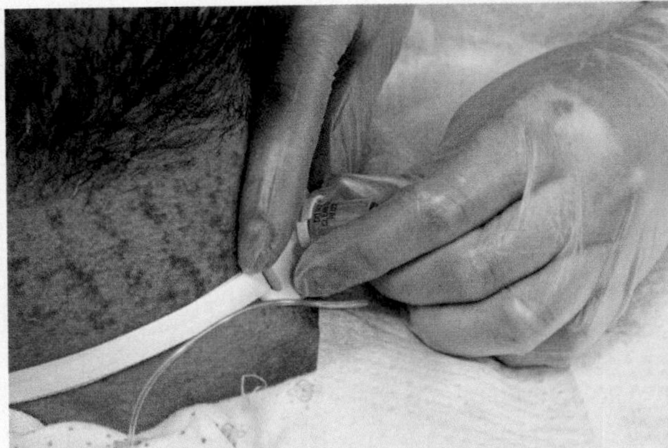

Figure B. Locking new inner cannula in place.

SKILL 14-14 Providing Tracheostomy Care *(continued)*

SKILL VARIATION Using Alternate Site Dressing if Commercially Prepared Sponge is Not Available

If a commercially prepared site dressing or drain sponge is not available, do not cut a gauze sponge to use at the tracheostomy site. Cutting the gauze can cause loose fibers, which can become lodged in the stoma, causing irritation or infection. Loose fibers could also be inhaled into the trachea, causing respiratory distress.

- Identify patient.
- Determine the need for tracheostomy care. Assess patient's pain and administer pain medication, if indicated.
- Explain what you are going to do and the reason to the patient, even if the patient does not appear to be alert. Reassure patient you will interrupt procedure if he or she indicates respiratory difficulty.
- Perform hand hygiene.
- Adjust bed to comfortable working position. Lower side rail closer to you. If patient is conscious, place him or her in a semi-Fowler's position. If patient is unconscious, place him or her in the lateral position, facing you. Move the overbed table close to your work area and raise to waist height. Place a trash receptacle within easy reach of work area.
- Remove oxygen source. Dip cotton-tipped applicator or gauze sponge in second basin with sterile saline and clean stoma under faceplate. Use each applicator or sponge only once, moving from stoma site outward.
- Pat skin gently with dry 4″ × 4″ gauze sponge.
- Fold two gauze sponges on the diagonal, to form triangles. Slide one triangle under the faceplate on each side of the stoma, with the longest side of the triangle against the tracheostomy tube.

SKILL VARIATION Securing a Tracheostomy With a Tracheostomy Collar Instead of Ties/Tape

Commercially prepared tracheostomy collars are available for use instead of cut twill tape for ties. Tracheostomy collars use a soft strap with Velcro strips on the ends that are inserted into the openings on the faceplate.

- Identify patient.
- Obtain the assistance of a second individual to hold the tracheostomy tube in place while the old collar is removed and the new collar is placed.
- Determine the need for tracheostomy care. Assess patient's pain and administer pain medication, if indicated.
- Explain what you are going to do and the reason to the patient, even if the patient does not appear to be alert. Reassure patient you will interrupt procedure if he or she indicates respiratory difficulty.
- Perform hand hygiene.
- Adjust bed to comfortable working position. Lower side rail closer to you. If patient is conscious, place him or her in a semi-Fowler's position. If patient is unconscious, place him or her in the lateral position, facing you. Move the overbed table close to your work area and raise to waist height. Place a trash receptacle within easy reach of work area.
- Open the package for the new tracheostomy collar.
- Both nurses should put on clean gloves.
- One nurse holds the faceplate to stabilize the tracheostomy while the other nurse pulls up the Velcro tabs to loosen the collar. Gently remove the collar.
- The first nurse continues to hold the tracheostomy faceplate, to prevent accidental extubation.
- The other nurse places the collar around the patient's neck and inserts first one tab, then the other, into the openings on the faceplate and secures the Velcro tabs to hold the tracheostomy in place.
- Remove gloves and perform hand hygiene.

SKILL 14-15 Providing Care of a Chest Drainage System

Chest tubes may be inserted to drain fluid (pleural effusion), blood (hemothorax), or air (pneumothorax) from the pleural space. A chest tube is a firm plastic tube with drainage holes in the proximal end that is inserted in the pleural space. Once inserted, the tube is secured with a suture and tape, covered with an airtight dressing, and attached to a drainage system that may or may not be attached to suction. Other components of the system may include a closed water-seal drainage system that prevents air from reentering the chest once it has escaped and a suction control chamber that prevents excess suction pressure from being applied to the pleural cavity. The suction chamber may be a water-filled or a dry chamber. A water-filled suction chamber is regulated by the amount of water in the chamber, while dry suction is automatically regulated to changes in the patient's pleural pressure (Lazzara, 2002). Many healthcare agencies use a molded plastic, three-compartment disposable chest drainage unit for management of chest tubes. There are also portable drainage systems that use gravity for drainage. Table 14-2 compares different types of chest drainage systems. The following procedure is based on the use of a traditional water seal, three-compartment chest drainage system (see Figure 1 for an example of this system). The Skill Variation following the procedure describes a technique for caring for a chest drainage system using dry seal or suction.

Equipment

- Bottle of sterile normal saline or water
- Two pairs of padded or rubber-tipped Kelly clamps
- Pair of clean scissors
- Disposable gloves
- Foam tape or bands
- Prescribed drainage system, if changing is required

TABLE 14-2 Comparison of Chest Drainage Systems

TYPE	DESCRIPTION	COMMENTS
Traditional water seal (also referred to as wet suction)	Has three chambers: a collection chamber, water-seal chamber (middle chamber), and wet suction-control chamber	• Requires that sterile fluid be instilled into water-seal and suction chambers • Has positive and negative pressure-release valves • Intermittent bubbling indicates that the system is functioning properly. • Additional suction can be added by connecting system to a suction source.
Dry-suction water seal (also referred to as dry suction)	Has three chambers: a collection chamber, water-seal chamber (middle chamber), and wet suction control	• Requires that sterile fluid be instilled in water-seal chamber at 2-cm level • No need to fill suction chamber with fluid • Suction pressure is set with a regulator. • Has positive and negative pressure-release valves • Has an indicator to signify that the suction pressure is adequate • Quieter than traditional water-seal systems
Dry suction (also referred to as one-way valve system)	Has a one-way mechanical valve that allows air to leave the chest and prevents air from moving back into the chest	• No need to fill suction chamber with fluid; can be set up quickly in an emergency • Works even if knocked over, making it ideal for patients who are ambulatory

(Used with permission from Smeltzer, S. and Bare, B. [2008]. *Brunner & Suddarth's Textbook of Medical Surgical Nursing* [11th ed.]. Philadelphia: Lippincott Williams & Wilkins.)

SKILL 14-15 Providing Care of a Chest Drainage System *(continued)*

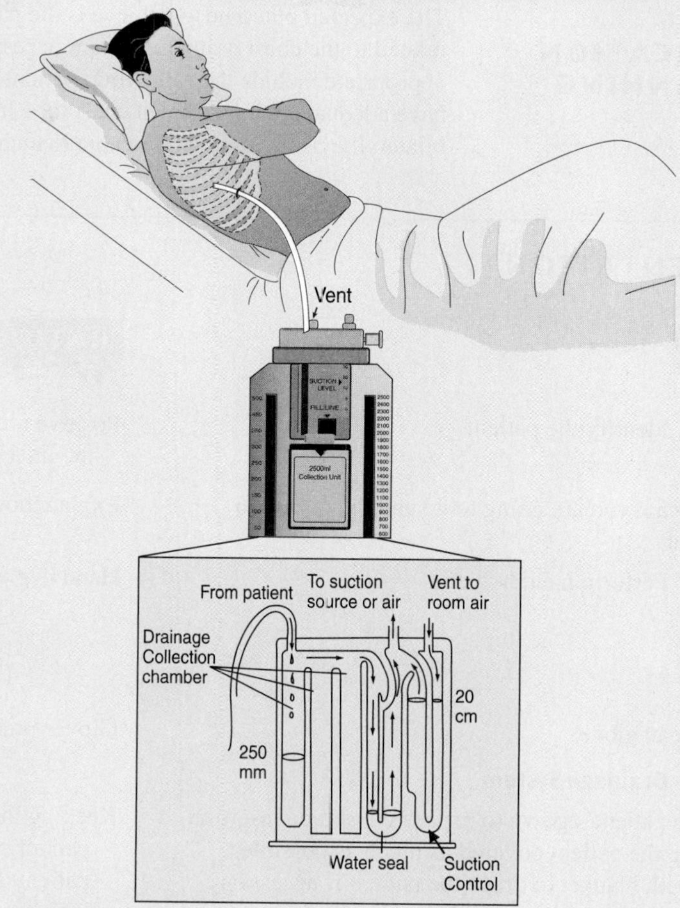

Figure 1. Chest drainage system

ASSESSMENT

Assess the patient's vital signs. Significant changes from baseline may indicate complications. Assess the patient's respiratory status, including oxygen saturation level. If chest tube is not functioning appropriately, the patient may become tachypneic and hypoxic. Assess the patient's lung sounds. The lung sounds over the chest tube site may be diminished due to the presence of fluid, blood, or air. Also assess the patient for pain. Sudden pressure or increased pain indicates potential complications. In addition, many patients report pain at the chest tube insertion site and request medication for the pain. Assess the patient's knowledge of the chest tube to ensure that he or she understands the rationale for the chest tube.

NURSING DIAGNOSIS

Determine the related factors for the nursing diagnosis based on the patient's current status. An appropriate nursing diagnosis is Risk for Impaired Gas Exchange. Other appropriate nursing diagnoses may include:

- Risk for Activity Intolerance
- Deficient Knowledge
- Acute Pain
- Anxiety

(continued)

SKILL 14-15 Providing Care of a Chest Drainage System *(continued)*

OUTCOME IDENTIFICATION AND PLANNING

The expected outcome to achieve is the patient will not experience any complications related to the chest drainage system or respiratory distress. Other outcomes that may be appropriate include the following: patient understands need for the chest tube; patient will have adequate pain control at chest tube insertion site; lung sounds will be clear and equal bilaterally; and patient will be able to increase activity tolerance gradually.

IMPLEMENTATION

ACTION	RATIONALE
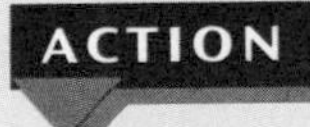 1. Identify the patient.	Positive identification of the patient is essential to ensure the intervention is administered to the correct patient.
2. Explain what you are going to do and the reason to the patient.	Explanation relieves anxiety and facilitates cooperation.
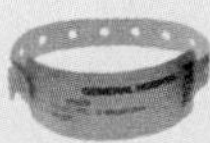 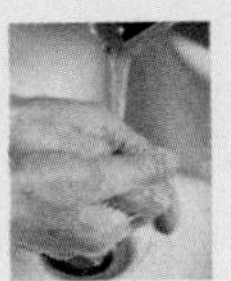 3. Perform hand hygiene.	Hand hygiene deters the spread of microorganisms.
4. Put on clean gloves.	Gloves prevent contact with contaminants and body fluids.
Assessing the Drainage System	
5. Move the patient's gown to expose chest tube insertion site. Keep the patient covered as much as possible, using a bath blanket to drape the patient if necessary. **Observe the dressing around the chest tube insertion site and ensure that it is dry, intact and occlusive (Figure 2).**	Keeping the patient as covered as possible maintains the patient's privacy and limits unnecessary exposure of the patient. If the dressing is not intact and occlusive, air can leak into the space, causing displacement of the lung tissue, and the site could be contaminated. Some patients experience significant drainage or bleeding at the insertions site, and the dressing needs to be replaced to maintain occlusion of the site.
6. Check that all connections are securely taped. Gently palpate around the insertion site, feeling for subcutaneous emphysema, a collection of air or gas under the skin. This may feel crunchy or spongy, or like "popping" under your fingers.	Small amounts of subcutaneous emphysema will be absorbed by the body after the chest tube is removed. If larger amounts or increasing amounts are present, it could indicate improper placement of the tube or an air leak and can cause discomfort to the patient.
7. Check drainage tubing to ensure that there are no dependent loops or kinks. The drainage collection device must be positioned below the tube insertion site.	Dependent loops or kinks in the tubing can prevent the tube from draining appropriately. The drainage collection device must be positioned below the tube insertion site so that drainage can move out of the tubing and into the collection device.
8. If the chest tube is ordered to be suctioned, note the fluid level in the suction chamber and check it with the amount of ordered suction. **Look for bubbling in the suction chamber.** Temporarily disconnect the suction to check the level of water in the chamber. Add sterile water or saline if necessary to maintain correct amount of suction.	Some fluid is lost due to evaporation. If suction is set too low, the amount needs to be increased to ensure that enough negative pressure is placed in the pleural space to drain the pleural space sufficiently. If suction is set too high, the amount needs to be decreased to prevent any damage to the fragile lung tissue. Gentle bubbling in the suction chamber indicates that suction is being applied to assist drainage.

SKILL 14-15 Providing Care of a Chest Drainage System *(continued)*

ACTION | **RATIONALE**

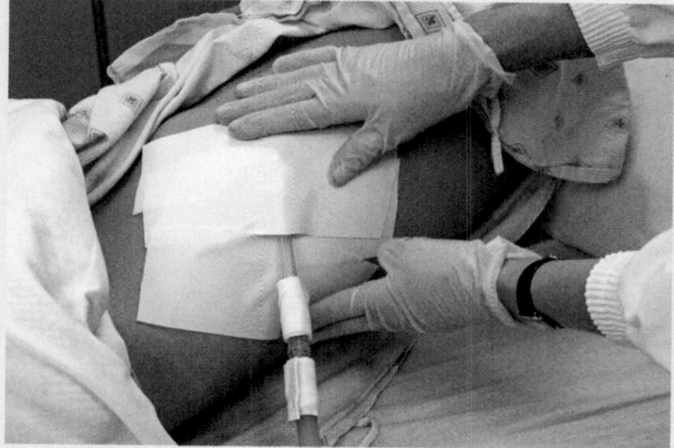

Figure 2. Assessing chest tube insertion site.

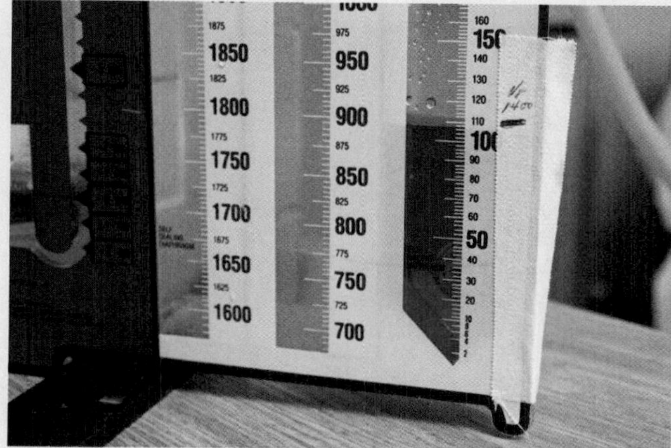

Figure 3. Drainage marked on device.

9. Observe the water-seal chamber for fluctuations of the water level with the patient's inspiration and expiration (tidaling). If suction is used, temporarily disconnect the suction to observe for fluctuation. Assess for the presence of bubbling in the water-seal chamber. Add water if necessary to maintain the level at the 2-cm mark, or the mark recommended by the manufacturer.

   Rationale: Fluctuations of the water level in the water-seal chamber with inspiration, and expiration is an expected and normal finding. Bubbles in the water-seal chamber after the initial insertion of the tube or when air is being removed are a normal finding. Constant bubbles in the water-seal chamber after initial insertion period indicate an air leak in the system. Leaks can occur within the drainage unit at the insertion site.

10. Assess the amount and type of fluid drainage. Measure drainage output at the end of each shift by marking the level on the container or placing a small piece of tape at the drainage level to indicate date and time (Figure 3). The amount should be a running total, because the drainage system is never emptied. If the drainage system fills, it is removed and replaced.

    Rationale: Measurement allows for accurate intake and output measurement, assessment of the effectiveness of therapy, and contributes to the decision to remove the tube. The drainage system would lose its negative pressure if it were opened.

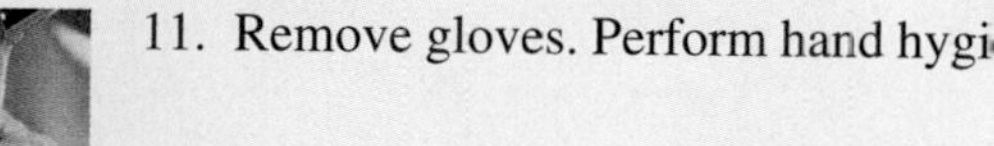

11. Remove gloves. Perform hand hygiene.

    Rationale: Hand hygiene deters the spread of microorganisms.

Changing the Drainage System

12. Obtain two padded Kelly clamps, a new drainage system, and bottle of sterile water. Add water to the water-seal chamber until it reaches the 2-cm mark or the mark recommended by the manufacturer. Follow manufacturer's directions to add water to suction system if suction is ordered.

    Rationale: Gathering equipment provides for an organized approach. Appropriate level of water in the water-seal chamber is necessary to prevent air from entering the chest. Appropriate level of water in the suction chamber provides the ordered suction.

13. Put on clean gloves.

    Rationale: Gloves prevent contact with contaminants and body fluids.

14. **Apply Kelly clamps 1.5″ to 2.5″ from insertion site and 1″ apart, going opposite directions (Figure 4).**

    Rationale: Clamp provides a more complete seal and prevents air from entering the pleural space through the chest tube.

(continued)

SKILL 14-15 Providing Care of a Chest Drainage System *(continued)*

ACTION	RATIONALE

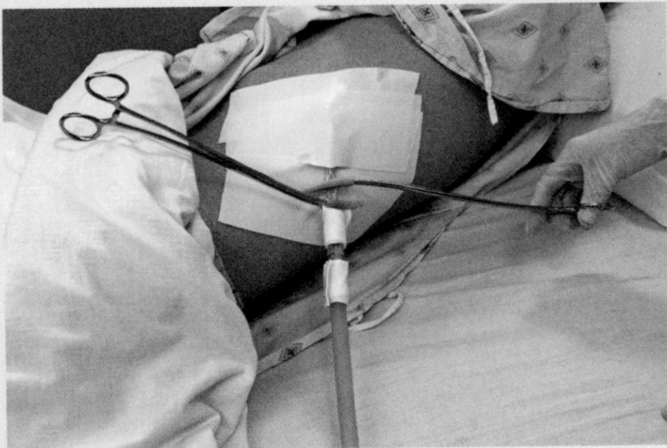

Figure 4. Using padded clamps on chest tube.

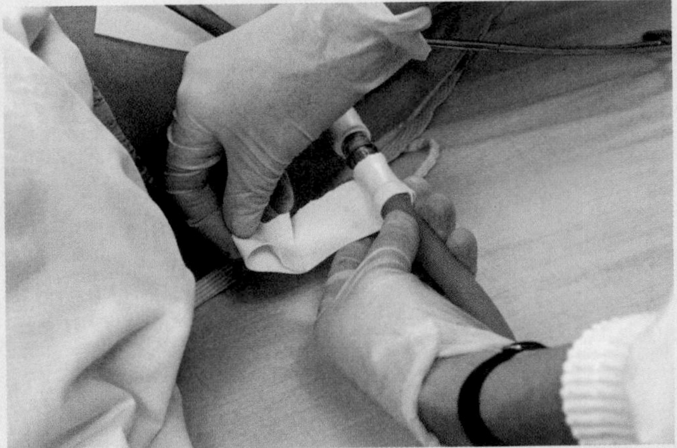

Figure 5. Unrolling the foam tape.

15. Remove the suction from the current drainage system. Unroll the band (Figure 5) or use scissors to carefully cut away (Figure 6) any foam tape on connection of chest tube and drainage system. Using a slight twisting motion, remove the drainage system. **Do not pull on the chest tube.**

Removing suction permits application to new system. In many institutions, bands or foam tape are placed where the chest tube meets the drainage system to ensure that the chest tube and the drainage system remain connected. Due to the negative pressure, a slight twisting motion may be needed to separate the tubes. The chest tube is sutured in place, so make sure you don't tug on the chest tube and dislodge it.

16. **Keeping the end of the chest tube sterile, insert the end of the new drainage system into the chest tube (Figure 7).** Remove Kelly clamps. Reconnect suction if ordered. Apply plastic bands or foam tape to chest tube/drainage system connection site.

Chest tube is sterile. Tube must be reconnected to suction to form a negative pressure and allow for re-expansion of lung or drainage of fluid. Prolonged clamping can result in a pneumothorax. Bands or foam tape help prevent the separation of the chest tube from the drainage system.

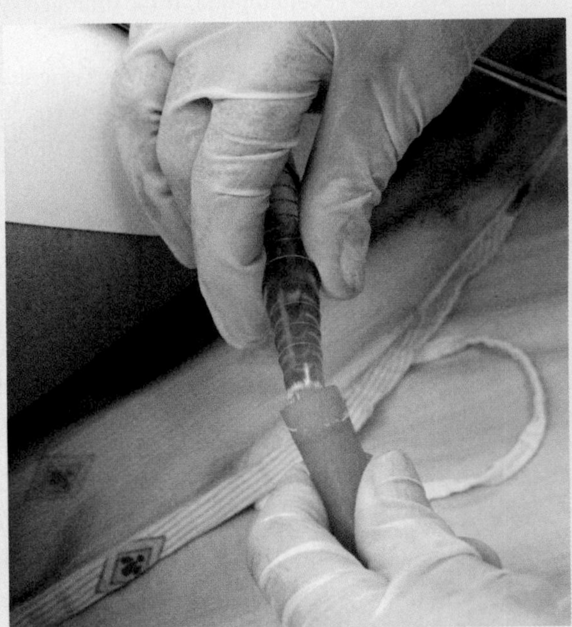

Figure 7. Attaching new drainage tube.

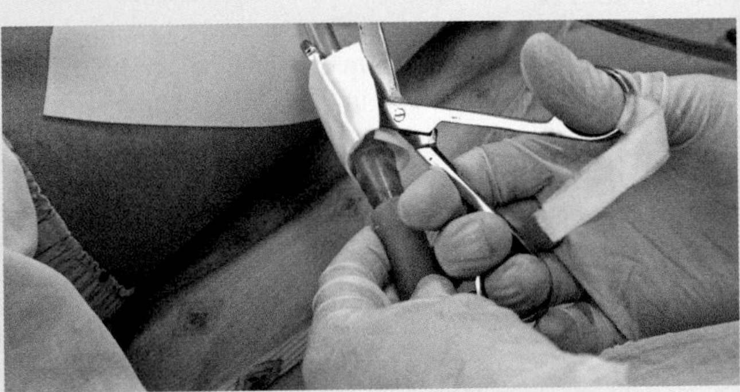

Figure 6. Cutting the foam tape.

SKILL 14-15 Providing Care of a Chest Drainage System *(continued)*

ACTION	RATIONALE
17. Assess the patient and the drainage system as outlined (Steps 5–10).	Assess for changes related to the manipulation of the system and placement of new drainage system.
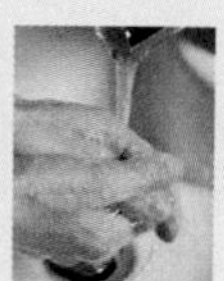 18. Remove gloves. Perform hand hygiene.	Hand hygiene deters the spread of microorganisms.

EVALUATION

The expected outcome is met when the chest drainage system is patent and functioning. In addition, the patient remains free of signs and symptoms of respiratory distress and complications related to the chest drainage system, verbalizes adequate pain relief, gradually increases activity tolerance, and demonstrates understanding of the need for the chest tube.

DOCUMENTATION

Guidelines

Document the site of the chest tube, amount and type of drainage, amount of suction applied, and any bubbling, tidaling, or subcutaneous emphysema noted. Document the type of dressing in place and the patient's pain level, as well as any measures performed to relieve the patient's pain.

Sample Documentation

9/10/08 1805 Chest tube present in right lower portion of rib cage at the axillary line. Draining moderate amount of serosanguineous fluid. Suction at 20 cm H_2O noted; gentle bubbling noted in suction chamber. Tidaling present in water-seal chamber, no air leak noted. Small amount of subcutaneous emphysema noted around insertion site, unchanged from previous assessment, patient denies any pain; occlusive dressing remains intact.—C. Bausler, RN

Unexpected Situations and Associated Interventions

- *The chest tube becomes separated from the drainage device:* Put on gloves. Open the sterile normal saline or water and insert the chest tube into the bottle while not contaminating the chest tube. This creates a water seal until a new drainage unit can be attached. Assess the patient for any signs of respiratory distress. Notify physician. Do not leave the patient. Anticipate the need for a new drainage system and a chest x-ray.
- *The chest tube becomes dislodged:* Put on gloves. Immediately apply an occlusive dressing to the site. There is a controversy in the literature over whether the occlusive dressing should be a sterile Vaseline-impregnated gauze covered with an occlusive tape or a sterile 4″ × 4″ folded and covered with an occlusive tape. (An example of an occlusive tape would be foam tape or the clear dressing used to cover IV insertion sites.) Assess the patient for any signs of respiratory distress. Notify physician. Anticipate the need for a chest x-ray. The physician will determine whether the chest tube needs to be replaced.
- *While assessing the chest tube, you notice a lack of drainage when there had been drainage previously:* Check for kinked tubing or a clot in the tubing. Note the amount of suction that the chest tube is set on. If there is a clot in the tubing, some institutions allow you to "milk" the tubing. To milk the tubing, start at the proximal end, grasp the tubing and gently squeeze quickly, then let go. Continue along the length of the tubing. "Stripping" the tubing, squeezing the length of the tube without releasing it, is not recommended. This intervention dangerously increases the negative pressure in the pleural space and causes damage to the fragile lung tissue. If the suction is not set appropriately, adjust until the ordered amount is achieved.

(continued)

SKILL 14-15 Providing Care of a Chest Drainage System *(continued)*

- *Drainage exceeds 100 mL/hr or becomes bright red:* Notify physician immediately. This can indicate fresh bleeding.
- *Chest tube drainage suddenly decreases and the water-seal chamber is not tidaling:* Notify physician immediately. This could signal that the tube is blocked.

Special Considerations

General Considerations

- Ensure that a bottle of sterile water or normal saline is at the bedside at all times. Chest tubes should never be clamped except to change the drainage system. If the chest tube becomes accidentally disconnected from the drainage system, place the end of the chest tube into the sterile solution. This prevents more air from entering the pleural space through the chest tube but allows for any air that does enter the pleural space, through respirations, to escape once pressure builds up.
- Two rubber-tipped clamps and additional dressing material should also be kept at the bedside for quick access if needed.
- If the patient has a small pneumothorax with little or no drainage and suction is not used, the tube may be connected to a Heimlich valve. A Heimlich valve is a water-seal chamber that allows air to exit from, but not enter, the chest tube. Check to assure that the valve is pointing in the correct direction. The blue end should be connected to the chest tube and the clear end is open as the vent. The arrow on the casing points away from the patient.
- The chest drainage system should be maintained in an upright position and lower than the level of the tube insertion site. This is necessary for proper function of the system and to aid drainage.
- Encourage the use of an incentive spirometer if ordered and/or frequent deep breathing and coughing by the patient. This helps drain the lungs, promotes lung expansion, and prevent atelectasis.

SKILL VARIATION Caring for a Chest Drainage System Using Dry Seal or Suction

- Identify the patient.
- Explain what you are going to do and the reason to the patient.
- Perform hand hygiene and put on gloves.
- Move the patient's gown to expose chest-tube insertion site. Keep the patient covered as much as possible, using a bath blanket to drape the patient if necessary. Observe the dressing around the chest tube insertion site and ensure that it is dry, intact, and occlusive.
- Check that all connections are securely taped. Gently palpate around the insertion site, feeling for subcutaneous emphysema, a collection of air or gas under the skin. This may feel crunchy or spongy, or like 'popping' under your fingers.
- Check drainage tubing to ensure that there are no dependent loops or kinks. The drainage collection device must be positioned below the tube insertion site.
- If the chest tube is ordered to be to suctioned, assess the amount of suction set on the chest tube against the amount of suction ordered. Assess for the presence of the suction control indicator, which is a bellows or float device, when adjusting the regulator to the desired level of suction, if prescribed.
- Assess for fluctuations in the diagnostic indicator with the patient's inspiration and expiration.
- Check the air-leak indicator for leaks in dry systems with a one-way valve.
- Assess the amount and type of fluid drainage. Measure drainage output at the end of each shift by marking the level on the container or placing a small piece of tape at the drainage level to indicate date and time. The amount should be a running total, because the drainage system is never emptied. If the drainage system fills, it is removed and replaced.
- Some portable chest drainage systems require manual emptying of the collection chamber. Follow the manufacturer's recommendations for timing of emptying. Typically, the unit should not be allowed to fill completely as drainage could spill out. Wear gloves, clean the syringe port with an alcohol wipe, use a 60-mL Luer-Lok syringe, screw the syringe into the port, and aspirate to withdraw fluid. Repeat as necessary to empty the chamber. Dispose of the fluid according to facility policy.
- Remove gloves. Perform hand hygiene.

SKILL 14-16 Assisting With Removal of a Chest Tube

Chest tubes are removed after the lung is re-expanded and drainage is minimal. Chest tube removal is usually performed by the physician, advance practice nurse, or physician's assistant. The practitioner will determine when the chest tube is ready for removal by evaluating the chest x-ray and assessing the patient and the amount of drainage.

Equipment

- Disposable gloves
- Suture removal kit (tweezers and scissors)
- Sterile Vaseline-impregnated gauze and 4 × 4 gauze dressings
- Occlusive tape, such as foam tape

ASSESSMENT

Assess the patient's respiratory status, including respiratory rate and oxygen saturation level. This provides a baseline for comparison after the tube is removed. If the patient begins to have respiratory distress, he or she will usually become tachypneic and hypoxic. Assess the patient's lung sounds. The lung sounds over the chest tube site may be diminished due to the tube. Assess the patient for pain. Many patients report pain at the chest tube insertion site and request medication for the pain. If the patient has not recently received pain medication, it may be given before the chest tube removal to decrease the pain felt with the procedure.

NURSING DIAGNOSIS

Determine the related factors for the nursing diagnosis based on the patient's current status. Appropriate nursing diagnoses may include:

- Deficient Knowledge
- Acute Pain
- Impaired Skin Integrity
- Risk for Impaired Gas Exchange

OUTCOME IDENTIFICATION AND PLANNING

The expected outcome to achieve when caring for a patient after removal of a chest tube is that the patient will remain free of respiratory distress. Other outcomes that may be appropriate include the following: the insertion site will remain clean and dry without evidence of infection; patient will experience adequate pain control during the chest tube removal; lung sounds will be clear and equal bilaterally; and patient will be able to increase activity tolerance gradually.

IMPLEMENTATION

ACTION	RATIONALE
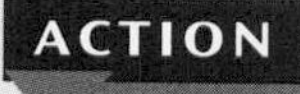 1. Identify the patient.	Positive identification of the patient is essential to ensure the intervention is administered to the correct patient.
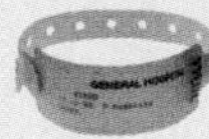 2. Explain what you are going to do and the reason to the patient.	Explanation relieves anxiety and facilitates cooperation.
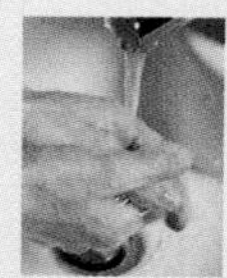 3. Perform hand hygiene.	Hand hygiene deters the spread of microorganisms.
4. Administer pain medication as prescribed. **Premedicate patient 10 to 15 minutes before chest tube removal.**	Most patients report discomfort during chest tube removal.

(continued)

SKILL 14-16 Assisting With Removal of a Chest Tube *(continued)*

ACTION	RATIONALE
5. Put on clean gloves.	Gloves prevent contact with contaminants and body fluids.
6. Provide reassurance to patient while physician removes dressing.	The removal of the dressing can increase the patient's anxiety level. Offering reassurance will help the patient feel more secure.
7. **After physician has removed chest tube and secured occlusive dressing, assess patient's lung sounds, respiratory rate, oxygen saturation, and pain level.**	In most institutions, physicians remove chest tubes, but some institutions train nurses to remove chest tubes. Once the tube is removed, the patient's respiratory status will need to be assessed to ensure that no distress is noted.
8. Anticipate the physician ordering a chest x-ray.	The physician may want a chest x-ray taken to evaluate the status of the lungs after chest tube removal.
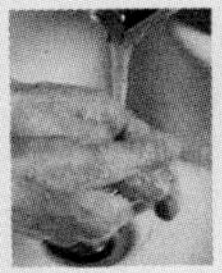 9. Dispose of equipment appropriately. Remove and dispose of gloves. Perform hand hygiene.	Hand hygiene deters the spread of microorganisms.

EVALUATION

The expected outcome is met when the patient exhibits no signs and symptoms of respiratory distress after the chest tube is removed. In addition, the patient verbalizes adequate pain control; lung sounds are clear and equal; and the patient's activity level gradually increases.

DOCUMENTATION

Guidelines

Document the patient's respiratory rate, oxygen saturation, lung sounds, total chest tube output, and status of insertion site and dressing.

Sample Documentation

9/16/08 1950 Procedure explained to patient. Morphine sulfate 2 mg intravenously given as ordered. Physician at bedside and R mid-axillary lower lobe chest tube removed. Vaseline gauze and gauze dressings applied over insertion site covered by foam tape. Lung sounds clear, slightly diminished over R lower lobe. Respirations unlabored at 16 breaths per min, pulse 88, blood pressure 118/64. Oxygen saturation 97% on room air. 322 mL of serosanguineous drainage noted in drainage device. Patient denies pain or respiratory distress.—C. Bausler, RN

Unexpected Situations and Associated Interventions

- *Patient experiences respiratory distress after chest tube removal:* Auscultate lung sounds. Diminished or absent lung sounds could be a sign that the lung has not fully reinflated or that the fluid has returned. Notify physician immediately. Anticipate an order for a chest x-ray and possible reinsertion of a chest tube.
- *Chest tube dressing becomes loosened:* The chest tube dressing should be changed at least every 24 hours or per agency policy so that the nurse can assess the site for erythema and drainage. Replace the occlusive dressing using a sterile technique. The dressing should remain occlusive for at least 3 days.

SKILL
14-17 Using a Bag and Mask (Handheld Resuscitation Bag)

If the patient is not breathing with an adequate rate and depth, or if the patient has lost the respiratory drive, a bag and mask may be used to deliver oxygen until the patient is resuscitated or can be intubated with an endotracheal tube. Bag and mask devices are frequently referred to as Ambu bags ("air mask bag unit") or BVMs ("bag-valve-mask" device). The bags come in infant, pediatric, and adult size. The bag consists of an oxygen reservoir (commonly referred to as the tail), oxygen tubing, the bag itself, a one-way valve to prevent secretions from entering the bag, an exhalation port, an elbow so that the bag can lie across the patient's chest, and a mask.

Equipment

- Handheld resuscitation device with a mask
- Oxygen source
- Disposable gloves
- Face shield or goggles and mask

ASSESSMENT

Assess the patient's respiratory effort and drive. If the patient is breathing <10 breaths per minute, is breathing too shallowly, or is not breathing at all, assistance with a BVM may be needed. Assess the oxygen saturation level. Patients who have decreased respiratory effort and drive may also have a decreased oxygen saturation level. Assess the heart rate and rhythm. Bradycardia may occur with a decreased oxygen saturation level, leading to a cardiac dysrhythmia. Many times the use of a BVM is in a crisis situation. Manual ventilation is also used during airway suctioning.

NURSING DIAGNOSIS

Determine the related factors for the nursing diagnosis based on the patient's current status. Appropriate nursing diagnoses may include:

- Ineffective Breathing Pattern
- Impaired Gas Exchange
- Decreased Cardiac Output
- Risk for Aspiration

Many other nursing diagnoses may require the use of this skill.

OUTCOME IDENTIFICATION AND PLANNING

The expected outcome is that the patient will exhibit signs and symptoms of adequate oxygen saturation. Other outcomes that may be appropriate include the following: patient will receive adequate volume of respirations with BVM; patient will maintain normal sinus rhythm.

IMPLEMENTATION

ACTION	RATIONALE
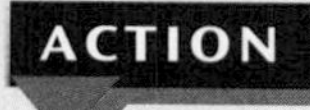 1. If not an emergency, identify the patient.	Positive identification of the patient is essential to ensure the intervention is administered to the correct patient.
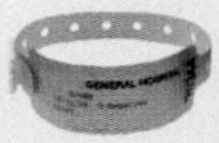 2. Explain what you are going to do and the reason to the patient, even if the patient does not appear to be alert.	Explanation alleviates fears. Even if patient appears unconscious, the nurse should explain what is happening.
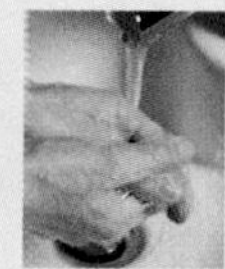 3. Perform hand hygiene, if not crisis situation. Put on disposable gloves. Put on face shield or goggles and mask.	Hand hygiene deters the spread of microorganisms. Personal protective equipment protects the nurse from pathogens.

(continued)

SKILL 14-17 Using a Bag and Mask (Handheld Resuscitation Bag) *(continued)*

ACTION	RATIONALE
4. **Ensure that the mask is connected to the bag device (Figure 1), the oxygen tubing is connected to the oxygen source, and the oxygen is turned on, at a flow rate of 10–15 liters/minute (Figure 2).** This may be done through visualization or by listening to the open end of the reservoir or tail: if air is heard flowing, the oxygen is attached and on.	Expected results may not be accomplished if the oxygen is not attached and on.

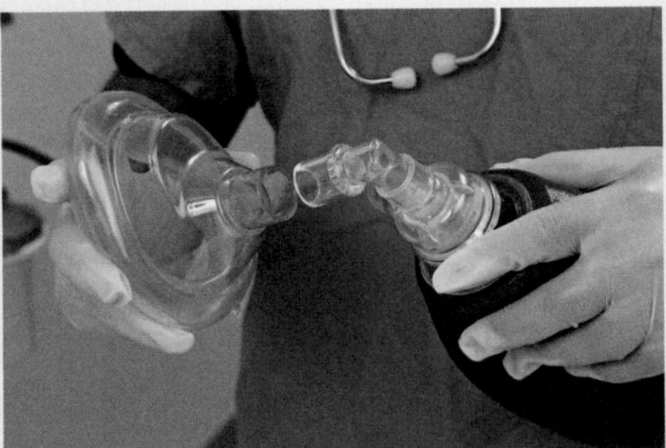

Figure 1. Connecting mask to bag-valve device.

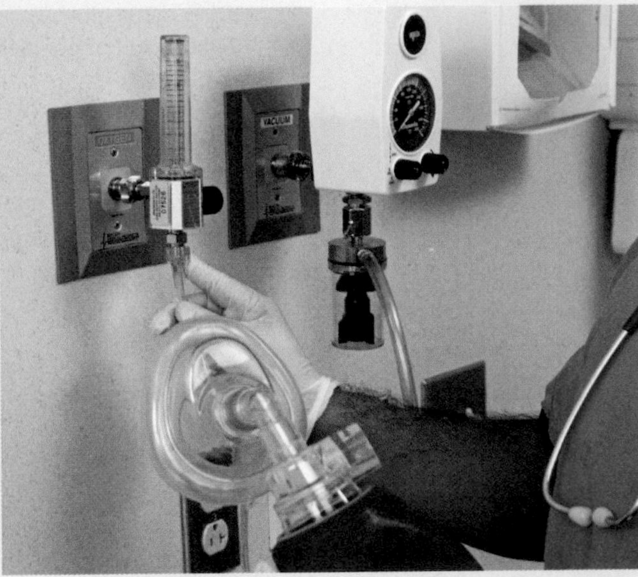

Figure 2. Connecting oxygen tubing on bag to oxygen source.

ACTION	RATIONALE
5. If possible, get behind head of bed and remove headboard. **Slightly hyperextend patient's neck (unless contraindicated). If unable to hyperextend, use jaw thrust maneuver to open airway.**	Standing at head of bed makes positioning easier when obtaining seal of mask to face. Hyperextending the neck opens the airway.
6. Place mask over patient's face with opening over oral cavity. If mask is teardrop-shaped, the narrow portion should be placed over the bridge of the nose.	This helps ensure an adequate seal so that oxygen may be forced into the lungs.
7. **With dominant hand, place three fingers on mandible, keeping head slightly hyperextended. Place thumb and one finger in C position around the mask, pressing hard enough to form a seal around patient's face (Figure 3).**	This helps ensure an adequate seal is formed so that oxygen may be forced into the lungs.
8. **Using nondominant hand, gently and slowly (over 2–3 seconds) squeeze the bag, watching chest for symmetric rise.** If two people are available, one person should maintain a seal on the mask with two hands while the other squeezes the bag to deliver the ventilation and oxygenation.	Volume of air needed is based on patient's size. Enough has been delivered if chest is rising. If air is introduced rapidly, it may enter the stomach.

SKILL 14-17

Using a Bag and Mask (Handheld Resuscitation Bag) *(continued)*

ACTION	RATIONALE
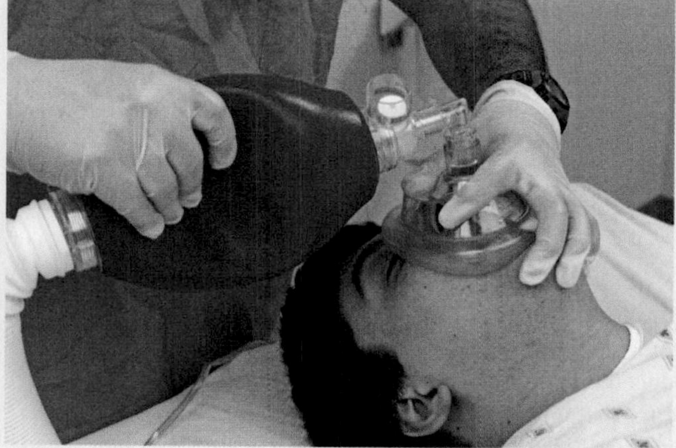 Figure 3. Creating a seal between mask and patient's face.	
9. Deliver the breaths with the patient's own inspiratory effort, if present. Avoid delivering breaths when the patient exhales. Deliver one breath every 5 seconds, if patient's own respiratory drive is absent. Continue delivering breaths until patient's drive returns or until patient is intubated and attached to mechanical ventilation.	Once patient's airway has been stabilized or patient is breathing on own, bag-mask delivery can be stopped.
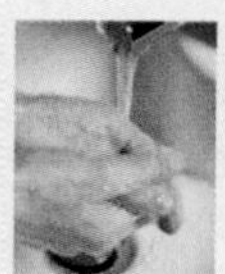 10. Remove face shield or goggles and mask. Remove gloves and perform hand hygiene.	Hand hygiene deters the spread of microorganisms.

EVALUATION

The expected outcome is met when the patient demonstrates improved skin color and nail beds without evidence of cyanosis, an oxygen saturation level >95%, and normal sinus rhythm. In addition, the patient maintains a patent airway and exhibits spontaneous respirations.

DOCUMENTATION

Guidelines

Document the incident, including patient's respiratory effort before initiation of bag-mask breaths; lung sounds; oxygen saturation; chest symmetry; and resolution of incident (ie, intubation or patient's respiratory drive returns).

(continued)

SKILL 14-17 Using a Bag and Mask (Handheld Resuscitation Bag) *(continued)*

Sample Documentation

9/1/08 2015 Patient arrived to emergency department with respiratory rate of 4 breaths per min; respirations shallow; manual breaths delivered using adult bag with mask and 100% oxygen, oxygen saturation increased from 78% to 100% after 8 breaths delivered; Dr. Alsup at bedside; patient sedated with 5 mg midazolam before intubation with 7.5 oral endotracheal tube, taped 10 cm at lips; lung sounds clear and equal all lobes; see graphics for ventilator settings. Nasogastric tube placed via R naris to low intermittent suction, small amount of dark green drainage noted, chest x-ray obtained.—C. Bausler, RN

Unexpected Situations and Associated Interventions

- *Breaths become increasingly difficult to deliver due to resistance:* Obtain order for placement of naso- or orogastric tube to remove air from the stomach (many institutions have policies that allow placement of a gastric tube during resuscitation). If air is delivered too fast, it may be introduced into the stomach. When the stomach fills with air, it decreases the space available for the lungs to inflate.
- *Chest is not rising when breaths are delivered, and resistance is felt:* Reposition the head or perform the jaw thrust maneuver. If the chest is not rising at all and resistance is being met, the tongue or another object is most likely obstructing the airway. If repositioning does not resolve the effort, consider performing the Heimlich maneuver.
- *Chest is rising asymmetrically:* Instruct assistant to listen to lung sounds bilaterally. Patient may need a chest tube placed due to pneumothorax. Anticipate the need for chest tube placement.
- *Oxygen saturation decreases from 100% to 80%:* Assess whether chest is rising. If chest is rising asymmetrically, the patient may have a pneumothorax. Anticipate the need for a chest tube. Check oxygen tubing. Someone may have stepped on the tubing, either kinking the tubing or pulling the tubing from the oxygen device.
- *A seal cannot be formed around the patient's face, and a large amount of air is escaping around mask:* Assess face and mask. Is the mask the correct size for the patient? If the mask size is correct, reposition fingers, or have a second person hold the mask while you compress the bag.

Special Considerations

General Considerations

- Air can be forced into the stomach during manual ventilation with a mask, causing abdominal distention. This distension can cause vomiting and possible aspiration. Be alert for vomiting; watch through the mask. If the patient starts to vomit, stop ventilating immediately, remove the mask, wipe and suction vomitus as needed, then resume ventilation.

The Taylor Suite offers these additional resources to enhance learning and facilitate understanding of this chapter:

- thePoint online resource, http://thepoint.lww.com/Lynn2E
- Student CD-ROM included with the book
- Skills Checklist to Accompany Taylor's Clinical Nursing Skills
- Taylor's Interactive Nursing
- Taylor's Video Guide to Clinical Nursing Skills: *Oxygenation and Tracheostomy Care*

Developing Critical Thinking Skills

1. Scott Mingus has a mediastinal chest tube in place after thoracic surgery. The chest tube has been draining 20 to 30 mL of serosanguineous fluid every hour. Suddenly, the chest tube output is 110 mL and the drainage is bright red. What should the nurse do?

2. Saranam Srivastava has a right-sided chest tube inserted due to a pneumothorax after a car accident. The water-seal chamber is noted to be continuously bubbling. What should the nurse do?

3. Paula Cunningham needs to be suctioned but begins to vomit during suctioning. What should the nurse do?

■ Bibliography

AARC. (2004). Clinical practice guideline: Nasotracheal suctioning—2004 revision & update. *Respiratory Care, 49*(9), 1080–1084.

Andrs, K. (2004). Chest drainage to go. *Nursing, 34*(5), 54–55.

Aschenbrenner, D. & Venable, S. (2006). *Drug therapy in nursing* (2nd ed.). Philadelphia: Lippincott Williams & Wilkins.

Buxton, L., Baldwin, J., Berry, J., et al. (2002). The efficacy of metered-dose inhalers with a spacer device in the pediatric setting. *Journal of the American Academy of Nurse Practitioners, 14*(9), 390–396.

Carroll, P. (2002). A guide to mobile chest drains. *RN, 65*(5), 56–62.

Carrol, P. (2002). Mobile chest drainage: Coming soon to a home near you. *Home Healthcare Nurse, 20*(7), 434–441.

Day, T., Farnell, S., Haynes, S., et al. (2002). Tracheal suctioning: An exploration of nurses' knowledge and competence in acute and high dependency ward areas. *Journal of Advanced Nursing, 39*(1), 35–45.

Deshpande, K., Tortolani, A., & Kvetan, V. (2003). Troubleshooting chest tube complications. *The Journal of Critical Illness, 18*(6), 275–280.

Dixon, B. & Tasota, F. (2003). Inadvertent tracheal decannulation. *Nursing, 33*(1), 96.

Dulak, S. (2004). Manual ventilation. *RN,* 67(12), 24ac1–4.

Dulak, S. (2005). Placing an oropharyngeal airway. *RN, 68*(2), 20ac1–3.

Gattoni, L., Tognoni, G., Pesenti, A., et al. (2001). Effect of prone positioning on the survival of patients with acute respiratory failure. *New England Journal of Medicine, 345*(8), 568–573.

Hockenberry, M. (2005). *Wong's essentials of pediatric nursing* (7th ed.). St. Louis, MO: Mosby.

Lazzara, D. (2002). Eliminate the air of mystery from chest tubes. *Nursing, 32*(6), 36–43.

McConnell, E. (2000). Suctioning a tracheostomy tube. *Nursing, 30*(1), 80.

McConnell, E. (2002a). Providing tracheostomy care. *Nursing, 32*(1), 17.

McConnell, E. (2002b). Teaching your patient to use a metered-dose inhaler. *Nursing, 32*(2), 73.

McConnell, E. (2002c). Using an automated external defibrillator. *Nursing, 32*(10), 18.

Mehta, M. (2003). Assessing respiratory status. *Nursing, 33*(2), 54–56.

Miracle, V. (2002). Action stat: Asthma attack. *Nursing, 32*(11), 104.

North American Nursing Diagnosis Association. (2005). *NANDA nursing diagnoses: Definitions and classification, 2005–2006.* Philadelphia: Author.

Pate, M. (2004). Placement of endotracheal and tracheostomy tubes. *Critical Care Nurse, 24*(3), 13.

Pate, M. & Zapata, T. (2002). Ask the experts: How deeply should I go when I suction an endotracheal or tracheostomy tube? *Critical Care Nurse, 22*(2), 130–131.

Pullen, R. (2003). Teaching bedside incentive spirometry. *Nursing2003, 33*(8), 24.

Roman, M. (2005). Tracheostomy tubes. *MEDSURG Nursing, 14*(2), 143–144.

Seay, S., Gay, S., & Strauss, M. (2002). Tracheostomy emergencies: Correcting accidental decannulation or displaced tracheostomy tube. *American Journal of Nursing, 102*(3), 59–63.

Smeltzer, S., Bare, B., Hinkle, J. H., & Cheever, K. H. (2008). *Brunner and Suddarth's textbook of medical–surgical nursing* (11th ed.). Philadelphia: Lippincott Williams & Wilkins.

Smith, T. (2004). Oxygen therapy for older people. *Nursing Older People, 16*(5), 22–28.

St. John, R. (2004). Protocols for practice: Airway management. *Critical Care Nurse, 24*(2), 93–96.

Tate, J. & Tasota, F. (2000). Using pulse oximetry. *Nursing, 30*(9), 30.

Togger, D. & Brenner, P. (2001). Metered dose inhalers. *American Journal of Nursing, 101*(10), 26–32.

CHAPTER 15

Fluid, Electrolyte, and Acid–Base Balance

Focusing on Patient Care

This chapter will help you develop some of the skills related to fluid, electrolyte, acid–base balance, and blood transfusions necessary to care for the following patients:

Simon Lawrence, age 3 years, has been admitted to the pediatric floor with dehydration after vomiting for 2 days. He needs intravenous fluids to become rehydrated.

Melissa Cohen, age 32, was just involved in a motor vehicle crash. She has lost a large amount of blood and needs a blood transfusion.

Jack Tracy, age 67, is undergoing chemotherapy. He is to be discharged and needs his port deaccessed.

Learning Objectives

After studying this chapter, you will be able to:

1. Start an IV infusion.
2. Change IV solution and tubing.
3. Monitor an IV site and infusion.
4. Change an IV dressing.
5. Cap a primary line for intermittent use.
6. Flush an IV line.
7. Administer a blood transfusion.
8. Change a CVAD line dressing.
9. Access an implanted port.
10. Deaccess an implanted port.

Key Terms

acid: substance containing a hydrogen ion that can be liberated or released

acidosis: condition characterized by a proportionate excess of hydrogen ions in the extracellular fluid or loss of a base, such as bicarbonate; pH falls below 7.35

active transport: movement of ions or molecules across cell membranes, usually against a pressure gradient, that requires metabolic energy

agglutinin: antibody that causes a clumping of specific antigens

alkalosis: condition characterized by a proportionate lack of hydrogen ions in the extracellular fluid concentration or the accumulation of bases; pH exceeds 7.45

anion: ion that carries a negative electric charge

antibody: immunoglobulin produced by the body in response to a specific antigen

antigen: foreign material capable of inducing a specific immune response

autologous transfusion: a blood transfusion donated by the patient in anticipation that he or she may need the transfusion during a hospital stay

base: substance that can accept or trap a hydrogen ion; synonym for alkali

buffer: substance that prevents body fluid from becoming overly acid or alkaline

cation: ion that carries a positive electric charge

colloid osmotic pressure: pressure exerted by plasma proteins, such as albumin on permeable membranes in the body; synonym for oncotic pressure

crossmatching: determining the compatibility of two blood specimens

dehydration: decreased fluid volume

diffusion: tendency of solutes to move freely throughout a solvent from an area of higher concentration to an area of lower concentration until equilibrium is established

edema: accumulation of fluid in body tissues

electrolyte: substance capable of breaking into ions and developing an electric charge when dissolved in solution

filtration: passage of a fluid through a permeable membrane whose spaces do not allow certain solutes to pass; passage is from an area of higher pressure to one of lower pressure

filtration pressure: difference between colloid osmotic pressure and blood hydrostatic pressure

hydrostatic pressure: force exerted by a fluid against the container wall

hypertonic: having a greater concentration of solutes than the solution with which it is being compared

hypervolemia: excess of isotonic fluid (water and sodium) in the extracellular space

hypotonic: having a lesser concentration than the solution with which it is being compared

hypovolemia: deficiency of isotonic fluid (water and sodium) from the extracellular space

ion: atom or molecule carrying an electric charge in solution

isotonic: having about the same solute concentration as the solution with which it is being compared

osmolarity: the concentration of solutes or particles in a solution, or a solution's pulling power

osmosis: passage of a solvent through a semipermeable membrane from an area of lesser concentration (less solutes) to an area of greater concentration (more solutes) until equilibrium is established

overhydration: increased fluid volume

pH: expression of hydrogen ion concentration and resulting acidity of a substance

solute: substance dissolved in a solution

solvent: liquid holding a substance in solution

typing: determining a person's blood type (A, B, AB, or O)

Because fluid is the main constituent of the body, the body's fluid balance is very important. Body fluid contains water (50%–60% of the human body by weight is water) and other dissolved substances in the form of electrolytes, nonelectrolytes, and gases. The balance, or homeostasis, of water and dissolved substances is maintained through the functions of almost every organ of the body. Fundamentals Review 15-1 provides the fluid intake and output requirements for a healthy state. Nurses routinely care for patients with minor to serious and even life-threatening fluid, electrolyte, and acid–base disturbances. One of nursing's most important roles is the prevention of these disturbances in high-risk populations, such as infants, older people, and patients with cardiac and renal disorders. Nurses must also monitor for complications associated with IV infusion (Fundamentals Review 15-2).

This chapter discusses the skills needed to care for patients with fluid, electrolyte, and acid–base balance needs. Please review Figure 15-1, which illustrates infusion sites.

Fundamentals Review 15-1

Balance of Fluid Intake and Output in a Healthy State

Fluid Intake (mL)	
Ingested water	1,300
Ingested food	1,000
Metabolic oxidation	300
Total	*2,600*
Fluid Output (mL)	
Kidneys	1,500
Skin	
Insensible loss	200–400
Sensible loss	300–500
Lungs	400
Gastrointestinal	100
Total	*2,500–2,900*

Fundamentals Review 15-2

Complications Associated with Intravenous Infusions

Complication/Cause	Signs and Symptoms	Nursing Considerations
Infiltration: the escape of fluid into the subcutaneous tissue Dislodged needle Penetrated vessel wall	Swelling, pallor, coldness, or pain around the infusion site; significant decrease in the flow rate	Check the infusion site several times per shift for symptoms. Discontinue the infusion if symptoms occur. Restart the infusion at a different site. Limit the movement of the extremity with the IV.
Sepsis: microorganisms invade the bloodstream through the catheter insertion site Poor insertion technique Multilumen catheters Long-term catheter insertion Frequent dressing changes	Red and tender insertion site Fever, malaise, other vital sign changes	Assess catheter site daily. Notify physician immediately if any signs of infection. Follow agency protocol for culture of drainage. Use scrupulous aseptic technique when starting an infusion.

(continued)

Complications Associated with Intravenous Infusions *(continued)*

Complication/Cause	Signs and Symptoms	Nursing Considerations
Phlebitis: an inflammation of a vein Mechanical trauma from needle or catheter Chemical trauma from solution Septic (due to contamination)	Local, acute tenderness; redness, warmth, and slight edema of the vein above the insertion site	Discontinue the infusion immediately. Apply warm, moist compresses to the affected site. Avoid further use of the vein. Restart the infusion in another vein.
Thrombus: a blood clot Tissue trauma from needle or catheter	Symptoms similar to phlebitis IV fluid flow may cease if clot obstructs needle	Stop the infusion immediately. Apply warm compresses as ordered by the physician. Restart the IV at another site. *Do not rub or massage the affected area.*
Speed shock: the body's reaction to a substance that is injected into the circulatory system too rapidly Too rapid a rate of fluid infusion into circulation	Pounding headache, fainting, rapid pulse rate, apprehension, chills, back pains, and dyspnea	If symptoms develop, discontinue the infusion immediately. Report symptoms of speed shock to the physician immediately. Monitor vital signs if symptoms develop. Use the proper IV tubing. A microdrip (60 gtt/mL) should be used on all pediatric patients. Carefully monitor the rate of fluid flow. Check the rate frequently for accuracy. A time tape is useful for this purpose.
Fluid overload: the condition caused when too large a volume of fluid infuses into the circulatory system Too large a volume of fluid infused into circulation	Engorged neck veins, increased blood pressure, and difficulty in breathing (dyspnea)	If symptoms develop, slow the rate of infusion. Notify the physician immediately. Monitor vital signs. Carefully monitor the rate of fluid flow. Check the rate frequently for accuracy.
Air embolus: air in the circulatory system Break in the IV system above the heart level allowing air in the circulatory system as a bolus	Respiratory distress Increased heart rate Cyanosis Decreased blood pressure Change in level of consciousness	Pinch off catheter or secure system to prevent entry of air. Place patient on left side in Trendelenburg position. Call for immediate assistance. Monitor vital signs and pulse oximetry.

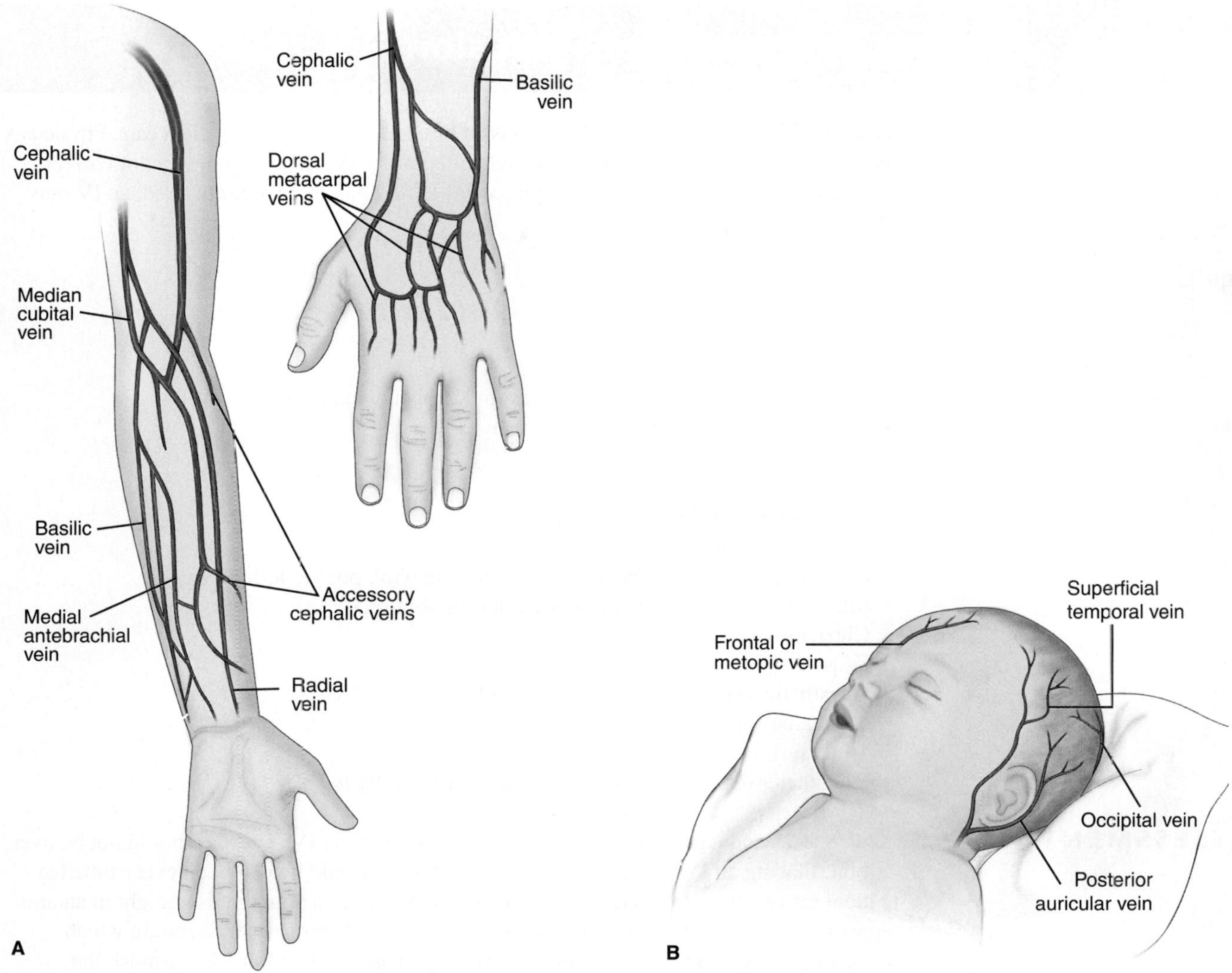

Figure 15-1. Infusion sites. (**A**) Ventral and dorsal aspects of lower arm and hand. (**B**) Scalp.

SKILL 15-1 Starting an Intravenous Infusion

Administering and monitoring IV fluids is an essential part of routine patient care. Physicians or other qualified healthcare professionals often order IV therapy to prevent or correct problems in fluid and electrolyte balance. For IV therapy to be administered, an IV must be inserted.

Equipment

- IV solution
- Towel or disposable pad
- Nonallergenic tape
- IV infusion set
- Gauze or transparent dressing (according to agency policy)
- Electronic infusion device (if ordered)
- IV tubing
- Tourniquet
- Time tape or label (for IV container)
- Armboard (if needed)
- Cleansing swabs (chlorhexidine preferred, alcohol, povidone-iodine
- Site protector or tube-shaped elastic netting (optional)
- Clean gloves
- IV pole
- Anesthetic (numbing) cream (if ordered)
- Lidocaine 1% injection (if ordered)
- 1-mL syringe (for lidocaine)
- IV catheter (over the needle, Angiocath) or butterfly needle

ASSESSMENT

Assess arms and hands for potential sites for initiating the IV. The site should not be over a joint. Placing an IV over a joint could mean the IV would be occluded every time the patient moves the extremity. Inspect the area, looking for a vein that is straight in an area approximately 5 cm long. Determine the type of IV catheter to use. Ascertain which extremity is the patient's dominant arm, and try to use the nondominant arm for the patient's comfort. Avoid using an upper extremity that has been compromised from previous conditions, for example, from a mastectomy or arteriovenous fistula. Review the patient's record for baseline data such as vital signs, intake and output balance, and pertinent laboratory values such as serum electrolytes.

NURSING DIAGNOSIS

Determine the related factors for the nursing diagnosis based on the patient's current status. Appropriate nursing diagnoses may include:

- Deficient Fluid Volume
- Impaired Skin Integrity
- Risk for Injury
- Risk for Infection
- Anxiety

Many other nursing diagnoses may require the use of this skill.

OUTCOME IDENTIFICATION AND PLANNING

The expected outcome to achieve when starting IV therapy is that the IV catheter is inserted using sterile technique on the first attempt. Also, the patient experiences minimal trauma, and the IV solution flows freely.

SKILL 15-1

Starting an Intravenous Infusion *(continued)*

IMPLEMENTATION

ACTION	RATIONALE
1. Verify IV order against the physician order. Clarify any inconsistencies. Check the patient's chart for allergies. Check for color, clarify, expiration date, etc.	This ensures that the correct IV solution and rate of infusion, and/or medication will be administered.
2. Know techniques for IV insertion, precautions, purpose of the IV administration, and medications if ordered	This knowledge and skill is essential for safe and accurate IV and medication administration.
3. Gather all equipment and bring to bedside.	Having equipment available saves time and facilitates accomplishment of task.
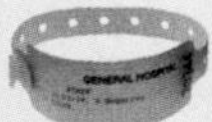 4. Identify the patient. Ask the patient if allergic to any medication, iodine, or tape, as appropriate. If considering using an anesthetic (numbing) cream or 1% lidocaine injection, check for allergies for these substances as well.	Identification of the patient ensures that the right patient receives the correct IV administration and medication as ordered. Possible allergies may exist related to medications, iodine, tape, anesthetic cream, or lidocaine injection. Injectable anesthetic can result in allergic reactions, tissue damage, and inadvertent injection into the vascular system.
5. Explain the need for the IV and procedure to patient.	Explanation allays anxiety.
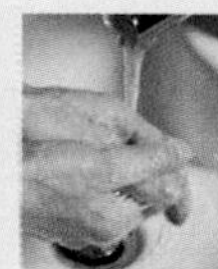 6. Perform hand hygiene. If using an anesthetic cream, apply the anesthetic cream to a few potential insertion sites.	Hand hygiene deters the spread of microorganisms. Anesthetic (numbing) cream decreases the amount of pain felt at the insertion site. Some of the numbing creams take up to an hour to become effective.
7. Prepare IV solution and tubing:	
a. **Maintain strict aseptic technique when opening sterile packages and IV solution. Remove administration set from package (Figure 1).**	Asepsis is essential for preventing the spread of microorganisms.
b. Clamp IV tubing, uncap spike on administration set, and insert into entry site on IV bag or bottle as manufacturer directs (Figure 2).	This punctures the seal in the IV bag or bottle. Clamping the IV tubing prevents air and fluid from entering the IV tubing at this time.
c. Squeeze drip chamber and allow it to fill at least halfway (Figure 3).	Suction causes fluid to move into drip chamber and prevents air from moving down the tubing.
d. Remove cap at end of the IV tubing and while maintaining its sterility, open the IV tubing clamp, and allow fluid to move through tubing. **Allow fluid to flow until all air bubbles have disappeared** and the entire length of the tubing is primed (filled) with IV solution. Close clamp and recap end of tubing, maintaining sterility of the setup.	This technique prepares for IV fluid administration and removes air from tubing. In large amounts, if air is not removed from the tubing, it can act as an embolus.
e. If an electronic device is to be used, follow manufacturer's instructions for inserting tubing and setting infusion rate.	This ensures correct flow rate and proper use of equipment.
f. Apply label if medication was added to container (pharmacy may have added medication and applied label). Label tubing with date and time that tubing was hung.	This provides for administration of correct solution with prescribed medication or additive. Labeling the tubing alerts nursing staff for need for IV tube changes. Consult hospital policy. In general, IV tubing is changed every 72 hours
g. Place time-tape on container and hang IV on pole.	This permits immediate evaluation of IV according to the time-taped schedule.

(continued)

SKILL 15-1 **Starting an Intravenous Infusion** *(continued)*

ACTION	RATIONALE

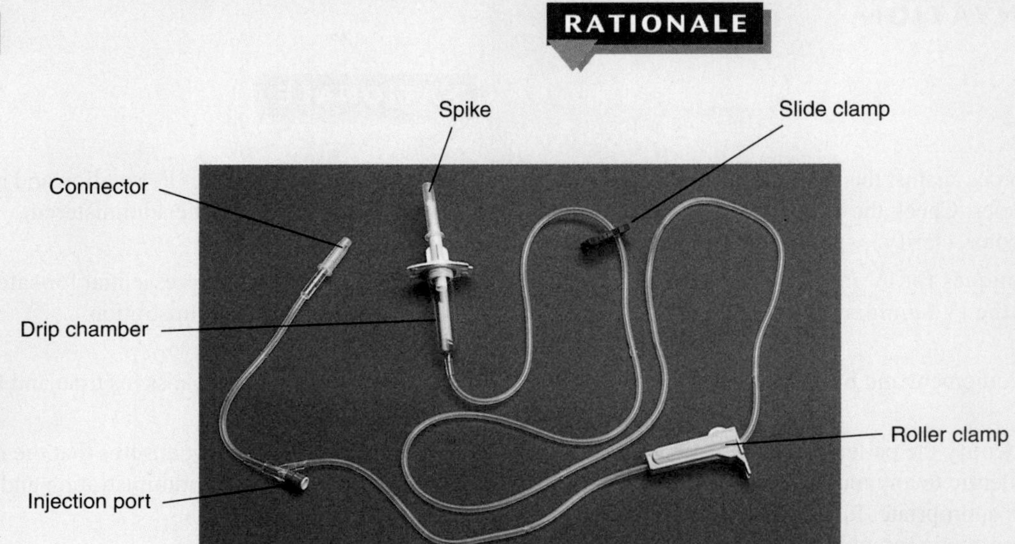

Figure 1. Basic administration set for intravenous therapy.

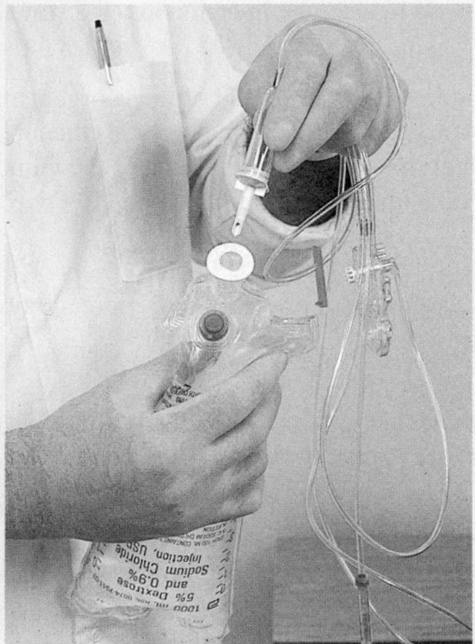

Figure 2. Inserting spike into IV bag.

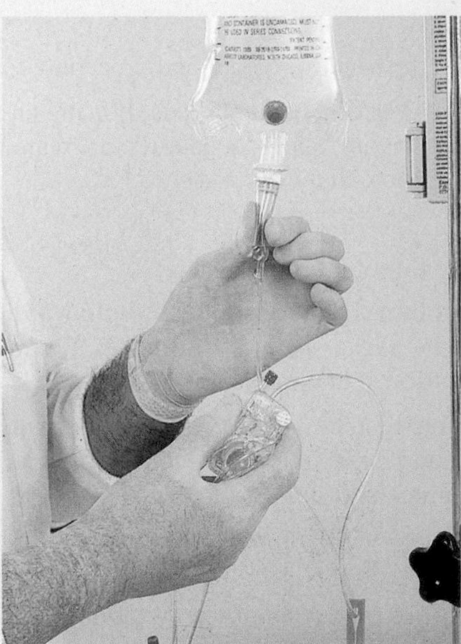

Figure 3. Squeezing drip chamber.

ACTION	RATIONALE
8. Place patient in low Fowler's position in bed. Place protective towel or pad under patient's arm. Close the door to the room or pull the bedside curtain.	The supine position permits either arm to be used and allows for good body alignment. Closing the door provides for patient privacy.
9. Provide emotional support as needed.	Patient may experience anxiety because he/she may fear needlestick or IV infusion in general.
10. **Select and palpate for an appropriate vein. Avoid an arm that has been compromised such as with presence of arteriovenous fistula.**	The use of an appropriate vein decreases discomfort for the patient and reduces the risk for damage to body tissues.
11. If the site is hairy and agency policy permits, clip a 2″ area around the intended site of entry.	Hair can harbor microorganisms.

SKILL 15-1 Starting an Intravenous Infusion *(continued)*

ACTION	RATIONALE
12. Apply a tourniquet 3″ to 4″ above the venipuncture site (Figure 4) to obstruct venous blood flow and distend the vein. Direct the ends of the tourniquet away from the site of entry. Make sure the radial pulse is still present.	Interrupting the blood flow to the heart causes the vein to distend. Distended veins are easy to see, palpate, and enter. The end of the tourniquet could contaminate the area of injection if directed toward the site of entry. Tourniquet may be applied too tightly so assessment for radial pulse is important.

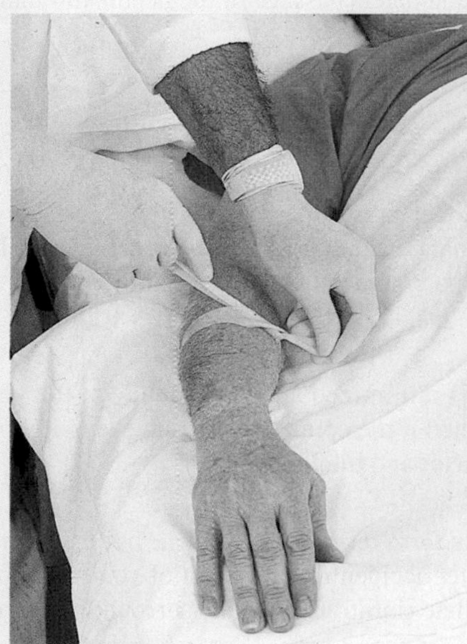

Figure 4. Applying tourniquet.

ACTION	RATIONALE
13. Instruct the patient to hold the arm lower than the heart.	Lowering the arm below the heart level helps distend the veins by filling them.
14. Ask patient to open and close fist. Observe and palpate for a suitable vein. Try the following techniques if a vein cannot be felt:	Contracting the muscles of the forearm forces blood into the veins, thereby distending them further.
a. Massage the patient's arm from proximal to distal end and gently tap over intended vein.	Massaging and tapping the vein help distend veins by filling them with blood.
b. Remove tourniquet and place warm, moist compresses over intended vein for 10 to 15 minutes.	Warm, moist compresses help dilate veins.
15. Put on clean gloves.	Gloves protect against transmission of HIV, hepatitis, and other bloodborne infections.
16. If using intradermal lidocaine, cleanse insertion site with alcohol using a circular motion. Inject a small amount (0.2–0.3 mL) of lidocaine into the area. If numbing cream was used, wipe cream off insertion site. **Cleanse site with an antiseptic solution such as chlorhexidine or according to agency policy. Use a circular motion to move from the center outward for several inches.**	The lidocaine numbs the skin and makes the insertion less painful. Cleansing that begins at the site of entry and moves outward in a circular motion carries organisms away from the site of entry. Organisms on the skin can be introduced into the tissues or the bloodstream with the needle. Chlorhexidine is the preferred antiseptic solution, but iodine, iodophor, and 70% alcohol are considered acceptable alternatives (Hadaway, 2003). If there is difficulty visualizing or palpating the intended vein for IV insertion, a tourniquet may be left in place.

(continued)

SKILL 15-1 Starting an Intravenous Infusion *(continued)*

ACTION	RATIONALE
17. Use the nondominant hand, placed about 1″ or 2″ below entry site, to hold the skin taut against the vein. **Avoid touching the prepared site.** Ask the patient to remain still while performing the venipuncture.	Pressure on the vein and surrounding tissues helps prevent movement of the vein as the needle or catheter is being inserted. The needle entry site and catheter must remain free of contamination from unsterile hands. Patient movement may prevent proper technique for IV insertion.
18. Enter the skin gently, holding the catheter by the hub in your dominant hand, bevel side up, at a 10- to 15-degree angle. Catheter may be inserted from directly over the vein or the side of the vein. While following the course of the vein, advance the needle or catheter into the vein. A sensation of "give" can be felt when the needle enters the vein.	This allows needle or catheter to enter vein with minimal trauma and deters passage of the needle through the vein.
19. When blood returns through the lumen of the needle or the flashback chamber of the catheter, advance either device ⅛″ to ¼″ farther into the vein. A catheter needs to be advanced until the hub is at the venipuncture site, but the exact technique depends on the type of device used.	The tourniquet causes increased venous pressure, resulting in automatic backflow. Placing the catheter well into the vein helps to prevent dislodgement.
20. Release the tourniquet as soon as possible. Quickly remove the protective cap from the IV tubing and attach the tubing to the catheter or needle. Stabilize the catheter or needle with your nondominant hand.	Bleeding is minimized and the patency of the vein is maintained if the connection is made smoothly between the catheter and tubing.
21. Start the flow of solution promptly by releasing the clamp on the tubing. Examine the tissue around the entry site for signs of infiltration.	Blood clots form readily if IV flow is not maintained. If catheter accidentally slips out of vein, solution will accumulate (infiltrate) into the surrounding tissue.
22. Secure the catheter with narrow nonallergenic tape (½″), placed sticky side up under the hub and crossed over the top of the hub.	The weight of the tubing is sufficient to pull it out of the vein if it is not well anchored. Nonallergenic tape is less likely to tear fragile skin.
23. **Place sterile dressing over venipuncture site.** Agency policy may direct nurse to use gauze dressing or transparent dressing. Apply tape to dressing if necessary. Loop the tubing near the site of entry, and anchor to dressing (Figure 5).	Transparent dressing allows easy visualization Gauze dressings are capable of absorbing drainage.

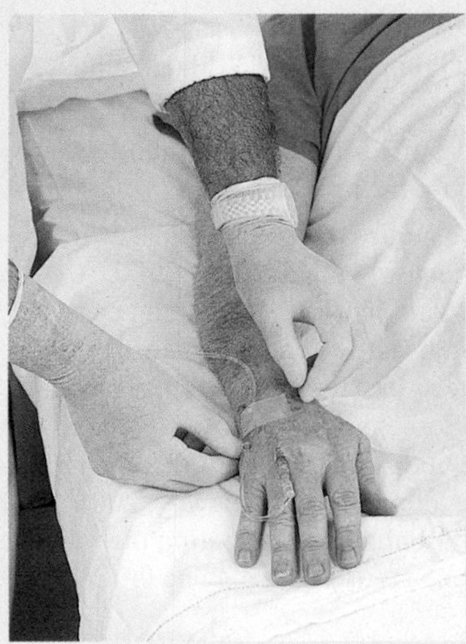

Figure 5. Securing the catheter.

SKILL 15-1 Starting an Intravenous Infusion *(continued)*

ACTION	RATIONALE
24. Label the IV dressing with the date, time, site, and type and size of catheter used for the infusion on the tape anchoring the tubing.	Other personnel working with the infusion will know what type of device is being used, the site, and when it was inserted. IV insertion sites are changed every 48 to 72 hours or according to agency policy. (Lavery, 2005)
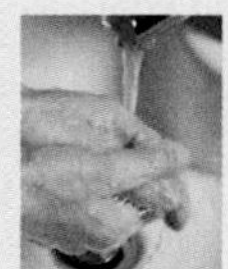 25. Remove all equipment and dispose of properly. Remove gloves and perform hand hygiene.	Hand hygiene deters the spread of microorganisms.
26. Anchor arm to an armboard for support if necessary, or apply a site protector or tube-shaped mesh netting over the insertion site. Explain to patient the purpose of the armboard and the importance of safeguarding the site when using the extremity.	An armboard or site protector helps to prevent the position of the catheter in the vein from changing.
27. Adjust the rate of solution flow according to the amount prescribed, or follow manufacturer's directions for adjusting flow rate on infusion pump.	The physician prescribes the rate of flow.
28. Document procedure and patient's response. Chart time, site, device used, and solution.	This provides accurate documentation and ensures continuity of care.
29. Return to check flow rate and observe IV site for infiltration 30 minutes after starting infusion. Ask the patient if experiencing any pain or discomfort related to the IV infusion.	This documents patient's response to infusion. Pain is a symptom often associated with IV complications such as infiltration and phlebitis.

EVALUATION

The expected outcome is met when the IV is started on the first attempt and fluid flows easily into the vein without any sign of infiltration. The patient verbalizes minimal discomfort related to insertion and demonstrates understanding of the reasons for the IV.

DOCUMENTATION

Guidelines

Document the location where the IV was started as well as the size of the IV catheter, the type of IV solution, and the rate of the IV infusion. Additionally, document the condition of the site, such as presence of redness, swelling, or drainage. Record the patient's reaction to the procedure and pertinent patient teaching, such as alerting the nurse if the patient experiences any pain from the IV or notices any swelling at the site. If necessary, document the IV fluid solution on the intake and output record.

Sample Documentation

11/02/09 0830 20G IV started in L hand. Dressing applied. Site without redness, drainage, or edema. D_5½ NS with 20 mEq KCl begun at 110 mL/hr. Patient instructed to call with any pain or swelling.—S. Barnes, RN

Unexpected Situations and Associated Interventions

- *Fluid does not easily flow into the vein:* Reposition the extremity because certain positions that the patient may assume may prevent the IV from infusing properly. If the IV is a free-flowing IV, raise the height of the IV pole. This may promote an increase in IV flow. Attempt to flush the IV with 3 mL of saline in a syringe. Check IV connector to ensure that clamp is fully open. If fluid still does not flow easily, or if resistance is met while flushing, the IV may be against a valve and may need to be restarted in a different location.

(continued)

SKILL 15-1 Starting an Intravenous Infusion *(continued)*

- *Fluid does not flow easily into the vein, and the skin around the insertion site is edematous and cool to the touch:* IV has infiltrated. Put on gloves and remove catheter. Pressure may need to be held with a sterile gauze pad. Apply a Band-Aid over insertion site and restart IV in a new location.
- *A small hematoma is forming at the site while you are inserting the catheter:* The vein is "blowing": a small hole has been made in the vein and blood is leaking out into the tissues. Remove and discard the catheter and choose an alternate insertion site.
- *Fluids are leaking around the insertion site:* Change dressing on IV. If site continues to leak, remove IV to decrease risk of infection and restart it in a new location.
- *IV infusion set becomes disconnected from IV:* Discard IV tubing to prevent infection. Attempt to flush IV with 3 mL of normal saline. If the IV is still patent, the site may still be used.
- *IV catheter is partially pulled out of insertion site:* Do not reinsert the catheter. Whether the IV is salvageable depends on how much of the catheter remains in the vein. If this catheter is not removed, it should be monitored closely for signs of infiltration.

Special Considerations

Infant and Child Considerations

- Scalp and feet can be used as alternate insertion sites. Palpate any scalp sites before insertion to ensure that an artery is not being used.
- Hand insertion sites should not be the first choice for children because nerve endings are very close to the surface of the skin, and it is more painful. Once the child can walk, do not use the feet as insertion sites.
- Do not replace peripheral catheters in children unless clinically indicated (Centers for Disease Control and Prevention, 2002).
- Catheter can be inserted with bevel side down if veins are blowing using the bevel-up technique.

Older Adult Considerations

- Avoid using vigorous friction and too much alcohol at the insertion site. Both can traumatize fragile skin and veins in the elderly.
- To decrease the risk for trauma to the vessel, experienced nurses may omit use of a tourniquet if the patient has prominent but especially fragile veins.
- To avoid an increased risk of phlebitis in adults, avoid inserting IV into the lower extremities (Rosenthal, 2004d).

SKILL 15-2 Changing IV Solution Container and Tubing

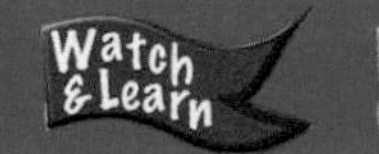

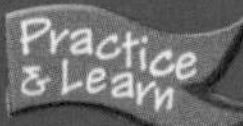

IV fluid administration frequently involves multiple bags or bottles of fluid infusion. A nursing responsibility in managing IV therapy is to monitor these fluid infusions and to replace the fluid containers as needed. Focus on the following points:

- If more than one IV solution or medication is ordered, check agency policy and appropriate literature to make sure that the additional IV solution can be attached to the existing tubing.
- As one bag is infusing, prepare the next bag so it is ready for a change when <50 mL of fluid remains in the original container.
- Ongoing verification of the IV solution and the infusion rate with the physician's order is essential.

SKILL 15-2 Changing IV Solution Container and Tubing *(continued)*

- Ongoing assessments related to the desired outcomes of the IV therapy as well as assessing for both local and systemic IV infusion complications are required.
- Before switching the IV solution containers, check the date and time of the infusion administration set to ensure it does not also need to be replaced. Check agency policy for guidelines for changing IV administration sets. For simple IV solutions, every 72 hours is recommended.

Different IV administration sets may have slightly different equipment. The accompanying Skill Variation details changing IV tubing connected directly into the hub of the IV access catheter.

Equipment

For solution change:

- IV solution as ordered by physician
- Sterile dressing and antiseptic solutions for possible need (according to agency policy)

For tubing change:

- Administration set
- Sterile gauze if needed
- Label with timing tape.

ASSESSMENT

Check the IV infusion. Observe the infusion solution and the label, confirming that it is the correct solution ordered. Inspect the rate of flow, checking the drip chamber and timing the drops if it is a gravity infusion, or checking the settings of an infusion pump, if used.

Inspect the IV site. The dressing should be intact, adhering to the skin on all edges. Check to see if there are any leaks or fluid under or around the dressing. Inspect the tissue around the IV entry site for swelling, coolness, or pallor. These are signs of fluid infiltration into the tissue around the IV catheter. Also inspect the site for redness, swelling, and warmth. These signs might indicate the development of phlebitis or an inflammation of the blood vessel at the site. Ask the patient if he/she is experiencing any pain or discomfort related to the IV line. Pain or discomfort is sometimes associated with both infiltration and phlebitis. Review the patient's intake and output balance, the patient's vital signs, results of any laboratory or diagnostic test results, and other assessments as appropriate.

NURSING DIAGNOSIS

Determine the related factors for the nursing diagnosis based on the patient's current status. An appropriate nursing diagnosis is Risk for Injury. Other nursing diagnoses that may be appropriate include:

- Risk for Infection
- Deficient Fluid Volume
- Excess Fluid Volume

Many other nursing diagnoses also may require the use of this skill.

OUTCOME IDENTIFICATION AND PLANNING

The expected outcome to achieve when changing IV solution and tubing is that the patient experiences minimal to no trauma when solution and tubing is changed. In addition, the IV infusion continues without interruption and no IV complications are identified.

(continued)

SKILL 15-2 Changing IV Solution Container and Tubing *(continued)*

IMPLEMENTATION

ACTION	RATIONALE
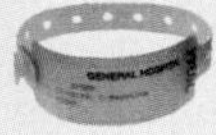 1. Identify the patient. Ask the patient if allergic to any medication, iodine, or tape, as appropriate.	Identification of the patient ensures that the right patient receives the correct IV administration and medication as ordered. Possible allergies may exist.
2. Gather all equipment and bring to bedside. Check IV solution and medication additives against physician's order. Label IV if medication is added. Include the date, time, and your name or initials.	Having equipment available saves time and facilitates accomplishment of task. Checking the physician's order and labeling ensures that patient receives the ordered IV solution and medication. Pharmacy may have added a medication label.
3. Explain procedure and reason for change to patient.	Explanation allays anxiety and facilitates compliance.
4. Perform hand hygiene.	Hand hygiene deters the spread of microorganisms.

To Change IV Solution Container

ACTION	RATIONALE
5. Carefully remove protective cover from new IV solution container and expose bag entry site.	This maintains sterility of IV solution.
6. **Close clamp on IV tubing (Figure 1). If using an electronic device, turn device to "hold" position.**	Clamping stops the flow of IV fluid during solution change.
7. Lift container off IV pole and invert it. **Quickly remove the spike from the old IV container, being careful not to contaminate it (Figure 2).**	This maintains sterility of IV setup.

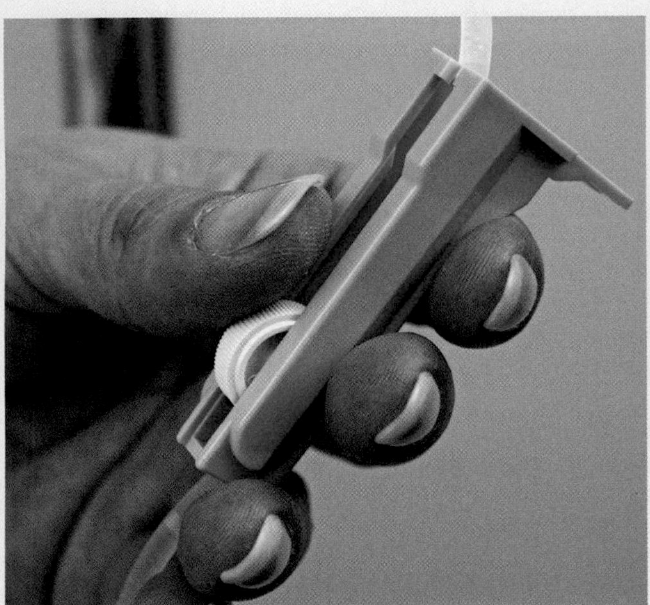
Figure 1. Clamping the tubing on administration set.

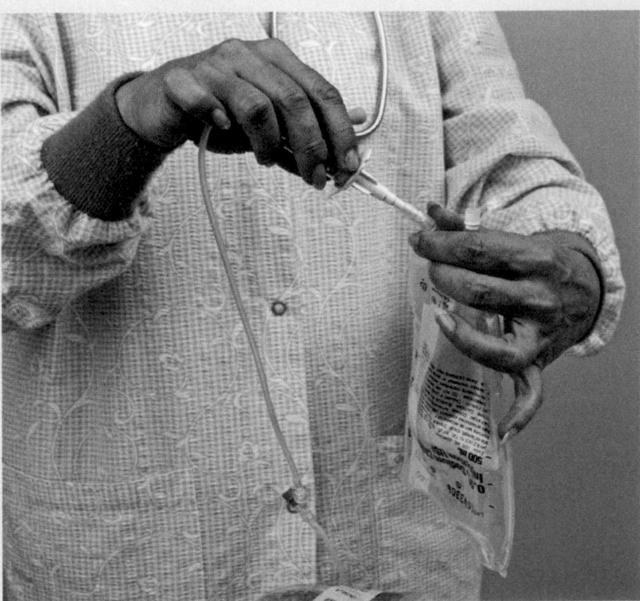
Figure 2. Inverting the solution bag and removing the spike.

SKILL 15-2 Changing IV Solution Container and Tubing *(continued)*

ACTION	RATIONALE
8. Steady new container and insert spike (Figure 3). Hang on IV pole.	This allows for uninterrupted flow of new solution.
9. Reopen clamp, check the drip chamber of the administration set on tubing, and adjust flow (Figure 4). Readjust electronic device by turning the device "ON" and verify the programmed flow rate. Inspect for air bubbles in the tubing. If using an electronic device, check that the device is operating correctly.	Opening clamp regulates flow rate into drip chamber. Electronic device regulates the milliliters per hour.

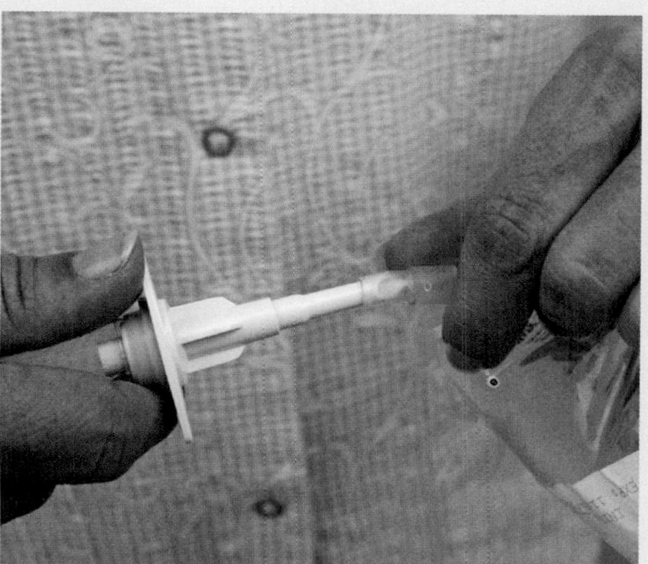

Figure 3. Spiking the new solution bag.

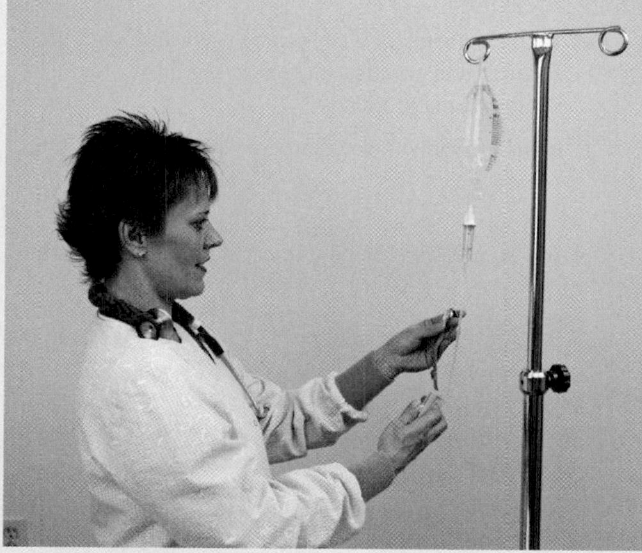

Figure 4. Reopening the clamp and adjusting the flow rate.

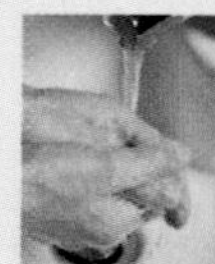

ACTION	RATIONALE
10. Label container according to agency policy. Record on intake and output record and document on chart according to agency policy. Discard used equipment properly. Perform hand hygiene.	This ensures accurate continuation and administration of correct IV solution. Hand hygiene deters the spread of microorganisms.

To Change IV Solution Container and Tubing

ACTION	RATIONALE
11. Prepare IV solution and tubing, checking IV order with the physician's order, and labeling the IV with date, time, and name or initials.	
a. **Maintain strict aseptic technique when opening sterile packages and IV solution.**	Asepsis is essential for preventing the spread of microorganisms.
b. Clamp IV tubing, uncap spike on administration set, and insert into entry site on IV bag or bottle as manufacturer directs (Figure 5).	Clamping the IV tubing prevents air and fluid from entering the IV tubing at this time. This punctures the seal in the IV bag or bottle.

(continued)

SKILL 15-2 Changing IV Solution Container and Tubing *(continued)*

ACTION / **RATIONALE**

c. Squeeze drip chamber and allow it to fill at least halfway.

Suction causes fluid to move into drip chamber and prevents air from moving down the tubing.

d. Remove cap at end of the IV tubing and while maintaining its sterility, open the IV tubing clamp, and allow fluid to move through tubing (Figure 6). **Allow fluid to flow until all air bubbles have disappeared** and the entire length of the tubing is primed (filled) with IV solution. Close clamp and recap end of tubing, maintaining sterility of the setup.

This technique prepares for IV fluid administration and removes air from tubing. In large amounts, if air is not removed from the tubing, it can act as an embolus.

e. If an electronic device is to be used, follow manufacturer's instructions for inserting tubing and setting infusion rate.

This ensures correct flow rate and proper use of equipment.

f. Label tubing with date and time that tubing was hung.

Labeling the tubing alerts nursing staff for need for IV tube changes. Consult hospital policy. In general, IV tubing is changed every 72 hours.

g. Place time-tape on container and hang IV on pole.

This permits immediate evaluation of IV according to the time-taped schedule.

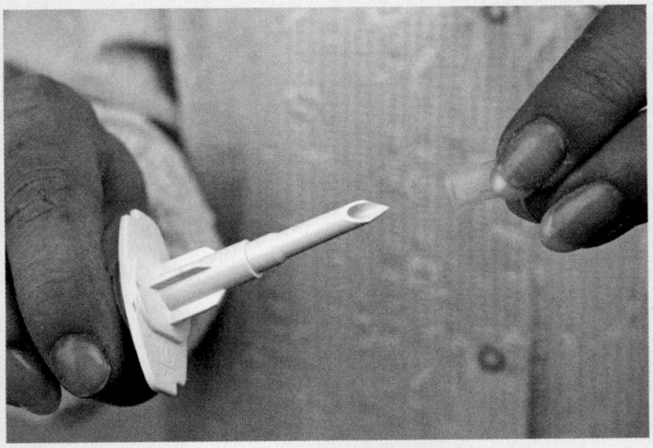

Figure 5. Removing protective cap from tubing.

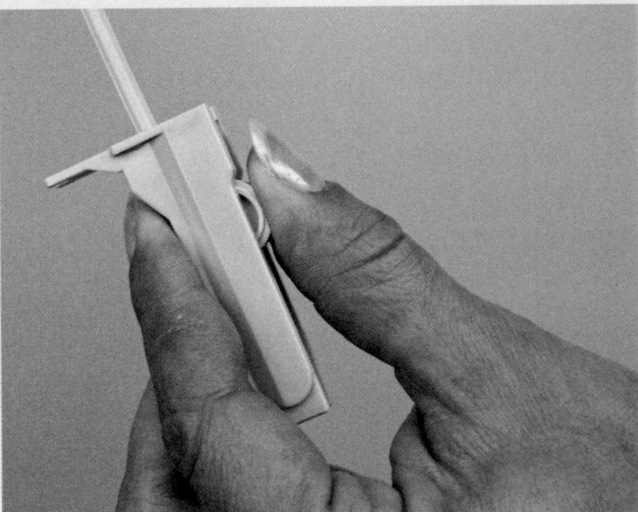

Figure 6. Releasing clamp to allow IV fluid through tubing.

12. Close the clamp on the existing IV tubing. Also, close the clamp on the short extension tubing connected to the IV catheter in the patient's arm.

A short, closed tubing set (extension set) with an injection port and closure clamp between the catheter or angiocath hub and the tubing reduces the risk for blood exposure. Clamping the existing IV tubing prevents leakage of fluid. Clamping the tubing on the extension set prevents introduction of air into the line.

SKILL 15-2 Changing IV Solution Container and Tubing *(continued)*

ACTION	RATIONALE
13. Remove the current infusion tubing from the resealable cap on the short extension IV tubing (Figure 7). Using an antimicrobial wipe, swab the resealable cap and insert the new IV tubing into the cap (Figure 8).	Cleansing the cap or port reduces the risk of contamination.

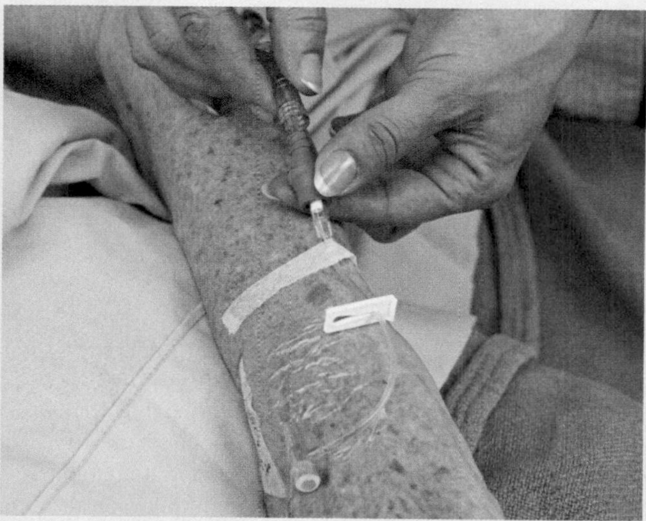

Figure 7. Removing old administration set tubing.

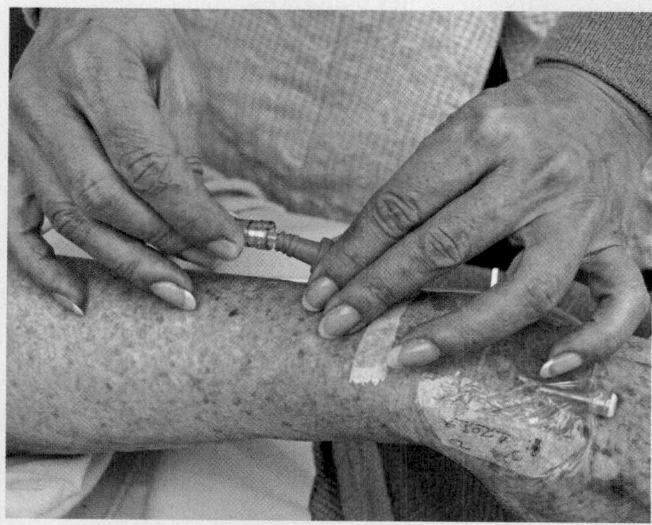

Figure 8. Inserting new IV tubing into extension tubing.

ACTION	RATIONALE
14. Open the clamp on the IV tubing and on the short extension tubing (Figure 9). Check the IV flow. Readjust electronic device as needed.	Opening clamp allows solution to flow to patient.

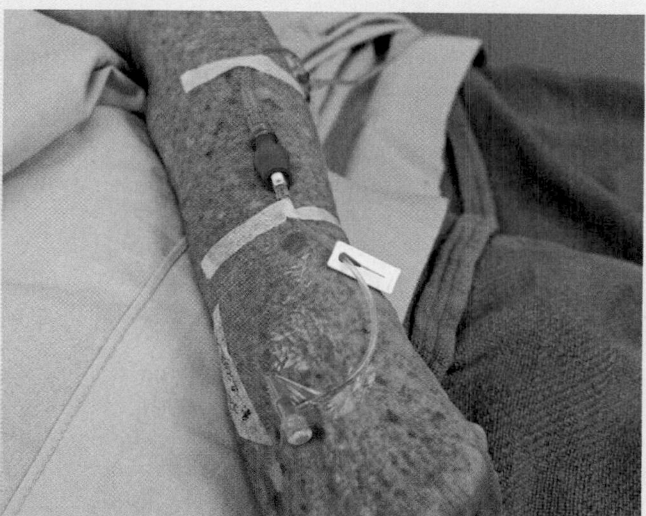

Figure 9. Making sure clamp is open on new tubing, with short extension tubing taped in place.

(continued)

SKILL 15-2 Changing IV Solution Container and Tubing *(continued)*

ACTION	RATIONALE
15. **Regulate IV flow according to physician's order.**	This ensures that patient receives IV solution at prescribed rate.
16. **Label IV tubing with date, time, and your initials. Label IV solution container and record procedure according to agency policy.** Discard used equipment properly and perform hand hygiene.	This documents IV tubing change. Hand hygiene deters the spread of microorganisms.
17. Record patient's response to IV infusion.	This ensures accurate documentation of patient's response.

EVALUATION

The expected outcome is achieved when the IV solution and tubing is changed without interrupting the ordered infusion therapy, and the patient experiences minimal to no trauma when solution and tubing is changed.

DOCUMENTATION

Guidelines

Document the type of IV solution, including if it is a change of solution from the previous type that was infusing. Also, record the assessment of the IV site, in particular, no signs of infiltration (swelling), redness, or drainage. Include patient's subjective response, such as denies pain from the IV infusion. Record any appropriate patient teaching related to the IV infusion and document on the intake and output record as appropriate.

Sample Documentation

11/3/09 1015 IV fluid changed from D_5½ NS with 20 mEq KCl/L to $D_5$0.9% NS with 20 mEq KCl/L. IV site intact; no swelling, redness or drainage noted.
—S. Barnes, RN

Unexpected Situations and Associated Interventions

- *Infusion does not flow or flow rate changes after bag and tubing is changed:* Make sure that the flow clamp is open and the drip chamber is approximately half full. Check the electronic device for proper functioning. Check the IV site for possible problems with the catheter, such as bending of the catheter or position of the patient's extremity, and inspect the IV site for signs and symptoms of complications. Readjust the flow rate.
- *After attaching new IV tubing, you note air bubbles in the tubing:* If the bubbles are above the roller clamp, you can easily remove them by closing the roller clamp, stretching the tubing downward, and tapping the tubing with your finger so the bubbles rise to the drip chamber. If there is a larger amount of air in the tubing, swab the medication port on the tubing below the air with an antimicrobial solution, allow it to dry, then insert a needle and syringe into the port below the air. Using the syringe, aspirate the air from the tubing. Remember that air bubbles in the tubing can be reduced if the tubing is primed slowly with fluid instead of allowing a wide-open flow of the solution.

SKILL 15-2 Changing IV Solution Container and Tubing *(continued)*

SKILL VARIATION Changing IV Tubing Connected Directly into the Hub of the IV Access Catheter

In certain situations, IV solution tubing does not have a short extension tubing. Instead, the IV tubing is connected directly into the hub of the IV access catheter. If available, it is good practice to add a short extension tubing to decrease the risk of contact with blood. However, on other occasions when the short extension tubing is not available, the nurse will proceed to change the IV tubing at the hub of the catheter.

After checking the physician's order, bring the primed IV tubing and the IV solution labeled with date, time, and your name or initials to the patient.

- Perform hand hygiene.
- Put on clean gloves.
- Place sterile gauze under catheter hub.
- Place new IV tubing close to IV site and slightly loosen protective cap.
- Clamp old IV tubing. Stabilize the needle hub with the nondominant hand until change is completed.
- Remove tubing with dominant hand using a twisting motion.
- Set old tubing aside. While maintaining sterility, carefully remove the covering or cap from the new administration set and insert end of tubing into catheter hub and twist to secure the tubing.
- Remove the gauze square under the hub.
- Retape the connection if necessary.
- Remove gloves.
- Open the clamp on the IV tubing and check the flow or readjust the electronic devise as needed.
- Reapply sterile dressing to site according to agency protocol (see Skill 15-4).
- Regulate IV flow according to physician's order.
- Discard used equipment properly.
- Perform hand hygiene.

SKILL 15-3 Monitoring an IV Site and Infusion

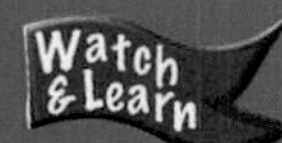

The nurse is responsible for monitoring the infusion rate and the IV site. This is routinely done as part of the initial patient assessment, at the beginning of a work shift, then at periodic intervals throughout the day. Monitoring the infusion rate is a very important part of the patient's overall management. If the patient does not receive the prescribed rate, he or she may experience a fluid volume deficit. In contrast, if the patient is administered too much fluid over a period of time, he or she may exhibit signs of fluid volume overload. Other responsibilities involve checking the IV site for possible complications and assessing for both the desired effects of an IV infusion as well as potential adverse reactions to IV therapy. IV sites are checked at specific intervals and each time an IV medication is given, as dictated by the institution's policies. It is common to check IV sites every hour, but be familiar with the requirements of your institution.

Equipment

- Clean gloves as needed
- Physical assessment equipment as needed

ASSESSMENT

Inspect the IV infusion solution for any particulates and the IV label. Confirm it is the solution ordered. Assess the current rate of flow by timing the drops if it is a gravity infusion or verifying the settings on the electronic infusion-control device (See Box 15-1). Check the tubing for kinks or anything that might clamp or interfere with the flow of solution. Inspect the IV site. The dressing should be intact, adhering to the skin on all edges. Assess fluid intake and output. Assess for complications associated with IV infusions. Assess the patient's knowledge of IV therapy.

(continued)

SKILL 15-3 Monitoring an IV Site and Infusion *(continued)*

BOX 15-1 Regulating IV Flow Rate

Follow agency's guidelines to determine if infusion should be administered by electronic pump or by gravity.

- Check physician's order for IV solution.
- Check patency of IV line and needle.
- Verify drop factor (number of drops in 1 mL) of the equipment in use.
- Calculate the flow rate:
  EXAMPLE—Administer 1000 mL D5W over 10 hours (set delivers 60 gtt/1 mL).

a. Standard formula

$$\text{gtt/min} = \frac{\text{volume (mL)} \times \text{drop factor (gtt/mL)}}{\text{time (in minutes)}}$$

$$\text{gtt/min} = \frac{1000 \text{ mL} \times 60}{600\ (60 \text{ min} \times 10 \text{ h})}$$

$$= \frac{60{,}000}{600}$$

$$= 100 \text{ gtt/min}$$

b. Short formula using milliliters per hour

$$\text{gtt/min} = \frac{\text{milliliters per hour} \times \text{drop factor (gtt/mL)}}{\text{time (60 min)}}$$

Find milliliters per hour by dividing 1000 mL by 10 hours:

$$\frac{1000}{10} = 100 \text{ mL/hr}$$

$$\text{gtt/min} = \frac{100 \text{ mL} \times 60}{60 \text{ min}}$$

$$= \frac{6{,}000}{60}$$

$$= 100 \text{ gtt/min}$$

NURSING DIAGNOSIS

Determine the related factors for the nursing diagnosis based on the patient's current status. Appropriate nursing diagnoses may include:

- Excess Fluid Volume
- Deficient Fluid Volume
- Risk for Infection
- Risk for Injury

In addition, many other nursing diagnoses also may require the use of this skill.

OUTCOME IDENTIFICATION AND PLANNING

The expected outcome to be met when monitoring the IV infusion and site is that the patient remains free from complications and demonstrates signs and symptoms of fluid balance.

IMPLEMENTATION

ACTION	RATIONALE
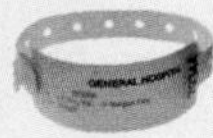 1. Identify the patient.	Identification of the patient ensures that the right patient receives the correct IV administration and medication as ordered.
2. **Monitor IV infusion every hour or per agency policy. More frequent checks may be necessary if medication is being infused.**	This promotes safe administration of IV fluids and medication.
a. Check physician's order for IV solution.	This ensures that the correct solution is being given at the correct rate and in the proper sequence with the correct medications.

SKILL 15-3 Monitoring an IV Site and Infusion *(continued)*

ACTION	RATIONALE
b. Check drip chamber and time drops (Figure 1), if IV is not regulated by an infusion-control device. Refer to Box 15-1 to review calculation of IV flow rates.	This ensures that flow rate is correct. The nurse will need to use watch with a second hand for counting the drops in regulating a gravity drip IV infusion.
c. Check tubing for anything that might interfere with flow (Figure 2). Be sure that clamp is in the open position. **Observe dressing for leakage of IV solution.**	Any kink or pressure on tubing may interfere with flow. Leakage may occur at the connection of the tubing with the hub of needle or catheter and allow for loss of IV solution.
d. Check settings, alarm, and indicator lights on infusion control device if one is being used (Figure 3). Educate patient related to alarm features on electronic infusion device.	Observation ensures that infusion control device is functioning and that alarm is in "on" position. Lack of knowledge about "alarms" may create anxiety for patient.

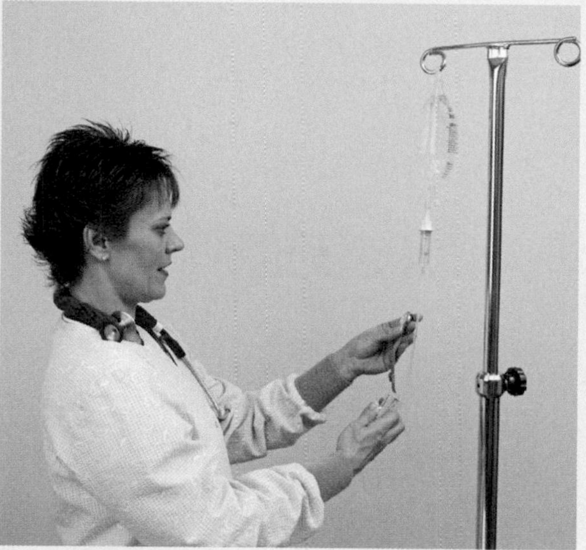

Figure 1. Checking drip chamber and time drops.

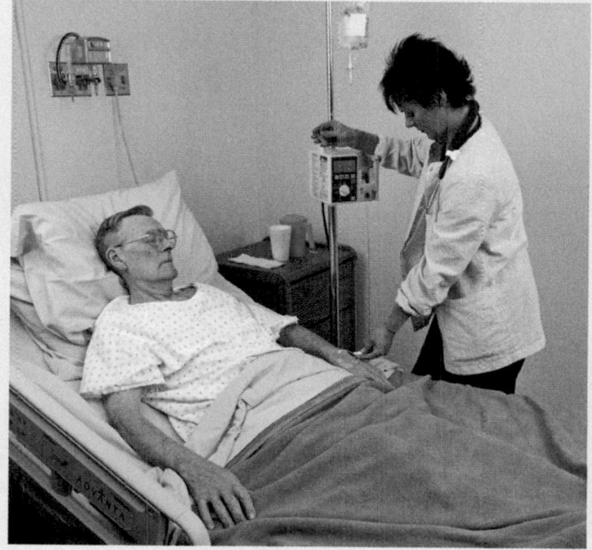

Figure 2. Checking tubing for anything that might interfere with flow rate.

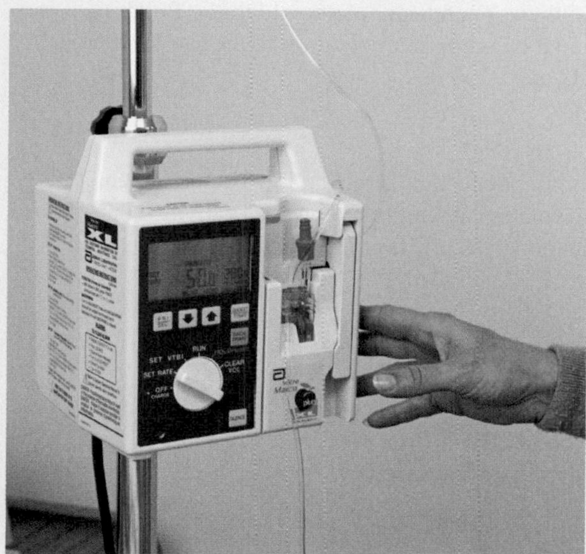

Figure 3. Checking the settings of the infusion device.

(continued)

SKILL 15-3 Monitoring an IV Site and Infusion *(continued)*

ACTION	RATIONALE
3. **Inspect site for swelling, leakage at the site, coolness, or pallor, which may indicate infiltration (Figure 4). Ask if patient is experiencing any pain or discomfort. This necessitates removing IV and restarting at another site. Check agency policy for treating infiltration** (See Fundamentals Review 15-2).	Catheter may become dislodged from vein, and IV solution may flow into subcutaneous tissue.

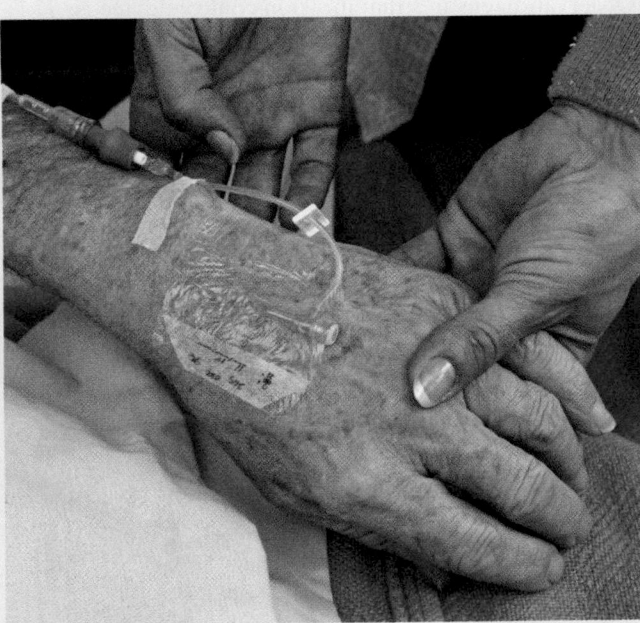

Figure 4. Inspecting IV site.

ACTION	RATIONALE
4. **Inspect site for redness, swelling and heat. Palpate for induration. Ask if patient is experiencing pain. These findings may indicate phlebitis. IV will need to be discontinued and restarted at another site. Notify physician if you suspect phlebitis. Check agency policy for treatment of phlebitis.**	Chemical irritation or mechanical trauma causes injury to the vein and can lead to phlebitis. Phlebitis is the most common complication related to IV therapy (Lavery, 2005).
5. **Check for local manifestations (redness, pus, warmth, induration, and pain) that may indicate an infection is present at the site, or systemic manifestations (chills, fever, tachycardia, hypotension) that may accompany local infection at the site. IV should be discontinued and physician notified. Be careful not to disconnect IV tubing when putting on patient's hospital gown.**	Poor aseptic technique may allow bacteria to enter the needle or catheter insertion site or tubing connection and may occur with manipulation of equipment.

SKILL 15-3

Monitoring an IV Site and Infusion *(continued)*

ACTION	RATIONALE
6. Be alert for additional complications of IV therapy.	
a. **Fluid overload can result in signs of cardiac and/or respiratory failure. Monitor intake and output and vital signs. Assess for edema and auscultate lung sounds. Ask if patient is experiencing any shortness of breath.**	Infusing too much IV solution results in an increased volume of circulating fluid volume. Elderly patients are most at risk for this complication due to possible decrease in cardiac and/or renal functions.
b. Bleeding at the site is most likely to occur when the IV is discontinued.	Bleeding may be caused by anticoagulant medication.
7. **If possible, instruct patient to call for assistance if any discomfort is noted at site, solution container is nearly empty, flow has changed in any way, or if the electronic pump alarm sounds.**	This facilitates cooperation of patient and safe administration of IV solution.

EVALUATION

The expected outcome is achieved when the patient remains free of injury (specifically, complications related to IV therapy) and exhibits an IV site that is pink, warm, dry, and pain-free. The IV solution infuses at the prescribed flow rate.

DOCUMENTATION

Guidelines

Document the type of IV solution as well as the infusion rate. Document the patient's reaction to the IV therapy as well as absence of subjective reports that he/she is not experiencing any pain or other discomfort, such as coolness or heat associated with the infusion. Additionally, record that the patient is not demonstrating any other IV complications, such as signs or symptoms of fluid overload. Record on the intake and output documents as needed.

Sample Documentation

11/6/09 1020 IV site is intact with no swelling, redness or drainage. D_5 0.9% NS with 20 mEq KCL continues to infuse at 110 mL/hr. Patient instructed to call nurse with any swelling or pain.—S. Barnes, RN

Unexpected Situations and Associated Interventions

- *Patient's lung sounds were previously clear, but now some crackles in the bases are auscultated:* Notify physician immediately. The patient may be exhibiting signs of fluid overload. Be prepared to tell the physician what the past intake and output totals were, as well as the vital signs and pulse oximetry findings of the patient.
- *IV is not flowing as easily as it previously had:* If there is no medication in the IV, open the clamp and see if the IV is patent (you may also flush with 3 mL of normal saline). If the IV does not flow with the clamp open, check all other clamps on the tubing and check tubing for any kinking. If the IV is over a joint, reposition the extremity and see if this helps the flow. An armboard may need to be applied. If the IV is painful or you meet resistance when attempting to flush, discontinue the IV and restart in another place.

SKILL 15-4 Changing a Peripheral IV Dressing

The IV site is a potential entry point for microorganisms into the bloodstream. To prevent this, sealed IV dressings are used to occlude the site and prevent complications. Whenever these dressings need to be changed, it is important to observe meticulous aseptic technique to minimize the possibility of contamination. As always, the institution's policies determine the type of dressing used and when these dressing are changed. IV site dressing changes often coincide with IV site rotations. However, dressing changes might be required more often, based on nursing assessment and judgment. Any IV dressing that is damp, loosened, or soiled should be changed immediately.

Equipment

- Sterile gauze (2 × 2 or 4 × 4) or transparent occlusive dressing
- 2% chlorhexidine, iodine, 70% alcohol
- Adhesive remover (optional)
- Alcohol swabs
- Tape
- Clean gloves
- Towel or disposable pad
- Masks for nurse and patient (optional)

ASSESSMENT

Assess IV site, looking for any drainage, redness, leakage, or other indications that the dressing needs to be changed. Also assess the patient's need to keep IV infusion. If patient does not need the IV, discuss with physician the possibility of capping for intermittent use or discontinuing it. Ask the patient about any allergies.

NURSING DIAGNOSIS

Determine the related factors for the nursing diagnosis based on the patient's current status. An appropriate nursing diagnosis is Risk for Infection. Many other nursing diagnoses also may require the use of this skill.

OUTCOME IDENTIFICATION AND PLANNING

The expected outcome to achieve when changing an IV dressing is that the patient will exhibit an IV site that is clean, dry, and without evidence of any signs and symptoms of infection, infiltration, or phlebitis. In addition, the dressing will be clean, dry, and intact.

IMPLEMENTATION

ACTION	RATIONALE
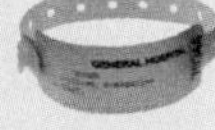 1. Identify the patient. Ask the patient if allergic to any medication, iodine, or tape, as appropriate.	Identification of the patient ensures that the right patient receives the correct nursing care. Possible allergies may exist related to medications, iodine, or tape.
2. Explain the need for the IV and procedure to patient.	Explanation allays anxiety.
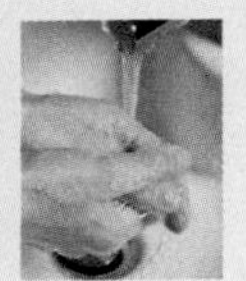 3. **Perform hand hygiene. Put on clean gloves.**	Hand hygiene deters the spread of microorganisms. Gloves prevent transmission of HIV and other bloodborne infections.

SKILL 15-4 Changing a Peripheral IV Dressing *(continued)*

ACTION | **RATIONALE**

4. Place towel or disposable pad under the arm with the IV site. **Carefully remove old dressing, but leave tape that anchors the IV needle or catheter in place (Figure 1).** Discard properly.

This prevents IV needle or catheter from becoming dislodged.

5. **Inspect IV site for presence of phlebitis (inflammation), infection, or infiltration (Figure 2). Discontinue and relocate IV if noted.**

Inflammation (phlebitis), infection, or infiltration cause trauma to tissues and necessitate removal of the IV needle or catheter.

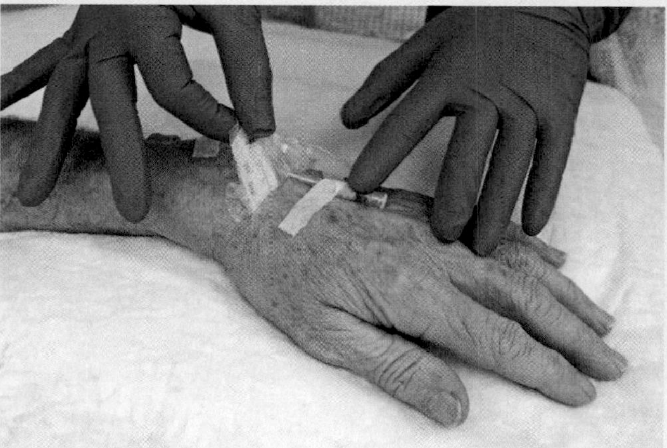

Figure 1. Removing the old dressing.

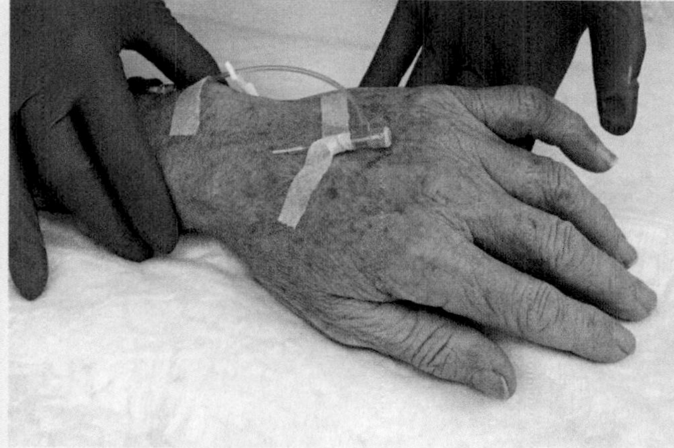

Figure 2. Inspecting the site.

6. Loosen and gently remove tape, being careful to steady catheter with one hand (Figure 3). Use adhesive remover if necessary.

Tape stabilizes needle and prevents it from becoming dislodged.

7. **Cleanse the entry site with a chlorhexidine solution, using a circular motion and moving from the center outward (Figure 4). Allow to dry.**

Cleaning in a circular motion while moving outward carries organisms away from the entry site. Use of antiseptic solutions reduces the number of microorganisms on the skin surface. Iodine and 70% alcohol are considered acceptable alternatives. Refer to agency policies.

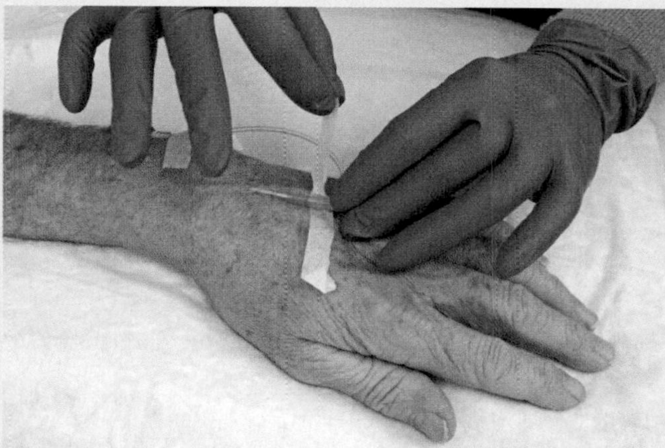

Figure 3. Loosening tape while stabilizing the catheter.

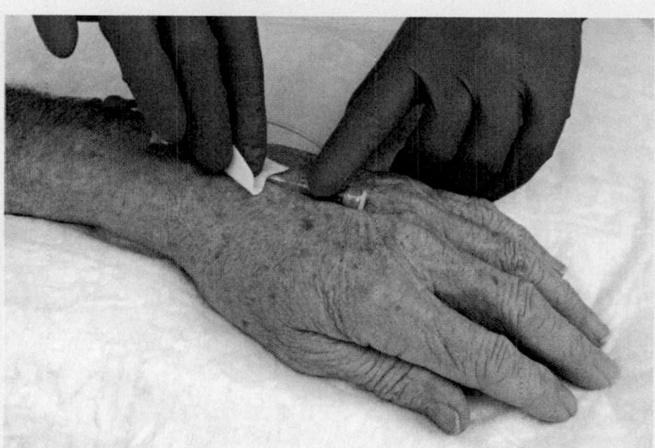

Figure 4. Cleaning site.

(continued)

SKILL 15-4 Changing a Peripheral IV Dressing *(continued)*

ACTION	RATIONALE
8. Reapply tape strip to needle or catheter at entry site (Figure 5).	Tape anchors needle or catheter to prevent dislodgement.
9. Apply transparent polyurethane dressing over entry site (Figure 6). Remove gloves and perform hand hygiene.	Dressing protects site and deters contamination with microorganisms. Hand hygiene deters the spread of microorganisms.

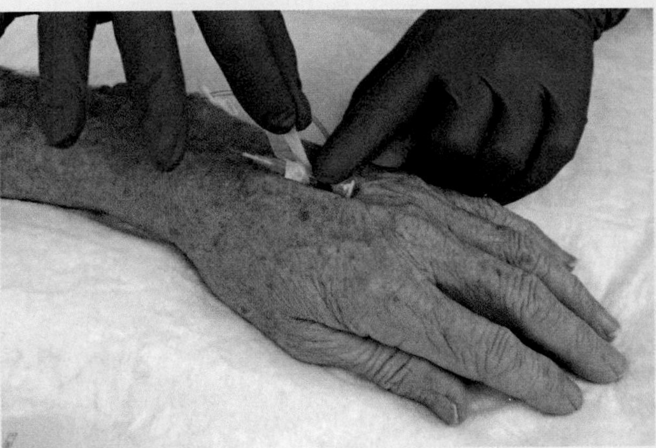

Figure 5. Reapplying a tape strip.

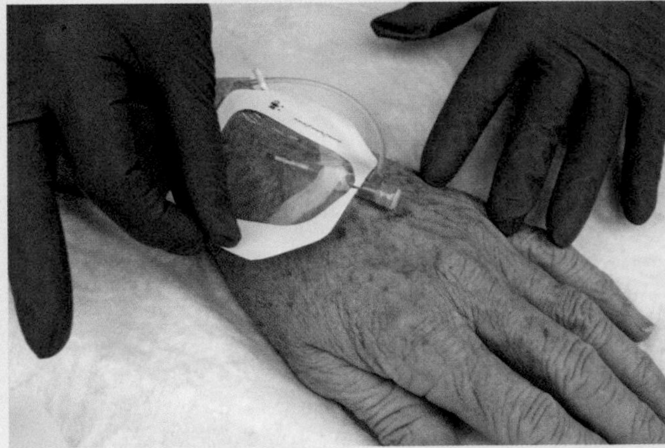

Figure 6. Applying a new dressing.

ACTION	RATIONALE
10. **Secure IV tubing with additional tape if necessary. Label dressing with date, time of change, and initials (Figure 7). Check that IV flow is accurate and system is patent.**	Labeling and documentation ensure communication about IV dressing change.

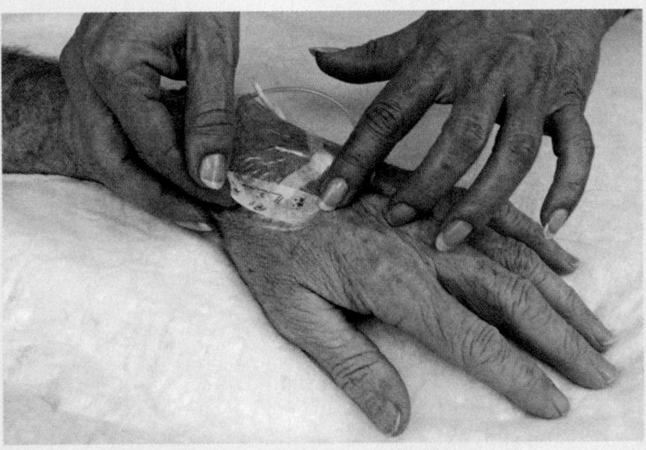

Figure 7. Labeling the dressing.

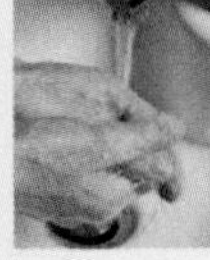

ACTION	RATIONALE
11. Discard equipment properly and perform hand hygiene.	Hand hygiene protects against spread of microorganisms.

SKILL 15-4 Changing a Peripheral IV Dressing *(continued)*

ACTION	RATIONALE
12. Record patient's response to dressing change and observation of site.	This provides accurate documentation and ensures continuity of care.

EVALUATION

The expected outcome is met when the patient remains free of any signs and symptoms of infection, phlebitis, or infiltration at the IV site. In addition, the IV dressing is clean, dry, and intact, and the patient has received the IV infusion at the correct rate.

DOCUMENTATION

Guidelines

Document the location of the IV site as well as the condition of this site. Include the presence or absence of signs of erythema or redness, swelling, or drainage. Record the subjective comments of the patient, that is, the absence or presence of pain at the IV site. Document the type of IV solution as well as the hourly rate. Note that the patient has been instructed to call for the nurse if he/she experiences any pain at the IV site or notices any swelling, redness, or leakage around the site.

Sample Documentation

11/15/09 1120 Dressing change to IV site in L hand complete. Site without erythema or redness, edema, or drainage. $D_5$0.9% NS infusing at 75 mL/hr. Patient instructed to call nurse with any pain, swelling, or questions.—S. Barnes, RN

Unexpected Situations and Associated Interventions

- *Patient complains that IV site feels "funny" and hurts:* Observe IV site for redness, edema, and warmth. If present, clamp the tubing to stop the IV solution flow, remove the catheter. and apply a gauze dressing. Start a new IV in a different site.

SKILL 15-5 Capping a Primary Line for Intermittent Use

Sometimes a continuous infusion of IV solution is no longer needed, but the patient still needs an access for the administration of IV medications or periodic fluid infusions. An IV line can then be capped, leaving the site as an access point for intermittent or emergency use. Basically, a capped line consists of the IV catheter connected to a short length of extension tubing sealed with a cap. Some facilities put the resealable cap directly into the IV catheter hub. Because there are different ways to cap an IV line, review your agency's policies. Capped lines are flushed at periodic intervals with normal saline or heparin to keep the IV catheter patent and to prevent clots from forming in the catheter. For simple peripheral capped lines, flushing with NSS is generally done once a shift, before and after administering an IV medication or as agency policy recommends.

The below skill describes capping a primary line when extension tubing is present; the accompanying skill variation describes capping a primary line when connecting directly to the hub of the IV access catheter.

(continued)

SKILL 15-5 Capping a Primary Line for Intermittent Use *(continued)*

Equipment

- Lock device
- Clean gloves
- 4″ × 4″ gauze pad
- Normal saline or heparin flush prepared in a syringe (1–3 mL) according to agency policy
- Antimicrobial wipe
- Tape
- Extension tubing (optional)

ASSESSMENT

Assess IV insertion site for local signs of any IV complications. Verify the physician's orders to ensure that continuous infusions are no longer necessary.

NURSING DIAGNOSIS

Determine the related factors for the nursing diagnosis based on the patient's current status. Appropriate nursing diagnoses may include Risk for Infection and Risk for Injury. Many other nursing diagnoses also may require the use of this skill.

OUTCOME IDENTIFICATION AND PLANNING

The expected outcome to achieve when capping a primary IV line is that the patient will remain free of injury and any signs and symptoms of IV complications. In addition, the capped IV device will remain patent.

IMPLEMENTATION

ACTION	RATIONALE
1. Gather equipment and verify physician's order. Fill syringe with normal saline or heparin flush according to agency policy. Recap syringe for use in Action 10.	Having equipment available saves time and facilitates the task. Checking the order ensures that the procedure has been ordered by the physician. Flushing maintains patency of lock and tubing. Some agencies use prefilled saline syringes.
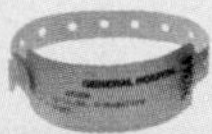 2. Identify the patient.	Identification of the patient ensures that the right patient receives the correct nursing care.
3. Explain procedure to patient.	Explanation allays anxiety and facilitates compliance.
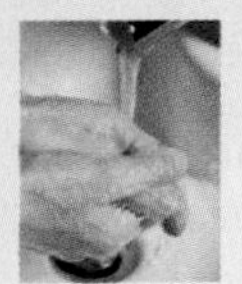 4. Perform hand hygiene.	Hand hygiene deters the spread of microorganisms.
5. Assess the IV site.	Complications such as infiltration, phlebitis, or infection necessitate discontinuation of the IV infusion at that site.
6. **Clamp off primary IV tubing (Figure 1).**	Clamping prevents inadvertent blood loss when IV and tubing are disconnected.

SKILL 15-5

Capping a Primary Line for Intermittent Use *(continued)*

ACTION | RATIONALE

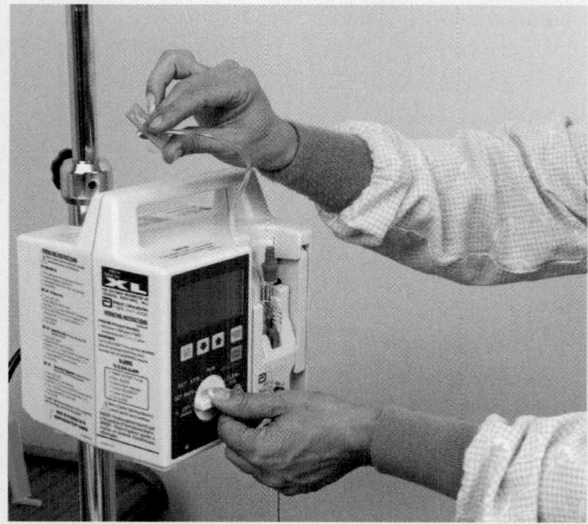

Figure 1. Clamping off the primary line.

7. Put on clean gloves according to hospital policy. Clamp the extension tubing if a clamp is present. Remove the primary IV tubing from the extension set (Figure 2) or adapter device. Cleanse adapter device with an antimicrobial swab (Figure 3).

Clamping prevents air from entering the line. Cleaning the cap reduces the risk for contamination.

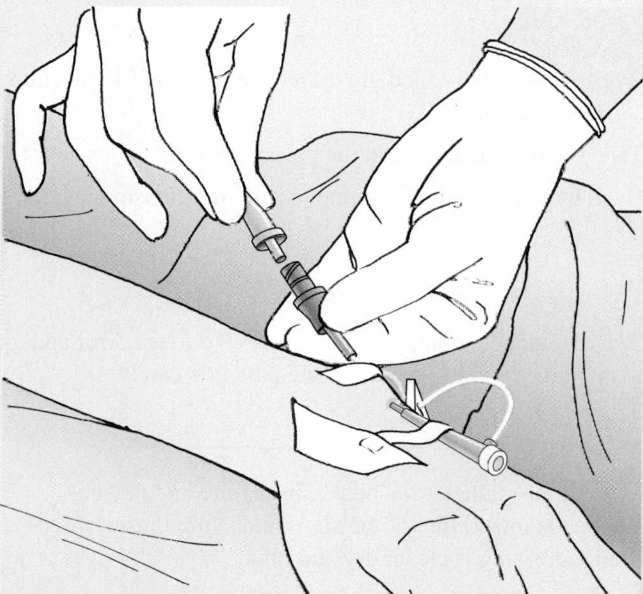

Figure 2. Removing IV tubing.

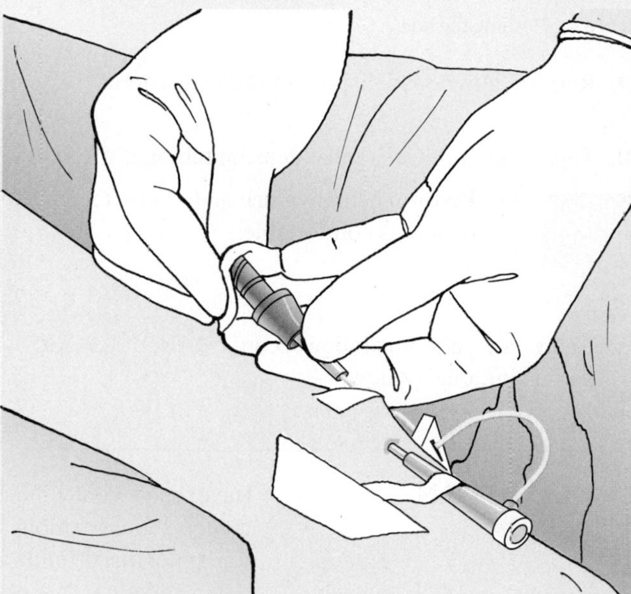

Figure 3. Cleaning the cap.

(continued)

SKILL 15-5 Capping a Primary Line for Intermittent Use *(continued)*

ACTION	RATIONALE
8. Unclamp the extension set and insert a saline or heparin flush syringe into the cap. Instill the solution over 1 minute or flush the line according to agency policy (Figure 4). Reclamp the extension tubing and remove the syringe.	Flushing maintains patency of the IV line.

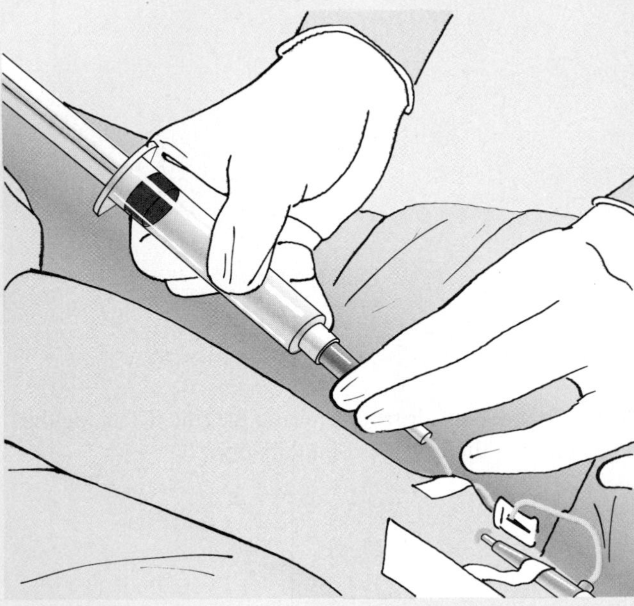

Figure 4. Flushing the line.

ACTION	RATIONALE
9. Remove gloves and dispose of them appropriately.	Proper disposal of soiled gloves reduces the risk for infection transmission.
10. Tape adapter device (and extension tubing if used).	Tape secures the device in the proper position.
11. Perform hand hygiene and ensure the patient is comfortable.	Hand hygiene deters the spread of microorganisms.
12. Chart on IV administration record, MAR, or CMAR per institutional policy.	Accurate documentation is necessary to prevent error and to maintain ongoing record of the patient's care.

EVALUATION

The expected outcome is met when the IV catheter flushes easily, indicating patency, and the patient exhibits an IV site that is intact, free of the signs and symptoms of infection, phlebitis, or infiltration. The IV dressing is clean, dry and intact.

DOCUMENTATION

Guidelines

Document the type of IV fluids that was discontinued. Record the condition of the IV site insertion as well as surrounding skin, such as "the IV is intact and free of redness, drainage, or swelling." Document the ease or difficulty in flushing the capped IV or saline lock. Record the patient's reaction to the procedure and any appropriate patient teaching that occurred.

SKILL 15-5 Capping a Primary Line for Intermittent Use *(continued)*

Sample Documentation

11/12/09 0615 IV fluids discontinued, IV flushes easily; site pink, warm, and dry without drainage; converted to saline lock.—S. Barnes, RN

Unexpected Situations and Associated Interventions

- *IV site leaks fluid whenever flushed:* To prevent infection and other complications, remove this IV and restart it in another location.
- *IV does not flush easily:* Check insertion site. The catheter may be blocked or clotted due to a kinked catheter at the insertion site. If the catheter has pulled out a short distance, do not reinsert it: it is no longer sterile. The catheter will most likely need to be removed and started in a new location.

SKILL VARIATION Capping a Primary Line When No Extension Tube is in Place

It is good practice to add a short extension tubing to decrease the risk of contact with blood, and for infection-control purposes. However, when this is not possible, the nurse will proceed to cap the IV tubing at the hub of the catheter. After checking the physician's order to cap the IV line, the nurse brings the IV cap-adapter device and the extension tubing, if available, to the bedside, as well as other needed equipment.

- Gather equipment and verify physician's order.
- Fill the adapter device and extension tubing if available with normal saline or heparin flush according to agency policy. Recap syringe for use.
- Explain the procedure to the patient.
- Perform hand hygiene.
- Assess IV site.
- Put on clean gloves.
- Place gauze 4 × 4 sponge underneath IV connection hub, between IV catheter and tubing.
- **Stabilize hub of IV catheter with nondominant hand. Use dominant hand to quickly twist and disconnect IV tubing from the catheter. Discard it. Attach the adapter device to the IV catheter hub using aseptic technique.**
- Cleanse cap with an antimicrobial solution.
- Insert the syringe with blunt cannula or standard syringe and gently flush with saline or heparin flush as per agency policy. Remove syringe carefully.
- Remove gloves and dispose of them appropriately.
- Tape adapter device.
- Perform hand hygiene and ensure the patient is comfortable.
- Chart on IV administration record, MAR, or CMAR per institutional policy.

SKILL 15-6 Administering a Blood Transfusion

A blood transfusion is the infusion of whole blood or a blood component such as plasma, red blood cells, or platelets into a patient's venous circulation (Table 15-1). Before a patient can receive blood, his or her blood must be typed to ensure that he or she receives compatible blood. Otherwise, a serious and life-threatening transfusion reaction may occur involving clumping and hemolysis of the red blood cells and death can occur (Table 15-2).

Equipment

- Blood product
- Blood administration set (tubing with in-line filter and Y for saline administration)
- 0.9% normal saline
- IV pole
- IV catheter (20 gauge or larger)
- Clean gloves
- Tape

(continued)

SKILL 15-6 Administering a Blood Transfusion *(continued)*

TABLE 15-1 Blood Products

BLOOD PRODUCT	FILTER	RATE OF ADMINISTRATION	ABO COMPATIBILITY	DOUBLE-CHECKED BY 2 PEOPLE
Packed red blood cells	Yes	1 unit over 2–3 hours; no longer than 4 hours	Yes	Yes
Platelets	Yes (in provided tubing)	As fast as patient can tolerate	No	Yes
Cryoprecipitate	No	IV push over 3 minutes	Recommended	Yes
Fresh-frozen plasma	No	200 mL/hr	Yes	Yes
Albumin	In tubing provided	1–10 mL/min (5%) 0.2–0.4 cc/min (25%)	No	No

TABLE 15-2 Transfusion Reactions

REACTION	SIGNS AND SYMPTOMS	NURSING ACTIVITY
Allergic reaction: allergy to transfused blood	Hives, itching Anaphylaxis	• Stop transfusion immediately and keep vein open with normal saline. • Notify physician stat. • Administer antihistamine parenterally as necessary.
Febrile reaction: fever develops during infusion	Fever and chills Headache Malaise	• Stop transfusion immediately and keep vein open with normal saline. • Notify physician. • Treat symptoms.
Hemolytic transfusion reaction: incompatibility of blood product	Immediate onset Facial flushing Fever, chills Headache Low back pain Shock	• Stop infusion immediately and keep vein open with normal saline. • Notify physician stat. • Obtain blood samples from site. • Obtain first voided urine. • Treat shock if present. • Send unit, tubing, and filter to lab. • Draw blood sample for serologic testing and send urine specimen to the lab.
Circulatory overload: too much blood administered	Dyspnea Dry cough Pulmonary edema	• Slow or stop infusion. • Monitor vital signs. • Notify physician. • Place in upright position with feet dependent.
Bacterial reaction: bacteria present in blood	Fever Hypertension Dry, flushed skin Abdominal pain	• Stop infusion immediately. • Obtain culture of patient's blood and return blood bag to lab. • Monitor vital signs. • Notify physician. • Administer antibiotics stat.

ASSESSMENT

Obtain a baseline assessment of the patient, including vital signs, heart and lung sounds, and urinary output. Review the most recent laboratory values, in particular, the complete blood count (CBC). Ask the patient about any previous transfusions, including the number he or she has had and any reactions experienced during a transfusion. Inspect the IV insertion site, noting that the gauge of the IV catheter is an 18 or larger, and check the type of solution being given.

SKILL 15-6 Administering a Blood Transfusion *(continued)*

NURSING DIAGNOSIS

Determine the related factors for the nursing diagnosis based on the patient's current status. Appropriate nursing diagnoses may include:

- Risk for Injury
- Deficient Fluid Volume
- Excess Fluid Volume
- Ineffective Peripheral Tissue Perfusion
- Decreased Cardiac Output

IMPLEMENTATION

ACTION	RATIONALE
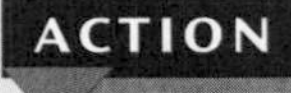 1. Identify the patient. Ask if the patient is allergic to any medication, iodine, tape, or if the patient has had a transfusion or transfusion reaction in the past.	Identification of the patient ensures that the right patient receives the correct blood transfusion. Possible allergies may exist related to medications, iodine, or tape.
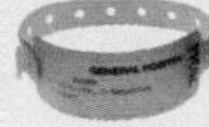 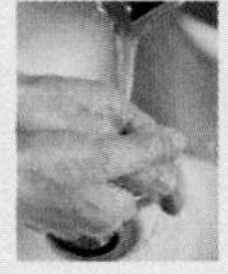 2. Determine whether patient knows reason for the blood transfusion. Explain to patient what will happen. Check for signed consent for transfusion if required by agency. Advise patient to report any chills, itching, rash, or unusual symptoms. If the physician has ordered any premedication, administer it now.	Explanation provides reassurance and facilitates cooperation. Any reaction to the transfusion necessitates stopping the transfusion immediately.
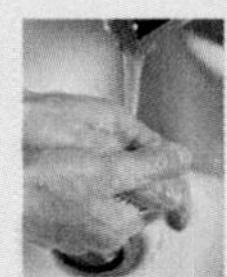 3. Perform hand hygiene and put on clean gloves.	Hand hygiene deters the spread of microorganisms. Gloves protect against accidental exposure to the patient's blood.
4. **Hang container of 0.9% normal saline with blood administration set to initiate IV infusion and follow administration of blood.**	Dextrose may lead to clumping of red blood cells and hemolysis. The filter in the blood administration set removes particulate material formed during storage of blood.
5. Start IV with 18- or 19-gauge catheter if not already present (see Skill 15-1). Keep IV open by starting flow of normal saline.	A large-bore needle or catheter is necessary for the infusion of blood products. The lumen must be large enough not to cause damage to red blood cells. IV should be started before obtaining blood in case the procedure takes longer than 30 minutes.
6. Obtain blood product from blood bank according to agency policy. Scan for bar codes on blood products if required.	Blood must be stored at a carefully controlled temperature (4°C). Bar codes on blood products are currently being implemented in some agencies to identify, track, and assign data to transfusions as an additional safety measure.
7. **Complete identification and checks as required by agency:** • **Identification number** • **Blood group and type** • **Expiration date** • **Patient's name** • **Inspect blood for clots.**	Most states/agencies require two registered nurses to verify information: unit numbers match; ABO group and Rh type are the same; expiration date (after 35 days, red blood cells begin to deteriorate). Blood is never administered to a patient without an identification band. If clots are present, blood should be returned to blood bank.

(continued)

SKILL 15-6 Administering a Blood Transfusion *(continued)*

ACTION	RATIONALE
8. **Take baseline set of vital signs before beginning transfusion.**	Any change in vital signs during the transfusion may indicate a reaction.
9. Start infusion of the blood product:	
a. Prime in-line filter with blood (Figure 1).	Priming is necessary for blood to flow properly.
b. **Start administration slowly (no more than 25–50 mL for the first 15 minutes). Stay with the patient for the first 5 to 15 minutes of transfusion (Figure 2).**	Transfusion reactions typically occur during this period, and a slow rate will minimize the volume of red blood cells infused.
c. **Assess vital signs at least every 15 minutes for the first half hour. Follow institution's recommendations for taking vital signs during the remainder of the transfusion (Figure 3).**	If there have been no adverse effects during this time, the infusion rate is increased. If complications occur, they can be observed and the transfusion can be stopped immediately.
d. Observe patient for flushing, dyspnea, itching, hives or rash, or any unusual comments.	These signs and symptoms may be early indication of a transfusion reaction.
e. Never warm blood in a microwave. Use a blood-warming device, if indicated or ordered, especially with rapid transfusions through a CVP catheter.	Rapid administration of cold blood can result in cardiac arrhythmias.

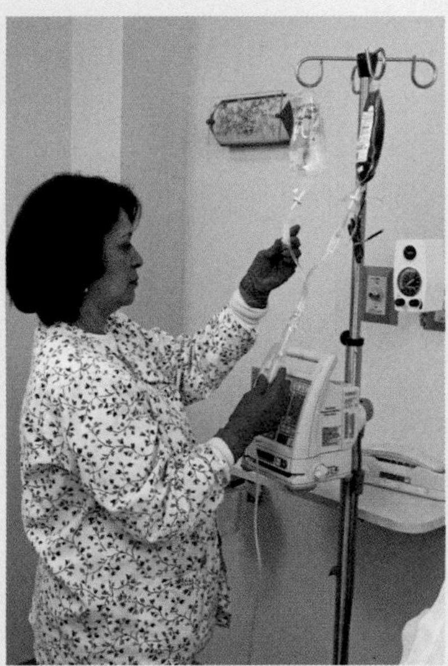

Figure 1. Priming in-line filter.

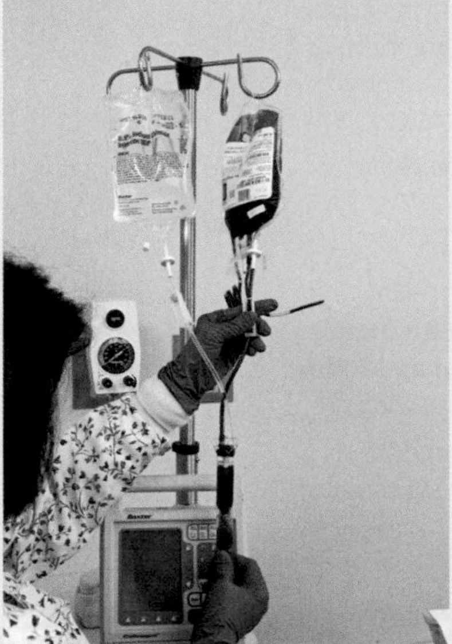

Figure 2. Starting transfusion slowly.

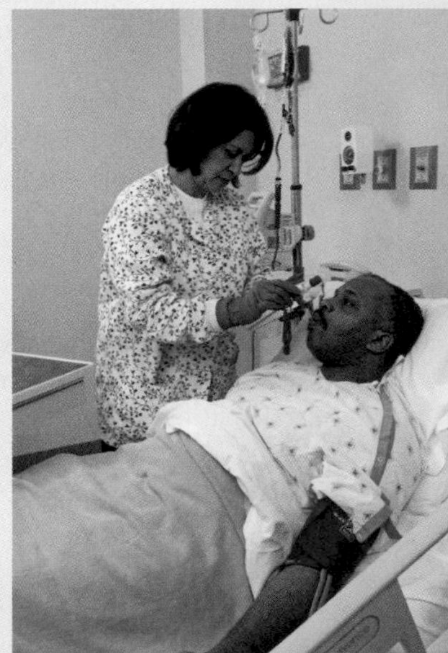

Figure 3. Assessing vital signs throughout the transfusion.

ACTION	RATIONALE
10. Maintain the prescribed flow rate as ordered or as deemed appropriate based on the patient's overall condition, keeping in mind the outer limits for safe administration. Ongoing monitoring is crucial throughout the entire duration of the blood transfusion for early identification of any adverse reactions. **Assess frequently for transfusion reaction. Stop blood transfusion if you suspect a reaction. Quickly replace the blood tubing with new tubing and 0.9% sodium chloride. Notify physician and blood bank.**	Rate must be carefully controlled, and patient's reaction must be monitored frequently. If a transfusion reaction is suspected, the blood must be stopped. Do not infuse the normal saline through the blood tubing because you would be allowing more of the blood into the patient's body, which could complicate a reaction. Besides a serious life-threatening blood transfusion reaction, the potential for fluid-volume overload exists in elderly patients and patients with decreased cardiac function.

SKILL 15-6 Administering a Blood Transfusion *(continued)*

ACTION	RATIONALE
11. When transfusion is complete, clamp off blood and begin to infuse 0.9% normal saline.	Saline prevents hemolysis of red blood cells and clears remainder of blood in IV line.
12. Record administration of blood and patient's reaction as ordered by agency. Return blood-transfusion bag to blood bank according to agency policy.	This provides for accurate documentation of patient's response to the transfusion.

EVALUATION

The expected outcome is met when the patient receives the blood transfusion without any evidence of a transfusion reaction or complication. The patient exhibits signs and symptoms of fluid balance, improved cardiac output, and enhanced peripheral tissue perfusion.

DOCUMENTATION

Guidelines

Document that the patient received the blood transfusion; include the type of blood product. Record the patient's condition throughout the transfusion, including pertinent data, such as vital signs, lung sounds, and the subjective response of the patient to transfusion. Document any complications or reactions or that the patient received the transfusion without any complications or reactions. Document the appearance of the IV site, and the presence or absence of redness, swelling, and pain.

Sample Documentation

11/2/09 1100 1 unit of packed blood red cells transfused into left forearm IV, 18-gauge needle, without difficulty. Vital signs remained stable throughout the transfusion. Pt states "no discomfort." IV site intact, no swelling, redness, or pain.—S. Barnes, RN

Unexpected Situations and Associated Interventions

- *Patient is becoming febrile but is exhibiting no other signs of a transfusion reaction:* Notify physician. The physician may have you pause the blood transfusion and medicate the patient with acetaminophen and an antihistamine before resuming the transfusion. If this is ordered, flush the IV with 3 mL of normal saline.
- *Patient reports shortness of breath, and on auscultation you note crackles bilaterally in the bases:* Compare vital signs to normal vital sounds for this patient. Obtain a pulse oximetry reading. Notify physician. The physician may order a dose of a diuretic or may have you slow the infusion Continue to assess the patients for signs and symptoms of fluid overload.
- *Patient is febrile, tachycardic, and complaining of back pain:* Patient is having a transfusion reaction. Stop the transfusion immediately. Obtain new IV tubing with 0.9% sodium chloride. Notify physician and blood bank. Send blood unit, tubing, and filter to the lab.
- *Blood is not infusing quickly enough:* Adjust the rate with the clamp. If this does not work, try flushing the IV with 3 mL of saline.

Special Considerations

- Electronic infusion devices may be used to maintain the prescribed rate but must be specifically designed for use with blood transfusions.

(continued)

SKILL 15-6 Administering a Blood Transfusion *(continued)*

Home Care Considerations

- Home care agencies evaluate patients who are candidates for a blood transfusion at home.
- Home transfusion is not appropriate for patients who are actively bleeding, require more than 4 hours for the transfusion, or recently had a reaction to a blood transfusion. Written consent must be obtained from the patient and the physician.
- The nurse transports the blood product to the patient's home in a special cooler. The nurse and the patient's caregiver check the serial number and other identification information together.

SKILL 15-7 Changing the Dressing and Flushing Central Venous Access Devices

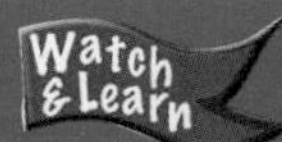

Central venous access devices (CVADs) can be inserted directly into the subclavian or the internal jugular veins for short-term use (Figure 1). CVADs can be tunneled through the subcutaneous skin to the subclavian vein when long-term placement is required. There are a variety of CVADs available. The type of CVAD catheter to be used depends upon the length of therapy, the patient's condition, and the type of solution or medication that is needed. A type of CVAD, the peripheral inserted central catheter (PICC) line, is frequently used in today's healthcare agencies, as well as in the home setting. A PICC line involves the insertion of a catheter into a peripheral vein instead of a central vein, but the catheter is long enough to terminate in the superior vena cava like the other CVADs (Figure 2). CVADs require the same meticulous dressing-change care as the PICC lines. When

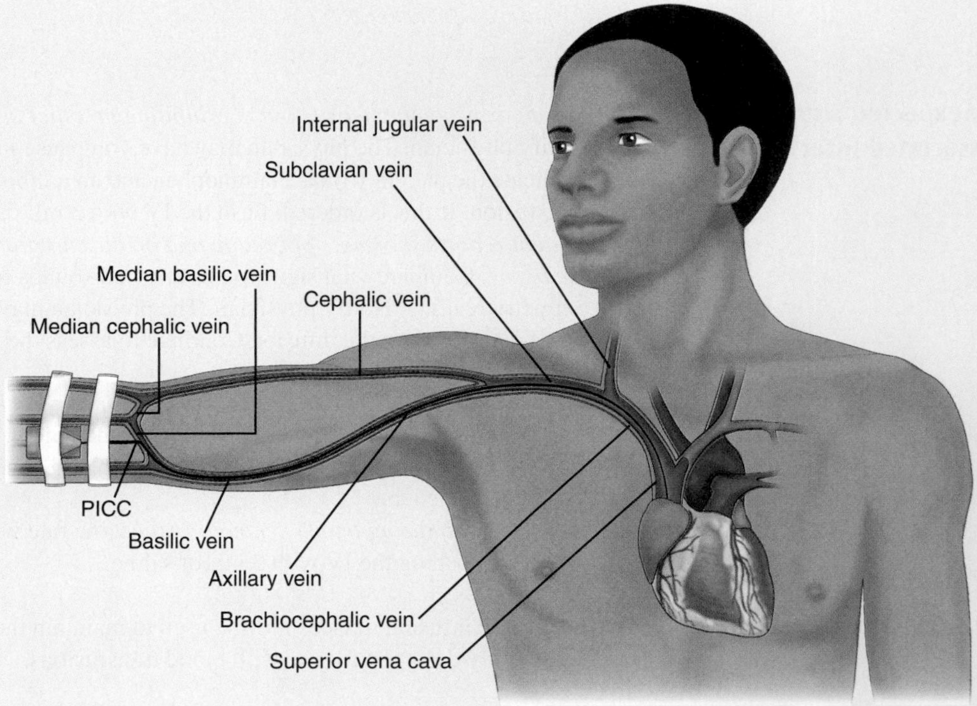

Figure 1. Placement of peripherally inserted central catheter (PICC).

SKILL 15-7

Changing the Dressing and Flushing Central Venous Access Devices *(continued)*

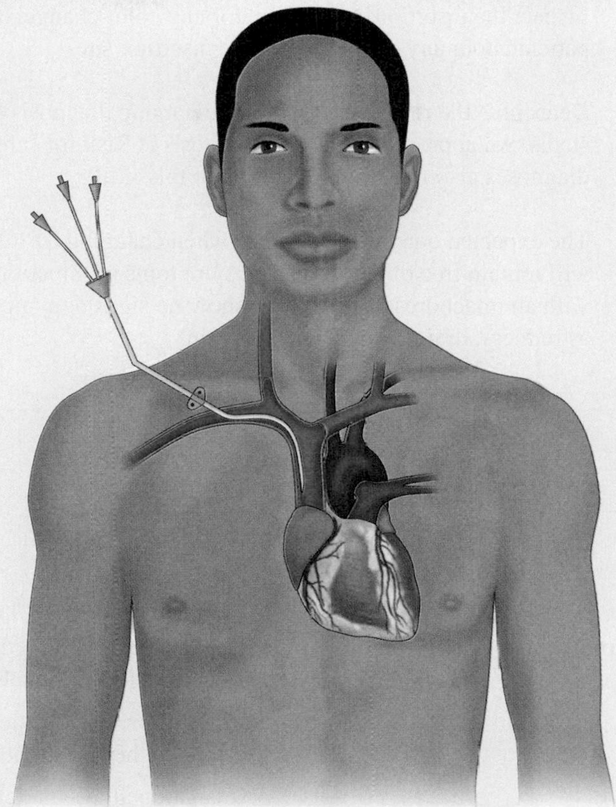

Figure 2. Placement of triple-lumen nontunneled percutaneous central venous catheter.

caring for a patient with a CVAD line, you must use sterile technique to prevent infection. Dressings are placed at the insertion site to occlude the site and prevent the introduction of microorganisms into the bloodstream. Scrupulous care of the site is required to control contamination. Agency policy generally determines the type of dressing used and the intervals for dressing change, but any dressing that is damp, loosened, or soiled should be changed immediately. One difference that may be encountered between a central line and PICC line dressing change relates to the assessment of sutures at the insertion site of the central line. PICC lines are generally not sutured into the patient.

Equipment

- Sterile tape or Steri-Strips
- Sterile semipermeable transparent dressing (or gauze dressing)
- Several 2 × 2s
- Sterile towel or drape
- 2% chlorhexidine solution
- NSS vial and 10-mL syringe or prefilled NSS syringe
- Heparin 100U/mL in 10-mL syringe
- Masks (2)
- Clean gloves
- Sterile gloves
- Sterile skin-protectant pad
- PICC injection caps

(continued)

SKILL 15-7 Changing the Dressing and Flushing Central Venous Access Devices *(continued)*

ASSESSMENT

Inspect the insertion site closely for any color change, drainage, swelling, or pain. Ask the patient about any complaints at the insertion site.

NURSING DIAGNOSIS

Determine the related factors for the nursing diagnosis based on the patient's current status. An appropriate nursing diagnosis is Risk for Infection. Many other nursing diagnoses also may require the use of this skill.

OUTCOME IDENTIFICATION AND PLANNING

The expected outcome to achieve when changing a PICC line dressing is that the patient will remain free of any signs and symptoms of infection. The site will be clean and dry, with an intact dressing, and will show no signs or symptoms of IV complications, such as redness, drainage, swelling, or pain.

IMPLEMENTATION

ACTION	RATIONALE
1. Gather equipment and verify physician's order (often this will be a standing protocol).	Having equipment available saves time and facilitates the task. Checking the order ensures that the procedure has been ordered by the physician.
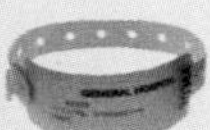 2. Identify the patient.	Identification of the patient ensures that the right patient receives the correct nursing care.
3. Explain procedure to patient.	Explanation allays anxiety.
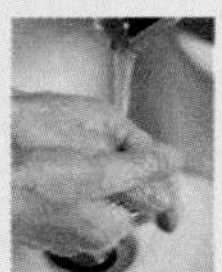 4. Perform hand hygiene.	Hand hygiene deters the spread of microorganisms. Unclean hands and improper technique are potential sources for infecting a CVAD.
5. Position the patient with the arm extended from body below heart level.	This position is recommended to reduce the risk of air embolism.
6. **Apply a mask and have patient also put on a mask.** Put on clean gloves. Set up sterile field on area to be used. Have patient place the arm in the middle of the sterile field. Open dressing kit using sterile technique and place on sterile towel.	Masks help to deter the spread of microorganisms. Gloves prevent transmission of HIV and other bloodborne infections and bacterial infections. Sterile towel gives the nurse a large clean area to work on. Most facilities have all sterile dressing supplies gathered in a single unit.
7. Assess CVAD insertion site (for inflammation, redness, etc.) through old dressing. Remove old dressing by lifting it distally and then working proximally, making sure to stabilize the catheter with thumb. Remove and dispose of gloves properly. Put on sterile gloves.	If the CVAD is a PICC line, note how PICC is secured. Most PICC lines are not sutured in but, rather, taped and are easy to dislodge when changing dressings.
8. Starting at insertion site and continuing in a circle, wipe off any old blood or drainage with a sterile antimicrobial wipe. **Cleanse according to agency policy. Move in a circular fashion, cleansing thoroughly from the insertion site outward (2″–3″ area). Allow to dry.**	*Coagulase–negative staphylococci and Staphylococcus aureus* are the most common causes of catheter-associated central-line infections. CDC recommends use of 2% chlorhexidine for antiseptic cleansing in the prevention of intravascular infections.

SKILL 15-7

Changing the Dressing and Flushing Central Venous Access Devices *(continued)*

ACTION	RATIONALE
9. **Reapply sterile dressing or securement device according to agency policy.** Secure tubing or lumens to prevent tugging on insertion site.	Dressing prevents contamination of the IV catheter and protects insertion site.
10. **Clamp all lines of the CVAD and remove injection caps. Cleanse the catheter ends with antimicrobial swab and then apply new injection caps (Figure 3). Tape the distal ends down securely.**	The catheter ends should be cleansed and injection caps changed to prevent infection. The distal ends are secured to prevent the catheter from becoming dislodged.

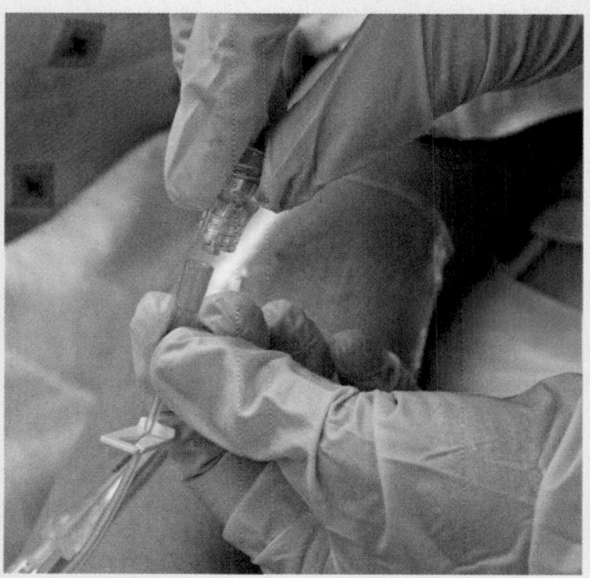

Figure 3. Applying new injection cap.

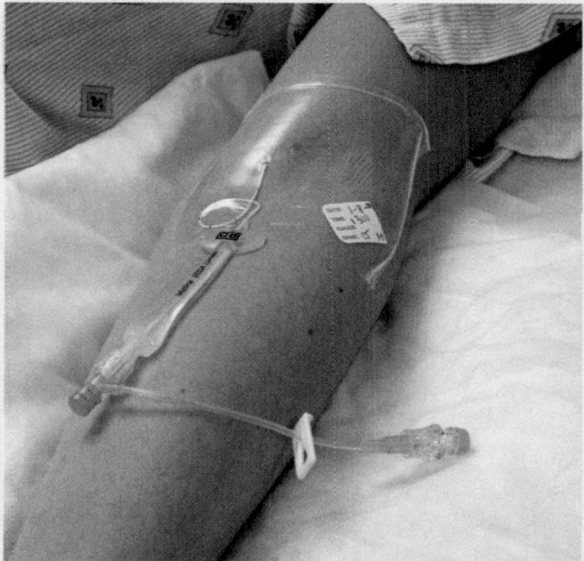

Figure 4. Noting date, time, size of catheter, and initials on dressing.

ACTION	RATIONALE
11. Some agency policies incorporate the flushing of the different lumens or injection port after the dressing change. Flush with 3 to 5 mL of NSS using a 10-mL syringe and 3 mL of heparin (100U/mL) after each use or as agency policy directs.	Flushing the injections ports helps maintain the patency of the CVAD line. Using a 10-mL syringe avoids exerting too great a pressure on the catheter.
12. Note date, time of dressing change, size of catheter, and initials on tape or dressing (Figure 4).	Data documents that dressing change occurred.
13. Discard equipment properly and perform hand hygiene.	Hand hygiene protects against spread of microorganisms.
14. Record patient's response to dressing change and observation of site.	This provides accurate documentation and ensures continuity of care.

EVALUATION

The expected outcome is met when the dressing is changed without any complications, including dislodgement of the PICC. The patient exhibits an insertion site that is clean and dry without redness or swelling. Dressing is clean, dry, and intact.

(continued)

SKILL 15-7 Changing the Dressing and Flushing Central Venous Access Devices *(continued)*

DOCUMENTATION

Guidelines

Document the location and appearance of the CVAD line-insertion site as well as the surrounding skin. The insertion site should be free of redness, drainage, or swelling. Record if the patient is experiencing any pain or discomfort related to the CVAD line. The CVAD line injection ports should flush without difficulty. Any abnormal findings such as dislodgement of the CVAD, abnormal insertion assessment findings, or inability to flush the injections ports of the CVAD should be reported to the physician.

Sample Documentation

11/12/09 0400 PICC line located in the right basilic vein. Old dressing removed, no drainage, redness, or swelling noted at site. NSS flush followed by heparin flush per protocol without difficulty. Patient denies pain or discomfort. Pt. instructed to inform nurse if any pain, swelling, or leakage related to PICC line.—S. Barnes, RN

Unexpected Situations and Associated Interventions

- *While dressing is being changed, PICC is inadvertently dislodged.* If PICC is not all the way out, notify physician. The physician will most likely want a chest x-ray to determine where the end of the PICC line is. Before the chest x-ray, reapply a dressing so that the PICC is not further dislodged.
- *When the dressing is removed, purulent drainage is noted at the insertion site:* Swab the drainage with a culture swab, clean the area, reapply a dressing, and then notify the physician. This prevents the PICC line from being open to air and unprotected while you are notifying the physician. If the physician does not want the culture, you can dispose of the culture kit.

Special Considerations

Home Care Considerations

Many patients and families have been taught how to care for CVAD in the home, especially PICC lines.

SKILL 15-8 Accessing an Implanted Port

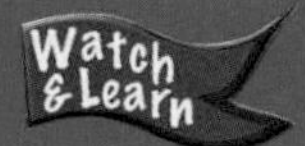

Totally implantable access devices allow long-term access without having a catheter protrude from the skin. The system includes the subcutaneous injection port and a catheter, which is usually inserted into the superior vena cava via the subclavian vein (Figure 1). When venous access is desired, the location of the injection port must be palpated. The system is accessed with a noncoring needle. Patency is maintained by periodic flushing. The length and gauge of the needle used to access the port should be selected based on the patient's anatomy and anticipated infusion requirements. In general, a ¾″ 20-gauge needle is most frequently used. If the patient has a significant amount of subcutaneous tissue, a longer length (1″ or 1.5″) may be selected. A larger gauge (19-gauge) is preferred for administration of blood products.

Equipment

- Sterile dressing kit
- Noncoring needle (Huber needle)
- Vial of sodium chloride or prefilled NSS syringe
- Blunt needles (2)

SKILL 15-8

Accessing an Implanted Port *(continued)*

- 10-mL syringes (2)
- Needleless injection cap
- Sterile gauze 2 × 2 (optional)
- Vial of heparin (as indicated by agency policy)
- Sterile gloves
- Clean gloves
- Mask

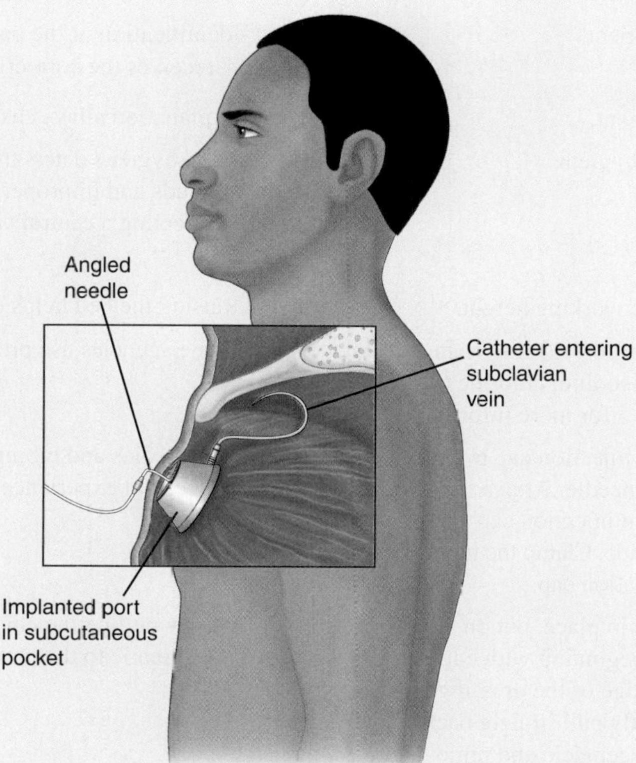

Figure 1. An implanted port with the catheter inserted in the subclavian vein and noncoring needle inserted into the port.

ASSESSMENT

Inspect the skin over port, looking for any swelling, redness, or drainage. Also assess site over port for any pain or tenderness. Review the patient's history for the length of time the port has been in place.

NURSING DIAGNOSIS

Determine the related factors for the nursing diagnosis based on the patient's current status. Appropriate nursing diagnose may include:

- Risk for Infection
- Acute Pain
- Risk for Injury
- Deficient Knowledge

OUTCOME IDENTIFICATION AND PLANNING

The expected outcome to achieve when accessing an implanted port is that the port is accessed with minimal to no discomfort to the patient. The patient experiences no trauma to the site.

(continued)

SKILL 15-8 Accessing an Implanted Port *(continued)*

IMPLEMENTATION

ACTION	RATIONALE
1. Gather equipment and verify physician's order (many times this will be a standing protocol).	Having equipment available saves time and facilitates the task. Checking the order ensures that the procedure has been ordered by the physician.
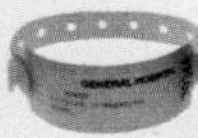 2. Identify the patient.	Identification of the patient ensures that the right patient receives the correct nursing care.
3. Explain procedure to patient.	Explanation allays anxiety.
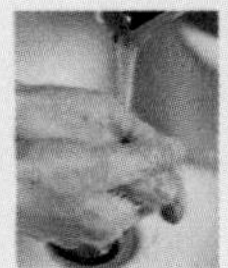 4. Perform hand hygiene.	Hand hygiene deters the spread of microorganisms. Unclean hands and improper technique are potential sources for infecting a central venous access device.
5. Raise bed to comfortable working height.	Raising the bed helps reduce strain on the nurse's back.
6. Attach the blunt needles to the 10-mL syringes. Withdraw 10 mL of .9% sodium chloride (NSS) from the vial (See Chap. 5 for more information).	Some agencies use prefilled saline syringes.
7. Connect the intermittent injection cap to the extension tubing on the noncoring needle. Attach the 10-mL syringe to the intermittent injection cap and flush the needle with sodium chloride. Clamp the tubing. Remove the syringe from the injection cap.	The needles and tubing must be free of air so that patient does not experience an air embolus.
8. If transparent dressing is in place, put on clean gloves and gently pull it back, beginning with edges and proceeding around the edge of the dressing. Once dressing is removed, gently pull straight back on needle. Discard in appropriate receptacle and remove gloves.	Gently pulling the edges of the dressing will be less traumatic to the patient.
9. **Open the kit using sterile technique. Put on the mask and sterile gloves. Set up your sterile field.** If port is not accessed, proceed to Action 10.	Improper technique is a potential source for infecting a central venous device.
10. **Cleanse according to agency policy. For example, using an antimicrobial swab, cleanse in a circular fashion from the insertion site outward (2″–3″ area). Use each swab once and discard. Allow site to dry.**	Coagulase-negative *staphylococci* and *Staphylococcus aureus* are the most common causes of catheter-related central line infections.
11. **Locate the port septum by palpation.** With your nondominant hand, hold the port stable, keeping the skin taut but without touching the port side (Figure 2).	The edges of the port must be palpated so that the needle can be inserted into the center of the port. Hold the port with your nondominant hand so that you can stick the port with your dominant hand.
12. Visualize the center of the port (Figure 3). **Push the Huber needle (noncoring 90-degree) through the skin into the portal septum until it hits the back of the port septum (Figure 4).**	To infuse fluids properly, the needle must be located in the middle of the port and inserted to the back of the port.

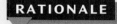

SKILL 15-8 Accessing an Implanted Port *(continued)*

ACTION

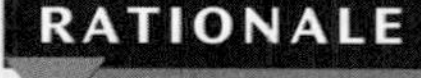
RATIONALE

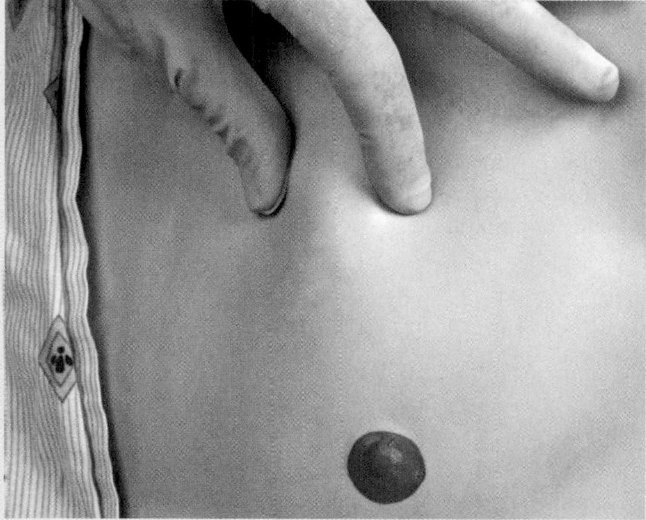

Figure 2. Stabilizing port with nondominant hand.

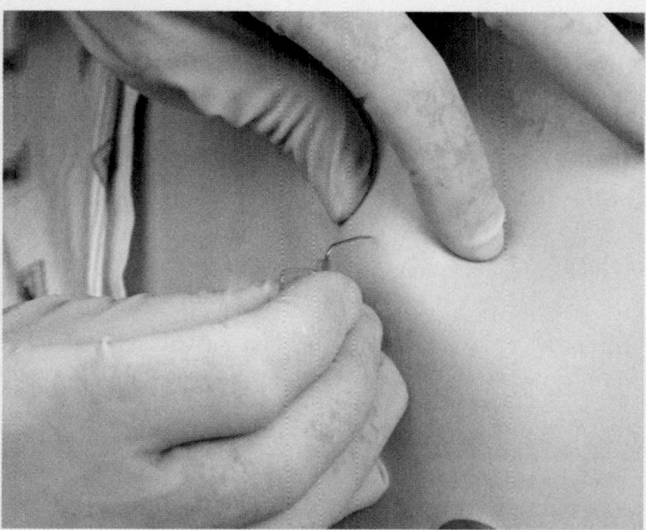

Figure 3. Preparing to push needle into port.

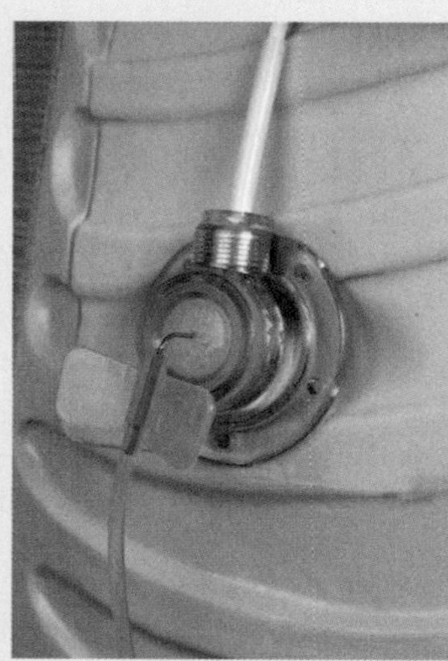

Figure 4. Huber (noncoring) needle in place.

13. Cleanse the injection cap with an antimicrobial swab and insert the syringe with normal saline.

Coagulase-negative *staphylococci* and *Staphylococcus aureus* are the most common causes of catheter-related central line infections.

14. **Open the clamp and push down on the syringe plunger, flushing the device with 3 to 5 mL of saline, while observing for fluid leak or infiltration. It should flush easily, without resistance.**

If needle is not inserted correctly, fluid will leak into tissue, causing the tissue to swell and producing signs of infiltration. Flushing without resistance is also a sign that the needle is inserted into the correct place.

(continued)

SKILL 15-8 Accessing an Implanted Port *(continued)*

ACTION	RATIONALE
15. Pull back on the syringe plunger to aspirate for blood return. Aspirate only a few milliliters of blood; do not allow blood to enter syringe.	The ability to withdraw blood is a sign that the port is patent. Not allowing blood to enter the syringe ensures that the needle will be flushed with pure saline.
16. Flush with the remainder of saline in syringe.	This ensures that the port will remain patent.
17. Clamp the tubing, remove the syringe, and attach the heparin-filled syringe (if appropriate for the institution). Clamp the tubing while maintaining positive pressure on the syringe barrel at the end of the flush.	Heparin ensures patency of the port. Flushing with positive pressure prevents blood from back-flowing into the port and clamping it off.
18. Remove the syringe. **If space exists between the skin and the needle, place a sterile folded 2 × 2 gauze in the space to support the needle.** If using a "Gripper" needle, remove the gripper portion from the needle by squeezing the sides together and lifting off the needle while holding the needle securely to the port with the other hand.	The 2 × 2 helps keep the needle from moving.
19. Apply tape or Steri-Strips in a starlike pattern over the needle to secure it.	The tape will help prevent the needle from accidentally pulling out.
20. Cover the entire needle and port with the transparent dressing, leaving the ports of the extension tubing uncovered for easy access.	Dressing prevents contamination of the IV catheter and protects insertion site.
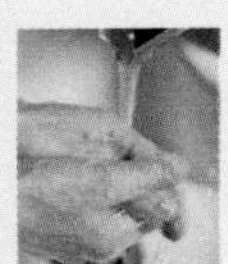 21. Remove gloves and discard. Perform hand hygiene.	Hand hygiene deters the spread of microorganisms.
22. Label the dressing with the date, time, size needle used, and your initials, according to agency policy.	This documents IV tubing change.
23. Document procedure, including time, date, type and location of port, condition of skin at site, size needle used, presence of blood return, and any difficulties encountered.	This provides accurate documentation and ensures continuity of care.

EVALUATION

The expected outcome is met when the port can be accessed without difficulty or pain, and the patient remains free of signs and symptoms of infection or trauma.

DOCUMENTATION

Guidelines

Document the location of the port and the size of Huber needle used to access the port. Record the ease of ability to flush the port and document the presence of a good blood return upon flushing. Document the patient's reaction to the procedure and if the patient is experiencing any pain or discomfort related to the port. Record if there was any drainage on the old dressing and its color if present. Document the condition of the skin surrounding the port. Record any appropriate patient teaching.

SKILL 15-8 Accessing an Implanted Port *(continued)*

Sample Documentation

11/22/09 1245 Implanted port R subclavian, old dressing removed, no drainage, swelling, or redness noted; 20G 3/4 Huber needle used to access port. Flushes easily with good blood return. Pt instructed to call nurse with any swelling, pain, or leaking.—S. Barnes, RN

Unexpected Situations and Associated Interventions

- *Port begins to swell when flushing with saline:* Stop flushing. Gently push on syringe and slowly begin to flush again. The needle may have become dislodged from the septum of the port. If the swelling continues, stop flushing and notify physician.
- *Port does not flush:* Check clamp to make sure tubing is open. Gently push down on needle and again try to flush. Ask the patient to perform a Valsalva maneuver. Try having the patient change position or place the affected arm over the head, or try raising or lowering the head of the bed. If the port still does not flush, notify physician.
- *Port flushes but does not draw blood:* Notify physician. Anticipate an order for a thrombolytic.

Special Considerations

- Groshong devices do not require the use of heparin for flushing.
- Some institutions call for a power flush (rapidly pushing the flush in small amounts).
- Implanted ports need to be accessed every 4 to 6 weeks (according to agency policy) to be flushed.

SKILL 15-9 Deaccessing an Implanted Port

When an implanted port will not be used for a period of time, such as when a patient is being discharged, the port can be deaccessed. Deaccessing a port involves removing the Huber (noncoring) needle from the port.

Equipment

- Clean gloves
- Syringe filled with 10 mL saline
- Syringe filled with 5 mL heparin (100 U/mL or institution's recommendations)
- Sterile gauze sponge
- Alcohol wipe
- Band-Aid

ASSESSMENT

Inspect the insertion site, looking for any swelling, redness, or drainage. Also assess site over port for any pain or tenderness. Review the patient's history for the length of time the port and Huber (noncoring) needle have been in place.

NURSING DIAGNOSIS

Determine the related factors for the nursing diagnosis based on the patient's current status. An appropriate nursing diagnosis is Risk for Injury. Many other nursing diagnoses, such as Acute Pain and Deficient Knowledge, also may require the use of this skill.

OUTCOME IDENTIFICATION AND PLANNING

The expected outcome to achieve when deaccessing an implanted port is that the needle is removed with minimal to no discomfort to the patient. The patient experiences no trauma to the site.

(continued)

SKILL 15-9 Deaccessing an Implanted Port *(continued)*

IMPLEMENTATION

ACTION	RATIONALE
1. Gather equipment and verify physician's order (many times this will be a standing protocol).	Having equipment available saves time and facilitates the task. Checking the order ensures that the procedure has been ordered by the physician.
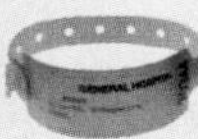 2. Identify the patient.	Identification of the patient ensures that the right patient receives the correct nursing care.
3. Explain procedure to patient.	Explanation allays anxiety.
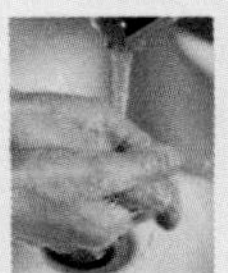 4. Perform hand hygiene.	Hand hygiene deters the spread of microorganisms. Unclean hands and improper technique are potential sources for infecting a central venous access device.
5. Raise bed to comfortable working height.	Raising the bed helps to reduce strain on the nurse's back.
6. Put on clean gloves.	Gloves prevent the transmission of HIV and other blood-borne diseases.
7. Gently pull back transparent dressing, beginning with edges and proceeding around the edge of the dressing. Carefully remove all the tape that is securing the needle in place.	Gently pulling the edges of the dressing is less traumatic to the patient.
8. Clean the injection cap and insert the saline-filled syringe. **Unclamp the catheter's extension tubing and begin to flush with a minimum of 10-mL normal saline.**	It is important to flush all substances out of the well of the implanted port, because it will be inactive for several weeks.
9. **Remove the syringe and insert the heparin-filled syringe, flushing with 5-mL heparin (100 U/mL or agency's policy). Clamp the extension tubing while maintaining positive pressure on the barrel of the syringe. Remove the syringe.**	Since the catheter will be inactive for several weeks, the heparin prevents clots from forming.
10. Secure the port on either side with the fingers of your nondominant hand. Grasp the needle/wings with the fingers of your dominant hand. Firmly and smoothly, pull the needle straight up at a 90-degree angle from the skin to remove it from the septum.	By grasping the port, the port is held in place while the needle is removed.
11. Apply gentle pressure with the gauze to the insertion site. A Band-Aid may be applied over the port if any oozing occurs.	A small amount of blood may form from the needlestick.
12. Remove gloves and place bed in the lowest position. Make sure that the patient is comfortable before you leave the room.	Placing the bed in the lowest position helps to prevent the patient from falling when trying to get out of bed.
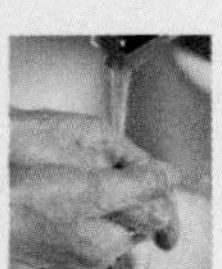 13. Perform hand hygiene.	Hand hygiene deters the spread of microorganisms.

SKILL 15-9 **Deaccessing an Implanted Port** *(continued)*

EVALUATION

The expected outcome is met when the port flushes easily, the needle is removed, and the site is clean, dry, and without evidence of redness, irritation, or warmth.

DOCUMENTATION

Document the location of the port and the ease or difficulty of flushing the port. Document removal of the access needle. Record the appearance of the site including if there is any drainage, swelling, or redness. Record any appropriate patient teaching.

Sample Documentation

11/13/09 1020 Implanted port flushed without resistance using 10 mL of saline and 5 mL of heparin. Positive pressure maintained. No hematoma noted. Access needle removed without difficulty. Site without redness, swelling, drainage, or heat.
—S. Barnes, RN

Unexpected Situations and Associated Interventions

- *Port does not flush:* Check clamp to make sure tubing is open. Gently push down on needle and again try to flush. Ask patient to perform a Valsalva maneuver. Have patient change position or place the affected arm over the head and raise or lower the head of the bed. If the port still does not flush, notify physician.
- *Site does not stop bleeding:* Continue to hold pressure. If the patient has some clotting disturbances, pressure may need to be applied for a slightly longer duration.

Special Considerations

- Groshong devices do not require heparin.
- Some institutions call for a power flush (rapidly pushing the flush in small amounts).

The Taylor Suite offers these additional resources to enhance learning and facilitate understanding of this chapter:

- thePoint online resource, http://thepoint.lww.com/Lynn2E
- Student CD-ROM included with the book
- Skills Checklist to Accompany Taylor's Clinical Nursing Skills
- Taylor's Interactive Nursing: *Fluid, Electrolyte, and Acid-Base Balance*
- Taylor's Video Guide to Clinical Nursing Skills: *Intravenous Therapy* and *Central Venous Access Devices*

Developing Critical Thinking Skills

1. Simon Lawrence's mother is asking about the risks associated with IV placement. What would you tell her about the risks associated with IV placement and rehydration?
2. During the first 7 minutes of Melissa Cohen's transfusion of packed red blood cells, she reports a headache and low back pain. When you assess her, you find that she has a temperature of 38.5°C and she is shivering. What actions would be most appropriate at this time?
3. Mr. Tracy asks about care of his new implanted port. What are some topics you should discuss with him before he is discharged?

Bibliography

Bagnall-Reeb, H. (2004). Evidence for the use of antibiotic lock technique. *Journal of Infusion Nursing 27*(2), 118–126.

Best practices: A guide to excellence in nursing care. (2002). Philadelphia: Lippincott Williams & Wilkins.

Biedrycki, B. (2004). Blood transfusions: Is "safest ever" safe enough? *Oncology Nursing Society News, 19*(11), 8–9.

Black, J., & Hawks, J. (2005). *Medical-surgical nursing* (7th ed.).:St. Louis, MO: Elsevier Saunders.

Centers for Disease Control and Prevention. (2002). Guidelines for the prevention of intravascular catheter-related infections. *Morbidity and Mortality Weekly Report, 51*(RR10), 1–32.

Centers for Disease Control and Prevention. (2003). Detection of West Nile virus in blood donations—United States, 2003. *Morbidity and Mortality Weekly Report, 52*(32), 769–772. Available at http://www.cdc.gov/mmwr/preview/mmwrhtml/mm5232a3.htm. Accessed February 16, 2004.

Chang, L., Tsai, J., Huang, S., & Shih, C. (2003). Evaluation of infectious complications of the implantable venous access system in a general oncologic population. *American Journal of Infection Control, 31*(1), 34–39.

Ellenberger, A. (2002). How to change a PICC dressing. *Nursing, 32*(2), 50–52.

Fischbach, F., & Dunning, M. (2006). Common laboratory values and diagnostic tests. Philadelphia: Lippincott Williams & Wilkins.

Fluids & electrolytes: A 2-in-1 reference for nurses. (2006). Philadelphia: Lippincott Williams & Wilkins.

Fluids & electrolytes made incredibly easy (3rd ed.). (2005). Philadelphia: Lippincott Williams & Wilkins.

Fitzpatrick, L. (2002). When to administer modified blood products. *Nursing, 32*(5), 36–42.

Gillies, D., O'Riordan, L., Wallen, M., Rankin, K., Morrison, A., Nagy, S. (2004). Timing of intravenous set changes: A systematic review. *Infection Control and Hospital Epidemiology, 25*(3), 240–250.

Gorski, L. (2004). Central venous access device outcomes in a homecare agency: A 7-year study. *Journal of Infusion Nursing 27*(2), 104–111.

Gorski, L., & Czaplewski, L. (2004). Peripherally inserted central catheters & midline catheters for the home care nurse. *Home Healthcare Nurse, 22*(11), 758–773.

Hadaway, L. (2003). Infusing without infecting. *Nursing, 33*(10), 58–63.

Hammond, T. (2004). Choice and use of peripherally inserted central catheters by nurses. *Professional Nurse, 19*(9), 493–497.

Johnson, A., & Criddle, L. (2004). Pass the salt: Indications for and implications of using hypertonic saline. *Critical Care Nurse, 24*(5), 36–46.

Joint Commission on Accreditation of Healthcare Organizations. (2003). *2004 National Patient Safety Goals.* Available at http://www.jcaho.org/accredited+organizations/patient+safety/04+npsg/04_npsg.htm.

Kagel, E., & Rayan, G. (2004). Intravenous catheter complications in the hand and forearm. *Journal of Trauma: Injury, Infection, and Critical Care, 56*(1), 123–127.

Lavery, I. (2005). Peripheral intravenous therapy: Key risks and implications for practice. *Nursing Standard, 19*(46), 55–64.

McCloskey, J., & Bulechek, G. (2004). *Nursing interventions classification* (4th ed.). St. Louis, MO: Mosby.

Miller, R. (2002). Blood component therapy. *Urologic Nursing, 22*(5), 331–339.

Moreau, N. (2002). IV rounds: How to remove a PICC with ease. *Nursing, 32*(5), 30.

Nebelkopf, H. (2004). Assessment of fluids and electrolytes. *American Association of Critical Care Nurses, 15*(4), 607–612.

North American Nursing Diagnosis Association. (2003). *NANDA nursing diagnoses: Definitions and classification, 2003–2004.* Philadelphia: Author.

Nouwairi, N. (2004). The risks of blood transfusions and the shortage of supply leads to the quest for blood substitutes. *American Association Nurse Anesthesia, 72*(5), 359–364.

O'Grady, N., Alexander, M., Dellinger, E., et al. (2002). Guidelines for the prevention of intravascular catheter related infections. *American Journal of Infection Control, 30*(8), 476–489.

Orr, M. (2002). The peripherally inserted central catheter: What are the current indications for its use? *Nutrition in Clinical Practice, 17*(2), 99–104.

Rosenthal, K. (2004a). The new look of IV therapy. *Nursing Management, 35*(12), 66–72.

Rosenthal, K. (2004b). Smart pumps help crack the safety code. *Nursing Management, 35*(5), 49–51.

Rosenthal, K. (2004c). What you should know about needleless systems, *Nursing 34*(9), 1457–1458.

Rosenthal, K. (2004d). Where did the patient's IV go wrong, *Nursing, 34*(5), 56–57.

Smeltzer, S., Bare, B., Hinkle, J. H., & Cheever, K. H. (2008). *Brunner and Suddarth's textbook of medical–surgical nursing* (11th ed.). Philadelphia: Lippincott Williams & Wilkins.

Tabloski, P. (2006). *Gerontological nursing.* Upper Saddle River, NJ: Pearson Prentice Hall.

Taylor, C., Lillis, C., LeMone, P., & Lynn, P. (2008). *Fundamentals of nursing: The art & science of nursing care* (6th ed.). Philadelphia: Lippincott Williams & Wilkins.

Ulrich, S. P., & Canale, S. W. (2005). *Nursing care planning guides: For adults in acute, extended, and home care settings* (6th ed.). St. Louis, MO: Elsevier Saunders.

Zerwekh, J. (2003). End-of-life hydration—benefit or burden? *Nursing, 33*(2), 32hn1–32hn3.

CHAPTER 16

Cardiovascular Care

Focusing on Patient Care

This chapter will help you develop some of the skills related to cardiovascular care necessary to care for the following patients:

Coby Pruder, age 40, is to undergo an electrocardiogram as part of his physical examination. Although he considers himself healthy, he is nervous.

Harry Stebbings, age 67, is admitted to the emergency department for chest pain and cardiac monitoring.

Ann Kribell, age 54, is a patient in the cardiac care unit. She has been diagnosed with heart failure and is receiving cardiac monitoring. She needs to have arterial blood samples drawn from her arterial line.

Learning Objectives

After studying this chapter, you will be able to:

1. Obtain a 12-lead ECG.
2. Apply a cardiac monitor.
3. Obtain an arterial blood sample from an arterial line-stopcock system.
4. Remove arterial and femoral lines.
5. Perform cardiopulmonary resuscitation (CPR).
6. Perform emergency automated external defibrillation.
7. Perform emergency manual external defibrillation (asynchronous).
8. Use an external pacemaker.

Key Terms

arterial blood gas (ABG): a laboratory test that evaluates the oxygen, carbon dioxide, bicarbonate, and pH of an arterial blood sample, determining metabolic or respiratory alkalosis or acidosis

cardiac arrest: sudden cessation of functional circulation of the heart (pulse), such as asystole or defibrillation, typically caused by the occlusion of one or more of the coronary arteries or cardiomyopathy

cardiac monitoring: visualization and monitoring of the cardiac electrical activity stimulating the heartbeat

cardiopulmonary resuscitation (CPR): also known as basic life support; revival in the absence of spontaneous respirations and heartbeat to preserve heart and brain function while waiting for defibrillation and advanced cardiac life support care. Achieved by manually pumping the heart by compressing the sternum and forcing oxygen into the lungs using mouth-to-mouth or rescue breathing.

cardioversion: conversion of a pathologic cardiac rhythm to normal sinus rhythm through low doses of electricity, using a device that applies synchronized countershocks to the heart

defibrillation: stopping fibrillation of the heart by using an electrical device that applies countershocks to the heart through electrodes on the chest wall. This countershock is given in an attempt to allow the heart's normal pacemaker to take over.

electrocardiogram (ECG/EKG): graphing of the electrical activity of the heart

The heart is an organ at the "heart" of the circulatory system. It provides the propulsive force (heartbeat) for circulating the blood through the vascular system. This four-chamber muscle pumps 3.5 to 8.0 liters of blood per minute (Porth, 2005). The pressure exerted is equal to lifting 80 pounds at 1 foot per minute. The heart averages 72 beats a minute or 38 million beats a year.

Assessment of heart function commonly involves noninvasive techniques such as auscultation, palpation, and sometimes percussion. Additional basic and important indicators of the heart's effectiveness are pulse rate, strength, and rhythm; blood pressure; skin color and temperature; and level of consciousness. Noninvasive heart monitoring involves electrocardiography and cardiac monitoring. Arterial blood gases (ABGs) are used to measure the oxygen level and pH of the blood, providing information about a patient's acid–base balance. Should the heart stop pumping, it can be manually pumped via cardiopulmonary resuscitation (CPR) until electrical defibrillation and additional medical support arrives. Skill 16-6 discusses defibrillation; other electrical therapy devices are discussed in Fundamentals Review 16-1.

Invasive techniques such as pulmonary artery monitoring, Swan-Ganz catheterization, cardiac output determination, and cardiac support via an intraaortic balloon pump (IABP) typically are used by trained critical care personnel to provide additional monitoring and support. These techniques are beyond the scope of this text.

This chapter will cover selected noninvasive skills to assist the nurse in providing cardiovascular care. Figure 16-1 provides an overview of cardiac anatomy, and Figure 16-2 provides a review of the cardiac conduction system. Figures 16-3 and 16-4 highlight cardiac landmark reference lines and auscultation areas.

Electrical Therapy Devices

In addition to defibrillation, electrical therapy may be delivered via the following devices:

- **Implantable cardioverter-defibrillator** (ICD) is a sophisticated device that automatically discharges an electric current when it senses ventricular tachyarrhythmias. Patients with a history of ventricular fibrillation, with poor ejection fraction (<35%), or with heart failure (New York Heart Association [NYHA] class III or IV) may be candidates for this type of device.
- **Synchronized cardioversion** is the treatment of choice for arrhythmias that do not respond to vagal maneuvers or drug therapy, such as atrial tachycardia, atrial flutter, atrial fibrillation, and symptomatic ventricular tachycardia. Cardioversion is performed similarly to defibrillation but is synchronized with the heart rhythm and uses fewer joules. Cardioversion works by delivering an electrical charge to the myocardium at the peak of the R wave. This causes immediate depolarization, interrupting reentry circuits and allowing the sinoatrial node to resume control. Synchronizing the electrical charge with the R wave ensures that the current will not be delivered on the vulnerable T wave and thus disrupt repolarization. It is usually performed in a critical care area, in the presence of a physician, an anesthesiologist, and emergency equipment. The patient is premedicated with pain medicine.
- **Pacemakers** are electronic devices that can be used to initiate the heartbeat when the heart's intrinsic electrical system cannot effectively generate a rate adequate to support cardiac output (Urden et al, 2002). Pacemakers can be temporary: placed on the skin (transcutaneous); via temporary epicardial pacing wires inserted during cardiac surgery; or transvenous, via a pacing electrode wire passed through a vein (often the subclavian or internal jugular) and into the right atrium or right ventricle. Pacemakers can also be permanent surgically implanted devices.
- **Biventricular pacemakers** (cardiac resynchronization) use electrical current to improve synchronization of left ventricular contraction. Biventricular pacemakers are used in patients with heart failure (NYHA class III or IV), with an intraventricular conduction delay (QRS >120 ms), and patients with left-ventricular ejection fraction ≤35%. These devices improve right and left ventricle contraction with a modest increase in left-ventricular ejection fraction (Ermis et al, 2004).

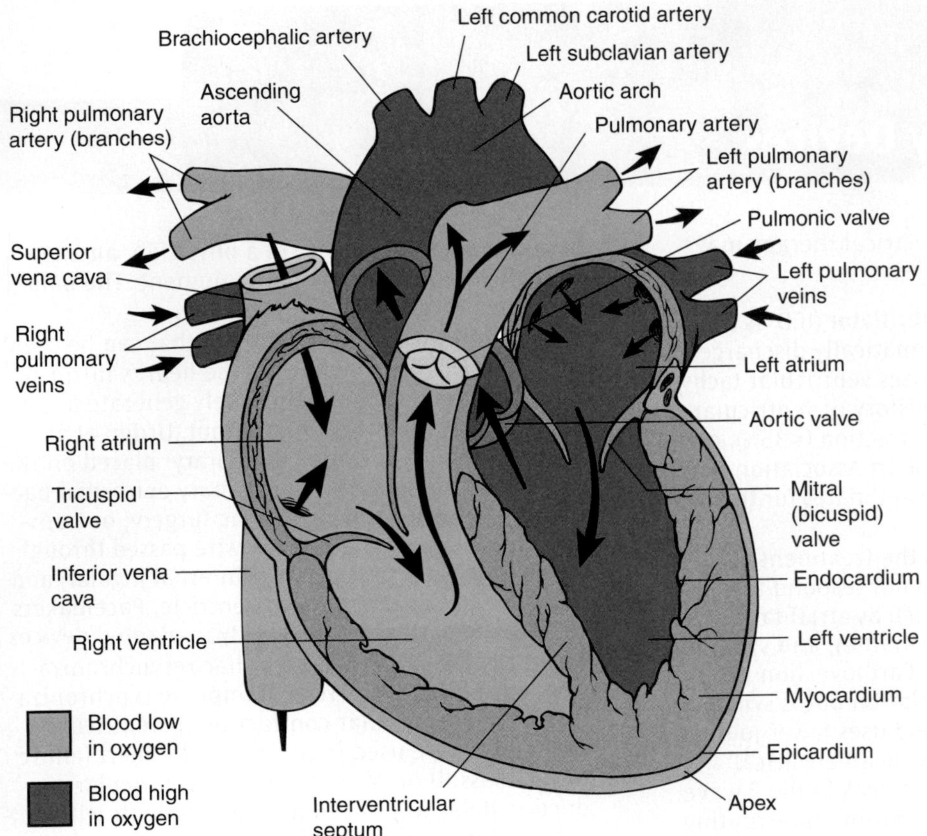
Left common carotid artery
Brachiocephalic artery
Left subclavian artery
Ascending aorta
Aortic arch
Right pulmonary artery (branches)
Pulmonary artery
Left pulmonary artery (branches)
Pulmonic valve
Superior vena cava
Left pulmonary veins
Right pulmonary veins
Left atrium
Aortic valve
Right atrium
Tricuspid valve
Mitral (bicuspid) valve
Inferior vena cava
Endocardium
Right ventricle
Left ventricle
Myocardium
Blood low in oxygen
Epicardium
Blood high in oxygen
Interventricular septum
Apex

Figure 16-1. Cardiac anatomy.

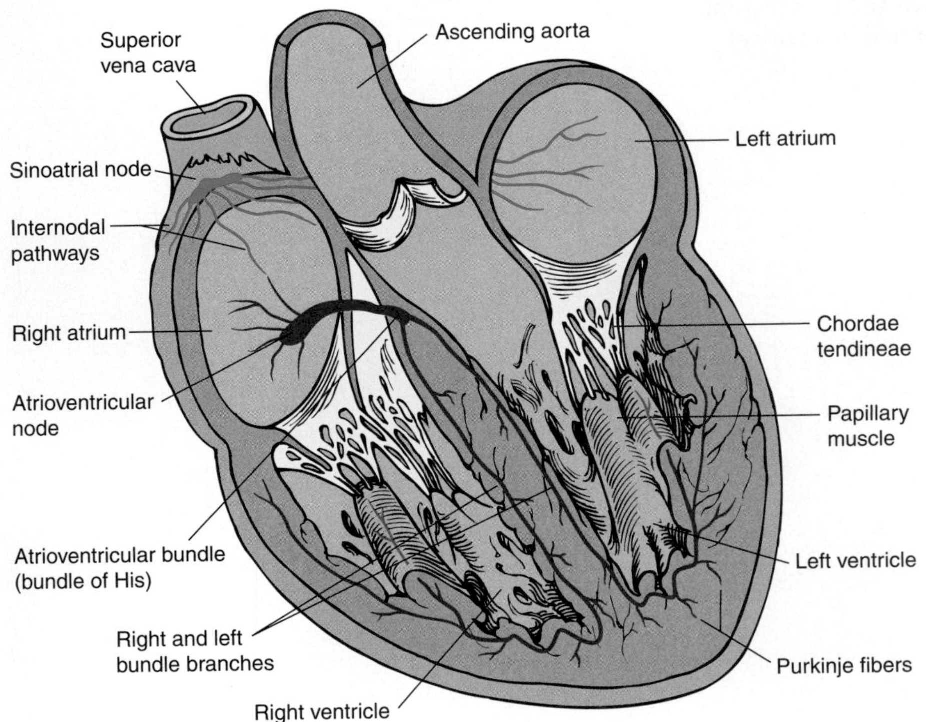
Superior vena cava
Ascending aorta
Left atrium
Sinoatrial node
Internodal pathways
Right atrium
Chordae tendineae
Atrioventricular node
Papillary muscle
Atrioventricular bundle (bundle of His)
Left ventricle
Right and left bundle branches
Purkinje fibers
Right ventricle

Figure 16-2. Cardiac conduction system.

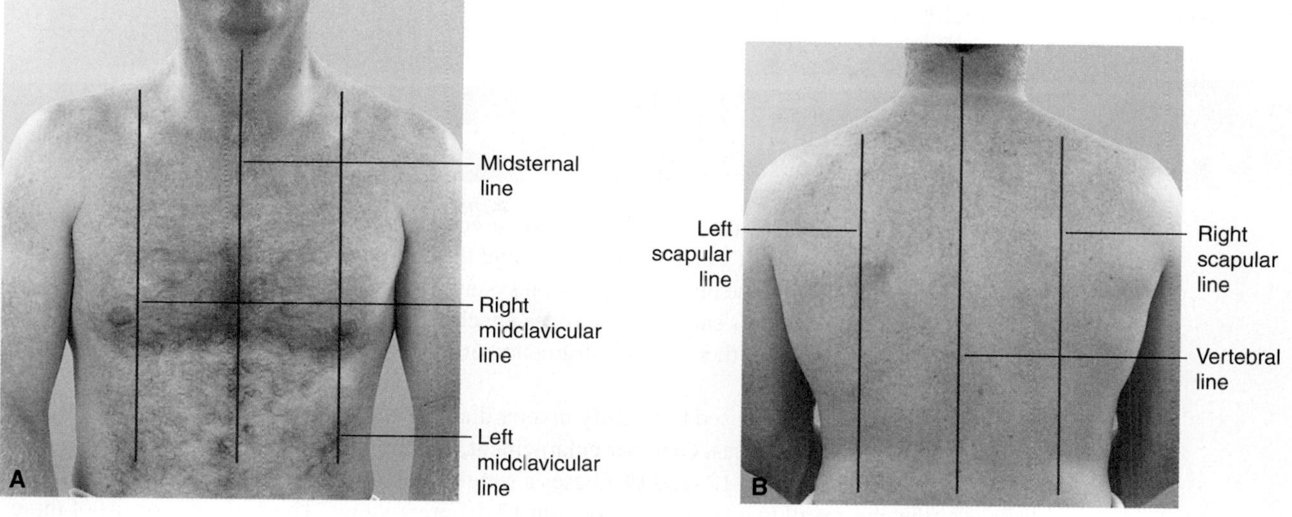

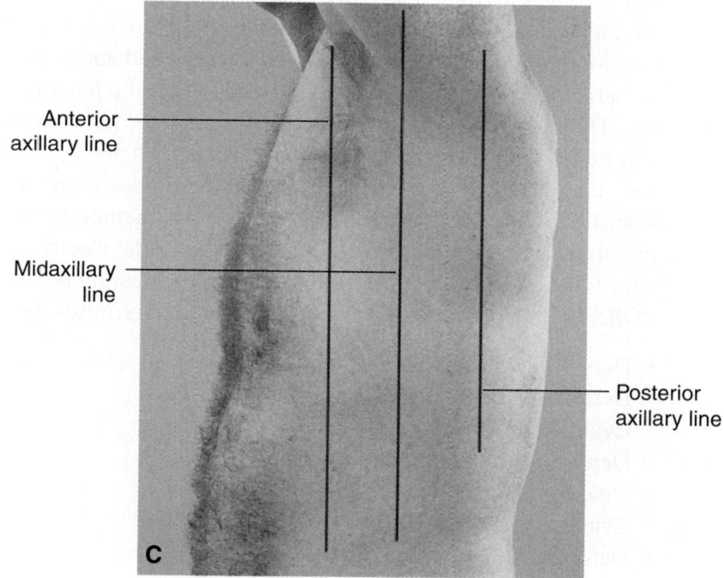

Figure 16-3. Cardiac landmarks: Reference lines. (**A**) Anterior chest. (**B**) Posterior chest. (**C**) Lateral chest.

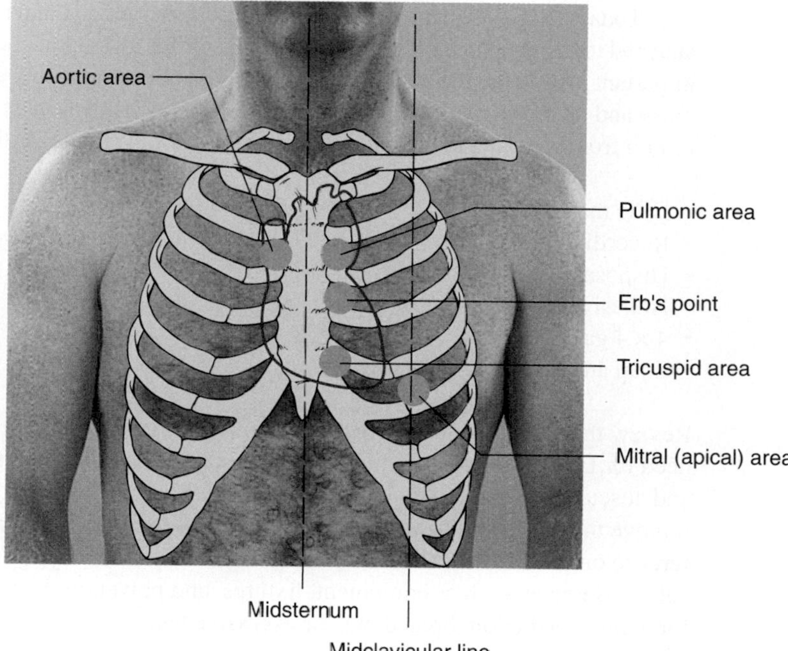

Figure 16-4. Cardiac landmarks: Auscultation areas.

SKILL 16-1 Obtaining an Electrocardiogram (ECG/EKG)

One of the most valuable and frequently used diagnostic tools, electrocardiography (ECG), measures the heart's electrical activity, and the data are graphed as waveforms. Impulses moving through the heart's conduction system create electric currents that can be monitored on the body's surface. Electrodes attached to the skin can detect these electric currents and transmit them to an instrument that produces a record (the electrocardiogram) of cardiac activity.

ECG can be used to identify myocardial ischemia and infarction, rhythm and conduction disturbances, chamber enlargement, electrolyte imbalances, and drug toxicity.

The standard 12-lead ECG uses a series of electrodes placed on the extremities and the chest wall to assess the heart from 12 different views. The 12 leads consist of three standard bipolar limb leads (designated I, II, III), three unipolar augmented leads (aV_R, aV_L, aV_F), and six unipolar precordial leads (V_1 to V_6). The exact location on the extremities does not matter as long as skin contact is good and bone is avoided (Urden, Stacy, & Lough, 2002). The chest leads are placed in specific locations to ensure accurate recording. The limb leads and augmented leads show the heart from the frontal plane. The precordial leads show the heart from the horizontal plane.

Each lead overlies a specific area of the myocardium and provides an electrographic snapshot of electrochemical activity of the cell membrane (Pyne, 2004). The ECG device measures and averages the differences between the electrical potential of the electrode sites for each lead and graphs them over time, creating the standard ECG complex, called PQRST (Box 16-1). Rhythm strip interpretation requires the following:

- Determine the rhythm.
- Determine the rate.
- Evaluate the P wave.
- Determine the duration of the PR interval.
- Determine the duration of the QRS complex.
- Evaluate the T waves.
- Determine the duration of the QT interval.
- Evaluate any other components.

Variations of standard ECGs include exercise ECG (stress ECG) and ambulatory ECG (Holter monitoring).

Today, ECG is typically accomplished using a multichannel method. All electrodes are attached to the patient at once and the machine prints a simultaneous view of all leads. It is important to reassure the patient that the leads do not transmit any electricity. The leads just sense and record (Urden, Stacy, & Lough, 2002). The patient must be able to lie still and refrain from speaking to prevent body movement from creating artifact in the ECG.

Equipment

- ECG machine
- Recording paper
- Disposable pregelled electrodes
- Adhesive remover swabs
- 4 × 4 gauze pads
- Soap and water, if necessary

ASSESSMENT

Review the patient's medical record and plan of care for information about the patient's need for ECG. Assess the patient's cardiac status, including heart rate, blood pressure, and auscultation of heart sounds. If the patient is already connected to a cardiac monitor, remove the electrodes to accommodate the precordial leads and minimize electrical interference on the ECG tracing. Keep the patient away from objects that might cause electrical interference, such as equipment, fixtures, and power cords. Inspect the patient's chest for areas of irritation, breakdown, or excessive hair that might interfere with electrode placement.

SKILL 16-1 **Obtaining an Electrocardiogram (ECG/EKG)** *(continued)*

BOX 16-1 ECG Complex

The ECG complex consists of five waveforms labeled with the letters P, Q, R, S, and T. In addition, sometimes a U wave appears.

- P wave: Represents atrial depolarization (conduction of the electrical impulse through the atria); the first component of ECG waveform
- PR interval: Tracks the atrial impulse from the atria through the AV node, from the SA node to the AV node. Measures from the beginning of the P wave to the beginning of the QRS complex. Normal PR is 0.12 to 0.2 seconds.
- QRS complex: Follows the PR interval and represents depolarization of the ventricles (the time it takes for the impulse to travel through the bundle branches to the Purkinje fibers) or impulse conduction and contraction of the myocardial cells (ventricular systole). The Q wave appears as the first negative deflection in the QRS complex, the R wave as the first positive deflection. The S wave appears as the second negative deflection or the first negative deflection after the R wave. Normal QRS is 0.06 to 0.1 seconds.
- ST segment: Represents the end of ventricular conduction or depolarization and the beginning of ventricular recovery or repolarization; the J point marks the end of the QRS complex and the beginning of the ST segment.
- T wave: Represents ventricular recovery or repolarization
- QT interval: Measures ventricular depolarization and repolarization; varies with the heart rate (ie, the faster the heart rate, the shorter the QT interval); extends from the beginning of the QRS complex to the end of the T wave. Normal QT is <0.4 seconds, but can vary with heart rate.
- U wave: Represents the recovery period of the Purkinje fibers or ventricular conduction fibers; not present on every rhythm strip

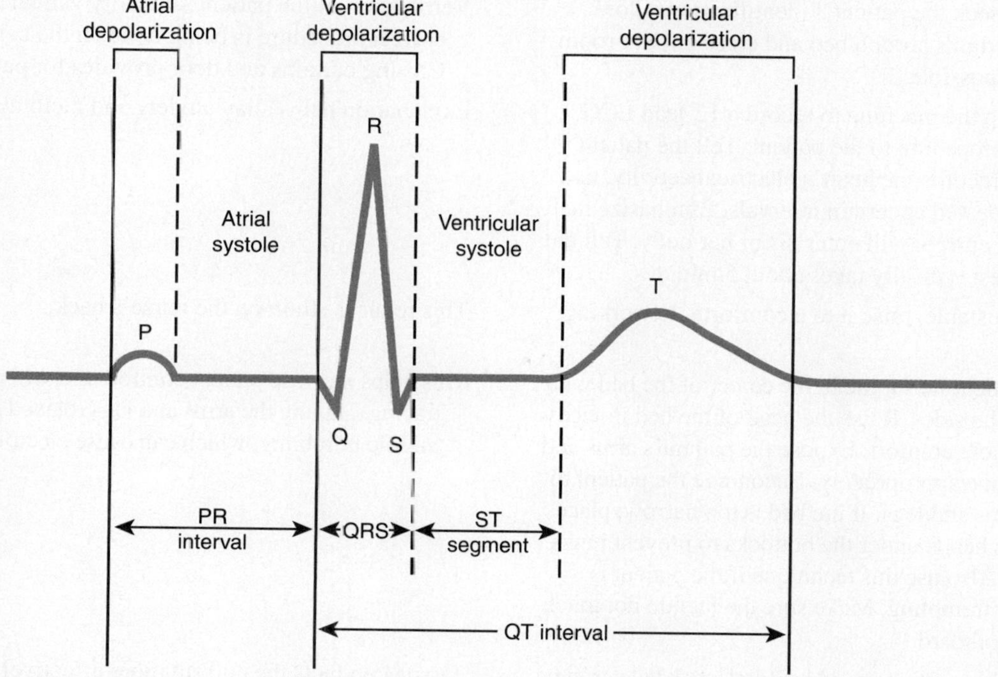

Normal ECG waveforms, intervals, and correlation with events of the cardiac cycle.

NURSING DIAGNOSIS

Determine the related factors for the nursing diagnoses based on the patient's current status. Appropriate nursing diagnoses may include:

- Decreased Cardiac Output
- Excess Fluid Volume
- Acute Pain
- Deficient Knowledge
- Ineffective Health Maintenance
- Activity Intolerance
- Anxiety

Many other nursing diagnoses may require the use of this skill.

(continued)

SKILL 16-1 Obtaining an Electrocardiogram (ECG/EKG) *(continued)*

OUTCOME IDENTIFICATION AND PLANNING

The expected outcome to achieve is that a cardiac electrical tracing is obtained without any complications. Other appropriate outcomes may include: the patient displays an increased understanding about the ECG, and the patient has reduced anxiety.

IMPLEMENTATION

ACTION	RATIONALE
1. Place the ECG machine close to the patient's bed, and plug the power cord into the wall outlet.	Having equipment available saves time and facilitates accomplishment of task.
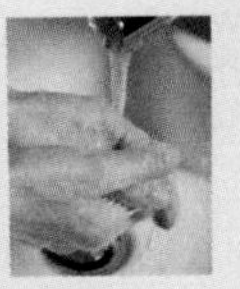 2. Perform hand hygiene.	Hand hygiene deters the spread of microorganisms.
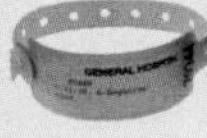 3. Check the patient's identification. Close curtains around bed and close door to room if possible.	Verification of the patient's identity validates that the correct procedure is being done on the correct patient. Closing curtains and door provides for patient privacy.
4. As you set up the machine to record a 12-lead ECG, explain the procedure to the patient. Tell the patient that the test records the heart's electrical activity, and it may be repeated at certain intervals. Emphasize that no electrical current will enter his or her body. Tell the patient the test typically takes about 5 minutes.	Explanation helps allay anxiety and facilitates compliance.
5. If bed is adjustable, raise it to a comfortable working height.	This reduces strain on the nurse's back.
6. Have the patient lie supine in the center of the bed with the arms at the sides. Raise the head of the bed if necessary to promote comfort. Expose the patient's arms and legs, and drape appropriately. Encourage the patient to relax the arms and legs. If the bed is too narrow, place the patient's hands under the buttocks to prevent muscle tension. Also use this technique if the patient is shivering or trembling. Make sure the feet do not touch the bed's footboard.	This helps increase patient comfort and will produce a better tracing. Having the arms and legs relaxed minimizes muscle trembling, which can cause electrical interference.
7. Select flat, fleshy areas on which to place the electrodes. Avoid muscular and bony areas. If the patient has an amputated limb, choose a site on the stump.	Tissue conducts the current more effectively than bone, producing a better tracing.
8. If an area is excessively hairy, clip the hair. Do not shave hair. Clean excess oil or other substances from the skin with soap and water and dry it completely.	Shaving causes microabrasions on the chest skin. Oils and excess hair interfere with electrode contact and function. Alcohol, benzoin, and antiperspirant are not recommended to prep skin (Del Monte, 2004).

SKILL 16-1

Obtaining an Electrocardiogram (ECG/EKG) *(continued)*

ACTION	RATIONALE
9. Refer to Figure 1 for lead placement (Figure 1). Apply the limb lead electrodes. The tip of each lead wire is lettered and color-coded for easy identification. The white or RA lead goes to the right arm; the green or RL lead to the right leg; the red or LL lead to the left leg; the black or LA lead to the left arm. Peel the contact paper off the self-sticking disposable electrode and apply directly to the prepared site, as recommended by the manufacturer (Figure 2). **Position disposable electrodes on the legs with the lead connection pointing superiorly.**	Having the lead connection pointing superiorly guarantees the best connection to the lead wire.

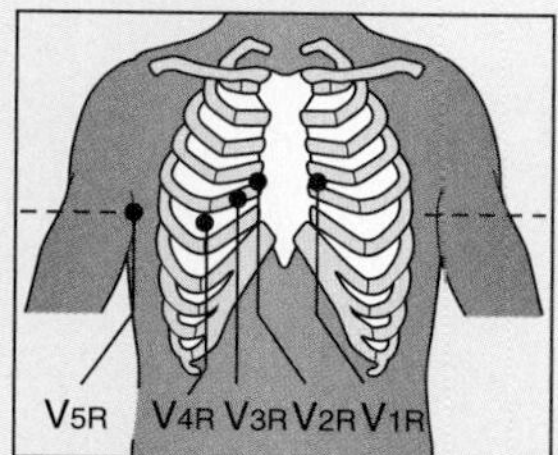

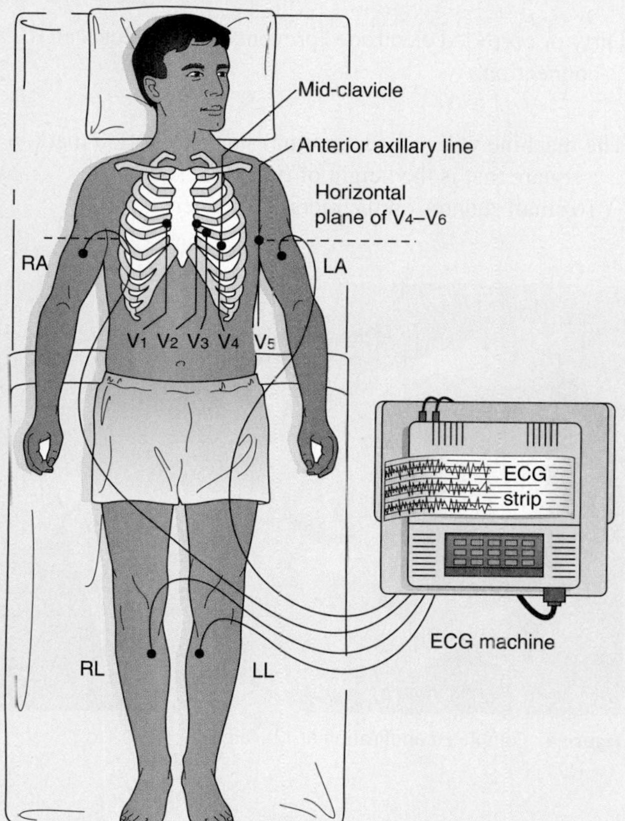

Figure 1. ECG lead placement. *Note:* V_6 (not shown) placed at mid-axillary line, level with V_4. From Smeltzer, S. C., Bare, B. G., et al. (2008). *Brunner and Suddarth's textbook of medical-surgical nursing* (11th ed). Philadelphia: Lippincott Williams & Wilkins.

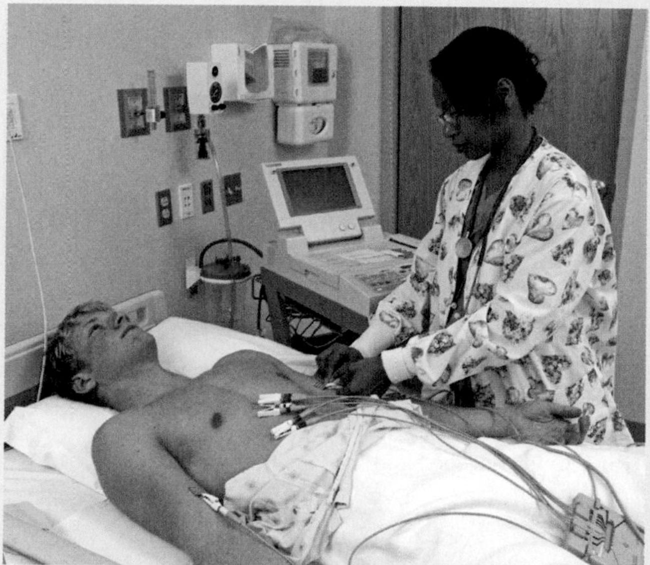

Figure 2. Applying limb lead.

(continued)

SKILL 16-1 Obtaining an Electrocardiogram (ECG/EKG) *(continued)*

ACTION	RATIONALE
10. Connect the limb lead wires to the electrodes. Make sure the metal parts of the electrodes are clean and bright.	Dirty or corroded electrodes prevent a good electrical connection.
11. Expose the patient's chest. Apply the precordial lead electrodes (Figure 3). The tip of each lead wire is lettered and color-coded for easy identification. The brown or V_1 to V_6 leads are applied to the chest. Peel the contact paper off the self-sticking disposable electrode and apply directly to the prepared site, as recommended by the manufacturer. Position chest electrodes as follows (Refer to Figure 1): • V_1: Fourth intercostal space at right sternal border • V_2: Fourth intercostal space at left sternal border • V_3: Halfway between V_2 and V_4 • V_4: Fifth intercostal space at the left midclavicular line • V_5: Fifth intercostal space at anterior axillary line (halfway between V_4 and V_6) • V_6: Fifth intercostal space at midaxillary line, level with V_4	Proper lead placement is necessary for accurate test results.
12. Connect the precordial lead wires to the electrodes. Make sure the metal parts of the electrodes are clean and bright.	Dirty or corroded electrodes prevent a good electrical connection.
13. After the application of all the leads (Figure 4), make sure the paper-speed selector is set to the standard 25 m/second and that the machine is set to full voltage.	The machine will record a normal standardization mark—a square that is the height of two large squares or 10 small squares on the recording paper.

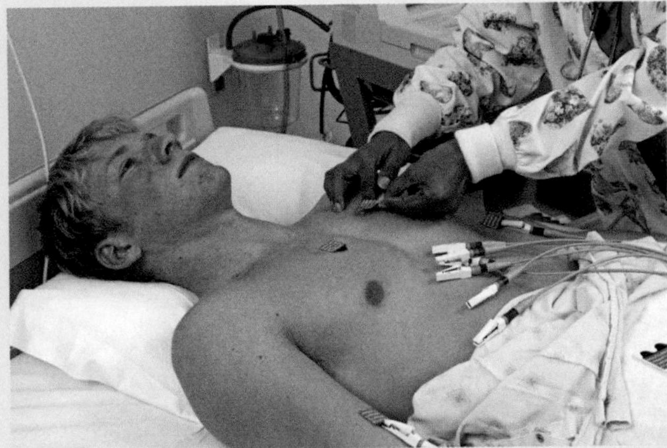

Figure 3. Applying chest lead.

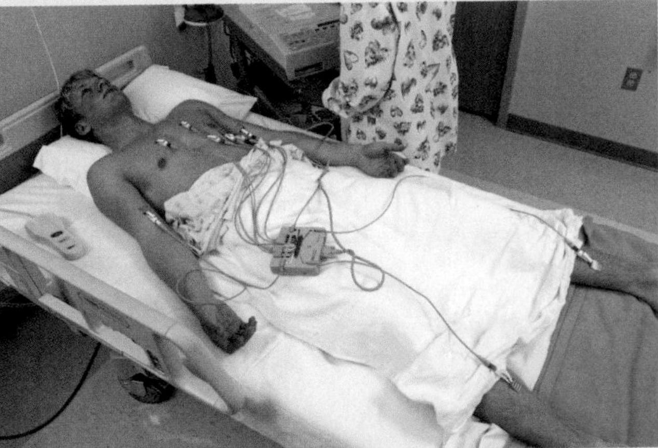

Figure 4. Completed application of 12-lead ECG.

ACTION	RATIONALE
14. If necessary, enter the appropriate patient identification data.	This allows for proper identification of the ECG strip.
15. Ask the patient to relax and breathe normally. **Tell him or her to lie still and not to talk while you record the ECG.**	Lying still and not talking produces a better tracing.

SKILL

16-1 Obtaining an Electrocardiogram (ECG/EKG) *(continued)*

ACTION	RATIONALE
16. Press the AUTO button. Observe the tracing quality (Figure 5). The machine will record all 12 leads automatically, recording three consecutive leads simultaneously. Some machines have a display screen so you can preview waveforms before the machine records them on paper. Adjust waveform if necessary. If any part of the waveform extends beyond the paper when you record the ECG, adjust the normal standardization to half-standardization and repeat. Note this adjustment on the ECG strip, because this will need to be considered in interpreting the results.	Observation of tracing quality allows for adjustments to be made if necessary. Notation of adjustments ensures accurate interpretation of results.

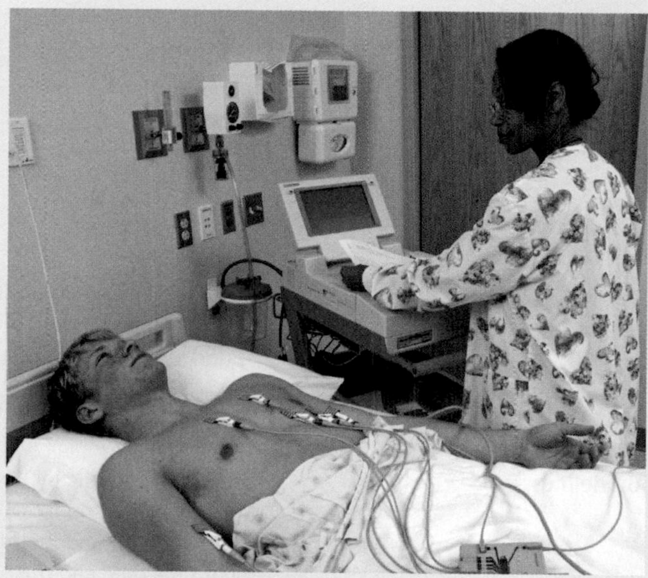

Figure 5. Observing tracing quality.

ACTION	RATIONALE
17. When the machine finishes recording the 12-lead ECG (Figure 6), remove the electrodes and clean the patient's skin, if necessary, with adhesive remover for sticky residue.	Removal and cleaning promote patient comfort.

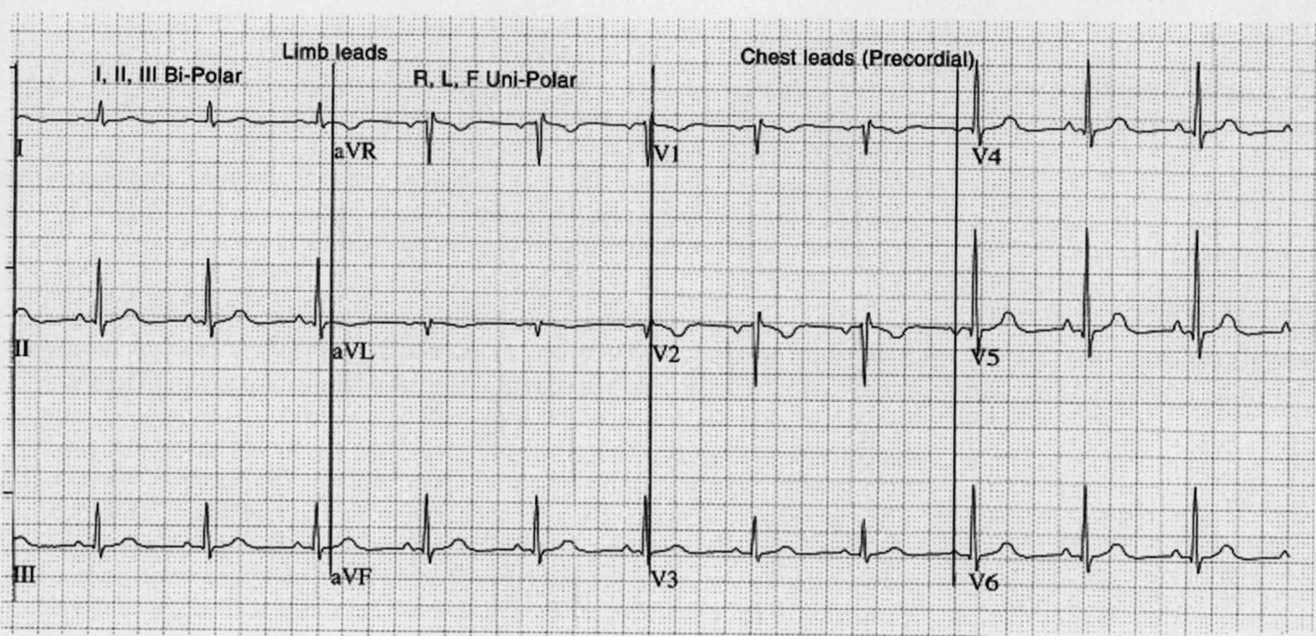

Figure 6. Normal 12-lead ECG configuration. From Diepenbrock, N. (2004). *Quick reference to critical care* (2nd ed.). Philadelphia: Lippincott Williams & Wilkins.

(continued)

SKILL 16-1 Obtaining an Electrocardiogram (ECG/EKG) *(continued)*

ACTION	RATIONALE
18. After disconnecting the lead wires from the electrodes, dispose of the electrodes.	Proper disposal deters the spread of microorganisms.
19. Return the patient to a comfortable position. Lower bed height and adjust head of bed to a comfortable position.	Promotes patient comfort. Promotes patient safety.
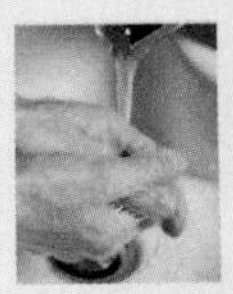 20. Remove any remaining equipment. Perform hand hygiene.	Hand hygiene deters the spread of microorganisms.

EVALUATION

The expected outcome is achieved when a quality ECG reading is obtained without any undue patient anxiety or complications or injury. In addition, the patient verbalizes an understanding of the reason for the ECG.

DOCUMENTATION

Guidelines

Document significant assessment findings, the date and time that the ECG was obtained, and the patient's response to the procedure. Label the ECG recording with the patient's name, room number, and facility identification number, if this was not done by the machine. Also record the date and time as well as any appropriate clinical information on the ECG, such as blood pressure measurement, if the patient was experiencing chest pain.

Sample Documentation

11/10/08 1745 Patient admitted to room 663. Denies pain, nausea, and shortness of breath. Apical heart rate 82 and regular. Blood pressure 146/88. ECG obtained as per admission orders. Copy faxed to Dr. Martin.—B. Clapp, RN

Unexpected Situations and Associated Interventions

- *An artifact appears on the tracing:* An artifact may be due to loose electrodes or patient movement. Reassess electrode connections and ask the patient to lie extremely still. Redo ECG, if necessary.
- *Minimal complexes are seen:* This may be due to extreme bradycardia. Run longer strips.
- *A wandering baseline is noted, and respirations distort the recording:* Ask the patient to hold his or her breath briefly to reduce baseline wander in the tracing.

Special Considerations

General Considerations

- If self-sticking disposable electrodes are not used, apply electrode paste or gel to the patient's skin at the appropriate sites. Rub the gel or paste into the skin. The paste or gel facilitates electrode contact and enhances tracing. Secure electrodes promptly after applying the paste or gel. This prevents drying of the medium, which could impair ECG quality. Never use alcohol or acetone pads in place of the electrode paste or gel. Acetone and alcohol impair electrode contact with the skin and diminish the transmission of electrical impulses. The use of alcohol as a conducting material can result in burns. After disconnecting the lead wires from the electrodes, dispose of or clean the electrodes, as indicated. Proper cleaning after use ensures that the machine will be ready for next use.

SKILL 16-1 Obtaining an Electrocardiogram (ECG/EKG) *(continued)*

- For female patients, place the electrodes below the breast tissue. In a large-breasted woman, you may need to displace the breast tissue laterally and/or superiorly.
- Small areas of hair on the patient's chest or extremities may be trimmed, but this usually is not necessary (Figure 7).

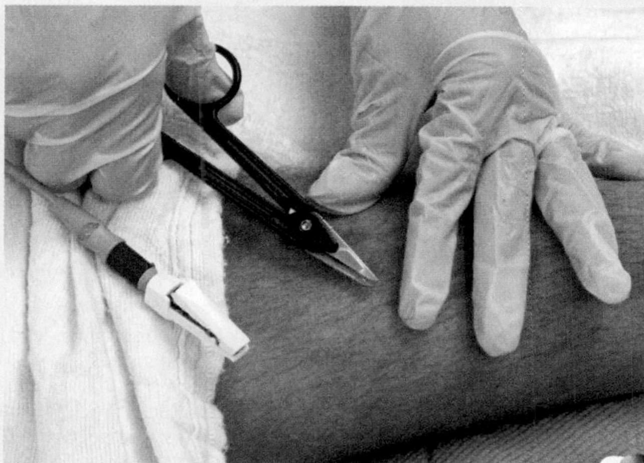

Figure 7. Trimming leg hair.

- If the patient's skin is exceptionally oily, scaly, or diaphoretic, rub the electrode site with a dry 4 × 4 gauze or soap and water before applying the electrode to help reduce interference in the tracing. Alcohol, benzoin, and antiperspirant are not recommended to prep skin (Del Monte, 2004).
- If the patient has a pacemaker, you can perform an ECG with or without a magnet, according to the physician's orders. Note the presence of a pacemaker and the use of the magnet on the strip.

SKILL 16-2 Applying a Cardiac Monitor

Bedside cardiac monitoring provides continuous observation of the heart's electrical activity. Cardiac monitoring is used for patients with conduction disturbances and for those at risk for life-threatening arrhythmias, such as postoperative patients and patients who are sedated. Like other forms of electrocardiography (ECG), cardiac monitoring uses electrodes placed on the patient's chest to transmit electrical signals that are converted into a tracing of cardiac rhythm on an oscilloscope. Three-lead or five-lead systems may be used (Figure 1). The three-lead–wire monitoring system of the patient in any of the limb leads. The five–lead-wire monitoring system facilitates monitoring of the patient in any one of the standard 12 leads.

(continued)

SKILL 16-2

Applying a Cardiac Monitor *(continued)*

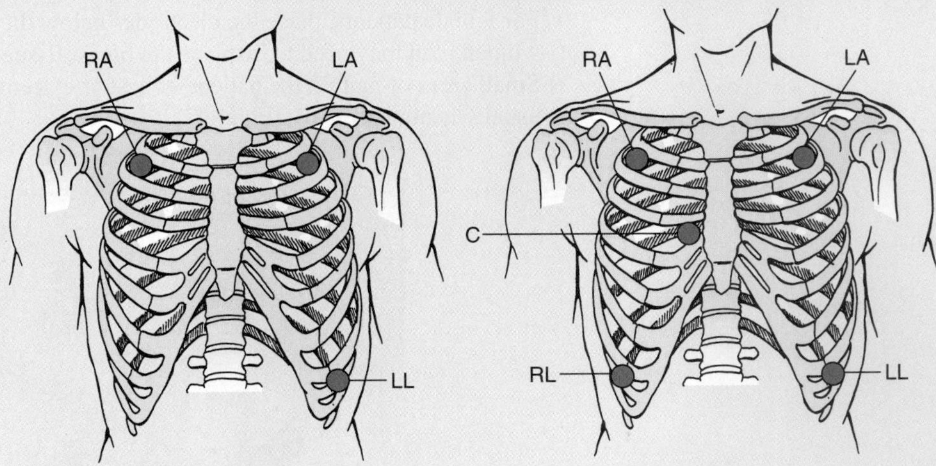

Figure 1. Electrode positions for three-lead (*left*) and five-lead systems (*right*).
Positions for the three-lead system:
RA (white electrode) below right clavicle, second ICS, right midclavicular line
LA (black electrode) below left clavicle, second ICS, left midclavicular line
LL (red electrode) left lower ribcage, eighth ICS, left midclavicular line
Positions for five-lead system:
RA (white electrode) below right clavicle, second ICS, right midclavicular line
RL (green electrode) right lower ribcage, eighth ICS, right midclavicular line
LA (black electrode) below left clavicle, second ICS, left midclavicular line
LL (red electrode) left lower ribcage, eighth ICS, left midclavicular line
Chest (brown electrode) any V lead position, usually V_1 (fourth ICS, right sternal border)

Two types of monitoring may be performed: hardwire or telemetry. In hardwire monitoring, the patient is connected to a monitor at the bedside. The rhythm display appears at the bedside but may also be transmitted to a console at a remote location. Telemetry uses a small transmitter connected to the ambulatory patient to send electrical signals to another location, where they are displayed on a monitor screen. Battery-powered and portable, telemetry frees patients from cumbersome wires and cables and lets them be comfortably mobile. Telemetry is especially useful for monitoring arrhythmias that occur during sleep, rest, exercise, or stressful situations.

Regardless of the type, cardiac monitors can display the patient's heart rate and rhythm, produce a printed record of cardiac rhythm, and sound an alarm if the heart rate exceeds or falls below specified limits. Monitors also recognize and count abnormal heartbeats as well as changes. For example, ST-segment monitoring helps detect myocardial ischemia, electrolyte imbalance, coronary artery spasm, and hypoxic events. The ST-segment represents early ventricular repolarization, and any changes in this waveform component reflect alterations in myocardial oxygenation. Any monitoring lead that views an ischemic heart region will reveal ST-segment changes. The monitor's software establishes a template of the patient's normal QRST pattern from the selected leads; then the monitor displays ST-segment changes. Some monitors display such changes continuously, while other monitors do this only on command.

Gel foam electrodes are commonly used. Electrodes should be changed every 24 hours, or according to facility policy, to prevent skin irritation. Hypoallergenic electrodes are available for patients with hypersensitivity to tape. Any loose or nonadhering electrode should be replaced immediately to prevent inaccurate or missing data.

Equipment

- Lead wires
- Pregelled (gel foam) electrodes (number varies from 3 to 5)
- Alcohol pads
- Gauze pads

SKILL 16-2 Applying a Cardiac Monitor *(continued)*

- Patient cable for hardwire cardiac monitor
- Transmitter, transmitter pouch, and telemetry battery pack for telemetry

ASSESSMENT

Review the patient's medical record and plan of care for information about the patient's need for cardiac monitoring. Assess the patient's cardiac status, including heart rate, blood pressure, and auscultation of heart sounds. Inspect the patient's chest for areas of irritation, breakdown, or excessive hair that might interfere with electrode placement. Electrode sites must be dry, with minimal hair. The patient may be sitting or supine, in a bed or chair.

NURSING DIAGNOSIS

Determine the related factors for the nursing diagnoses based on the patient's current status. Appropriate nursing diagnoses may include:

- Decreased Cardiac Output
- Excess Fluid Volume
- Impaired Gas Exchange
- Acute Pain
- Deficient Knowledge
- Activity Intolerance
- Anxiety (related to unknown procedure)

Many other nursing diagnoses may require the use of this skill.

OUTCOME IDENTIFICATION AND PLANNING

The expected outcome to achieve when performing cardiac monitoring is that a clear waveform, free from artifact, is displayed on the cardiac monitor. Other appropriate outcomes may include: the patient displays understanding of the reason for monitoring, and the patient experiences reduced anxiety.

IMPLEMENTATION

ACTION	RATIONALE
1. Gather all equipment and bring it to the bedside.	Having equipment available saves time and facilitates accomplishment of task.
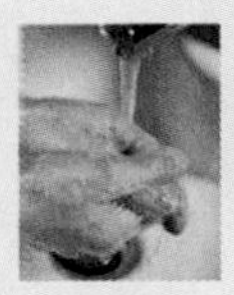 2. Perform hand hygiene.	Hand hygiene deters the spread of microorganisms.
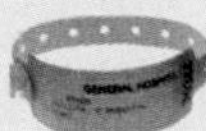 3. Check the patient's identification. Explain the procedure to the patient. Close curtains around bed and close door to room if possible.	Verification of the patient's identity validates that the correct procedure is being done on the correct patient. Explanation helps allay anxiety and promotes compliance. Closing curtains provides for patient privacy.
4. Plug the cardiac monitor into an electrical outlet and turn it on to warm up the unit while preparing the equipment and the patient. For telemetry monitoring, insert a new battery into the transmitter. Match the poles on the battery with the polar markings on the transmitter case. Press the button at the top of the unit, test the battery's charge, and test the unit to ensure that the battery is operational.	Proper setup ensures proper functioning. Not all models have test button. Test according to manufacturer's directions.

(continued)

SKILL 16-2 Applying a Cardiac Monitor *(continued)*

ACTION	RATIONALE
5. Insert the cable into the appropriate socket in the monitor.	Proper setup ensures proper functioning.
6. Connect the lead wires to the cable. In some systems, the lead wires are permanently secured to the cable. For telemetry, if the lead wires are not permanently affixed to the telemetry unit, attach them securely. If they must be attached individually, connect each one to the correct outlet.	Proper setup ensures proper functioning.
7. Connect an electrode to each of the lead wires, carefully checking that each lead wire is in its correct outlet.	Proper setup ensures proper functioning.
8. Expose the patient's chest and determine electrode positions, based on which system and leads are being used (refer to Figure 1). If necessary, clip the hair from an area about 10 cm in diameter around each electrode site. Clean the area with soap and water and dry it completely to remove skin secretions that may interfere with electrode function.	These actions allow for better adhesion of the electrode and thus better conduction. Alcohol, benzoin, and antiperspirant are not recommended to prep skin (Del Monte, 2004).
9. Remove the backing from the pregelled electrode. Check the gel for moistness. If the gel is dry, discard it and replace it with a fresh electrode. **Apply the electrode to the site and press firmly to ensure a tight seal.** Repeat with the remaining electrodes to complete the three-lead or five-lead system (Figures 2 and 3).	Gel acts as a conduit and must be moist and secured tightly.

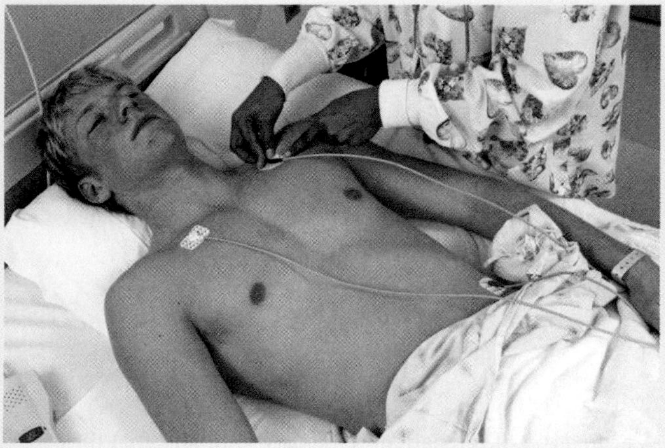

Figure 2. Applying the electrodes for three-lead monitoring system.

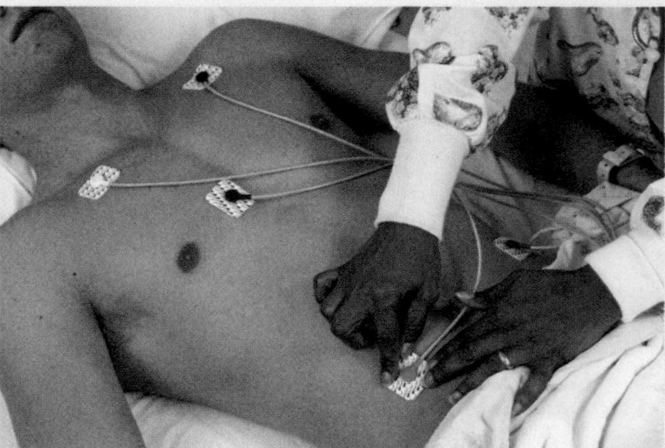

Figure 3. Applying electrodes for five-lead monitoring system.

ACTION	RATIONALE
10. When all the electrodes are in place, connect the appropriate lead wire to each electrode. Check waveform for clarity, position, and size. **To verify that the monitor is detecting each beat, compare the digital heart rate display with an auscultated count of the patient's heart rate.** If necessary, use the gain control to adjust the size of the rhythm tracing, and use the position control to adjust the waveform position on the monitor.	This ensures accuracy of reading.

SKILL 16-2 Applying a Cardiac Monitor *(continued)*

ACTION	RATIONALE
11. Set the upper and lower limits of the heart rate alarm, based on the patient's condition or unit policy.	Setting the alarm allows for audible notification if the heart rate is beyond limits. The default setting for the monitor automatically turns all alarms on; limits should be set for each patient.
12. For telemetry, place the transmitter in the pouch in the hospital gown. If not available in gown, use a portable pouch. Place transmitter in pouch. Tie the pouch strings around the patient's neck and waist, making sure that the pouch fits snugly without causing discomfort. If no pouch is available, place the transmitter in the patient's bathrobe pocket.	Patient comfort leads to compliance.
13. To obtain a rhythm strip, press the RECORD key either at the bedside for monitoring or at the central station for telemetry. Label the strip with the patient's name and room number, date, time, and rhythm identification. Place the rhythm strip in the appropriate location in the patient's chart. Analyze strip as appropriate.	A rhythm strip provides a baseline.
14. Return the patient to a comfortable position.	Promotes patient comfort.
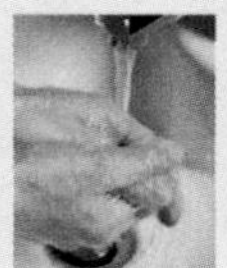 15. Remove any remaining equipment. Perform hand hygiene.	Hand hygiene deters the spread of microorganisms.

EVALUATION

The expected outcome is achieved when the cardiac monitoring waveform displays the patient's cardiac rhythm, with a waveform that is detecting each beat, and is appropriate for clarity, position, and size. In addition, the patient demonstrates no undue anxiety and remains free of complications or injury.

DOCUMENTATION

Guidelines

Record the date and time that monitoring begins and the monitoring lead used in the medical record. Document a rhythm strip at least every 8 hours and with any changes in the patient's condition (or as stated by your facility's policy). Label the rhythm strip with the patient's name and room number, date, and time.

Sample Documentation

12/3/08 1615 Patient admitted to room. Cardiac telemetry monitor in place; monitoring in lead II. See flow sheet for assessment data and initial rhythm strip.—T. Shah, RN

Unexpected Situations and Associated Interventions

- *False high-rate alarm sounds:* Assess for monitor that is interpreting large T waves as QRS complexes, thus doubling the rate, or skeletal muscle activity. Reposition electrodes to a lead where the QRS complexes are taller than the T waves, and place electrodes away from major muscle masses. Change lead view on monitor. Use "relearn" feature, if available, to identify where the normal complexes are.

(continued)

SKILL 16-2 Applying a Cardiac Monitor *(continued)*

- *False low-rate alarm sounds:* Assess for a shift in the electrical axis due to patient movement, making QRS complexes too small to register; low amplitude of QRS; or poor contact between skin and electrode. Reapply electrodes. Set gain so that the height of complex is greater than 1 millivolt.
- *Low amplitude:* Assess for gain dial set too low; poor contact between skin and electrodes; dried gel; broken or loose lead wires; poor connection between patient and monitor; or malfunctioning monitor. Check connections on all lead wires and monitoring cable. Replace electrodes as necessary. Reapply electrodes, if required.
- *Wandering baseline:* Assess for poor position or contact between electrodes and skin, or thoracic movement with respirations. Reposition or replace electrodes.
- *Artifact (waveform interference):* Assess for patient movement, improperly applied electrodes, or static electricity. Attach all electrical equipment to a common ground. Check plugs to make sure prongs are not loose.
- *Skin excoriation under electrodes:* Assess for allergic reaction to electrode adhesive or electrodes being left on the skin too long. Remove electrodes and apply hypoallergenic electrodes and hypoallergenic tape, or remove electrode, clean site, and reapply electrode at new site.

Special Considerations

General Considerations

- Make sure all electrical equipment and outlets are grounded to avoid electric shock and interference (artifacts).
- Avoid opening the electrode packages until just before using to prevent the gel from drying out.
- Avoid placing the electrodes on bony prominences, hairy locations, areas where defibrillator pads will be placed, or areas for chest compression.
- If the patient's skin is very oily, scaly, or diaphoretic, rub the electrode site with a dry 4 × 4 gauze pad before applying the electrode to help reduce interference in the tracing.
- Assess skin integrity and examine the leads every 8 hours. Replace and reposition the electrodes as necessary.
- If the patient is being monitored by telemetry, show him or her how the transmitter works. If applicable, identify the button that will produce a recording of the ECG at the central station. Instruct the patient to push the button whenever symptoms occur; this causes the central console to print a rhythm strip. Also, advise patient to notify nurse immediately.
- If medical order is in place, tell the patient to remove the transmitter during showering or bathing, if appropriate, but stress that he or she should let you know the unit is being removed.

SKILL 16-3 Obtaining an Arterial Blood Sample From an Arterial Line–Stopcock System

Obtaining an arterial blood sample requires percutaneous puncture of the brachial, radial, or femoral artery (see Chapter 18: Specimen Collection). However, an arterial blood sample can also be obtained from an arterial line. When collected, the sample can be analyzed to determine arterial blood gas (ABG), laboratory specimens, or other values.

The below procedure describes obtaining a sample from an open system. For information on obtaining an arterial blood sample from a closed reservoir system, please see the Skill Variation at the end of the skill.

Equipment

- Arterial blood gas (ABG) syringe with needleless cannula, if ABG is ordered
- Gloves
- Goggles
- Two 5-mL syringes

SKILL 16-3

Obtaining an Arterial Blood Sample From an Arterial Line–Stopcock System *(continued)*

- Vacutainer® with needleless adapter and appropriate blood collection tubes for ordered tests
- Alcohol swabs or chlorhexidine, per facility policy
- Rubber cap for ABG syringe hub
- Ice-filled plastic bag or cup
- Label with patient identification information and test order number
- Laboratory request form, if necessary
- Biohazard bag

ASSESSMENT

Review the patient's medical record and plan of care for information about the patient's need for an arterial blood sample. Assess the patient's cardiac status, including heart rate, blood pressure, and auscultation of heart sounds. Also assess the patient's respiratory status, including respiratory rate, excursion, lung sounds, and use of oxygen if ordered. Check the patency and functioning of the arterial line. Determine the dead-space volume of the arterial line system immediately before withdrawing the laboratory sample (see Step 8). A sufficient amount of discard volume needs to be withdrawn before obtaining the blood sample to be tested in the laboratory. The dead space is the volume of the space from the tip of the catheter to the sampling port of the stopcock. The dead-space volume will depend on the gauge and length of the catheter, the length of the connecting tubing, and the number of stopcocks in the system. If an insufficient amount of discard volume is withdrawn, the specimen may be diluted and contaminated with flush solution. If an excessive amount of discard volume is withdrawn, the patient may experience an iatrogenic (treatment-induced) blood loss (Mims et al, 2004). Assess the patient's understanding about the need for specimen collection.

NURSING DIAGNOSIS

Determine the related factors for the nursing diagnoses based on the patient's current status. Appropriate nursing diagnoses may include:

- Impaired Gas Exchange
- Decreased Cardiac Output
- Ineffective Airway Clearance
- Risk for Injury
- Risk for Infection
- Excess Fluid Volume
- Anxiety

In addition, many other nursing diagnoses also may require the use of this skill.

OUTCOME IDENTIFICATION AND PLANNING

The expected outcome to achieve when obtaining an arterial blood sample is that a specimen is obtained without compromise to the patency of the arterial line. In addition, the patient experiences minimal discomfort and anxiety, remains free from infection, and demonstrates an understanding about the need for the specimen collection.

IMPLEMENTATION

ACTION	RATIONALE
1. Gather all equipment and bring it to the bedside.	Having equipment available saves time and facilitates accomplishment of task.
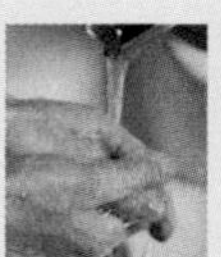 2. Perform hand hygiene.	Hand hygiene deters the spread of microorganisms.

(continued)

SKILL 16-3 Obtaining an Arterial Blood Sample From an Arterial Line–Stopcock System *(continued)*

ACTION	RATIONALE
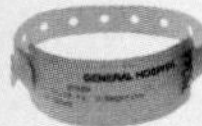 3. Check the patient's identification. Compare the specimen label with the patient's identification. Explain the procedure to the patient. Close curtains around bed and close door to room if possible.	Verification of the patient's identity validates that the correct procedure is being done on the correct patient, and the specimen is accurately labeled. Explanation helps allay anxiety and promotes compliance. Closing curtains provides for patient privacy.
4. If bed is adjustable, raise it to a comfortable working height.	Reduces strain on the nurse's back
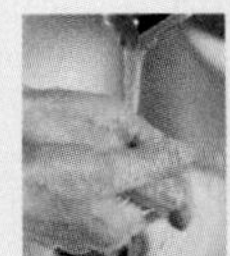 5. Perform hand hygiene and put on gloves and goggles.	Hand hygiene deters the spread of microorganisms. Gloves and goggles prevent contact with blood and body fluids.
6. Turn off or temporarily silence the arterial pressure alarms, depending on your facility's policy (some facilities require that alarms be left on).	The integrity of the system is being altered, which will cause the system to sound an alarm.
7. Locate the stopcock nearest the arterial line insertion site. Use the alcohol swab or chlorhexidine to scrub the sampling port on the stopcock. Allow to air dry.	Prevents contamination from microorganisms on infusion plug
8. Attach a 5-mL syringe into the sampling port on the stopcock to obtain the discard volume (Figure 1). Turn the stopcock off to the flush solution. Aspirate slowly until blood enters the syringe. Stop aspirating. Note the volume in the syringe, which is the dead-space volume. Continue to aspirate until the dead-space volume has been withdrawn a total of 3 times. For example, if the dead-space volume is 0.8 mL, aspirate 2.4 mL of blood.	A sufficient amount of discard volume needs to be withdrawn prior to obtaining the blood sample to be tested in the laboratory. This sample is discarded because it is diluted with flush solution, possibly leading to inaccurate test results. The dead space is the volume of the space from the tip of the catheter to the sampling port of the stopcock. The dead-space volume will depend on the gauge and length of the catheter, the length of the connecting tubing, and the number of stopcocks in the system. If an insufficient amount of discard volume is withdrawn, the specimen may be diluted and contaminated with flush solution. If an excessive amount of discard volume is withdrawn, the patient may experience an iatrogenic (treatment-induced) blood loss (Mims et al, 2004).

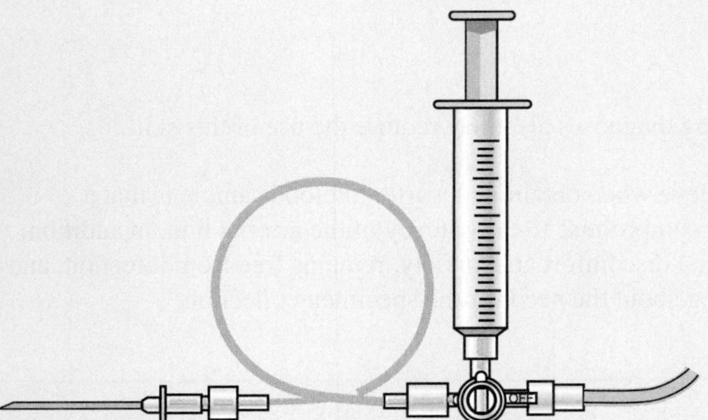

Figure 1. Attaching a 5-mL syringe to the sampling port on the stopcock.

ACTION	RATIONALE
9. Turn the stopcock to the halfway position between the flush solution and the sampling port to close the system in all directions.	Turning the stopcock off maintains the integrity of the system.
10. Remove the discard syringe and dispose of appropriately.	Observe Standard Precautions. Diluted blood still poses a risk for infection transmission.
11. Place the syringe for the laboratory sample or the Vacutainer in the sampling port of the stopcock. Turn the stopcock off to the flush solution, and slowly	Turning the stopcock off to the flush solution prevents dilution from the flush device.

SKILL 16-3

Obtaining an Arterial Blood Sample From an Arterial Line–Stopcock System *(continued)*

withdraw the required amount of blood. For each additional sample required, repeat this procedure. If the physician has ordered coagulation tests, obtain blood for this sample from the final syringe.

12. Turn the stopcock to the halfway position between the flush solution and the sampling port to close the system in all directions. Remove the syringe or Vacutainer. Apply the rubber cap to the ABG syringe hub, if necessary.

    Turning the stopcock off maintains the integrity of the system.

13. Insert a 5-mL syringe into the sampling port of the stopcock. Turn the stopcock off to the patient. Activate the in-line flushing device. Flush through the sampling port into the syringe to clear the stopcock and sampling port of any residual blood.

    This maintains the integrity of the system, preventing clotting and infection.

14. Turn off the stopcock to the sampling port; remove the syringe. Remove sampling port cap and replace with new sterile one. Intermittently flush the arterial catheter with the in-line flushing device until the tubing is clear of blood.

15. Reactivate the monitor alarms. Attach needles to the filled syringes and transfer the blood samples to the appropriate containers, if necessary. Record date and time the samples were obtained on the labels, as well as the required information to identify the person obtaining the samples. If ABG was collected, record oxygen flow rate (or room air) on label. Apply labels to the specimens, according to facility policy. Place in biohazard bags; place ABG sample in bag with ice.

    Reactivating the system ensures proper functioning. Proper labeling prevents error. Recording oxygen flow rate ensures accurate interpretation of results of ABG. Use of biohazard bag prevents contact with blood and body fluids. Ice maintains integrity of sample.

16. Check the monitor for return of the arterial waveform and pressure reading.

    This ensures proper functioning and integrity of the system.

17. Return the patient to a comfortable position. Lower bed height and adjust head of bed to a comfortable position.

    Promotes patient comfort. Promotes patient safety.

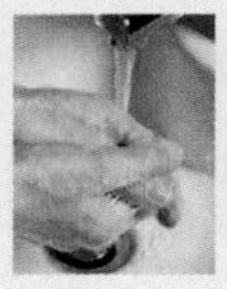

18. Remove any remaining equipment. Perform hand hygiene. Send specimens to the lab immediately.

    Hand hygiene deters the spread of microorganisms. Specimens must be processed in a timely manner to ensure accuracy.

EVALUATION

The expected outcome to achieve when obtaining an arterial blood sample is that a specimen is obtained without compromise to the patency of the arterial line. In addition, the patient experiences minimal discomfort and anxiety, remains free from infection, and demonstrates an understanding about the need for the specimen collection.

DOCUMENTATION

Guidelines

Document any pertinent assessments, the laboratory specimens obtained, date and time specimens were obtained, and disposition of specimens.

(continued)

SKILL 16-3 Obtaining an Arterial Blood Sample From an Arterial Line–Stopcock System *(continued)*

Sample Documentation

10/20/08 0230 Continuous heparin IV infusion at 900 units via left subclavian central catheter. Blood specimens for repeat PT/PTT, CBC, and BMP obtained via right radial arterial line per order. Line flushed per policy; specimens sent to lab. —R. Chin, RN

Unexpected Situations and Associated Interventions

- *The specimen obtained is dark:* Dark blood means a vein may have been accessed, or the blood may be poorly oxygenated. Ensure that the line from which you are obtaining the specimen is indeed an arterial line. Also, check the patient's oxygen saturation level to evaluate for possible hypoxemia. Make sure that the artery was punctured before sending the specimen to the laboratory.
- *When retracting the syringe for the discarded sample, you feel resistance.* Reposition the affected extremity and check the insertion site for obvious problems (such as catheter kinking). Then attempt to obtain the sample to be discarded. If resistance is still felt, notify the physician or primary care professional.
- *After obtaining the specimen and reactivating the arterial pressure monitoring system, no waveform is noted.* Check the stopcock to make sure that it is open to the patient and recheck all connections and components of the system to ensure proper set up. If necessary, rebalance the transducer or replace the system as necessary. If problem persists, suspect a clotted catheter tip. Follow facility policy to troubleshoot a potentially clotted arterial line and notify the physician or primary care professional.

Special Considerations

General Considerations

- If the patient is receiving oxygen, make sure that this therapy has been underway for at least 15 minutes before collecting an arterial blood sample for ABG analysis. Indicate on the laboratory request slip the amount and type of oxygen therapy the patient is receiving. Also note the patient's current temperature, most recent hemoglobin level, and current respiratory rate. If the patient is receiving mechanical ventilation, note the fraction of inspired oxygen and tidal volume.
- If the patient is not receiving oxygen, indicate that he or she is breathing room air.
- If the patient has just received a nebulizer treatment, wait about 20 minutes before collecting the sample for ABG analysis.

SKILL VARIATION Obtaining an Arterial Blood Sample From a Closed Reservoir System

- Gather all equipment and bring it to the bedside.
- Perform hand hygiene. Check the patient's identification. Compare the specimen label with the patient's identification.
- Explain the procedure to the patient. Close curtains around bed and close door to room if possible.
- If bed is adjustable, raise it to a comfortable working height.
- Perform hand hygiene and put on gloves and goggles.
- Locate the closed-system reservoir and blood-sampling site. Deactivate or temporarily silence monitor alarms (some facilities require that alarms be left on).
- Clean the sampling site with an alcohol swab or chlorhexidine.
- Holding the reservoir upright, grasp the flexures, and slowly fill the reservoir with blood over a 3- to 5-second period. If you feel resistance, reposition the affected extremity and check the catheter site for obvious problems (such as kinking). Then resume blood withdrawal.
- Turn the one-way valve off to the reservoir by turning the handle perpendicular to the tubing. Using a syringe with attached cannula, insert the cannula into the sampling site. (Make sure the plunger is depressed to the bottom of the syringe barrel.) Slowly fill the syringe. Then grasp the cannula near the sampling site and remove the syringe and cannula as one unit. Repeat the procedure as needed to fill the required number of syringes. If the physician has ordered coagulation tests, obtain blood for those tests from the final syringe.
- After filling the syringes, turn the one-way valve to its original position, parallel to the tubing. Now smoothly

SKILL 16-3 Obtaining an Arterial Blood Sample From an Arterial Line–Stopcock System *(continued)*

SKILL VARIATION Obtaining an Arterial Blood Sample From a Closed Reservoir System *(continued)*

and evenly push down on the plunger until the flexures lock in place in the fully closed position and all fluid has been reinfused. The fluid should be reinfused over a 3- to 5-second period. Then activate the fast-flush release.

- Clean the sampling site with an alcohol swab. Reactivate the monitor alarms. Using the blood transfer unit, transfer blood samples to the appropriate specimen tubes, if necessary. Record on the labels the date and time the samples were obtained, as well as the required information to identify the person obtaining the samples. Apply labels to the specimens according to facility policy. Place in biohazard bags; place ABG sample in bag with ice.
- Check the monitor for return of the arterial waveform and pressure reading.
- Remove any remaining equipment. Perform hand hygiene. Send specimens to the lab immediately.

SKILL 16-4 Removing Arterial and Femoral Lines

Arterial and femoral lines are used for intensive and continuous cardiac monitoring and intraarterial access. Once the lines are no longer necessary or have become ineffective, they will need to be removed. Consult facility policy to determine whether you are permitted to perform this procedure. Two nurses should be at the bedside until bleeding is controlled and available to give emergency medications if necessary. The patient should be kept NPO until catheter is removed in case of nausea with a vasovagal response.

Equipment

- Sterile gloves
- Clean gloves
- Impervious gown
- Mask
- Protective eyewear
- Box of sterile 4 × 4 gauze pads
- Sheet protector
- Sterile suture removal set
- Tegaderm dressing
- Alcohol pads
- Hypoallergenic tape
- For femoral line: small sandbag (5–10 pounds), wrapped in towel or pillowcase
- Emergency medications (such as atropine, for a vasovagal response with femoral line removal) for emergency response, per facility policy and guidelines
- Marker

ASSESSMENT

Review the patient's medical record and plan of care for information about discontinuation of the arterial or femoral line. Assess the patient's coagulation status, including laboratory studies, to reduce the risk of complications secondary to impaired clotting ability. Assess the patient's understanding of the procedure. Inspect the site for leakage, bleeding, or hematoma. Assess skin color and temperature and assess distal pulses for strength and quality. Mark distal pulses with an 'X' for easy identification postprocedure. Assess patient's blood pressure; systolic blood pressure should be less than 180 mm Hg before catheter removed.

(continued)

SKILL 16-4 Removing Arterial and Femoral Lines *(continued)*

NURSING DIAGNOSIS

Determine the related factors for the nursing diagnoses based on the patient's current status. Appropriate nursing diagnoses may include:

- Risk for Injury
- Impaired Skin Integrity
- Risk for Infection
- Anxiety

Many other nursing diagnoses also may require the use of this skill.

OUTCOME IDENTIFICATION AND PLANNING

The expected outcome to achieve when removing an arterial or femoral line is that the line is removed intact and without injury to the patient. In addition, the site remains clean and dry, without evidence of infection, bleeding, or hematoma.

IMPLEMENTATION

ACTION	RATIONALE
1. Gather all equipment and bring it to the bedside.	Having equipment available saves time and facilitates accomplishment of task.
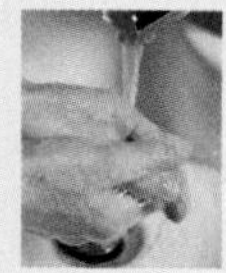 2. Perform hand hygiene.	Hand hygiene deters the spread of microorganisms.
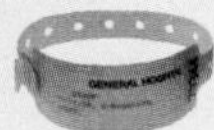 3. Check the patient's identification. Explain the procedure to the patient. Close curtains around bed and close door to room if possible.	Verification of the patient's identity validates that the correct procedure is being done on the correct patient. Explanation helps allay anxiety and promotes compliance. Closing curtains provides for patient privacy.
4. Ask patient to empty bladder. Maintain an IV infusion of normal saline during procedure, as per medical orders or facility guidelines.	This ensures patient comfort. Maintains IV access in case of hypotension or bradycardia.
5. Put on clean gloves, goggles, and gown.	These prevent contact with blood and body fluids.
6. Use Doppler ultrasound to locate femoral artery, if line being removed is in a femoral site, 1″ to 2″ above entrance site of femoral line. Mark with 'X' using special marker for skin.	This ensures accurate location of femoral artery.
7. Turn off the monitor alarms and then turn off the flow clamp to the flush solution. Carefully remove the dressing over the insertion site. Put on sterile gloves. Remove any sutures using the suture removal kit; make sure all sutures have been removed.	These measures help prepare for withdrawal of line.
8. **Withdraw the catheter using a gentle, steady motion. Keep the catheter parallel to the blood vessel during withdrawal. Watch for hematoma formation during catheter removal by gently palpating surrounding tissue. If hematoma starts to form, reposition hands until optimal pressure is obtained to prevent further leakage of blood.**	Using a gentle, steady motion parallel to the blood vessel reduces the risk for traumatic injury.

SKILL 16-4 Removing Arterial and Femoral Lines *(continued)*

ACTION	RATIONALE
9. **Immediately after withdrawing the catheter, apply pressure 1″ or 2″ above the site at the previously marked spot with a sterile 4 × 4 gauze pad. Maintain pressure for at least 10 minutes, or per facility policy (longer if bleeding or oozing persists).** Apply additional pressure to a femoral site or if the patient has coagulopathy or is receiving anticoagulants.	If sufficient pressure is not applied, a large, painful hematoma may form.
10. Assess distal pulses every 3 to 5 minutes while pressure is being applied. Note: dorsalis pedis and posterior tibial pulses should be markedly weaker from baseline if enough pressure is applied to femoral artery.	Assesses blood flow to extremity. Pulses should return to baseline after pressure is released.
11. Cover the site with an appropriate dressing and secure the dressing with tape. If stipulated by facility policy, make a pressure dressing for a femoral site by folding four sterile 4 × 4 gauze pads in half, and apply the dressing. Cover the dressing with a tight adhesive bandage, per policy, and then cover the femoral bandage with a sandbag. Maintain the patient on bed rest, with the head of the bed <30°, for 6 hours with the sandbag in place.	Sufficient pressure is needed to prevent continued bleeding and hematoma formation.
12. Remind the patient not to lift his/her head while on bed rest. Use log roll to assist patient in using bedpan, if needed.	Raising head increases intraabdominal pressure, which could lead to bleeding from site.
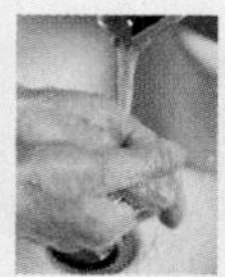 13. Remove and properly dispose of gloves and personal protective equipment. Perform hand hygiene.	Proper removal and disposal of equipment and hand hygiene deter the spread of microorganisms.
14. Observe the site for bleeding. Assess circulation in the extremity distal to the site by evaluating color, pulses, and sensation. Repeat this assessment every 15 minutes for the first 1 hour, every 30 minutes for the next 2 hours, hourly for the next 2 hours, then every 4 hours, or according to facility policy.	Continued assessment allows for early detection and prompt intervention should problems arise.

EVALUATION

The expected outcome is met when the patient exhibits an arterial or femoral line site that is clean and dry without evidence of injury, infection, bleeding, or hematoma. In addition, the patient demonstrates intact peripheral circulation and verbalizes a reduction in anxiety.

DOCUMENTATION

Guidelines

Document the time the line was removed and how long pressure was applied. Document site assessment every 5 minutes while pressure is being applied (second nurse can do this). Document assessment of peripheral circulation, appearance of site, type of dressing applied, the timed assessments, patient's response, and any medications given.

(continued)

SKILL 16-4 Removing Arterial and Femoral Lines *(continued)*

Sample Documentation

12/20/08 1830 Right arterial line removed per order. Pressure applied to site for 10 minutes. Site intact without signs of hematoma; radial pulse present, +2 and regular. Hand warm and dry; hand skin tone consistent with left hand. Pressure dressing applied to site. Patient denies pain, nausea, shortness of breath. Vital signs stable before, during and after procedure. See flow sheet.—B. Clapp, RN

Unexpected Situations and Associated Interventions

- *You note fresh blood on the site dressing:* Apply pressure. If bleeding continues, notify the physician or primary care professional.
- *The patient has a history of peripheral vascular disease:* Assess the peripheral circulation for changes; if necessary, apply slightly decreased pressure at the insertion site.
- *Affected extremity is cold and/or pulseless:* Immediately notify physician or primary care professional.
- *Patient complains of severe back pain or noted to be hypotensive:* Symptoms may be due to retroperitoneal bleeding. Notify physician or primary care professional immediately.

Special Considerations

General Considerations

- If the physician has ordered a culture of the catheter tip (to diagnose a suspected infection), gently place the catheter tip on a 4 × 4 sterile gauze pad. When the bleeding is under control, hold the catheter over the sterile container. Using sterile scissors, cut the tip so it falls into the sterile container. Label the specimen and send it to the laboratory.

SKILL 16-5 Performing Cardiopulmonary Resuscitation (CPR)

Cardiopulmonary resuscitation (CPR), also known as basic life support, is used in the absence of spontaneous respirations and heartbeat to preserve heart and brain function while waiting for defibrillation and advanced cardiac life-support care. It is a combination of "mouth-to-mouth" or rescue breathing, which supplies oxygen to the lungs, and chest compressions, which manually pump the heart to circulate blood to the body systems.

Assess the patient, activate the emergency response system, and perform the ABCDs. Remember the ABCs of CPR—airway, breathing, and circulation—followed by the 'D' of defibrillation to manage sudden cardiac death (American Heart Association [AHA], 2005).

In the hospital setting, it is imperative that personnel be aware of the patient's stated instructions regarding a wish not to be resuscitated. This should be clearly expressed and documented in the patient's medical record.

Equipment

- Personal protective equipment such as a face shield or one-way valve mask and gloves, if available
- Ambu-bag and oxygen, if available

ASSESSMENT

Assess the patient's vital parameters and determine the patient's level of responsiveness. Check for partial or complete airway obstruction. Assess for the absence or ineffectiveness of respirations. Assess for the absence of signs of circulation and pulses.

NURSING DIAGNOSIS

Determine the related factors for the nursing diagnoses based on the patient's current status. Appropriate nursing diagnoses may include:

SKILL 16-5

Performing Cardiopulmonary Resuscitation (CPR) *(continued)*

- Decreased Cardiac Output
- Ineffective Airway Clearance
- Impaired Gas Exchange
- Inability to Sustain Spontaneous Ventilation
- Ineffective Tissue Perfusion
- Risk for Aspiration
- Risk for Injury

Many other nursing diagnoses may require the use of this skill.

OUTCOME IDENTIFICATION AND PLANNING

The expected outcome to achieve when performing CPR is that CPR is performed effectively without adverse effect to the patient. Additional outcomes include: the patient regains a pulse and respirations; the patient's heart and lungs maintain adequate function to sustain life; and advanced cardiac life support is initiated. Another appropriate outcome may be that the patient does not experience injury.

IMPLEMENTATION

ACTION	RATIONALE
1. Assess responsiveness. If the patient is not responsive, call for help, pull call bell, and call the facility emergency response number. Call for the automated external defibrillator (AED).	Assessing responsiveness prevents starting CPR on a conscious victim. Activating the emergency response system initiates a rapid response.
2. Put on gloves, if available. Position the patient supine on his or her back on a firm, flat surface, with arms alongside the body. If the patient is in bed, place a backboard or other rigid surface under the patient (often the footboard of the patient's bed).	Gloves prevent contact with blood and body fluids. Position required for resuscitative efforts and evaluation to be effective. If the patient must be rolled, move as a unit so the head, shoulders, and torso move simultaneously without twisting.
3. Use the head tilt–chin lift maneuver to open the airway (Figure 1). Place one hand on the victim's forehead and apply firm, backward pressure with the palm to tilt the head back. Place the fingers of the other hand under the bony part of the lower jaw near the chin and lift the jaw upward to bring the chin forward and the teeth almost to occlusion. If trauma to the head or neck is present or suspected, use the jaw-thrust maneuver to open the airway (Figure 2). Place one hand on each side of the patient's head. Rest elbows on the flat surface under the patient, grasp the angle of the patient's lower jaw and lift with both hands.	This maneuver may be enough to open the airway and promote spontaneous respirations.
4. Look, listen, and feel for air exchange.	These techniques provide information about the patient's breathing and the need for rescue breathing.
5. If the patient resumes breathing or adequate respirations and signs of circulation are noted, place the patient in the recovery position.	Maintains alignment of the back and spine while allowing for continued observation and maintains access to the patient.

(continued)

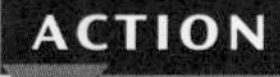

SKILL 16-5 Performing Cardiopulmonary Resuscitation (CPR) *(continued)*

ACTION | **RATIONALE**

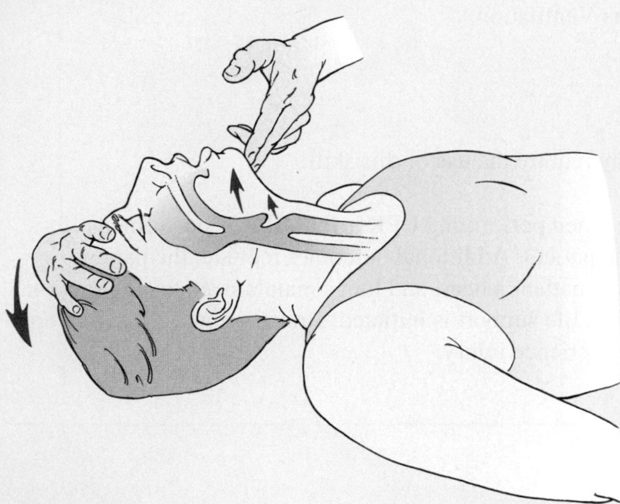

Figure 1. Using the head tilt–chin lift method to open the airway.

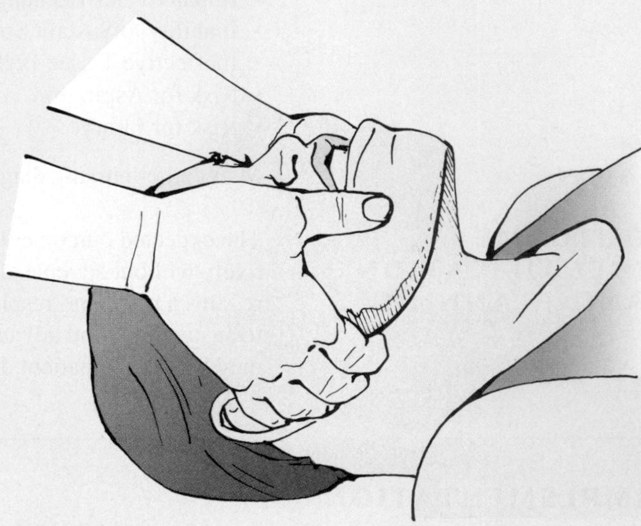

Figure 2. Using the jaw-thrust maneuver to open the airway.

6. If no spontaneous breathing is noted, seal the patient's mouth and nose with the face shield, one-way valve mask, or Ambu-bag (resuscitation bag), if available (Figures 3 and 4). If not available, seal mouth with your mouth.

Sealing the patient's mouth and nose prevents air from escaping. Devices such as masks reduce the risk for transmission of infections.

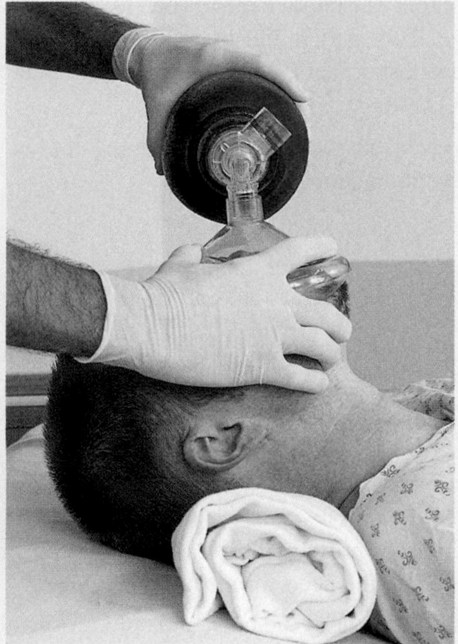

Figure 3. Using hand-held resuscitation bag. *(Photo © B. Proud.)*

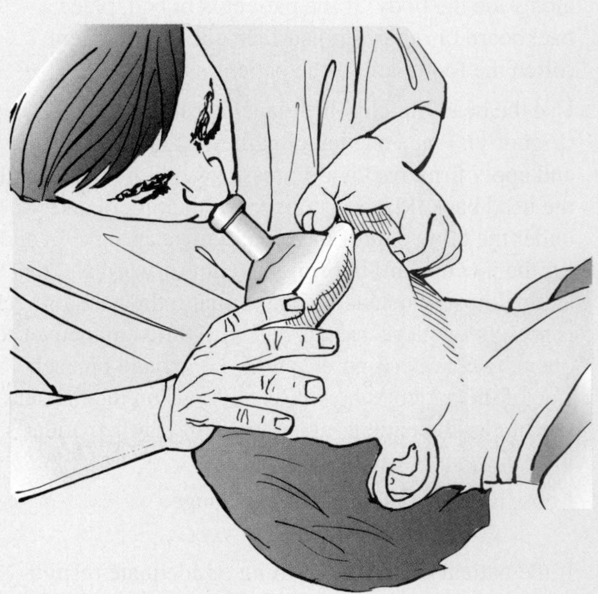

Figure 4. One-way valve mask.

SKILL 16-5 Performing Cardiopulmonary Resuscitation (CPR) *(continued)*

ACTION	RATIONALE
7. Instill two breaths, each lasting 1 second, making the chest rise.	Breathing into the patient provides oxygen to the patient's lungs. Hyperventilation results in increased positive chest pressure and decreased venous return. Blood flow to the lungs during CPR is only about 25%–33% normal; patient requires less ventilation to provide oxygen and remove carbon dioxide. Longer breaths reduce the amount of blood that refills the heart, reducing blood flow generated by compressions. Delivery of large, forceful breaths may cause gastric inflation and distension.
8. If you are unable to ventilate or the chest does not rise during ventilation, reposition the patient's head and reattempt to ventilate. If still unable to ventilate, inspect oral airway. Remove any foreign matter or vomitus that is visible in the mouth. Use suction to remove material, if available. Perform five abdominal thrusts to remove the obstruction (Figure 5). If patient is obese or pregnant, perform five chest thrusts. Chest thrusts are delivered with the hands in the same position, using the same technique, as that for chest compressions during CPR. Attempt to ventilate. Repeat this cycle as necessary.	Inability to ventilate indicates that the airway may still be obstructed. These maneuvers may be enough to open the airway and promote spontaneous respirations. Abdominal thrusts help to move the obstruction.

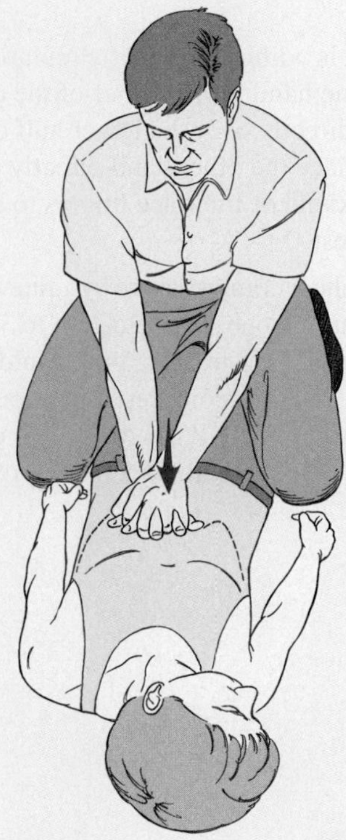

Figure 5. Attempting to clear an obstruction using abdominal thrusts.

ACTION	RATIONALE
9. Check the carotid pulse, simultaneously evaluating for breathing, coughing, or movement. This assessment should take no more than 10 seconds. Place the patient in the recovery position if breathing resumes (Figure 6).	Pulse and other assessments evaluate cardiac function. The femoral pulse may be used for the pulse check.

(continued)

SKILL 16-5 Performing Cardiopulmonary Resuscitation (CPR) *(continued)*

ACTION	RATIONALE

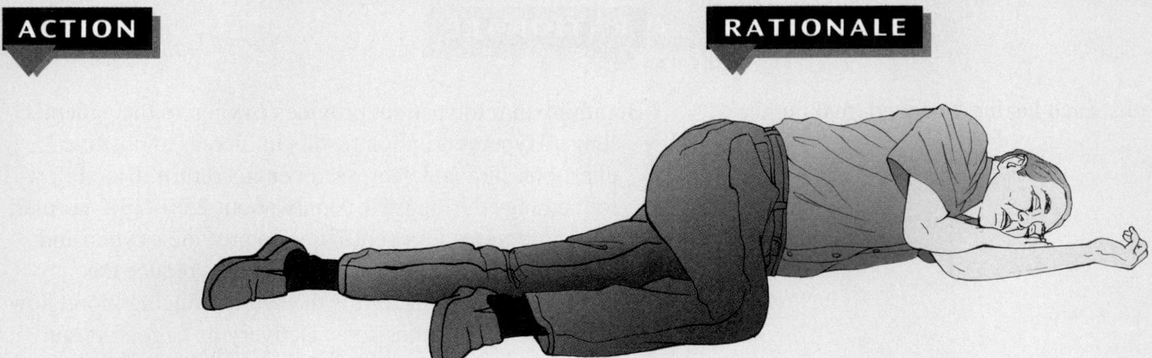

Figure 6. Recovery position.

ACTION	RATIONALE
10. If patient has a pulse, but remains without spontaneous breathing, continue rescue breathing at a rate of one breath every 5–6 seconds, for a rate of 10–12 breaths per minute.	Rescue breathing maintains adequate oxygenation.
11. If the patient is without signs of circulation, position the heel of one hand in the center of the chest between the nipples, directly over the lower half of the sternum (Figure 7). Place the other hand directly on top of the first hand. Extend or interlace fingers to keep fingers above the chest.	A backboard provides a firm surface on which to apply compressions. Proper hand positioning ensures that the force of compressions is on the sternum, thereby reducing the risk of rib fracture, lung puncture, or liver laceration.
12. Perform 30 chest compressions at a rate of 100 per minute, counting "one, two, etc." up to 30, keeping elbows locked, arms straight, and shoulders directly over the hands. Chest compressions should depress the sternum approximately ⅓ to ½ the depth of the chest. Allow full chest recoil after each compression (Figure 8).	Direct cardiac compression and manipulation of intrathoracic pressure supply blood flow during CPR. Compressing the chest ⅓ to ½ the depth of the chest ensures that compressions are not too shallow and provides adequate blood flow. Full chest recoil allows adequate venous return to the heart.

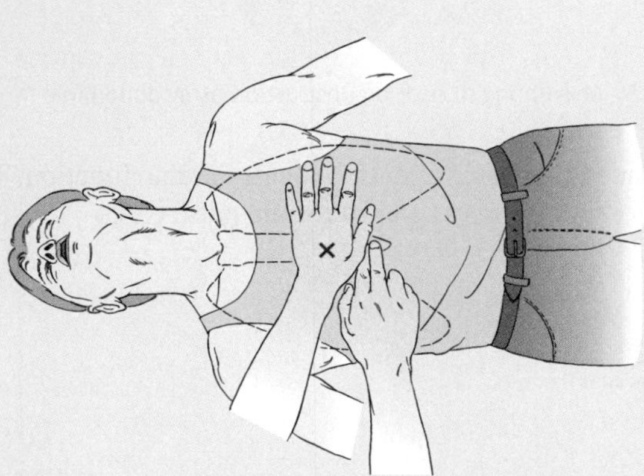

Figure 7. Using correct hand placement for chest compressions.

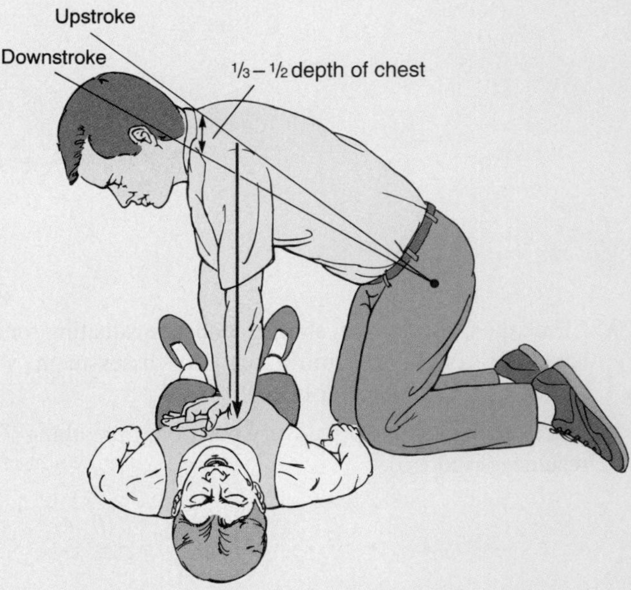

Figure 8. Using correct body alignment for chest compressions. Depressing sternum approx. ⅓ to ½ depth of chest.

SKILL 16-5 **Performing Cardiopulmonary Resuscitation (CPR)** *(continued)*

ACTION	RATIONALE
13. Give two rescue breaths after each set of 30 compressions. Do five complete cycles of 30 compressions and two ventilations.	Breathing and compressions simulate lung and heart function, providing oxygen and circulation.
14. Reassess breathing and circulation after each set of five compression/breathing cycles. Take no more than 10 seconds to do this.	Reassessment determines the need for continued CPR.
15. Defibrillation should be provided at the earliest possible moment, as soon as AED available. Refer to Skill 16-6: Automated External Defibrillation and Skill 16-7: Manual External Defibrillation.	The interval from collapse to defibrillation is the most important determinant of survival from cardiac arrest (AHA, 2005; Mims et al, 2004).
16. Continue CPR until the patient resumes spontaneous breathing and circulation, medical help arrives, you are too exhausted to continue, or a physician discontinues CPR.	Once started, CPR must continue until one of these conditions is met. In a hospital setting, help should arrive within a few minutes.

EVALUATION

The expected outcome is achieved when CPR is performed effectively without adverse effect to the patient; the patient regains a pulse and respirations; the patient's heart and lungs maintain adequate function to sustain life; advanced cardiac life support is initiated; and the patient does not experience injury.

DOCUMENTATION

Guidelines

Document the time you discovered the patient unresponsive and started CPR. Continued intervention, such as by the code team, is typically documented on a code form, which identifies the actions and drugs provided during the code. Provide a summary of these events in the patient's medical record.

Sample Documentation

07/06/08 2230 Called to patient's room by wife. Patient noted to be without evidence of respirations or circulation. Emergency response system activated, CPR initiated. See code sheet.—B. Clapp, RN

Unexpected Situations and Associated Interventions

- *When performing chest compression, you hear something crack:* Most commonly this sound indicates cracking of the ribs. Recheck your hand position. Then continue compressions.
- *You come upon a patient lying on the floor:* Determine the patient's level of responsiveness. If the patient is unresponsive, quickly clear an area, call for assistance and AED, and begin CPR.

Special Considerations

General Considerations

- For a choking conscious patient exhibiting signs of severe obstruction (inability to speak), perform the Heimlich maneuver until the obstruction is removed. If the patient is obese or pregnant, use chest thrusts.

(continued)

SKILL 16-5 Performing Cardiopulmonary Resuscitation (CPR) *(continued)*

- Perform CPR in the same manner if the patient is obese.
- Perform CPR for pregnant patients using the same guidelines, with a few additional measures. Before initiating chest compressions, the uterus is displaced to decrease aortocaval compression and subsequent hypotension (Martin, 2003). This is accomplished in one of two ways. Place a rolled towel or a wedge under the woman's right hip to tip the uterus toward her left hip. Care must be taken to avoid tilting her shoulder as well, resulting in decreased effectiveness of chest compressions. Alternately, the uterus can be manually displaced. Stand on the patient's left side. Use both arms to pull the uterus toward the left. Use additional pressure with chest compressions. Pregnancy-related decreased chest-wall compliance decreases the efficiency of chest compressions (Martin, 2003).
- If you cannot completely seal the patient's mouth for reasons such as oral trauma, perform mouth-to-nose breathing. If the patient has a tracheostomy, provide ventilations through the tracheostomy instead of the mouth.

Infant and Child Considerations

- As soon as it is determined that an infant or child is unresponsive, shout for help. If you are alone, CPR should be initiated immediately and provided for approximately 2 minutes at the rate of 100 compressions per minute (compression-to-ventilation ratio 30 to 2), before leaving the infant/child to activate the emergency response system. If the child is small and it is safe to do so, consider carrying the child with you to activate the emergency response system.
- If the victim is under 12 to 14 years of age, use the heel of one or two hands to provide chest compressions, based on child's body size. Depth of compressions remains the same; ⅓ to ½ depth of chest.
- For an infant under 1 year of age, use two or three fingers placed in the midline one fingerbreadth below the nipple line and compress ⅓ to ½ depth of chest.
- To open the airway of a child, place one hand on the child's forehead and gently lift the chin with the other hand (called the sniffing position in infants). If head or neck injury is suspected, use the jaw-thrust method.
- If available, use a one-way valve mask over the child's nose and mouth when performing CPR.
- Rescue breathing for infants and children with a pulse are provided at a rate of one breath every 3 to 5 seconds, to deliver 12 to 20 breaths per minute.

SKILL 16-6 Performing Emergency Automated External Defibrillation

The most frequent initial cardiac rhythm in witnessed sudden cardiac arrest is ventricular fibrillation (AHA, 2005). Electrical defibrillation is the most effective treatment for ventricular fibrillation and early defibrillation is critical to increase patient survival (AHA, 2005; Dwyer et al, 2004). Electrical therapy can be administered by defibrillation, cardioversion, or a pacemaker (see Fundamentals Review 16-1 at the beginning of the chapter). Defibrillation delivers large amounts of electric current to a patient over brief periods of time. It is the standard treatment for ventricular fibrillation (VF) and is also used to treat pulseless ventricular tachycardia (VT). The goal is to temporarily depolarize the irregularly beating heart and allow more coordinated contractile activity to resume. It does so by completely depolarizing the myocardium, producing a momentary asystole. This provides an opportunity for the natural pacemaker centers of the heart to resume normal activity. The automated external defibrillator (AED) is a portable exter-

SKILL 16-6
Performing Emergency Automated External Defibrillation *(continued)*

nal defibrillator that automatically detects and interprets the heart's rhythm and informs the operator if a shock is indicated (Dwyer et al, 2004). AEDs are appropriate for use in situations where the patient is unresponsive, not breathing and has no pulse (AHA, 2005; Dwyer et al, 2004; *Nursing procedures* . . . , 2005). The defibrillator responds to the patient information by advising 'shock' or 'no shock.' Fully automatic models automatically perform rhythm analysis and shock if indicated. These are usually found in out-of-hospital settings (Mims et al, 2004; Vines, 2004). Semiautomatic models require the operator to press an 'Analyze' button to initiate rhythm analysis and then press a 'Shock' button to deliver the shock if indicated. Semiautomatic models are usually found in the hospital setting (Mims et al, 2004; Vines, 2004). AEDs will not deliver a shock unless the electrode pads are correctly attached and a shockable rhythm is detected. Some AEDs have motion-detection devices that ensure the defibrillator will not discharge if there is motion, such as motion from personnel in contact with the patient. The strength of the charge is preset. Once the pads are in place and the device is turned on, follow the prompts given by the device. The following guidelines are based on the American Heart Association (AHA, 2005) guidelines. AHA guidelines state that these recommendations may be modified for the in-hospital setting, where continuous electrocardiographic or hemodynamic monitoring may be in place. Current recommendations call for the application of the AED as soon as it is available, allowing for analysis of cardiac status and delivery of an initial shock, if indicated, for adults and children. After initial shock, deliver 5 cycles of chest compressions/ventilations (30/2), and then reanalyze cardiac rhythm. Provide sets of 1 shock alternating with 2 minutes of CPR until the AED indicates a 'no shock indicated' message or until ACLS is available (AHA, 2005).

In the hospital setting, it is imperative that personnel be aware of the patient's stated instructions regarding a wish not to be resuscitated. This should be clearly expressed and documented in the patient's medical record.

Equipment

- Automated external defibrillator (AED)
- Self-adhesive pregelled monitor-defibrillator pads (6)
- Cables to connect the pads and AED
- Razor
- Towel

Some models have the pads, cables, and AED preconnected.

ASSESSMENT

Assess the patient for unresponsiveness, effective breathing, and signs of circulation. Assess the patient's vital parameters and determine the patient's level of responsiveness. Check for partial or complete airway obstruction. Assess for the absence or ineffectiveness of respirations. Assess for the absence of signs of circulation and pulses. AEDs should be used only when a patient is unresponsive, not breathing, and without signs of circulation (pulseless, lack of effective respirations, coughing, moving). Determine whether special situations exist that require additional actions before the AED is used or contraindicate its use. Refer to Box 16-2, Special Situations Related to AED, for details of these situations and appropriate actions.

(continued)

SKILL 16-6 Performing Emergency Automated External Defibrillation *(continued)*

BOX 16-2 Special Situations Related to Automated External Defibrillation (AED)

- ***The patient is less than 8 years of age or weighs less than approximately 55 lbs (25 kg).*** Currently available AEDs deliver energy doses that exceed the recommended pediatric dose of 2 to 4 joules/kg in most children less than 8 years old. In hospital situations, weight-based manual defibrillation should be administered. Weight-based manual dosing: First shock—2 joules/kg; second—4 joules/kg; third—4 joules/kg (AHA, 2005; Urden et al, 2002).
- ***The patient is in or near standing water.*** Water is a good conductor of electricity. Defibrillation administered to a patient in water could result in shocking the AED operator and bystanders. Another possible effect is that water on the patient's skin will provide a direct path for the electrical current from one electrode to the other. The arcing of the electrical current between the electrodes bypasses the heart, resulting in the delivery of inadequate current to the heart. Patients should be removed from standing water and the chest quickly dried before initiating AED.
- ***The patient has an implanted pacemaker.*** Place the AED electrode pad at least 1″ to the side of the implanted device. If an AED electrode pad is placed directly over an implanted device, the device may block delivery of the shock to the heart. If the implanted device is delivering shocks to the patient (observed external chest muscle contractions), wait 30 to 60 seconds for the device to complete the treatment cycle before delivering a shock from the AED.
- ***A transdermal medication patch or other object is located on the patient's skin where the electrode pads are to be placed.*** Remove the patch and wipe the area clean before attaching the electrode pads. Do not place the electrode pad directly on top of a medication patch. The patch may block the delivery of energy to the heart.

(Adapted from American Heart Association. [2002]. *BLS for healthcare providers.* Dallas, TX: Author.)

NURSING DIAGNOSIS

Determine the related factors for the nursing diagnoses based on the patient's current status. Appropriate nursing diagnoses may include:

- Decreased Cardiac Output
- Ineffective Airway Clearance
- Impaired Gas Exchange
- Inability to Sustain Spontaneous Ventilation
- Ineffective Tissue Perfusion
- Risk for Injury

Many other nursing diagnoses may require the use of this skill.

OUTCOME IDENTIFICATION AND PLANNING

The expected outcome to achieve when performing automatic external defibrillation is that it is performed correctly without adverse effect to the patient, and the patient regains signs of circulation, with organized electrical rhythm and pulse. Additional outcomes include: the patient regains respirations; the patient's heart and lungs maintain adequate function to sustain life; the patient does not experience injury; and advanced cardiac life support is initiated.

IMPLEMENTATION

ACTION	RATIONALE
1. Assess responsiveness. If the patient is not responsive, call for help and pull call bell, and call the facility emergency response number. Call for the AED. Perform cardiopulmonary resuscitation (CPR) until the defibrillator and other emergency equipment arrive.	Assessing responsiveness prevents starting CPR on a conscious victim. Activating the emergency response system initiates a rapid response. Initiating CPR preserves heart and brain function while awaiting defibrillation.

SKILL 16-6

Performing Emergency Automated External Defibrillation *(continued)*

ACTION	RATIONALE
2. Prepare the AED. Power on the AED. Push the power button. Some devices will turn on automatically when the lid or case are opened.	Proper setup ensures proper functioning.
3. Attach AED connecting cables to the AED (may be preconnected). Attach AED cables to the adhesive electrode pads (may be preconnected).	Proper setup ensures proper functioning.
4. Stop chest compressions. Peel away the covering from the electrode pads to expose the adhesive surface. Attach the electrode pads to the patient's chest. Place one pad on the upper right sternal border, directly below the clavicle. Place the second pad lateral to the left nipple, with the top margin of the pad a few inches below the axilla (Figure 1).	Proper setup ensures proper functioning. The use of self-adhesive pads allows hands-free defibrillation and excellent skin–electrode contact, which provides lower impedance, less artifact, and greater user safety (Dwyer et al, 2004).
5. Once the pads are in place and the device is turned on, follow the prompts given by the device. Clear the patient and analyze the rhythm. Ensure no one is touching the patient. Loudly state a 'Clear the patient' message. Press 'Analyze' button to initiate analysis, if necessary. Some devices automatically begin analysis when the pads are attached. Avoid all movement affecting the patient during analysis.	Movement and electrical impulses cause artifact during analysis. Avoidance of artifact ensures accurate rhythm analysis and accidental shock to personnel.
6. If ventricular tachycardia or ventricular fibrillation is present, the device will announce that a shock is indicated and begin charging. Once the AED is charged, a message will be delivered to shock the patient.	Shock message is delivered through a written message or visual on the AED screen, an auditory alarm, or a voice-synthesized statement.

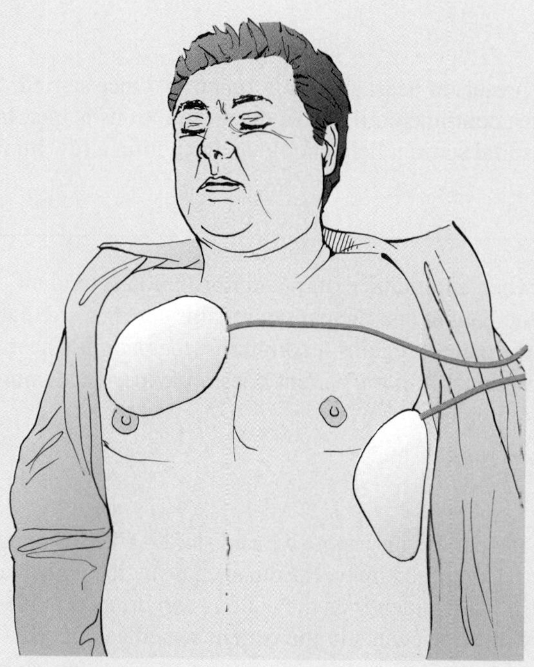

Figure 1. AED electrode pad placement.

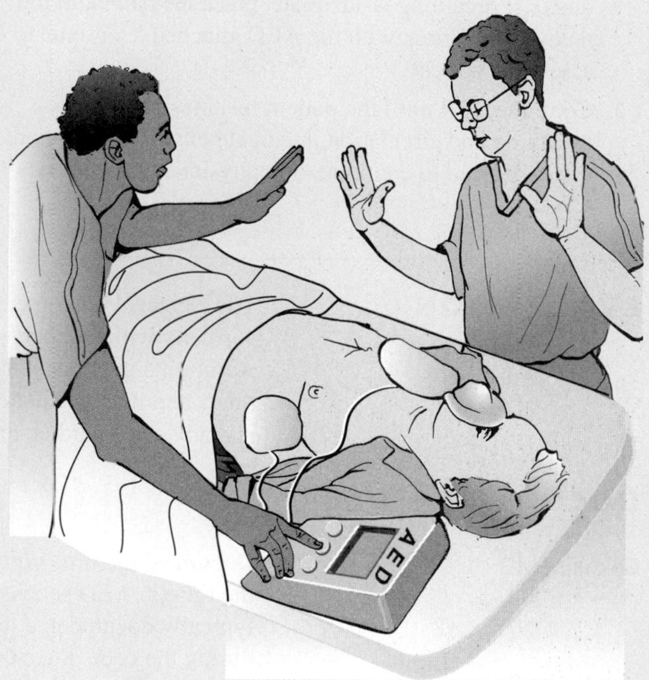

Figure 2. Clearing the patient.

(continued)

SKILL 16-6 Performing Emergency Automated External Defibrillation *(continued)*

ACTION	RATIONALE
7. Before pressing the 'Shock' button, loudly state a 'Clear the patient' message. Visually check that no one is in contact with the patient (Figure 2). Press the 'Shock' button. If the AED is fully automatic, a shock will be delivered automatically.	Avoids accidental shocking of personnel.
8. After the first shock, check the patient for signs of circulation, including a pulse. If the patient is without signs of circulation, resume CPR for 2 minutes. Rhythm checks should be performed every 2 minutes.	Provides optimal treatment. This is based on AHA 2005 recommended guidelines. Some AEDs in the community for use by lay persons are automatically programmed to cycle through three analysis/shock cycles in one set. Be familiar with type of AED available for use.
9. After any 'no shock indicated' message, or 2 minutes, check the patient for signs of circulation, including a pulse. If no signs of circulation are present, press 'Analyze' on the AED. Defibrillate if indicated by the AED. Continue with CPR and AED interpretation until the AED gives a 'no shock indicated' message, the patient exhibits signs of circulation, or until ACLS is available. If signs of circulation do not return after an additional shock, resume CPR for 2 minutes.	Reassessment determines the need for continued intervention. Provides optimal treatment. CPR preserves heart and brain function.
10. Continue with CPR and AED interpretation until the AED gives a 'no shock indicated' message, the patient exhibits signs of circulation, or until ACLS is available.	Reassessment determines the need for continued intervention. Provides optimal treatment.
11. When 'no shock indicated' message is received, check for signs of circulation. If signs of circulation are present, check breathing. If breathing is inadequate, assist breathing. Start rescue breathing (1 breath every 5 seconds). If breathing is adequate, place the patient in the recovery position, with the AED attached. Continue to assess the patient.	Reassessment determines the need for continued intervention. Provides optimal treatment.
12. Continue CPR until the patient resumes spontaneous breathing and circulation, medical help arrives, you are too exhausted to continue, or a physician discontinues CPR.	CPR preserves heart and brain function. Once started, CPR must continue until one of these conditions is met. In a hospital setting, help should arrive within a few minutes.

EVALUATION

The expected outcome is achieved when automatic external defibrillation is applied correctly without adverse effect to the patient and the patient regains signs of circulation. Additional outcomes may include: the patient regains respirations; the patient's heart and lungs maintain adequate function to sustain life; the patient does not experience injury; and advanced cardiac life support is initiated.

DOCUMENTATION

Guidelines

Document the time you discovered the patient unresponsive and started CPR. Document the time(s) AED shocks are initiated. Continued intervention, such as by the code team, is typically documented on a code form, which identifies the actions and drugs provided during the code. Provide a summary of these events in the patient's medical record.

SKILL 16-6 Performing Emergency Automated External Defibrillation *(continued)*

Sample Documentation

07/06/08 2230 Called to patient's room by wife. Patient noted to be without evidence of respirations or circulation. Emergency response system activated, CPR initiated. AED applied at 2232. See code sheet.—B. Clapp, RN

Unexpected Situations and Associated Interventions

- *A 'Check pads' or 'Check electrodes' message appears on the AED:* The electrode pads are not securely attached to the chest or the cables are not securely fastened. Check that the pads are firmly and evenly adhered to the patient's skin. Verify connections between the cables and the AED and the cables and electrode pads. Check that the patient is not wet or diaphoretic, or has excessive chest hair. See actions below for appropriate interventions in these situations.
- *The patient has a hairy chest:* The adhesive electrode pads may stick to the hair of the chest instead of the skin, preventing adequate contact with the skin. Press firmly on the current pads to attempt to provide sufficient adhesion. If unsuccessful, briskly remove the current pads to remove a good portion of the chest hair. Apply a second set of electrode pads over the same sites. Attempt rhythm analysis. If error message appears again, remove the second set of pads. Clip or shave the area. Apply a third set of pads. Continue with the procedure.
- *The patient is noticeably diaphoretic or the skin is wet:* The electrode pads will not attach firmly to wet or diaphoretic skin. Dry the chest with a cloth or towel before attaching the electrode pads.

Special Considerations

General Considerations

- Appropriate maintenance of the AED is critical for proper operation. Check the AED for any visible signs of damage. Check the 'ready for use' indicator on the AED daily. Perform maintenance according to the manufacturer's recommendations and facility policy.

Infant and Child Considerations

- Automatic external defibrillators effectively detect ventricular fibrillation and ventricular tachycardia in children, but the preset energy levels are inappropriate for use with children under 8 years of age or under approximately 55 lbs (25 kg) (AHA, 2005; Dwyer, 2004).

SKILL 16-7 Performing Emergency Manual External Defibrillation (Asynchronous)

Electrical therapy is used to quickly terminate or control potentially lethal arrhythmias. Electrical therapy can be administered by defibrillation, cardioversion, or a pacemaker. Defibrillation delivers large amounts of electric current to a patient over brief periods of time. It is the standard treatment for ventricular fibrillation (VF) and is also used to treat ventricular tachycardia (VT), in which the patient has no pulse. The goal is to temporarily depolarize the irregularly beating heart and allow more coordinated contractile activity to resume. It does so by completely depolarizing the myocardium, producing a momentary asystole. This provides an opportunity for the natural pacemaker centers of the heart to resume normal activity. The electrode paddles delivering the current may be placed on the patient's chest or, during cardiac surgery, directly on the myocardium. Because ventricular fibrillation leads to death if not corrected, the success of defibrillation depends on early recognition and quick treatment of this arrhythmia.

Manual defibrillation depends upon the operator for analysis of rhythm, charging, proper application of the paddles to the patient's thorax, and delivery of countershock. It

(continued)

SKILL 16-7 Performing Emergency Manual External Defibrillation (Asynchronous) *(continued)*

requires the user to have immediate and accurate arrhythmia recognition skills (Dwyer et al, 2004; Vines, 2004). The following guidelines are based on the American Heart Association 2005 guidelines. AHA guidelines state that these recommendations may be modified for the in-hospital setting, where continuous electrocardiographic or hemodynamic monitoring may be in place.

In the hospital setting, it is imperative that personnel be aware of the patient's stated instructions regarding a wish not to be resuscitated. This should be clearly expressed and documented in the patient's medical record.

Equipment

- Defibrillator (monophasic or biphasic)
- External paddles (or internal paddles sterilized for cardiac surgery)
- Conductive medium pads
- Electrocardiogram (ECG) monitor with recorder (often part of the defibrillator)
- Oxygen therapy equipment
- Hand-held resuscitation bag
- Airway equipment
- Emergency pacing equipment
- Emergency cardiac medications

ASSESSMENT

Assess the patient for unresponsiveness, effective breathing, and signs of circulation. Assess the patient's vital parameters and determine the patient's level of responsiveness. Check for partial or complete airway obstruction. Assess for the absence or ineffectiveness of respirations. Assess for the absence of signs of circulation and pulses. Call for help and perform cardiopulmonary resuscitation (CPR) until the defibrillator and other emergency equipment arrive.

NURSING DIAGNOSIS

Determine the related factors for the nursing diagnoses based on the patient's current status. Appropriate nursing diagnoses may include:

- Decreased Cardiac Output
- Ineffective Airway Clearance
- Impaired Gas Exchange
- Inability to Sustain Spontaneous Ventilation
- Ineffective Peripheral Tissue Perfusion
- Risk for Injury

Many other nursing diagnoses may require the use of this skill.

OUTCOME IDENTIFICATION AND PLANNING

The expected outcome to achieve when performing manual external defibrillation is that it is performed correctly without adverse effect to the patient, and the patient regains signs of circulation. Additional outcomes may include: the patient regains respirations; the patient's heart and lungs maintain adequate function to sustain life; the patient does not experience injury; and advanced cardiac life support is initiated.

IMPLEMENTATION

ACTION	RATIONALE
1. Assess responsiveness. If the patient is not responsive, call for help and pull call bell, and call the facility emergency response number. Call for the AED. Perform cardiopulmonary resuscitation (CPR) until the defibrillator and other emergency equipment arrive.	Assessing responsiveness prevents starting CPR on a conscious victim. Activating the emergency response system initiates a rapid response. Initiating CPR preserves heart and brain function while awaiting defibrillation.

SKILL 16-7 Performing Emergency Manual External Defibrillation (Asynchronous) *(continued)*

ACTION	RATIONALE
2. Turn on the defibrillator.	Charging and placement prepare for defibrillation.
3. If the defibrillator has "quick-look" capability, place the paddles on the patient's chest. Otherwise, connect the monitoring leads of the defibrillator to the patient and assess the cardiac rhythm.	Connecting the monitor leads to the patient allows for a quick view of the cardiac rhythm.
4. Expose the patient's chest, and apply conductive pads at the paddle placement positions. For anterolateral placement, place one paddle to the right of the upper sternum, just below the right clavicle, and the other over the fifth or sixth intercostal space at the left anterior axillary line (Figure 1). 'Hands-free' defibrillator pads can be used with the same placement positions, if available. For anteroposterior placement, place the anterior paddle directly over the heart at the precordium, to the left of the lower sternal border. Place the flat posterior paddle under the patient's body beneath the heart and immediately below the scapulae (but not on the vertebral column) (Figure 2).	This placement ensures that the electrical stimulus needs to travel only a short distance to the heart.

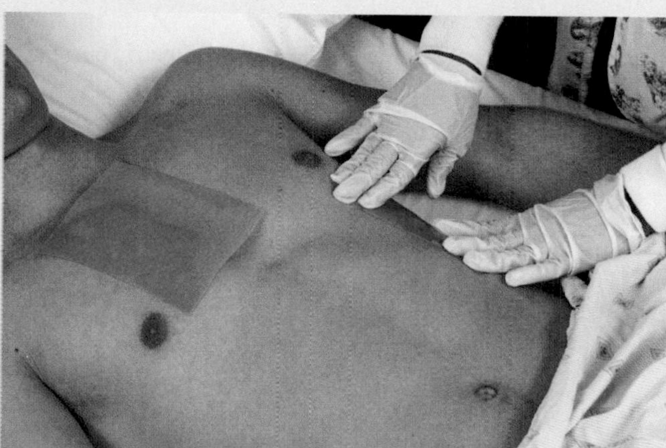

Figure 1. Anterolateral placement of defibrillator pads.

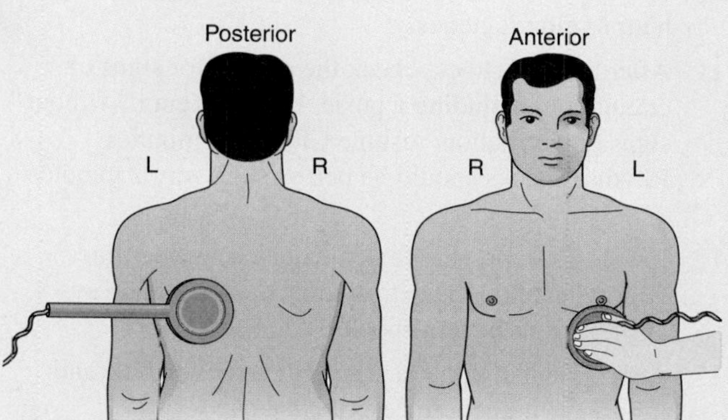

Figure 2. Anteroposterior placement of defibrillator pads. From Smeltzer, S. C., Bare, B. G., et al. (2008). *Brunner and Suddarth's Textbook of medical-surgical nursing* (11th ed.). Philadelphia: Lippincott Williams & Wilkins.

ACTION	RATIONALE
5. Set the energy level for 360 joules for an adult patient when using monophasic defibrillator. Use clinically appropriate energy levels for biphasic defibrillators, beginning with 150 to 200 J (AHA, 2005).	Proper setup ensures proper functioning.
6. Charge the paddles by pressing the charge buttons, which are located either on the machine or on the paddles themselves.	Proper setup ensures proper functioning.
7. **Place the paddles over the conductive pads (Figure 3) and press firmly against the patient's chest, using 25 lb (11 kg) of pressure.**	Proper setup ensures proper functioning. Solid adhesion is necessary for conduction.

(continued)

SKILL 16-7 Performing Emergency Manual External Defibrillation (Asynchronous) *(continued)*

ACTION	RATIONALE
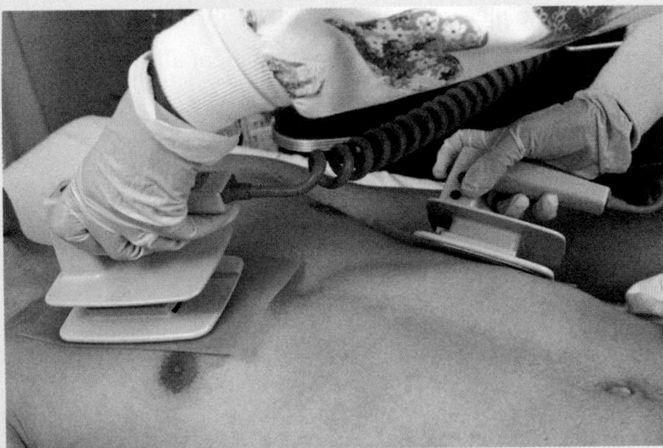 Figure 3. Placing paddles on the patient's chest.	
8. Reassess the cardiac rhythm.	The rhythm may have changed during preparation.
9. **If the patient remains in VF or pulseless VT, instruct all personnel to stand clear of the patient and the bed, including the operator.**	Standing clear of the bed and patient helps prevent electrical shocks to personnel.
10. Discharge the current by pressing both paddle charge buttons simultaneously.	Pressing the charge buttons discharges the electric current for defibrillation.
11. After the first shock, check the patient for signs of circulation, including a pulse. If the patient is without signs of circulation, resume CPR for 2 minutes. Rhythm checks should be performed every 2 minutes.	Provides optimal treatment. This is based on AHA 2005 recommended guidelines. Some AEDs in the community for use by lay persons are automatically programmed to cycle through three analysis/shock cycles in one set. Be familiar with type of AED available for use.
12. If necessary, prepare to defibrillate a second time. Energy level on the defibrillator should remain at 360 J for subsequent shocks (AHA, 2005).	Additional shocking may be needed to stimulate the heart.
13. Announce that you are preparing to defibrillate and follow the procedure described above.	
14. Reassess the patient.	Reassessment is necessary to determine whether perfusion has returned and to evaluate the effectiveness of treatment.
15. Reassess the patient for signs of circulation, including a pulse. If no signs of circulation are present, reassess heart rhythm. Defibrillate if indicated. Continue with CPR and rhythm interpretation until the patient exhibits adequate cardiac rhythm, signs of circulation, or until ACLS is available. If signs of circulation do not return after an additional shock, resume CPR for 2 minutes.	Reassessment determines the need for continued intervention. Provides optimal treatment. CPR preserves heart and brain function.
16. If defibrillation restores a normal rhythm:	The patient will need continuous monitoring to prevent further problems. Continuous monitoring helps provide for early detection and prompt intervention should additional problems arise.
a. Check for signs of circulation; check the central and peripheral pulses, and obtain a blood pressure reading, heart rate, and respiratory rate.	

SKILL 16-7

Performing Emergency Manual External Defibrillation (Asynchronous) *(continued)*

ACTION	RATIONALE
b. If signs of circulation are present, check breathing. If breathing is inadequate, assist breathing. Start rescue breathing (1 breath every 5 seconds).	Reassessment determines the need for continued intervention. Provides optimal treatment.
c. If breathing is adequate, place the patient in the recovery position. Continue to assess the patient.	
d. Assess the patient's level of consciousness, cardiac rhythm, breath sounds, and skin color and temperature.	
e. Obtain baseline ABG levels and a 12-lead ECG, if ordered.	
f. Provide supplemental oxygen, ventilation, and medications as needed.	
17. Check the chest for electrical burns and treat them, as ordered, with corticosteroid or lanolin-based creams. If using 'hands-free' pads, keep pads on in case of recurrent ventricular tachycardia or ventricular fibrillation.	
18. Prepare the defibrillator for immediate reuse.	

EVALUATION

The expected outcome is achieved when manual external defibrillation is performed correctly without adverse effect to the patient and the patient regains signs of circulation. Additional outcomes may include: the patient regains respirations; the patient's heart and lungs maintain adequate function to sustain life; the patient does not experience injury; and advanced cardiac life support is initiated.

DOCUMENTATION

Guidelines

Document the time you discovered the patient unresponsive and started CPR. Document the procedure, including the patient's ECG rhythms both before and after defibrillation; the number of times defibrillation was performed; the voltage used during each attempt; whether a pulse returned; the dosage, route, and time of drug administration; whether CPR was used; how the airway was maintained; and the patient's outcome. Continued intervention, such as by the code team, is typically documented on a code form, which identifies the actions and drugs provided during the code. Provide a summary of these events in the patient's medical record.

Sample Documentation

07/06/08 2230 Called to patient's room by wife. Patient noted to be without evidence of respirations or circulation. Emergency response system activated, CPR initiated. Manual defibrillation initiated at 2230. See code sheet.—B. Clapp, RN

Unexpected Situations and Associated Interventions

- *The defibrillator fails to fire:* Check that the power is turned on. If the defibrillator is not plugged in, check if the battery is low. Check that it is fully charged.
- *The patient develops a skin burn at the site of the pad placement:* In most cases, an insufficient amount of conductive medium is the cause. Prepare to treat the burn area as ordered, such as with corticosteroid or lanolin-based creams.

(continued)

SKILL 16-7 Performing Emergency Manual External Defibrillation (Asynchronous) *(continued)*

Special Considerations

General Considerations

- Defibrillation can cause accidental electric shock to those providing care.
- Defibrillators vary from one manufacturer to the next, so familiarize yourself with your facility's equipment. Defibrillator operation should be checked at least every 8 hours, or per facility policy, and after each use.
- Defibrillation can be affected by several factors, including paddle size and placement, condition of the patient's myocardium, duration of the arrhythmia, chest resistance, and the number of countershocks.

Infant and Child Considerations

- Weight-based manual defibrillation dosing is required for children under 8 years of age or 55 pounds (25 kg). First shock—2 joules/kg; second—4 joules/kg; third—4 joules/kg (Urden et al, 2002; American Heart Association, 2005).

SKILL 16-8 Using an External (Transcutaneous) Pacemaker

A temporary pacemaker consists of an external, battery-powered pulse generator and a lead or electrode system to electrically stimulate heartbeat. Transcutaneous pacing can temporarily supply an electrical current in the heart when electrical conduction is abnormal. In a life-threatening situation, when time is critical, a transcutaneous pacemaker is the best choice. This device works by sending an electrical impulse from the pulse generator to the patient's heart by way of two electrodes, which are placed on the front and back of the patient's chest. This stimulates the contraction of cardiac muscle fibers through electrical stimulation (depolarization) of the myocardium. Transcutaneous pacing is quick and effective but is usually used as short-term therapy until the situation resolves or the physician can institute transvenous pacing. Transcutaneous pacing is contraindicated in patients with severe hypothermia and prolonged brady-asystolic cardiac arrest (Craig, 2005).

Equipment

- Transcutaneous pacing generator
- Transcutaneous pacing electrodes
- Cardiac monitor

ASSESSMENT

Review the patient's medical record and plan of care for information about the patient's need for pacing. Transcutaneous pacing is generally an emergency measure. Assess the patient's initial cardiac rhythm, including a rhythm strip and 12-lead ECG. Monitor heart rate, respiratory rate, level of consciousness, and skin color. If pulselessness occurs, initiate CPR.

NURSING DIAGNOSIS

Determine the related factors for the nursing diagnoses based on the patient's current status. Appropriate nursing diagnoses include:

- Decreased Cardiac Output
- Ineffective Cardiopulmonary Tissue Perfusion
- Anxiety
- Deficient Knowledge
- Ineffective Peripheral Tissue Perfusion
- Risk for Injury

Many other nursing diagnoses also may require the use of this skill.

SKILL 16-8 Using an External (Transcutaneous) Pacemaker *(continued)*

OUTCOME IDENTIFICATION AND PLANNING

The expected outcome to achieve when using an external transcutaneous pacemaker is that it is applied correctly without adverse effect to the patient, and the patient regains signs of circulation, including the capture of at least the minimal set heart rate. Additional outcomes may include: the patient's heart and lungs maintain adequate function to sustain life; and the patient does not experience injury.

IMPLEMENTATION

ACTION	RATIONALE
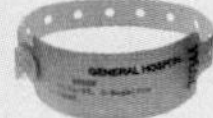 1. If patient is responsive, explain the procedure to the patient. Explain that it involves some discomfort and that you'll administer medication to keep him comfortable and help him relax. Perform hand hygiene. Check the patient's identification, if not an emergency situation.	External pacemakers are typically used with unconscious patients because most alert patients cannot tolerate the uncomfortable sensations produced by the high energy levels needed to pace externally. If responsive, the patient will most likely be sedated. Hand hygiene deters the spread of microorganisms. Verification of the patient's identity validates that the correct procedure is being done on the correct patient.
2. Close curtains around bed and close door to room if possible.	This provides for patient privacy.
3. If necessary, clip the hair over the areas of electrode placement. **However, do not shave the area.**	Shaving can cause tiny nicks in the skin, causing skin irritation. Also, the current from the pulse generator could cause discomfort.
4. Attach cardiac monitoring electrodes to the patient in the lead I, II, and III positions. Do this even if the patient is already on telemetry monitoring. If you select the lead II position, adjust the LL (left leg) electrode placement to accommodate the anterior pacing electrode and the patient's anatomy.	Connecting the telemetry electrodes to the pacemaker is required.
5. Attach the patient monitoring electrodes to the ECG cable and into the ECG input connection on the front of the pacing generator. Set the selector switch to the MONITOR ON position.	These actions ensure that the equipment is functioning properly.
6. Note the ECG waveform on the monitor. Adjust the R-wave beeper volume to a suitable level and activate the alarm by pressing the ALARM ON button. Set the alarm for 10 to 20 beats lower and 20 to 30 beats higher than the intrinsic rate.	These actions ensure that the equipment is functioning properly.
7. Press the START/STOP button for a printout of the waveform.	Initiates printout.
8. Apply the two pacing electrodes. Make sure the patient's skin is clean and dry to ensure good skin contact. Briskly rubbing the skin with your hand before placing the electrodes may improve monitor signal quality (Del Monte, 2004). Pull the protective strip from the posterior electrode (marked BACK) and apply the electrode on the left side of the thoracic spinal column, just below the scapula (Figure 1).	This placement ensures that the electrical stimulus must travel only a short distance to the heart.

(continued)

SKILL 16-8 Using an External (Transcutaneous) Pacemaker *(continued)*

ACTION | **RATIONALE**

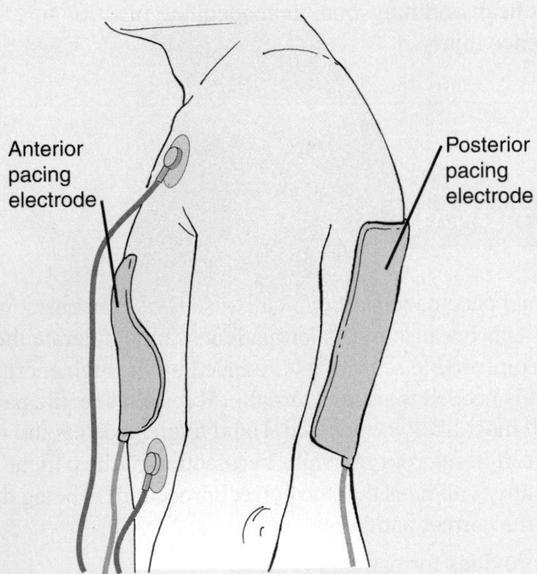

Figure 1. Transcutaneous pacemaker pads in place.

9. Apply the anterior pacing electrode (marked FRONT), which has two protective strips: one covering the gelled area and one covering the outer rim. Expose the gelled area and apply it to the skin in the anterior position, to the left side of the sternum in the usual V_2 to V_5 position, centered close to the point of maximal cardiac impulse (Figure 1). Move this electrode around to get the best waveform. Then expose the electrode's outer rim and firmly press it to the skin.

   Rationale: This placement ensures that the electrical stimulus must travel only a short distance to the heart.

10. Prepare to pace the heart. After making sure the energy output in milliamperes (mA) is on 0, connect the electrode cable to the monitor output cable.

    Rationale: This sets the pacing threshold.

11. Check the waveform, looking for a tall QRS complex in lead II.

12. Check the selector switch to PACER ON. Select synchronous (demand) or asynchronous (fixed-rate or nondemand) mode, per medical orders. **Tell the patient he or she may feel a thumping or twitching sensation. Reassure the patient you will provide medication if the discomfort is intolerable.**

    Rationale: Asynchronous pacing delivers a stimulus at a set (fixed) rate regardless of the occurrence of spontaneous myocardial depolarizations. Synchronous pacing delivers a stimulus only when the heart's intrinsic pacemaker fails to function at a predetermined rate (Urden et al, 2002).

13. Set the pacing rate dial to 10 to 20 beats higher than the intrinsic rhythm. Look for pacer artifact or spikes, which will appear as you increase the rate. If the patient does not have an intrinsic rhythm, set the rate at 80 beats/minute (Craig, 2005).

SKILL 16-8 Using an External (Transcutaneous) Pacemaker *(continued)*

ACTION	RATIONALE
14. Set the pacing current output (in milliamperes [mA]). For patients with bradycardia, start with the minimal setting and **slowly increase the amount of energy delivered to the heart by adjusting the OUTPUT mA dial. Do this until electrical capture is achieved: you will see a pacer spike followed by a widened QRS complex and a tall broad T wave that resembles a premature ventricular contraction.**	
15. Increase output by 2 mA or 10%. **Do not go higher because of the increased risk of discomfort to the patient.**	Increasing the output ensures consistent capture. With full capture, the patient's heart rate should be approximately the same as the pacemaker rate set on the machine. The usual pacing threshold is 40 to 80 mA. Thresholds may vary due to recent cardiothoracic surgery, pericardial effusions, cardiac tamponade, acidosis, and hypoxia. These conditions may require higher thresholds (Del Monte, 2004).
16. Assess for mechanical capture: Presence of a pulse and signs of improved cardiac output (increased blood pressure, improved level of consciousness, improved body temperature).	Both electrical and mechanical capture must occur to benefit the patient (Del Monte, 2004).
17. For patients with asystole, start with the full output. If capture occurs, slowly decrease the output until capture is lost, then add 2 mA or 10% more.	Increasing the output ensures consistent capture. With full capture, the patient's heart rate should be approximately the same as the pacemaker rate set on the machine. The usual pacing threshold is 40 to 80 mA.
18. Secure the pacing leads and cable to the patient's body.	Prevents accidental displacement of the electrode, resulting in failure to pace or sense.
19. Monitor the patient's heart rate and rhythm to assess ventricular response to pacing. Assess the patient's vital signs, skin color, level of consciousness, and peripheral pulses. Take blood pressure in both arms.	Assessment helps determine the effectiveness of the paced rhythm. If the blood pressure reading is significantly higher in one arm, use that arm for measurements.
20. Assess the patient's pain and administer analgesia/sedation as ordered to ease the discomfort of chest wall muscle contractions (Craig, 2005).	Promotes patient comfort.
21. Perform a 12-lead ECG and perform additional ECGs daily or with clinical changes.	ECG monitoring provides a baseline for further evaluation.
22. Continually monitor the ECG readings, noting capture, sensing, rate, intrinsic beats, and competition of paced and intrinsic rhythms. If the pacemaker is sensing correctly, the sense indicator on the pulse generator should flash with each beat.	Continuous monitoring helps evaluate the patient's condition and determine the effectiveness of therapy.
23. Perform hand hygiene.	Hand hygiene deters the spread of microorganisms.

(continued)

SKILL 16-8 Using an External (Transcutaneous) Pacemaker *(continued)*

EVALUATION

The expected outcome is achieved when using an external transcutaneous pacemaker when it is applied correctly without adverse effect to the patient; the patient regains signs of circulation, including the capture of at least the minimal set heart rate; the patient's heart and lungs maintain adequate function to sustain life; and the patient does not experience injury. The expected outcome is met with the capture of at least the minimal set heart rate, with minimal patient complications.

DOCUMENTATION

Guidelines

Document the reason for pacemaker use, time that pacing began, electrode locations, pacemaker settings, patient's response to the procedure and to temporary pacing, complications, and nursing actions taken. Document the patient's pain-intensity rating, analgesia or sedation administered, and the patient's response. If possible, obtain a rhythm strip before, during, and after pacemaker placement; any time that pacemaker settings are changed; and whenever the patient receives treatment because of a complication due to the pacemaker.

Sample Documentation

1/2/08 1218 Baseline rhythm strip obtained, sinus bradycardia at 43 bpm; see flow sheet. External temporary pacemaker placed by Dr. Goodman. Cardiac monitoring electrodes placed in the lead I, II, and III positions. Pacer set in synchronous mode at rate of 80 bpm; pacing current output 72 mA. Patient with strong femoral pulses; see flow sheet for vital signs. Patient reports chest discomfort of 4/10. Medicated with morphine 2 mg IV per order. Pacer alarms set at 50 and 90 bpm, per order. —R. Robinson, RN

1/2/08 1250 Patient reports decreased pain, 1/10.—R. Robinson, RN

Unexpected Situations and Associated Interventions

- *Failure to pace:* This happens when the pacemaker either doesn't fire or fires too often. The pulse generator may not be working properly, or it may not be conducting the impulse to the patient. If the pacing or sensing indicator flashes, check the connections to the cable and the position of the pacing electrode in the patient (by x-ray). The cable may have come loose, or the electrode may have been dislodged, pulled out, or broken. If the pulse generator is turned on but the indicators still aren't flashing, change the battery. If that does not help, use a different pulse generator. Check the settings if the pacemaker is firing too rapidly. If they are correct, or if altering them (according to your facility's policy or the physician's order) does not help, change the pulse generator.
- *Failure to capture:* Here, you see pacemaker spikes but the heart is not responding. The most common reason is failure to increase the current sufficiently. It may also be caused by changes in the pacing threshold from ischemia, an electrolyte imbalance (high or low potassium or magnesium levels), acidosis, an adverse reaction to a medication, a perforated ventricle, fibrosis, or the position of the electrode. If the patient's condition has changed, notify the physician and ask him or her for new settings. If pacemaker settings have been altered by the patient (or family members), return them to their correct positions and then make sure the face of the pacemaker is covered with a plastic shield. Tell the patient and family members not to touch the dials. If the heart is not responding, try any or all of these suggestions:
  - Carefully check all connections, making sure they are placed properly and securely.
  - Increase the milliamperes slowly (according to your facility's policy or the physician's order).
  - Turn the patient on his or her left side, then on the right side (if turning to the left did not help).
  - Schedule an anteroposterior or lateral chest x-ray to determine the position of the electrode.

SKILL 16-8 **Using an External (Transcutaneous) Pacemaker** *(continued)*

- *Failure to sense intrinsic beats:* This could cause ventricular tachycardia or ventricular fibrillation if the pacemaker fires on the vulnerable T wave. This could be caused by the pacemaker sensing an external stimulus as a QRS complex, which could lead to asystole, or by the pacemaker not being sensitive enough, which means it could fire anywhere within the cardiac cycle. If the pacing is undersensing, turn the sensitivity control completely to the right. If it is oversensing, turn it slightly to the left. If the pacemaker is not functioning correctly, change the battery or the pulse generator. Remove items in the room causing electromechanical interference (eg, razors, radios, cautery devices). Check the ground wires on the bed and other equipment for obvious damage. Unplug each piece and see if the interference stops. When you locate the cause, notify the staff engineer and ask him or her to check it. If the pacemaker is still firing on the T wave and all else has failed, turn off the pacemaker and notify the physician. Make sure atropine is available in case the patient's heart rate drops. Be prepared to call a code and institute cardiopulmonary resuscitation if necessary.

Special Considerations

General Considerations

- Patients should not be left unattended during noninvasive pacing. It is safe to touch the patient and perform procedures during pacing (CPR, for example). Gloves should be worn.
- Monitor for changes in the patient's underlying rhythm. Ventricular fibrillation requires immediate defibrillation.
- Check the skin where the electrodes are placed for skin burns or tissue damage. Reposition as needed.
- Avoid using the carotid pulse to confirm mechanical capture. Electrical stimulation can cause jerky muscle contractions that may be interpreted as carotid pulsations. Assess the femoral pulse.
- If the patient needs emergency defibrillation, make sure the pacemaker can withstand the procedure. If you are unsure, disconnect the pulse generator to avoid damage.
- Do not place the electrodes over a bony area, because bone conducts current poorly.
- With a female patient, place the anterior electrodes under the patient's breast but not over her diaphragm.
- Do not use electrical equipment that is not grounded, such as telephones, electric shaver, television, or lamps; otherwise, the patient may experience microshock.

The Taylor Suite offers these additional resources to enhance learning and facilitate understanding of this chapter:

- thePoint online resource, http://thepoint.lww.com/Lynn2E
- Student CD-ROM included with the book
- Skills Checklist to Accompany Taylor's Clinical Nursing Skills

Developing Critical Thinking Skills

1. Coby Pruder becomes visibly anxious when you bring in the ECG machine and begin to open the supplies. What could you do to help alleviate his anxiety?
2. You go in to assess Harry Stebbings and find him unresponsive. How should you respond?
3. You meet resistance while attempting to draw the discard sample from Ann Kribell's arterial line. Should you use excessive pressure to try to obtain the discard sample? Discuss the appropriate actions to problem solve this unexpected situation.

Bibliography

American Heart Association (AHA). (2002). *BLS for healthcare providers.* Dallas, TX: Author.

American Heart Association. (2005). Highlights of the 2005 American Heart Association guidelines for cardiopulmonary resuscitation and emergency cardiovascular care. *Currents in Emergency Cardiovascular Care, 16*(4), 1–27.

Asselin, M. E., & Cullen, H. A. (February 2002). A new beat for BLS and ACLS guidelines. *Nursing Management, 33*(2), 31–38.

Automated external defibrillator algorithm. (2005). *Nursing, 35*(5), 28.

Craig, K. (2005). How to provide transcutaneous pacing. *Nursing, 35*(10), 52–53.

Del Monte, L. (2004). *Medtronic. Noninvasive pacing: What you should know.* Educational Series. Redmond, WA: Medtronic Emergency Response Systems, Inc.

Diepenbrock, N. (2004). *Quick reference to critical care* (2nd ed.). Philadelphia: Lippincott Williams & Wilkins.

Dries, D. J., & Sample, M. A. (March 2002). Recent advances in emergency life support. *Nursing Clinics of North America, 37*(10), 1–10.

Dulak, S. (2005). In-hospital CPR: Building on success. *RN, 68*(7), 53–57.

Dwyer, T., Williams, L., & Jacobs, I. (2004). The benefits and use of shock advisory defibrillators in hospitals. *International Journal of Nursing Practice, 10*(2), 86–92.

Ermis, C., Lurie, K., Zhu, A., et al. (2004). Biventricular implantable cardioverter defibrillators improve survival compared with biventricular pacing alone in patients with severe left ventricular dysfunction. *Journal of Cardiovascular Electrophysiology, 15*(8), 862–866.

Freeman, J. J., & Hedges, C. H. (June 2003). Cardiac arrest: The effect on the brain. *American Journal of Nursing, 103*(6), 50–55.

Gullick, J. (2004). A study into safe and efficient use of defibrillators by nurses. *Nursing Times, 100*(44), 42–44.

Hockenberry, M. (2005). *Wong's essentials of pediatric nursing* (7th ed.). St. Louis, MO: Elsevier Mosby.

Mair, M. (August 2003). Monophasic and biphasic defibrillators. *American Journal of Nursing, 103*(8), 58–60.

Martin, P. (2003). CPR when the patient's pregnant. *RN, 66*(8), 34–40.

Mastering ACLS (2002). Springhouse, PA: Springhouse Corp.

McCance, K., & Huether, S. (2002). *Pathophysiology: The biologic basis for disease in adults and children* (4th ed.). St. Louis, MO: Mosby.

Mims, B., Toto, K., Luecke, L., et al. (2004). *Critical care skills: A clinical handbook* (2nd ed.). St. Louis, MO: Saunders.

Nursing procedures made incredibly easy. (2002). Springhouse, PA: Springhouse Corp.

Porth, C. (2005). Pathophysiology: Concepts of altered health states (7th ed.). Philadelphia: Lippincott Williams & Wilkins.

Pyne, C. (2004). Classification of acute coronary syndromes using the 12-lead electrocardiogram as a guide. *American Association of Critical-Care Nurses Clinical Issues Advanced Practice in Acute Critical Care, 15*(4), 558–567.

Skillbuilders: Expert ECG interpretation. (2003). Philadelphia: Lippincott Williams & Wilkins.

Smeltzer, S., Bare, B., Hinkle, J. H., & Cheever, K. H. (2008). *Brunner & Suddarth's textbook of medical-surgical nursing* (11th ed.). Philadelphia: Lippincott Williams & Wilkins.

Urden, L., Stacy, K., & Lough, M. (2002). *Thelan's critical care nursing: Diagnosis and management* (4th ed.). St. Louis, MO: Mosby.

Vines, D. (2004). AARC clinical practice guideline: Resuscitation and defibrillation in the health care setting—2004 revision & update. *Respiratory Care, 49*(9), 1085–1099.

Weber, J., & Kelley, J. (2007). *Health assessment in nursing* (3rd ed.). Philadelphia: Lippincott Williams & Wilkins.

CHAPTER 17

Neurological Care

Focusing on Patient Care

This chapter will help you develop some of the skills related to neurologic care necessary to care for the following patients:

Aleta Jackson, age 68, was involved in a head-on collision. She has been prescribed a cervical collar to stabilize her neck.

Yuka Chong, age 16, has received spinal rods to resolve her scoliosis. The nurse must logroll Ms. Chong to change her position.

Nikki Gladstone, 19, is in your intensive care unit following surgery related to a cranial malignancy. She has an external ventriculostomy device in place to monitor intracranial pressure.

Learning Outcomes

After studying this chapter, you will be able to:

1. Logroll a patient.
2. Apply a two-piece cervical collar.
3. Care for patient in halo traction.
4. Care for a patient with an external ventriculostomy device.
5. Care for a patient with a fiberoptic intracranial catheter.

Key Terms

cerebral perfusion pressure (CPP): a way of calculating cerebral blood flow; the formula is MAP (mean arterial pressure) minus ICP (intracranial pressure) equals CPP; normal CPP for an adult is 60 to 90 mm Hg (Hickey, 2003)

consciousness: the degree of wakefulness or ability to be aroused

intracranial pressure (ICP): pressure within the cranial vault; normal ICP is less than 10 to 15 mm Hg (Arbour, 2004).

ventriculostomy: a catheter inserted through a hole made in the skull into the ventricular system of the brain; can be used to monitor ICP and or drain cerebrospinal fluid

Many patients experience injury to the head, neck, or spinal column. In addition, numerous disorders, such as infections and tumors, can affect the brain and spinal cord, interfering with neurologic function. Specialized devices may be used to monitor and control intracranial pressure. Meticulous care is needed after injury or trauma to ensure that further injury does not occur.

This chapter will cover skills to assist the nurse in providing neurologic care. Fundamentals Review 17-1, 17-2, and 17-3 provide a review of important knowledge to assist you in understanding the skills related to neurologic care. In addition, refer to Chapter 2, Health Assessment, for a review of the components of a neurologic assessment.

Fundamentals Review 17-1

Glasgow Coma Scale

The Glasgow Coma Scale (GCS) evaluates three key categories of behavior that most closely reflect activity in the higher centers of the brain: eye opening, verbal response, and motor response (Waterhouse, 2005). Within each category, each level of response is given a numerical value. The maximum score is 15, indicating a fully awake, alert, and oriented patient; the lowest score is 3, indicating deep coma (Hickey, 2003). The Glasgow coma scale is used in conjunction with other neurological assessments, including pupillary reaction and vital sign measurement to evaluate a patient's status (Waterhouse, 2005).

Component	Score	Response
Eye opening	4	Opens eyes spontaneously when someone approaches
	3	Opens eyes in response to speech (normal tone or shouting)
	2	Opens eyes only to painful stimuli (apply pressure with a pen to the lateral outer aspect of the second or third finger, up to 10 seconds, then release)
	1	No response to painful stimuli
Motor response	6	Accurately responds to instructions; obeys a simple command, such as "Lift your left hand off the bed"
	5	Localizes (move hand to point of stimulation) to painful stimuli and attempts to remove source.
	4	Flexion reflex action, but unable to locate the source of pain; purposeless movement in response to pain
	3	Flexes elbows and wrists while extending lower legs to pain; decorticate posturing
	2	Extends upper and lower extremities to pain; decerebrate posturing
	1	No motor response to pain on any limb
Verbal response	5	Converses; oriented to time, place, and person
	4	Converses; disoriented to time, place, or person; any one or all indicators
	3	Converses only in words or phrases that make little sense in the context of the questions
	2	Responds with incomprehensible sounds; no understandable words and/or moaning, groaning or crying in response to painful stimuli
	1	No response

(Adapted from Waterhouse, C. [2005]. The Glasgow Coma Scale and other neurological observations. Nursing Standard, *19[33], 56–64c; and Hickey, J. V. [2003].* The clinical practice of neurological and neurosurgical nursing *(5th ed.). Philadelphia: Lippincott Williams & Wilkins)*

Interpreting ICP Waveforms

Three waveforms—A, B, and C—are used to monitor intracranial pressure (ICP). A waves are an ominous sign of intracranial decompensation and poor compliance. B waves correlate with changes in respiration, and C waves correlate with changes in arterial pressure.

Normal Waveform

A normal ICP waveform typically shows a steep upward systolic slope followed by a downward diastolic slope with a dicrotic notch. In most cases, this waveform occurs continuously and indicates an ICP between 0 and 15 mm Hg—normal pressure.

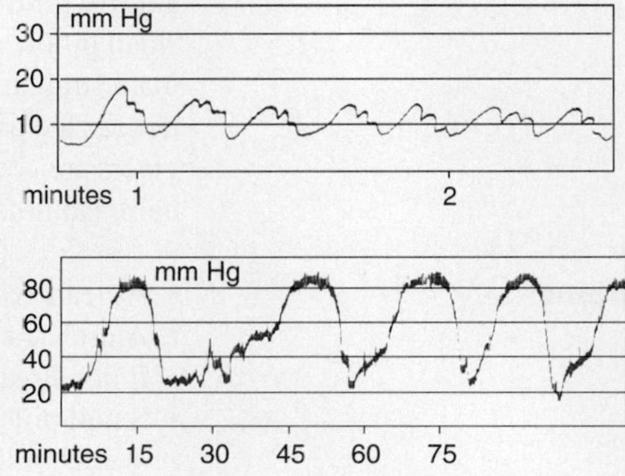

A Waves

The most clinically significant ICP waveforms are A waves, which may reach elevations of 50 to 100 mm Hg, persist for 5 to 20 minutes, then drop sharply—signaling exhaustion of the brain's compliance mechanisms. A waves may come and go, spiking from temporary rises in thoracic pressure or from a condition that increases ICP beyond the brain's compliance limits. Such activities as sustained coughing or straining during defecation can cause temporary elevations in thoracic pressure.

B Waves

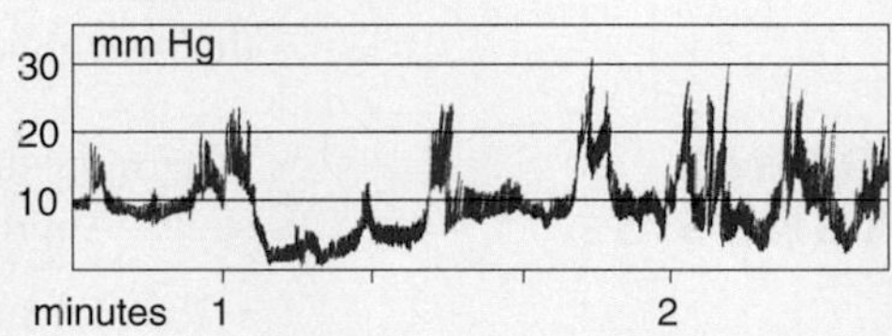

B waves, which appear sharp and rhythmic with a sawtooth pattern, occur every 1½ to 2 minutes and may reach elevations of 50 mm Hg. Their clinical significance isn't clear, but the waves correlate with respiratory changes and may occur more frequently with decreasing compensation. Because B waves sometimes precede A waves, notify the doctor if B waves occur frequently.

C Waves

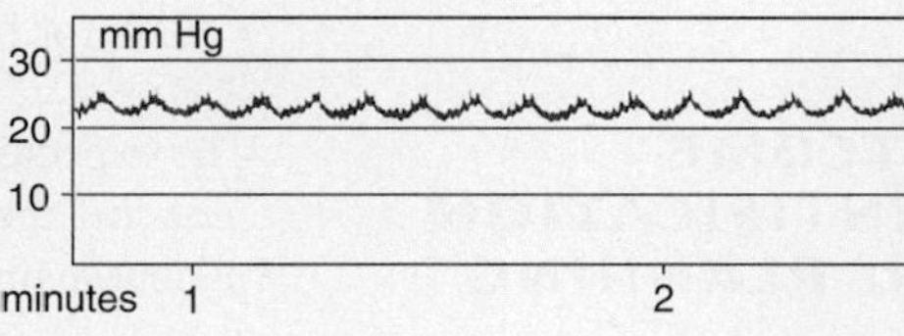

Like B waves, C waves are rapid and rhythmic, but they aren't as sharp. Clinically insignificant, they may fluctuate with respirations or systemic blood pressure changes.

Signs and Symptoms of Increased Intracranial Pressure

- Decreased level of consciousness
- Changes in mental status
- Lethargy
- Confusion
- Coma
  - Confusion
  - Restlessness
  - Irritability
- Hypoactive reflexes
- Slowed response time
- Ataxia
- Aphasia
- Slowed speech
- Progressively severe headache
- Nausea and vomiting (usually projectile vomiting)
- Seizures
- Changes in pupil size; unequal pupils
- Slowed or lack of pupillary response to light
- Widening of pulse pressure
- Respiratory pattern changes
- Leakage of clear yellow or pinkish fluid from ear or nose

SKILL 17-1 Logrolling a Patient

The "logrolling" technique is a maneuver that involves moving the patient's body as one unit so that the spine is kept in alignment, without twisting or bending. This technique is commonly used to reposition patients who have had spinal or back surgery or who have suffered back or neck injuries. If the patient is being logrolled due to a neck injury, do not use a fluffy pillow under the patient's head. However, the patient may need a bath blanket or small pillow under the head to keep the spinal column straight. The patient's neck should remain straight during the procedure and after positioning. The use of logrolling when repositioning the patient helps to maintain the alignment of the neck and spine. Two or three caregivers are needed to accomplish this safely. Do not try to logroll the patient without enough help. Do not twist the patient's head, spine, shoulders, knees, or hips while logrolling.

Equipment

- At least two additional persons to help
- A drawsheet and/or friction-reducing sheets, if possible, to facilitate smooth movement, if not already in place
- Small pillow for placement between the legs
- Wedge pillow or two pillows for behind the patient's back

ASSESSMENT

Assess for conditions that would contraindicate logrolling such as unstable neurologic status, severe pain, or the presence of drains. Assess the patient's baseline neurologic status. Assess for paresthesia and pain. If the patient is complaining of pain, consider medicating the patient before repositioning.

NURSING DIAGNOSIS

Determine the related factors for the nursing diagnoses based on the patient's current status. Appropriate nursing diagnoses may include:

- Risk for Injury
- Acute Pain
- Impaired Physical Mobility
- Risk for Impaired Skin Integrity

OUTCOME IDENTIFICATION AND PLANNING

The expected outcome is that the patient's spine remains in proper alignment, thereby reducing the risk for injury. Other outcomes may include: patient verbalizes relief of pain, patient maintains joint mobility, and patient remains free of skin breakdown.

IMPLEMENTATION

ACTION	RATIONALE
1. Review the medical record and nursing plan of care for conditions that may influence the patient's ability to move or to be positioned. Assess for tubes, IV lines, incisions, or equipment that may alter the positioning procedure. Identify any movement limitations.	Reviewing the medical record and care plan validates the correct patient and correct procedure. Checking for equipment and limitations reduces the risk for injury during the transfer.
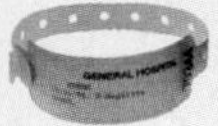 2. Identify the patient. Explain the procedure to the patient.	Patient identification validates the correct patient and correct procedure. Discussion and explanation allay anxiety and prepare the patient for what to expect.
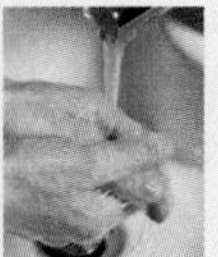 3. Perform hand hygiene and put on gloves, if necessary.	Hand hygiene and gloving prevent the spread of microorganisms.

SKILL 17-1 Logrolling a Patient *(continued)*

ACTION	RATIONALE
4. Close the door to the room or draw the bedside curtains.	Closing the door and curtain provides for privacy.
5. Adjust the bed to a comfortable working height.	Having the bed at the proper height prevents back and muscle strain.
6. Stand on one side of the bed and have two assistants stand on the opposite side of the bed. Lower the side rails. Place the bed in flat position. Place a small pillow between the patient's knees.	Using three or more people to turn the patient helps ensure that the spinal column will remain in straight alignment. A pillow placed between the knees helps keep the spinal column aligned.
7. If a drawsheet or friction-reducing sheet is not in place under the patient, take the time to place one, to facilitate future movement of the patient. See the Unexpected Situations below for information on placing a drawsheet or friction-reducing sheet.	Use of a drawsheet or friction-reducing sheet facilitates smooth movement in unison and minimizes pulling on patient's body.
8. If the patient can move the arms, ask the patient to cross the arms on the chest. Roll or fanfold the drawsheet or friction-reducing sheet close to the patient's sides and grasp it. In unison, gently slide the patient to the side of the bed opposite to that which the patient will be turned.	Crossing arms across the chest keeps the arms out of the way while rolling the patient. This also encourages patient not to help by pulling on the side rails. Moving the patient to the side opposite to that which the patient will be turned prevents the patient from being uncomfortably close to the side rail. If the patient is large, more assistants may be needed to prevent injury to the patient.
9. Make sure the drawsheet and sheet under the patient are straightened and wrinkle free. Reroll the drawsheet on the side from which the patient is being turned, if necessary, after straightening the sheets.	Drawsheet should be wrinkle free to prevent skin breakdown. Rolling the drawsheet strengthens the sheet and helps the nurse hold onto the sheet.
10. If necessary, reposition personnel to ensure two nurses stand on the side of the bed to which the patient is turning. The third helper stands on the other side. **Grasp the drawsheet at hip and shoulder level; have assistants on the opposite side grasp the drawsheet above and below your area.**	Proper positioning of personnel provides even division of support and pulling forces on the patient to maintain alignment.

(continued)

SKILL 17-1 Logrolling a Patient *(continued)*

ACTION	RATIONALE
11. Have everyone face the patient. On a predetermined signal, move the patient by holding the rolled draw-sheet taut to support the body. Turn the patient as a unit in one smooth motion toward the side of the bed with the two nurses. The patient's head, shoulders, spine, hips, and knees should turn simultaneously (Figure 1).	The patient's spine should not twist during the turn. The spine should move as one unit.

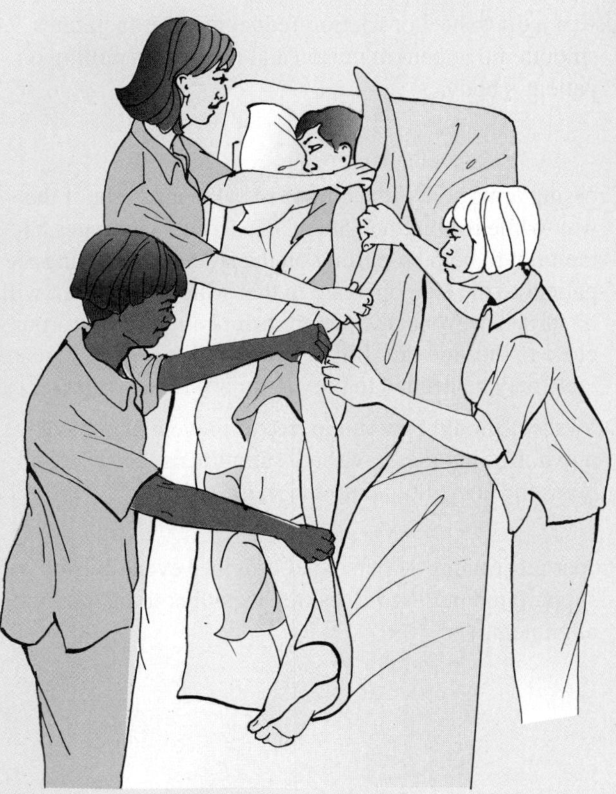

Figure 1. Turning patient as one unit.

ACTION	RATIONALE
12. **Once the patient has been turned, use pillows to support the patient's back, buttocks, and legs in straight alignment in a side-lying position. Raise the side rails, if necessary.**	The pillows or wedge provide support and ensure continued spinal alignment after turning.
13. **Stand at the foot of the bed and assess the spinal column. It should be straight, without any twisting or bending.** Ensure that the call bell and telephone are within reach. Replace covers. Lower bed height. Raise side rails as appropriate	Inspection of the spinal column ensures that the patient's back is not twisted or bent. Lowering the bed ensures patient safety.
14. Reassess the patient's neurologic status and comfort level.	Reassessment helps to evaluate the effects of movement on the patient.

SKILL 17-1 **Logrolling a Patient** *(continued)*

ACTION	RATIONALE
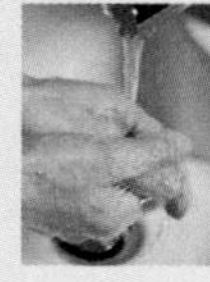 15. Place the bed in lowest position. Make sure the call bell is in reach. Remove gloves, if worn, and perform hand hygiene.	Bed in lowest position and access to call bell contribute to patient safety. Hand hygiene deters the spread of microorganisms.

EVALUATION

The expected outcome is met when the patient remains free of injury during and after turning and exhibits proper spinal alignment in the side-lying position. Other expected outcomes are met when the patient states that pain was minimal on turning, the patient demonstrates adequate joint mobility, and the patient exhibits no signs and symptoms of skin breakdown.

DOCUMENTATION

General Guidelines

Document the time of the patient's change of position, use of supports, and any pertinent observations, including neurologic and skin assessments. Document the patient's tolerance of the position change. Many facilities provide areas on bedside flow sheet to document repositioning.

Sample Documentation

11/15/08 1120 Patient logrolled with 3-person assist. Placed on left side. Patient pushed PCA button prior to turning. Dressing over middle of back from base of neck to lumbar region clean, dry, and intact; no redness noted on back or buttocks.
—B. Traudes, RN

Unexpected Situations and Associated Interventions

- *Patient requires repositioning using logrolling, but a drawsheet or friction-reducing sheet is not in place under the patient:* Placement of a drawsheet or friction-reducing sheet will facilitate future patient movement and should be put into place before the patient occupies the bed. If this was not done, take time to put one in place. This requires careful movement using logrolling and a minimum of three caregivers. Stabilize the cervical spine by holding the patient's head firmly on either side directly above the ears.
- *Patient requires repositioning using logrolling, but you are working alone:* If assistance is not available, wait for at least one additional caregiver for assistance. Do not attempt to reposition the patient alone. At least two caregivers are necessary to perform logrolling to reposition a patient; three caregivers for a large patient (Pullen, 2004).

SKILL 17-2 Applying a Two-Piece Cervical Collar

Patients suspected of having injuries to the cervical spine must be immobilized with a cervical collar to prevent further damage to the spinal cord. A cervical collar maintains the neck in a straight line, with the chin slightly elevated and tucked inward. Care must be taken when applying the collar not to hyperflex or hyperextend the patient's neck.

Equipment

- Nonsterile gloves
- Tape measure
- Cervical collar of appropriate size
- Washcloth
- Soap
- Towel

ASSESSMENT

Assess for a patent airway. If airway is occluded, try repositioning using the jaw thrust–chin lift method, which helps open the airway without moving the patient's neck. Inspect and palpate the cervical spine area for tenderness, swelling, deformities, or crepitus. Do not ask the patient to move the neck if a cervical spinal cord injury is suspected. Assess the patient's level of consciousness and ability to follow commands to determine any neurologic dysfunction. If the patient is able to follow commands, instruct him or her not to move the head or neck. Ideally, have a second person stabilize the cervical spine by holding the patient's head firmly on either side directly above the ears.

NURSING DIAGNOSIS

Determine the related factors for the nursing diagnoses based on the patient's current status. Appropriate nursing diagnoses may include:

- Risk for Injury
- Acute Pain
- Risk for Aspiration
- Ineffective Breathing Pattern

OUTCOME IDENTIFICATION AND PLANNING

The expected outcome is that the patient's cervical spine is immobilized, preventing further injury to the spinal cord. Other outcomes that may be acceptable include: patient maintains head and neck without movement, patient experiences minimal to no pain, and patient demonstrates an understanding about the need for immobilization.

IMPLEMENTATION

ACTION	RATIONALE
1. Review the medical record and nursing plan of care to determine need for placement of a cervical collar. Identify any movement limitations.	Reviewing the record and care plan validates the correct patient and correct procedure. Identification of limitations prevents injury.
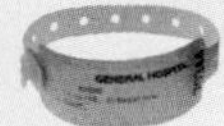 2. Identify the patient. Explain the procedure to the patient.	Patient identification validates the correct patient and correct procedure. Discussion and explanation allay anxiety and prepare the patient for what to expect.
3. Assess patient for any changes in neurologic status. (See Chapter 2 for assessment details.)	Patients with cervical spine injuries are at risk for problems with the neurologic system.
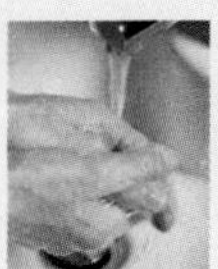 4. Perform hand hygiene and put on gloves, if necessary.	Hand hygiene and gloving prevent the spread of microorganisms.
5. Close the door to the room or draw the bedside curtains.	Closing the door and curtain provides for privacy.

SKILL 17-2 Applying a Two-Piece Cervical Collar *(continued)*

ACTION	RATIONALE
6. Adjust the bed to a comfortable working height. Lower the side rails if necessary.	Having the bed at the proper height and lowering the side rails prevents back and muscle strain.
7. Gently clean the face and neck with a mild soap and water. If the patient has experienced trauma, inspect the area for broken glass or other material that could cut the patient or the nurse. Pat the area dry.	Blood, glass, leaves, and twigs may be present on the patient's neck. The area should be clean before applying the cervical collar to prevent skin breakdown.
8. With a second person stabilizing the cervical spine, measure from the bottom of the chin to the top of the sternum, and measure around the neck. Match these height and circumference measurements to the manufacturer's recommended size chart.	To immobilize the cervical spine and to prevent skin breakdown under the collar, the correct size of collar must be used.
9. Slide the flattened back portion of the collar under the patient's head. **The center of the collar should line up with the center of the patient's neck. Do not allow the patient's head to move when passing the collar under the head.**	Stabilizing the cervical spine is crucial to prevent the head from moving which could cause further damage to the cervical spine. Placing the collar in the center ensures that the neck is aligned properly.
10. Place the front of the collar centered over the chin, while ensuring that the chin area fits snugly in the recess. Be sure that the front half of the collar overlaps the back half. Secure Velcro straps on both sides (Figure 1). Check to see that at least one finger can be inserted between collar and patient's neck.	The collar should fit snugly to prevent the patient from moving the neck and causing further damage to the cervical spine. Velcro will help hold the collar securely in place. Collar should not be too tight to cause discomfort.

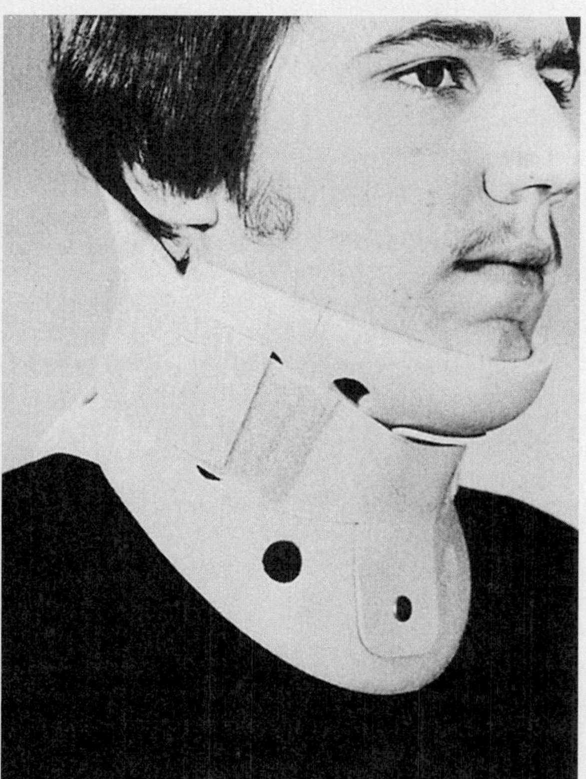

Figure 1. Cervical collar in place (From: Hickey, J. [2003]. *The clinical practice of neurological and neurosurgical nursing* [5th ed.] Philadelphia: Lippincott Williams & Wilkins, p. 414.)

(continued)

SKILL 17-2 Applying a Two-Piece Cervical Collar *(continued)*

ACTION	RATIONALE
11. Place the bed in lowest position. Make sure the call bell is in reach. Raise the side rails. Remove gloves and perform hand hygiene.	Bed in lowest position and access to call bell contribute to patient safety. Hand hygiene deters the spread of microorganisms.
12. **Check the skin under the cervical collar at least every 4 hours for any signs of skin breakdown.** Remove the top half of the collar daily and cleanse the skin under the collar. **When the collar is removed, have a second person immobilize the cervical spine.**	Skin breakdown may occur under the cervical collar if the skin is not inspected and cleansed.

EVALUATION

The expected outcomes are met when the patient's cervical spine is immobilized without further injury. The patient verbalizes minimal to no pain and demonstrates an understanding of the rationale for cervical spine immobilization.

DOCUMENTATION

Guidelines

Document the application of the collar, including size and any skin care necessary prior to the application, condition of skin under the cervical collar, and patient's pain level, neurologic assessments and any other assessment findings.

Sample Documentation

11/22/08 0900 Patient arrived on unit; cervical spine immobilized; medium cervical collar applied. Patient awake, alert, and oriented. Admits to right neck pain; denies other pain. See flow sheet for neuro assessment. Skin pink, warm, and dry. 3-cm laceration noted on R anterior side of neck. Wound cleansed and antibiotic ointment applied. Patient instructed to refrain from moving without assistance; call bell placed in right hand.—B. Clapp, RN

Unexpected Situations and Associated Interventions

- *The height and neck circumference measurements are between two sizes:* Start with the smaller size. If the collar is too large, the neck may not be immobilized.
- *Skin breakdown is noted on the shoulder, neck, or ear:* Apply a protective dressing over the area and continue to assess for further skin breakdown.
- *Patient complains that the collar is "choking" him:* If not contraindicated, place the patient in the reverse Trendelenburg position to see if this helps. Assess the tightness of the cervical collar; you should be able to slide at least one finger under the collar.
- *Patient is able to move head from side to side with cervical collar on:* Tighten the cervical collar if possible. If the collar is as tight as possible, apply a collar one size smaller and evaluate for a better fit.

SKILL 17-3 Caring for a Patient in Halo Traction

Halo traction provides immobilization to patients with spinal cord injury. Halo traction consists of a metal ring that fits over the patient's head, connected with skull pins into the skull, and metal bars that connect the ring to a vest that distributes the weight of the device around the chest. It immobilizes the head and neck after traumatic injury to the cervical vertebrae and allows early mobility. Although most injuries are treated with surgical intervention followed by halo application to stabilize the spinal cord while healing takes place, halo traction can be used alone.

Nursing responsibilities include reassuring the patient, maintaining the device, monitoring neurovascular status, monitoring respiratory status, promoting exercise, preventing complications from the therapy, preventing infection by providing pin-site care, and providing teaching to ensure compliance and self-care. Pin-site care is performed frequently in the first 48 to 72 hours after application, when drainage may be heavy. Thereafter, pin-site care may be done daily or weekly. Dressings are often applied for the first 48 to 72 hours, and then sites may be left open to air. There is little research evidence on which to base the management of pin sites (Baird-Holmes & Brown, 2005). Pin-site care varies based on physician and facility policy. Refer to specific patient medical orders and facility guidelines.

Nurses play a major role in preparing the patient psychologically for the application of the device. Patients are often unsettled by the appearance of the device and may have feelings of claustrophobia. Misconceptions regarding pain and discomfort associated with the device also must be addressed.

Equipment

- Basin of warm water
- Bath towels
- Medicated skin powder or cornstarch, per physician order or facility policy
- Sterile applicators
- Cleansing solution, usually sterile normal saline or chlorhexidine, per physician order or facility policy
- Sterile gauze or dressing per order or policy
- Antimicrobial ointment, per physician's order or facility policy
- Analgesic, per physician's order
- Clean gloves, if appropriate, for bathing under the vest
- Sterile gloves for performing pin care, depending on facility policy

ASSESSMENT

Review the patient's medical record, physician's orders, and nursing plan of care to determine the type of device being used and prescribed care. Assess the halo traction device to ensure proper function and position. Perform respiratory, neurologic, and skin assessments. Inspect the pin-insertion sites for inflammation and infection, including swelling, cloudy or offensive drainage, pain, or redness. Assess the patient's knowledge regarding the device and self-care activities and responsibilities, and his or her feelings related to treatment.

NURSING DIAGNOSIS

Determine the related factors for the nursing diagnoses based on the patient's current status. Appropriate nursing diagnoses may include:

- Anxiety
- Disturbed Body Image
- Risk for Falls
- Ineffective Coping
- Deficient Knowledge
- Impaired Gas Exchange
- Risk for Infection
- Risk for Injury
- Self-Care Deficit (toileting, bathing or hygiene, dressing or grooming)

(continued)

SKILL 17-3 Caring for a Patient in Halo Traction *(continued)*

- Impaired Physical Mobility
- Acute Pain
- Impaired Skin Integrity
- Disturbed Sleep Pattern

OUTCOME IDENTIFICATION AND PLANNING

The expected outcome to achieve when caring for a patient with halo traction is that the patient maintains cervical alignment. Additional outcomes that may be appropriate include that the patient shows no evidence of infection; the patient is free from complications such as respiratory impairment, orthostatic hypotension, and skin breakdown; the patient experiences relief from pain; and the patient is free from injury.

IMPLEMENTATION

ACTION	RATIONALE
1. Review the medical record and the nursing plan of care to determine the type of device being used and prescribed care.	Reviewing the medical record and care plan validate the correct patient and correct procedure.
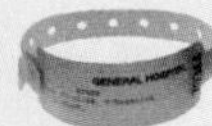 2. Identify the patient. Explain the procedure to the patient.	Patient identification validates the correct patient and correct procedure. Discussion and explanation help allay anxiety and prepare the patient for what to expect.
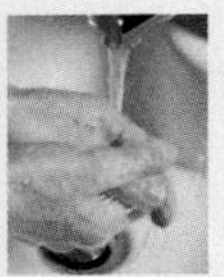 3. Perform hand hygiene.	Hand hygiene prevents the spread of microorganisms.
4. Close the room door or curtains. Place the bed at a comfortable working height or have the patient sit up if appropriate.	Closing the door or curtains promotes privacy. Proper bed height helps prevent muscle strain.
5. Monitor vital signs and perform a neurologic assessment, including level of consciousness, motor function, and sensation, per facility policy. This is usually at least every 2 hours for 24 hours, or possibly every hour for 48 hours.	Changes in the neurologic assessment could indicate spinal cord trauma, which would require immediate intervention.
6. Examine the halo vest unit every 8 hours for stability, secure connections, and positioning (Figure 1). Make sure the patient's head is centered in the halo without neck flexion or extension. Check each bolt for loosening.	Assessment ensures correct function of the device and patient safety.
7. Check the fit of the vest. With the patient in a supine position, you should be able to insert one or two fingers under the jacket at the shoulder and chest.	Checking the fit prevents compression on the chest, which could interfere with respiratory status.
8. Put on unsterile gloves, if appropriate. Wash the patient's chest and back daily. Place the patient on his or her back or sitting up if appropriate. Loosen the bottom Velcro straps.	Gloves prevent contact with blood and body fluids. Daily cleaning prevents skin breakdown and allows assessment. Loosening the straps allows access to the chest and back.
9. Wring out a bath towel soaked in warm water. Pull the towel back and forth in a drying motion beneath the front. Do not use soap or lotion under the vest.	Using an overly wet towel could lead to skin maceration and breakdown. Soaps and lotions can cause skin irritation.

SKILL 17-3 **Caring for a Patient in Halo Traction** *(continued)*

ACTION	RATIONALE
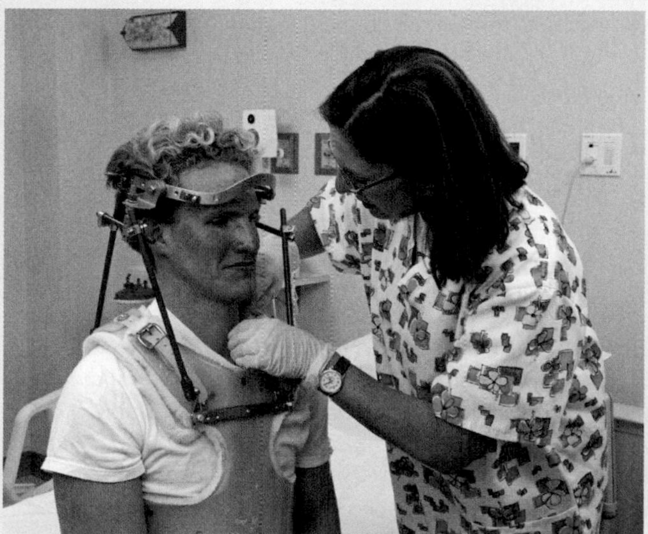 **Figure 1.** Examining the halo vest for stability, secure connections, and positioning.	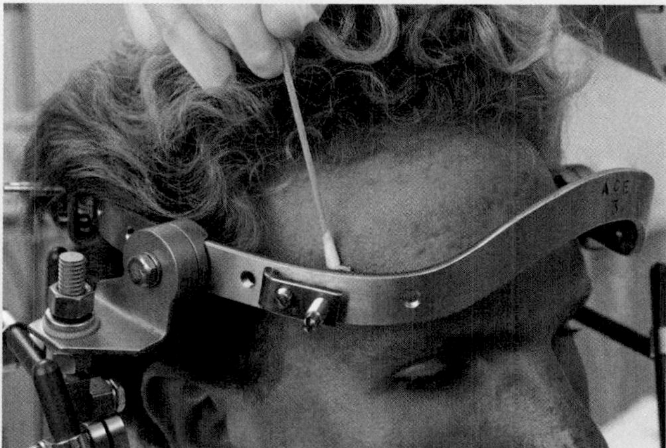 **Figure 2.** Cleansing around pin sites with normal saline and an applicator.
10. Thoroughly dry the skin in the same manner with a dry towel. Inspect the skin for tender, reddened areas or pressure spots. Lightly dust the skin with a prescribed medicated powder or cornstarch.	Drying and using powder or cornstarch, which helps absorb moisture, prevent skin breakdown.
11. Turn the patient on his or her side, less than 45 degrees if lying supine, and repeat the process on the back. Close the Velcro straps. Assist the patient with changing the shirt.	Doing so prevents skin breakdown. Soaps and lotions can cause skin irritation.
12. Perform a respiratory assessment. Check for respiratory impairment, such as absence of breath sounds, the presence of adventitious sounds, reduced inspiratory effort, or shortness of breath.	The halo vest limits chest expansion, which could lead to alterations in respiratory function. Pulmonary embolus is a common complication associated with spinal cord injury.
13. Assess the pin sites for redness, tenting of the skin, prolonged or purulent drainage, swelling, and bowing, bending, or loosening of the pins. Monitor body temperature.	Pin sites provide an entry for microorganisms. Assessment allows for early detection and prompt intervention should problems arise.
14. Perform pin-site care (Figure 2). (See Skills 9-18 and 9-19.)	Pin-site care reduces the risk of infection and subsequent osteomyelitis.
15. Depending on physician order and facility policy, apply the antimicrobial ointment to pin sites and apply a dressing.	Antimicrobial ointment helps prevent infection. Dressing provides protection and helps contain any drainage.
16. Remove gloves and dispose of them appropriately. Place the bed in the lowest position.	Disposing of gloves reduces the risk of microorganism transmission. Proper bed height ensures patient safety.
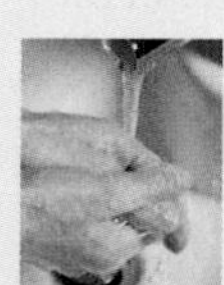 17. Perform hand hygiene	Hand hygiene prevents the spread of microorganisms.

(continued)

SKILL 17-3 Caring for a Patient in Halo Traction *(continued)*

EVALUATION

The expected outcome is met when the patient maintains cervical alignment. Additional outcomes are met when the patient shows no evidence of infection; the patient is free from complications such as respiratory impairment, orthostatic hypotension, and skin breakdown; the patient experiences relief from pain; and the patient is free from injury

DOCUMENTATION

Guidelines

Document the time, date, and type of device in place. Include the skin assessment, pin-site assessment, and pin-site care. Document the patient's response to the device and the neurologic assessment and respiratory assessment.

Sample Documentation

11/10/08 2030 Halo traction in place. Skin care provided under jacket; two fingers fit at shoulders and chest. Skin intact without redness or irritation. Pin-site care performed. Pin sites cleaned with normal saline and open to the air. Sites without redness, swelling, and drainage. Neurovascular status intact. Patient reports pain at pin sites 4/10. Medicated with ibuprofen 600 mg per order. Will reevaluate pain in 1 hour.—M. Leroux, RN

Unexpected Situations and Associated Interventions

- *Your patient, being treated with halo traction, complains of a headache after the physician or advanced practice professional has tightened the skull pins:* This is a common complaint; obtain an order for and administer an analgesic. However, if the pain is associated with jaw movement, notify the physician immediately, as the pins may have slipped onto the temporal plate.

Special Considerations

General Considerations

- Wrenches specific for the vest should always be kept at the bedside for emergency removal of the anterior portion of the vest should it be necessary to perform CPR.
- Patient teaching to prevent injury is very important. Patients need to learn to turn slowly and refrain from bending forward to avoid falls.
- Stress to the frame could cause misalignment of the spine and straining or tearing of the skin.

SKILL 17-4 Caring for an External Ventriculostomy (Intraventricular Catheter–Closed Fluid-Filled System)

An external ventriculostomy is one method used to monitor intracranial pressure (ICP). It is part of a system that includes an external drainage system and an external transducer. This device is inserted into a ventricle of the brain, most commonly the nondominant lateral ventricle, through a hole drilled into the skull. The dura is incised or punctured, and the catheter is passed through the cerebral tissue into the ventricle (Arbour, 2004). The ventriculostomy can be used to measure the ICP, to drain cerebrospinal fluid (CSF), such as removing excess fluid associated with hydrocephalus, or to decrease the volume in the cranial vault, thereby decreasing the ICP, and to instill medications. ICP measurement is used to calculate cerebral perfusion pressure (CPP), an estimate of the adequacy of cerebral blood supply. CPP is the pressure difference across the brain. It is the difference between the incoming systemic mean arterial pressure (MAP) and the ICP. It is calculated by finding the difference between the MAP and the ICP (Josephson, 2004).

SKILL 17-4 Caring for an External Ventriculostomy (Intraventricular Catheter–Closed Fluid-Filled System) *(continued)*

Equipment

- Flashlight
- Ventriculostomy setup

ASSESSMENT

Assess the color of the fluid draining from the ventriculostomy. Normal CSF is clear or straw colored. Cloudy CSF may suggest an infection. Red or pink CSF may indicate bleeding. Assess vital signs, because changes in vital signs can reflect a neurologic problem. Assess the patient's pain level. The patient may be experiencing pain at the ventriculostomy insertion site.

Assess the patient's level of consciousness. If the patient is awake, assess for his or her orientation to person, place, and time. If the patient's level of consciousness is decreased, note the patient's ability to respond and be aroused. Inspect pupil size and response to light. Pupils should be equal and round and should react to light bilaterally. Any changes in level of consciousness or pupillary response may suggest a neurologic problem. If the patient can move the extremities, assess strength of hands and feet (see Chapter 2 for detailed instructions on assessing muscle strength). A change in strength or a difference in strength on one side compared to the other may indicate a neurologic problem.

NURSING DIAGNOSIS

Determine the related factors for the nursing diagnoses based on the patient's current status. Appropriate nursing diagnoses may include:

- Risk for Injury
- Risk for Infection
- Pain
- Activity Intolerance

OUTCOME IDENTIFICATION AND PLANNING

The expected outcome to achieve is that the patient maintains intracranial pressure at less than 10 to 15 mm Hg (Arbour, 2004) and cerebral perfusion pressure at 60 to 90 mm Hg (Hickey, 2003). Other outcomes that may be appropriate include: patient is free from infection, patient is free from pain, and patient/significant others understand the need for the ventriculostomy.

IMPLEMENTATION

ACTION	RATIONALE
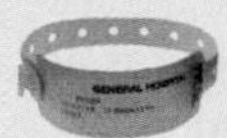 1. Identify the patient. Explain procedure to patient. Review physician's order for specific information about parameters.	Patient identification validates the correct patient and correct procedure. Explanation relieves anxiety and facilitates cooperation. The nurse needs to know the most recent order for the height of the ventriculostomy. For example, if the health care practitioner has ordered that the ventriculostomy is to be at 10 cm, this means the patient's ICP must rise above 10 cm before the ventriculostomy will drain CSF.
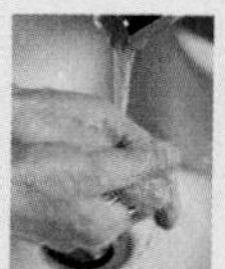 2. Perform hand hygiene; apply gloves if indicated.	Hand hygiene and gloving deter the spread of microorganisms.
3. Assess patient for any changes in neurologic status (See Chapter 2 for details of assessment).	Patients with ventriculostomies are at risk for problems with the neurologic system.

(continued)

SKILL 17-4 Caring for an External Ventriculostomy (Intraventricular Catheter–Closed Fluid-Filled System) *(continued)*

ACTION

4. **Assess the height of the ventriculostomy system to ensure that the stopcock is at the level of midpoint between the outer canthus of the patient's eye and the tragus of the patient's ear or external auditory canal (Littlejohns, 2005), using carpenter level's, bubble-line level, or laser level, according to facility policy.** Adjust the height of the system if needed. **Move the drip chamber to the ordered height (Figure 1).** Assess the amount of CSF in the drip chamber if the ventriculostomy is draining.

RATIONALE

For measurements to be accurate, the stopcock must be at the level of the location of the foramen of Monro, which is the actual level for measurements. If the transducer and extraventricular drain (EVD) are not referenced to the foramen of Monro correctly, using a carpenter level's, bubble-line level, or laser level, there can be a significant error (March, 2005). If the ventriculostomy is used just to measure the ICP and not to drain CSF, the stopcock will be turned off to the drip chamber. If the ventriculostomy is to drain CSF, the nurse must turn the stopcock off to the drip chamber. After the ICP value is obtained, remember to turn the stopcock back off to the transducer so that CSF is allowed to drain.

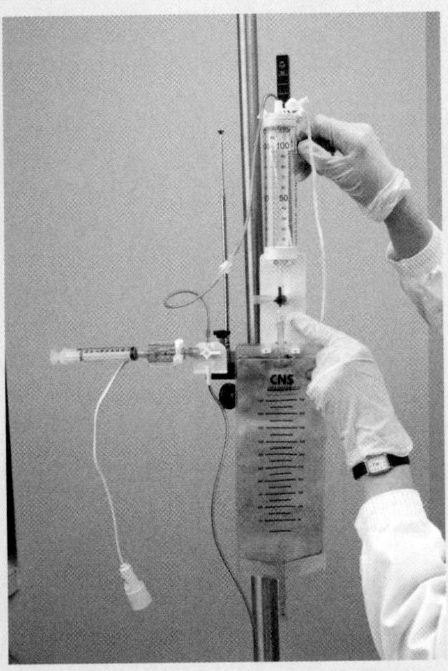

Figure 1. Adjusting drip chamber.

ACTION

5. **Zero the transducer.** Turn stopcock off to the patient. Remove the cap from the transducer, being careful not to touch the end of the cap. Press and hold the calibration button on the monitor until the monitor beeps. Return the cap to the transducer. **Turn the stopcock off to the drip chamber to obtain an ICP reading. After transducer.**

RATIONALE

The readings would not be considered accurate if the transducer had not been recently zeroed. If the stopcock is not turned off to the patient, when opened to room air, CSF will flow out of the stopcock. The end of the cap must remain sterile to prevent an infection. The stopcock must be off to the drip chamber (open to the transducer) to obtain an ICP. If the ventriculostomy is to drain CSF, the nurse must turn the stopcock off to the drip chamber. After the ICP value is obtained, remember to turn the stopcock back off to the transducer so that CSF is allowed to drain.

SKILL 17-4

Caring for an External Ventriculostomy (Intraventricular Catheter–Closed Fluid-Filled System) *(continued)*

ACTION	RATIONALE
6. **Move the ventriculostomy to prevent too much drainage, too little drainage, or inaccurate ICP readings.**	If the patient's head is lower than the ventriculostomy, the drainage of CSF will slow or stop. If the patient's head is higher than the ventriculostomy, the drainage of CSF will increase. Any ICP readings taken when the ventriculostomy is not level with the outer canthus of the eye would be inaccurate.
7. Care for the insertion site according to the institution's policy. Assess the site for any signs of infection, such as purulent drainage, redness, or warmth. Ensure the catheter is secured at site per facility policy.	Site care varies, possibly ranging from leaving the site open to air to applying antibiotic ointment and gauze. Securing the catheters after insertion prevents dislodgement and breakage of the device.
8. Calculate the CPP, if necessary. Calculate the difference between the systemic mean arterial pressure and the ICP.	CPP is an estimate of the adequacy of the blood supply to the brain.
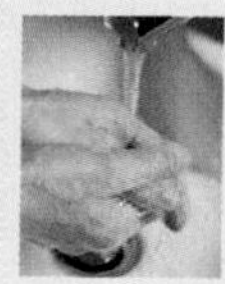 9. Remove gloves, if worn. Perform hand hygiene.	Hand hygiene deters the spread of microorganisms.

EVALUATION

The expected outcome is met when the patient demonstrates a CPP and an ICP within identified parameters; remains free from infection; understands the need for the ventriculostomy; and reports no pain.

DOCUMENTATION

General Guidelines

Document the following information: amount and color of CSF; ICP; CPP; pupil status; motor strength bilaterally; orientation to time, person, and place; level of consciousness; vital signs; pain; appearance of insertion site; and height of ventriculostomy.

Sample Documentation

11/2/08 1410 External ventriculostomy zeroed; transducer level with outer canthus of eye, drip chamber 10 cm; draining cloudy, straw-colored CSF (12 cc), physician notified of clarity. ICP 10 mm Hg, CPP 83 mm Hg. Ventriculostomy insertion site with small amount of serosanguineous drainage; open to air. Strong equal grip bilaterally. Patient awake, alert, and oriented to person, place, and time. Pupils equal round and reactive to light 6/4 bilaterally. See graphics for vital signs. Patient denies pain.—B. Traudes, RN

Unexpected Situations and Associated Interventions

- *CSF stops draining:* Assess for any kinks or narrowing of tubing. Assess that all connections on the tubing are well connected and that CSF is not leaking anywhere from the tubing. Assess the height of the system and the height of the drip chamber. If the system is too high, the CSF drainage will taper off. Assess for any liquid on the sheets around the patient's head. If the ventriculostomy has become clogged, the CSF may begin to leak around the insertion site. Assess the patency of the ventriculostomy catheter. Raise and lower the system. If the ventriculostomy catheter is patent, the fluid in the tube will tidal, or rise and fall with the position change. If CSF still is not draining or if you believe that tube is clogged, notify the physician. The tube may need to be flushed sterilely to ensure patency.

(continued)

SKILL 17-4 Caring for an External Ventriculostomy (Intraventricular Catheter–Closed Fluid-Filled System) *(continued)*

- *The amount of CSF drainage increases:* Assess the height of the system and the height of the drip chamber. If the system is too low, the amount of CSF drainage will increase. If CSF continues to drain at an increased amount, notify the physician. The height of the drip chamber may need to be increased.
- *CSF has changed from clear to cloudy:* Notify the physician immediately. This can signify an infection, and antibiotics may need to be started.
- *CSF has changed from straw colored to pink tinged or serosanguineous:* Notify the physician immediately. This can signify bleeding in the ventricles of the brain.
- *Catheter is accidentally dislodged:* Notify the physician immediately. Put on sterile gloves and cover the insertion site with sterile gauze. Monitor for color and amount of CSF if draining from site.

Special Considerations

General Considerations

- Securing the catheters according to facility policy after insertion and using care when moving patients will prevent dislodgement and breakage of these devices (March, 2005).
- Several independent nursing activities, such as turning and positioning, have been shown to increase ICP. Care should be taken when caring for patients with ICP monitoring to manage factors known to increase ICP. Turn and position the patient in proper body alignment, avoiding angulation of body parts. Extreme hip flexion or flexion of upper legs can increase intra-abdominal pressure, leading to increased ICP. Logrolling should be used. Maintain the neck in neutral position at all times to avoid neck vein compression, which can interfere with venous return. Maintain the head of the bed in the flat position or elevated to 30 degrees, depending on medical orders and facility procedure. Avoid noxious stimuli, using soft voices or music and a gentle touch. Plan care to avoid grouping activities and procedures known to increase ICP. Bathing, turning, and other routine care often have a cumulative effect to increase ICP when performed in succession. Allow rest periods between procedures and carefully assess the patient's response to interventions (Hickey, 2003; Hockenberry, 2005).

SKILL 17-5 Caring for a Fiber Optic Intracranial Catheter

Fiber optic catheters are another method used to monitor intracranial pressure (ICP). Fiber optic catheters directly monitor ICP using an intracranial transducer located in the tip of the catheter. A miniature transducer in the catheter tip is coupled by a long, continuous wire or fiber optic cable to an external electronic module. This device can be inserted into the lateral ventricle, subarachnoid space, subdural space, or brain parenchyma, or under a bone flap. The dura is perforated, and the transducer probe is threaded through the cerebral tissue to the desired depth and fixed in position (Hickey, 2003). Fiber optic catheters can be used to monitor the ICP and cerebral perfusion pressure (CPP). Some versions of catheters can also be used to drain cerebral spinal fluid (CSF). These devices are calibrated by the manufacturer and zero-balanced only once at the time of insertion.

ICP measurement is used to calculate CPP, an estimate of the adequacy of cerebral blood supply. CPP is the pressure difference across the brain. It is the difference between the incoming systemic mean arterial pressure (MAP) and the ICP. It is calculated by finding the difference between the MAP and the ICP (Josephson, 2004).

SKILL 17-5 Caring for a Fiber Optic Intracranial Catheter *(continued)*

Equipment

- None needed

ASSESSMENT

Perform a neurologic assessment. Assess the patient's level of consciousness. If the patient is awake, assess the patient's orientation to person, place, and time. If the patient's level of consciousness is decreased, note the patient's ability to respond and be aroused. Inspect pupil size and response to light. Pupils should be equal and round and should react to light bilaterally. Any changes in level of consciousness or pupillary response may suggest a neurologic problem. If the patient can move the extremities, assess strength of hands and feet (see Chapter 2 for detailed instructions on assessing muscle strength). A change in strength or a difference in strength on one side compared to the other may indicate a neurologic problem. Assess vital signs, because changes in vital signs can reflect a neurologic problem. Assess the patient's pain level. The patient may be experiencing pain at the fiber optic catheter insertion site.

NURSING DIAGNOSIS

Determine the related factors for the nursing diagnoses based on the patient's current status. Appropriate nursing diagnoses may include:

- Risk for Infection
- Risk for Injury
- Pain

Many other nursing diagnoses also may require the use of this skill.

OUTCOME IDENTIFICATION AND PLANNING

The expected outcome to achieve is that the patient maintains ICP less than 10 to 15 mm Hg (Arbour, 2004) and CPP 60 to 90 mm Hg (Hickey, 2003). Other outcomes that may be appropriate include: patient is free from infection and injury, patient is free from pain, and patient/significant others understand the need for the catheter and monitoring.

IMPLEMENTATION

ACTION	RATIONALE
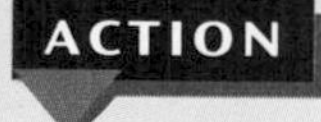 1. Identify the patient. Explain procedure to patient. Review physician's order.	Patient identification validates the correct patient and correct procedure. Explanation relieves anxiety and facilitates cooperation. Nurse needs to know the most recent order for acceptable ICP and CPP values.
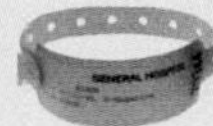 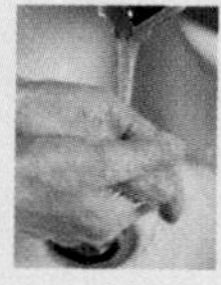 2. Perform hand hygiene.	Hand hygiene deters the spread of microorganisms.
3. Assess patient for any changes in neurologic status. (See Chapter 2 for details of assessment.)	Patients with intracranial catheters are at risk for problems with the neurologic system.
4. **Assess ICP, MAP, and CPP at least hourly. Note ICP waveforms as shown on the monitor. Notify the physician if A or B waves are present.**	Frequent assessment provides valuable indicators for identifying subtle trends that may suggest developing problems.

(continued)

SKILL 17-5 Caring for a Fiber Optic Intracranial Catheter *(continued)*

ACTION	RATIONALE
5. Care for the insertion site according to the institution's policy. Assess the site for any signs of infection, such as drainage, redness, or warmth. Ensure the catheter is secured at site per facility policy.	Site care varies, possibly ranging from leaving the site open to air to applying antibiotic ointment and gauze. Site care aids in reducing the risk for infection. Securing the catheters after insertion prevents dislodgement and breakage of the device.
6. Calculate the CPP, if necessary. Calculate the difference between the systemic mean arterial pressure and the ICP.	CPP is an estimate of the adequacy of the blood supply to the brain.
7. Perform hand hygiene.	Hand hygiene deters the spread of microorganisms.

EVALUATION

The expected outcome is met when the patient demonstrates a CPP and an ICP within identified parameters; remains free from infection; understands the need for the catheter and monitoring; and reports no pain.

DOCUMENTATION

General Guidelines

Document the following information: neurologic assessment; ICP; CPP; vital signs; pain; appearance of insertion site.

Sample Documentation

11/2/08 1710 Patient sedated; disoriented and combative when awake. Pupils equal round and reactive to light 6/4 bilaterally. See graphics for vital signs. ICP 22 mm Hg, CPP 61 mm Hg; physician notified. Dopamine drip increased to 8 mcg/kg/min. Insertion site with small amount of serosanguineous drainage; site open to air.—B. Traudes, RN

Unexpected Situations and Associated Interventions

- *Fiber optic catheter is accidentally dislodged:* Notify the physician immediately. Put on sterile gloves and cover the site with sterile gauze. Observe for any CSF leakage from site.
- *Waveforms are not changing with procedures known to cause an increase in the ICP (suctioning):* Fiber optic catheter may be damaged. Check the manufacturer's instructions for troubleshooting. Notify the physician.
- *CSF is leaking from insertion site:* Notify the physician. CSF is a prime medium for bacteria, and leakage can lead to an infection. Follow your institution's policy. Some institutions may have the nurse apply a sterile dressing around the insertion site; others may have the nurse cleanse the area more frequently.

Special Considerations

General Considerations

- Securing the catheters according to facility policy after insertion and using care when moving patients will prevent dislodgement and breakage of these devices (March, 2005).
- Several independent nursing activities, such as turning and positioning, have been shown to increase ICP. Care should be taken when caring for patients with ICP monitoring to manage factors known to increase ICP. Turn and position the patient in proper

SKILL 17-5 **Caring for a Fiber Optic Intracranial Catheter** *(continued)*

body alignment, avoiding angulation of body parts. Extreme hip flexion or flexion of upper legs can increase intra-abdominal pressure, leading to increased ICP. Logrolling should be used. Maintain the neck in neutral position at all times to avoid neck vein compression, which can interfere with venous return. Maintain the head of the bed in the flat position or elevated to 30 degrees, depending on medical orders and facility procedure. Avoid noxious stimuli, using soft voices or music and a gentle touch. Plan care to avoid grouping activities and procedures known to increase ICP. Bathing, turning, and other routine care often have a cumulative effect to increase ICP when performed in succession. Allow rest periods between procedures and carefully assess the patient's response to interventions (Hickey, 2003; Hockenberry, 2005).

The Taylor Suite offers these additional resources to enhance learning and facilitate understanding:

- thePoint online resource, http://thepoint.lww.com/Lynn2E
- Student CD-ROM included with the book
- Skills Checklist to Accompany Taylor's Clinical Nursing Skills

Developing Critical Thinking Skills

1. Aleta Jackson, age 68, was involved in a head-on collision. She has begun to complain that the cervical collar is hurting her neck. What should you do?
2. Yuka Chong had spinal surgery yesterday and is to be logrolled every 2 hours. The nurse caring for Yuka had her push her patient-controlled analgesia button 10 minutes prior to turning. When you go to turn Yuka and change her bed linens, you find that Yuka's dressing has a small saturated spot that has soiled the sheet. What should you do?
3. Mr. and Mrs. Gladstone ask about "the tube coming out of Nikki's head," referring to her ventriculostomy. What will you tell them regarding the rationale for the ventriculostomy? What guidelines regarding positioning and turning Nikki will you keep in mind when caring for her and include in your teaching with her parents?

Bibliography

Allen, L. (2005). Neurosurgical emergency care. *Australian Nursing Journal, 12*(11), 38.

Arbour, R. (2004). Intracranial hypertension. Monitoring and nursing assessment. *Critical Care Nurse, 24*(5), 19–32.

Baird-Holmes, S., & Brown, S. (2005). Skeletal pin site care. National Association of Orthopaedic Nurses: Guidelines for orthopaedic nursing. *Orthopaedic Nursing, 24*(2), 99–106.

Elkin, M. K., et al. (2004). *Nursing interventions and clinical skills* (3rd ed.). St. Louis, MO: Mosby.

Gupta, A. K. (2002). Monitoring the injured brain in the intensive care unit. *Journal of Post-Graduate Medicine, 48*(3), 218–225.

Hickey, J. V. (2003). *The clinical practice of neurological and neurosurgical nursing* (5th ed.). Philadelphia: Lippincott Williams & Wilkins.

Hockenberry, M. (2005). *Wong's essentials of pediatric nursing* (7th ed.). St. Louis, MO: Elsevier Mosby.

Josephson, L. (2004). Management of increased intracranial pressure. *Dimensions of Critical Care Nursing, 23*(5), 194–207.

Littlejohns, L. R. (2005). Ask the experts . . . external ventricular drainage (EVD) systems. *Critical Care Nurse, 25*(3), 57–59.

Lower, J. (2002). Facing neuro assessment fearlessly. *Nursing, 32*(2), 58–64.

Lynn-McHale, D., & Carlson, K. K. (2001). *AACN procedure manual for critical care* (4th ed.). Philadelphia: W. B. Saunders.

March, Karen. (2005). Intracranial pressure monitoring: Why monitor? *AACN Clinical Issues: Advanced Practice in Acute & Critical Care, 16*(4), 456–475.

Porth, C. (2005). *Pathophysiology: Concepts of altered health states* (7th ed.). Philadelphia: Lippincott Williams & Wilkins.

Pullen, R. (2004). Logrolling a patient. *Nursing, 34*(2), 22.

Shoemaker, W., et al. (2002). *Procedures and monitoring for the critically ill.* Philadelphia: W. B. Saunders.

Sirven, J., & Malamut, B. (2002). *Clinical neurology of the older adult.* Philadelphia: Lippincott Williams & Wilkins.

Smeltzer, S. C., Bare, B. G., Hinkle, J. H., & Cheever, K. H. (2008). *Brunner and Suddarth's textbook of medical-surgical nursing* (11th ed.). Philadelphia: Lippincott Williams & Wilkins.

Taylor, C., Lillis, C., LeMone, P, & Lynn, P. (2008). *Fundamentals of nursing: The art & science of nursing care* (6th ed.). Philadelphia: Lippincott Williams & Wilkins

Waterhouse, C. (2005). The Glasgow Coma Scale and other neurological observations. *Nursing Standard, 19*(33), 56–64.

CHAPTER 18

Laboratory Specimen Collection

Focusing on Patient Care

This chapter will help you develop some of the skills related to collecting specimens of body fluids when caring for the following patients:

Joseph Conklin, age 90, has been admitted to the hospital due to confusion related to a suspected urinary tract infection. You are to obtain a urine specimen for urinalysis and culture.

Huana Yon, age 67, has made an appointment to see her primary physician for a yearly exam. She is to collect a stool specimen for occult blood testing.

Catherine Yeletsky, age 54, is a patient in the cardiac care unit. She has been diagnosed with heart failure and is receiving cardiac monitoring. She also has diabetes and requires peripheral capillary (fingerstick) blood sampling to monitor her blood glucose levels.

Learning Objectives

After studying this chapter, you will be able to:

1. Test a stool specimen for occult blood.
2. Collect a stool specimen for culture.
3. Obtain a capillary blood sample for glucose testing.
4. Collect a sputum specimen (expectorated) for culture.
5. Obtain a urine specimen (clean catch, midstream) for urinalysis and culture.
6. Obtain a urine specimen from indwelling urinary catheter.
7. Collect a venous blood specimen by venipuncture for routine laboratory testing.
8. Obtain a venous blood specimen for culture and sensitivity.
9. Obtain an arterial blood specimen for blood gas analysis.

Key Terms

arterial blood gas (ABG): a laboratory test that evaluates the adequacy of oxygenation, ventilation and acid–base status

expectorate: expel from the mouth; spit

lancet: a small, sharp device for piercing the skin

occult blood: blood that is hidden in a stool specimen or cannot be seen on gross examination

protocol: written plan that details the nursing activities to be executed in specific situations

standard: acceptable, expected level of performance established by authority, custom, or consent

Standard Precautions: precautions used in the care of all hospitalized individuals, regardless of their diagnosis or possible infection status; these precautions apply to blood, all body fluids, secretions and excretions (except sweat), nonintact skin, and mucous membranes

sterile technique: involves practices used to render and keep objects and areas free from microorganisms

Specimens are collected to aid in the screening and diagnosing of patient health problems, directing treatment, and monitoring the effectiveness of treatments. The most commonly collected specimens are blood, urine, stool, and sputum (Fishbach & Dunning, 2006). Follow facility protocol to collect, handle, and transport specimen. Always observe standard precautions and use sterile technique where appropriate. It is very important to adhere to protocols and standards, collect the appropriate amount, use appropriate containers and media, and store and transfer the specimen within specified timelines (Fishbach & Dunning). It is also extremely important to ensure accurate labeling of any specimen collected, according to facility policy. These measures prevent invalid and inaccurate test results.

Patient teaching is an important part of specimen collection. Explain the rationale for the sample collection and the process for obtaining the specimen. Evaluate the patient's ability to follow the specific procedure for collecting the specimen.

When collecting a specimen, take care to prevent the outside of the container from becoming contaminated with any secretions or body fluids. Place all laboratory specimens in plastic bags marked "Biohazard" and seal the bags to prevent leakage during transportation.

This chapter will review methods to obtain specimens for common laboratory tests. Nurses also must be knowledgeable about normal and abnormal findings associated with these laboratory tests. Fundamentals Review 18-1 and 18-2 highlight the normal findings associated with stool and urine specimens.

Fundamentals Review 18-1

Characteristics of Stool

Characteristic	Normal Findings	Special Considerations for Observation
Volume	Variable	Volume of the stool depends on the amount the person eats and the nature of the diet. For example, a diet high in roughage produces more feces than a soft, bland diet. Consistently large diarrheal stools suggest a disorder in the small bowel or proximal colon; small, frequent stools with urgency to pass them suggest a disorder of the left colon or rectum.
Color	Infant: Yellow to brown Adult: Brown	The brown color of the stool is due to stercobilin, a bile pigment derivative. The rapid rate of peristalsis in the breastfed infant causes the stool to be yellow. The color of the stool is influenced by diet. For example, the stool will be almost black if the person eats red meat and dark green vegetables, such as spinach. The stool will be light brown if the diet is high in milk and milk products and low in meat. The absence of bile may cause the stool to appear white or clay colored. Certain drugs influence the color of the stool. For example, iron salts cause the stool to be black. Antacids cause it to be whitish. Bleeding high in the intestinal tract causes a stool to be black due to the digestion of the blood. Bleeding low in the intestinal tract results in fresh blood in the stool. The stool darkens with standing.
Odor	Pungent; may be affected by foods ingested	The characteristic odor of the stool is due to indole and skatole, caused by putrefaction and fermentation in the lower intestinal tract. The odor of the stool is influenced by its pH value, which normally is neutral or slightly alkaline. Excessive putrefaction causes a strong odor. The presence of blood in the stool causes a unique odor.
Consistency	Soft, semisolid, and formed	The consistency of the stool is influenced by fluid and food intake and gastric motility. The less time stool spends in the intestine (or the shorter the intestine), the more liquid the stool. Many pathologic conditions influence consistency.
Shape	Formed stool is usually about 1" (2.5 cm) in diameter and has the tubular shape of the colon, but may be larger or smaller, depending on the condition of the colon.	A gastrointestinal obstruction may result in a narrow, pencil-shaped stool. Rapid peristalsis thins the stool. Increased time spent in the large intestine may result in a hard, marble-like fecal mass.

(continued)

Characteristics of Stool *(continued)*

Characteristic	Normal Findings	Special Considerations for Observation
Constituents	Waste residues of digestion: bile, intestinal secretions, shed epithelial cells, bacteria, and inorganic material (chiefly calcium and phosphates); seeds, meat fibers, and fat may be present in small amounts.	Internal bleeding, infection, inflammation, and other pathologic conditions may result in abnormal constituents. These include blood, pus, excessive fat, parasites, ova, and mucus. Foreign bodies also may be found in the stool.

Characteristics of Urine

Characteristic	Normal Findings	Special Considerations
Color	A freshly voided specimen is pale yellow, straw-colored, or amber, depending on its concentration.	Urine is darker than normal when it is scanty and concentrated. Urine is lighter than normal when it is excessive and diluted. Certain drugs, such as cascara, L-dopa, and sulfonamides, alter the color of urine. Some foods can alter the color; for example, beets can cause urine to appear red in color.
Odor	Normal urine smell is aromatic. As urine stands, it often develops an ammonia odor because of bacterial action.	Some foods cause urine to have a characteristic odor; for example, asparagus causes urine to have a strong, musty odor. Urine high in glucose content has a sweet odor. Urine that is heavily infected has a fetid odor.
Turbidity	Fresh urine should be clear or translucent; as urine stands and cools, it becomes cloudy.	Cloudiness observed in freshly voided urine is abnormal and may be due to the presence of red blood cells, white blood cells, bacteria, vaginal discharge, sperm, or prostatic fluid.
pH	The normal pH is about 6.0, with a range of 4.6 to 8. (Urine alkalinity or acidity may be promoted through diet to inhibit bacterial growth or urinary stone development or to facilitate the therapeutic activity of certain medications.) Urine becomes alkaline on standing when carbon dioxide diffuses into the air.	A high-protein diet causes urine to become excessively acid. Certain foods tend to produce alkaline urine, such as citrus fruits, dairy products, and vegetables, especially legumes. Certain foods, such as meats, tend to produce acidic urine. Certain drugs influence the acidity or alkalinity of urine; for example, ammonium chloride produces acidic urine, and potassium citrate and sodium bicarbonate produce alkaline urine.

Characteristics of Urine *(continued)*

Characteristic	Normal Findings	Special Considerations
Specific gravity	This is a measure of the concentration of dissolved solids in the urine. The normal range is 1.015 to 1.025.	Concentrated urine will have a higher-than-normal specific gravity, and diluted urine will have a lower-than-normal specific gravity. In the absence of kidney disease, a high specific gravity usually indicates dehydration and a low specific gravity indicates overhydration.
Constituents	*Organic* constituents of urine include urea, uric acid, creatinine, hippuric acid, indican, urene pigments, and undetermined nitrogen. *Inorganic* constituents are ammonia, sodium, chloride, traces of iron, phosphorus, sulfur, potassium, and calcium.	*Abnormal constituents* of urine include blood, pus, albumin, glucose, ketone bodies, casts, gross bacteria, and bile.

SKILL 18-1 Testing Stool for Occult Blood

Certain conditions, such as ulcer disease, inflammatory bowel disorders, and colon cancer, place the patient at high risk for intestinal bleeding, which can be detected in the stool. Occult blood (hidden blood or blood that cannot be seen on gross examination) in the stool can be detected with simple screening tests. These tests, which may be performed quickly by nurses within an institution or by patients at home, use reagent substances to detect the enzyme peroxidase in the hemoglobin molecule. The Hematest and guaiac test are chemical tests commonly used to identify occult blood in the stool.

Ingestion of certain substances before the specimen collection can result in false-positive results. These substances include red meat, animal liver and kidneys, salmon, tuna, mackerel and sardines, tomatoes, cauliflower, horseradish, turnips, melon, bananas, and soybeans. Certain medications, such as a salicylate intake of more than 325 mg daily, steroids, iron preparations, and anticoagulants, also may lead to false-positive readings (Ahmed, Karch, & Karch, 2000; Kyle & Prynn, 2004). The ingestion of vitamin C can produce false-negative results even if bleeding is present. The following are recommendations for the patient preparing for a fecal occult blood test:

- Before stool testing, avoid the foods (for 4 days) and drugs (for 7 days) that may alter test results.
- In a woman who is menstruating, postpone the test until 3 days after her period has ended.
- Postpone the test if hematuria or bleeding hemorrhoids are present.
- Postpone the test if the patient has had a recent nose or throat bleed.
- Caution a person who is color-blind to the color blue not to attempt to interpret the test results.

In clinical settings, these restrictions are usually not practical. Be sure to note the presence of any of the aforementioned conditions in the clinical setting.

(continued)

SKILL 18-1 Testing Stool for Occult Blood *(continued)*

The below procedure describes collecting a specimen from a bedpan, commode, or plastic receptacle in toilet. Performing a digital rectal examination to obtain a stool specimen for occult blood is described in the Skill Variation at the end of the skill.

Equipment

- Disposable gloves
- Wooden applicator
- Hemoccult testing card and developer
- Bedpan or plastic collection receptacle for toilet
- Biohazard bag
- Appropriate label for specimen, based on facility policy and procedure

ASSESSMENT

Assess the patient's understanding of the collection procedure and ability to cooperate. Assess the patient for a history of gastrointestinal bleeding. Review prescribed restrictions for medications and diet, and evaluate patient compliance with required restrictions. Assess patient for any blood in perineal area, including hemorrhoids, menstruation, urinary tract infection, or vaginal or rectal tears. Blood may be from a source other than the gastrointestinal tract.

NURSING DIAGNOSIS

Determine the related factors for the nursing diagnoses based on the patient's current status. Several nursing diagnoses may be appropriate, including:

- Deficient Knowledge
- Constipation
- Diarrhea
- Bowel Incontinence
- Anxiety
- Pain

OUTCOME IDENTIFICATION AND PLANNING

The expected outcome to achieve is that an uncontaminated stool sample is obtained, following collection guidelines, and transported to the laboratory within the recommended time frame, without adverse effect. Other outcomes may include the following: the patient demonstrates accurate understanding of testing instructions; the patient verbalizes a decrease in anxiety; and the specimen is obtained with minimal discomfort or embarrassment.

IMPLEMENTATION

ACTION	RATIONALE
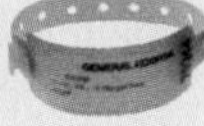 1. Identify the patient. Discuss with patient the need for a stool sample. Explain to patient the process by which the stool will be collected, either from a bedpan, commode, or plastic receptacle in toilet.	Identifying the patient ensures the right patient receives the intervention and helps prevent errors. Discussion and explanation help to allay some of the patient's anxiety and prepare the patient for what to expect. Organization facilitates performance of tasks.
2. Close curtains around bed or close door to room if possible.	Closing the door or curtain provides for patient privacy.
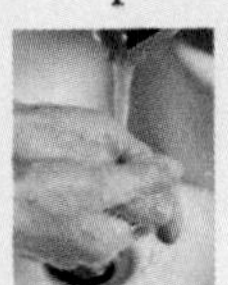 3. Perform hand hygiene.	Hand hygiene deters the spread of microorganisms.

SKILL 18-1 Testing Stool for Occult Blood *(continued)*

ACTION	RATIONALE
4. Place the plastic collection receptacle in the toilet, if applicable. Assist the patient to the bathroom or onto the bedside commode, or assist the patient onto the bedpan. Instruct patient not to urinate or discard toilet paper with the stool, which may contaminate the specimen.	Proper collection into an appropriate receptacle for stool prevents inaccurate results. Urine or toilet paper can contaminate the specimen, interfering with accurate results.
5. After the patient defecates, assist the patient out of the bathroom, off the commode, or remove the bedpan. Perform hand hygiene and put on disposable gloves.	Hand hygiene deters the spread of microorganisms. Gloves protect nurse from microorganisms in feces.
6. **With wooden applicator, apply a small amount of stool from the center of the bowel movement onto one window of Hemoccult testing card. With opposite end of wooden applicator, obtain another sample of stool from another area and apply a small amount of stool onto second window of Hemoccult card (Figure 1).**	Two separate areas of the same stool sample are tested in case there is trace blood from a hemorrhoid or fissure. By using opposite ends of the wooden applicator, cross-contamination is avoided.

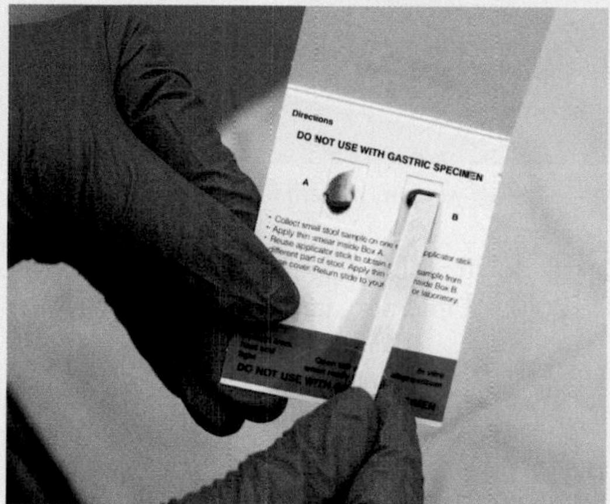

Figure 1. Using a wooden applicator to transfer stool specimen to window of testing card.

ACTION	RATIONALE
7. Close flap over stool samples.	Closing the flap prevents contamination of the samples.
8. If sending to laboratory, check specimen label with patient identification bracelet. Label should include patient's name and identification number, time specimen was collected, route of collection, identification for person obtaining sample, and any other information required by agency policy. Label the specimen card per facility policy. Place in sealable plastic biohazard bag and send to laboratory immediately.	Facilities may allow point-of-service testing (at bedside or on unit) or specimen may have to be sent to laboratory for testing. Confirmation of patient identification information ensures specimen is labeled correctly for the right patient. Packaging the specimen in a biohazard bag prevents the person transporting the container from coming in contact with stool.

(continued)

SKILL 18-1 Testing Stool for Occult Blood *(continued)*

ACTION	RATIONALE
9. If testing at bedside, open flap on opposite side of card and **place two drops of developer over each window and wait the time stated in the manufacturer's instructions (Figure 2).**	The developer will react with any blood in the stool. Following the manufacturer's instructions promotes accuracy of results.
10. Observe card for any blue areas (Figure 3).	Any blue coloring on the card indicates a positive test result for blood.

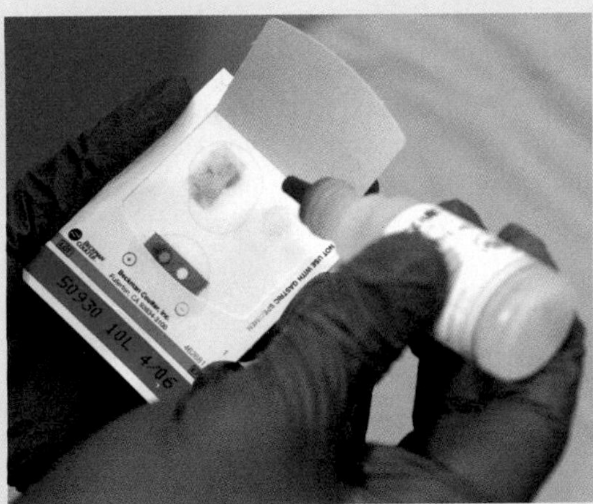

Figure 2. Applying developer to card windows.

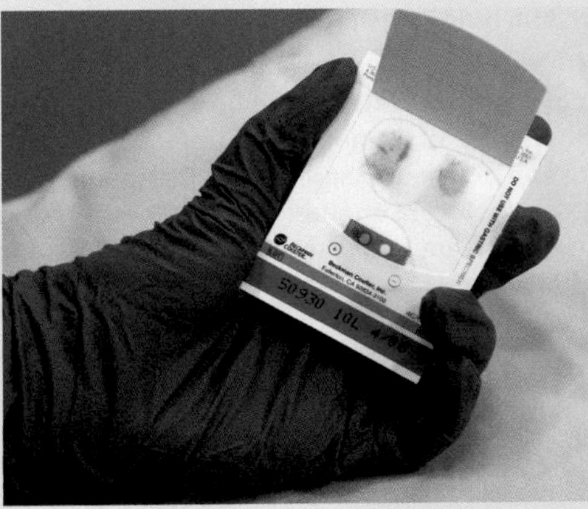

Figure 3. Observing windows on card for blue areas.

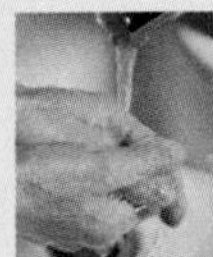

ACTION	RATIONALE
11. Discard Hemoccult testing slide appropriately, according to facility policy. Remove gloves and perform hand hygiene.	Hand hygiene and proper disposal of equipment reduces the transmission of microorganisms.

EVALUATION

The expected outcome is met when a stool sample is obtained following collection guidelines and transported to the laboratory within the recommended time frame, without adverse effect; the patient demonstrates accurate understanding of testing instructions; the patient verbalizes decreased anxiety; and the specimen is obtained with minimal discomfort and embarrassment. If the patient is to obtain the stool sample on his or her own, another outcome is met when the patient is able to collect the stool and place it correctly on the card.

DOCUMENTATION

Guidelines

Document method used to obtain specimen and transport to laboratory. If testing done by nurse, document results and communication of results to healthcare provider.

Sample Documentation

07/12/08 1040 Stool sample obtained from bowel movement. Labeled and sent to lab for occult blood testing.—K. Sanders, RN

Unexpected Situations and Associated Interventions

- *One window tests positive, while the second window tests negative:* This could indicate that the blood is from a source other than the gastrointestinal tract. These results should be documented and the primary care provider notified.

SKILL 18-1 Testing Stool for Occult Blood *(continued)*

Special Considerations

General Considerations

- Specimen should be obtained from formed bowel movement. Liquid stool may cause false-negative results.
- To ensure validity, test should be repeated three to six times on different samples on different days.
- Specimen can be collected from ostomy appliance. Apply a clean ostomy appliance and obtain sample as soon as patient passes stool into the appliance.

Infant and Child Considerations

- Stool can be collected from the diaper of an infant or child, as long as the specimen is not contaminated with urine.

Home Care Considerations

- Patients are often instructed on how to collect stool specimens for occult blood at home and bring the samples to the office, clinic, or laboratory. Patients should understand that it is important to follow instructions carefully to ensure validity of results. Patients are responsible only for obtaining a sample of stool and applying to collection card. Testing is done at the clinic, office, or laboratory.

SKILL VARIATION Performing a Digital Rectal Exam to Obtain a Stool Specimen for Occult Blood

- Identify the patient. Discuss with patient the need for a stool sample. Explain to patient the process by which the stool will be collected, as a result of a digital rectal examination.
- Perform hand hygiene and put on nonsterile gloves.
- If patient is able to stand, instruct patient to bend over examination table or bed placed at a comfortable height. If patient is bedridden, place in Sims' or side-lying position.
- **Generously lubricate 1″ to 1.5″ of finger with water-soluble lubricant to be inserted into anus to collect stool sample.**
- Ask patient to take a large, deep breath through the nose and exhale through the mouth.
- After separating buttocks with nondominant hand, gently insert lubricated finger of dominant hand 1″ to 2″ into rectum while lightly palpating for any stool (Figure 1).
- Remove finger. **Apply stool to one window of Hemoccult testing card. Apply stool to second window of Hemoccult testing card from different place on glove than first sample.**
- Close flap over stool samples.
- Depending on facility policy, actual testing of stool may take place at bedside or the specimen may be sent to the laboratory.
- If sending to laboratory, label the specimen card per facility policy. Place in sealable plastic biohazard bag and send to laboratory immediately.
- If testing at bedside, open flap on opposite side of card and **place two drops of developer over each window and wait the time stated in the manufacturer's instructions.**
- Observe card for any blue areas.
- Discard Hemoccult testing slide. Remove disposable gloves from inside out and discard. Perform hand hygiene.
- Document method used to obtain sample and testing results.

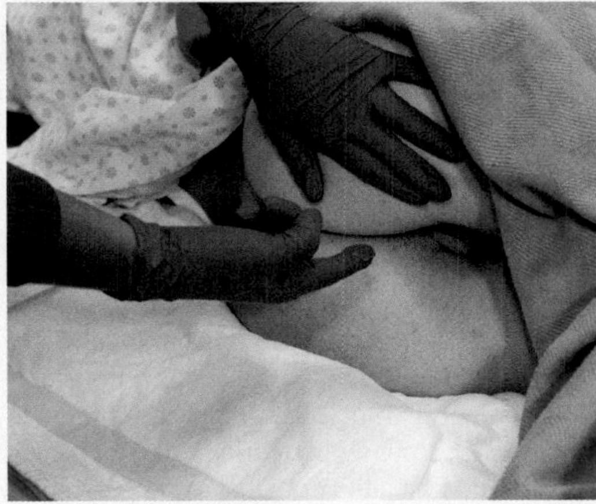

Figure 1. Separating buttocks with nondominant hand and inserting lubricated finger into rectum.

SKILL 18-2 Collecting a Stool Specimen for Culture

A stool specimen may be ordered to screen for pathogenic organisms, such as *c. difficile* or ova and parasites, electrolytes, fat, and leukocytes. The nurse is responsible for obtaining the specimen according to agency procedure, labeling the specimen, and ensuring that the specimen is transported to the laboratory in a timely manner. The institution's policy and procedure manual or laboratory manual identifies specific information about the amount of stool needed, the time frame during which stool is to be collected, and the type of specimen container to use.

Usually, 1″ (2.5 cm) of formed stool or 15 to 30 mL of liquid stool is sufficient. If portions of the stool include visible blood, mucus, or pus, include these with the specimen. Also be sure that the specimen is free of any barium or enema solution. Because a fresh specimen produces the most accurate results, send the specimen to the laboratory immediately. If this is not possible, refrigerate it unless contraindicated, such as when testing for ova and parasites. Refrigeration will affect parasites. Ova and parasites are best detected in warm stool. Some institutions require ova and parasite specimens to be placed in container filled with preservatives; check institutional policy.

Equipment

- Tongue blade (2)
- Clean specimen container (or container with preservatives for ova and parasites)
- Biohazard bag
- Nonsterile gloves
- Appropriate label for specimen, based on facility policy and procedure

ASSESSMENT

Assess the patient's understanding of the need for the test and the requirements of the test. Ask the patient when his or her last bowel movement was, and check the patient's medical record for this information.

NURSING DIAGNOSIS

Determine the related factors for the nursing diagnoses based on the patient's current status. Appropriate nursing diagnoses include:

- Deficient Knowledge
- Diarrhea
- Anxiety

OUTCOME IDENTIFICATION AND PLANNING

The expected outcome to achieve is that an uncontaminated specimen is obtained and sent to the laboratory promptly. Additional outcomes that may be appropriate include the following: the patient demonstrates ability to collect stool specimen and verbalizes a decrease in anxiety related to stool collection.

IMPLEMENTATION

ACTION	RATIONALE
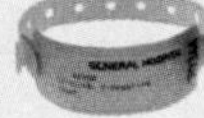 1. Gather necessary equipment. Identify the patient. Place disposable collection container (hat) in toilet or bedside commode to catch stool without urine. Instruct patient to void first and not to discard toilet paper with stool. Tell patient to call you as soon as bowel movement is completed.	Organization facilitates performance of task. Identifying the patient ensures the right patient receives the intervention and helps prevent errors. The patient should void first because the laboratory study may be inaccurate if the stool contains urine. Placing a container in the toilet or bedside commode aids in obtaining a clean stool specimen uncontaminated by urine. Explanation helps to alleviate anxiety and facilitate cooperation.
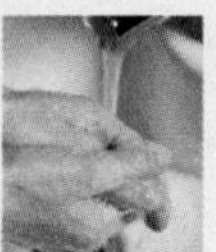 2. Perform hand hygiene and put on gloves.	Hand hygiene deters the spread of microorganisms. Gloves protect nurse from microorganisms in feces.

SKILL 18-2 Collecting a Stool Specimen for Culture *(continued)*

ACTION	RATIONALE
3. After patient has passed a stool, use the tongue blades to obtain a sample, free of blood or urine, and place it in a dry, clean container.	Due to the nature of the testing, no preservatives are needed for the stool. The container does not have to be sterile, since stool is not sterile. To ensure accurate results, the stool should be free of urine or menstrual blood.
4. Collect as much of the stool as possible to send to the laboratory.	Different tests and laboratories require different amounts of stool. Collecting as much as possible helps to ensure that the laboratory has an adequate amount of specimen for testing.
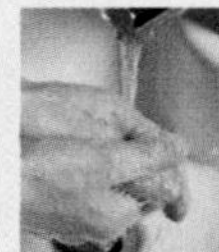 5. Place lid on container. Remove gloves and perform hand hygiene.	Hand hygiene deters the spread of microorganisms.
6. Check specimen label with patient identification bracelet. Label should include patient's name and identification number, time specimen was collected, route of collection, identification for person obtaining sample, and any other information required by agency policy. Place label on the container per facility policy. Place container in plastic sealable biohazard bag.	Confirmation of patient identification information ensures specimen is labeled correctly for the right patient. Packaging the specimen in a biohazard bag prevents the person transporting the container from coming in contact with stool.
7. **Transport specimen to laboratory while stool is still warm. If immediate transport is impossible, check with laboratory personnel or policy manual as to whether refrigeration is contraindicated.**	Most tests have better results with fresh stool. Different tests may require different preparation if the test is not immediately completed. Some tests will be compromised if the stool is refrigerated.

EVALUATION

The expected outcome is met when the patient passes a stool that is not contaminated by urine or menstrual blood and is placed in a clean container. The specimen is transported appropriately to the laboratory. The patient participates in stool collection and verbalizes feelings of diminished anxiety related to the procedure.

DOCUMENTATION

Guidelines

Document amount, color, and consistency of stool obtained, time of collection, and specific test for which the specimen was collected.

Sample Documentation

7/12/08 2045 Large amount of pasty, green stool sent to laboratory for ova and parasite testing.—K. Sanders, RN

Unexpected Situations and Associated Interventions

- *Patient is menstruating or has discarded toilet paper into commode with stool:* Call laboratory to discuss possible effects on test results. Not all tests will be affected by contaminants. The laboratory may accept the specimen even with the contaminant. Make notation on order card that goes to laboratory with specimen.
- *Specimen is inadvertently left on counter instead of being sent to laboratory:* Call laboratory to discuss possible effects on test results. Not all tests will be affected by leaving the specimen on the counter for a period of time. The laboratory may accept the specimen even though it has been sitting out. Make sure that the time on the card is the actual time the specimen was obtained.

(continued)

SKILL 18-2 Collecting a Stool Specimen for Culture *(continued)*

Special Considerations

General Considerations

- If patient is wearing a diaper, the stool may be collected from diaper, as long as it is not contaminated with urine.
- Barium procedures and laxatives should be avoided for 1 week before specimen collection to ensure valid results.
- Specimen can be collected from ostomy appliance. Apply a clean ostomy appliance and obtain sample as soon as patient passes stool into the appliance.
- If a timed stool test is ordered, such as fecal fat, the entire amount of stool produced for 24 to 72 hours is sent to the laboratory. Be sure to follow instructions for storage while collection is ongoing.

Infant and Child Considerations

- Stool can be collected from the diaper of an infant or child, as long as the specimen is uncontaminated with urine.

Home Care Considerations

- Patients are often instructed on how to collect stool specimens at home and bring the samples to the office, clinic, or laboratory. Patients should understand that it is important to follow instructions carefully to ensure validity of results. Ensure the patient understands the proper procedure for sample storage before bringing to laboratory or office.

SKILL 18-3 Obtaining a Capillary Blood Sample for Glucose Testing

Blood glucose monitoring provides information about how the body is controlling glucose metabolism. Controlling patient's blood glucose levels reduces complications, saves lies, shortens hospital stays, and reduces healthcare costs (Levetan, 2005). It is indicated in the care of patients with many conditions, including diabetes, seizures, enteral and parenteral feeding, liver disease, pancreatitis, head injury, stroke, alcohol and drug intoxication, and sepsis. Point-of-care testing (testing done at the bedside, where samples are not sent to the laboratory) provides a convenient, rapid, and accurate measurement of blood glucose (Ferguson, 2005). Blood samples are commonly obtained from the edges of the fingers for adults, but samples can be obtained from the earlobe, forearm, and anterior thigh, depending on the monitor used. Avoid fingertips, because they are more sensitive. Rotate sites to prevent skin damage. It is important to be familiar with and follow the manufacturer's guidelines and facility policy and procedure to ensure accurate results. Normal fasting glucose is 60 to 110 mg/dL (Levetan, 2005).

Equipment

- Blood glucose meter
- Sterile lancet
- Cotton balls or gauze squares
- Testing strips for meter
- Nonsterile gloves
- Alcohol swab or soap and water

ASSESSMENT

Assess the patient's history for indications necessitating the monitoring of blood glucose levels, such as high-carbohydrate feedings, history of diabetes mellitus, or corticosteroid therapy. In addition, assess the patient's knowledge about monitoring blood glucose. Assess the area of the skin to be used for testing. Avoid bruised and open areas.

SKILL 18-3

Obtaining a Capillary Blood Sample for Glucose Testing *(continued)*

NURSING DIAGNOSIS

Determine the related factors for the nursing diagnoses based on the patient's current status. Possible nursing diagnoses may include:

- Risk for Injury
- Deficient Knowledge
- Anxiety

OUTCOME IDENTIFICATION AND PLANNING

The expected outcome to achieve is that the blood glucose level is measured accurately without adverse effect. In addition, the patient remains free of injury, the patient demonstrates a blood glucose level within acceptable parameters, the patient demonstrates ability to participate in monitoring, and the patient verbalizes increased comfort with the procedure.

IMPLEMENTATION

ACTION	RATIONALE
1. Check the patient's medical record or nursing plan of care for monitoring schedule. You may decide that additional testing is indicated based on nursing judgment and the patient's condition.	This confirms scheduled times for checking blood glucose. Independent nursing judgment may lead to the decision to test more frequently, based on the patient's condition.
2. Gather equipment.	This provides an organized approach to the task.
3. Close curtains around bed and close door to room if possible.	Closing the curtain or door provides for patient privacy.
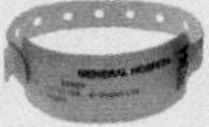 4. Identify the patient. Explain procedure to patient and instruct patient about the need for monitoring blood glucose.	Identifying the patient ensures the right patient receives the intervention and helps prevent errors. Explanation helps to alleviate anxiety and facilitate cooperation.
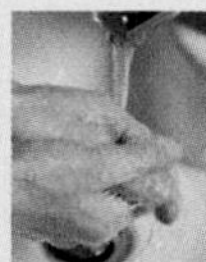 5. Perform hand hygiene. Put on nonsterile gloves.	Hand hygiene deters the spread of microorganisms. Gloves protect nurse from exposure to blood or body fluids.
6. Turn the monitor on.	Allows monitor to be used.
7. Enter the patient's identification number, if required, according to facility policy.	Allows for electronic storage and accurate identification of patient data.
8. Prepare lancet using aseptic technique.	Aseptic technique maintains sterility.
9. Remove test strip from the vial. **Recap container immediately.** Test strips also come individually wrapped. Turn monitor on. **Check that code number for the strip matches code number on monitor screen.**	Immediately recapping protects strips from exposure to humidity, light, and discoloration. Matching code numbers on the strip and glucose monitor ensures that the machine is calibrated correctly.
10. Insert strip into the meter according to directions for that specific device.	Correctly inserted strip allows meter to read blood glucose level accurately.
11. For adult, massage side of finger toward puncture site.	Massage encourages blood to flow to the area.
12. **Have patient wash hands with soap and warm water and dry thoroughly. Alternately, the skin may be cleansed with an alcohol swab. Allow skin to dry completely.**	Washing with soap and water or alcohol cleanses the puncture site. Warm water also helps to cause vasodilation. Alcohol can interfere with accuracy of results if not completely dried.

(continued)

SKILL 18-3 Obtaining a Capillary Blood Sample for Glucose Testing *(continued)*

ACTION	RATIONALE
13. Hold lancet perpendicular to skin and pierce site with lancet (Figure 1).	Holding lancet in proper position facilitates proper skin penetration.

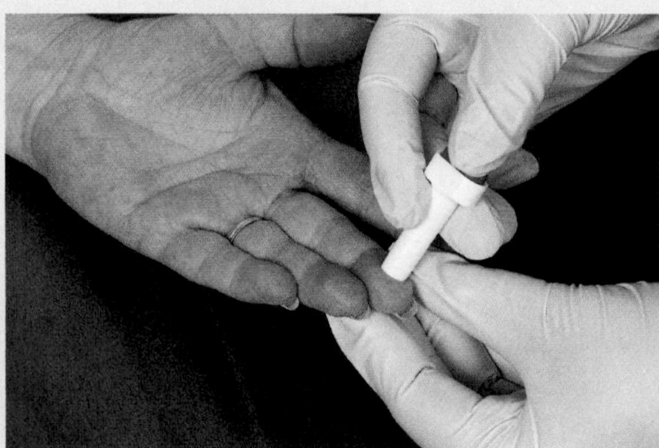

Figure 1. Piercing patient's finger with lancet.

ACTION	RATIONALE
14. **Wipe away first drop of blood with gauze square or cotton ball if recommended by manufacturer of monitor.**	Manufacturers recommend discarding the first drop of blood, which may be contaminated by serum or cleansing product, producing an inaccurate reading.
15. Encourage bleeding by lowering hand, making use of gravity. Lightly stroke the finger, if necessary, until sufficient amount of blood has formed to cover the sample area on the strip, based on monitor requirements (check instructions for monitor). Take care not to squeeze the finger, not to squeeze at puncture site, or not to touch puncture site or blood.	An appropriate-sized droplet facilitates accurate test results. Squeezing can cause injury to the patient and alter the test result (Ferguson, 2005).
16. **Gently touch drop of blood to pad on test strip without smearing it (Figure 2).**	Smearing blood on strip may result in inaccurate test results.

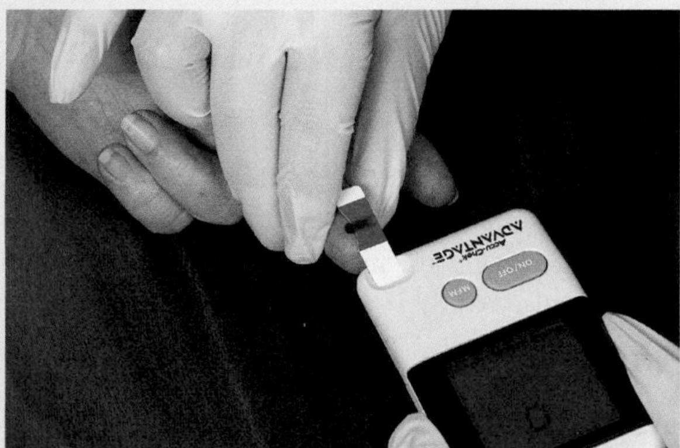

Figure 2. Applying blood to test strip.

ACTION	RATIONALE
17. Press time button if directed by manufacturer.	Correct timing produces accurate results.
18. Apply pressure to puncture site with a cotton ball. **Do not use alcohol wipe.**	Pressure causes hemostasis. Alcohol stings and may prolong bleeding.

SKILL 18-3

Obtaining a Capillary Blood Sample for Glucose Testing *(continued)*

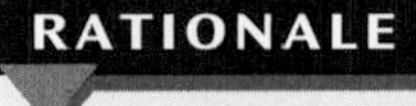

ACTION	RATIONALE
19. Read blood glucose results and document appropriately at bedside. Inform patient of test result.	Timing depends on type of meter.
20. Turn meter off, remove test strip and dispose of supplies appropriately. Place lancet in sharps container.	Proper disposal prevents exposure to blood and accidental needlesticks.
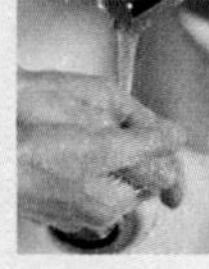 21. Remove gloves and perform hand hygiene.	Hand hygiene prevents the spread of microorganisms.

EVALUATION

The expected outcome is met when the patient's blood glucose level is measured accurately without adverse effect; the blood glucose level is within acceptable limits; the patient participates in monitoring; and the patient verbalizes comfort with the procedure.

DOCUMENTATION

Guidelines

Document blood glucose level in medical record for flow sheet, according to facility policy. Document pertinent patient assessments, any intervention related to glucose level, and any patient teaching. Report abnormal results and/or significant assessments to primary healthcare provider.

Sample Documentation

11/1/08 0800 Patient performed own fingerstick blood glucose test with minimal guidance. Verbalized rationale for fasting measurement and able to state symptoms of hypoglycemia. Patient's fingerstick blood glucose level 168. 4 units regular humulin insulin given per sliding scale, in addition to 10 units NPH humulin insulin scheduled for 0800. Patient encouraged to review written guidelines for subcutaneous insulin administration; will review procedure and plan to have patient administer insulin at dinnertime. Patient verbalized an understanding.—B. Clapp, RN

Unexpected Situations and Associated Interventions

- *Extremity is pale and cool to the touch:* Begin by warming the extremity. Have adult patients warm their hands by rubbing them together. Warm moist compresses also may be used.
- *Blood glucose level results are above or below normal parameters:* Assess the patient for signs of hypoglycemia or hyperglycemia. Check medical record for ordered interventions, such as insulin dosage or carbohydrate administration. Notify healthcare provider of results and assessment.

Special Considerations

General Considerations

- Meters require calibration at least monthly or according to the manufacturer's recommendation, and when a new bottle of test strips is opened. Manufacturer's directions for calibration should be followed. After calibration, the meter is checked for accuracy by testing a control solution containing a known amount of glucose.
- Inadequate sampling can cause errors in the results. It is very important to be aware of requirements for specific monitor used.

(continued)

SKILL 18-3 Obtaining a Capillary Blood Sample for Glucose Testing *(continued)*

- Monitors that measure glucose collected from the skin have recently become available. One of these devices use electrical stimulation to draw interstitial fluid through intact skin into a transdermal pad worn like a watch and provides a reading every 20 minutes. Another device is a monitor worn on a belt that uses a fine needle worn in the subcutaneous tissue to measure interstitial fluid glucose levels and transmit the results to a computer (Corbett, 2004).

Infant and Child Considerations

- In infants and young children, use the heel to obtain the blood specimen. In an infant, use the outer aspect of the heel.
- If the heel is cool, place a warm compress on the foot.

Older Adult Considerations

- Meters are available with large digital readouts or audio components for patients with visual impairments.

Home Care Considerations

- Patients monitor blood glucose levels routinely at home.
- There are many different types of monitors available. Assist patients to identify desirable features for individual use.

SKILL 18-4 Collecting a Sputum Specimen for Culture

Sputum analysis is used to diagnose disease, test for drug sensitivity, and guide patient treatment. Sputum may be obtained to identify pathogenic organisms, determine if malignant cells are present, and assess for hypersensitivity states. A sputum specimen may be ordered if a bacterial, viral, or fungal infection of the pulmonary system is suspected. Sputum can be collected by having the patient expectorate into a sterile container. A sputum specimen can also be obtained by endotracheal suctioning, during bronchoscopy, and via transtracheal aspiration. Collecting an expectorated sputum specimen first thing in the morning when the patient rises is desired, as secretions have accumulated during the night, aiding in the collection process (Smeltzer et al, 2008).

The below procedure describes collecting an expectorated sample. Collecting a sputum specimen by suctioning via an endotracheal tube is discussed in the Skill Variation at the end of the skill.

Equipment

- Sterile sputum specimen container
- Nonsterile gloves
- Goggles or safety glasses
- Biohazard bag
- Appropriate label for specimen, based on facility policy and procedure

ASSESSMENT

Assess patient's lung sounds. Patients with a productive cough may have coarse, wheezing, or diminished lung sounds. Monitor oxygen saturation levels, because patients with excessive pulmonary secretions may have decreased oxygen saturation. Assess patient's level of pain. Consider administering pain medication before obtaining the sample, since patient will have to cough. Assess the characteristics of the sputum; color, quantity, presence of blood, and viscosity.

SKILL 18-4 Collecting a Sputum Specimen for Culture *(continued)*

NURSING DIAGNOSIS

Determine the related factors for the nursing diagnoses based on the patient's current status. Appropriate nursing diagnoses may include:

- Risk for Infection
- Acute Pain
- Ineffective Airway Clearance
- Impaired Gas Exchange

OUTCOME IDENTIFICATION AND PLANNING

The expected outcome to achieve when collecting a sputum specimen is that the patient produces an adequate sample from the lungs. Other outcomes that may be appropriate include the following: airway patency is maintained; oxygen saturation increases; the patient demonstrates understanding about the need for specimen collection; and the patient demonstrates improved respiratory status.

IMPLEMENTATION

ACTION	RATIONALE
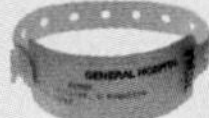 1. Identify the patient. Explain procedure to patient. If patient may have pain with coughing, administer pain medication if ordered. If patient can perform task without assistance after instruction, leave container at bedside with instructions to call nurse as soon as specimen is produced.	Identifying the patient ensures the right patient receives the intervention and helps prevent errors. Explanation provides reassurance and promotes cooperation. Pain relief facilitates compliance.
2. Assemble equipment.	This provides for organized approach.
3. Close curtains around bed and close door to room if possible.	Closing curtain or door provides for patient privacy.
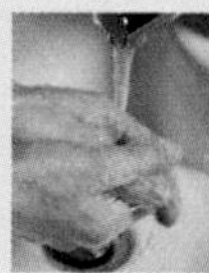 4. Perform hand hygiene. Put on disposable gloves and goggles.	Hand hygiene deters the spread of microorganisms. The gloves and goggles prevent contact with blood and body fluids.
5. Adjust bed to comfortable working position. Lower side rail closer to you. Place patient in semi-Fowler's position. **Have patient clear nose and throat and rinse mouth with water before beginning procedure.**	The semi-Fowler's position will help the patient to cough and expectorate the sputum specimen. Water will rinse the oral cavity of saliva and any food particles.
6. **Instruct patient to inhale deeply and cough.** If patient has had abdominal surgery, assist patient to splint abdomen.	The specimen will need to come from the lungs; saliva is not acceptable. Splinting helps to reduce the pain in the abdominal incision.
7. If patient produces sputum, open the lid to the container and have patient expectorate specimen into container.	The specimen needs to come from the lungs; saliva is not acceptable.
8. If patient believes he or she can produce more specimen, have patient repeat the procedure.	This ensures that there is an adequate amount of specimen for analysis.
9. Close lid to container. Offer oral hygiene to patient.	Closing the container prevents contamination of the specimen and possible infection transmission. Oral hygiene helps to remove pathogens from the oral cavity.

(continued)

SKILL 18-4 Collecting a Sputum Specimen for Culture *(continued)*

ACTION	RATIONALE
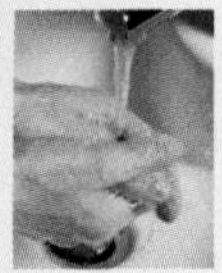 10. Remove goggles and gloves. Perform hand hygiene.	Hand hygiene deters the spread of microorganisms.
11. Check specimen label with patient identification bracelet. Label should include patient's name and identification number, time specimen was collected, route of collection, identification for person obtaining sample, and any other information required by agency policy. Place label on the container per facility policy. Place container in plastic sealable biohazard bag. Immediately transport to laboratory.	Confirmation of patient identification information ensures specimen is labeled correctly for the right patient. Packaging the specimen in a biohazard bag prevents the person transporting the container from coming in contact with stool.

EVALUATION

The expected outcome is met when the patient expectorates sputum, and it is collected in a sterile container and sent to the laboratory as soon as possible. In addition, the patient maintains a patent airway, oxygen saturation level is within expected parameters, and the patient demonstrates understanding about the rationale for the specimen collection.

DOCUMENTATION

Guidelines

Record the time the specimen was collected and sent, and the characteristics and amount of secretions. Document the tests for which the specimen was collected. Note the respiratory assessment pre and post collection. Note antibiotics administered in the past 24 hours on the laboratory request form, if required by the facility.

Sample Documentation

9/13/08 1015 Respirations unlabored; lungs with decreased breath sounds at posterior bases. Sputum specimen obtained; patient has moderate amount of thick, yellow sputum; specimen sent to lab for culture and sensitivity.—C. Bausler, RN

Unexpected Situations and Associated Interventions

- *Patient produced a specimen but did not tell you, so you don't know how long the specimen has been sitting at the bedside:* Unless the patient is able to tell you when the specimen was produced, discard the sample and recollect. Most specimens should be sent to the laboratory as soon as possible to ensure valid results.
- *Patient spits saliva into container, without specimen from lungs:* Instruct patient that specimen needs to come from the lungs. Review procedure for collection. Discard contaminated container and place new container at the bedside.

Special Considerations

General Considerations

- Sputum specimens for AFB (to test for tuberculosis) should be collected for 3 days in a row, in the morning.
- If patient understands directions and is able to cooperate, specimen-collection container may be left at bedside for patient to collect sputum when available. Instruct patient to call to inform staff as soon as sputum is produced, so it can be transported to laboratory in a timely manner.

SKILL 18-4 Collecting a Sputum Specimen for Culture *(continued)*

Home Care Considerations

- If the patient is to collect specimen at home, ensure that he or she has a clear understanding of collection procedure and that the specimen needs to be transported immediately to the laboratory. Reinforce the fact that they cannot touch the inside of the collection container. Sputum specimens usually cannot be refrigerated (Fischbach & Dunning, 2006).

SKILL VARIATION Collecting Sputum Specimen via Endotracheal Suctioning

Sputum specimens can be collected by suctioning an endotracheal tube or tracheostomy tube. A sterile collection receptacle is attached between the suction catheter and the suction tubing to trap sputum as it is removed from the patient's airway, before reaching the suction collection canister.

- Refer to Skill 14-18 for the procedure for endotracheal suctioning.
- After checking suction pressure (Step 7), attach a sterile specimen trap to the suction tubing, taking care to avoid contaminating the open ends (see Figure 1).
- Continue with Step 8, taking care to handle the suction tubing and sputum trap with your nondominant hand. Proceed with suction procedure.
- After first suction pass, if 1 to 2 mL of sputum has been obtained, disconnect specimen container, and set aside. If <1 mL has been collected, suction patient again, after waiting the appropriate amount of time for the patient to recover.
- If secretions are extremely thick or tenacious, flush the catheter with a small amount (1–2 mL) of sterile normal saline to aid in moving the secretions into the trap.
- Once sputum trap is removed, connect suction tubing to the suction catheter. The catheter may then be flushed with normal saline before suctioning again. Continue with suctioning procedure, if necessary, based on remaining steps in Skill 14-18.
- When suctioning is completed, check specimen label with patient identification bracelet. Label should include patient's name and identification number, time specimen was collected, route of collection, and any other information required by agency policy. Place label on the container per facility policy. Place container in plastic sealable biohazard bag and send to the laboratory immediately.

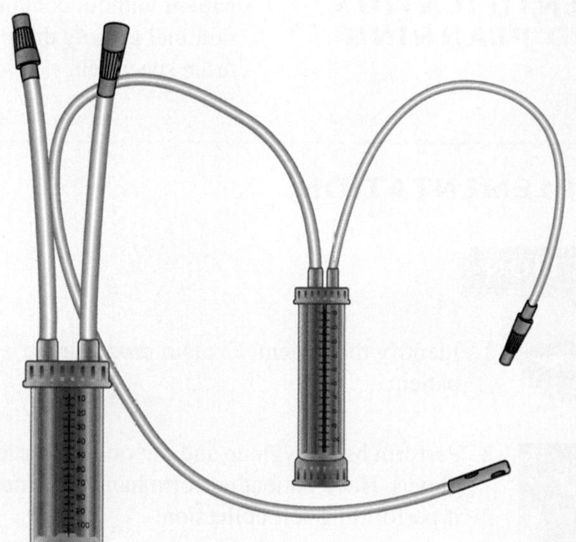

Figure 1. Suction trap for sputum collection.

SKILL 18-5 Collecting a Urine Specimen (clean catch, midstream) for Urinalysis and Culture

Collecting a urine specimen for urinalysis and culture is an assessment measure to determine the characteristics of a patient's urine. A voided urine specimen for culture is collected midstream to provide a specimen that most closely reflects the characteristics of the urine being produced by the body. If patient is able to understand and follow the procedure, the patient may collect sample for self.

Equipment

- Moist cleansing towelettes or soap, water, and washcloth
- Nonsterile gloves

(continued)

SKILL 18-5 Collecting a Urine Specimen (clean catch, midstream) for Urinalysis and Culture *(continued)*

- Sterile specimen container
- Biohazard bag
- Appropriate label for specimen, based on facility policy and procedure

ASSESSMENT

After verifying the physician's order for specimen collection, ask patient about any medications that he or she is taking, because medications may affect the results of the test. Assess for any signs and symptoms of a urinary tract infection, such as burning, pain (dysuria), or frequency. Assess the patient's ability to cooperate with the collection process. Assess need for assistance from nurse to obtain specimen correctly.

NURSING DIAGNOSIS

Determine the related factors for the nursing diagnoses based on the patient's current status. Possible nursing diagnoses may include:

- Altered Urinary Elimination
- Anxiety
- Deficient Knowledge

OUTCOME IDENTIFICATION AND PLANNING

The expected outcome to be met is that an adequate amount of urine is obtained from the patient without contamination. Other outcomes include the following: the patient exhibits minimal anxiety during specimen collection and demonstrates ability to collect a clean urine specimen.

IMPLEMENTATION

ACTION	RATIONALE
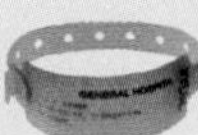 1. Identify the patient. Explain procedure to patient.	Identifying the patient ensures the right patient receives the intervention and helps prevent errors. Explanation provides reassurance and promotes cooperation.
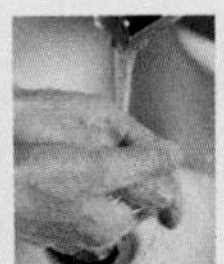 2. Perform hand hygiene and put on nonsterile gloves. Have patient perform hand hygiene, if performing self collection.	Hand hygiene prevents the transmission of microorganisms. Gloves prevent contact with blood and body fluids.
3. Close curtains around bed and close door to room if possible.	Closing door or curtain provides for patient privacy.
4. Assist the patient to the bathroom, onto the bedside commode or bedpan. Instruct patient not to defecate or discard toilet paper into the urine, which may contaminate the specimen (Figure 1).	

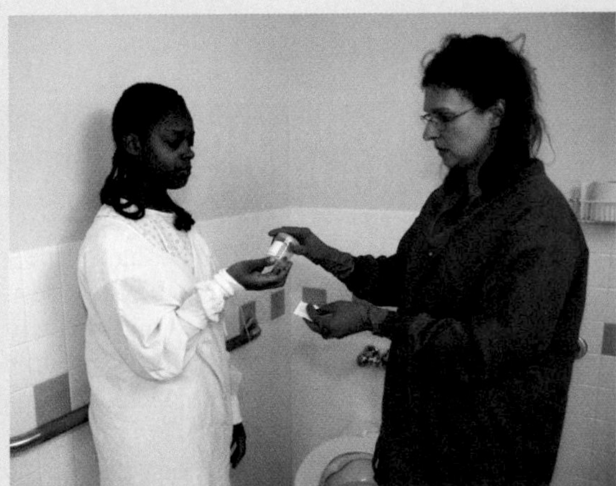

Figure 1. Instructing patient about the procedure for urine collection.

SKILL 18-5

Collecting a Urine Specimen (clean catch, midstream) for Urinalysis and Culture *(continued)*

ACTION	RATIONALE
5. Instruct the female patient to separate the labia for cleaning of the area and during collection of urine. Female patients should use the towelettes or wet washcloth to clean each side of the urinary meatus, then the center over the meatus, from front to back, using a new wipe for each stroke (Figure 2). Male patients should use a towelette to clean the tip of the penis, wiping in a circular motion away from the urethra. Instruct male patient who is not circumcised to retract foreskin before cleaning and during collection (Figure 3).	Cleaning the perineal area or penis reduces the risk for contamination of the specimen.

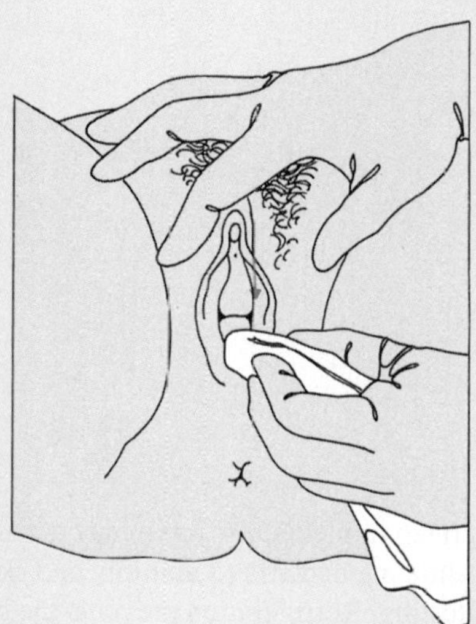

Figure 2. Cleaning female perineum. Separating labia and cleansing from front to back.

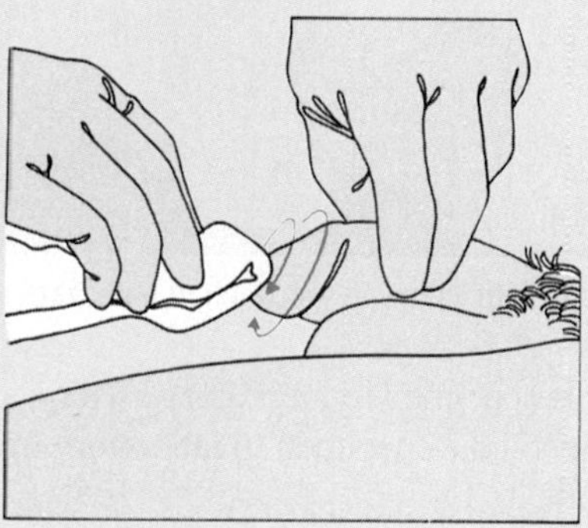

Figure 3. Cleaning male perineum. Wiping in a circular motion away from urethra.

ACTION	RATIONALE
6. **Have patient void about 25 mL into toilet, bedpan, or commode. The patient should then stop urinating briefly, then void into collection container. Collect specimen (10–20 mL is enough), and then finish voiding. Do not touch the inside of the container or the lid.**	Collecting a midstream specimen ensures that fresh urine is analyzed. Some urine may have collected in the urethra from the last void. By voiding a little before collecting the specimen, the specimen will contain only fresh urine.
7. Place lid on container. If necessary, transfer specimen to appropriate containers for ordered test, according to facility policy.	Placing lid on container helps to keep specimen clean and prevents spills.
8. Assist the patient from the bathroom, off the commode, or off the bedpan. Provide perineal care if necessary.	Perineal care promotes patient comfort and hygiene.
9. Remove gloves. Perform hand hygiene.	Hand hygiene deters the spread of microorganisms.

(continued)

SKILL 18-5 Collecting a Urine Specimen (clean catch, midstream) for Urinalysis and Culture *(continued)*

ACTION	RATIONALE
10. Check specimen label with patient identification bracelet. Label should include patient's name and identification number, time specimen was collected, route of collection, identification for person obtaining sample, and any other information required by agency policy. Place label on the container per facility policy. Place container in plastic sealable biohazard bag (Figure 4).	Confirmation of patient identification information ensures specimen is labeled correctly for the right patient. Labeling the container provides valuable information to the laboratory and ensures accurate reporting of results. Packaging the specimen in a biohazard bag prevents the person transporting the container from coming in contact with stool.

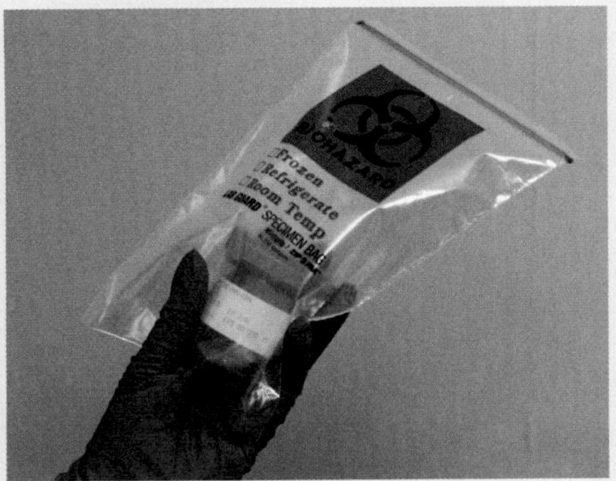

Figure 4. Placing labeled urine specimen in biohazard transport bag.

ACTION	RATIONALE
11. Transport specimen to laboratory as soon as possible. If unable to take specimen to laboratory immediately, refrigerate it.	If not refrigerated immediately, urine may act as a culture medium, allowing bacteria to multiply and skewing the results of testing. Refrigeration prevents the bacteria from multiplying.

EVALUATION

The expected outcome is met when an uncontaminated urine specimen is collected and sent to the laboratory. Other outcomes may include the following: the patient demonstrated the proper technique for specimen collection and stated that anxiety is lessened.

DOCUMENTATION

Guidelines

Document specimen sent, odor, amount (if known), color, and clarity of urine. Note significant patient assessments.

Sample Documentation

7/10/08 2200 Patient instructed to collect midstream urine sample. Verbalized understanding of directions. 70 mL of cloudy, odorless, yellow urine sent to laboratory. Patient denies pain or discomfort on urination.—A. Blitz, RN

SKILL 18-5

Collecting a Urine Specimen (clean catch, midstream) for Urinalysis and Culture *(continued)*

Unexpected Situations and Associated Interventions

- *Patient cannot provide a large enough urine sample:* Offer patient fluids to drink, although drinking too much fluid may dilute the urine, invalidating the test. Patient may return later in day to supply sample. Offer patient assistance with the next void.
- *When checking urine collection bag on an infant, nurse notes that bag has fallen off and the child has voided into the diaper:* Remove the bag, perform perineal care, and apply a new collection bag.
- *The patient missed voiding into the specimen container but did void into the specimen hat:* Do not use this urine as a sample for a culture; it could be heavily contaminated with bacteria and give a misleading result. Attempt to collect urine with next void. Offer patient assistance when trying to collect sample.

Special Considerations

General Considerations

- For many urine tests, such as a urinalysis, drug testing, or diabetes testing, the specimen does not need to be sterile and does not need to be collected as a midstream specimen. However, in the case of urinalysis, if the specimen shows nitrates and white blood cells, a culture of a urine specimen may be ordered.
- Since the first voiding of the day contains the highest bacterial counts, this sample should be collected whenever possible.
- Urine specimens may also be obtained by direct urethral catheterization. Refer to Skills 12-5 and 12-6 for catheterization procedure.

Infant and Child Considerations

- The most reliable method to obtain a urine specimen is to perform a suprapubic aspiration or transurethral catheterization for infants and children 2 months to 2 years of age (Dulczak, 2005). Discuss sampling options with primary care provider and patient's parents.
- Midstream collection can be accomplished with children older than 2 years of age, provided the child is able to follow direction and will cooperate with the nurse. Try having the child sit facing the back of the toilet, straddling the toilet seat. The nurse or parent can position them self behind the child, holding the sterile container for urine collection (Dulczak, 2005).
- A bagged specimen can be used for urinalysis, but not for urine culture. See the accompanying Skill Variation for the steps to obtain a bagged urine specimen for an infant or young child. If the urinalysis of the bagged specimen suggests the presence of a urinary tract infection, a second specimen must be obtained for culture, either by urethral catheterization or suprapubic aspiration, to verify the diagnosis and identify the causative microorganism.
- Familiar terms, such as "pee-pee" or "tinkle" may be used with young children, to ensure they understand what is being explained (Hockenberry, 2005). Enlist the assistance of the patient's parents or significant others to identify appropriate terms.

Home Care Considerations

- If the patient is to collect specimen at home, ensure they have a clear understanding of collection procedure, and that the specimen needs to be transported immediately to the laboratory. Reinforce the fact that they cannot touch the inside of the collection container. Urine specimens must be refrigerated until they can be brought to the laboratory.

(continued)

SKILL 18-5 Collecting a Urine Specimen (clean catch, midstream) for Urinalysis and Culture *(continued)*

SKILL VARIATION Obtaining a Bagged Urine Specimen for Urinalysis From an Infant or Young Child

- Identify the patient. Explain steps to a young child, if old enough, and to the parents. Talk to child at child's level, stressing that no pain will be involved.
- Perform hand hygiene and put on nonsterile gloves.
- Remove the diaper or underwear. Perform thorough perineal care with soap and water: for girls, spread labia and cleanse area; for boys, retract foreskin if intact and cleanse glans of penis. Pat skin dry.
- Remove paper backing from adhesive faceplate. Apply faceplate over labia or over penis. Gently push faceplate so that seal forms on skin (see Figure 1).
- Apply clean diaper or underwear over bag to help prevent dislodgement. Remove gloves and perform hand hygiene. **Check bag every 15 minutes to see whether child has voided.**
- As soon as the patient has voided, perform hand hygiene and put on nonsterile gloves. Gently remove bag by pushing skin away from bag. Transfer urine to appropriate container.
- Perform perineal care and reapply diaper or clothing.
- Remove gloves. Perform hand hygiene.
- Check specimen label with patient identification bracelet. Label should include patient's name and identification number, time specimen was collected, route of collection, and any other information required by agency policy. Place label on the container per facility policy. Place container in plastic sealable biohazard bag.
- Transport specimen to laboratory as soon as possible. If unable to take specimen to laboratory immediately, refrigerate it.
- If voiding does not occur within 15 minutes after applying the bag, the bag must be removed and reapplied following the same cleaning routine. The bag must be checked every 15 minutes until the patient voids (Dulczak, 2005).

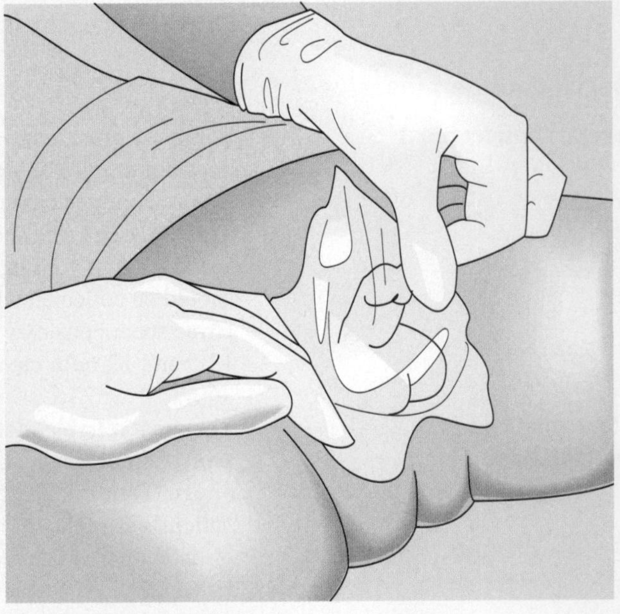

Figure 1. Applying infant urine collection bag.

SKILL 18-6 Obtaining a Urine Specimen From an Indwelling Urinary Catheter

Collecting a urine specimen for urinalysis and culture is an assessment measure to determine the characteristics of a patient's urine. Indwelling catheter drainage tubes have special sampling ports in the tubing for removal of urine for testing. Some ports require the use of a needle or blunt cannula to access the sampling port; others are needleless systems. The drainage tubing below the access port may be bent back on itself or clamped so that urine collects near the port, unless contraindicated, based on the patient's condition. Do not open the drainage system to obtain urine specimens. Urine specimens should never be taken from the catheter drainage bag because the urine is not fresh.

Equipment

- 10-mL sterile syringe
- 18-gauge needle or blunt cannula, if needed, based on specific catheter in use
- Nonsterile gloves

SKILL 18-6

Obtaining a Urine Specimen From an Indwelling Urinary Catheter *(continued)*

- Sterile specimen container
- Biohazard bag
- Appropriate label for specimen, based on facility policy and procedure

ASSESSMENT

After verifying the physician's order for specimen collection, review the medical record for information about any medications that the patient is taking, because medications may affect the results of the test. Assess the characteristics of the urine draining from the catheter. Assess the catheter tubing to identify type of sampling port.

NURSING DIAGNOSIS

Determine the related factors for the nursing diagnoses based on the patient's current status. Possible nursing diagnoses may include:

- Altered Urinary Elimination
- Anxiety
- Deficient Knowledge

OUTCOME IDENTIFICATION AND PLANNING

The expected outcome to be met is that an adequate amount of urine is obtained from the patient without contamination or adverse effect, and the patient experiences minimal anxiety during the collection process.

IMPLEMENTATION

ACTION	RATIONALE
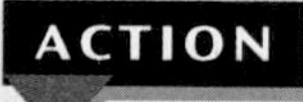 1. Identify the patient. Explain procedure to patient. Organize equipment at bedside.	Identifying the patient ensures the right patient receives the intervention and helps prevent errors. Explanation provides reassurance and promotes patient cooperation. Organization improves efficiency.
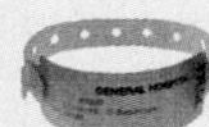 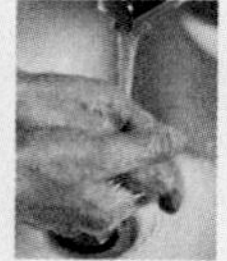 2. Perform hand hygiene and put on nonsterile gloves.	Hand hygiene deters the spread of microorganisms. Gloves protect nurse from any microorganisms in urine.
3. Close curtains around bed and close door to room if possible.	Closing curtain or door provides for patient privacy.
4. Clamp the catheter drainage tubing or bend it back on itself distal to the port. If an insufficient amount of urine is present in the tubing, allow tubing to remain clamped up to 30 minutes, to collect sufficient amount of urine, unless contraindicated. Remove lid from specimen container, keeping the inside of the container and lid free from contamination.	Clamping tubing ensures the collection of an adequate amount of fresh urine. Clamping for extended period of time leads to overdistention of the bladder. Clamping may be contraindicated based on patient's condition (after bladder surgery, for example). The container needs to remain sterile so as not to contaminate the urine.
5. **Cleanse aspiration port with alcohol wipe and allow port to air dry.**	Cleaning with alcohol deters entry of microorganisms when the needle punctures the port.

(continued)

SKILL 18-6

Obtaining a Urine Specimen From an Indwelling Urinary Catheter *(continued)*

ACTION	RATIONALE
6. Insert the blunt-tipped needle into the port, or attach the syringe to the needleless port. Slowly aspirate enough urine for specimen (usually 10 mL is adequate; check facility requirements) (Figure 1). Remove needle or syringe from port. Engage needle guard. **Unclamp drainage tubing.**	Using a blunt-tipped needle prevents a needlestick. Collecting urine from the port ensures that the specimen will contain fresh urine. Unclamping catheter drainage tubing prevents overdistention of and injury to the patient's bladder.

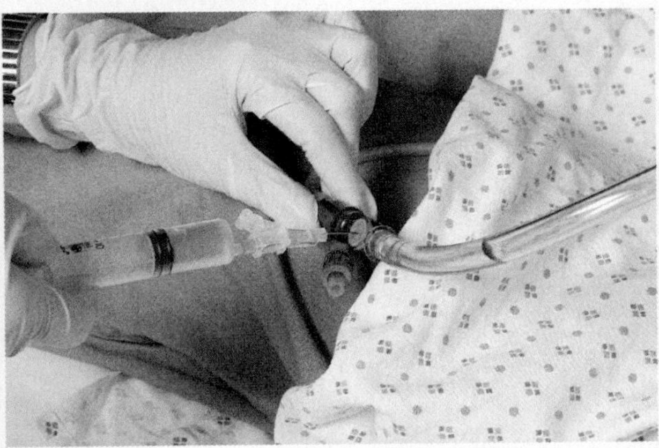

Figure 1. Inserting the needle in aspiration port and slowly withdrawing urine specimen.

ACTION	RATIONALE
7. If a needle was used on the syringe, remove the needle from the syringe before emptying the urine from the syringe into the specimen cup. Slowly inject urine into specimen container. Replace lid on container. Dispose of needle and syringe appropriately.	If the urine is injected quickly into the container, it may splash out of the container or into the nurse's eyes. Forcing urine through the needle breaks up cells and impedes accurate results of microscopic urinalysis.
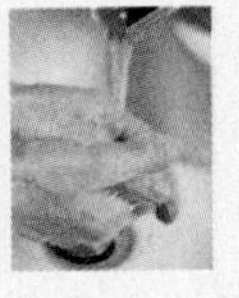 8. Remove gloves. Perform hand hygiene.	Hand hygiene deters the spread of microorganisms.
9. Check specimen label with patient identification bracelet. Label should include patient's name and identification number, time specimen was collected, route of collection, identification for person obtaining sample, and any other information required by agency policy. Place label on the container per facility policy. Place container in plastic sealable biohazard bag.	Confirmation of patient identification information ensures specimen is labeled correctly for the right patient. Packaging the specimen in a biohazard bag prevents the person transporting the container from coming in contact with stool.
10. Transport specimen to laboratory as soon as possible. If unable to take specimen to laboratory immediately, refrigerate it.	If not refrigerated immediately, urine may act as a culture medium, allowing bacteria to multiply and skewing the results of testing. Refrigeration prevents the bacteria from multiplying.

SKILL 18-6 Obtaining a Urine Specimen From an Indwelling Urinary Catheter *(continued)*

EVALUATION

The expected outcome is met when an uncontaminated urine specimen is collected and sent to the laboratory without adverse effect. Additionally, the patient does not experience increased anxiety during the collection process.

DOCUMENTATION

Guidelines

Document the method used to obtain the specimen; type of specimen sent; characteristics of urine. Note any significant patient assessments. Record urine volume on intake and output record, if appropriate.

Sample Documentation

10/20/08 1515 Patient with indwelling urinary catheter in place. Urine noted to be dark yellow and cloudy. Patient's temperature 103° F, pulse 96, respirations 18, BP 118/64. Dr. Burning notified. Specimen for urine culture obtained from indwelling catheter and catheter removed per order. Patient due to void by 2115.—B. Clapp, RN

Unexpected Situations and Associated Interventions

- *No urine or insufficient amount noted in catheter tubing:* Clamp tubing below access port for up to 30 minutes, according to facility policy, unless contraindicated by patient condition.

Special Considerations

General Considerations

- It is very important to remove clamp from drainage tubing as soon as the specimen is collected, unless there is a specific order to leave clamped, to prevent overdistention of the patient's bladder and injury.

SKILL 18-7 Using Venipuncture to Collect a Venous Blood Sample for Routine Testing

A venipuncture is used to obtain a venous blood sample. A venipuncture involves piercing a vein with a needle and collecting blood in a syringe or evacuated tube. The superficial veins of the arm are typically used for venipuncture; specifically, the vessels in the antecubital fossa. However, venipuncture can be performed on a vein in the dorsal forearm, the dorsum of the hand, or another accessible location. Do not use the inner wrist because of the high risk for damage to underlying structures. Avoid areas that are edematous, paralyzed, or are on the same side as a mastectomy, arteriovenous shunt, or graft. Areas of infection or with abnormal skin conditions should be avoided (Fischbach & Dunning, 2006). Do not draw blood form the same extremity being used for administration of intravenous medications, fluids, or blood transfusions. Some facilities will allow use of such sites as a 'last resort,' after the infusion has been held for a period of time. If necessary, choose a site distal to the intravenous access site. Check facility policy and procedure (Corbett, 2004; Fischbach & Dunning).

Explanation and communication with patients about the need for venipuncture can reduce anxiety. Information on the need for blood tests should be carefully explained to ensure patient understanding.

Measures to reduce the risk of infection are an important part of venipuncture. Hand hygiene, aseptic technique, the use of personal protective equipment, and safe disposal of sharps are key to providing safe venipuncture (Lavery & Ingram, 2005).

(continued)

SKILL 18-7 Using Venipuncture to Collect a Venous Blood Sample for Routine Testing *(continued)*

Equipment

- Tourniquet
- Nonsterile gloves
- Antimicrobial swab, such as chlorhexidine or alcohol
- Sterile needle, gauge appropriate to the vein and sampling needs, using the smallest possible
- Vacutainer needle adaptor
- Blood-collection tubes appropriate for ordered tests
- Appropriate label for specimen, based on facility policy and procedure
- Biohazard bag
- Gauze pads (2 × 2)
- Adhesive bandage

ASSESSMENT

Review the patient's medical record and physician order for the blood specimens to be obtained. Ensure that the necessary computerized laboratory request has been completed. Assess the patient for any allergies, especially to the topical antimicrobial to be used for skin cleansing. Assess for presence of any conditions or use of medications that may prolong bleeding time, necessitating additional application of pressure to puncture site. Ask the patient about any previous laboratory testing that he or she may have had, including any problems, such as difficulty with venipuncture, fainting, or complaints of dizziness, lightheadedness, or nausea. Assess the patient's anxiety level and understanding about the reasons for the blood test.

NURSING DIAGNOSIS

Determine the related factors for the nursing diagnoses based on the patient's current status. Appropriate nursing diagnoses may include:

- Deficient Knowledge
- Anxiety
- Risk for Injury
- Risk for Infection

Many other nursing diagnoses also may require the use of this skill.

OUTCOME IDENTIFICATION AND PLANNING

The expected outcome to achieve is that an uncontaminated specimen will be obtained without the patient experiencing undue anxiety and injury. Other outcomes may be appropriate depending on the patient's nursing diagnosis.

IMPLEMENTATION

ACTION	RATIONALE
1. Gather the necessary supplies. Check product expiration dates. Identify ordered tests and select the appropriate blood-collection tubes.	Organization facilitates efficient performance of the procedure. Ensures proper functioning of equipment. Using correct tubes ensures accurate blood sampling.
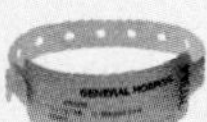 2. Identify the patient. Explain the procedure. Allow the patient time to ask questions and verbalize concerns about the venipuncture procedure.	Identifying the patient ensures the right patient receives the intervention and helps prevent errors. Explanation provides reassurance and promotes cooperation.
3. Close curtains around bed and close door to room if possible.	Closing the door or curtain provides for patient privacy.

SKILL 18-7

Using Venipuncture to Collect a Venous Blood Sample for Routine Testing *(continued)*

ACTION	RATIONALE
4. Provide for good light. Artificial light is recommended. Place a trash receptacle within easy reach.	Good lighting is necessary to perform the procedure properly.
5. Assist the patient to a comfortable position, either sitting or lying. If the patient is lying in bed, raise the bed to a comfortable working height. Expose the arm, supporting it in an extended position on a firm surface, such as a table top.	Proper positioning allows easy access to site and promotes patient comfort and safety. Having the bed in the high position reduces strain on the nurse's back while performing the procedure.
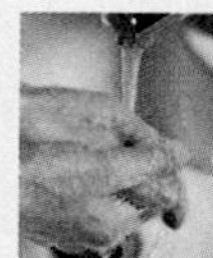 6. Perform hand hygiene.	Hand hygiene reduces the spread of microorganisms.
7. Determine the patient's preferred site for the procedure based on his or her previous experience. Apply a tourniquet to the upper arm on the chosen side approximately 3″ to 4″ above the potential puncture site. Apply enough pressure to impede venous circulation but not arterial blood flow.	Allows patient to be involved in treatment and gives the nurse information that may aid in site selection (Lavery & Ingram, 2005). Use of tourniquet increases venous pressure to aid in vein identification. Tourniquet should remain in place no more than 90 seconds to prevent injury (Lavery & Ingram, 2005).
8. Assess the veins to determine the best puncture site. Observe the skin for the vein's blue color, or palpate the vein for a firm rebound sensation.	Using the best site reduces the risk of injury to the patient. Identification of vein's course and depth aids in entry. Palpation allows for making distinction between other structures, such as tendons and arteries, in area to avoid injury.
9. Release the tourniquet. Check that the vein has decompressed (Lavery & Ingram, 2005).	Releasing the tourniquet reduces the length of time the tourniquet is applied. Tourniquet should remain in place no more than 90 seconds to prevent injury. Thrombosed veins will remain firm and palpable and should not be used for venipuncture (Lavery & Ingram, 2005).
10. Attach the needle to the Vacutainer device. Place first blood-collection tube into the Vacutainer, but not engaged in the puncture device in the Vacutainer.	Prepares device for use.
11. Put on nonsterile gloves. Clean the patient's skin at the selected puncture site with the antimicrobial swab. If using chlorhexidine, use a back-and-forth motion, applying friction for 30 seconds to site, or procedure recommended by the manufacturer. If using alcohol, wipe in a circular motion spiraling outward. Allow the skin to dry before performing the venipuncture.	Gloves prevent contact with blood and body fluids. Cleaning the patient's skin reduces risk for transmission of microorganisms. Allowing the skin to dry maximizes antimicrobial action and prevents contact of the substance with the needle on insertion, thereby reducing the sting associated with insertion.

(continued)

SKILL 18-7 Using Venipuncture to Collect a Venous Blood Sample for Routine Testing *(continued)*

ACTION	RATIONALE
12. Reapply the tourniquet approximately 3″ to 4″ above the identified puncture site (Figure 1). Apply enough pressure to impede venous circulation but not arterial blood flow.	Use of tourniquet increases venous pressure to aid in vein identification. Tourniquet should remain in place no more than 90 seconds to prevent injury (Lavery & Ingram, 2005).

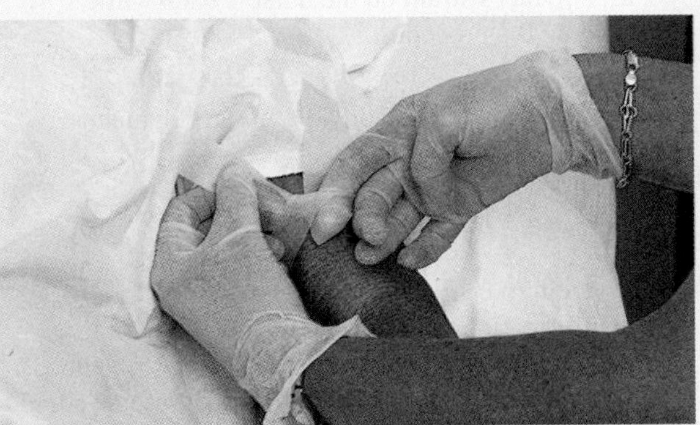

Figure 1. Applying the tourniquet.

ACTION	RATIONALE
13. Hold the patient's arm in a downward position with your nondominant hand. Align the needle and Vacutainer device with the chosen vein, holding the Vacutainer and needle in your dominant hand. Use the thumb or first finger of nondominant hand to apply pressure and traction to the skin just below the identified puncture site.	Applying pressure helps immobilize and anchor the vein. Taut skin at entry site aids smooth needle entry.
14. Inform the patient that he or she is going to feel a pinch. With the bevel of the needle up, insert the needle into the vein at a 15-degree angle to the skin (Fischbach & Dunning, 2006) (Figure 2).	Warning the patient prevents reaction related to surprise. Positioning the needle at the proper angle reduces the risk of puncturing through the vein.

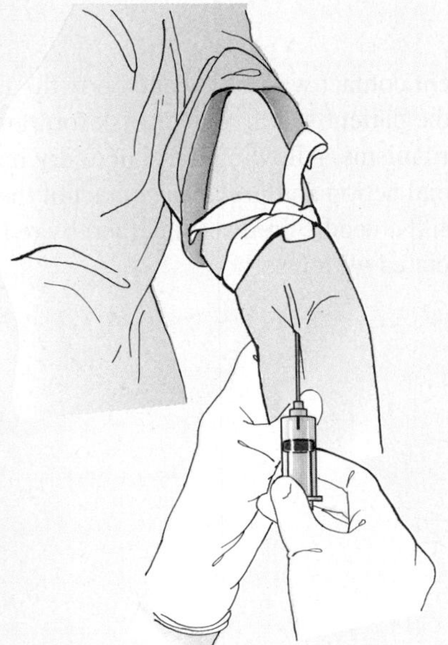

Figure 2. Inserting the needle at a 15-degree angle, with the bevel up.

SKILL 18-7 Using Venipuncture to Collect a Venous Blood Sample for Routine Testing *(continued)*

ACTION	RATIONALE
15. Grasp the Vacutainer securely to stabilize it in the vein with your nondominant hand, and push the first collection tube into the puncture device in the Vacutainer, until the rubber stopper on the collection tube is punctured. You will feel the tube push into place on the puncture device. Blood will flow into the tube automatically (Figure 3).	The collection tube is a vacuum; negative pressure within the tube pulls blood into the tube.

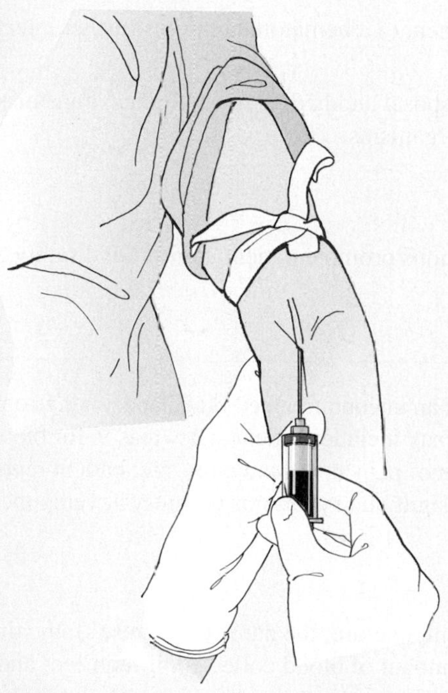

Figure 3. Observing blood flowing into the collection tube.

ACTION	RATIONALE
16. **Remove the tourniquet as soon as blood flows adequately into the tube.**	Tourniquet removal helps to prevent stasis and hemoconcentration, which can impair test results.
17. Continue to hold Vacutainer in place in the vein and continue to fill the required tubes, removing one and inserting another. Gently rotate each tube as you remove it.	Filling the required tubes ensures that the sample is accurate. Gentle rotation helps to mix any additive in the tube with the blood sample.
18. **After you have drawn all required blood samples, remove the last collection tube from the Vacutainer. Place a gauze pad over the puncture site and slowly and gently remove the needle from the vein. Engage needle guard.** Do not apply pressure to site until the needle has been fully removed.	Slow, gentle needle removal prevents injury to the vein. Releasing vacuum before withdrawing needle prevents injury to vein and hematoma formation. Use of needle guard prevents accidental needlestick injuries. Applying pressure to site after needle removal prevents injury.
19. Apply gentle pressure to the puncture site for 2 to 3 minutes or until bleeding stops.	This prevents bleeding and extravasation into the surrounding tissue, which can cause a hematoma.
20. After bleeding stops, apply an adhesive bandage.	The bandage protects the site and aids in applying pressure.

(continued)

SKILL 18-7 Using Venipuncture to Collect a Venous Blood Sample for Routine Testing *(continued)*

ACTION	RATIONALE
21. Check specimen labels with patient identification bracelet. Label should include patient's name and identification number, time specimen was collected, route of collection, identification for person obtaining sample, and any other information required by agency policy. Place label on the tubes per facility policy. Place tubes in plastic sealable biohazard bag. Immediately transport to laboratory.	Confirmation of patient identification information ensures specimen is labeled correctly for the right patient. Packaging the specimen in a biohazard bag prevents the person transporting the samples from coming in contact with blood.
22. Check the venipuncture site to see if a hematoma has developed.	Development of a hematoma requires further intervention.
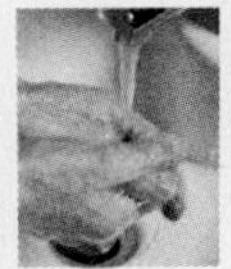 23. Discard Vacutainer and needle in sharps container. Remove gloves and perform hand hygiene.	Proper disposal and hand hygiene reduce transmission of microorganisms.
24. Assist the patient to a comfortable position. If patient's bed was raised, place the bed in the lowest position.	These actions promote patient comfort and safety.

EVALUATION

The expected outcome is achieved when an uncontaminated blood specimen is obtained without adverse event. Other outcomes may include: patient states reason for blood test; patient verbalizes minor if any complaint of pain at venipuncture site; patient reports decreased anxiety; and patient exhibits no signs and symptoms of injury at venipuncture site.

DOCUMENTATION

Guidelines

Record the date, time, and site of the venipuncture; the name of the test(s); the time the sample was sent to the laboratory; the amount of blood collected, if required; and any significant assessments or patient reactions.

Sample Documentation

6/10/08 0945 Blood specimen for CBC with differential obtained from right antecubital space. Approximately 8 cc of blood collected and sent to laboratory.
—C. Lewis, RN

Unexpected Situations and Associated Interventions

- *After applying the tourniquet, you have trouble finding a distended vein:* Have the patient make a fist, or try tapping the skin over the vein lightly several times. If unsuccessful, remove the tourniquet and try lowering the patient's arm to allow blood to pool in the veins. If necessary, apply warm compresses for about 10 minutes before reapplying the tourniquet.
- *The patient has large, distended, highly visible veins:* Perform venipuncture without a tourniquet to minimize the risk for hematoma.
- *Patient has a clotting disorder or is receiving anticoagulant therapy:* Maintain firm pressure on the venipuncture site for at least 5 minutes after withdrawing the needle to prevent hematoma formation.

SKILL 18-7 Using Venipuncture to Collect a Venous Blood Sample for Routine Testing *(continued)*

- *Oozing or bleeding continues from the puncture site for more than a few minutes:* Elevate the area and apply a pressure dressing. If bleeding is excessive or persists for longer than 10 minutes, notify the primary healthcare provider.
- *A hematoma develops at the venipuncture site:* Apply pressure until you are sure bleeding has stopped (about 5 minutes). Notify the patient's primary healthcare provider. Document size and appearance of hematoma, notification of primary healthcare provider, and any ordered interventions.
- *Patient reports feeling lightheaded and says she is going to faint:* Stop the venipuncture. If the patient is in bed, have the patient lie flat and elevate the feet. If the patient is in a chair, have the patient put her head between her knees. Encourage the patient to take slow, deep breaths. Call for assistance and stay with the patient. Obtain vital signs if possible.

Special Considerations

General Considerations

- Be aware of the facility's policy regarding order of collection of multiple tubes of blood to ensure accurate results.
- If the flow of blood into the collection tube or syringe is sluggish, leave the tourniquet in place longer, but always remove it before withdrawing the needle. Don't leave the tourniquet on for more than 90 seconds.
- Avoid collecting blood from edematous areas, arteriovenous shunts, an upper extremity on the same side as a previous lymph node dissection or mastectomy, infected sites, same extremity as an intravenous infusion, and sites of previous hematomas or vascular injury.
- Veins in the lower extremities should not be used for venipuncture, because of an increased risk of thrombophlebitis. Some facilities allow collection from lower extremities with a physician's order to collect blood from a leg or foot vein. Check your facility's policies.
- Warm compresses applied to the selected site 15 to 20 minutes before venipuncture can aid in distending veins that are difficult to locate.
- Consider the use of topical anesthetic creams to minimize discomfort and pain for the patient, based on facility policy. Be familiar with requirements and specifications for particular product available for use. Application needs to occur far enough in advance to allow enough time to become effective.
- Distraction has been shown to be of benefit in reducing anxiety related to venipuncture, especially with children. Asking the patient to concentrate on relaxing, and performing deep breathing may help. Asking the patient to cough at the time of venipuncture is another technique that has shown to be effective in reducing pain with venipuncture (Usichenko et al, 2004).

Infant and Child Considerations

- Use smaller-gauge needles with infants and children because their veins are smaller and more fragile.
- Consider automatically applying warm compresses to distend the small veins of infants and young children before attempting any venipuncture (Fischbach & Dunning, 2006).
- Use scalp vein (or "butterfly") needles as appropriate for obtaining blood in infants and small children.
- Be aware of alternative sites for venipuncture in infants and small children, including the scalp, hand, and foot. Use the lateral aspect of the heel to avoid the plantar artery.
- Keep in mind that the femoral vein may also be used for venipuncture for infants (Hockenberry, 2004).

Older Adult Considerations

- Keep in mind that the veins of an older adult are fragile and may collapse easily. In addition, the skin is less elastic and may be more difficult to pull taut.
- Consider performing venipuncture without a tourniquet for older patients to prevent rupture of capillaries. Instruct the patient to make a tight fist before needle insertion. Do not have the patient pump the fist, as this may increase plasma potassium levels (Fischbach & Dunning, 2006).

SKILL 18-8 Obtaining a Venous Blood Specimen for Culture and Sensitivity

Normally bacteria-free, blood is susceptible to infection through infusion lines as well as from thrombophlebitis, infected shunts, and bacterial endocarditis due to prosthetic heart-valve replacements. Bacteria may also invade the vascular system from local tissue infections through the lymphatic system and the thoracic duct.

Blood cultures are performed to detect bacterial invasion (bacteremia) and the systemic spread of such an infection (septicemia) through the bloodstream. In this procedure, a venous blood sample is collected by venipuncture into two bottles, one containing an anaerobic medium and the other an aerobic medium. Special collection bottles that are treated to neutralize antibiotics in the blood sample also are available. These special bottles can be used for patients who have received antibiotics before the cultures are obtained (Corbett, 2004; Rushing, 2004). The bottles are incubated, encouraging any organisms that are present in the sample to grow in the media. Ideally, two to three sets of cultures, 1 hour apart or from separate sites, should be obtained.

The main problem encountered with blood-culture testing is that the specimen is easily contaminated with bacteria from the environment. Care must be taken to properly clean the skin at the venipuncture site to prevent contamination with skin flora, and aseptic technique must be used during the procedure. The blood-culture bottle access ports must be properly cleaned before access.

Equipment

- Tourniquet
- Nonsterile gloves
- Antimicrobial swabs, such as chlorhexidine, per facility policy, for cleaning skin and culture bottle tops
- Vacutainer needle adaptor
- Sterile butterfly needle, gauge appropriate to the vein and sampling needs, using the smallest possible, with extension tubing
- Two blood-culture collection bottles for each set being obtained; one anaerobic bottle and one aerobic bottle
- Appropriate label for specimen, based on facility policy and procedure
- Biohazard bag
- Nonsterile gauze pads (2 × 2)
- Sterile gauze pads (2 × 2)
- Adhesive bandage

ASSESSMENT

Review the patient's medical record and the medical orders for the number and type of blood cultures to be obtained. Ensure that the appropriate computer laboratory request has been completed. Assess the patient for signs and symptoms of infection, including vital signs, and note any antibiotic therapy being administered. Inspect any invasive monitoring insertion sites or incisions for indications of infection. Assess the patient for any allergies, especially related to the topical antimicrobial used for skin cleansing. Assess for presence of any conditions or use of medications that may prolong bleeding time, necessitating additional application of pressure to puncture site. Ask the patient about any previous laboratory testing that he or she may have had, including any problems, such as difficulty with venipuncture, fainting, or complaints of dizziness, lightheadedness, or nausea. Assess the patient's anxiety level and understanding about the reasons for the blood test.

NURSING DIAGNOSIS

Determine the related factors for the nursing diagnoses based on the patient's current status. Appropriate nursing diagnoses may include:

- Hyperthermia
- Deficient Knowledge
- Anxiety
- Risk for Injury
- Risk for Infection

Many other nursing diagnoses also may require the use of this skill.

SKILL 18-8 Obtaining a Venous Blood Specimen for Culture and Sensitivity *(continued)*

OUTCOME IDENTIFICATION AND PLANNING

The expected outcome to achieve is that an uncontaminated specimen will be obtained without the patient experiencing undue anxiety and injury. Other outcomes may be appropriate depending on the patient's nursing diagnosis.

IMPLEMENTATION

ACTION	RATIONALE
1. Gather the necessary supplies. Check product expiration dates. Identify ordered tests and select the appropriate blood-collection tubes. If tests are ordered in addition to the blood cultures, collect the blood-culture specimens before other specimens (Rushing, 2004).	Organization facilitates efficient performance of the procedure. Use of equipment before expiration date ensures proper functioning of equipment. Using correct tubes ensures accurate blood sampling.
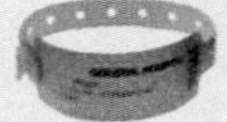 2. Identify the patient. Explain the procedure. Allow the patient time to ask questions and verbalize concerns about the venipuncture procedure.	Identifying the patient ensures the right patient receives the intervention and helps prevent errors. Explanation provides reassurance and promotes cooperation.
3. Close curtains around bed and close door to room if possible.	Closing the door or curtain provides for patient privacy.
4. Provide for good light. Artificial light is recommended. Place a trash receptacle within easy reach.	Good lighting is necessary to perform the procedure properly.
5. Assist the patient to a comfortable position, either sitting or lying. If the patient is lying in bed, raise the bed to a comfortable working height. Expose the arm, supporting it in an extended position on a firm surface, such as a table top.	Proper positioning allows easy access to site and promotes patient comfort and safety. Having the bed in the high position reduces strain on the nurse's back while performing the procedure.
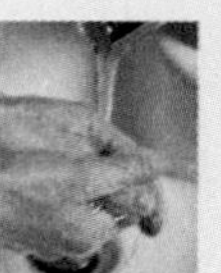 6. Perform hand hygiene.	Hand hygiene reduces the spread of microorganisms.
7. Determine the patient's preferred site for the procedure based on his or her previous experience. Apply a tourniquet to the upper arm on the chosen side approximately 3″ to 4″ above the potential puncture site. Apply enough pressure to impede venous circulation but not arterial blood flow.	Patient preference promotes patient participation in treatment and gives the nurse information that may aid in site selection (Lavery & Ingram, 2005). Use of tourniquet increases venous pressure to aid in vein identification. Tourniquet should remain in place no more than 90 seconds to prevent injury (Lavery & Ingram, 2005).
8. Assess the veins to determine the best puncture site. Observe the skin for the vein's blue color, or palpate the vein for a firm rebound sensation.	Using the best site reduces the risk of injury to the patient. Identification of vein's course and depth aids in entry. Observation and palpation allow for making distinction between other structures, such as tendons and arteries, in area to avoid injury.
9. Release the tourniquet. Check that the vein has decompressed (Lavery & Ingram, 2005).	Releasing the tourniquet reduces the length of time the tourniquet is applied. Tourniquet should remain in place no more than 90 seconds to prevent injury. Thrombosed veins will remain firm and palpable and should not be used for venipuncture (Lavery & Ingram, 2005).

(continued)

SKILL 18-8 Obtaining a Venous Blood Specimen for Culture and Sensitivity *(continued)*

ACTION	RATIONALE
10. Attach the butterfly-needle extension tubing to the Vacutainer device.	Connection prepares device for use.
11. Move collection bottles to a location close to arm, with bottles sitting upright on table top.	Bottles must be close enough to reach with extension tubing on butterfly needle to fill after venipuncture is completed. Bottles should remain upright to prevent backflow of contents to patient.
12. Put on nonsterile gloves. Clean the patient's skin at the selected puncture site with the antimicrobial swab. If using chlorhexidine, use a back-and-forth motion, applying friction for 30 seconds to site, or procedure recommended by the manufacturer. Allow the site to dry.	Gloves prevent contact with blood and body fluids. Cleaning the patient's skin reduces risk for transmission of microorganisms. Allowing the skin to dry maximizes antimicrobial action and prevents contact of the substance with the needle on insertion, thereby reducing the sting associated with insertion.
13. Using a new antimicrobial swab, clean the stoppers of the culture bottles with the appropriate antimicrobial, per facility policy. Cover bottle top with sterile gauze square, based on facility policy.	Cleaning the bottle top reduces risk for transmission of microorganisms into bottle. Covering top reduces risk of contamination.
14. Reapply the tourniquet approximately 3″ to 4″ above the identified puncture site (Figure 1). Apply enough pressure to impede venous circulation but not arterial blood flow.	Use of tourniquet increases venous pressure to aid in vein identification. Tourniquet should remain in place no more than 90 seconds to prevent injury (Lavery & Ingram, 2005).

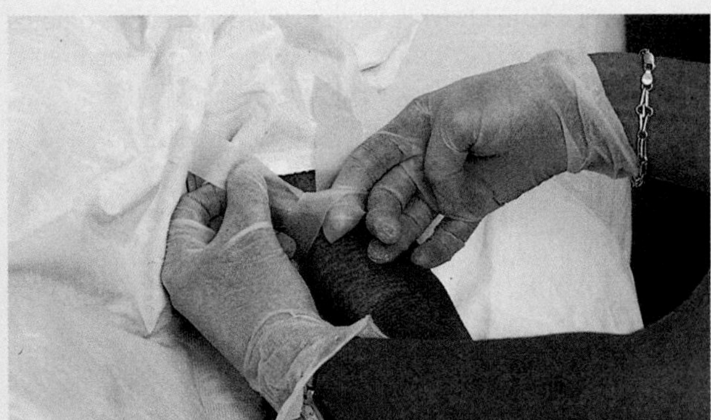

Figure 1. Applying the tourniquet.

ACTION	RATIONALE
15. Hold the patient's arm in a downward position with your nondominant hand. Align the butterfly needle with the chosen vein, holding the needle in your dominant hand. Use the thumb or first finger of nondominant hand to apply pressure and traction to the skin just below the identified puncture site. Do not touch the insertion site.	Applying pressure helps immobilize and anchor the vein. Taut skin at entry site aids smooth needle entry. Not touching the insertion site helps to prevent contamination.
16. Inform the patient that he or she is going to feel a pinch. With the bevel of the needle up, insert the needle into the vein at a 15-degree angle to the skin (Fischbach & Dunning, 2006). You should see a flash of blood in the extension tubing close to the needle when the vein is entered.	Warning the patient prevents reaction related to surprise. Positioning the needle at the proper angle reduces the risk of puncturing through the vein. Flash of blood indicates entrance into the vein.

SKILL 18-8 Obtaining a Venous Blood Specimen for Culture and Sensitivity *(continued)*

ACTION	RATIONALE
17. Grasp the butterfly securely to stabilize it in the vein with your nondominant hand, and push Vacutainer onto the first collection bottle (aerobic bottle), until the rubber stopper on the collection bottle is punctured. You will feel the bottle push into place on the puncture device. Blood will flow into the bottle automatically.	The collection bottle is a vacuum; negative pressure within the bottle pulls blood into the bottle. In case difficulties arise with blood draw, it is better to fill the aerobic bottle first because most septicemias are caused by aerobic organisms or anaerobes that can tolerate aerobic conditions (Corbett, 2004).
18. **Remove the tourniquet as soon as blood flows adequately into the bottle.**	Tourniquet removal helps to prevent stasis and hemoconcentration, which can impair test results.
19. Continue to hold butterfly needle in place in the vein. Once first bottle is filled, remove the Vacutainer and place on second bottle. After the blood culture specimens are obtained, continue to fill any additional required tubes, removing one and inserting another. Gently rotate each bottle and tube as you remove it.	Filling the required tubes ensures that the sample is accurate. Gentle rotation helps to mix any additive in the tube with the blood sample.
20. **After you have drawn all required blood samples, remove last collection tube from the Vacutainer. Place a gauze pad over the puncture site and slowly and gently remove the needle from the vein. Engage needle guard.** Do not apply pressure to site until the needle has been fully removed.	Slow, gentle needle removal prevents injury to the vein. Releasing vacuum before withdrawing needle prevents injury to vein and hematoma formation. Use of needle guard prevents accidental needlestick injuries. Applying pressure to site after needle removal prevents injury.
21. Apply gentle pressure to the puncture site with the gauze pad for 2 to 3 minutes or until bleeding stops.	This prevents bleeding and extravasation into the surrounding tissue, which can cause a hematoma.
22. After bleeding stops, apply an adhesive bandage.	The bandage protects the site and aids in applying pressure.
23. Check specimen labels with patient identification bracelet. Label should include patient's name and identification number, time specimen was collected, route of collection, identification for person obtaining sample, and any other information required by agency policy Place label on the culture bottles per facility policy. Place culture bottles and any other collection tubes in plastic sealable biohazard bags, according to facility policy. Immediately transport to laboratory.	Confirmation of patient identification information ensures specimen is labeled correctly for the right patient. Packaging the specimen in a biohazard bag prevents the person transporting the samples from coming in contact with blood.
24. Check the venipuncture site to see if a hematoma has developed.	Development of a hematoma requires further intervention.
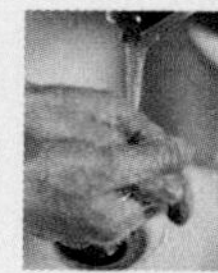 25. Discard Vacutainer and butterfly needle in sharps container. Remove gloves and perform hand hygiene.	Proper disposal and hand hygiene reduce transmission of microorganisms.
26. If a second set of blood cultures is ordered, repeat the procedure, collecting from another site or wait the specified time to obtain the specimen.	Drawing more than one set increases the chance of detection of any organisms.
27. Assist the patient to a comfortable position. If patient's bed was raised, place the bed in the lowest position.	Positioning promotes patient comfort and safety.

(continued)

SKILL 18-8

Obtaining a Venous Blood Specimen for Culture and Sensitivity *(continued)*

EVALUATION

The expected outcome is achieved when an uncontaminated blood specimen is obtained without adverse event. Other outcomes may include: patient states reason for blood test; patient verbalizes minor if any complaint of pain at venipuncture site; patient reports decreased anxiety; and patient exhibits no signs and symptoms of injury at venipuncture site.

DOCUMENTATION

Guidelines

Record the date, time, and site of the venipuncture; the name of the test(s); the time the sample was sent to the laboratory; the amount of blood collected, if required; and any significant assessments or patient reactions.

Sample Documentation

6/6/08 1710 Patient's temperature increased to 104.2° F. Patient very lethargic, pale, diaphoretic, with cool clammy skin. Bradycardic with pulse rate of 56 beats per minute and hypotensive with blood pressure of 90/50 mm Hg. Physician notified. Blood cultures × 2 ordered and obtained from two different sites; left and right antecubital veins.—B. Pearson, RN

Unexpected Situations and Associated Interventions

- *Your patient has had one set of blood cultures obtained but now requires another set. You expect to obtain the blood cultures from the patient's right antecubital site. When you are applying the tourniquet, the patient tells you, "That's where they got blood the last time":* Clarify if the patient is referring to the last set of blood cultures or other blood specimens. If the site was used for the previous blood cultures, use another site. If the site was used for routine blood specimens, ask the patient if the site is causing discomfort; if it is, choose another site for the venipuncture. If not, prepare the site for venipuncture.
- *After applying the tourniquet, you have trouble finding a distended vein:* Have the patient make a fist, or try tapping the skin over the vein lightly several times. If unsuccessful, remove the tourniquet and try lowering the patient's arm to allow blood to pool in the veins. If necessary, apply warm compresses for about 10 minutes before reapplying the tourniquet.
- *The patient has large, distended, highly visible veins:* Perform venipuncture without a tourniquet to minimize the risk for hematoma.
- *Patient has a clotting disorder or is receiving anticoagulant therapy:* Maintain firm pressure on the venipuncture site for at least 5 minutes after withdrawing the needle to prevent hematoma formation.
- *Oozing or bleeding continues from the puncture site for more than a few minutes:* Elevate the area and apply a pressure dressing. If bleeding is excessive or persists for longer than 10 minutes, notify the primary healthcare provider.
- *A hematoma develops at the venipuncture site:* Apply pressure until you are sure bleeding has stopped (about 5 minutes). Notify the patient's primary healthcare provider. Document size and appearance of hematoma, notification of primary healthcare provider, and any ordered interventions.
- *Patient reports feeling lightheaded and says she is going to faint:* Stop the venipuncture. If the patient is in bed, have the patient lie flat and elevate the feet. If the patient is in a chair, have the patient put her head between her knees. Encourage the patient to take slow, deep breaths. Call for assistance and stay with the patient. Obtain vital signs if possible.

SKILL 18-8

Obtaining a Venous Blood Specimen for Culture and Sensitivity *(continued)*

Special Considerations

General Considerations

- Be aware that the size of the culture bottles may vary according to facility policy, but the sample dilution should always be 1:10.
- Avoid using existing blood lines for cultures unless the sample is drawn when the line is inserted or catheter sepsis is suspected.
- Avoid collecting blood from edematous areas, arteriovenous shunts, an upper extremity on the same side as a previous lymph node dissection or mastectomy, infected sites, same extremity as an intravenous infusion, and sites of previous hematomas or vascular injury.
- Veins in the lower extremities should not be used for venipuncture, because of an increased risk of thrombophlebitis. However, some facilities do allow collection from lower extremities with a physician's order to collect blood from a leg or foot vein. Check your facility's policies.
- Apply warm compresses to the selected site 15 to 20 minutes before venipuncture to aid in distending veins that are difficult to locate.
- Consider the use of topical anesthetic creams to minimize discomfort and pain for the patient, based on facility policy. Be familiar with requirements and specifications for particular product available for use. Application needs to occur far enough in advance to allow enough time to become effective.
- Use distraction, which has been shown to be of benefit in reducing anxiety related to venipuncture, especially with children. Asking the patient to concentrate on relaxing, and performing deep breathing may help. Asking the patient to cough at the time of venipuncture is another technique that has shown to be effective in reducing pain with venipuncture (Usichenko et al, 2004).

Infant and Child Considerations

- Consider automatically applying warm compresses to distend the small veins of infants and young children before attempting any venipuncture (Fischbach & Dunning, 2006).
- Keep in mind alternative sites for venipuncture in infants and small children, including the scalp, hand, and foot. Use the lateral aspect of the heel to avoid the plantar artery.
- Be aware that the femoral vein may also be used for venipuncture for infants (Hockenberry, 2004).

SKILL 18-9

Obtaining an Arterial Blood Specimen for Blood Gas Analysis

Arterial blood gases (ABGs) are obtained to determine the adequacy of oxygenation and ventilation, to assess acid–base status, and to monitor the effectiveness of treatment. The most common site for sampling arterial blood is the radial artery; other arteries may be used, but most institutions require a physician's order to obtain the sample from another artery.

ABG analysis evaluates ventilation by measuring blood pH and the partial pressures of arterial oxygen (PaO_2) and partial pressure of arterial carbon dioxide ($PaCO_2$). Blood pH measurement reveals the blood's acid–base balance. PaO_2 indicates the amount of oxygen that the lungs deliver to the blood, and $PaCO_2$ indicates the lungs' capacity to eliminate carbon dioxide. ABG samples can also be analyzed for oxygen content and saturation, and for bicarbonate values. Table 18-1 highlights the normal values for ABGs. A respiratory technician or specially trained nurse can collect most ABG samples, but a physician usually performs collection from the femoral artery, depending on facility

(continued)

SKILL 18-9 Obtaining an Arterial Blood Specimen for Blood Gas Analysis *(continued)*

policy. An Allen's test should always be performed before using the radial artery to determine whether the ulnar artery delivers sufficient blood to the hand and fingers, in case there is damage to the radial artery during the blood sampling.

TABLE 18-1 Arterial Blood Gas: Normal Values

PARAMETER	NORMAL VALUE
pH	7.35–7.45
$PaCO_2$	35–45 mm Hg
HCO_3	22–26 mEq/L
SaO_2	Oxygen saturation >95%
PaO_2	>80–100 mm Hg (normal value decreases with age; subtract 1 mm Hg from 80 mm Hg for every year over 60 years of age up to age 90 (Fischbach & Dunning, 2006)
Base excess or deficit	+/– 2 mEq/L

Equipment

- ABG kit, *or* heparinized self-filling 10-mL syringe with 22G 1″ needle attached
- Airtight cap for hub of syringe
- 2″ × 2″ gauze pad
- Band-Aid
- Antimicrobial swab, such as chlorhexidine
- Biohazard bag
- Appropriate label for specimen, based on facility policy and procedure
- Cup or bag of ice
- Nonsterile gloves
- Rolled towel

ASSESSMENT

Review the patient's medical record and plan of care for information about the need for an ABG specimen. Assess the patient's cardiac status, including heart rate, blood pressure, and auscultation of heart sounds. Also assess the patient's respiratory status, including respiratory rate, excursion, lung sounds, and use of oxygen, including the amount being used, if ordered. Determine the adequacy of peripheral blood flow to the extremity to be used by performing the Allen's test (detailed below). If Allen's test reveals no or little collateral circulation to the hand, do not perform an arterial stick to that artery. Assess the patient's radial pulse. If you are unable to palpate the radial pulse, consider using the other wrist.

Assess the patient's understanding about the need for specimen collection. Ask the patient if he or she has ever felt faint, sweaty, or nauseated when having blood drawn.

NURSING DIAGNOSIS

Determine the related factors for the nursing diagnoses based on the patient's current status. Appropriate nursing diagnoses may include:

- Acute Pain
- Risk for Injury
- Impaired Gas Exchange
- Decreased Cardiac Output
- Ineffective Airway Clearance
- Anxiety
- Fear

Many other nursing diagnoses may require the use of this skill.

SKILL 18-9

Obtaining an Arterial Blood Specimen for Blood Gas Analysis *(continued)*

OUTCOME IDENTIFICATION AND PLANNING

The expected outcome to achieve is that the blood sample is obtained from the artery without damage to the artery. Other outcomes that may be appropriate include: the patient experiences minimal pain and anxiety during the procedure, and the patient demonstrates understanding of the need for the ABG specimen.

IMPLEMENTATION

ACTION	RATIONALE
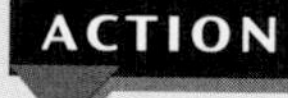 1. Check the patient's identification and confirm the patient's identity. Tell the patient you need to collect an arterial blood sample, and explain the procedure. Tell the patient that the needlestick will cause some discomfort but that he or she must remain still during the procedure. Check the chart to make sure the patient hasn't been suctioned within the past 15 minutes.	Explanation facilitates cooperation and provides reassurance for patient. Suctioning may change the oxygen saturation and is a temporary change not to be confused with baseline for the patient.
2. Gather equipment and provide privacy.	This provides for an organized approach to the task.
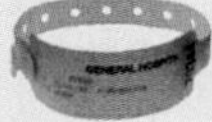 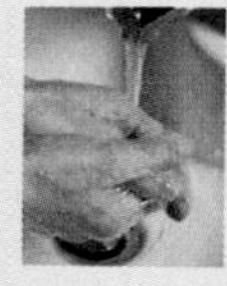 3. Perform hand hygiene.	Hand hygiene deters the spread of microorganisms.
4. If the patient is on bed rest, ask him or her to lie in a supine position, with the head slightly elevated and the arms at the sides. Ask the ambulatory patient to sit in a chair and support the arm securely on an armrest or a table. Place a waterproof pad under the site and a rolled towel under the wrist.	Positioning the patient comfortably helps minimize anxiety. Using a rolled towel under the wrist provide for easy access to the insertion site.
5. **Perform Allen's test (Figure 1) before obtaining a specimen from the radial artery:**	Allen's testing assesses patency of the ulnar and radial arteries.
a. Have the patient clench the wrist to minimize blood flow into the hand.	
b. Using your index and middle fingers, press on the radial and ulnar arteries (Figure 1A). Hold this position for a few seconds.	
c. Without removing your fingers from the arteries, ask the patient to unclench the fist and hold the hand in a relaxed position (Figure 1B). The palm will be blanched because pressure from your fingers has impaired the normal blood flow.	
d. Release pressure on the ulnar artery (Figure 1C). If the hand becomes flushed, which indicates that blood is filling the vessels, it is safe to proceed with the radial artery puncture. If the hand doesn't flush, perform the test on the other arm.	

(continued)

SKILL 18-9 Obtaining an Arterial Blood Specimen for Blood Gas Analysis *(continued)*

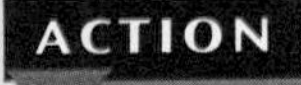

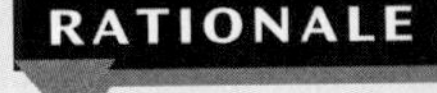

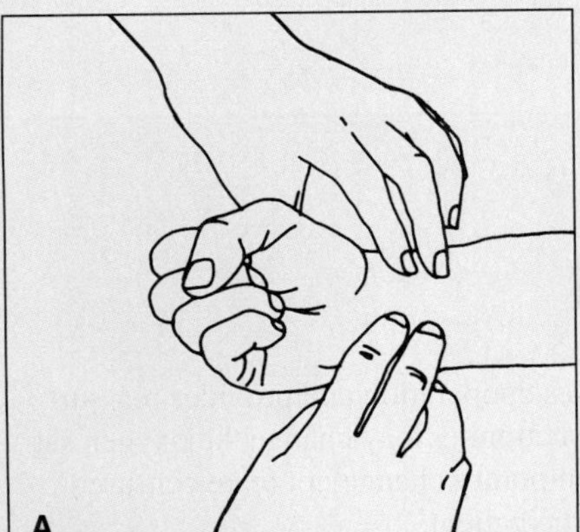

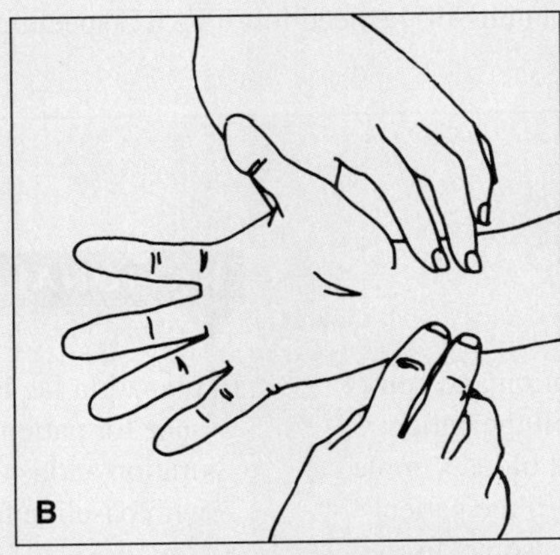

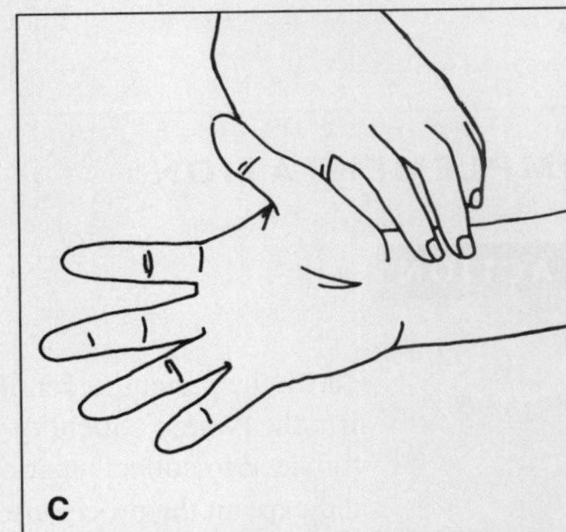

Figure 1. Performing Allen's Test. (**A**) Compressing the arteries with the patient's fist closed. (**B**) Maintaining compression as patient unclenches fist. (**C**) Compressing only the radial artery.

ACTION	RATIONALE
6. Perform hand hygiene again and put on gloves.	Hand hygiene and gloving deter the spread of microorganisms.
7. Locate the radial artery and lightly palpate it for a strong pulse.	If you push too hard during palpation, the radial artery will be obliterated and hard to palpate.
8. Clean the site with the antimicrobial swab. If using chlorhexidine, use a back-and-forth motion, applying friction for 30 seconds to site, or procedure recommended by the manufacturer. Allow the site to dry.	Site cleansing prevents potentially infectious skin flora from being introduced into the vessel during the procedure.
9. Stabilize the hand with the wrist extended over the rolled towel, palm up. Palpate the artery with the index and middle fingers of your nondominant hand while holding the syringe over the puncture site with your dominant hand. **Do not directly touch the area to be stuck.**	Stabilizing the hand and palpating the artery with one hand while holding the syringe in the other provides better access to the artery. Palpating the area to be stuck would contaminate the clean area.
10. Hold the needle bevel up at a 45-degree angle at the site of maximal pulse impulse, with the shaft parallel to the path of the artery. (When puncturing the brachial artery, hold the needle at a 60-degree angle.)	The proper angle of insertion ensures correct access to the artery. The artery is shallow and does not require a deeper angle to penetrate.
11. Puncture the skin and arterial wall in one motion. Watch for blood backflow in the syringe (Figure 2). The pulsating blood will flow into the syringe. Do not pull back on the plunger. Fill the syringe to the 5-mL mark.	The blood should enter the syringe automatically due to arterial pressure.

SKILL 18-9

Obtaining an Arterial Blood Specimen for Blood Gas Analysis *(continued)*

ACTION	RATIONALE
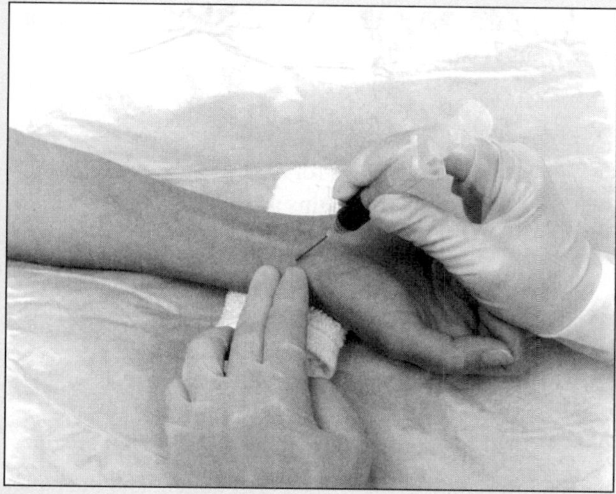 Figure 2. Observing blood flow into syringe.	
12. After collecting the sample, withdraw the syringe while your nondominant hand is beginning to place pressure proximal to the insertion site with the 2″ × 2″ gauze. Press a gauze pad firmly over the puncture site until the bleeding stops—at least 5 minutes. **If the patient is receiving anticoagulant therapy or has a blood dyscrasia, apply pressure for 10 to 15 minutes; if necessary, ask a coworker to hold the gauze pad in place while you prepare the sample for transport to the laboratory, but do not ask the patient to hold the pad.**	If insufficient pressure is applied, a large, painful hematoma may form, hindering future arterial puncture at the site.
13. When the bleeding stops and the appropriate time has lapsed, apply a small adhesive bandage or small pressure dressing (fold a 2″ × 2″ gauze into fourths and firmly apply tape, stretching the skin tight).	Applying a dressing also prevents arterial hemorrhage and extravasation into the surrounding tissue, which can cause a hematoma.
14. Once the sample is obtained, check the syringe for air bubbles. If any appear, remove them by holding the syringe upright and slowly ejecting some of the blood onto a 2″ × 2″ gauze pad.	Air bubbles can affect the laboratory values.
15. Engage the needle guard and remove the needle. Place the airtight cap on the syringe. Gently rotate the syringe to ensure that heparin is well distributed. Do not shake. Insert the syringe into a cup or bag of ice.	This prevents the sample from leaking and keeps air out of the syringe, because blood will continue to absorb oxygen and will give a false reading if allowed to have contact with air. Heparin prevents blood from clotting. Ice prevents the blood from degrading. Vigorous shaking may cause hemolysis.
16. Check specimen labels with patient identification bracelet. Label should include patient's name and identification number, time specimen was collected, route of collection, identification for person obtaining sample, amount of oxygen patient is receiving, and any other information required by agency policy. Place label on the syringe per facility policy. Place iced syringe in plastic sealable biohazard bag. Immediately transport to laboratory.	Confirmation of patient identification information ensures specimen is labeled correctly for the right patient. Packaging the specimen in a biohazard bag prevents the person transporting the samples from coming in contact with blood.

(continued)

SKILL 18-9

Obtaining an Arterial Blood Specimen for Blood Gas Analysis *(continued)*

ACTION	RATIONALE
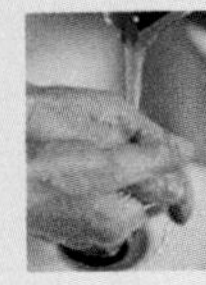 17. Discard needle in sharps container. Remove gloves and perform hand hygiene.	Proper disposal and hand hygiene reduce transmission of microorganisms.
18. Continue to monitor the patient's vital signs, and monitor the extremity for signs and symptoms of circulatory impairment such as swelling, discoloration, pain, numbness, or tingling. Watch for bleeding at the puncture site. Advise the patient not to use the affected extremity for vigorous activity for at least 24 hours.	Frequent monitoring allows for early detection and prompt intervention should problems arise.

EVALUATION

The expected outcome is met when an arterial blood specimen is obtained, and the patient reports minimal pain during the procedure. In addition, the site remains free of injury, without evidence of hematoma formation, and the patient verbalizes the rationale for the specimen collection.

DOCUMENTATION

Guidelines

Document results of Allen's test, time the sample was drawn, arterial puncture site, amount of time pressure was applied to the site to control bleeding, type and amount of oxygen therapy, if any, the patient was receiving, pulse oximetry, respiratory rate, respiratory effort, and any other significant assessments.

Sample Documentation

9/22/08 1245 Allen's test positive. ABG obtained using R radial artery. Pressure applied to site for 5 minutes. Patient receiving 3 L/NC oxygen, pulse ox 94%, respirations even/unlabored, respiratory rate 18 breaths per minute, patient denies dyspnea.—C. Bausler, RN

Unexpected Situations and Associated Interventions

- *While you are attempting to puncture the artery, the patient complains of severe pain:* Using too much force may cause the needle to touch bone, causing the patient pain. Too much force may also result in advancing the needle through the opposite wall of the artery. If this happens, slowly pull the needle back a short distance and check to see if blood returns. If blood still fails to enter the syringe, withdraw the needle completely and restart procedure.
- *You cannot obtain a specimen after two attempts from the same site:* Stop. Do not make more than two attempts from the same site. Probing the artery may injure it and the radial nerve.
- *Blood won't flow into the syringe:* Typically, this occurs as a result of arterial spasm. Replace the needle with a smaller one and try the puncture again. A smaller-bore needle is less likely to cause arterial spasm.
- *After inserting the needle, you note that the syringe is filling sluggishly with dark red/purple blood:* If the patient is in critical condition, this may be arterial blood. But if the patient is awake and alert with a pulse oximeter reading within normal parameters, you have most likely obtained a venous sample. Discard the sample and redraw.

SKILL 18-9

Obtaining an Arterial Blood Specimen for Blood Gas Analysis *(continued)*

- *The patient is on warfarin (Coumadin) therapy:* Expect to hold pressure on the puncture site for at least 10 minutes. If pressure is not held long enough, a hematoma may form, place pressure on the artery, and decrease the flow of blood.
- *The patient cannot keep the wrist extended or lying flat:* Obtain a small armboard, as used for securing an IV, and a roll of gauze. Place the roll of gauze under the patient's wrist. Tape the fingers and forearm to the armboard. This will keep the wrist in an extended position during the blood draw.
- *Blood was drawn without incident, but now, 2 hours later, the patient is complaining of tingling in the fingers and the hand is cool and pale:* Notify the physician. An arterial thrombosis may have formed. If not treated, the thrombosis can lead to necrosis of tissue on the extremity.
- *Puncture site continues to ooze:* If the site is not actively bleeding, consider placing a small pressure bandage on the insertion site. This will prevent the artery from continuing to ooze. Continually check the site for bleeding and assess the extremity to ensure that blood flow is adequate.
- *The Allen's test is negative:* Try the other extremity. If the other extremity has a positive result (collateral circulation), use that extremity. If the Allen's test is negative in both extremities, notify the physician.

Special Considerations

General Considerations

- Be aware that use of a particular arterial site is contraindicated for the following reasons: absence of a palpable radial artery pulse; Allen's test showing only one artery supplying blood to the hand; Allen's test showing obstruction in the ulnar artery; cellulitis or infection at the site; presence of arteriovenous fistula or shunt; severe thrombocytopenia (platelet count 20,000/mm^3 or less, or based on facility policy), and a prolonged prothrombin time or partial thromboplastin time.
- A Doppler probe or finger pulse transducer may be used to assess circulation and perfusion in patient's with dark skin tones or uncooperative patients (Fischbach & Dunning, 2006).
- If the patient is receiving oxygen, make sure that this therapy has been underway for at least 15 minutes before collecting an arterial blood sample. Also be sure to indicate on the laboratory request and the specimen label the amount and type of oxygen therapy the patient is receiving. If the patient is receiving mechanical ventilation, note the fraction of inspired oxygen and tidal volume.
- If the patient isn't receiving oxygen, indicate that he or she is breathing room air.
- If the patient has just received a nebulizer treatment, wait about 20 minutes before collecting the sample.
- Consider obtaining an order for the use of a local anesthetic (1% lidocaine solution) to minimize discomfort and pain for the patient, based on facility policy. Be familiar with requirements and specifications for particular product available for use. Application needs to occur far enough in advance to allow enough time to become effective, which may be contraindicated by the patient's condition. Consider such use of lidocaine carefully because it can delay the procedure. The patient may be allergic to the drug, or the resulting vasoconstriction may prevent successful puncture.
- If the femoral site is used for the procedure, apply pressure for a minimum of 10 minutes.
- Arterial blood and other blood samples may be obtained from an arterial line. Refer to Chapter 16, Cardiovascular Care. When sampling from arterial lines, record amount of blood drawn for each sampling. Frequent sampling can result in significant amount of blood being removed.

The Taylor Suite offers these additional resources to enhance learning and facilitate understanding of this chapter:

- thePoint online resource, http://thepoint.lww.com/Lynn2E
- Student CD-ROM included with the book
- Skills Checklist to Accompany Taylor's Clinical Nursing Skills

Developing Critical Thinking Skills

1. The nurse explained to Mr. Conklin the procedure for obtaining the required urine specimens. Unfortunately, it becomes clear that the patient is too confused at this time to follow the directions and obtain the specimen by himself. How would you handle this situation? How would you successfully obtain an uncontaminated specimen from a patient who is unable to cooperate?
2. Huana Yon's primary care provider provides pre- and post-appointment education and information for the patients in the practice. Part of the nurse's responsibilities when contacting patients before their scheduled visit is to provide information related to anticipated laboratory tests and any necessary patient preparation. What information would you include if you were calling this patient before her visit in relation to collecting a stool specimen for occult blood? What medications, dietary habits, or other habits would you question her about? What information would you give her to prepare for the test?
3. The nurse assigned to Mrs. Yeletsky questions her about her blood glucose testing at home. Mrs. Yeletsky states, "I never really figured out how to work the machine they gave me the last time I saw the doctor. The buttons are too small, and I can't see the writing on the screen very well. Besides, I'm only a little diabetic." What additional information would you want to obtain from this patient? How would you address her possible lack of understanding regarding diabetes? What interventions could you attempt to aid her in managing her blood glucose levels? What other aspects of her health habits would you want to assess?

Bibliography

Ahmed, D., Karch, A., & Karch, F. (2000). Hidden factors in occult blood testing. *American Journal of Nursing, 100*(12), 25.

Calfee, D. P., & Farr, B. M. (2002). Comparison of four antiseptic preparations for skin in the prevention of contamination of percutaneously drawn blood cultures: A randomized trial. *Journal of Clinical Microbiology, 40*(5):1660–1665.

Corbett, J. (2004). *Laboratory tests and diagnostic procedures* (6th ed.). Upper Saddle River, NJ: Pearson Prentice Hall.

Dulczak, S. (2005). Overview of the evaluation, diagnosis, and management of urinary tract infections in infants and children. *Urologic Nursing, 25*(3), 185–192.

Fain, J. (2004). Blood glucose meters: Different strokes for different folks. *Nursing, 34*(11), 48–51.

Ferguson, A. (2005). Blood glucose monitoring. *Nursing Times, 101*(38), 28–29.

Fischbach, F., & Dunning, M. (2006). *Common laboratory & diagnostic tests* (4th ed.). Philadelphia: Lippincott Williams & Wilkins.

Hockenberry, M. (2005). *Wong's essentials of pediatric nursing* (7th ed.). St. Louis, MO: Elsevier Mosby.

Kyle, G., & Prynn, P. (2004). Guidelines for patients undergoing faecal occult blood testing. *Nursing Times, 100*(48), 62–64.

Lavery, I., & Ingram, P. (2005). Venipuncture: Best practice. *Nursing Standard, 19*(49), 55–65.

Levetan, C. (2005). Blood glucose in the hospital. *Diabetes Forecast 58*(9), 49–50.

Mitchell, S., Schaefer, D., & Dubagunta, S. (2004). A new view of occult and obscure gastrointestinal bleeding. *American Family Physician, 69*(4), 875–881.

North American Nursing Diagnosis Association. (2005). *NANDA nursing diagnosis: Definitions & classification 2005–2006.* Philadelphia: Author.

Rushing, J. (2004). Drawing blood culture specimens for reliable results. *Nursing, 34*(12), 20.

Smeltzer, S., Bare, B., Hinkle, J. H., & Cheever, K. H. (2008). *Brunner and Suddarth's textbook of medical–surgical nursing* (11th ed.). Philadelphia: Lippincott Williams & Wilkins.

Taylor, C., Lillis, C., LeMone, P., et al. (2008). *Fundamentals of nursing* (6th ed.). Philadelphia: Lippincott Williams & Wilkins.

Usichenko, T., Pavlovic, D., Foellner, S., et al. (2004). Reducing venipuncture pain by a cough trick: A randomized crossover volunteer study. *Anesthesia & Analgesia, 98*(2), 343–345.

Woodrow, P. (2004). Arterial blood gas analysis. *Nursing Standard, 18*(21), 45–52.

U • N • I • T

III

Integrated Case Studies

These case studies are designed to focus on integrating concepts. They are not meant to be all-inclusive. The critical thinking questions should guide your discussions of related issues. The discussion within the integrated nursing care section represents possible nursing care solutions to problems; you may find other solutions that are equally acceptable.

Basic Case Studies

Case Study

Abigail Cantonelli

Abigail Cantonelli, age 80, injured her left knee and wrist when she fell on an icy sidewalk. She has been on your orthopedic and neurologic unit for several days. She has an extended history of cardiomyopathy, for which she receives furosemide (Lasix). Her vital signs are stable and she rates her pain as a 2 on a scale of 1 to 10 (10 = worst pain). Since Mrs. Cantonelli has an increased risk of falling, her physician has ordered physical therapy and cane-walking instructions before discharge. Although the physical therapy staff has already initiated the cane-walking instructions, you will need to ambulate Mrs. Cantonelli with her cane during your shift. While you are ambulating down the hall, she says, "Oh, dear! I feel dizzy." She begins to lose her balance and falls toward you.

Medical Orders

Physical therapy for cane-walking instruction
Ambulate every shift with cane assistance
Lasix 20 mg PO every morning
Potassium chloride 10 mEq PO every day
Lortab 5 one tab PO q 4–6 hours prn pain

Critical Thinking Questions

- Identify Mrs. Cantonelli's risk factors for falling.
- Describe the actions you would implement when Mrs. Cantonelli begins to fall.

(continued)

Case Study

Abigail Cantonelli (continued)

- Considering these risk factors, what special assessments and precautions should you implement before assisting her to ambulate? While assisting with ambulation?

Integrated Nursing Care

Falls are the leading cause of accidental death in people over age 79. Because of Mrs. Cantonelli's age, past history of falls, and impaired mobility, she continues to be at risk for falls. Her weakness and pain from her injuries also contribute to this risk. In addition, she is taking Lortab for pain and Lasix, which is a diuretic. These medications contribute to an increased risk for falling and subsequent injury (Taylor et al., 2008).

Before ambulating Mrs. Cantonelli, you could implement several assessments and precautions to prevent orthostatic hypotension. Have her sit on the side of the bed for a few minutes and make sure she does not feel dizzy, weak, or lightheaded (see Chapter 9). Since she has a history of cardiomyopathy, assess for shortness of breath and chest pain. If she cannot tolerate sitting up on the side of the bed without having these symptoms, then she will not tolerate standing up or ambulating. Assess her pain level immediately before ambulation. If you have to medicate her for pain, then wait until the pain medicine has had time to take effect before ambulating. Since she is weaker on her left side, assess strength on her right side to ensure she will be able to support her weight with the cane (see Chapter 9). If she has difficulty maintaining her balance, apply a special safety belt (gait belt) before she begins to ambulate with the cane (some institutions require the use of a safety belt).

While Mrs. Cantonelli is ambulating with her cane, observe her closely. Assess her technique with the cane. Observe for symptoms such as dizziness, chest pain, and shortness of breath. As she continues ambulating, evaluate how she tolerates this activity. Before she is discharged from the hospital, assess her self-confidence as well as her overall ability to use the cane.

When Mrs. Cantonelli begins to fall, it is important to protect her while also protecting yourself. As you feel her start to fall, maintain a wide base of support, grasp the safety belt firmly, and place her weight against your body. You can then gently and slowly guide her down toward the floor (see Chapter 9). Assess her orientation and stay with her while waiting for help from another nurse. Take her vital signs to determine if there is a change from baseline. Thoroughly explore other factors that may have contributed to her fall, and plan interventions that will prevent future falls. If Mrs. Cantonelli continues to have problems with falling, a walker may need to be considered.

Case Study

Tiffany Jones

Tiffany Jones, age 17, is scheduled to undergo an ovarian cyst biopsy under local anesthesia. She has been NPO since midnight. Her ID bracelet is on and her consent form is signed. Her mother is in the waiting room. You are to provide her preoperative care. You place an IV in her left hand without difficulty. The next procedure is to insert an indwelling urinary (Foley) catheter. You set up the sterile field between her legs. As you clean the urinary meatus, Tiffany keeps drawing her legs closer together. When you remind her, she opens her legs and says, "Sorry, I didn't mean to move." As you insert the catheter into the urethra, Tiffany is startled and slams her knees together. When she opens her knees, the catheter appears to be inserted, but there is no urine flowing.

Medical Orders

Intravenous fluids: D5 ½ NS @ 50 mL/hr

Foley catheter to straight drainage

Critical Thinking Questions

- Where is the urinary catheter, and should you advance the catheter further?
- How could you have set up a more stable sterile field?
- Describe methods of responding to Tiffany's nervousness.
- How do you determine whether the catheter and the sterile field are still sterile?
- Identify issues that are of concern to patients before surgery.

(continued)

Case Study

Tiffany Jones (continued)

Integrated Nursing Care

Concepts

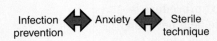

Infection prevention ⟺ Anxiety ⟺ Sterile technique

The female urethra is short, only about 1.5″ to 2.5″ long. If the catheter is advanced that far and no urine is flowing, the catheter may be in the vagina. Do not remove the catheter; it will serve as a guide to locate the urethral opening, which is just above the vagina (see Chapter 12). You would not advance the catheter further even if it were in the urethra, because it is probable that when Tiffany closed her legs, the catheter came into contact with her skin and is no longer sterile. Advancing a nonsterile catheter into the urethra would increase her risk for developing a urinary tract infection. Since you are not certain whether her legs touched the sterile field, the sterile field is also no longer considered sterile (see Chapter 12).

You will need to obtain another complete catheter insertion kit. Cover Tiffany and verify that she understands your plans. As you set up the new kit, place it on the bedside table, not between her legs, to prevent accidental contamination (see Chapter 12).

Teenagers are generally uncomfortable with urinary catheterization because in this procedure, the nurse must look at and touch a very private area. Teenage girls may have "nervous legs": as you touch their inner thighs or labia, the knees slam shut almost involuntarily. Such an invasion of privacy is traumatic at an age when girls are easily embarrassed. Have a second nurse or a relative attend to the teenager. The nurse or relative can distract and soothe the teen, minimizing the unpleasantness of the experience, and can also keep a "reminder" hand on Tiffany's open knee to help you maintain sterility.

Like most preoperative patients, Tiffany has several reasons to feel nervous. She is facing surgery, an unknown and anxiety-producing experience. The preoperative procedures, such as IV insertion and urinary catheterization, are unpleasant and uncomfortable. There are several strategies you can implement to reduce preoperative patients' anxiety. Have a familiar person stay with the patient. Tell the patient your name. Clearly explain procedures, and provide instructions to the patient before you begin. Instructions should include the rationale and the length of time the procedure will take. For urinary catheterization, the patient may also want to know how long he or she will have the catheter in place. Emphasize to the patient that it is all right to ask questions. Describe how the procedure will feel to the patient—for example, "when I clean you, it will feel cold and wet." Keep your voice calm and very matter-of-fact throughout the procedure (see Chapter 6).

Case Study

James White

James White is a patient with an exacerbation of COPD on your medical-surgical unit. You need to obtain his vital signs per the MD order and give him a bath. His vital signs at 8 a.m. were as follows: temperature, 98.4°F; pulse, 86 beats/minute and regular; respirations, 18/minute; blood pressure, 130/68 mm Hg. The physical therapist who is working with this patient on conditioning therapy has just brought him back from his exercises. You notice that his breathing is labored, with audible expiratory wheezes. While you are obtaining his oral temperature and vital signs, you continue

Case Study

James White (continued)

to hear audible expiratory wheezing. His vital signs now are as follows: temperature, 96.8°F; pulse, 106 beats/minute and irregular; respirations, 26/minute; blood pressure, 140/74 mm Hg.

Medical Orders

Daily physical therapy for conditioning
Vital signs q 4 hr
Oxygen at 2 L via nasal prongs prn for pulse oximetry <90%
Oxygen saturation levels via pulse oximeter every shift and prn

Critical Thinking Questions

- Did you take the second set of vital signs at the most appropriate time? Why or why not?
- Describe the timing and type of bath you think Mr. White requires and the degree of assistance he will need. Explain your rationale.
- How have Mr. White's exercises affected the accuracy of his vital signs?
- What would be your course of action in response to his labored breathing?

Integrated Nursing Care

Concepts

Vital signs ⟷ Oxygenation ⟷ Activity

Always compare vital signs with the baseline before making further clinical decisions (see Chapter 1). As you compare the previous vital signs with the ones you just obtained, you notice that Mr. White's pulse rate, respiratory rate, and blood pressure are elevated. Your assessment of his pulse also indicates that his pulse is now irregular. Mr. White has just experienced a significant increase in activity, and waiting until he has recovered from the exertion would be more appropriate in order to obtain a resting set of vital signs.

What does the very low temperature indicate? Remember that you continued to hear Mr. White's heavy breathing while obtaining the remainder of the vital signs. Mr. White could not keep his lips pursed in a seal around the thermometer, and this often gives an inaccurate temperature. Mouth breathing and respiratory distress are contraindications for obtaining an oral temperature. As a nurse, you are responsible for determining the most appropriate site to obtain the temperature (see Skill 1-1).

Does Mr. White's elevated respiratory rate and noisy breathing indicate respiratory distress or a

(continued)

Case Study

James White (continued)

need for oxygen? Obtain an oxygen saturation level via pulse oximetry; an order already exists for this intervention. If the oxygen saturation level is satisfactory for Mr. White, then you can be confident his body is compensating for the increased oxygen demand. Allow him to rest, with the head of his bed elevated, and retake his vital signs in 15 to 30 minutes. Take vital signs as often as the patient's condition warrants. If Mr. White's oxygen saturation and vital signs continue to deviate from baseline after a rest period, notify the physician (see Chapter 1).

A bath represents another increase in activity. Mr. White needs time to recover from the exercises before attempting the bath. He should be able to sit in a chair and, in fact, will breathe more comfortably sitting up than lying down. Having him lie flat could make him decompensate, so you should not perform occupied bed-making. If encouraged to sit up, he will probably be able to complete much of his bath by himself.

Case Study

Naomi Bell

Naomi Bell, age 90, was admitted to the hospital yesterday after experiencing chest pain. She wears a hearing aid in her left ear. In report you were told that she is "confused" and "doesn't answer questions appropriately." Her night vital signs were as follows: temperature, 98.0°F; pulse, 62 beats/minute; respirations, 18/minute; blood pressure, 132/86 mm Hg. She is due for her AM medications. As you give Mrs. Bell her medications and state their purpose, she points to the Lanoxin and says, "Honey, I don't take that pill."

Medical Orders

Lanoxin 0.125 mg PO every morning
Lasix 20 mg PO every morning
Potassium chloride 10 mEq PO every morning
ECASA 1 tab PO every day
Pepcid 20 mg PO BID
Captopril 50 mg PO TID

Critical Thinking Questions

- How would you respond to Mrs. Bell's statement, "Honey, I don't take that pill"?
- Suggest ways in which you can confirm you are giving Mrs. Bell the correct medications.

Case Study

Naomi Bell (continued)

- Identify the medications that require assessment prior to administration.
- Describe factors that can contribute to inappropriate answers, and identify nursing actions to diminish these factors.
- How would you determine Mrs. Bell's level of confusion?

Integrated Nursing Care

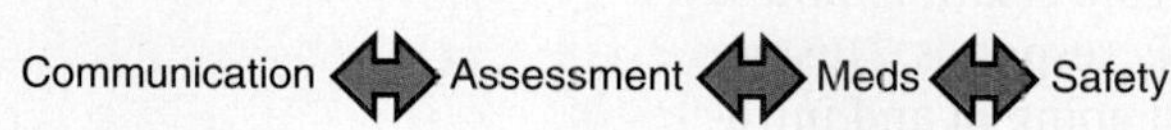

When patients question you regarding their medications, listen to them. Questions like this should send a "red flag" to the nurse. Often patients are familiar with what they normally take and can alert you that this may not be the right medication. Do not insist that Mrs. Bell take the Lanoxin until you confirm the accuracy of the order. In this case, it could be that Mrs. Bell just didn't hear what you said. Always confirm what patients say to you by restating it back to them. It could also be that she is more familiar with this drug's other name, which is digoxin.

To give medications safely, there are many safety checks you can use. Some measures include researching the drug before giving it and double-checking all of the five "rights." Compare the Medication Administration Record to the physician's order. If the order still remains unclear to you, call the physician to clarify it (see Chapter 5).

Some medications require assessment before you administer them to the patient. In this case, Mrs. Bell takes four medications that will require assessment prior to administration. Lanoxin, Lasix, and captopril will affect pulse and blood pressure. In addition, laboratory test results should be available on potassium and digoxin levels. If Mrs. Bell has a low pulse rate, low blood pressure, or a toxic laboratory value, you will not administer these medications and will notify the physician (see Chapter 5).

Sometimes elderly patients become confused in the hospital. However, do not assume this is always the case. The nurse who gave you report may have assumed that Mrs. Bell's inappropriate answers were due to confusion, when in fact they may be related to Mrs. Bell's hearing problem. When patients with hearing impairment are admitted to the hospital, encourage them to wear their hearing aids and help them check their batteries to ensure they are working. If you are still unclear whether Mrs. Bell is confused, perform a standard mental status examination used by your institution. This will establish a baseline assessment of her mental status that you can use to individualize her nursing plan of care.

If you determine she is confused, assess the source of confusion. Given Mrs. Bell's cardiac condition, assess her respiratory status and oxygen saturation level via pulse oximetry to determine whether she is experiencing hypoxia or ischemia. If the cause is physiologic, notify the physician immediately. Another source contributing to confusion could be isolation caused by hearing loss. One way to reduce possible confusion for Mrs. Bell is to improve communication. Ensure that her hearing aid battery is operating and that the unit is placed correctly. Other ways to improve communication include talking to her at eye level, facing her directly when speaking, or even speaking into her unaffected ear. If Mrs. Bell's vision is better than her hearing, you can also give her pertinent information in writing.

Case Study

John Willis

You are a nursing student in your first semester of nursing school and your second week of clinical. Your assigned patient has been discharged before your arrival. Your instructor provides you with the name of another patient to care for, based on the recommendation of the staff. Before you can review the information about the patient with her, she is called to consult with another student and a physician about an emergent patient situation. You read the clinical pathway for John Willis and find that he has methicilllin-resistant *staphylococcus aureus* (MRSA) in his sputum and suspected pulmonary tuberculosis (TB). You remember reviewing these topics in class and in the learning resource center. Because your instructor is still occupied with the patient emergency, you decide to begin caring for your new patient, instead of wasting time waiting to review the information with her. When you go to your patient's room, you see the isolation cart containing the infection-control–precaution supplies outside the room, with the hospital's policy and procedure posted for precautions to use for TB and MRSA. You see there are individual masks in plastic bags with different people's names on them, as well as masks with protective eye shields. You recall something from class about wearing a specially fitted mask when implementing these precautions, but realize you don't remember as much as you thought you did. You are unsure of exactly what you need to do. You find the staff nurse assigned to the patient in another patient's room, interrupt his conversation, and say, "I don't have a mask to care for my patient." The nurse sharply responds, "Just go get started. I'm in the middle of something." You consider just going in and introducing yourself and checking on the patient's status. Should you "borrow" a mask from one of the bags? You think it is your duty to care for this patient, but think you may need more information to be safe.

Medical Orders

Airborne precautions
Contact precautions
Sputum specimen for culture and sensitivity
Vital signs every shift

Critical Thinking Questions

- Compare the mode of transmission for TB and MRSA.
- Identify the appropriate protective equipment needed to care for a patient with TB and a patient with MRSA.
- What may have led to the nurse's abrupt and sharp response?
- Describe another way in which you could have approached this situation.

Case Study

John Willis (continued)

- What can occur if you do not take the appropriate transmission-based precautions and enter other patient rooms?

Integrated Nursing Care

Concepts

Safety ⟷ Isolation ⟷ Communication

Pulmonary TB transmission occurs through airborne respiratory droplets. MRSA transmission can occur through contact with contaminated blood or body fluids. MRSA can be spread by direct or indirect contact. In this case, MRSA could be transmitted indirectly by coming into contact with any soiled items, such as the mask (CDC, 2003, p. 3).

Agencies will require the use of gowns, gloves, and masks when caring for patients with TB and MRSA. Unique to the airborne precautions needed for TB is the use of specially fitted masks called high-efficiency particulate air (HEPA) masks that prevent the inspiration of airborne microorganisms (see Chapter 4). There are also disposable masks available, but they usually require fit-testing as well. If a fit-tested mask is required by your agency, you would either need to be fit-tested for a mask (often done by employee health) or reassigned to another patient. In addition, to protect yourself whenever there is the potential for contamination to your eyes, such as coughing, you should wear goggles or a mask with a face shield (Taylor et al., 2008). Institutions vary greatly in their supplies. If you do not take the appropriate transmission-based precautions, you put yourself at risk for exposure to disease; in this case, tuberculosis and MRSA. In addition, entering other patient rooms results in the potential for transmission of a nosocomial infection. It is always your responsibility, even as a student, to follow the policy and procedure of the agency where you are placed for clinical.

Hospitals are stressful places. Understanding when and how to communicate with others is an invaluable set of skills. Waiting for the nurse to complete his conversation and task before asking for guidance would have been the ideal situation. Nurses have to prioritize the care they provide. Asking, "Do you have a moment to review something with me?" is a good way to ensure getting the time and attention you need. Since there was no emergency to obtain the vital signs and sputum specimen, they can wait until you are sure you can provide safe care.

You were right to question the appropriateness of caring for this patient. In this situation, waiting to review the patient information with your instructor is the ideal solution. Your instructor did not have all the information about the patient before being called away to an emergency. She would not have assigned this patient to you after reviewing his diagnosis, realizing that you would need a specially fitted mask to care for the patient. While waiting for your instructor, you should obtain as much information as possible. Background research and knowledge are powerful tools. Examples of resources you can access include the hospital policy-and-procedure manual, the infection-control manual, the infection-control nurse, and experienced staff members, provided they are able to take time out from their patient care responsibilities. Then, when your instructor is available, you can share this information with her to plan your care for that day.

Case Study

Claudia Tran

Claudia Tran, age 84, has been on your skilled nursing floor for several weeks following a cerebral vascular accident (CVA). She had previously been a resident of a long-term care facility. Her neuro checks and vital signs are unchanged from her baseline admission. Her CVA has impaired her ability to chew and swallow. She has left-sided weakness with flaccidity of her left hand. She is emaciated and her skin is very fragile. She has reddened areas on her coccyx, heels, and elbows. She is receiving weekly vitamin B_{12} injections for pernicious anemia. Over the past week, Mrs. Tran has become increasingly confused and incontinent. She constantly pulls at her feeding tube and has had to have it reinserted after pulling it out. Because of this, soft wrist restraints have been ordered. She has a nasogastric tube for tube feedings, which she receives every 8 hours. During your shift, Mrs. Tran is due for a tube feeding. You check the residual and it is 380 mL.

Medical Orders

Soft wrist restraints for safety
Vitamin B_{12} injection 1,000 mcg IM weekly
Hold feeding for gastric residual ≥300 mL and notify MD.
Nasogastric tube feedings q 8 hr
Physical therapy daily, passive and active range of motion (ROM) as tolerated

Critical Thinking Questions

- Considering Mrs. Tran's condition, what special safety measures should be implemented with her restraints?
- What are the risks of falling for this patient?
- Identify the risks associated with tube feeding for this patient.
- Identify risk factors and preventive measures for Mrs. Tran's skin breakdown.
- Identify appropriate sites for the vitamin B_{12} injections in Mrs. Tran. Develop a schedule of rotating sites for this injection.

Case Study

Claudia Tran (continued)

Integrated Nursing Care

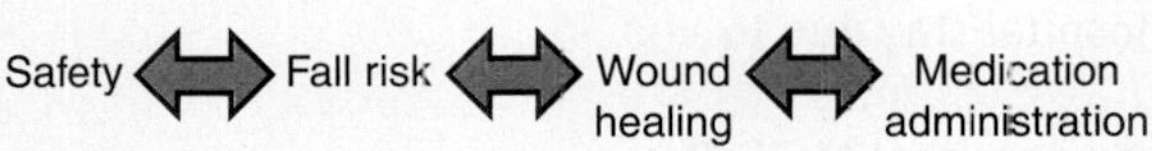

Restraints should be used only as a last resort after all other measures have failed. Other measures could include placing her bed in a low position, having a family member sit with her, and placing her in a room near the nurses' station. Restraints must be used only with a physician's order, and you must follow strict guidelines to protect the patient. Since Mrs. Tran already has skin breakdown, pad the restraints and make sure they are the correct size. An additional safety measure would be performing frequent neurovascular checks, such as checking warmth, sensation, and capillary refill. Restraints are released at specified frequencies. This will improve the circulation to her extremities, reduce the chance of skin breakdown, and give you an opportunity to assess the site. Mrs. Tran has left-sided weakness; therefore, applying a restraint on her flaccid arm could cause harm and is not needed (see Chapter 3).

Mrs. Tran has many risk factors for skin breakdown, including immobilization, malnutrition, altered mental status, age, incontinence, and positioning for tube feedings. To reduce these risk factors and prevent further skin breakdown will require a multifaceted approach. Development of a schedule for repositioning is essential. She could benefit from a special type of mattress, such as a pressure-reducing surface. Implementing a physical therapy program of active and passive ROM exercises would be helpful. A nutritional consult would be of utmost importance to ensure she will receive adequate protein, as well as other vitamins and minerals essential for skin integrity.

What skin breakdown complications could result from immobilization and incontinence? You and the doctor could consider the risks versus benefits of placement of a urinary retention catheter for Mrs. Tran. A noninvasive way to reduce the chance of recurrent incontinence is to offer Mrs. Tran a bedpan at regular intervals.

Since Mrs. Tran is confused and in a restraint, her risk for falling is high. Her bed should be in a low position at all times and her call light within reach. Frequently check on patients such as Mrs. Tran to decrease isolation and provide orientation.

Mrs. Tran is receiving tube feedings and has an excessive residual. She is at increased risk for aspiration of tube feedings into her lungs if positioned supine. To decrease the risk for aspiration, check the residual amount before every feeding. In this situation, Mrs. Tran's gastric residual was greater than 300 mL. Therefore, her head should remain elevated, her tube feeding will be held, and her physician should be contacted as soon as possible (see Chapter 11).

When giving Mrs. Tran vitamin B_{12} injections, use larger muscles and rotate sites. Implement the rotation schedule for this injection in her plan of care. This is particularly important since Mrs. Tran is emaciated and does not have good muscle mass. Avoid areas that are reddened or have palpable nodules and scars. Since vitamin B_{12} injections can be irritating, inject the medication slowly to minimize pain, trauma, and discomfort (see Chapter 5).

Case Study

Joe LeRoy

Joe LeRoy, age 60, was brought in by his daughter and admitted to your small rural hospital. He has had the stomach flu at home for several days and is suffering from dehydration. He has right-sided hemiplegia due to a cerebral vascular accident (CVA) 3 years ago. Mr. LeRoy has been remaining in bed during his hospital stay due to extreme weakness and fatigue.

You received report on your seven patients. From report, you note that Mr. LeRoy continues to have frequent liquid stools (averaging about three or four times/shift). The doctor has ordered a stool sample for culture and sensitivity. When entering his room, you notice his sheets are very dirty and he has a body odor.

Medical Orders

Intravenous fluids: D5 ½ NS IV at 125 mL/hr
Stool sample for culture and sensitivity
VS every shift

Critical Thinking Questions

- **Develop your priorities and rationales for the following nursing care for Mr. LeRoy:**
  - **Changing his sheets**
  - **Completing the AM assessment**
  - **Obtaining vital signs**
  - **Collecting the sample**
  - **Giving a bath**
- **What considerations should be taken into account when collecting the stool sample?**
- **Are there any assessments that you would want to pay particular attention to during your nursing care?**
- **Describe how your attitude and nonverbal behavior could affect Mr. LeRoy's hospital experience.**

Case Study

Joe LeRoy (continued)

Integrated Nursing Care

Concepts

Diarrhea ⟷ Skin integrity ⟷ Personal care

Prioritizing care is a difficult but important skill for all nurses. Determine whether Mr. LeRoy can provide his own morning care, although this is unlikely due to his hemiplegia and weakness. If you need to assist him with his personal care, determine the needs of your other patients before beginning this task. Before leaving Mr. LeRoy, let him know your plan and the time he can expect to have assistance with his bath. Another alternative is letting a nursing assistant (if you have one on your unit) know of Mr. LeRoy's need for a bath and linen change. On your initial assessment of Mr. LeRoy, cover any very obviously dirty areas of his sheets with a blue waterproof pad or a clean sheet. You could also offer him a wet, warm washcloth and a dry towel for initial cleaning while you are completing his assessment. You should also inform him of the need for a stool specimen.

If your floor has no nursing aide, return to his room after your other patient assessments are complete. First obtain the warm stool sample, give the bath, and then change his linens. This sequence saves time and energy for both the nurse and the patient, because when providing a bed bath or assisting a patient on a bedpan, you can easily soil the linens.

While wearing gloves, collect and send the stool specimen promptly to the laboratory. Specimens should be sent while still warm, as the microorganisms present at body temperature may die when the specimen temperature changes, and this would produce a false-negative result (see Chapter 13).

During your assessment, pay particular attention to his skin. Mr. LeRoy is at risk for pressure ulcers due to his age, diarrhea, altered nutrition, and immobility. Assist Mr. LeRoy to turn over so that you can inspect his back and bony prominences, the most likely areas for skin breakdown. If you notice any skin breakdown, notify the physician so that treatment can begin promptly.

A nurse's nonverbal behavior can have a dramatic impact on a patient's hospital experience. Projecting a positive attitude and providing nonjudgmental care help a patient cope with hospitalization. You may be offended by Mr. LeRoy's body odor and the smell of his stool, but as a nurse you will need to learn strategies to manage strong odors and make sure that your facial expressions or body language do not convey discomfort or disgust.

Case Study

Kate Townsend

Kate Townsend, a 70-year-old patient with chronic obstructive pulmonary disease (COPD), has just returned to your medical-surgical unit from surgery for excision of a nonmalignant intestinal polyp. She has a midline abdominal transverse incision secured with sutures and covered with a dry sterile dressing. She has a right peripheral IV with D5 ½ NS @ 75 mL/hr. She has a history of long-term steroid use for her COPD. She has a nasogastric tube in her right naris, which is clamped at this time. The physician orders oxygen 2 L via nasal cannula. This is your first semester, fourth

(continued)

Case Study

Kate Townsend (continued)

week in school, and the nurse asks you to place the patient on oxygen. When you attempt to place the cannula in the patient's naris with the nasogastric (NG) tube, you think it is uncomfortable and a little odd. For comfort, you decide to place a simple oxygen mask on Mrs. Townsend instead. Her vital signs are as follows: temperature, 99.6°F; pulse, 76 beats/minute; respirations, 24 breaths/minute; blood pressure, 110/70 mm Hg; oxygen saturation, 92%.

Medical Orders

Nasogastric tube clamped
Morphine sulfate 2–4 mg q 4 hr prn pain
Intravenous fluid: D5 ½ NS @ 75 mL/hr
Incentive spirometry prn
Oxygen 2 L via nasal cannula

Critical Thinking Questions

- What is the difference between oxygen given in a nasal cannula and that given via a simple oxygen mask?
- What is a complication that could occur with Mrs. Townsend when changing her to a simple oxygen mask?
- Considering Mrs. Townsend's chronic lung disease, what are the complications that can occur, and what nursing interventions could decrease these complications?
- What comfort measures would you want to provide for Mrs. Townsend?
- Develop a discharge plan for Mrs. Townsend.

Case Study

Kate Townsend (continued)

Integrated Nursing Care

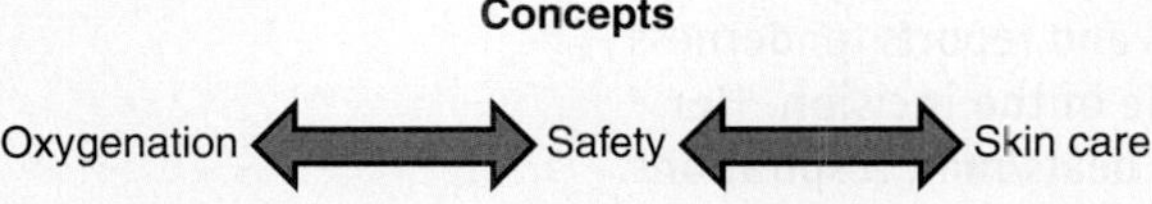

Several delivery systems exist to provide oxygen to patients, and they deliver varying amounts of oxygen. Oxygen delivered via a nasal cannula set at 2 L would deliver about 28% oxygen, whereas oxygen delivered in a simple mask could deliver 40% to 60% oxygen, depending on the flow meter setting (see Chapter 14). Oxygen is considered a medicine, so it is not a nursing order but a medical order. The oxygen concentration and delivery system are adjusted according to orders or parameters from a physician or other advanced practice professional.

For people without chronic lung disease, breathing is driven by the buildup of carbon dioxide levels in the blood (hypercapnia). The drive to breathe for patients with COPD is a lack of oxygen (hypoxia). Because of this, increasing oxygen levels in patients with COPD will decrease their respiratory drive. Therefore, when changing Mrs. Townsend for comfort reasons from the nasal cannula to the mask, you could have increased her oxygen anywhere from 12% to 32%, and even a small increase in oxygen has the potential to stop her breathing. Although it is not entirely comfortable to have a NG tube, much less another tube in the naris, it is not unusual for this to occur. Both will fit with some manipulation by the nurse.

Patients with chronic lung disease are at increased risk after surgery for pulmonary complications, including atelectasis and pneumonia. General anesthesia alters all of the muscles involved in breathing and clearing the airway. COPD is a restrictive lung disease, meaning that the patient's lungs lose their elasticity and become less compliant. For Mrs. Townsend, this combination of underlying disease and the effects of surgery results in a decreased ability to mobilize secretions, which could lead to atelectasis and possibly pneumonia. Mrs. Townsend may be experiencing atelectasis due to her temperature of 99.6°F. Other signs of atelectasis would be decreased breath sounds in the lung bases, shortness of breath, increased respiratory rate, and decreased oxygen saturation of pulse oximetry. Without nursing intervention, atelectasis could lead to pneumonia. Measures to facilitate lung expansion and mobilization of secretions will minimize atelectasis. These nursing measures include elevation of the head of her bed, deep-breathing exercises, incentive spirometry, adequate pain control, and early ambulation.

Long-term steroid use can make the skin very fragile, increase the potential for skin breakdown, and delay wound healing. To prevent this, observe the skin under her NG and oxygen cannula tubing. The pressure of the tubes on her face and behind her ears could cause a break in skin integrity. Repositioning the tape that is holding the NG tube may make it more comfortable. If needed, you may need to protect the skin under the cannula tubing with a hydrocolloid dressing (see Chapter 8), especially if the skin becomes reddened. There are many commercial products to hold oxygen nasal cannulas, as well as NG tubes, which may also increase her comfort.

Discharge plans for Mrs. Townsend would need to address both her underlying lung disease as well as her recent intestinal surgery. Patient education should focus on measures that enable Mrs. Townsend to improve her lung compliance and increase her oxygenation. Incentive spirometry and a daily activity schedule will be imperative. Due to her prolonged use of steroids, she may also have delayed wound healing at her incision site. Patient education should address optimal nutrition and prevention of infection. Before discharge, validate Mrs. Townsend's knowledge of measures to prevent pulmonary and wound complications.

Case Study

Tula Stillwater

Tula Stillwater is a 36-year-old Native American who has had diabetes since age 26. She weighs 218 lb. She is gravida 1 para 1 and delivered a 9 lb, 6 oz boy via cesarean section 3 days ago. She has a transverse abdominal incision with staples and reports tenderness on the right side of the incision but acute pain on the left side of the incision. Her 8 a.m. vital signs are as follows: temperature, 101.6°F; pulse 76 beats/min; respirations, 18 per minute; blood pressure, 134/78 mm Hg. Her blood sugar before breakfast is 185 mg/dL; her blood sugars on previous days had ranged from 90 to 124 mg/dL.

On your assessment, you find her incision is open to air and the staples are intact. The incision is well approximated and without erythema on the right side. However, the left side of the incision is pulling apart and is edematous and warm to the touch, with a scant amount of purulent drainage.

Medical Orders

Vital signs q 4 hr
Fingerstick blood sugar AC & QHS
Regular insulin per sliding scale

Standing order: Remove staples before discharge.
Standing order: Discharge on third day if stable.

Critical Thinking Questions

- What is your interpretation of her vital signs? Who should be notified and when?
- What is the relationship between Mrs. Stillwater's diabetes and her postsurgical condition?
- How should you respond to her fingerstick blood sugar?
- How would you determine whether Mrs. Stillwater meets the criteria for discharge?
- What factors affect her staple removal?
- What nursing interventions would you foresee performing?

Case Study

Tula Stillwater (continued)

- Describe the timing and the technique for administering her insulin.

Integrated Nursing Care

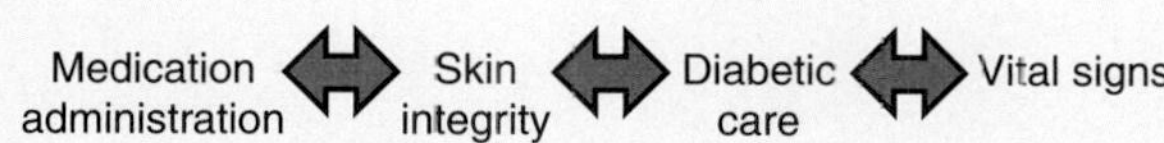

Mrs. Stillwater's vital signs should alert you to a potential complication. She may have an infection related to her incision, as evidenced by her increased temperature and her subjective report of acute pain at the incision. Her blood pressure could be a result of her pain, but it should be compared to her baseline and monitored. You inspected the incision carefully for signs of infection. Her physician needs to be notified immediately of this potential complication.

Wound healing may be impaired in people with diabetes, so any patient with diabetes requires vigilant wound assessment. Additionally, the stress of surgery usually results in increased blood sugar levels. Mrs. Stillwater's fingerstick blood sugar is elevated from her baseline, another symptom of a possible infection. When you see a dramatic increase in blood sugar in a patient with diabetes, consider the possible etiologies.

Despite the urgency of this new complication of wound infection, Mrs. Stillwater should receive her insulin and breakfast as she usually would. Administer her insulin in a subcutaneous site; she can help you identify the site where she should receive her insulin. Patients who are accustomed to managing their diabetes at home will have preferences when in the hospital, and these preferences should be honored.

Many women who have had cesarean sections are discharged on the third day. One of the expected outcomes for discharge would include being free of infection. Mrs. Stillwater is not free of infection: she has pain at her incision site, a fever, and an elevated fingerstick blood sugar. When you notify the physician of these symptoms, she orders a complete blood count, a wound culture, incision site care, and cancellation of the discharge.

Given the delayed discharge and impaired wound healing, you would not want to remove the staples from this incision because removing the staples at this time could place Mrs. Stillwater at risk for dehiscence. Another factor affecting the risk for dehiscence and impaired wound healing is Mrs. Stillwater's increased subcutaneous fat (Taylor et al., 2008).

Did you foresee obtaining a complete blood count and a wound culture and performing incision site care? Did you also anticipate that this patient should not be discharged nor have her staples removed? In addition, although her physiologic care is very important, you will also need to relieve anxiety related to this infection and acknowledge her disappointment that she cannot go home today.

Intermediate Case Studies

Case Study

Olivia Greenbaum

Olivia Greenbaum is a 9-month-old infant admitted with respiratory syncytial virus (RSV). She was born prematurely at 30 weeks' gestation. Her complications at birth included respiratory distress syndrome (RDS), suspected sepsis ×1, and formula intolerance. She was discharged home after 5 weeks on soy-based formula. This is her first hospitalization since her birth. Olivia is Mr. and Mrs. Greenbaum's only child, and they are very anxious. Mrs. Greenbaum is her primary care provider.

Olivia is receiving supplemental humidified oxygen administered via oxygen tent at 40%. She is very fussy and is not tolerating separation from her mother well. She has a peripheral IV inserted in her right hand with D5 ¼ NS infusing at 20 mL/hr. It is covered with a sock puppet. She is wearing a T-shirt and a disposable diaper. She is quite active within the crib. Her previous vital signs were as follows: temperature, 36.4°C ax; pulse, 84 beats/min; respirations, 38/minute; blood pressure, 94/58 mm Hg.

Mrs. Greenbaum spent the night and is currently sleeping in the recliner in Olivia's room. You enter the room and observe Olivia sleeping. She is pale with circumoral cyanosis. Her respiratory rate is 40/minute with an audible expiratory wheeze. Her heart rate on the monitor is 86 bpm; her pulse rate is 62 bpm. The pulse oximeter is currently showing an oxygen saturation level of 68%, and the alarm is turned off.

Medical Orders

Vital signs q 4 hr
Oxygen via tent at 40%
Continuous pulse oximetry when quiet; may obtain q hr intermittent pulse oximeter readings when active
Intravenous fluids: D5 ¼ NS @ 20 mL/hr
Encourage coughing.
Maintain O_2 saturation 93% to 97%. Adjust O_2 in increments of 2% up to a max of 50%.
Isomil 6–8 oz q 4 hr when awake
Heart rate/resp. monitor

Critical Thinking Questions

- What is your first priority after observing Olivia sleeping?
- Should you increase the oxygen being administered?

(continued)

Case Study

Olivia Greenbaum (continued)

- **What is your interpretation of her vital signs and oxygen saturation?**

- **Identify factors that affect the accuracy of the oxygen saturation reading.**

- **How do you encourage coughing in a 9-month-old baby?**

- **Give examples of how to manage thermoregulation within an oxygen tent.**

- **How frequently should Olivia's IV site be assessed? What is the function of the sock puppet?**

Integrated Nursing Care

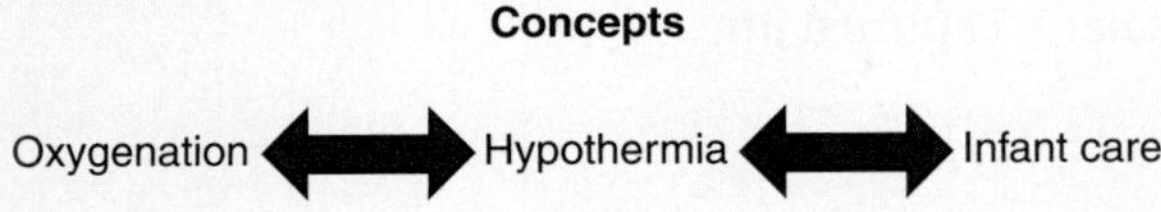

Your first priority is to establish whether Olivia is hypoxic. You noted a rapid respiratory rate and circumoral cyanosis, both potential symptoms of hypoxia. The pulse oximeter heart rate does not match the cardiac monitor heart rate. Gently, without disturbing Olivia, you begin to reattach the pulse oximeter.

Your preliminary assessment is that the pulse oximeter is not accurately assessing her oxygenation. You are able to hold the probe to her toe and get a reading of 95%. Olivia begins to wake up. Take her apical heart rate, which is the most reliable site for infants and small children (see Chapter 1). Compare her apical pulse rate to the heart rate on the pulse oximeter as well as the heart rate on the cardiac monitor. Nurses must always verify that the equipment is accurately reflecting the patient's status. Next, you take her temperature, which is 36.2°C. The humidified oxygen is also cooling Olivia, making her hands, feet, and lips appear cold, blue, and dusky (see Chapter 14).

Once Olivia is awake, she will not tolerate having the pulse oximeter probe on her toe and keeps pulling it off. You will need to check the oxygen saturation intermittently. Your next priority is to warm her up. When children become chilled, they have increased energy expenditure. When infants are stressed beyond aerobic metabolism, they use anaerobic metabolism. This produces lactic acid, which increases the acidity of the blood, exacerbating respiratory distress. Urge her mother to bring in more clothes and to layer her clothes to keep Olivia

Case Study

Olivia Greenbaum (continued)

thermoregulated within the humidified tent. You do not need to increase the oxygen level; what at first looked like hypoxia is in fact hypothermia!

The accuracy of a pulse oximetry reading is affected by several factors, including patient perfusion and peripheral vasoconstriction. Other factors that prevent the detection of oxygen saturation may be as simple as nail polish or artificial nails (see Chapter 14).

Encouraging coughing in an infant is accomplished either through crying or laughing. If the infant is periodically crying vigorously, that is sufficient. You can try tickling or playing peek-a-boo to get a 1-year-old to laugh. Crying and laughing require deep breaths and will cause a patient to cough, thus promoting airway clearance.

Check this patient's IV site every hour to ensure there are no signs of infiltration. The sock puppet is one way to disguise the IV site dressing while leaving it accessible for examination. If a young child can see the IV site dressing, he or she will often persist in trying to remove the tape and dressing despite all your efforts. If you cover the site, the child will not remember it is there. Piaget's theory of cognitive development includes the concept of object permanence (Taylor et al., 2008). At 9 months old, a child cannot imagine what he or she cannot see—in other words, what is out of sight is out of mind.

Case Study

Victoria Holly

Victoria Holly, age 68, is newly admitted to the hospital due to anemia and severe dehydration. To treat the dehydration she has an IV of D5 ½ NS infusing into the right hand. To treat the anemia, she has a medication or IV lock in her left arm to be used for blood administration only. She recently received 2 units of packed red blood cells. You have medical orders to draw a complete blood count and a complete metabolic profile. Mrs. Holly also has an ileostomy, which she has managed for several years on her own. Upon your initial physical assessment of Mrs. Holly, you find her vital signs are as follows: temperature, 97.2°F; pulse, 96 beats/min; respirations, 18/minute; blood pressure, 88/50 mm Hg. Her skin is "tenting" and you are having difficulty palpating her peripheral pulses. Her lips are dry and cracked. The skin around her stoma site is bright red and open in areas. You notice that her ostomy pouch was cut much larger than the stoma site. She reports she is very tired and "lacks energy." Her family informs you that she has always been a very independent person but in the last couple of months she just "hasn't been herself."

Medical Orders

Intravenous fluids: D5 ½ NS IV @ 125 mL/hr
Daily weights
Strict I&O
Complete blood count (CBC) and Complete metabolic profile (CMP) stat

(continued)

Case Study

Victoria Holly (continued)

Critical Thinking Questions

- **Identify appropriate sites and equipment needed to draw the blood.**
- **What concerns you about Mrs. Holly's present condition in relationship to performing her activities of daily living (ADLs) independently?**
- **What are measurable physical parameters you can use to determine whether fluid replacement therapy and blood administration are sufficient?**
- **Describe how you would assess Mrs. Holly's peripheral circulation.**
- **What is alarming about her ileostomy? Identify possible explanations for the stoma's condition.**
- **Develop a discharge teaching plan for Mrs. Holly related to her ostomy care.**

Integrated Nursing Care

Concepts

Blood sampling ⟷ ADLs ⟷ Hypotension ⟷ Stoma care

You cannot draw blood specimens from a dedicated line such as the one Mrs. Holly has for blood administration. You also cannot obtain the specimen from above the IV in her right hand because the specimen will be diluted with the D5 ½ NS solution and will, thus, be inaccurate. It is not considered best practice to draw laboratory specimens from an IV site unless absolutely necessary, according to facility policy. Mrs. Holly's laboratory work should be collected from her left arm, avoiding the right arm, due to the IV infusion, via venipuncture. Equipment you will need to draw the blood includes syringes, needles, alcohol swabs, laboratory tubes, gloves, and a tourniquet.

Mrs. Holly's vital signs are disconcerting because her blood pressure is low. Because of her hypotension, ADLs may unduly tax her. Until you see a positive change in her vital signs, you should provide assistance with her ADLs (see Chapter 7). In addition, Mrs. Holly has an IV in each arm. It would be difficult for her to care for the ostomy while attempting to keep the IV sites free from infection.

One outcome to anticipate with Mrs. Holly would be an increase in blood pressure. Other outcomes include palpable peripheral pulses and normal skin turgor. Subjectively, Mrs. Holly should report that she

Case Study

Victoria Holly (continued)

has an increase in energy. Her family may also comment that she is becoming more "like herself." Sometimes healthcare workers make judgments about elderly people, thinking that they are always tired. Since the healthcare workers are often unfamiliar with their patients' normal conditions, comments made by family members can often be very helpful in determining progress. This is especially true if your patient cannot communicate. Objectively, one outcome would be that Mrs. Holly becomes more active in her own care.

When a patient has no peripheral pulses, you must investigate further. Never ignore the absence of pulses, as this could signal a life-threatening condition. Have another nurse check the pulses, or you can use a Doppler. Upon checking Mrs. Holly's pulses with a Doppler device, you were able to hear them and marked them with an "x" to facilitate future assessments. In your initial assessment, you were not surprised that Mrs. Holly's pulses were nonpalpable, as she has a very low circulating volume (see Chapter 1).

Mrs. Holly's ileostomy site is very red and excoriated. You are alarmed, as this could place her at risk for infection; the physician will need to be notified. Do not assume that a physician has seen the excoriation around the ostomy site. If the patient came into the hospital with more pressing matters such as decreased blood pressure, the physician may not have observed the ileostomy. Mrs. Holly may lack knowledge about the appropriate method for sizing and cutting her ostomy appliance. You suspect that she may be cutting the faceplate in such a way as to leave her skin exposed to the liquid stool, which is then causing the excoriation (see Chapter 13).

One area you should investigate is Mrs. Holly's ability to care for the ostomy before she came to the hospital. It is possible that her skin around the stoma site has looked like this for a period of time. Before her hospital discharge, evaluate her knowledge through return demonstration to ensure that she can care for the stoma and can identify possible family resources. She may benefit from a home health referral to ensure she is caring for her stoma properly.

Case Study

Tula Stillwater

It is now day 5 in the hospital for Mrs. Stillwater. She has developed a staphylococcal infection in her cesarean section incision. This is the second time you have cared for this patient. You are familiar with her diabetic status, baseline vital signs, and routine postpartum care. She is currently receiving an IV antibiotic. Her vital signs are as follows: temperature, 99.2°F; pulse, 74 beats/min; respirations, 18/minute; blood pressure, 130/80 mm Hg. Her fingerstick blood sugar (FSBS) before breakfast is 120 mg/dL.

You learned in report that her incision is intact and healing on the right side, but the far left side of her incision is being packed with iodoform strips, requiring about half a bottle to fill the wound. The open part of the incision is approximately 1″ long, 0.5″ wide, and 1″ deep. This part of her incision is draining copious amounts of foul-smelling, yellow to green purulent drainage. The incision is very painful. Mrs. Stillwater reports her pain at a 6 on a scale of 1 to 10 (10 = worst) before her pain medication is administered.

(continued)

Case Study

Tula Stillwater (continued)

Mrs. Stillwater's 5-day-old boy is now bottle-feeding regularly. He is taking 3 oz of Similac with Iron every 4 hours. Mrs. Stillwater is eager to assume the majority of his care.

Medical Orders

Medication or IV lock; flush every shift and prn
Vancomycin 1.0 g IV q 12 hr
Sterile dressing change with iodoform packing every shift
Irrigate wound with NS with dressing change
Fingerstick blood sugar every ac and every hs
Regular insulin per sliding scale
Vital signs q 4 hr
Lortab 7.5 mg, 2 tabs q 4 to 6 hr prn pain

Critical Thinking Questions

- How will you plan her dressing change, and what equipment will you need?
- Describe your assessment and interventions for this wound.
- Identify factors that will promote wound healing in Mrs. Stillwater.
- How will you organize your nursing care to provide uninterrupted time for Mrs. Stillwater to care for her 5-day-old son?
- What techniques can you show Mrs. Stillwater to improve her mobility and ability to hold and care for her infant?
- Describe the procedure you will use to administer the IV antibiotic.

Case Study

Tula Stillwater (continued)

Integrated Nursing Care

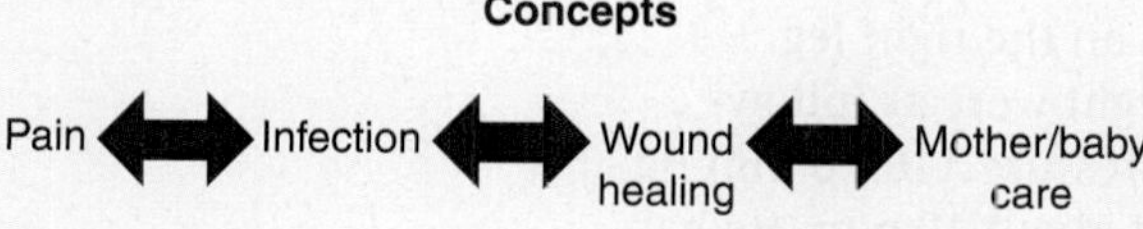

Mrs. Stillwater's dressing change will be stressful and uncomfortable. To manage the pain, the dressing change should be performed after she has taken her pain medication and you have allowed enough time for it to be effective. Given her diabetic status, she should be allowed to eat her breakfast and receive her insulin before you begin her dressing change. Mrs. Stillwater's focus is probably on her son. Encourage her to give him his morning bottle and to be satisfied that he is comfortable before you begin the dressing change.

Review Chapter 8 to develop the list of equipment you will need for the dressing change. You will need to set up a sterile field and maintain the sterility during the dressing change. Mrs. Stillwater can be positioned supine and rotated slightly to her left to promote drainage of the wound during irrigation.

Your assessment of the wound will include the size, the presence of granulation tissue, a description of the drainage, wound color, the presence of edema and erythema, and temperature (see Chapter 7). Note the condition of the skin at the wound edges as well as the skin where the wound dressing is taped. Look for changes in the condition of the wound and note how Mrs. Stillwater is tolerating the dressing change. If she will be taught to care for this wound and perform the dressing changes at home, instruction and return demonstration would become part of her discharge planning.

For Mrs. Stillwater's wound to heal, the infection must be resolved and the wound edges will need to become approximated. To optimize wound healing, Mrs. Stillwater will need a diet high in protein and minerals. You should obtain a nutritional consultation (Taylor et al., 2008).

The care of her infant son is a priority for Mrs. Stillwater. Cluster your nursing care such as wound dressings, vital signs, and medication administration to allow her sufficient time to provide care for her son.

Make sure Mrs. Stillwater knows how to use a splint, such as a pillow, across her abdomen to give support to her abdominal musculature when moving or coughing. Spending time in a comfortable chair may be preferable to getting in and out of bed. Assess that Mrs. Stillwater is using the "football hold" to feed and comfort her son. The advantage of this position is that the infant does not rest on the mother's abdomen. Mrs. Stillwater should have several pillows available to provide support for her arms when holding her infant.

To give the IV antibiotic, assess the IV site for patency, flush the IV per hospital policy prior to administration, administer the antibiotics according to the pharmacy or manufacturer's guidelines, and then flush the medication or IV lock after the antibiotic is infused.

Case Study

Jason Brown

Jason Brown is a 21-year-old college football player. It is the second postop day following surgical repair of a fracture of his right tibia and fibula. He has sutures over the anterior knee and lateral malleolus and a posterior splint on the right leg. He continues to report considerable pain. His vital signs at midnight were as follows 98.3°F; pulse, 58 beats/min; respirations, 12/minute; blood pressure 118/70 mm Hg. He reported his pain as a 3 on a scale of 1 of 10 (10 = worst) at about 10 p.m. He has a peripheral IV in his left forearm infusing D5 ½ NS at a keep-vein-open (TKO) rate of 20 mL/hr. He is using a PCA pump for pain relief. The nursing care for the morning includes routine a.m. care, cast care, and a trip to PT. You are on the day shift. Shortly after morning report, the unit clerk catches you and says, "Jason says he needs a nurse. He is in terrible pain."

You enter the room. Jason is pale and diaphoretic. His sheets are damp with some wet spots. He says, "My leg hurts. It really hurts." You ask him to rate his pain, and he answers, "At least an 8. I've been pushing my pain pump but I'm still in pain." His IV site looks okay. You say, "I'm going to find out why it is hurting. I need to get your vital signs first." His vital signs now are as follows: temperature, 98.9°F; pulse, 72 beats/min; respirations, 20/minute; blood pressure, 124/78 mm Hg.

Medical Orders

Vital signs q 4 hr
Intravenous fluids: D5 ½ NS TKO
Ambien 5 mg every HS
PCA—Morphine sulfate 1 mg q 6 min lockout, max 10 mg in 1 hr
Physical therapy for weight-bearing as tolerated

Critical Thinking Questions

- What is the significance of the changes in Jason's vital signs?
- What interventions for Jason's pain must occur immediately before administering nursing care and PT?
- How do you assess the following:
  - Infection versus inflammation?
  - Neurovascular compromise?
  - IV patency?

Case Study

Jason Brown (continued)

Integrated Nursing Care

Always compare vital signs to a comparable baseline and the previous vital signs (see Chapter 1). While Jason's temperature is elevated slightly, it has not increased dramatically, as it would be with an infection. His respiratory rate and pulse rate were quite low at midnight. Since he is a young, healthy athlete, his resting pulse rate may be lower than what is often considered as the norm. You notice that his resting pulse rates on the night shift have been running from 56 to 60 beats/min. Another factor contributing to his decreased pulse rate is the effect of the Ambien that he took at 9 p.m. to help him sleep. Therefore, while his morning respiratory rate and pulse rate are still within normal range, they represent a significant increase from his resting baseline. These are objective assessments supporting his assertion of increased pain.

One reason for an increase in pain with any postsurgical patient is the possibility of infection. Quickly assess all surgical incision sites and observe for redness, swelling, or a foul odor (Chapter 8). Due to short hospital stays, signs and symptoms of infection do not usually appear until after the patient is discharged (Taylor et al., 2008).

In addition to infection, Jason is at risk for neurovascular compromise because of the trauma to his right leg as well as from the splint and dressing. Assess for neurovascular compromise and perform cast care (see Chapter 9). Jason's fracture has been placed in a splint rather than a cast, which is a more current surgical practice, but nurses still refer to the care of the affected extremity as "cast care." Determine whether there are any signs of compartment syndrome (see Chapter 9). You need no additional equipment for this assessment, and it should take very little time; do this immediately.

Upon assessment, you find that Jason's foot and leg are pink and warm with 2+ pulses, no edema, full sensation, motion, and capillary refill measuring less than 3 seconds. The incision sites show no redness, swelling, drainage, or foul odor.

Another possible reason for his pain is that his IV may no longer be patent and, therefore, he would not be receiving any pain medication. You remember the wet spots on the bed as you begin systematically checking each of the IV administration-set connections. Your assessment of the IV site shows no swelling, and he reports no pain at the site. Your next check should be from the IV site to the IV tubing. You find that the connection of the IV tubing to the IV insertion catheter is loose and leaking. Determine whether the IV site is still patent (see Chapter 15). If the IV is still patent, replace the IV tubing (see Chapter 5). Check the medication in the PCA pump to ensure it is the correct medication. You will be required to check the PCA history to determine the amount of medication used as well as the amount remaining every 4 hours or according to facility policy (see Chapter 10).

Contact the physician to explain that the PCA pain medication was infusing onto the sheets, and obtain an order for an appropriate bolus dose so that Jason can obtain immediate pain relief. After 30 minutes, obtain another set of vital signs and perform a pain assessment. Document the evaluation of your interventions. Jason's pain will need to be controlled before initiating additional nursing care. Coordinating with PT to reschedule his therapy until his pain is resolved is a nursing responsibility.

Case Study

Kent Clark

Kent Clark, age 29, was admitted 24 hours ago for observation related to a suspected closed head injury following a motor vehicle accident (MVA). Mr. Clark's baseline vital signs are stable. He has a cervical collar and is scheduled to undergo a MRI to determine if he has a cervical spine injury. The physician has asked you to reduce his activity until cervical spinal injuries are ruled out.

Currently, Mr. Clark is awake, alert, and oriented (to person, place, and time); his pupils are equally round and reactive to light and accommodation (PERRLA). He moves all four extremities bilaterally. His head is elevated 30 degrees to minimize increased intracranial pressure (ICP) and edema. A peripheral IV in his right arm is infusing D5 ½ NS at 20 mL/hr.

Just before you are scheduled to take him to Special Procedures, Mr. Clark becomes restless and anxious. During the neuro check you notice that his right pupil is sluggish. Although he denies pain, he says, "I don't care what the doctors say. I am not going to stay in this bed any longer!" When you call the physician, he orders Valium 5 mg IV push. However, as you give the IV push medication to Mr. Clark, you notice a cloudy substance forming in the IV line and he reports a slight burning at his IV insertion site.

Medical Orders

Bedrest
HOB elevated 30 degrees
Cervical collar
Intravenous fluids: D5 ½ NS at 20 mL/hr
Neuro checks q 2 hr
Valium 5 mg IV push now

Critical Thinking Questions

- What clinical symptoms alert you that Mr. Clark's condition is changing, and what additional assessments will you do?
- Describe special positioning and transfer techniques to be followed for Mr. Clark.
- Identify the source of the pain at the IV insertion site and the cloudy substance in the IV tubing.
- What could you have done to prevent these complications, and how will you intervene now?

Case Study

Kent Clark (continued)

- How will you handle Mr. Clark's anger and prevent him from getting out of bed?

Integrated Nursing Care

Concepts

Neuro assessment ⟷ IV push ⟷ Safety

In a patient with a closed head injury, bleeding or swelling may occur within the confines of the skull, leading to increased ICP. This increased ICP could cause extensive brain damage. Mr. Clark became increasingly restless and anxious, which could be a subtle sign of increased ICP. Even slow bleeding inside the cranium can cause changes. When you observe a change, immediately complete a neuro assessment to determine if there are further neurologic alterations. When Mr. Clark became restless, you found that his right pupil was more sluggish to light than the left, which is another sign of increased ICP. Complete neuro checks as often as his condition warrants, and immediately report subtle changes in neuro checks to the physician. Meticulous documentation of baseline neuro checks and subsequent assessments is important to detect subtle neurologic changes (see Chapter 17).

Cervical spinal injuries can vary in severity, and even hairline fractures can become unstable if the patient is not positioned and transferred correctly. Mr. Clark has a cervical collar and the physician has asked you to minimize his movement. If you need to turn Mr. Clark, keep his head lowered and then logroll him as a unit without flexing or turning his neck. Obtain help from additional staff so that you can stabilize his head, neck, and torso in straight alignment while he is being turned (Taylor et al., 2008). When Mr. Clark is transferred from the bed to a stretcher, use a drawsheet to gently and carefully move him as a unit. Even though he has a cervical collar, do not assume that it is safe for him to sit up further in the bed or get up and move around.

Mr. Clark is angry and wants to get out of bed. Restraints would be the least desirable option for him. At this time, placing restraints on him could increase his agitation and make him feel more trapped, and this could increase his ICP (see Chapter 3). For Mr. Clark, careful pharmacologic sedation may be a better option. The physician has ordered Valium to reduce his agitation and anxiety. Another possible intervention is to help Mr. Clark feel more in control of his environment. This could be as simple as having a family member stay with him, and checking on his needs frequently.

Pain at the IV site could mean that the IV is not patent. Carefully observe the IV site for any signs of phlebitis or infiltration before and while giving the IV push. If you determine that Mr. Clark's IV has a good blood return and is not infiltrated, the burning sensation at his IV site may be from the Valium administration. Valium as well as other medications can be irritating. Give the medication and the flush that follows at a slower rate. If not contraindicated, some medications can also be diluted if ordered (Karch, 2004).

The most probable cause for the cloudy appearance in Mr. Clark's IV line is precipitation of the drug due to chemical incompatibility of the Valium and the IV fluid of D5 ½ NS. When giving any medication through an IV line, you must know whether the drug and IV solution are chemically compatible (see Chapter 5). When IV drugs are not compatible, a reaction immediately occurs that may not be visible to the eye but nevertheless can be dangerous. To prevent this, flush the IV line before and after medication administration per institution policy. Since a precipitate has already formed, clamp the tubing off closest to Mr. Clark and make sure that the cloudy substance does not reach him (see Chapter 5). Some hospitals require discontinuing the IV and restarting another IV with new IV tubing; other hospitals require changing only the IV tubing. If signs of incompatibility occur, notify the physician and continue to assess Mr. Clark's need for further medication.

Case Study

Lucille Howard

Lucille Howard, age 78, is in the hospital for a severe urinary tract infection (UTI). She has a history of urinary retention and UTIs. She is overweight, has a history of heart failure, and is allergic to many medications, including several antibiotics. Twenty-four hours ago she had severe nausea and vomiting and was ordered nothing by mouth (NPO). She has an IV catheter inserted in her left arm, infusing D5 ½ NS @ 75 mL/hr. Mrs. Howard just had a triple-lumen urinary retention catheter inserted for continuous bladder irrigation with amphotericin B. The catheter was inserted at 6:30 a.m. and your shift started at 6:45 a.m. During your shift, you notice that she begins to have some coarse audible breath sounds and difficulty breathing. She reports pain in her abdomen.

Medical Orders

Amphotericin B 50 mg in 1,000 mL sterile H_2O irrigating in bladder at 40 mL/hr for 5 days
Strict I&O

Intravenous fluids: D5 ½ NS @ 75 mL/hr
NPO

Critical Thinking Questions

- What are possible causes of Mrs. Howard's current symptoms?
- How would you identify the source of her current symptoms?
- What actions will you take?

Integrated Nursing Care

Concepts

Fluid overload ⟷ Allergic reactions ⟷ I & Os

There are several potential causes for Mrs. Howard's symptoms. In light of her drug sensitivities, she may be allergic to the amphotericin B. Allergic responses can include difficulty breathing as well as itching and a rash. Another source of her symptoms could be related to her heart problems. People with heart problems can easily become overloaded with fluid. Symptoms of fluid overload, a common problem for patients with heart failure, include crackles in the lungs, abnormal heart sounds, and possibly edema. A final possibility is that her catheter is placed incorrectly in the vagina rather than the bladder.

To determine the cause of Mrs. Howard's symptoms, you need to perform several assessments. First, auscultate her heart and lung sounds and palpate her

Case Study

Lucille Howard (continued)

abdomen. Also assess for a rash on her skin, and ask her if she has any itching. If her heart and lung sounds are normal but her lower abdomen is hard, check for the position of the catheter. Sometimes it is difficult to tell if the catheter is in the right position just by looking, especially if the area around the catheter is swollen or if your patient is overweight. You can also check inputs to see if they match outputs. Currently, Mrs. Howard is getting 75 mL/hr of IV fluid and 40 mL/hr of the amphotericin B irrigant. She should be putting out in her urine at least 70 mL/hr: the hourly output of the urinary irrigant (40 cc) plus the least amount of urine you would expect to see in an hour (30 mL). If the catheter is in the correct place and her overall input is higher than the output, you are placing Mrs. Howard at risk for overload. If the catheter is not in the correct place, then you are giving her a vaginal irrigation and not the bladder irrigation that is ordered (see Chapter 12).

If Mrs. Howard is having an allergic reaction, stop the irrigant immediately, follow anaphylactic protocol, and notify the physician. If she is beginning to have problems with fluid overload due to her heart problems, reduce the IV rate to TKO, stop the irrigant, and notify the physician for further orders. If you discover that the catheter was not placed correctly, stop the irrigant, leave the catheter in place, and obtain another catheter kit. Insert the new triple-lumen urinary retention catheter into the urinary meatus and then remove the other catheter. Begin your irrigations once the new catheter is in place, and notify the physician. Continue to monitor Mrs. Howard until you are certain she is stabilized and her symptoms have resolved.

Case Study

Janice Romero

Janice Romero, age 24, has recently been diagnosed with acute lymphocytic leukemia (ALL). To provide long-term venous access, she was admitted to have an implanted port placed. She had a 21-gauge peripheral IV inserted in her right arm prior to surgery. After her port was placed, Mrs. Romero's physician ordered 2 units of packed red blood cells (PRBCs). Once you obtain the PRBCs from the blood bank, you note to the nursing aide that the blood seems very cold. She says, "Oh, that isn't a problem; it's just like warming up lunch." When you talk to Mrs. Romero about the blood transfusion, she tells you that the last time she received blood she had chills and fever during the transfusion.

Medical Orders

2 units packed RBCs stat

Intravenous fluids: D5 ½ NS at 50 mL/hr

(continued)

Case Study

Janice Romero (continued)

Critical Thinking Questions

- Identify the site you will use to administer blood to Mrs. Romero. Why did you choose this site?
- Identify the purposes for warming blood, and describe the safest way to warm blood.
- Describe the technique you will use to administer blood to Mrs. Romero.
- Considering Mrs. Romero's history and diagnosis, describe the precautions you will implement before giving her blood.

Integrated Nursing Care

Concepts

Safety ⟷ Blood administration

Before Mrs. Romero can receive blood, you must select an appropriate site (see Chapter 15). Site selection depends on the gauge of the IV and the fluid infusing in the IV. Blood must be given through a large-bore catheter to prevent red blood cell damage. Since dextrose will cause hemolysis, blood can be administered only with normal saline. For these two reasons, the optimal site for blood administration is her implanted port. Before you give her blood through the port, be certain that the port is not dedicated for other infusions, such as chemo.

Since the implanted port is new, ensure that it is working properly prior to use. Check the medical record for a medical order allowing use of the port. Depending on your hospital policy, wear a mask and sterile gloves when accessing the port, particularly since she has leukemia and may be immunocompromised. In addition, a larger-gauge (19) Huber needle is recommended for giving blood (see Chapter 15). Check the port for patency and blood return per hospital policy. Infuse the normal saline slowly while you observe the implanted port site for signs of swelling. If the port shows any sign of infiltration, notify the physician, and choose another site to give her blood.

Some patients may need to have their blood warmed before it is administered. This includes patients who are at risk for cardiac arrhythmias, patients with unusual immune responses, as well as neonatal and pediatric patients. A medical order is required for the warming of blood products during transfusion. Various devices exist to warm blood. Do not use the microwave to warm any blood product: it coagulates the proteins of the blood and causes severe hemolysis that could be fatal. Whenever you need to warm blood, always use a blood warmer that has been approved by your institution.

Mrs. Romero's past history of chills and fever are signs of a possible transfusion reaction; thus, she is at increased risk for a transfusion reaction. Ensure that she has a signed consent form and that she fully understands her need for the blood. The physician needs to be aware of this history of a transfusion reaction. The physician may order premedication with diphenhydramine (Benadryl), acetaminophen (Tylenol), or hydrocortisone prior to blood administration to reduce the risk for developing another reaction. Stay with her for at least 15 minutes at the beginning of the transfusion. Continue to monitor her vital signs frequently per hospital policy. When you leave her room, make sure her call light is available, and instruct her to contact you if she has any unusual symptoms.

Case Study

Gwen Galloway

Mrs. Galloway, age 64, had a left-sided mastectomy and is now receiving follow-up chemotherapy for recurrent breast cancer with axillary node involvement. She has been hospitalized for 48 hours. She reports pain on her left side and under her left arm. She has a right double-lumen Hickman catheter inserted. Recent laboratory work shows a low white blood cell count of 1.8 μL and a low platelet count of 39,000/μL. She also bleeds and bruises very easily. You have to obtain vital signs and provide a.m. care. You also need to draw a complete blood count and change the dressing on her central line.

Medical Orders

Vital signs q 4 hr
Complete blood count (CBC) now and every a.m.
Morphine sulfate IV 6–8 mg q 2 hr prn pain
Cefazolin sodium (Ancef) 1 g IV q 8 hr
Change central line dressing q 72 hr

Critical Thinking Questions

- What special precautions should you take while obtaining Mrs. Galloway's vital signs?
- Explain why some sites would be contraindicated when taking Mrs. Galloway's temperature.
- Describe the special precautions you would take when drawing blood from Mrs. Galloway; identify the site where you would draw the blood.
- Identify your interventions when changing Mrs. Galloway's central line dressing and the rationale for these interventions.
- Discuss the equipment used, restrictions, and concerns regarding Mrs. Galloway's personal care.

(continued)

Case Study

Gwen Galloway (continued)

Integrated Nursing Care

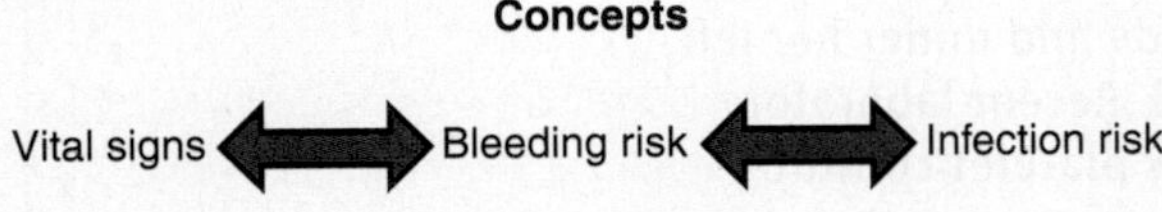

To individualize care, always assess your patient's condition and special needs. When a patient undergoes a mastectomy, she will often have lymph nodes removed from the affected side. Taking a blood pressure reading in the affected arm could interfere with circulation and harm the extremity (see Chapter 1). In Mrs. Galloway's case, her affected side is on the left, so take her blood pressure on the right side.

Mrs. Galloway has a low platelet count, which places her at risk for bleeding (see Chapter 1). In addition, her low white blood cell count places her at risk for infection and other complications. Therefore, taking a rectal temperature would be contraindicated for Mrs. Galloway. It would also be contraindicated to take a left-sided axillary temperature on Mrs. Galloway because she is still having some discomfort due to her recent mastectomy.

Given Mrs. Galloway's risk for bleeding, would a peripheral venipuncture be the best choice to obtain her CBC? Due to the risk for prolonged bleeding, her central line may provide the best access for a blood specimen (see Chapter 15). Determine whether her physician has restricted her central line for chemotherapy. If her central line is dedicated to chemotherapy only, obtain a blood specimen by doing a venipuncture. If you needed to do a venipuncture, using Mrs. Galloway's left side would be contraindicated due to the mastectomy. You will need to apply pressure to the site for a longer period of time because of her increased risk for bleeding.

When changing Mrs. Galloway's central line dressing, use sterile technique due to her increased risk for infection. Depending on agency policy, you may also need to place a mask on yourself and Mrs. Galloway. To prevent bleeding and bruising at the central line site, do not move or pull on the catheter as you are manipulating the central line dressing.

Several restrictions could apply when performing Mrs. Galloway's personal care. Patients at risk for bleeding should avoid shaving. Another concern is the potential for bleeding from the mucous membranes when using a hard-bristled toothbrush and dental floss. Use mouth rinses and very soft toothettes to minimize trauma (see Chapter 7).

Case Study

George Patel

George Patel, age 64, was admitted to your floor 3 days ago following surgical insertion of a tracheostomy tube. His diagnosis prior to surgery was acute upper airway obstruction. He has a left IV or medication lock. Currently, he is receiving oxygen via his trach at 40%. His pulse oximetry readings have been consistently running in the low 90s. He quickly becomes short of breath when his oxygen is interrupted during suctioning. During your shift, you will have to suction Mr. Patel as needed and provide routine trach care. You will also need to transport him with portable oxygen to radiology for his AP and lateral chest x-rays.

Case Study

George Patel (continued)

Medical Orders

Morphine sulfate 2–6 mg IV q 2 hr prn for pain
Pulse oximetry every shift and prn
Tracheostomy care every shift and prn
Tracheal suctioning prn
AP and lateral chest x-rays
Oxygen via trach Venturi mask at 40%
Medication or IV lock flush every shift

Critical Thinking Questions

- How would you determine when Mr. Patel needs to be suctioned?
- How would you determine when Mr. Patel needs to have trach care?
- Describe expected outcomes when suctioning and providing trach care.
- When transporting Mr. Patel to the radiology department, what precautions should you implement to ensure his safety?

Integrated Nursing Care

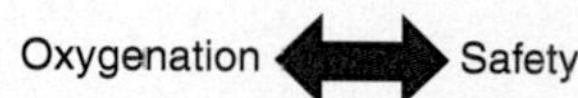

To evaluate the need for suctioning, first assess Mr. Patel's respiratory status. Examine his oxygen saturation and compare it to his baseline. If his oxygen saturation is decreased from his baseline, this may be an indication that he needs to be suctioned. If you have a physician's order to hyperoxygenate, this would be the time to do so. Observe his respirations to determine if they are more labored than usual. Listen to his lung sounds for crackles or wheezes. Also, listen around his trach for gurgling. Does he have a productive cough? All of these signs and symptoms are indications that he needs to be suctioned.

To assess the need for trach care (see Chapter 14), closely examine his trach as well as the trach ties and precut gauze dressing. If it appears wet or moist, trach care would be indicated. If his trach dressing appears dry and intact, you may want to wait until later in your shift to do trach care. Suctioning and subsequent coughing will often soil the trach dressings, so wait until after suctioning to change the trach dressing.

Your expected outcomes when suctioning a tracheostomy include minimizing hypoxia, discomfort, and fatigue. Hypoxia may be reduced by hyperoxygenating the patient before suctioning according to facility policy. When you suction Mr. Patel, limit the length of suction time to 10 to 15 seconds and allow him to rest before suctioning him again (see Skill 14-13). During trach care or repeat suctioning, quickly replace his oxygen source and limit the time his oxygen is interrupted. Since Mr. Patel has a new trach, it is very likely he will

(continued)

Case Study

George Patel (continued)

need to be premedicated with morphine for pain. Morphine depresses respirations, so continually assess Mr. Patel's respiratory status after administering the pain medication. In addition, adequate rest periods are needed to minimize fatigue from suctioning. Mr. Patel may require a rest period between suctioning the trach and his trach care.

The precautions you would take when transporting Mr. Patel focus on providing adequate oxygenation. First, assess Mr. Patel's oxygen saturation and respiratory status prior to transport. If indicated, suction Mr. Patel before he leaves his room. You must also check that the portable oxygen tank is full and the label says "oxygen." Before turning off his wall oxygen, make sure the portable oxygen tank is working properly and that the equipment is ready. This avoids interruption of his oxygenation while placing him on the portable oxygen.

Advanced Case Studies

Case Study

Cole McKean

Cole McKean is a 4-year-old boy in the pediatric intensive care unit (PICU). He weighs 22 kg. He was admitted 3 days ago after nearly drowning in a neighbor's pool. He was submerged for 5 to 10 minutes. The neighbor initiated CPR and the rescue team had a heart rate established within 10 minutes of their arrival. The aspirated pool water caused a severe inflammatory response resulting in pulmonary edema. Cole is intubated with an endotracheal tube (ETT) and is on a mechanical ventilator. The past 2 days he produced copious bronchial secretions and required suctioning about every 2 hours. Today his breath sounds are clearer and he requires less frequent suctioning. He is being weaned off oxygen. The plan for today is possible extubation. An arterial line is in place in his left radial artery, infusing NS at 2 to 3 mL/hr. A PICC line with an infusion of D5 ½ NS @ 75 mL/hr is inserted into his right arm. His heart rate, respiratory rate, and arterial waveform are being monitored. The pulse oximeter sensor is applied to his right toe. He has an indwelling urinary (Foley) catheter to gravity drainage and a nasogastric tube in place to low intermittent suction. He is receiving sedation but is opening his eyes at times and moving his extremities. He is becoming more active.

The alarm goes off on the ventilator. You look at Cole. His eyes are open and he is making crying sounds. You know when a child is properly intubated he or she cannot make sounds. You notice that his oxygen saturation level has dropped to 81% and his color is dusky. He is breathing on his own around the tube; his abdomen is rounded. You are assessing Cole's respiratory status and oxygenation when the physician comes to the bedside. The physician tells you to remove the ET tube and begin oxygen at 40% via face mask. When you place Cole on the face mask, his oxygen saturation returns to the mid-90s. The physician says, "This little fellow was ready to get rid of his tube." She orders a follow-up ABG to be drawn in 15 minutes.

Medical Orders

Continuous pulse oximetry
Maintain O_2 saturation 92%–98%
Vent settings: 36% O_2, IMV 36, Pressures 26/6
Vital signs q 1 hr
Neuro checks q 1 hr
Endotracheal suctioning prn
Foley to gravity
I&O
Nasogastric tube to low intermittent suction
Arterial blood gases q 2 hr
Intravenous fluids: D5 ½ NS @ 75 mL/hr
Arterial line: NS 2–3 mL/hr

(continued)

Case Study

Cole McKean (continued)

Critical Thinking Questions

- Describe your initial actions in response to a possible extubation.
- How can the technique of drawing ABGs be adapted for a pediatric patient?
- How will Cole's response be evaluated now that he is on an oxygen mask?
- Develop a plan of care that will allow Cole rest and sleep periods but also allow hourly assessments.
- Identify the nursing skills involved in monitoring Cole's respiratory status.

Integrated Nursing Care

Concepts

Oxygenation ⟷ Ventilation ⟷ Comfort

When a patient is intubated, the patency of this airway is a critical priority. When you hear Cole cry, you must determine if his ETT is in the proper place. Listen with your stethoscope over the lung fields and abdomen. If you do not hear ventilator-induced breath sounds over the lung fields, then the ETT is not in place. Because a child's neck is so short, it is not difficult to displace a tracheal tube into the esophagus. If this occurs, you may hear ventilator-cycled sounds in the abdomen. Signs that an ETT is not in the correct position include unstable oxygen saturation levels, cyanosis, and abdominal distention. In Cole's situation, you determine that the ETT is no longer in the lungs. All patients on mechanical ventilation must have an Ambu bag and a mask of the correct size at the bedside. Cole did not require mask-bag respirations at this time, but he has the potential for this need.

When you are evaluating Cole's response, the ABG results will guide clinical decision making regarding oxygen delivery. In Cole's case, 10 to 15 minutes after changing to the 40% oxygen mask, you draw an ABG (see Chapter 16). The results come back as follows: PaO_2, 82 mm Hg; $PaCO_2$, 46 mm Hg; pH, 7.34; HCO_3, 20 mEq/L. This ABG shows that Cole's oxygen level is acceptable and there is no indication for immediate reintubation. ABGs will continue to be drawn periodically to evaluate Cole's response to treatment.

To monitor his respiratory status, observe his work of breathing, count his respiratory rate, observe

Case Study

Cole McKean (continued)

his color, and auscultate breath sounds. If he shows no significant respiratory distress and has a stable respiratory rate and clear breath sounds, he is responding well to the change in his oxygen source. In addition, continuously monitor the oxygen saturation level via pulse oximetry. Immediately report to the physician any increases or decreases in oxygen saturation.

Because children have a small total blood volume, the blood drawn back in the arterial line is usually not discarded but returned to the patient after the laboratory sample is drawn. Smaller volumes of blood are sent to the laboratory in pediatric specimen tubes. The setup for a pediatric arterial line delivers a smaller volume of fluid when the fast-flush release is activated (ie, the pigtail is pulled).

When a patient, especially a child, is critically ill, cluster your hands-on care so that the patient will have a significant amount of sleep and rest between hourly interventions. One of the initial assessments a nurse makes in an intensive care setting is to determine that each of the monitoring devices is accurately displaying the patient's status (see Chapters 14 and 16). After you determine that the monitors accurately reflect the patient's vital signs, obtaining alternating sets of vital signs from the patient and from the monitor may be permitted, according to hospital policy. Maintain a quiet environment. Because of the noise and activity of the intensive care unit, many infant and child intensive care units dim the lights at night to create day/night cycles for the children.

Case Study

Dewayne Wallace

Dewayne Wallace, age 19, was admitted to the emergency department approximately 4 hours ago with a stab wound that he received in a knife fight while intoxicated. You are asked to care for Dewayne while his nurse attends to a new emergency. She gives you the following report: He was admitted in respiratory distress and bleeding from the stab wound. His wound is on the right side at the sixth intercostal space and is approximately 1″ in length, sutured and intact. The chest x-ray confirmed a right hemothorax, and as a result the physician inserted a chest tube. The chest tube is connected to a disposable drainage system and placed to suction at –20 cm H_2O. The chest tube is draining a small amount of dark-red blood. There has not been any new drainage for the past 2 hours.

Dewayne's most recent vital signs were as follows: temperature, 98.4°F; pulse, 88 beats/min; respirations, 24/minute; blood pressure, 112/74 mm Hg. He is receiving oxygen via face mask at 30% and is on continuous pulse oximetry. The oxygen saturation level is currently 96%. He says he feels short of breath. He does not have labored breathing and is not using accessory muscles. He reports pain at the chest tube insertion site and stab wound site. He has a patent IV infusing in his left forearm. His lab work reported a blood alcohol level of 0.12. The nurse giving report says, "Good luck with that delinquent. He says he's in pain, but I think he already drank his pain medication from a bottle."

(continued)

Case Study

Dewayne Wallace (continued)

Dewayne turns on his call light. When you approach him, you notice his breathing is labored with subclavicular retractions. The pulse oximeter reads 95%. Dewayne says, "This thing in my side really hurts."

You take another set of vital signs: temperature, 98.6°F; pulse, 90 beats/min; respirations, 37/minute; blood pressure, 118/78 mm Hg. You find the breath sounds are diminished on the right. The chest drainage tubing is in the bed without a dependent loop, and Dewayne has been lying on a segment of the tubing. You ask him to rate his pain on a scale of 1 to 10 (10 = worst), and he says, "About a 5." You ask if the medicine he got earlier helped with the pain, and he answers that he didn't get any pain medicine. When you check the chart you find that an order for hydrocodone bitartrate 5 mg/acetaminophen 500 mg (Lortab 5/500) was written about 3 hours ago, but when you look over the medication Kardex you do not see that any has been administered. You find his nurse and ask if the Lortab was given. The response you get is, "Are you kidding? If he's tough enough to drink and fight, he's tough enough for a little chest tube. He made his bed; he can just lie in it."

Medical Orders

Chest tube with drainage system to suction @ –20 cm H_2O
Oxygen at 30% via face mask
Continuous pulse oximetry
Intravenous fluids: NS at 100 mL/hr
Lortab 5/500, 1 or 2 tabs q 4 hr PO prn pain

Critical Thinking Questions

- Which of Dewayne's needs is your first priority? Describe your assessments related to your first priority.
- Describe the purpose of a chest tube drainage system for a hemothorax.
- How would you troubleshoot his chest tube drainage system? What could be the source of his respiratory distress?
- Discuss valid reasons a nurse might not give a pain medication when there is a prn order.

Case Study

Dewayne Wallace *(continued)*

- Discuss prejudices nurses may have that may prohibit adequate pain management.

Integrated Nursing Care

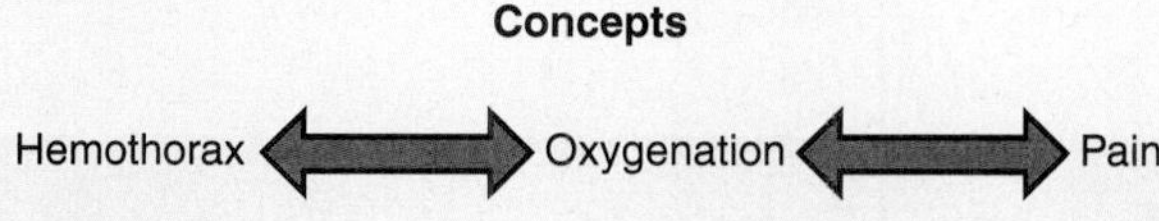

Your first priority is Dewayne's increased respiratory distress. While the change in oxygen saturation levels is very small, this is only because Dewayne's body is compensating for it now. Dewayne's work of breathing has dramatically changed, signaling a change in his respiratory status. Your preliminary assessment showed a respiratory rate of 37 breaths/minute, up significantly from his earlier respiratory rate of 24. When you inspected the chest you found subclavicular retractions; this indicates that Dewayne is using his intercostal muscles to breathe. When you auscultated breath sounds you found decreased air movement on the right, indicating a hemothorax.

In a hemothorax, blood collects in the pleural space and compresses a lung. The purpose of the chest tube is to evacuate the blood and allow the lung to expand fully. In Dewayne's case, the stab wound created a puncture in the pleura, allowing blood to accumulate within the pleural space. The right lung will need to be evaluated on a routine basis to make sure the blood in the pleural space has been removed so that the lung can re-expand. Any change in respiratory status may indicate a problem with the chest tube drainage system.

As you noted in this case, Dewayne has had a change in his respiratory status. Since you have completed his physical assessment, now begin inspecting the equipment. As with any equipment check, begin inspection at the patient and move to the equipment. Start your inspection at the insertion site of the chest tube. Observe the dressing to ensure it is occlusive and inspect the tubing for leaks, kinks, and dependent loops. Compare the amount of recent drainage in the drainage system to the volume of old drainage, and check the amount of suction (see Chapter 14). In this case, Dewayne has been lying on his tubing, which would prevent it from draining properly. When you reposition Dewayne's tubing, approximately 60 mL of dark old blood flows into the drainage set. His respiratory status improves quickly. Thus, this accumulated blood in the pleural space was the source of his respiratory distress.

There are several situations in which giving a narcotic analgesic is contraindicated. During a life-saving procedure, pain is not always a priority. In this case, Dewayne did not receive pain medication before the insertion of his chest tube as he was at risk for respiratory arrest. Narcotics are also contraindicated when it is critical to assess alertness, because the narcotic might mask neurologic changes. Narcotic analgesics also are associated with the side effects of respiratory depression and vital sign changes. Patients sometimes do not receive the pain medication ordered because the nurse is worried about these side effects. Because of this, controversy exists as to whether the benefit of pain control outweighs the risk of side effects. Many hospitals have committees that can assist with these ethical decisions. A dialog among nurses, doctors, and pharmacists can result in optimal pain control with minimal side effects. Speak with the physician before independently deciding to withhold pain medication to prevent side effects.

Another reason nurses may withhold medication is their own preconception of the patient's pain and their own prejudices. Some nurses are not even aware

(continued)

Case Study

Dewayne Wallace *(continued)*

that they have these feelings. As a nursing student, you need to understand how you will respond to patients, and you need to explore your own beliefs and prejudices. The accepted standard in nursing is that a patient defines his or her own pain and that it is the nurse's responsibility to manage it properly. Guidelines for pain management have been written by state Boards of Nursing, the U.S. Department of Health and Human Services, the World Health Organization, as well as other professional organizations.

Case Study

Robert Espinoza

Robert Espinoza, age 44, has just had exploratory abdominal surgery. The post-anesthesia recovery room (PACU) nurse calls at 2:10 p.m. to report on Mr. Espinoza and tells you he has a peripheral IV inserted in his right arm, infusing NS at 50 mL/hour. He has a midline abdominal dressing that is dry and intact with two Jackson-Pratt (JP) drains in place. He also has a nasogastric (NG) tube and an indwelling urinary (Foley) to gravity drainage. She reports that his NG tube has been checked for placement and has been draining moderate amounts of yellow-green contents. His vital signs in the PACU are as follows: temperature, 98.0°F; pulse, 86 beats/min; respirations, 16/minute; blood pressure, 134/80 mm Hg. At 2 p.m., he received 6 mg morphine sulfate IV for a pain rating of 6 on a scale of 1 to 10 (10 = worst).

At 3 p.m., you receive Mr. Espinoza on your medical-surgical unit via stretcher by a hospital transporter. The NG tube tape that secured the NG to his nose is no longer in place. You also notice that the urinary drainage bag lying on top of his legs has a small amount of amber urine in the reservoir. While you are in his room, Mr. Espinoza says, "Hey, it feels like there's something wet under my back." His vital signs on arrival are as follows: temperature, 98.0°F; pulse, 130 beats/min; respirations, 18/minute; and blood pressure, 100/68 mmHg. His respirations are regular and unlabored and his skin color is pink. He now rates his pain as a 2 on a scale of 1 to 10 (10 = worst). Mr. Espinoza's family is anxiously waiting in the waiting room on your floor.

Medical Orders

Indwelling urinary catheter (Foley) to gravity
Strict I&O
Nasogastric tube to intermittent suction
Intravenous fluids: NS @ 50 mL/hr
Routine JP drain care
Routine postop VS
Morphine sulfate 4–10 mg IV q 2 hr prn for pain

Case Study

Robert Espinoza (continued)

Critical Thinking Questions

- Considering Mr. Espinoza's immediate postop status, describe how you would transfer him from the stretcher to his bed.
- Prioritize, with rationales, your assessments and nursing care for Mr. Espinoza in the following areas:
  - Immediate physical assessments and interventions
  - Assessment and management of tubes
  - Pain management and comfort level
  - Care of his family

Integrated Nursing Care

When transferring Mr. Espinoza to his bed, consider the following factors: minimizing his pain level, protecting his incision, and protecting the patency of his tubes. Excessive strain from moving can cause disruption and bleeding to his abdominal incision. Per hospital policy, carefully transfer him with the assistance of others. During transfer, be careful not to disrupt his tubes or dressings. Once Mr. Espinoza is in his bed, place his urinary drainage bag on the bed frame so that it hangs below the level of his bladder. This position will allow the urine to drain by gravity and decrease the possibility of a urinary tract infection (see Chapter 12).

Since Mr. Espinoza is a new postoperative patient, your first priority is to perform an assessment based on the ABC criteria (airway, breathing, and circulation). Compare his vital signs upon arrival to his baseline vital signs. Mr. Espinoza's respiratory rate has not changed significantly from his baseline. If not contraindicated, elevate his head to facilitate deep breathing and continue to assess his airway and respiratory status (see Chapter 6).

Circulation is the next immediate priority. In Mr. Espinoza's case, his blood pressure has decreased and his heart rate has increased from his baseline in the PACU. Both of these changes could indicate decreased blood volume related to bleeding. Therefore, assess Mr. Espinoza's abdominal dressing to evaluate if it is dry and intact. Never assume that an incision is dry just because you cannot see any blood on top of the dressing. If the abdominal dressing is covered by foam tape, blood underneath the tape may not be easily visualized. Look under the patient to see if blood has trickled underneath the dressing. Mr. Espinoza said that he felt something "wet" under his back, and when turning him, you discover that there is a large puddle of bright-red blood underneath him that is caused by acute bleeding from his abdominal incision. Do not remove the abdominal dressing. You may, however, reinforce the dressing if you have a physician's order.

Identify all other possible sources of bleeding. When you assess the JP drains, note the color, amount, and consistency of blood. Assess his abdomen for signs of internal bleeding such as abdominal distention. Also check for decreased urine output, another sign indicating a possible decrease in blood volume. A urine output of less than 30 mL/hr may be a sign of hypovolemic shock. Although Mr. Espinoza is bleeding and has signs of decreased blood volume, he is not yet in hypovolemic shock. If Mr. Espinoza's blood pressure continues to drop, elevate his feet to increase venous return. Report all indications of internal and/or external bleeding to the physician. Acute postop bleeding requires surgical repair.

Your next priority is to ensure that all of his tubes are intact and working properly. One of the first tubes

(continued)

Case Study

Robert Espinoza (continued)

you want to assess for patency is his IV, particularly since he may be returning to surgery. The next tubes you want to examine are the JP drains. To maintain suction, a JP drain must be less than half full. Assess the color and other characteristics of the JP drainage (see Chapter 8). Next, assess his NG tube. Mr. Espinoza's NG tube tape is not secure, so you cannot assume that the tube is still in his stomach. Check the NG for placement, assess the color and amount of the return, and then place the NG to intermittent suction (see Chapter 11). Next, evaluate his urinary catheter to determine it is draining properly (see Chapter 12).

The next priority is to monitor Mr. Espinoza's pain level. If he is in acute pain, immediately consider incisional disruption. Because Mr. Espinoza is bleeding, you may need to give small increments as opposed to large amounts of morphine to prevent a further drop in his blood pressure. In addition to his physical comfort, attend to his possible anxiety about returning to the operating room. Maintain a calm voice and demeanor when caring for Mr. Espinoza.

Do not forget Mr. Espinoza's family, who are anxious to see him. It is helpful to send another staff nurse to keep them updated while you are busy in his room. When his condition stabilizes and before the family visits him, tell them about the tubes that they will see, including the reason for and function of each of the tubes. Be flexible when allowing the family to come in and visit Mr. Espinoza.

Case Study

Jason Brown, Gwen Galloway, Claudia Tran, and James White

This is your first week as an RN in a small rural hospital. You work the night shift on a medical-surgical unit. Tonight your only aide and a nurse have called in sick, which makes the unit short-staffed. You have notified the night supervisor that you need help, and she sends an aide from another floor to assist you. She tells you she can get someone on the floor to help you in about an hour, and instructs you to take care of the priority cases until that time.

You have six relatively uncomplicated patients, and you need to check their vital signs and give medications. You have four other patients about whom you are concerned:

- Jason Brown, a 64-year-old patient with a tracheostomy, has gurgling sounds coming from his trach and a frequent, nonproductive cough. His oxygen saturation level via pulse oximetry is 88%. You have orders to suction his trach prn.
- Gwen Galloway had been receiving chemotherapy and has now come back to the hospital with gastroenteritis. When you arrive on your shift, she is experiencing bouts of nausea and vomiting.
- Claudia Tran, an 84-year-old patient from a nursing home, is post-CVA. She has a stage III pressure ulcer on her coccyx and a stage I ulcer on her left hip. She needs to be turned every 15 minutes because of rapidly developing erythema on bony prominences. She is confused and has fallen the past 2 nights when left unattended, even when restrained. Her family is visiting her now but plans to leave in 30 minutes.
- James White has COPD. The aide reports that the blood pressure from the automatic cuff is 168/100 mm Hg; his baseline is usually 130/70 mm Hg. The aide also reports that he has a severe headache but no other complaints.

Case Study

Jason Brown, Gwen Galloway, Claudia Tran, and James White (continued)

Critical Thinking Questions

- Identify the order in which you would provide care to these patients. Explain your rationales as well as your interventions.

Integrated Nursing Care

Concepts

Oxygenation → Perfusion → Safety → Wound prevention → Comfort

Mr. Brown is having difficulty with airway clearance and oxygenation, so he will be your first priority. Nursing priorities always follow the "ABCs": airway, breathing, and circulation. He will require prompt tracheal suctioning and further evaluation of his respiratory status (see Chapter 14). When his oxygen saturation levels have stabilized, you can then attend to the other patients.

Next, address the dramatic change in vital signs that Mr. White is experiencing. Mr. White is at risk for a stroke if his blood pressure continues to stay elevated and is not controlled immediately. Before planning any other interventions, verify the blood pressure by taking it yourself with a manual cuff (see Chapter 1). Initial nursing assessment includes assessing the accuracy of the equipment as well as the accuracy of the information reported to you by an aide. The blood pressure you obtain is 190/110 mm Hg. Check for the physician's orders regarding possible prn blood pressure medications. Call the physician right away and notify him or her of the change in Mr. White's status.

You know that Mrs. Tran is at high risk for falls if left unattended, and she may injure herself seriously if this occurs. Reducing her risk for injury is your next priority (see Chapter 3). In Mrs. Tran's case, you could ask a family member to stay the night, or at least until you get more help on the unit. Many families are willing to help if you make them aware of such situations. If the family leaves, ask the aide to remove the restraint, place the bed in a low position, and stay with Mrs. Tran until you get further help. You can delegate Mrs. Tran's positioning schedule to the aide.

Despite the obvious distress of vomiting, this is not a life-threatening situation for Mrs. Galloway; therefore, her condition is a lower priority than that of the other three patients. Mrs. Galloway requires comfort. Check if an antiemetic medication has been ordered; if not, call the physician and obtain an order. Other

Concepts

Prioritization ↔ Delegation

interventions you can perform until her medication takes effect are lowering the lights, applying a cool cloth to the neck, decreasing noises, removing substances that may have a strong odor (eg, food and vomitus), and keeping her head elevated.

When prioritizing and delegating care, here are some questions that might help guide your decision-making process:

- Is the situation life-threatening?
- How rapidly could this patient deteriorate?
- How quickly can you remedy the problem?
- Who can provide assistance?

Whenever a patient's airway, breathing, or circulation is jeopardized, this is a life-threatening emergency. Base your priorities on the ABC criteria. Mr. Brown is your first priority because his airway and oxygenation are a problem. When a patient's condition has the potential to deteriorate rapidly, this is also a

(continued)

Case Study

Jason Brown, Gwen Galloway, Claudia Tran, and James White (continued)

priority. In Mr. White's case, because of the spike in his blood pressure, he has the potential for a stroke. Preventing this life-threatening event requires immediate action. When two patients have problems of similar urgency such as oxygenation, respond to the problem that you can remedy the quickest. Sometimes when you have many activities to accomplish in a short period of time, it is difficult to take time to seek additional help. Many hospitals will have night supervisors to assist you with problem solving. Additionally, physicians are available by phone or in the hospital. Nonlicensed personnel such as aides are sometimes available to assist with noncritical tasks. A nursing skill to develop is prioritization of nursing care and delegation of noncritical tasks.

Case Study References

Centers for Disease Control and Prevention (CDC). (1999; updated 2004). Information about MRSA (methicillin-resistant *Staphylococcus aureus*) for healthcare personnel. Accessed September 2, 2006. Available at www.cdc.gov/ncidod/dhqp/ar_mrsa_healthcareFS.html.

Joint Commission on Accreditation of Healthcare Organizations. (2005). *Patient safety. The official "Do not use" list.* Available at www.jointcommission.org/PatientSafety/DoNotUseList/. Accessed May 15, 2006.

Karch, A. M. (2007). *2007 Lippincott's nursing drug guide*. Philadelphia: Lippincott Williams & Wilkins.

Taylor, C., Lillis, C., LeMone, P., & Lynn, P. (2008). *Fundamentals of nursing: The art and science of nursing care* (6th ed.). Philadelphia: Lippincott Williams & Wilkins.